PSYCHO…
D…
DI…
2…

THE PROFESSIONALS' POCKET HANDBOOK AND AIDE MEMOIRE

PSYCHOTROPIC DRUG DIRECTORY 2016

THE PROFESSIONALS' POCKET HANDBOOK AND AIDE MEMOIRE

STEPHEN BAZIRE

LRP Lloyd-Reinhold Publications

Lloyd-Reinhold Publications Limited

British Library Cataloguing-in-Publication Data
A catalogue record is available for this book

ISBN-13 978-0-9569156-3-4

Printed in the UK by Page Bros Ltd, Mile Cross Lane, Norwich, Norfolk, NR6 6SA

CONTENTS

INTRODUCTION ix

CHAPTER 1: DRUG TREATMENT OPTIONS IN PSYCHIATRIC ILLNESS 1

1.1 Acute psychiatric emergency 2
1.2 Aggression 7
1.3 Agoraphobia 9
1.4 Alcohol dependence and abuse 10
1.5 Alcohol withdrawal syndrome 17
1.6 Anxiety disorder 21
1.7 Attention deficit hyperactivity disorder 26
1.7.1 ADHD in children and adolescents 26
1.7.2 ADHD in adults 33
1.8 Autistic spectrum disorders 36
1.9 Benzodiazepine dependence and withdrawal 40
1.10 Bipolar mood disorder 42
1.10.1 Prophylaxis and maintenance 42
1.10.2 Mania and hypomania 48
1.10.3 Bipolar depression 54
1.10.4 Rapid-cycling bipolar disorder 59
1.11 Borderline personality disorder 61
1.12 Catatonia 64
1.13 Dementia 66
1.13.1 Treatment of Alzheimer's disease 67
1.13.2 BPSD/BPSSD 72
1.13.3 Vascular dementia 77
1.13.4 Parkinson's disease dementia 78
1.13.5 Prophylaxis and prevention 79
1.14 Depression 85
1.14.1 Unipolar depression 85
1.14.2 Postpartum depression 107
1.14.3 Depression in Parkinson's disease 110
1.14.4 Dysthymia 112
1.15 Eating disorders 114
1.15.1 Anorexia nervosa 114
1.15.2 Bulimia nervosa 115
1.15.3 Binge-eating disorder 117
1.16 Insomnia 119
1.17 Narcolepsy 124
1.18 Obsessive-compulsive disorders 126
1.18.1 OCD 126
1.18.2 Body dysmorphic disorder 131
1.19 Panic disorder 132
1.20 Post-traumatic stress disorder 135
1.21 Psychosis and schizophrenia 140
1.21.1 Psychosis and schizophrenia 143
1.21.2 First episode 167
1.21.3 Cognitive impairment 171
1.21.4 Negative symptoms 174
1.21.5 Psychosis in Parkinson's disease 176
1.22 Seasonal affective disorder 178
1.23 Self-injurious behaviour 179
1.24 Sexual deviancy disorders 180
1.25 Social anxiety disorder 181
1.26 Tourette's syndrome 184
1.27 Trichotillomania 186
1.28 Caffeinism 187
1.29 Electroconvulsive therapy 189

CHAPTER 2: SELECTING DRUGS, DOSES AND PREPARATIONS 193

2.1 Relative side-effects of:
2.1.1 Hypnotics 194
2.1.2 Antidepressants 195
2.1.3 Antidepressants — pharmacokinetics and receptor effects 197
2.1.4 Antipsychotics 199
2.1.5 Antipsychotics — pharmacokinetics and receptor effects 201
2.1.6 Anxiolytics 203
2.2 Switching or discontinuing psychotropics 204
2.2.1 Antipsychotics 205
2.2.1.1 General advice 205
2.2.1.2 Specific drug switches 206
2.2.1.3 Antipsychotic dose equivalents 213
2.2.1.4 Post-switching antipsychotic issues 214
2.2.1.5 Depot and LAI injections 216
2.2.2 Benzodiazepines 216
2.2.3 Anticholinergics 216
2.2.4 Drugs of abuse 216
2.2.5 ADHD treatments 226
2.2.6 Anticholinesterases 226
2.2.7 Antidepressants 228

CHAPTER 3: PSYCHOTROPICS IN PROBLEM AREAS 237

3.1 Bariatric surgery 238
3.1.1 Antipsychotics 238
3.1.2 Antidepressants 238
3.1.3 Mood and bipolar 239
3.1.4 Anxiolytics and hypnotics 239
3.1.5 Anticonvulsants 239
3.1.6 Others 239
3.2 Cardiovascular disease 240
3.2.1 Antipsychotics 241
3.2.2 Antidepressants 245
3.2.3 Mood and bipolar 247
3.2.4 Anxiolytics and hypnotics 248
3.2.5 Anticonvulsants 248

3.2.6 Others 248
3.3 Diabetes 251
3.3.1 Antipsychotics 252
3.3.2 Antidepressants 253
3.3.3 Mood and bipolar 254
3.3.4 Anxiolytics and hypnotics 254
3.3.5 Anticonvulsants 254
3.3.6 Others 255
3.4 Epilepsy 256
3.4.1 Antipsychotics 257
3.4.2 Antidepressants 257
3.4.3 Mood and bipolar 258
3.4.4 Anxiolytics and hypnotics 259
3.4.5 Anticonvulsants 259
3.4.6 Others 259
3.5 Glaucoma 260
3.5.1 Antipsychotics 261
3.5.2 Antidepressants 261
3.5.3 Mood and bipolar 262
3.5.4 Hypnotics 262
3.5.5 Anticonvulsants 262
3.5.6 Others 262
3.6 Hepatic impairment 263
3.6.1 Antipsychotics 264
3.6.2 Antidepressants 265
3.6.3 Mood and bipolar 266
3.6.4 Anxiolytics and hypnotics 266
3.6.5 Anticonvulsants 266
3.6.6 Others 267
3.7 Old age 268
3.7.1 Antipsychotics 269
3.7.2 Antidepressants 271
3.7.3 Mood and bipolar 273
3.7.4 Anxiolytics and hypnotics 274
3.7.5 Anticonvulsants 275
3.7.6 Others 275
3.8 Parkinson's disease 276
3.8.1 Antipsychotics 277
3.8.2 Antidepressants 277
3.8.3 Mood and bipolar 277
3.8.4 Anxiolytics and hypnotics 277
3.8.5 Anticonvulsants 278
3.8.6 Others 278
3.9 Perinatal 280
3.9.1 Antipsychotics 284
3.9.2 Antidepressants 289
3.9.3 Mood and bipolar 299
3.9.4 Anxiolytics and hypnotics 303
3.9.5 Anticonvulsants 307
3.9.6 Others 310
3.10 Renal impairment 316
3.10.1 Antipsychotics 317
3.10.2 Antidepressants 318
3.10.3 Mood and bipolar 319
3.10.4 Anxiolytics and hypnotics 320
3.10.5 Anticonvulsants 320
3.10.6 Others 321
3.11 Sleep apnea 322
3.11.1 Antipsychotics 323
3.11.2 Antidepressants 323
3.11.3 Mood and bipolar 324
3.11.4 Anxiolytics and hypnotics 324
3.11.5 Anticonvulsants 324
3.11.6 Others 324

CHAPTER 4: DRUG INTERACTIONS 326

4.1 Anxiolytics and hypnotics 327
4.1.1 Benzodiazepines 327
4.1.2 Buspirone 330
4.1.3 Chloral hydrate 331
4.1.4 Melatonin 332
4.1.5 Pregabalin 332
4.1.6 Zaleplon 333
4.1.7 Zolpidem 333
4.1.8 Zopiclone 334
4.2 Antipsychotics 335
4.2.1 General antipsychotics 335
4.2.2 Aripiprazole 338
4.2.3 Asenapine 339
4.2.4 Clozapine 339
4.2.5 Lurasidone 342
4.2.6 Olanzapine 343
4.2.7 Quetiapine 345
4.2.8 Risperidone 346
4.2.9 Ziprasidone 348
4.3 Antidepressants 348
4.3.1 Tricyclic anti-depressants 348
4.3.2 SSRIs 352
4.3.2.1 Citalopram/escitalopram 352
4.3.2.2 Fluoxetine 354
4.3.2.3 Fluvoxamine 357
4.3.2.4 Paroxetine 360
4.3.2.5 Sertraline 362
4.3.3. Other antidepressants 364
4.3.3.1 Agomelatine 364
4.3.3.2 Duloxetine 365
4.3.3.3 Mianserin 366
4.3.3.4 Mirtazapine 366
4.3.3.5 Moclobemide 368
4.3.3.6 Reboxetine 369
4.3.3.7 Trazodone 370
4.3.3.8 Venlafaxine 371
4.3.3.9 Vortioxetine 373
4.3.3.10 St John's wort 373
4.3.4 MAOIs 376
4.4 Mood stabilisers 381
4.4.1 Carbamazepine 381
4.4.2 Lamotrigine 387
4.4.3 Lithium 389
4.4.4 Valproate 393
4.5 Anticonvulsants 395
4.5.1 Gabapentin 395
4.5.2 Levetiracetam 396
4.5.3 Oxcarbazepine 396
4.5.4 Phenobarbital and primidone 397
4.5.5 Phenytoin 400
4.5.6 Topiramate 405
4.6 Other drugs 406
4.6.1 Acamprosate 406
4.6.2 Anticholinergics 406
4.6.3 Anticholinesterases 407
4.6.3.1 Donepezil 407
4.6.3.2 Galantamine 408
4.6.3.3 Rivastigmine 408
4.6.4 Atomoxetine 408
4.6.5 Buprenorphine 409
4.6.6 Bupropion 410
4.6.7 Clomethiazole 412
4.6.8 Disulfiram 412
4.6.9 Guanfacine 413
4.6.10 Lisdexamfetamine 413
4.6.11 Memantine 413
4.6.12 Methadone 414
4.6.13 Methylphenidate 417
4.6.14 Modafinil 417
4.6.15 Nalmefene 418
4.6.16 Naltrexone 419
4.6.17 Pirenzepine 419
4.6.18 Sodium oxybate 419
4.7 Non-prescribed drugs 420
4.7.1 Alcohol 420
4.7.2 Cannabis 423
4.7.3 Cocaine 423
4.7.4 Smoking 424
4.8 Cytochrome P450 drug metabolism 426
4.8.1 CYP1A2 427
4.8.2 CYP2B6 428
4.8.3 CYP2C9 429
4.8.4 CYP2C19 430
4.8.5 CYP2D6 431
4.8.6 CYP3A3/4 433

CHAPTER 5: DRUG-INDUCED PSYCHIATRIC DISORDERS 436

5.1 Agitation, anxiety and nervousness 437
5.2 Aggression 440
5.3 Behavioural changes 440
5.4 Delirium and confusion 441
5.5 Depression 446
5.6 Hallucinations 452
5.7 Mania, hypomania or euphoria 456
5.8 Movement disorders 462
5.8.1 Pseudoparkinsonism 462
5.8.2 Akathisia 464
5.8.3 Dystonias 466
5.8.4 Dyskinesias 469
5.8.5 Other movement disorders 471
5.8.5.1 Catatonia 471
5.8.5.2 Cataplexy 472
5.8.5.3 Choreas 472
5.8.5.4 Rabbit syndrome 473
5.8.5.5 Tics 474
5.9. Neuroleptic malignant syndrome 475
5.10 Obsessive-compulsive symptoms 477
5.11 Panic attacks 478
5.12 Paranoid or schizo-phrenic-like psychoses 480
5.13 Serotonin syndrome 490
5.14 Sleep problems 493
5.14.1 Sleep disturbances 493
5.14.2 Vivid dreams and nightmares 495
5.15 Suicidal ideation 496

CHAPTER 6: MANAGEMENT OF SIDE-EFFECTS 503

6.1 Anticholinergic and related side-effects 505
~ blurred vision 505
~ constipation 505
~ dry mouth 505
~ urinary retention 506
~ urinary hesitancy 506
~ urinary incontinence 506
6.2 Blood disorders 506
~ bleeding 506
~ blood dyscrasias; neutropenia, agranulocytosis 506
~ eosinophilia 507
6.3 Cardiac effects 507
~ hypertension 507
~ hypotension 507
~ myocarditis 508
~ postural hypotension 508
~ QTc prolongation 508
~ tachycardia 509
6.4 Central adverse effects 509
~ abnormal dreams 509
~ anorexia 509
~ ataxia 509
~ delirium 509
~ drowsiness 510
~ dysphoria 510
~ fatigue 510
~ hypomania 511
~ insomnia 511
~ irritability, jitteriness or agitation 511
~ nausea 512
~ nocturnal enuresis 512
~ OCD 513
~ psychosis 513
~ sedation 513
~ seizures 513
6.5 Dermatological effects 514
~ acne 514
~ alopecia and hair loss 514
~ Darier's disease 515
~ exfoliative dermatitis 515
~ folliculitis 515
~ maculopapular eruption 515
~ photosensitivity 515
~ pigmentation 515
~ psoriasis 516
~ rash 516
~ seborrheic dermatitis 519
~ sweating 519
6.6 Endocrine effects 519
~ diabetes insipidus 519
~ diabetes mellitus 520
~ hepatotoxicity 520
~ hyperammonaemia 520
~ hypercalcemia 521
~ hypercholesterolaemia 521
~ hyperglycaemia 521
~ hyperlipidaemia 521
~ hyperprolactinaemia 522
~ hyperthyroidism 524
~ hyponatraemia 524
~ hypothyroidism 525
~ polyuria and renal impairment 526
~ weight gain 526
6.7 Movement disorders 533
~ blepharospasm 533
~ bruxism 533
~ dysphagia 534
~ EPSE, akathisia 534
~ EPSE, dyskinesias 536
~ EPSE, Parkinsonism 538
~ EPSE, dystonia 539
~ laryngospasm 540
~ myoclonus 540
~ Pisa syndrome 541
~ restless legs 541
6.8 Neuroleptic malignant syndrome 542
~ neuroleptic rechallenge 542
6.9 Serotonin syndrome 544
~ Sternbach's diagnostic criteria 544
6.10 Sexual side-effects 544
~ libido 547
~ arousal 547
~ anorgasmia 548
~ ejaculation problems 550
~ priapism 551
6.11 Others, side-effects 551
~ gastric irritation or nausea 551
~ glaucoma 551
~ hypersalivation 551
~ incontinence 551
~ jaundice 552
~ mastalgia 552
~ megaloblastic anaemia 552
~ oedema 552
~ osteopenia 552
~ osteoporosis 552
~ pain at site of injection 552
~ raised LFTs 552
~ sialorrhoea 552
~ tremor 554
~ vomiting 554

CHAPTER 7: PSYCHOTROPIC DRUGS 555

New drugs expected 565

INDEX AND ABBREVIATIONS 569

INTRODUCTION

Why the *Psychotropic Drug Directory (PDD) 2016*? Well, the title tries to describe the contents, and how you should use them. The 'directory' part is because the book contains general principles, lists, issues, advice and references to help you make decisions but then directs you where to go to get the further information you might need, since it would be virtually impossible to convey all the subtleties of a research paper, case report or review in a couple of lines. I have, for instance, again added well over 2000 new references to the text in this edition. If I spent a couple of hours thoroughly reading and analysing each and every paper, I'd never be able to finish the book. So, you really should check papers before making important decisions. I would be hugely grateful for any advice or tips about papers that I may have taken at face value and inadvertently missed the errors, hidden bias or multiple publication.

It may be worth pointing out that this book is an entirely independent publication. There is no commercial sponsorship, support or influence on the content, which remains entirely my own work.

How to use the book...

The *PDD 2016* is arranged in a problem-solving way to aid optimum medication use:

- *Chapter 1*: select a mental health problem needing medication management and consider the pharmacological options from the BNF, combination and unlicensed lists.
- *Chapter 2* aids choosing a drug and dose, where a choice exists or is necessary.
- *Chapter 3* aids drug choice in a compromised patient.
- *Chapter 4* allows checking for drug–drug interactions.
- *Chapter 5* is an important check that the mental health problem is not drug-induced.
- *Chapter 6* helps to guide you where a drug works, but side-effects limit effectiveness.
- *Chapter 7* has got historical and other information I couldn't think where else to put.

A minimum level of knowledge is assumed and information given should be followed up in the appropriate sources when time allows. References, where quoted, are either of good recent review articles or of specific information.

Further information can be obtained by referring to the main paper or papers cited and also to the reference sections of those main papers. Lists and references are as comprehensive as viable but could never claim to be fully complete, nor could this book ever be as comprehensive as a MedLine search on a chosen topic. **The listing of a drug use in this book does not in any way imply that it is licensed in your country or safe for this use,** and all information is presented in good faith. Throughout, I have tried to be as objective as possible. The reader should make up his or her own mind on a topic, but I hope that the statements and references point you in the right direction and the time saved in looking papers up will allow more thought. It is inevitable that some papers are from specialist journals but, where possible, I have always quoted more accessible journals in preference. If the only paper published on the use of a drug is from an obscure or ancient source, this may well indicate the status of the paper.

Changes to this edition

Updates have been made to all chapters (marked with * as ever). Major developments include adding aripiprazole LAI, guanfacine, vortioxetine and lurasidone in full, a section on negative symptoms of schizophrenia, and antidepressant equivalent doses and receptor affinity. *Chapter 3* has had psychotropics in bariatric surgery added, drugs are now grouped more practically, and finally the breast feeding and pregnancy sections have been merged and expanded into a comprehensive perinatal section.

Acknowledgements

Writing and continually updating a book since the first tentative and amateur editions back in 1989 has been a tremendous challenge and drain on my stamina and enthusiasm, not to mention those of the people around me. Subsequently, the continued help, encouragement, constructive criticism and advice I have received from colleagues and correspondents throughout the world has, as ever, been utterly invaluable, not to mention very rewarding. It is wonderful to know that the book has helped improve the pharmaceutical care of many people with mental health needs. I would thus like to thank the many active members of the College of Mental Health Pharmacy (CMHP) and BAP (British Association for Psychopharmacology) for their continued enthusiasm, encouragement and support. Thanks as ever must go to many pharmacy and other former colleagues in NSFT Trust for continuing to humour me. Special thanks to the University of East Anglia's top-rated School of Pharmacy for the renewed honour. I also wish to thank the many people who have fed back on the book's contents and/or spotted ambiguities in the quarter of a million words, e.g. Robin Saadvandi, Bob Flanagan, Ariel Hubbert, Audrey Purcell, Graham Parton, Alison Marshall (numerous times), Camilla Sowerby, Wojciech Kusz, Dennis Liew and Richard Owen.

Thanks as ever to John Tams, Pink Floyd and Absolute Radio for the company; to Ossi's (01603-927459) on Prince of Wales Road, Norwich for my Monday night veggie pizzas; and, of course, Binkie, for being so amazing to work with; my parents and my Godmother Kate Baxter for continuing to show interest; and Jill for putting up with me.

Stephen Bazire *BPharm, FRPharmS, DipPsychPharm, FCMHP, MBE*
Honorary Professor, School of Pharmacy, University of East Anglia, Norwich NR4 7TJ, England
Director, Mistura Enterprise and Informatics, Ashington, Northumberland
Trustee, Norwich and Central Norfolk Mind
E-mail: steve.bazire@choiceandmedication.org.uk
Websites to aid service user choice of medication: www.choiceandmedication.org

Revised January 2016

1 DRUG TREATMENT OPTIONS IN PSYCHIATRIC ILLNESS

Contents

1.1 Acute psychiatric emergency 2
1.2 Aggression 7
1.3 Agoraphobia 9
1.4 Alcohol dependence and abuse 10
1.5 Alcohol withdrawal syndrome 17
1.6 Anxiety disorder 21
1.7 Attention deficit hyperactivity disorder 26
1.7.1 ADHD in children and adolescents 26
1.7.2 ADHD in adults 33
1.8 Autistic spectrum disorders 36
1.9 Benzodiazepine dependence and withdrawal 40
1.10 Bipolar mood disorder 42
1.10.1 Prophylaxis and maintenance 42
1.10.2 Mania and hypomania 48
1.10.3 Bipolar depression 54
1.10.4 Rapid-cycling bipolar disorder 59
1.11 Borderline personality disorder 61
1.12 Catatonia 64
1.13 Dementia 66
1.13.1 Alzheimer's disease 67
1.13.2 BPSD/BPSSD 72
1.13.3 Vascular dementia 77
1.13.4 Parkinson's disease dementia 78
1.13.5 Prophylaxis and prevention 79
1.14 Depression 85
1.14.1 Unipolar depression 85
1.14.2 Postpartum depression 107
1.14.3 Depression in Parkinson's disease 110
1.14.4 Dysthymia 112
1.15 Eating disorders 114
1.15.1 Anorexia nervosa 114
1.15.2 Bulimia nervosa 115
1.15.3 Binge-eating disorder 117
1.16 Insomnia 119
1.17 Narcolepsy 124
1.18 Obsessive-compulsive disorders 126
1.18.1 OCD 126
1.18.2 Body dysmorphic disorder 131
1.19 Panic disorder 132
1.20 Post-traumatic stress disorder 135
1.21 Psychosis and schizophrenia 140
1.21.1 Psychosis and schizophrenia 143
1.21.2 First episode 167
1.21.3 Cognitive impairment 171
1.21.4 Negative symptoms * 174
1.21.5 Psychosis in Parkinson's disease 176
1.22 Seasonal affective disorder 178
1.23 Self-injurious behaviour 179
1.24 Sexual deviancy disorders 180
1.25 Social anxiety disorder 181
1.26 Tourette's syndrome 184
1.27 Trichotillomania 186
1.28 Caffeinism 187
1.29 Electroconvulsive therapy 189

Chapter One lists medicines that are indicated for, or have been used in, the conditions listed. The author would welcome suggestions for further inclusions. References should be consulted for fuller details of non-approved uses. In some cases, drugs not available in the UK have been included as possible options if available, and for non-UK readers.

Drugs are classified as follows:

BNF listed

BNF listed drugs are listed in the *British National Formulary* and licensed in the UK for that condition, although there are a few drugs listed in the BNF for which no full licence has been granted. See the appropriate section in the BNF for a review of a drug's role in therapy and its prescribing details. Much information provided here is in addition to that in the standard texts.

+ Combinations

The combinations section includes some combinations that have been used, but carry the risks of additive side-effects and interactions.

● Unlicensed/some efficacy

This section includes drugs shown to have some clinical efficacy (e.g. in at least one RCT) or are strategies which can be used, but where no product licence exist at the time of writing.

■ Unlicensed/possible efficacy

Drugs of minor or as yet unproven importance or efficacy. No product licence exists.

✹ Case reports

Single cases or case series awaiting further reports to confirm an early signal, or not, as the case may be.

◆ Others

This section includes drugs tried, but where no significant data exists since the original reports. The lack of positive follow-up data suggests a lack of efficacy although, if you know otherwise, the author would like to hear.

□ No efficacy

Drugs in this section are not thought to be of clinical use.

Information in these last four categories is given to provide help once all recognised and evidence-based treatments have been tried. These classifications are to some extent arbitrary, and the information is based on data presently available.

It is the prescriber's responsibility to ensure that all precautions are taken when prescribing a drug for any licensed or unlicensed use.

1.1 ACUTE PSYCHIATRIC EMERGENCY (APE) including RAPID TRANQUILLISATION

see Aggression (*1.2*), Mania and hypomania (*1.10.2*) and Psychosis and schizophrenia (*1.21*)

Violent patients (usually either schizophrenic, manic or substance abusers) present a risk to themselves and others. Swift, safe and effective treatment is often needed. Rapid tranquillisation (RT) is the term used to describe the procedure of giving varying amounts of antipsychotic medication, usually with benzodiazepines, over brief intervals of time to help control agitated, threatening and potentially destructive patients.

Routes: The IM route should be preferred except in exceptional circumstances as it carries additional dangers, albeit quicker-acting than IM and can allow physical restraint to be removed more quickly. Parenteral doses generally have a higher potency than oral doses. 'When required' or regular doses prescribed as 'IM/PO' are entirely inappropriate. All 'PRN' doses should be checked daily to ensure maximum doses are not being exceeded in any 24 hours. Antipsychotics can be fatal in moderate doses in drug-naïve people.

Doses: The need for high doses of antipsychotics is unnecessary, as higher doses may, in fact, be less effective, e.g. inducing akathisia. Use of concomitant benzodiazepines is safer and more effective than using high doses of antipsychotics as monotherapy.

General principles of the management of an acute psychiatric emergency (APE)

1. Obtain a drug history and carry out a physical examination if possible. Unless known previous exposure to psychotropics, use doses at the lower end of the ranges.
2. Antipsychotics in combination with benzodiazepines are preferred.
3. Parenteral administration should be reserved **only** for when the person cannot be persuaded to take drugs orally.
4. No anticholinergics should be used routinely, as this may confuse the clinical picture.
5. Switch to oral doses as soon as possible.
6. Check BP, pulse and temperature frequently.
7. Although APE management can be carried out in the community, great care is needed and it is not recommended.

Potential complications of antipsychotics in APE:

1. Cardiovascular complications and sudden death — drugs causing QTc prolongation are contraindicated in people with pre-existing cardiac problems, and great care is needed in adrenaline-driven excited patients.
2. Respiratory depression.
3. Extrapyramidal symptoms, especially acute dystonia (may occur in 10–30% of patients within the first 24 hours and later in up to 50% of young males). Akathisia should be considered if agitation occurs, worsens or recurs, as it may be drug-induced and exacerbate the disturbed behaviour (see *C6.7*).
4. Seizures, especially in non-compliant epileptics.
5. Neuroleptic malignant syndrome (see *C6.8* for risk factors). Close observation of temperature should be carried out, especially in the early stages. Check CPK as well.
6. Local bruising, pain or extravasations (common, in up to 30% patients).
7. In people already taking antipsychotics, additional acute doses may reach toxic levels.
8. Acute hypotension (minimised if the patient can lie down) can occur, especially with phenothiazines and in the elderly.
9. Mega-colon (rare), aspiration.

Review: use of BDZs and antipsychotics in emergency departments (Rund *et al, J Emerg Med* 2006;**31**:317–24).

BNF listed

Drugs in this section are licensed for emergency, short-term or adjunct therapy of, e.g. acute psychosis, mania, anxiety or exacerbations of chronic psychosis, violent or impulsive behaviour, psychomotor agitation and excitement, or violent or dangerously impulsive behaviour.

ANTIPSYCHOTICS

Aripiprazole *

Aripiprazole is licensed for rapid control of agitation and disturbed behaviour in people with schizophrenia or mania. The initial IM dose is 9.75 mg (range 5.25–15 mg). A second injection can be given after two hours, with no more than three doses in any 24 hours (maximum daily dose 30 mg, including all formulations). The IM onset is 30 minutes, peaks at 90 minutes and sustained until 24 hours, with an 84% response rate at 2 hours (n=201, open, 1/7, De Filippis *et al, Pharmacotherapy* 2013;**33**:603–14). In acute psychotic agitation, aripiprazole (15–30 mg/d, n=298) is as effective as olanzapine (20 mg/d, n=306) (n=604, RCT, d/b, 5/7, Kinon *et al, J Clin Psychopharmacol* 2008;**28**:601–7) and haloperidol (n=448, RCT, d/b, p/c, Andrezina *et al, Psychopharmacol (Berl)* 2006:**188**:281–92). The effect may be a specific anti-agitation effect rather than just a non-specific sedation (s=3, Currier *et al, J Psychiatr Pract* 2007;**13**:159–69). Benzodiazepines can be given concomitantly, but the patient must be monitored for excessive sedation and postural hypotension.

Review: consensus statement on use of IM aripiprazole (Gonzalez *et al, Curr Med Res Opin* 2013;**29**:241–50).

Chlorpromazine

Chlorpromazine is licensed for adjunctive short-term treatment of anxiety, agitation, violence or dangerously impulsive behaviour. The IM injection is 2–4 times as potent, on a mg for mg basis, as oral chlorpromazine, so must not be prescribed as '100 mg po/im'. Cochrane concludes that chlorpromazine is as effective as haloperidol, but causes serious postural hypotension and so should be avoided (s=1, n=30, Ahmed *et al, Cochrane Database Syst Rev* 2010;**4**:CD007445).

Haloperidol (see also combinations)

Haloperidol is licensed for adjunctive short-term treatment of moderate-to-severe agitation, violence or dangerously impulsive behaviour. It can be used at BNF doses, e.g. up to 20mg/d orally or 18mg/d by IM injection only (SmPC). Due to potential QTc prolongation the SmPC now recommends cardiac assessment and an ECG before starting treatment (see also *C3.2.1*). Akathisia may exacerbate disturbed behaviour. Cochrane concludes that haloperidol (o, IM, IV) can be lifesaving, the evidence for adjunctive benzodiazepines is not strong but the evidence for newer drugs is no better (s=32, RCTs, Powney *et al, Cochrane Database Syst Rev* 2012;**11**:CD009377).

Loxapine (not available in UK as of 2016)

Loxapine nasal spray rapidly reduces agitation in acute mania (n=314, RCT, d/b, p/c, 24/24, Kwentus *et al, Bipolar Disorder* 2012;**14**:31–40) and schizophrenia (n=344, RCT, d/b, p/c, Lesem *et al, Br J Psychiatry* 2011;**198**:51–8; n=129, RCT, d/b, p/c, Allen *et al, J Clin Psychiatry* 2011;**72**:1313–21), with 5–10mg acting in around 10 minutes. The hand-held single-dose inhalator (Adasuve®) is approved in the EU and could be launched in the UK in 2016.

Olanzapine

Olanzapine IM can be used to rapidly control agitation and disturbed behaviours in acute schizophrenia or bipolar mania when oral is inappropriate. Olanzapine IM 10mg is at least as effective as haloperidol 7.5mg IM in acute agitation (in schizophrenia), possibly with a slightly quicker onset of action (e.g. at 30 minutes), no QT prolongation and significantly fewer EPS, including dystonia and akathisia. The following are the main recommendations:

Use of olanzapine IM in APE:

- The initial dose should be 10mg as a single injection (use lower doses in elderly people and in renal or hepatic impairment)
- A maximum of three injections of olanzapine IM may be administered in any 24 hours, with a minimum of two hours between each injection
- Olanzapine IM is intended for short-term use, maximum of three consecutive days.
- The maximum combined daily dose of oral and IM olanzapine is 20mg
- People with significant alcohol before olanzapine IM have decreased oxygen saturation after injection, more marked in people who also had BDZs at the same time (n=25, Wilson *et al, J Emerg Med* 2012;**43**:771–2)
- **IM benzodiazepines** should not be given within an hour of olanzapine IM. Of 160 cases of ADRs reported to Lilly in USA, there were 29 fatalities of which 66% had concomitant BDZs and 76% had concomitant other antipsychotics (Marder *et al, J Clin Psychiatry* 2010;**71**:433–41)
- **Orodispersible olanzapine** produce a plasma level profile similar to oral tablets. IM peak plasma levels are five times higher than oral, peaking after a few minutes. Aggressive oral dosing strategies (e.g. up to 40mg/d) appear reasonably well tolerated and effective in acutely agitated people with a variety of diagnoses (n=148, RCT, p/c, 4/7, Baker *et al, J Clin Psychopharmacol* 2003;**23**:342–8;MS).

A systematic review and meta-analysis has concluded that olanzapine IM is preferable to haloperidol IM but comparator information with other treatments was inadequate (s=13, n=2724, RCTs, Kishi *et al, J Psychiatr Res* 2015;**68**:198–209). Cochrane also noted the manufacturer's involvement, poor and incomplete reporting and the borderline ethical nature of the trials (s=4, n=769, Belgamwar and Fenton, *Cochrane Database Syst Rev* 2005;**2**:CD003729).

Reviews: general (n=1945, Perrin *et al, Eur Psychiatry* 2012;**27**:234–9).

Quetiapine

Quetiapine is licensed for the treatment of acute manic episodes, and 100–200mg stat may have some efficacy as a sedative in emergency settings, but with no clear dose-response pattern (n=20, s/b, Currier *et al, J Psychiatr Pract* 2006;**12**:223–8).

Risperidone (see also combinations)

Risperidone is licensed for acute mania. A prospective study suggested risperidone orodispersible was as effective and tolerable as

IM haloperidol in acute psychotic agitation (n=124, RCT, open, Lim *et al*, *Neuropsychobiology* 2010;**62**:81–6).

Trifluoperazine

Trifluoperazine is licensed as an adjunctive therapy for acute anxiety and agitated states.

Zuclopenthixol acetate (Clopixol Acuphase®)

Clopixol Acuphase® (Lundbeck) can be given at a dose of 50–150mg stat, then repeated after 2–3 days (maximum every 1–2 days) after the first injection. The maximum cumulative dose is 400mg, i.e. four injections or over two weeks, whichever comes first. The onset of action is at about eight hours (peaking at about 36 hours; see psychosis *1.21*), and so should only be used when initial control has been established with other agents. The maximum single dose in the elderly is 100mg. It appears as effective and more sedating than haloperidol in APE and there is an advantage of the need for fewer injections. Several reviews have suggested that more data is needed to prove an advantage over standard therapies (e.g. Gibson *et al*, *Cochrane Database Syst Rev* 2012;**4**:CD000525; FFT). Care is needed with Acuphase® to avoid it being given into a vein of a struggling or over-active patient.

BENZODIAZEPINES (see also combinations)*

Cochrane concludes that the evidence does not show benzodiazepines are superior to placebo monotherapy or with antipsychotics for psychosis-induced aggression or agitation, although practical experience suggests otherwise (s=21, n=1968, RCTs, Gillies *et al*, *Cochrane Database Syst Rev* 2013;**4**:CD003079). Disinhibition may occur with benzodiazepines, especially in people with poor impulse control or impulsivity, high-potency drugs, young or older age, developmental disabilities and/or pre-existing CNS damage. This remains controversial and probably over-rated (review by Paton, *Psychiatr Bull* 2002;**26**:460–2 noting the actual incidence may be lower than 1%).

Diazepam (see also combinations)

The recommended dose of diazepam is 10mg IV or IM, repeated after not less than four hours. IV diazepam is much more consistently absorbed than IM which, in turn, is little faster than oral and slower than the rectal route but should only be used in exceptional circumstances by trained clinicians (see SmPC). Mechanical ventilation and flumazenil should be available in case of respiratory depression, as hypoxic drive can be affected. Diazepam has a long half-life and active metabolites, and so accumulation and toxic delirium (especially in the elderly or in hepatic impairment) must be avoided by use of decreased doses later on. A wide safety margin makes diazepam and lorazepam drugs of choice.

Lorazepam (see also combinations)

Lorazepam IM absorption is as slow as oral administration, but more rapid in an active patient and IM carries less risk than IV. IM lorazepam alone was as effective as lorazepam IM plus either risperidone or haloperidol (both oral) in acute agitation and/or psychosis, although the combination was numerically superior (n=30, RCT, d/b, d/b, Veser *et al*, *J Psychiatr Pract* 2006;**12**:103–8). The dose in acute anxiety is 0.025–0.05mg/kg (1.75–3.5mg for a 70kg person), repeated six-hourly. Some services use 0.5–2mg PO/IM every 1–2 hours until symptoms are controlled, omitting doses when excessive sedation occurs. This can be a highly effective therapy, albeit unlicensed. Lorazepam does not accumulate with repeated doses or in hepatic impairment; distinct advantages over diazepam.

+ Combinations

Antipsychotic + benzodiazepine
(see also separate drugs) *

Combinations of antipsychotics and benzodiazepines are effective, more rapid and predictable and patients are less likely to need a second injection. In a prospective comparison of olanzapine, ziprasidone, haloperidol plus promethazine, haloperidol, and haloperidol and midazolam (all IM), all were equally effective although haloperidol plus midazolam had the worst results (n=150, d/b, 12 hours, Baldaçara *et al*, *Rev Bras Psiquiatr* 2011;**33**:30–9; FFT).

Clonazepam + haloperidol syrup appears more effective and better tolerated than IM haloperidol monotherapy (n=205, 47/7, Fang *et al, Int Clin Psychopharmacol* 2012;**27**:107–13).

Diazepam 10mg IM/IV is a suitable BDZ.

Lorazepam+haloperidol is a widely used combination, with 2mg IM plus haloperidol IM 5-10mg being significantly better than lorazepam alone after 60–180 minutes (n=98, RCT, Battaglia *et al, Am J Emerg Med* 1997;**15**:335–40).

Lorazepam+risperidone (both 2mg orally)was as effective and well tolerated as haloperidol 5mg IM plus lorazepam 2mg IM over two hours (n=162, RCT, s/b, Currier *et al, J Clin Psychiatry* 2004;**65**:386–94). Oro-dispersible risperidone tablets may be useful to ensure administration, and as the peak plasma level occurs at 1.4–1.8 hours (the same as plain tablets) it can be as effective as an alternative to IM antipsychotics (n=191, open, Normann *et al, Pharmacopsychiatry* 2006;**39**:209–12).

Lorazepam+zuclopenthixol oral (20–50mg/d) was inferior to risperidone 2–6mg/d with lorazepam in acute psychosis (n=75, open, 14/7, Hovens *et al, J Psychopharmacol* 2005;**19**:51–7).

Midazolam+haloperidol is another alternative. Haloperidol 2.5mg + midazolam 7.5mg (HAL-MID) was compared to haloperidol 2.5mg + promethazine 25mg (HAL-PRO), ziprasidone 10mg (ZIP) and olanzapine 10mg (OLZ). All four reduced agitation, although agitation was reduced less with ZIP and HAL-PRO, with the latter having the higher risk of EPSE (n=100, RCT, s/b, 1/7, Mantovani *et al, J Clin Psychopharmacol* 2013;**33**:306–12).

Haloperidol + promethazine (HAL-PRO)

Three large trials have shown IM promethazine 25–50mg to be an effective adjunct to haloperidol 10mg IM and as effective as lorazepam IM 4mg, with 96% patients in each group 'tranquil or asleep' after four hours (cf. 76% asleep with HAL-PRO and 45% with lorazepam IM monotherapy; n=200, RCT, Alexander *et al, Br J Psychiatry* 2004;**185**:63–9; favourable comment by McAllister-Williams, *EBMH* 2005;**8**:7; see also n=316[c=311], open, Huf *et al, Br Med J* 2007;**335**:839). HAL-PRO was as effective as olanzapine IM alone in agitated and violent people with mental health problems and needed fewer additional medical interventions at four hours (n=300[c=298], RCT, open, 2/52, Raveendran *et al, Br Med J* 2007;**335**:865). Cochrane concludes that:

- 1% of people given any haloperidol treatment experience a seizure
- After 20 minutes, HAL-PRO is more tranquillising than haloperidol alone
- After 15 minutes olanzapine is as tranquillising as HAL-PRO but does not have an enduring effect and more people need additional treatment at four hours (s=4, n=1117, Huf *et al, Cochrane Database Syst Rev* 2009;**3**:CD005146).

• Unlicensed/some efficacy

Asenapine *

A single dose study concluded asenapine 10mg had equivalent efficacy to IM anti-psychotics (n=120, RCT, d/b, p/c, 1/7, Pratts *et al, Acta Psychiatr Scand* 2014;**130**:61-8).

Clonazepam (see also combinations)

Clonazepam is licensed only for status epilepticus but can be used as an alternative to diazepam and lorazepam, albeit slower-acting. The dose is 1mg (1mL) by slow (1mg per 30 seconds) IV injection, which is strongly recommended to be into the large vein of the antecubital fossa with, if possible, the patient in a supine position to minimise the incidence of hypotension (see SmPC).

Midazolam (see also combinations)

Midazolam may be useful for short-term sedation, with a quick onset and offset. IV is too dangerous in non-specialist mental health settings due to the potential for acute respiratory depression, but 2.5–10mg IM may be rapidly effective (6–20 minutes) in controlling acute agitation, repeated every 20 minutes up to 20mg per sedation event and monitored for at least four hours after the last dose. In a pragmatic real-world trial, with a simple end-point and only 1% drop-outs, IM midazolam was superior to HAL-PRO at 20 and 40 minutes in aggressive or agitated emergency room patients, with few side-effects (n=301, RCT, TREC-CG, *Br Med J* 2003;**317**:708–13 comment by Waraich, *EBMH* 2004;**7**:42). Midazolam IM 5mg was also as effective as (and much quicker acting than) lorazepam IM

2mg or haloperidol IM 5mg in acute agitation, but the effects were shorter-lived (82 minutes vs 217 minutes vs 126 minutes respectively; n=111, RCT, d/b, Nobay *et al*, *Acad Emerg Med* 2004;**11**:744–9).

Buccal midazolam is a non-invasive option, and has an onset of action of 10–15 minutes (n=8, Haschke *et al*, *Br J Clin Pharmacol* 2010;**69**:607–16), peaking at 30 minutes and lasting for at least an hour, with no serious adverse reactions or over-sedation (n=25, 115 doses, open, Taylor *et al*, *Int J Psychiatr Clin Pract* 2008;**12**:309–11).

■ Unlicensed/possible efficacy

Topiramate

A retrospective study suggested topiramate might have some efficacy for the control of aggression in psychosis (n=45, Gobbi *et al*, *J Clin Psychopharmacol* 2006;**26**:467–73).

Valproate

Valproate IV 20mg/kg was better tolerated and as effective as haloperidol IM 5mg at 30minutes (n=80, RCT, d/b, Asadollahi *et al*, *Int Clin Psychopharmacol* 2015;**30**:142-50). Loading doses have an antimanic effect over 48–72 hours (n=7, open, Phroloiv *et al*, *J Clin Psychiatry* 2004;**65**:68–70). See also entry under mania (*1.10.2*).

Ziprasidone IM (not UK)

Ziprasidone 10mg IM every two hours or 20mg IM every four hours is effective (n=79, RCT, d/b, Daniel *et al*, *Psychopharmacol* 2001;**155**:128–34). Lorazepam can be given at the same time, but not in the same syringe.

1.2 AGGRESSION

see also Acute psychiatric emergency (*1.1*), Borderline personality disorder (*1.11*) and Self-injurious behaviour (*1.23*)

Aggression is defined as behaviour accompanied by verbal or physical threats which, if carried out, would cause harm to others, self or property and can include situational (provoked), non-situational (unprovoked), passive, physical or interictal aggression (especially in temporal lobe epilepsy). Aggression is not a diagnosis in itself, but can be a symptom of many conditions, e.g. dementia, personality disorders, PTSD, PMS, trauma, drug withdrawal or intoxication, or as an expression of emotional or behavioural motivations. Low GABA and serotonin levels are associated with aggressive behaviour, and higher noradrenaline and dopamine levels in the brain are associated with increased aggression.

Role of drugs

Drugs may be useful in helping control some cases where suppression of aggression is considered important on safety grounds.

Reviews: pharmacotherapy (Comai *et al*, *J Clin Psychopharmacol* 2012;**32**:237–60), AEDs for aggression and impulsivity (s=14, n=672, Huband *et al*, *Cochrane Database Syst Rev* 2010;**2**:CD003499), in children (Parikh *et al*, *J Child Adolesc Psychopharmacol* 2008;**18**:157–78).

BNF listed

Lithium

Lithium has been shown to reduce aggression and the frequency of episodes in learning disabilities, reducing impulsive aggression with organic brain damage and in children with aggression or conduct disorder, albeit poorly tolerated (e.g. n=86, RCT, d/b, p/c, Malone *et al*, *Arch Gen Psychiatry* 2000;**57**:649–54). A two-month trial at 0.6–1.0mmol/L may be justified in people unmanageable by environmental factors but the potential adverse consequences of sudden discontinuation (accidental or deliberate) should be considered and managed.

■ Unlicensed/some efficacy

Antipsychotics *

Raised dopamine levels may be associated with aggression, so dopamine-blockers may have some rationale. Higher doses are likely to be effective only via a sedating effect. Despite regular use in challenging behaviour in LD, clinical trials show little difference between haloperidol, risperidone and placebo for aggression, and the placebo groups at no point showed a worse response than the antipsychotics (n=86, RCT, d/b, p/c, 26/52, Tyrer *et al*, *Lancet* 2008;**371**:57–63). However, they may still have a role if used carefully.

Clozapine is not easy to use but a large review concludes that clozapine has anti-aggressive effects in schizophrenia and other mental health disorders, particularly TRS (s=4 RCT, s=34 others, Frogley *et al, Int J Neuropsychopharmacol* 2012;**15**:1351–71).

Olanzapine (mean 19mg/d) has reduced impulsive and psychotic symptoms in violent aggressive people with schizophrenia (n=15, RCT, open, 10/52, Gobbi *et al, Neuropsychiatr Dis Treat* 2014;**10**:757–65).

Quetiapine 25–300mg/d may help aggression due to traumatic brain injury (n=7, open, 6/52, Kim and Bijlani, *J Neuropsychiatry Clin Neurosci* 2006;**18**:547–9), and at higher doses (mean 525mg/d) for violent, aggressive behaviour in schizophrenia, with impulsive and psychotic symptoms (n=15, RCT, open, 10/52, Gobbi *et al, Neuropsychiatr Dis Treat* 2014;**10**:757–65).

Risperidone can be useful for treating aggression in a range of behavioural disorders, agitation and dementia (s=19, De Deyn and Buitelaar, *Eur Psychiatry* 2006;**21**:21–8), especially at lower dose, e.g. for severe, primary aggressive behaviour in adolescents with disruptive behaviours compounded by sub-average cognitive abilities (n=38, RCT, p/c, 6/52, Buitelaar *et al, J Clin Psychiatry* 2001;**62**:239–48).

Zuclopenthixol has limited evidence for aggression in learning disabilities (n=39, RCT, d/b, p/c, Hässler *et al, Pharmacopsychiatry* 2008;**41**:232–9), but a discontinuation study suggested lower aggression in treated vs non-treated people (n=39[c=31], two years, Hässler *et al, Pharmacopsychiatry* 2011;**44**:339–43), so it either works and/or there can be rebound aggression on withdrawal.

Benzodiazepines

Benzodiazepines are reported to be effective in episodic behavioural disorders by aborting aggression in the prodromal stage. Use should normally be limited to only a few weeks to minimise the incidence of disinhibition or paradoxical reactions (review by Paton, *Psychiatr Bull* 2002;**26**:460–2, although the actual incidence may be lower than 1%).

Valproate

Valproate may exert an effect by increasing any abnormally low GABA levels. Several studies have shown a rapid effect, e.g. compared to quetiapine (n=33, RCT, d/b, 28/7, Barzman *et al, J Child Adolesc Psychopharmacol* 2006;**16**:665–70) and oxcarbazepine (n=31, retrospective, MacMillan *et al, J Psychiatr Pract* 2006;**12**:214–22), although earlier open studies were less than encouraging (s=17, n=164, Lindenmayer and Kotsaftis, *J Clin Psychiatry* 2000;**61**:123–8).

■ Unlicensed/possible efficacy

Aromatherapy

Lavender can reduce agitation in people with dementia (n=70, RCT, c/o, 3+3/52, Lin *et al, Int J Geriatr Psychiatry* 2007;**22**:405–10).

Beta-blockers

Beta-blockers have been reported to help manage aggression in learning disabilities, autism, schizophrenia and in intermittent explosive disorders, but have potential effects on bp and heart-rate (review by Haspel, *Harv Rev Psychiatry* 1995;**2**:274–81).

Buspirone

A 30mg/d trial is necessary, and an initial transient worsening may occur (n=20, 3/12, Stanislav *et al, J Clin Psychopharmacol* 1994;**14**:126–30) with up to 90mg/d successful for aggressive behaviour in profound LD (n=1, Brahm *et al, Ann Pharmacother* 2008;**42**:131–7).

Carbamazepine

Evidence for carbamazepine in aggression is largely anecdotal, based on an association with TLE or other EEG abnormalities. Carbamazepine 600mg/d has reduced aggressive behaviour in schizophrenia, paroxysmal behaviour disorder and dementia (n=51, RCT. 6/52, Tariot *et al, Am J Psychiatry* 1998;**155**:54–61) and 200mg/d has been successful for BDZ-resistant impulsive aggression (eg. n=1, Pae, *Psychiatry Clin Neurosci* 2008;**62**:483). Beware of an interaction with antipsychotics.

Estrogens (estrogens) See dementia (*1.13*).

Gabapentin

Gabapentin has been used in episodic agitation in severely mentally ill in-patients (n=11, 6/12,

Megna *et al*, *Ann Pharmacother* 2002;**36**:12–6).

Lamotrigine See dementia (*1.13*).

Oxcarbazepine

Oxcarbazepine has improved impulsive aggressiveness (n=48 [c=45], RCT, d/b, p/c, 4–10/52, Mattes, *J Clin Psychopharmacol* 2005;**25**:575–9), including in prison (Mattes, *J Am Acad Psychiatry Law* 2012;**40**:234–8).

Phenytoin

Phenytoin 300 mg/d may reduce impulsive aggressive acts but not premeditated attacks in prisoners (n=60, d/b, p/c, Barratt *et al*, *J Clin Psychopharmacol* 1997;**17**:341–9).

SSRIs

Low serotonin levels have been associated with aggression so the use of SSRIs may be rational. Aggression in learning disabilities may also be associated with unrecognised mood disorders, e.g. depression. **Citalopram** 20–60 mg/d (e.g. n=25, open, 8/52, Reist *et al*, *J Clin Psychiatry* 2003;**64**:81–5) and **sertraline** 50–200 mg/d (open, Kavoussi *et al*, *J Clin Psychiatry* 1994;**55**:137–41) have reduced aggressive incidents with no deterioration or significant side-effects. **Fluoxetine** seems to have a clear anti-aggressive effect in intermittent explosive disorder, although less than 50% achieve a full or partial remission (n=100, RCT, d/b, p/c, Coccaro *et al*, *J Clin Psychiatry* 2009;**70**:653–62), but 20–60 mg/d was ineffective in reducing abuse and aggression by men against intimate-partners (n=26, RCT, p/c, Lee *et al*, *Int Clin Psychopharmacol* 2008;**23**:337–41). Trials may need to be longer to see the full effect.

Vitamins

Nutritional supplements (containing vitamins, minerals and fatty acids) dramatically reduced antisocial behaviour and violent incidents of young offenders within just two weeks (n=231, RCT, p/c, Gesch *et al*, *Br J Psychiatry* 2002;**181**:22–8).

◆ Case reports *

- **Guanfacine** (n=1, Prader-Willi syndrome, Singh *et al*, *J Child Adolesc Psychopharmacol* 2015;**25**:376–7)
- **Topiramate** (Farinde, *J Pharm Pract* 2011;**24**:568–70).

☐ No efficacy

Levetiracetam

Levetiracetam was of no efficacy for impulsive aggression (n=40 [c=34], RCT, d/b, p/c, 10/52, Mattes, *J Clin Psychiatry* 2008;**69**:310–5).

1.3 AGORAPHOBIA

see also Anxiety disorder (*1.6*), Panic disorder (*1.19*) and Social anxiety (*1.25*)

Agoraphobia is an overwhelming and disabling anxiety provoked by being alone or in places where escape might be difficult or embarrassing and so these situations are avoided. Panic attacks may accompany the phobia and depression may be present in up to a half of patients. A link with serotonin deficiency has been shown.

Role of drugs

Pharmacotherapy may be effective in many people, with psychotherapy often being a component of any treatment package. A meta-analysis concluded that symptoms are improved by tricyclics and high potency benzodiazepines and, although there may be a short-term deterioration, this usually turns to a longer-term improvement (s=43, n=2367, Bakker *et al*, *Acta Psychiatr Scand* 2002;**106**:163–7). Exposure therapy can be enhanced by antidepressants. Adding a CBT package to SSRIs for panic (with or without agoraphobia) seems of little additional benefit, with SSRIs more effective than CBT alone (n=150, 9/12, van Apeldoorn *et al*, *Acta Psychiatr Scand* 2008;**117**:260–70).

Reviews: general (Perugi *et al*, *CNS Drugs* 2007;**21**:741–64), epidemiology (Goodwin *et al*, *Eur Neuropsychopharmacol* 2005;**15**:435–43).

BNF listed

Citalopram

Citalopram is licensed for the symptoms of panic disorder, with or without agoraphobia (see also *1.19*). The dose is 10mg/d for a week, increasing to 20–30mg/d, with a maximum of 40mg/d. The maximal effect may take three months to develop.

Escitalopram

Escitalopram is licensed for the symptoms of panic disorder, with or without agoraphobia (see also *1.19*). The dose is 5mg/d for a week, then 10mg/d (maximum 20mg/d). Maximal effects may take three months to develop.

Paroxetine

Paroxetine is licensed for the symptoms and prevention of relapse of panic disorder, with or without agoraphobia. See panic disorder (*1.19*).

● Unlicensed/some efficacy

Benzodiazepines

Alprazolam, diazepam and **clonazepam** have shown significant efficacy (eg. n=24, RCT, p/c, 6/52, Valenca *et al*, *Arq Neuropsiquiatr* 2000;**58**:1025–9).

Review: general (Bruce *et al*, *Am J Psychiatry* 2003;**160**:1432–8).

Tricyclics

While SSRIs are now first choice, tricyclics are still effective in 70% but with high (30%) drop-out rates and 20% may worsen. **Clomipramine** (up to 300mg/d) has been shown to be effective (n=108, d/b, p/c, 8/52, Johnson *et al*, *Arch Gen Psychiatry* 1988;**45**:453–9), with a continuous improvement shown over many weeks. See also panic (*1.19*).

■ Unlicensed/possible efficacy

Buspirone

Buspirone can enhance the effect of CBT (n=41, d/b, 68/52, Cottraux *et al*, *Br J Psychiatry* 1995;**167**:635–41), but an open study was unable to replicate this (open, p/c, Bouvard *et al*, *Psychother Psychosom* 1997;**66**:27–32).

◆ Cases

- **Tranylcypromine** (n=1, Boerner and Lühring, *Psychiatr Prax* 2010;**37**:350–2).

1.4 ALCOHOL DEPENDENCE AND ABUSE

see also Alcohol withdrawal syndrome (*1.5*)

Symptoms

The main diagnostic symptoms of alcohol dependence are a primacy of drinking over other activities, increased tolerance of alcohol, symptoms of repeated withdrawal, stereotyped pattern of drinking, compulsion to drink and relief drinking.

Drinking risk level (DRL)	Total consumption (g/day)	
	Men	Women
Very high risk	>100	64%
High risk	61–100	26%
Medium	41–60	9%
Low risk	1–40	6%

Role of drugs *

Pharmacological treatment can play a significant role in an overall package. Any vitamin deficiency needs correcting (see AWS, *1.5*). Drugs may be useful to treat associated psychiatric morbidity, such as withdrawal, affective disorders, suicidal thoughts and hallucinations. The COMBINE study concluded that acamprosate is ineffective, but that naltrexone, CBI (combined behavioural intervention), or both performed best over the short-term (n=1383, RCT, p/c, 16/52 and follow-up, Anton *et al*, *JAMA* 2006;**295**:2003–17), there is a significant placebo effect in large trial from pills, AA and seeing a healthcare professional (n=1383 Weiss *et al*, *J Stud Alcohol Drugs* 2008;**69**:878–84). CBI had little practical effect (Zweben *et al*, *Alcohol Clin Exp Res* 2008;**32**:1661–9).

In the longer term **disulfiram** probably has limited efficacy but thrice-weekly supervised consumption may be superior to unsupervised daily acamprosate (n=353, retrospective, Diehl *et al*, *Alcohol Alcohol* 2010;**45**:271–7).

A systematic review and meta-analysis (s=123, n=22803, RCT, >12/52, Jonas *et al*, *JAMA* 2014;**311**:1889–900) concluded that acamprosate and oral naltrexone are associated with reduced return to drinking and a comparison between the two showed no significant differences in NNTs:

Preventing return to:	Any drinking	Heavy drinking
Acamprosate	NNT = 12	(NNT = 12)
Naltrexone	NNT = 20	NNT = 12

Reviews: * general (Addolorato *et al*, *CNS Drugs* 2013;**27**:287–99; Leeman *et al*, *Curr Addict Rep* 2014;**1**:41–52; Müller *et al*, *Expert Opin Pharmacother* 2014;**15**:471–81; Lev-Ran *et al*, *Can J Psychiatry* 2012;**57**:342–9), drinking reduction drug strategies (Aubin and Daeppen, *Drug Alcohol Depend* 2013;**133**:15–29), in adolescents (Clark, *CNS Drugs* 2012;**26**:559–69), genetics (Kranzler and Edenberg, *Curr Pharm Des* 2010;**16**:2141–8), anticonvulsants in alcohol dependence (Pani *et al*, *Cochrane Database Syst Rev* 2014;**2**:CD008544).

BNF listed

Acamprosate *

Acamprosate is licensed for abstinence maintenance therapy for up to one year in motivated alcohol-dependent people. It is a GABA analogue and may act to reduce the severity and frequency of relapse by enhancing GABA inhibitory neurotransmission and antagonising glutamate excitation by antagonising mGluR5 receptors, reducing reward and craving, or by increasing plasma calcium levels (Spanagel *et al*, *Neuropsychopharmacology* 2014;**39**:783–91). It takes about seven days to reach therapeutic levels and so can be started soon after detoxification (n=40, RCT, d/b, p/c, 2/52 plus 10/52, Kampman *et al*, *Addict Behav* 2009;**34**:581–6). Continued alcohol consumption negates the therapeutic effect, but occasional lapses do not necessarily do this. Many RCTs have shown clinical effect and a meta-analysis concluded that acamprosate has a significant beneficial effect in enhancing abstinence in recently detoxified alcohol-dependent individuals and as part of a therapeutic approach targeted at achieving abstinence (s=33, Carmen *et al*, *Addiction* 2004;**99**:811–28), although COMBINE was not too encouraging. There appear to be no predictors of the likelihood of efficacy (s=7, n=1485, RCT, p/c, Verheul *et al*, *Psychopharmacol [Berl]* 2005;**178**:167–73), but may have no effect when craving is high (n=169, RCT, d/b, p/c, 12/52, Richardson *et al*, *Addiction* 2008;**103**:953–9). Its efficacy may be enhanced in combination with disulfiram, and as an adjunct to psychosocial and behavioural therapies including counselling (see combinations). Cochrane concluded that acamprosate was effective and safe, albeit with a modest effect size, and an NNT of 9 (s=24, n=6915, RCT, d/b, Rösner *et al*, *Cochrane Database Syst Rev* 2010;**9**:CD004332; see also n=327, RCT, d/b, p/c, 24/52, Higuchi *et al*, *J Clin Psychiatry* 2015;**76**:181–8).

Reviews: * general (Mason, *J Clin Psychiatry* 2015;**76**:e224–5; FFT; Plosker, *Drugs* 2015;**75**:1255–68), pharmacology (Kalk and Lingford-Hughes, *Br J Clin Pharmacol* 2014;**77**:315–23; FFT), mode of action (Mason and Heyser, *CNS Neurol Disord Drug Targets* 2010;**9**:23–32; FFT).

Disulfiram *

Disulfiram irreversibly inhibits ALDH (hepatic Aldehyde-NAD reductase) leading to accumulation of acetaldehyde from incomplete alcohol metabolism. It acts as a negative reinforcer for abstinence via the potential for the disulfiram-alcohol inter-

Disulfiram test dose

A test dose is now considered dangerous due to the risks involved and because the mode of action is via a conditioning process. If considered necessary, wait five days after starting treatment for full enzyme block to occur.

1. Give 10–15ml of 95% alcohol (or 15–25ml spirits).
2. Reaction should start in 5–15 minutes.
3. Repeat in 30 minutes if no reaction. Reaction shows as flushed face, tachycardia, nausea, vomiting, fall in blood pressure. (Have crash box plus personnel available.)

The usual cause of no reaction is too low a dose of disulfiram.
Bronchospasm has also been reported (Berti *et al*, *Br Med J* 1993;**306**:396).

action, i.e. an adversive/conditioning and maintenance therapy in alcoholics although experiencing the Antabuse Reaction may lead to earlier treatment discontinuation (n=46, retrospective, Mutschler *et al*, *Clin Neuropharmacol* 2011;**34**:161–5). Some published advice tends to underestimate doses needed, e.g. <250 mg/d has only a minor interaction with alcohol (Malcolm *et al*, *Expert Opin Drug Saf* 2008;**7**:459–72), so it is suggested to start with a loading dose of 400 mg/d, with 365 mg/d the average dose used (n=33, retrospective, Mueser *et al*, *Am J Addict* 2003;**12**:242–52). A recent review concluded that only open trials show efficacy and that blinded RCTs show no efficacy over controls (s=22, Skinner *et al*, *PLoS One* 2014;**9**:e87366; see also n=109, RCT, s/b, p/c, 26/52, Yoshimura *et al*, *Alcohol Clin Exp Res* 2014;**38**:572–8). 'Antabuse®' (Alpharma) tablets are dispersible and so can be given as a liquid in a supervised setting. It can also be given as a two or three times a week dose (i.e. daily dose x 7 divided by 2), as the enzyme inhibition is irreversible and the clinical effect lasts about 7–10 days.

Review: thorough and positive (Krampe and Ehrenreich, *Curr Pharm Des* 2010;**16**:2076–90).

Nalmefene *

Nalmefene is an opioid receptor antagonist licensed in the UK for the reduction of alcohol consumption in people who have a high drinking risk level without withdrawal symptoms and who do not need detoxification. Other opiate antagonists (e.g. naltrexone) are only licensed for maintenance of abstinence probably by blocking reward pathways. Three major studies have shown efficacy. ESENSE 1 showed 'when required' use of nalmefene 18 mg taken 1–2 hours before alcohol exposure is effective for significantly reducing heavy drinking days (12–13 fewer HDDs per month) and total alcohol consumption (by 58–70 g/d) over six months (n=604[c=347], RCT, d/b, p/c, 24/52, Mann *et al*, *Biol Psychiatry* 2013;**73**:706–13). ESENCE 2 showed that in alcohol dependence (>6 heavy drinking days in the last 4/52) nalmefene significantly reduced heavy drinking days with a non-significant reduction in total intake, the effect being better in people unable to reduce drinking in the 4/52 between referral and randomisation (n=718, RCT, d/b, p/c, 24/52, Gual *et al*, *Eur Neuropsychopharmacol* 2013;**23**:1432–42). Long-term efficacy has been shown (n=675[c=422], RCT, p/c, 12/12, SENSE trial, van den Brink *et al*, *J Psychopharmacol* 2014;**28**:733–44). In an analysis of these three key studies (nalmefene n=1134, placebo n=789), nalmefene was on average taken on 51% days, and 56% (4 days per week) for the licensed target patient group, with an NNT=7 for dropping two WHO drinking categories over 6/12 (ESENSE 1 and 2 combined). Sub-analysis of ESENCE 1 and 2 shows nalmefene to be superior to placebo and with a greater effect in people with at least high drinking risk level at both screening and randomisation (s=2, n=667, RCT, p/c, 6/12, François *et al*, *PloS One* 2015;**10**:e0129289; FFT). The main side-effects are transient nausea, dizziness, headache and insomnia.

Reviews: * general (Paille and Martini, *Subst Abuse Rehabil* 2014;**5**:87–94; FFT; Soyka, *Int J Neuropsychopharmacol* 2014;**17**:675–84; Gual *et al*, *Drugs Today [Barc]* 2014;**50**:347–55).

Naltrexone (UK Adepend® and Naltrexone Accord® brands only at time of writing) *

Naltrexone may be effective through blocking the pleasure (or 'high') caused by alcohol and reducing alcohol-seeking behaviour or reducing craving. A systematic review concluded that naltrexone reduces the risk of heavy drinking to 83% and decreases drinking days by 4%, with mainly GI and sedative ADRs (s=50, n=7793, RCT, d/b, Rösner *et al*, *Cochrane Database Syst Rev* 2010;**12**:CD001867). Sweet taste preference has a strong correlation with response to naltrexone (n=78, p/c, 32/52, Laaksonen *et al*, *Alcohol Alcohol* 2011;**46**:308–11; FFT). The efficacy may be enhanced by limited psychosocial interventions, brief interventions, psychotherapy, prescribing with an antidepressant or by targeted naltrexone, i.e. before situations that might have a high risk of heavy drinking (n=153, RCT, p/c, 8/52, Kranzler *et al*, *J Clin Psychopharmacol* 2003;**23**:294–304). High-dose naltrexone 150 mg/d significantly reduced alcohol consumption cf 50 mg/d and was well tolerated (n=24, open, 8/52, Yoon *et al*, *Hum Psychopharmacol* 2011;**26**:125–32).

Reviews: * general (Hester, *J Clin Psychiatry* 2015;**76**:e226–7; FFT; Ray *et al*, *CNS Neurol Disord Drug Targets* 2010;**9**:13–22).

Vitamin B_1 (thiamine) *

Vitamin deficiency occurs after chronic alcohol abuse due to inadequate diet, impaired absorption, increased metabolic demand and impaired utilisation. Thiamine (B_1) maintenance may be necessary to help reverse the mental confusion secondary to thiamine deficiency where 250 mg IM for 3–5 days will minimise the risk of Wernicke's encephalopathy (Thompson and Marshall, *Alcohol Alcohol* 2006;**41**:159–67; FFT). The usual daily requirement is around 1.5 mg and the most absorbed from the GI tract is around 4.5 mg/d regardless of the dose taken. In alcoholics, absorption is highly variable, can even be none and also very low if alcohol is consumed shortly beforehand (Agabio, *Alcohol Alcohol* 2005;**40**:155–6). Cochrane concludes that thiamine is essential but that the data for dose, frequency, duration and route is lacking (s=1, n=107, RCT, Day *et al*, *Cochrane Database Syst Rev* 2013;**7**:CD004033). See AWS *1.5*.

Review: * reinforcing the need for thiamine (n=100, Rees and Gowing, *Alcohol Alcohol* 2013;**48**:88–92).

+ Combinations

The COMBINE study provides some guidance, but combining drugs with different modes of action may be useful.

Acamprosate + disulfiram

Disulfiram has improved the effectiveness of acamprosate, but a high drop-out did not allow full analysis (n=118, RCT, p/c, 12/12, Besson *et al*, *Alcohol Clin Exp Res* 1998;**22**:573–9).

Acamprosate + naltrexone

The combination was slightly superior to monotherapy and significantly superior to placebo for time to first drink and time to relapse (n=160, RCT, d/b, p/c, 12/52, Kiefer *et al*, *Arch Gen Psychiatry* 2003;**60**:92–9).

Naltrexone + disulfiram

The combination has no advantage over either agent individually for craving or abstinence (n=254, RCT, p/c, 12/52, Petrakis *et al*, *Biol Psychiatry* 2005;**57**:1128–37).

Naltrexone + gabapentin

Gabapentin (≤1200 mg/d) plus naltrexone (50 mg/d) was superior to naltrexone for drinking outcomes at six weeks (n=150, RCT, d/b, p/c, 6/52, Anton *et al*, *Am J Psychiatry* 2011;**168**:709–17; FFT).

Naltrexone + ondansetron

Augmentation of naltrexone 50 mg/d by ondansetron 0.5 mg/d can decrease alcohol craving (n=90, RCT, d/b, p/c, 7/7, Myrick *et al*, *Arch Gen Psychiatry* 2007;**64**:466–75).

Naltrexone + sertraline

Sertraline 200 mg/d plus naltrexone 100 mg/d was superior to either drug separately and to placebo for depression and alcohol dependence (n=170, RCT, d/b, p/c, 14/52, Pettinati *et al*, *Am J Psychiatry* 2010;**167**:668–75).

Oxybate (GHB) + disulfiram

In the 60–70% who maintain alcohol abstinence with GHB, adding disulfiram can enhance the effect (n=52[c=34], 6/52, Maremmani *et al*, *Int J Environ Res Public Health* 2011;**8**:2816–27; FFT).

● Unlicensed/some efficacy

Aripiprazole

Aripiprazole 5–15 mg/d was equivalent in efficacy to naltrexone 50mg/d (n=57 [c=43], RCT, d/b, 16/52, Martinotti *et al*, *J Psychopharmacol* 2009;**23**:123–9), reducing the reward and euphoria from alcohol (n=18, RCT, 3/7, p/c, c/o, Kranzler *et al*, *Alcohol Clin Exp Res* 2008;**32**:573–9).

Baclofen *

There is growing evidence for the use of baclofen. One review concluded that 30 mg/d is safe, well tolerated, significantly improves abstinence and with a low addiction liability (s=3, Muzyk *et al*, *CNS Drugs* 2012;**26**:69–78) although another concluded the evidence was variable and inconclusive (s=3, n=203, RCTs, Brennan *et al, Clin Pharmacol* 2013;**5**:99–107).

Dose: A dose-response seems highly likely as 60 mg/d can be more effective (e.g. n=42, RCT, d/b, p/c, 12/52, Addolorato *et al, Alcohol Alcohol* 2011;**46**:312–7). Its pharmacokinetics are linear from 30–240 mg/d but there is significant interindividual variation (n=37, Marsot *et al, Alcohol Clin Exp Res* 2014;**38**:316–21). A mean dose of 129±71 mg/d produced a marked reduction in alcohol intake, with 52% abstinent (n=181[c=132], one year, Rigal *et al, Alcohol Alcohol* 2012;**47**:439–42; FFT) and doses of 83±57 mg/d can be used with the main ADRs being insomnia in 63% (n=116[c=108], Rigal *et al, Alcohol Alcohol* 2015;**50**:551–7). Individually titrated high doses of 30–270 mg/d have been used and 68% maintained total abstinence over 12/52 cf. 24% with placebo (NNT=3?), without adverse consequences (n=56, RCT, d/b, p/c, 12/52, Müller *et al, Eur Neuropsychopharmacol* 2015;**25**:1167–77). A retrospective case review even showed high doses 300–630mg/d can be used, can be highly effective in resistant cases but is not without risk (n=100, de Beaurepaire, *Front Psychiatry* 2014;5:**143**; FFT). Beware of a Baclofen Withdrawal Syndrome (BWS) which, with symptoms of confusion, agitation, seizures and delirium, looks similar to AWS (n=3, Rolland *et al, J Clin Psychopharmacol* 2014;**34**:153–6).

Reviews: * general (Gorsane *et al, Subst Abus* 2012;**33**:336–49; Leggio *et al, CNS Neurol Disord Drug Targets* 2010;**9**:33–44).

Carbamazepine

An old study showed a significant long-term increase in the time to the first drink and survival rates (n=29, RCT, 12/12, Mueller *et al, Alcohol Clin Exp Res* 1997;**21**:86–92).

Gabapentin (see also combinations) *

Gabapentin 600 mg/d monotherapy post-detox has significantly reduced consumption and craving, improving outcomes, and was well tolerated (n=60, RCT, d/b, p/c, 4/52, Furieri *et al, J Clin Psychiatry* 2007;**68**:1691–1700), and it may help insomnia (n=21, RCT, d/b, p/c, 8/52, Brower *et al, Alcohol Clin Exp Res* 2008;**32**:1429–38).

Dose	Abstinence	No heavy drinking
0 mg/d	4%	23%
900 mg/d	11%	30%
1800 mg/d	17%	45%

In alcohol dependence (see table above), gabapentin was safe and effective, especially at the 1800 mg/d dose (n=150[c=85], RCT, d/b, p/c, 12/52, Mason *et al, JAMA Intern Med* 2014;**174**:70–7).

Gamma-hydroxybutyrate (GHB) see Oxybate

LSD (Lysergic acid diethylamide)

Surprisingly, to me at least, a meta-analysis concludes that a single dose of LSD reduces alcohol misuse (s=6, n=536, RCT, Krebs and Johansen, *J Psychopharmacol* 2012;**26**:994–1002).

Naltrexone depot injection (import only, UK license delayed)

A long-acting naltrexone injection (Vivitrex®, Alkermes) may be effective within two days and have a sustained action over at least 6/12 (n=624, RCT, d/b, p/c, 24/52, Ciraulo *et al, J Clin Psychiatry* 2008;**69**:190–5; review by Gastfriend, *Ann N Y Acad Sci* 2011;**1216**:144–66).

Olanzapine *

Olanzapine 5mg/d reduces alcohol craving and 2.5mg/d decreased drinking days and increased control over drinking, and both doses were well tolerated (n=129, RCT, p/c, 12/52, Littlewood *et al, Psychopharmacology (Berl)* 2015;**232**:1261–8).

Ondansetron (see also combinations)

Ondansetron 8 mcg/kg/d was superior to placebo in increasing drink-free days, especially for pre-25 years onset alcoholism (n=271, RCT, Johnson *et al, JAMA* 2000;**284**:963–71).

Pregabalin *

Pregabalin 150–450 mg/d was as effective as naltrexone for drinking indices and craving, but its effect may be more related to management of comorbid psychiatric symptoms (n=71 [c=48], RCT, d/b, 16/52, Martinotti *et al, J*

Psychopharmacol 2010;**24**:1367–74), although it may help prevent relapse (s=5, Guglielmo *et al*, *Adv Ther* 2012;**29**:947–57).

Review: general (Oulis and Kostantakopoulos, *Expert Opin Investig Drugs* 2012;**21**:1019–29).

Quetiapine

Quetiapine can significantly improve response inhibition to alcohol exposure, a potentially novel mode of action (n=20, RCT, d/b, p/c, c/o, Moallem and Ray, *Pharmacol Biochem Behav* 2012;**100**:490–3; FFT). Quetiapine as monotherapy in dual diagnosis (alcohol dependence and bipolar) markedly reduced alcohol consumption, craving and symptoms (review by Ray *et al*, *Drug Alcohol Rev* 2010; **29**:568–75). However, 25–200mg/d had no additional effect as an adjunct to naltrexone (n=62[c=47], RCT, d/b, p/c, 12/52, Guardia *et al*, *Addict Behav* 2011;**36**:265–9).

Topiramate *

The most recent analysis suggests 150–450mg/d has a small to moderate effect on helping prevent relapse (s=7, n=1125, RCT, p/c, Blodgett *et al*, *Alcohol Clin Exp Res* 2014; **38**:1481–8). Low-dose topiramate (<75mg/d) seems well tolerated and effective in reducing craving as an adjunct to psychotherapy (n=90, open, 6/52 + 4/12, Paparrigopoulos *et al*, *BMC Psychiatry* 2011;**11**:41; FFT).

Valproate

Valproate augmentation of TAU has decreased heavy drinking in people with bipolar I with comorbid alcohol dependence (n=59, RCT, d/b, p/c, 24/52, Salloum *et al*, *Arch Gen Psychiatry* 2005;**62**:37–45; enthusiastic review by Le Fauve, *EBMH* 2005;**8**:79) and successfully treated alcoholic hallucinosis (n=40, RCT, d/b, 10/7, Aliyev and Aliyev, *Alcohol Alcohol* 2008;**43**:456–9).

Varenicline *

Varenicline can reduce alcohol consumption in smokers and non-smokers, reducing overall alcohol consumption and craving, but probably not abstinence rates (s=7, RCT, p/c, Erwin and Slaton, *Ann Pharmacother* 2014; **48**:1445–55).

■ **Unlicensed/possible efficacy**

Agomelatine *

Agomelatine is not prone to abuse so has been used safely for insomnia in abstinent alcohol-dependent people (n=9, 6/52, Grosshans *et al*, *Clin Neuropharmacol* 2014;**37**:6–8).

Benzodiazepines

Although not recommended in alcoholics for the very real fear of dependence, benzodiazepines have been advocated if they are able to reduce alcohol dependence (as a 'lesser of two evils' strategy). Any use should be well-documented in the patient's notes.

Buspirone

Anxious alcoholics have shown reduced anxiety, alcohol consumption and drinking days (e.g. n=61, 12/52, Kranzer *et al*, *Arch Gen Psychiatry* 1994;**51**:720–31), but robust trials show no effect on drinking or anxiety (e.g. n=156, RCT, Fawcett *et al*, *Alcohol Clin Exp Res* 2000;**24**:666–74). It may need four weeks at full therapeutic dose to achieve the effect and so a proper trial is necessary.

Memantine *

There are conflicting data on memantine, e.g. 20–40mg/d dose-dependently attenuated alcohol cue-induced craving (n=38, RCT, 3/7, Krupitsky *et al*, *Am J Psychiatry* 2007;**164**:519–23), but had no effect on any measures in treatment-seeking alcoholic-dependent people (n=34[c=27], d/b, p/c, 16/52, Evans *et al*, *Alcohol Clin Exp Res* 2007;**31**:775–82). It may be effective in alcohol-misuse related dementia or Wernicke-Korsakoff syndrome (n=1, Bonnet *et al*, *Ann Pharmacother* 2014;**48**:1371–5).

Oxcarbazepine

Oxcarbazepine may be as effective and well tolerated as acamprosate in preventing alcohol relapse (n=30, RCT, open, 24/52, Croissant *et al*, *Alcohol Clin Exp Res* 2006;**30**:630–5).

Oxybate, gamma-hydroxybutyrate (GHB) *

Oxybate, licensed in some countries for alcohol and opiate withdrawal, is the approved name for pharmaceutical quality and marketed GHB, whereas GHB is the chemical name, generally used to describe illicit formulations (of highly variable quality and concentrations) for non-medical uses (review by Carter *et al, Drug Alcohol Dependence* 2009;**104**:1–10). The doses for alcohol dependence are 50–100mg/kg/d (usually a 1.75g vial 3–4 times a day). For alcohol dependence the most recent data suggests mid/long-term use is positive but of poor quality (s=7, RCTs, Brambilla *et al, Riv Psichiatr* 2012;**47**:269–80). Its greater abuse potential cf. alcohol is due to lack of delayed adversive effects cf. alcohol, which has e.g. headache (n=14, d/b, c/o, p/c, Johnson and Griffiths, *Exp Clin Psychopharmacol* 2013;**21**:112–23).

Review: * general (Skala *et al, Expert Opin Pharmacother* 2014;**15**:245–57).

SSRIs (see also SSRIs, no efficacy) *

Some SSRIs have produced a modest (16–17%) but significant reduction in alcoholic drink intake and increase in drink-free days in studies of alcoholics, possibly by decreasing desire or reducing the reward eg. **fluoxetine** (n=51, RCT, d/b, p/c, 12/52, Cornelius *et al, Arch Gen Psychiatry* 1997;**54**:700–5), but a larger study failed to reproduce these findings (n=101, RCT, p/c, 6/12, Kranzler *et al, Am J Psychiatry* 1995;**152**:391–7).

Tiagabine

Adjunctive tiagabine (mean 17mg/d) showed improved craving and lower relapse (7% vs 14%) than placebo (n=120, open, RCT, 6/12, Paparrigopoulos *et al, J Psychopharmacol* 2010;**24**:1375–80), although not by attenuating alcohol-induced activation of the reward system (n=20, Fehr *et al, Psychopharmacol (Berl)* 2007;**191**:975–83).

Zonisamide

Two unrepeated pilot studies showed up to 300mg/d was well tolerated and improved craving and alcohol intake (n=22, open, 12/52, Rubio *et al, Clin Neuropharmacol* 2010;**33**:250–3; n=10, open, d/b, p/c, 13/52, Knapp *et al, Am J Drug Alcohol Abuse* 2010;**36**:102–5).

• Case reports

- **Mirtazapine** (n=1, Crockford and White, *J Clin Psychiatry* 2005;**66**:540).

□ No efficacy

Antipsychotics * (see also some efficacy)

A meta-analysis of trials on antipsychotics including amisulpride (e.g. n=274, open, 6/12, Flórez *et al, Adicciones* 2011;**23**:149–56), aripiprazole, flupentixol decanoate (n=281, RCT, d/b, 12/12, Weisbeck *et al, Alcohol Alcohol* 2001;**36**:329–34), olanzapine (n=60, RCT, d/b, 12/52, Guardia *et al, Alcohol Clin Exp Res* 2004;**28**:736–45) and quetiapine, for primary alcohol dependence concluded there was no improvement and in many cases were detrimental, with the exception of a small study with aripiprazole (s=13, n=1593, RCT, d/b, Kishi *et al, J Clin Psychiatry* 2013;**74**:642–54).

Donepezil

High dose donepezil may help the memory deficits from Korsakoff's psychosis (n=2, Codina *et al, Rev Neurol* 2002;**35**:341–5) but not reverse the process (n=7, s/b, p/c, c/o, 30/7, Sahin *et al, Clin Neuropharmacol* 2002;**25**:16–20).

Levetiracetam

Two robust RCTs have shown no efficacy (n=130, RCT, d/b, p/c, 16/52, Fertig *et al, Alcohol Clin Exp Res* 2012;**36**:1421–30; FFT), or on relapse prevention (n=201, RCT, d/b, p/c, 16/52, Richter *et al, J Clin Psychopharmacol* 2012;**32**:558–62).

Lithium

Three trials have shown no advantage over placebo (e.g. n=156, RCT, 6/12, Fawcett *et al, Alcohol Clin Exp Res* 2000;**24**:666–74).

SSRIs (see also SSRIs, possible efficacy)

Fluvoxamine was worse than placebo (n=493, RCT, d/b, p/c, 12/12, Chick *et al, Drug Alcohol Depend* 2004;**74**:61–70), **sertraline** was ineffective (n=113, RCT, d/b, p/c, 10/52, Farren *et al, Drug Alcohol Depend* 2009;**99**:317–21) and **citalopram** was actually worse than placebo on some measures (n=265, RCT, d/b, p/c, 12/52, Charney *et al, Alcohol Clin Exp Res* 2015;**39**:1756–65).

1.5 ALCOHOL WITHDRAWAL SYNDROME (AWS)

see also Alcohol dependence and abuse (*1.4*)

Symptoms *

AWS presents as psychological (e.g. anxiety, insomnia and restlessness), psychotic and physical symptoms (e.g. hallucinations, tremor, sweating, tachycardia, gastrointestinal), GTC seizures, hallucinations and illusions, clouding of consciousness, delirium tremens (DT) and Wernicke's encephalopathy (WE). WE is the acute phase, lasting for about 48 hours after the last drink, and results from thiamine (B1) deficiency. If untreated it can become chronic (Korsakoff psychosis, KP) characterised by severe short-term memory loss. Fits may start within 6–8 hours of the last drink and peak at 12–24 hours (chronic alcohol consumption causes adaptation and down-regulation of GABA and upregulation of NMDA receptors, so sudden withdrawal leads to hyperexcitability and hence seizures). In DT, seizures may occur either primary or secondary to hypoglycaemia, hypomagnesaemia, hyperkalaemia (n=190, Ignjatovic-Ristic *et al*, *Ann Gen Psychiatry* 2013;**12**:39) or hyponatraemia, as may suicidal ideation, gross disorientation, delusions, violence and marked tremor. DT peaks on the third or fourth day, and physical complications are common, e.g. pulmonary infection and hepatic encephalopathy. Risk factors for alcohol withdrawal delirium include concurrent infection, tachycardia, symptoms of withdrawal with blood alcohol levels above 1g/L, and a history of epileptic seizures or delirious episodes.

Role of drugs

Seizures and psychiatric disturbances are serious problems and adequate treatment of severe AWS is essential. Cochrane concludes that benzodiazepines are protective against seizures and other outcomes, but the data is inconclusive, and there is insufficient evidence for the use of anticonvulsants, baclofen and oxybate (s=114, n=7333, Amato *et al*, *Cochrane Database Syst Rev* 2011;**6**:CD008537).

NICE recommended (June 2010):

For alcohol withdrawal syndrome:

1. First-line therapy is benzodiazepines (diazepam and chlordiazepoxide are licensed) or carbamazepine — dosage should be individualised according to withdrawal severity, comorbidity and history of withdrawal seizures.
2. Clomethiazole is an alternative for in-patients.
3. Do not offer phenytoin for AWS.

For delirium tremens:

1. Use lorazepam orally (unlicensed). If refused or ineffective try lorazepam injection, haloperidol or olanzapine (all unlicensed).

For prevention of Wernicke's encephalopathy:

1. Offer prophylactic thiamine at the top end of BNF range, orally or parenterally.
2. If WE is suspected, offer IM thiamine for at least five days, then maintenance oral thiamine.

Reviews: * pharmacotherapy (s=14, Ungur *et al*, *Alcohol Clin Exp Res* 2013;**37**:675–86; Franck and Jayaram-Lindström, *Curr Opin Neurobiol* 2013;**23**:692–9), seizures (Hughes, *Epilepsy Behav* 2009;**15**:92–7), anticonvulsants in AWS (s=56, n=4076, Minozzi *et al*, *Cochrane Database Syst Rev* 2010;**3**:CD005063), in-patient management (Perry, *CNS Drugs* 2014;**28**:401–10).

BNF listed

Benzodiazepines *

Benzodiazepines are the first-line drugs for acute AWS, e.g. **chlordiazepoxide** (n=108, Wiseman *et al*, *J Clin Psychiatry* 1998;**59**:289–93) and **diazepam**, where loading doses are rapidly successful and reduce seizures and duration of DTs (s=4, RCT, Muzyk *et al*, *Am J Addict* 2013;**22**:113–8). **Lorazepam** starting at 8mg/d (n=100, RCT, d/b, 12/7, Kumar *et al*, *J Stud Alcohol Drugs* 2009;**70**:457–74) and **oxazepam** (n=117, RCT, Daeppen *et al*, *Arch Intern Med* 2002;**162**:1117–21) have also been used, as they have an intermediate half-life, no active metabolites and may be safer in lower doses in impaired liver function. In symptom-triggered use of lorazepam (n=33), the mean dose of 9.5mg was lower and used for a shorter time (48 hours) than fixed dose lorazepam (20mg; 146 hours) (n=63, RCT, d/b, a/c, Sachdeva *et al*, *Alcohol Alcohol* 2014;**49**:287–91; FFT). **Clonazepam** has been used (n=74, open, Bonnet *et al*, *Alcohol Alcohol* 2011;**46**:68–73). Higher doses of benzodiazepines may reduce the need for mechanical ventilation in acute DTs (n=54, Gold *et al*, *Crit Care Med* 2007;**35**:724–30). Beware of an extended metabolism in liver damage (see *3.6*), and respiratory depression. **Review:** BDZs in AWS (s=64, n=4309, Amato *et al*, *Cochrane Database Syst Rev* 2010;**3**:CD005063).

Clomethiazole (chlormethiazole)

Clomethiazole is effective for AWS at up to 16 capsules/d, reducing over 5–9 days. It has a low addictive potential, although dependence (mainly psychological) can be seen in some people on longer-term therapy. Clomethiazole is as effective as carbamazepine for AWS, with less risk of premature discharge (n=168, Hillemacher *et al*, *Pharmacopsychiatry* 2008; **41**:134–7), albeit markedly suppressing REM sleep (n=20, RCT, p/c, d/b, 13/7, Gann *et al*, *Pharmacopsychiatry* 2004;**37**:228–35).
Reviews: home detoxification schedules, and discussion that clomethiazole may not be as toxic as reputed (Sowerby and Hunter, *J Substance Misuse* 1997;**2**:62–3;114–7), general (Duncan and Taylor, *Psychiatr Bull* 1996;**20**:157–9).

Vitamin B (inc. thiamine) supplementation *

Despite its obvious need, it seems thiamine is still not being used enough for WE (n=217, Isenberg-Grzeda *et al*, *J Addict Med* 2014;**8**:1–5). Classic signs of vitamin deficiency may only occur in extreme depletion and so are easily missed, being interpreted as intoxication. B vitamins act as co-enzymes for essential carbohydrate metabolism and deficiency of nicotinamide, riboflavin (B_2) and pyridoxine (B_6) can cause neuropathies. Thiamine (B_1) supplementation must be primary and priority treatment to reverse the mental confusion secondary to thiamine deficiency (Wernicke's encephalopathy). Oral thiamine has a saturable absorption and only about 4.5 mg of an oral dose is absorbed. Thiamine 100 mg TDS allows about 13.5 mg to be absorbed, adequate only for mild deficiency. In chronic alcohol misusers, oral absorption can be reduced by 70%. Large oral doses are thus futile and adequate parenteral therapy should be routine, and is essential to treat or prevent KP/WE (review, Thompson, *Alcohol Alcohol* 2000;**35**[Suppl 1]:S2–S7). Indeed, only 16% of people with WE recovered when given low parenteral thiamine doses (50–100 mg/d) and 20% died (see Thompson *et al*, *Alcohol Alcohol* 2002;**37**:513–21). The parenteral dose necessary is about 500–1000 mg for 3–5 days (Thompson and Marshall, *Alcohol Alcohol* 2006;**41**:159–67). Although anaphylaxis has been reported with 'Parentrovite®' (Link), the incidence is about one report for every 5,000,000 IM ampoules used, somewhat less than the risk from WE. It may be necessary to administer glucose after thiamine when administering thiamine to prevent WE. Cochrane concludes that thiamine is essential but that the data for dose, frequency, duration and route is lacking (Day *et al*, *Cochrane Database Syst Rev* 2013;**7**:CD004033).
Reviews: * Reinforcing the need for thiamine (n=100, Rees and Gowing, *Alcohol Alcohol* 2013;**48**:88–92), general and recommendations (Latt and Dore, *Intern Med J* 2014;**44**:911–5; Thompson *et al*, *Alcohol Alcohol* 2002;**37**:513–21).

+ Combinations

Carbamazepine + tiapride

These were more effective than either drug separately (n=56, RCT, open, Croissant *et al*, *Pharmacopsychiatry* 2009;**42**:175–81).

• Unlicensed/some efficacy

Antipsychotics

Decreased dopamine activity may occur in DT so care is needed with anti-dopaminergic drugs (despite NICE's recommendations), as these may aggravate symptoms and lower the seizure threshold. NMS may also occur and not be recognised. Temperature regulation and liver function pose further difficulties.

Baclofen *

Baclofen 30 mg/d (n=18) may be as effective as diazepam (n=19) in uncomplicated AWS (n=37, RCT, 10/7, Addolorato *et al*, *Am J Med* 2006;**119**:13–8). A more recent trial showed baclofen 30 mg/d significantly reduced the need for high-dose lorazepam use for AWS (n=44[c=31], RCT, p/c, 3/7, Lyon *et al*, *J Hosp*

Med 2011;**6**:469–74). Cochrane concludes that there is still insufficient evidence for efficacy (s=2, n=81, RCTs, Liu and Wang, *Cochrane Database Syst Rev* 2015;**4**:CD008502).

Carbamazepine

Carbamazepine appears safe, tolerable and effective for moderate-to-severe AWS in inpatient settings, but is unproven for seizures and DTs compared to BDZs (s=7, n=612, Barrons and Roberts, *J Clin Pharm Ther* 2010;**35**:153–67). It is non-addictive and its metabolism is generally little affected by liver dysfunction, but may be inhibited by higher doses of alcohol. It has also been used for outpatient detoxifications due to its safety and lack of abuse potential (n=76[c=60], open, Collins *et al*, *Br J Psychiatry* 1990;**156**:871–4).

Dexmedetomidine *

In severe AWS adjunctive dexmedetomidine infusion can be used in an ITU for sedation and autonomic symptoms (s=13, Wong *et al Am J Drug Alcohol Abuse* 2015;**41**:82–91; n=41, Lizotte *et al*, *Clin Pharmacol* 2014;**6**:171–7; FFT). It can have a BDZ-sparing effect (n=61, open, Crispo *et al*, *Pharmacotherapy* 2014;**34**:910–7) in the short-term, but not in the long-term (Mueller *et al*, *Crit Care Med* 2014;**42**:1131–9).

■ Unlicensed/possible efficacy

Alcohol IV

In an acute setting, IV alcohol had no advantage over diazepam for acute AWS (n=50, RCT, 4/7, Weinberg *et al*, *J Trauma* 2008;**64**:99–104).

Beta-blockers

Beta-blockers, such as atenolol and propranolol, have been used in treating some symptoms of mild-to-moderate AWS, e.g. tachycardia and tremor, and to reduce craving, but are generally not recommended. Propranolol has variable kinetics in cirrhosis (e.g. Worner, *Am J Drug Alcohol Abuse* 1994;**20**:115–24).

Gabapentin *

Gabapentin (1200mg/d tapering down) may be as effective as lorazepam (n=100, RCT, d/b, 12/7, Myrick *et al*, *Alcohol Clin Exp Res* 2009;**33**:1582–8) and chlordiazepoxide (n=26, RCT, d/b, 6/7, Stock *et al*, *Ann Pharmacother* 2013;**47**:961–9) for AWS and reduce post-withdrawal drinking, with less sedation and craving. Higher doses of up to 3200mg in the first 24 hours may be helpful in less severe and uncomplicated AWS, but not for more severe AWS (n=37, open, Bonnet *et al*, *Alcohol Alcohol* 2010;**45**:143–5).

Lamotrigine

Lamotrigine may help DTs but does not decrease mortality (n=240, RCT, 4/52, Djokic *et al*, *Srp Arh Celok Lek* 2011;**139**(Suppl 1):41–5).

Lofexidine

Lofexidine (e.g. 0.4mg qds for 2–3 days) is superior to placebo in controlling AWS (e.g. n=23, RCT, d/b, p/c, Cushman and Sowers, *Alcohol Clin Exp Res* 1989;**13**:361–4), but it was ineffective as an adjunct to chlordiazepoxide, with more adverse effects and poorer retention (n=72, RCT, Keaney *et al*, *Alcohol Alcohol* 2001;**36**:426–30).

Mirtazapine

Adjunctive mirtazapine 30–60mg/d can reduce anxiety and depressive symptoms during detox (n=68, 4/52, Liappas *et al*, *J Psychopharmacol* 2004;**18**:88–93).

Oxcarbazepine

Oxcarbazepine may be more effective than carbamazepine, with less craving (n=29, RCT, s/b, Schik *et al*, *Addict Biol* 2005;**10**:283–8).

Oxybate, gamma-hydroxybutyrate (GHB) *

GHB 50mg is effective for AWS and may be available in the UK under a special license as Alcover® for uncomplicated AWS. GHB counteracts the increased CNS excitability during alcohol withdrawal and, although oxybate has anticonvulsant activity, this is unquantified so during withdrawal it is appropriate to use BDZs for about five days. GHB can be started before the blood alcohol level would have reached zero, as the onset is 20 minutes after the first dose. It has a short half-life (four hours; eight-hour action), so it may be needed 4–6 times a day initially for craving. A duration of 7–10 days is recommended for alcohol withdrawal, with longer for dependence Efficacy has been shown against e.g. oxazepam (similar outcomes and highly tolerable; n=126, RCT, d/b, a/c, 10/7, Caputo *et al, CNS Drugs* 2014;**28**:743–52), superior to diazepam (n=42, RCT, open, 3/52, Nava *et al, Am J Drug Alcohol Abuse* 2007;**33**:379–92) and as effective as clomethiazole (n=98[c=65], RCT, d/b, p/c, 8/7, Nimmerrichter *et al, Alcohol Alcohol* 2002;**37**:67–73). The main ADR is slight 'subjective dizziness' in most people after the first dose, which resolves in 15–30 minutes and does not occur with subsequent administrations. GHB risks abuse and dependence in polysubstance misuse.

Reviews: general (Addolorato *et al Expert Opin Investig Drugs* 2009;**18**:675–86), mode of action (Ameisen, *Alcohol Alcohol* 2007;**42**:506).

Oxytocin *

Intranasal oxytocin 24iu BD can block alcohol withdrawal symptoms, rather than just sedating (n=11, RCT, d/b, p/c, 3/7, Pedersen *et al, Alcohol Clin Exp Res* 2013;**37**:484–9).

Phenobarbital *

Phenobarbital IV (mean 509mg/d) can be as effective as lorazepam oral (mean 4.2mg/d) for mild-to-moderate AWS at 48 hours (n=44, RCT, Hendey *et al, Am J Emerg Med* 2011;**29**:382–5), an alternative to diazepam (n=194, Hjermø *et al, Dan Med Bull* 2010;**57**:A4169). A single IV dose of phenobarbital added to a lorazepam alcohol withdrawal protocol has reduced ICU admissions (n=102, RCT, d/b, p/c, Rosenson *et al, J Emerg Med* 2013;**44**:592–8). In BDZ-resistant AWS, phenobarbital IV 65mg with 130mg 15 minutes later was effective (n=1, Hayner *et al, Pharmacotherapy* 2009;**29**:875–8). For the academically minded, the seizures had failed to respond to lorazepam at over 40mg/hr IV, so that indisputably classifies as BDZ-resistant.

Pregabalin

Pregabalin up to 200–450mg/d was as effective as lorazepam in uncomplicated AWS (n=111, RCT, s/b, 14/7, Martinotti *et al, Addiction* 2010;**105**:288–99) and might be an alternative for out-patient detoxification (n=40, open, Di Nicola *et al, Hum Psychopharmacol* 2010;**25**:268–75). However, one study concluded that pregabalin >300mg/d was not superior to placebo (n=42, RCT, d/b, p/c, 6/7, Förg *et al, Alcohol Alcohol* 2012;**47**:149–55; FFT).

Propofol *

BDZ-refractory AWS adjunctive propofol infusion can be used in an ITU for sedation with no bradycardia (n=184, Wong *et al, J Crit Care* 2015;**30**:405–9; n=41, Lizotte *et al, Clin Pharmacol* 2014;**6**:171–7; FFT).

Tiapride

A study concluded that tiapride has potential efficacy (n=140, Franz *et al, Eur Arch Psychiatry Clin Neurosci* 2001;**251**:185–92).

Trazodone

A systematic review concluded that trazodone is the drug of choice for insomnia in alcohol recovery, albeit with some qualifications (Kolla *et al, Alcohol Alcohol* 2011;**46**:578–85).

Valproate

Only a third of the available studies show a significant effect for valproate in AWS (s=6, Lum *et al, Ann Pharmacother* 2006;**40**:441–8), although it may be a suitable alternative to BDZs due to its lack of abuse potential (n=16, RCT, 6/52, Longo *et al, J Addict Dis* 2002;**21**:55–64) and may be more tolerable, with lower seizures and shorter treatment duration than carbamazepine as an adjunct to clomethiazole and clonidine (n=827, retrospective, Eyer *et al, Alcohol Alcohol* 2011;**46**:177–84; FFT).

Zonisamide

Zonisamide ≤600mg/d (reducing to 100–300mg/d) was superior to diazepam ≤130mg/d (reducing to 5–15mg/d) for AWS (n=40, RCT, 3/52, Rubio *et al, Pharmacopsychiatry* 2010;**43**:257–62).

◆ Others *

Other drugs tried include **magnesium sulphate** (Cochrane concludes the evidence is insufficient to show whether it is harmful or beneficial, s=4, n=317, RCT, Sarai *et al, Cochrane Database Syst Rev* 2013;**6**:CD008358) and **nitrous oxide** (s=6, Prince and Turpin, *Am J Health Syst Pharm* 2008;**65**:1039–47).

☐ No efficacy

Fluvoxamine

Fluvoxamine has no role in alcoholic Korsakoff (n=8, p/c, d/b, c/o, 4/52, O'Carroll *et al, Psychopharmacology (Berl)* 1994;**116**:85–8).

Levetiracetam

A prospective study showed no apparent efficacy (n=106, RCT, d/b, p/c, 6/7, Richter *et al, J Clin Psychopharmacol* 2010;**30**:720–5).

ALZHEIMER'S DISEASE

see Dementia (*1.13*)

ANOREXIA AND BULIMIA NERVOSA

see Eating disorders (*1.15*)

1.6 ANXIETY DISORDER

(generalised) — Generalised Anxiety disorder (GAD) includes also panic disorder (*1.19*) with or without agoraphobia (*1.3*), OCD (*1.18*) and social phobia (*1.25*)

Symptoms *

The many numerous symptoms of generalised anxiety disorder (also a symptom of many conditions) can be placed into two main groups:

- Psychological symptoms include fearful apprehension, irritability, poor concentration, restlessness, fatigue, noise sensitivity, disturbed sleep and poor memory and concentration.
- Physical symptoms, mainly sympathetic system overactivity or increased muscle tension, e.g. GI (dry mouth, difficulty swallowing, wind, loose motions, etc), CNS (tinnitus, blurred vision, dizziness), respiratory (difficulty inhaling, overbreathing), cardiovascular (palpitations, heart pain, missed or ectopic beats, neck throbbing), genitourinary (increased micturition, lack of libido and impotence), muscular tension (headache, tremor) and panic attacks.

The lifetime prevalence is about 17% in USA (s=46, Somers *et al, Can J Psychiatry* 2006;**51**:100–13), with a 90% lifetime comorbidity and only about 25% of GAD cases present without any comorbidity (Maier *et al, Acta Psychiatr Scand* 2000;**101**:29–36).

Role of drugs *

Benzodiazepines used as a 'first-line' measure are quite appropriate, but longer-term effectiveness is difficult to assess as anxiety tends to fluctuate regardless of treatment. The decision for longer-term treatment must be considered on an individual basis, with the risk:benefit analysis varying with the disability caused, the age of the person and the risk of self-management strategies such as alcohol. The SSRIs and venlafaxine are effective across a range of anxiety disorders and generally considered first-line treatment. Initial worsening and rare suicidal ideation can occur, so specific monitoring is needed early in treatment. BDZs are effective, but use is not recommended by NICE and should only be used in the short-term if anxiety is treatment-resistant. Low-dose trifluoperazine is about the only antipsychotic shown to be effective for GAD. There is unlikely to be a response if there is no evidence of onset of an effect within four weeks. Treatment should be continued for at least 12 months if successful (Baldwin *et al, Int J Neuropsychopharmacol* 2011; **14**:697–710).

The most recent systematic review and meta-analysis concluded that the top ranking drugs in mixed states were **fluoxetine** (response and remission) and **sertraline** (tolerability); and for pure GAD, the top drugs were duloxetine (response), **escitalopram** (remission) and **pregabalin** (tolerability), with venlafaxine and paroxetine lower ranked (s=27, RCT, Baldwin *et al, Br Med J* 2011;**342**:d1199; FFT). A meta-analysis of psychological therapies for GAD noted that most used CBT, with waiting list controls, with some element of publication bias and low to moderate heterogeneity (s=41, n=2132, Cuijpers *et al, Clin Psychol Rev* 2014;**34**:130–40).

Reviews: * new approaches (Buoli *et al, Expert Opin Pharmacother* 2013;**14**:175–84), pharmacological alternatives to antidepressants and BDZs (s=36, Huh *et al, Prim Care Companion CNS Disorders* 2011;**13**:PCC.08r00709), BAP Guidelines (Baldwin *et al, J Psychopharmacol* 2014;**28**:403–39), new approaches (Buoli *et al, Expert Opin Pharmacother* 2013;**14**:175–84), strategies for refractory GAD (Samuel *et al,*

Int Clin Psychopharmacol 2011;**26**:63–8), meta-analysis (s=234, n=37,333, Bandelow *et al*, *Int Clin Psychopharmacol* 2015;**30**:183–92).

BNF listed

BENZODIAZEPINES

Benzodiazepines may be extremely useful for chronic anxiety and should not be overlooked. Indiscriminate benzodiazepine prescribing is inappropriate, but they have a distinct role as safe and effective treatments, and that long-term use will not inevitably lead to dose escalation or other dependence. A systematic review and meta-analysis of benzodiazepines showed robust evidence for efficacy if later, more rigorous, trials are favoured (s=23, RCT, p/c, Martin *et al*, *J Psychopharmacol* 2007;**21**:774–82). Use of benzodiazepines can be restricted to short-term (up to four weeks) or intermittent courses.

Risks of benzodiazepines:

- All benzodiazepines can be fatal in overdose (especially combined with alcohol) and should not be prescribed for people at high risk of overdose, particularly temazepam, alprazolam and flurazepam (303 overdose study by Buckley *et al*, *Br Med J* 1995;**310**:219–21)
- Significantly greater risk of road accidents, possibly due to a greater difficulty in maintaining road position (s=27, Rapoport *et al*, *J Clin Psychiatry* 2009; **70**:663–73)
- Increased risk of hip fractures by 50% with doses of >3 mg/d diazepam (or equivalent), especially after initiation and after more than a month of treatment. Shorter half-life BDZs did not appear to reduce this risk (n=6110, Wang *et al*, *Am J Psychiatry* 2001;**158**:892–8).

Reviews: general (Cloos and Ferreira, *Curr Opin Psychiatry* 2009;**22**:90–5), withdrawing BDZs (Lader *et al*, *CNS Drugs* 2009;**23**:19–34).

Alprazolam

Alprazolam (review, Verster and Volkerts, *CNS Drug Rev* 2004;**10**:45–76) is a widely-used BDZ (except in UK).

Chlordiazepoxide

Chlordiazepoxide has a slower onset of action and many active metabolites.

Clobazam

Clobazam is licensed for the short-term (two to four weeks) treatment of anxiety.

Diazepam

Diazepam is the standard longer-acting benzodiazepine, with sedative, anxiolytic and muscle relaxant properties (among others). It has a long half-life and many active metabolites.

Lorazepam

Lorazepam is a shorter-acting benzodiazepine with a higher receptor affinity.

Oxazepam

Oxazepam is a shorter-acting benzodiazepine (the ultimate metabolite of diazepam and some others) with no active metabolites.

Non-benzodiazepines

Beta-blockers

Propranolol at 20–60 mg/d may be useful for somatic symptoms such as tachycardia, sweating and tremor (n=120, open, c/o, Milanov, *Electromyogr Clin Neurophysiol* 2007; **7**:3–9). It appears most effective in people presenting with autonomic complaints, e.g. palpitations and shortness of breath, but not if they have asthma.

Buspirone

Buspirone is a non-benzodiazepine anxiolytic with negligible sedative, cognitive, hypnotic, anticonvulsant and muscle relaxant properties. Buspirone possibly acts on 5-HT_{1A} receptors and

> Benzodiazepines are indicated for short-term relief of severe anxiety. Other treatment methods should then be started, e.g. relaxation, psychotherapy, treating any underlying depression, etc. Caution is advised for the use of benzodiazepines, e.g. short-term use, and avoid in depression and personality disorders.

has no effect on withdrawal in benzodiazepine-dependent people. Buspirone has a slow onset of action and may be underused, as it needs four weeks at 10mg TDS for full efficacy. It is not well tolerated and slower acting in people stopping benzodiazepines (n=735, DeMartinis *et al, J Clin Psychiatry* 2000;**61**:91–4). Cochrane concludes that buspirone is superior to placebo but less effective than BDZs (s=36, n=5908, Chessick *et al, Cochrane Database Syst Rev* 2006;**3**:CD006115).

Reviews: general (Loane and Politis, *Brain Res* 2012;**1461**:111–8), pharmacokinetics (Salazar *et al, J Clin Pharmacol* 2001;**41**:1351–8).

Duloxetine

Duloxetine is licensed for GAD, with a starting dose of 30mg/d, increasing up to 60mg/d and a maximum dose of 120mg/d. Data from three independent trials showed duloxetine 60–120mg/d to consistently improve functioning in GAD (s=3, n=1163, RCT, d/b, p/c, 9–10/52, Endicott *et al, J Clin Psychiatry* 2007;**68**:518–24) and 120mg/d is non-inferior to venlafaxine (s=2, n=984, RCT, d/b, p/c, 10/52, Allgulander *et al, J Psychopharmacol* 2008;**22**:417–25). In non-responders to 60mg/d for 6/52 there was some benefit from a further 18/52, but not from increasing the dose to 120mg/d (n=39 [c=22], RCT, d/b, p/c, 24/52, Simon *et al, CNS Spectr* 2010;**15**:367–73). In responders, relapse with duloxetine 60–120mg/d was 14% vs 42% with placebo (n=405, RCT, d/b, p/c, 26/52, Davidson *et al, Eur Neuropsychopharmacol* 2008;**18**:673–81), and higher in people with co-morbid pain (n=429, open, Bodkin *et al, Hum Psychopharmacol* 2011:**26**:258–66).

Reviews: general (s=4, d/b, p/c, 9–10/52, Kornstein *et al, Expert Rev Neurother* 2009; **9**:155–65), use in comorbid depression (Mancini *et al, Expert Opin Pharmacother* 2010; **11**:1167–81).

Escitalopram

Escitalopram is licensed for GAD, starting at 10mg/d up to a 20mg/d maximum. There may be a significant improvement as early as the first week, and the majority of people respond by week eight with a significant improvement in functioning (n=315, RCT, d/b, p/c, 8/52, Davidson *et al, Depress Anxiety* 2004;**19**:234–40), but a trial should last at least four weeks before any changes are considered (s=40, Baldwin *et al, Hum Psychopharmacol* 2009;**24**:269–75). Several large studies have shown that 10–20mg/d are equally effective for GAD and superior to paroxetine (suggesting that perhaps not all SSRIs are the same in GAD) and placebo (n=681, RCT, d/b, 12/52, Baldwin *et al, Br J Psychiatry* 2006;**189**:264–72;n=3, RCT, p/c, Stein *et al, Ann Clin Psychiatry* 2005;**17**:71–5). It also seems effective in the long-term, with relapse on escitalopram (20%) less than placebo (50%) (s=4, RCT, d/b, 24/52, Bech *et al, J Clin Psychiatry* 2010;**71**:121–9).

Hydroxyzine *

Hydroxyzine (still licensed for anxiety but omitted from the BNF) is an antihistamine related to the phenothiazines and may have slight efficacy. Cochrane is scathing about the available studies and does not think it possible to recommend hydroxyzine as a reliable anxiolytic in GAD (s=5, n=884, Guaiana *et al, Cochrane Database Syst Rev* 2011;**12**:CD006815).

Paroxetine *

Paroxetine is licensed for GAD and a series of RCTs have shown 20–50mg/d to be rapidly effective but 20mg/d may be adequate (e.g. n=278, RCT, d/b, p/c, 12/52, Baldwin *et al, Br J Psychiatry* 2006;**189**:264–72), and 40mg/d may be only slightly more effective than 20mg/d (n=566, RCT, p/c, d/b, 8/52, Rickels *et al, Am J Psychiatry* 2003;**160**:749–56). Relapse prevention has been shown (n=652, d/b, p/c extension, 32/52, Stocchi *et al, J Clin Psychiatry* 2003;**64**:250–8;MS). PLoS One is less than enthusiastic, stating only a modest advantage over placebo for anxiety (Sugarman *et al, PLoS One* 2014;**9**:e106337).

Review: overview of studies (s=4, n=1800, RCT, d/b, p/c, Rickels *et al, J Clin Psychiatry* 2006;**67**:41–7).

Pregabalin *

Pregabalin is licensed for GAD and two meta-analyses and reviews concluded it is effective (s=7, n=1352, p/c, Boschen, *Can J Psychiatry* 2011;**56**:558–66; s=8, Wensel *et al, Ann Pharmacother* 2012;**46**:424–9). Pregabalin

200–450 mg/d appears the optimal dose range, with 450-600mg/d possible (s=3, RCTs, p/c, Kawalec *et al*, *Expert Opin Investig Drugs* 2015;**24**:585–94). It may also be highly effective as an adjunct to SSRIs/SNRIs in partial response of GAD (n=356, RCT, d/b, p/c, 8/52, Rickels *et al*, *Int Clin Psychopharmacol* 2012;**27**:142–50). In GAD, improvement at 2/52 (i.e. >20% reduction in symptoms) predicts long-term response, but lack of response at 2/52 does not predict non-response (s=4, d/b, p/c, Baldwin *et al*, *Eur Neuropsychopharmacol* 2012;**22**:137–42). In responders, relapse prevention (42% vs 65%) has been shown (n=624, open, 8/52; then n=338, RCT, p/c, d/b, 6/12, Feltner *et al*, *Int Clin Psychopharmacol* 2008;**23**:18–28, MS), with no significant withdrawal symptoms over 12–24/52 in responders to 12 weeks treatment for GAD (RCT, d/b, p/c, a/c, 6/12, Kasper *et al*, *Int J Neuropsychopharmacol* 2014;**17**:685–95), although tapering over a week is recommended (s=11, RCTs, d/b, Baldwin *et al*, *J Psychopharmacol* 2015;**29**:1047–60).

Reviews: * general (Baldwin *et al*, *Neuropsychiatr Dis Treat* 2013;**9**:883–92; Both *et al*, *Expert Rev Neurother* 2014;**14**:29–38), use in adults (Frampton, *CNS Drugs* 2014;**28**:835–54), kinetics and pharmacodynamics (Schulze-Bonhage, *Expert Opin Drug Metab Toxicol* 2013;**9**:105–15), ADRs (Zaccara *et al*, *Epilepsia* 2011;**52**:826–36).

Venlafaxine XL

Venlafaxine is licensed for GAD, with 75 mg/d considered the optimum dose, but 37.5mg is ineffective (n=541, p/c, d/b, 24/52, Allgulander *et al*, *Br J Psychiatry* 2001;**179**:15–22, MS). Venlafaxine 75 mg/d was equipotent with pregabalin (400–600 mg/d) but less well tolerated and possibly with a slower onset (n=426, RCT, d/b, 6/52, Montgomery *et al*, *J Clin Psychiatry* 2006;**67**:771–82). Higher doses are not routinely recommended but can be used, e.g. venlafaxine 150–225 mg/d was superior to placebo in non-depressed outpatients with GAD (n=251, RCT, 6/52, Gelenberg *et al*, *JAMA* 2000;**283**:3082–8). In a pooled analysis, venlafaxine was as well tolerated and effective in older adults as in younger adults (s=5, n=1839, RCT, Katz *et al*, *J Am Geriatr Soc* 2002;**50**:18–25).

• Unlicensed/some efficacy

Agomelatine *

Agomelatine 25–50 mg/d appears effective and well tolerated for pure GAD (s=2, d/b, RCT, Levitan *et al*, *Exp Clin Psychopharmacol* 2012;**20**:504–9), can reduce relapse cf. placebo (20% vs 31%) (n=227, RCT, d/b, p/c, 6/12, Stein *et al*, *J Clin Psychiatry* 2012;**73**:1002–8) and has equivalent efficacy to escitalopram in GAD, but is better tolerated (n=412, RCT, d/b, p/c, a/c, 12/52, Stein *et al*, *J Clin Psychiatry* 2014;**75**:362–8).

Reviews: * general (De Berardis *et al*, *Int J Immunopathol Pharmacol* 2013;**26**:299–304; Demyttenaere, *Expert Opin Investig Drugs* 2014;**23**:857–64), pharmacokinetics in GAD (Buoli *et al*, *Expert Opin Drug Metab Toxicol* 2014;**10**:885–92).

Antipsychotics *

Antipsychotics are often used but the actual published evidence is scarce and akathisia can be a confounding side-effect, so they should be used carefully and only for infrequent, sustained agitation. Cochrane concludes that the evidence for olanzapine and risperidone is too limited but quetiapine monotherapy seems effective, but with a lower tolerability (s=11, n=4144, Depping *et al*, *Cochrane Database Syst Rev* 2010;**12**:CD008120).

Quetiapine 150 mg/d monotherapy was shown by a systematic review and meta-analysis to be superior to placebo but that augmentation was not superior to placebo in refractory anxiety (s=9, Kreys and Phan, *Pharmacotherapy* 2015;**35**:175–88) but not at 300 mg/d (n=951, RCT, d/b, p/c, 10/52, Khan *et al*, *J Clin Psychopharmacol* 2011;**31**:418–28). The onset of action can be as quick as day four (n=854, RCT, d/b, p/c, 8/52, Merideth *et al*, *Int Clin Psychopharmacol* 2012;**27**:40–54). It may have some limited efficacy as an adjunct in inadequate responders to SSRIs/SNRIs (n=409, RCT, d/b, p/c, 11/52, Khan *et al*, *Ann Clin Psychiatry* 2014;**26**:3–18), in resistant GAD (n=40, open, 12/52, Katzman *et al*, *J Anxiety Disord* 2008;**22**:1480–6) and in over the 65s (n=450, RCT, d/b, p/c, 11/52, Mezhebovsky *et al*, *Int J Ger Psychiatry* 2013;**28**:615–25). Relapse prevention has been shown, e.g. 10% relapsed on quetiapine vs 54% placebo after 6/12 (e.g. n=432, RCT, d/b, p/c, Katzman *et al*, *Int Clin Psychopharmacol* 2011;**26**:11–24) and after a year (n=432, RCT, d/b, p/c, one year, Sheehan *et al*, *J Affect Disord* 2013;**151**:906–13).

Aripiprazole may be useful as an adjunct in resistant GAD (n=13, open, 8/52, Hoge *et al*, *CNS Spectr* 2008;**13**:522–7; review by Katzman, *J Aff Disord* 2011;**128**[Suppl 1]:S11–20).

Risperidone 0.5–1.5mg/d may have a role as add-on to existing anxiolytics (n=40, RCT, d/b, p/c, 5/52, Brawman-Mintzer *et al*, *J Clin Psychiatry* 2005;**66**:1321–5) and at up to 3mg/d in refractory anxiety disorders (n=30[c=21], open, 8/52, Simon *et al*, *J Clin Psychiatry* 2006;**67**:381–5), but not for anxiety comorbid with bipolar disorder (n=111, RCT, d/b, p/c, 8/52, Sheehan *et al*, *J Affect Disord* 2009:**115**:376–85).

Trifluoperazine 2–6mg/d may be superior to placebo (review by Gao *et al*, *J Clin Psychiatry* 2006;**67**:1327–40).

Ziprasidone has limited efficacy as an adjunct (n=62[c=47], RCT, d/b, p/c, 8/52, Lohoff *et al*, *J Clin Psychopharmacol* 2010;**30**:185–9).

Review: antipsychotics as adjuncts (Lorenz *et al*, *Pharmacotherapy* 2010;**30**:942–51).

Mirtazapine

Mirtazapine (15–45mg/d) may be effective within a week for the symptoms of GAD with comorbid depression and 30mg produced response in 78% and remission in 36% in a pilot study (n=44, open, 12/52, Gambi *et al*, *J Psychopharmacol* 2005;**19**:483–7).

SSRIs (see also paroxetine and escitalopram)

SSRIs have some efficacy in anxiety, with paroxetine and escitalopram licensed. Use lower doses initially, as SSRIs may exacerbate symptoms over the first 1–2 weeks of treatment. **Citalopram** may be effective even in some people who have failed with other SSRIs (n=13, 12/52, Varia and Rauscher, *Int Clin Psychopharmacol* 2002;**17**:103–7). **Fluvoxamine** CR was superior to placebo for anxiety in adults, with few sexual side-effects (n=300, RCT, d/b, p/c, 12/52, Westenberg *et al*, *J Clin Psychopharmacol* 2004;**24**:49–55). **Sertraline** 50–150mg/d was superior to placebo (n=370, RCT, d/b, p/c, 12/52, Allgulander *et al*, *Am J Psychiatry* 2004;**161**:1642–9), including for acute symptoms (n=326, RCT, d/b, p/c, 10/52, Brawman-Mintzer *et al*, *J Clin Psychiatry* 2006;**67**:874–81).

Tricyclic antidepressants

Although not generally recommended, tricyclics such as imipramine (n=230, d/b, p/c, 8/52, Rickels *et al*, *Arch Gen Psychiatry* 1993;**50**:884–95) may be effective for persistent or disabling anxiety.

Vortioxetine *

A meta-analysis and systematic review suggests vortioxetine may have some efficacy in GAD, particularly severe GAD (s=4, RCT, Pae *et al*, *J Psychiatr Res* 2015;**64**:88–98).

■ Unlicensed/possible efficacy

Acamprosate

Acamprosate 1998mg/d had a 62% remission rate when used as an adjunct to SSRIs/SNRIs (n=13, open, 8/52, Schwartz *et al*, *Ann Pharmacother* 2010;**44**:1930–2).

Gabapentin *

Gabapentin 100–900mg/d may produce a sustained clinical improvement in symptoms of anxiety and 800mg has reduced public-speaking provoked anxiety (n=32, d/b, p/c, de-Paris *et al*, *J Psychopharmacol* 2003;**17**:184–8) and in post-breast cancer survival anxiety (n=420, RCT, d/b, p/c, 8/52, Lavigne *et al*, *Breast Cancer Res Treat* 2012;**136**:479–86).

Galphimia glauca

Galphimia glauca (a traditional Mexican herbal medicine) may be as effective and better tolerated than lorazepam 1mg/d in GAD (eg. n=191[c=104], RCT, d/b, 15/52, Herrera-Arellano *et al*, *Planta Med* 2012;**78**:1529–35).

Kava kava

Although Kava kava has been reported to be effective (n=129, RCT, 8/52, d/b, Boerner *et al*, *Phytomedicine* 2003;**10**[Suppl 4]:S38–S49), it was compared with sub-therapeutic buspirone and opipramol, with a 75% response rate for all treatment arms, which must say something about the illness severity in the trial.

Levetiracetam

Levetiracetam (mean 2g/d) may have some effect in resistant GAD (n=40, open, 9/52, Kinrys *et al*, *J Clin Psychiatry* 2007;**68**:1010–3), but the only RCT failed to show any efficacy (n=217, RCT, d/b, p/c, 12/52, Stein *et al*, *J Clin Psychiatry* 2010;**71**:627–31).

Memantine *

A small study suggested some efficacy as an adjunct in treatment-resistant anxiety (n=15, open, Schwartz *et al*, *Case Rep Psychiatry* 2012; **2012**:749796).

Omega-3 fatty acids

There is no clear evidence as yet for efficacy (Ross, *Prostaglandins Leukot Essent Fatty Acids* 2009;**81**:309–12).

Passionflower (*Passiflora*)

Passionflower may have an anxiolytic effect, but Cochrane concludes the data is too sparse to draw any conclusions (s=2, n=198, Miyasaka *et al*, *Cochrane Database Syst Rev* 2007:**1**:CD004518).

Riluzole

Riluzole 100mg/d was rapidly effective in 80%, producing remission in 53% over 2–3 weeks (n=18 [c=15], open, 8/52, Mathew *et al*, *Am J Psychiatry* 2005;**162**:2379–81).

Trazodone

Trazodone may have some efficacy, albeit with more ADRs than benzodiazepines (n=230, d/b, p/c, 8/52, Rickels *et al*, *Arch Gen Psychiatry* 1993;**50**:884–95).

*** Case reports**

- **Testosterone** injections (n=1, Cooper and Ritchie, *Am J Psychiatry* 2000;**157**:1884).

□ No efficacy

Caffeine

Caffeine consumption should be calculated in GAD (see *1.28*), as higher intakes can cause nervousness, anxiety, restlessness, irritability and palpitations (Broderick and Benjamin, *J Okla State Med Assoc* 2004;**97**:538–42).

Homeopathy

Classical homeopathy was equivalent to placebo (n=44, RCT, d/b, p/c, 10/52, Bonne *et al*, *J Clin Psychiatry* 2003;**64**:282–7).

Ondansetron

Ondansetron 4mg/d was no better than placebo (n=97, RCT, Romach *et al*, *J Clin Psychopharmacol* 1998;**18**:121–31).

Tiagabine

A systematic review shows no significant efficacy (s=3, RCT, p/c, d/b, 10/52, Pollack *et al*, *J Clin Psychopharmacol* 2008;**28**:308–16).

Yohimbine

Yohimbine actually increases self-rated anxiety in anxiety-prone children (n=32, Sallee *et al*, *Am J Psychiatry* 2000;**157**:1236–42).

1.7 ATTENTION DEFICIT HYPERACTIVITY DISORDER (ADHD), including HYPERKINETIC DISORDER

1.7.1 ADHD IN CHILDREN AND ADOLESCENTS

Symptoms:

Attention deficit hyperactivity disorder (ADHD) is characterised by a developmentally inappropriate degree of gross motor activity, impulsivity, inattention to detail and temper outbursts. Children with ADHD have persistent restlessness, sustained and prolonged motor activity, difficulty in organising and maintaining attention to work or play. They are careless, reckless, impulsive, reward seeking, prone to accidents, can have learning difficulties (partly due to poor concentration), sleep problems (n=466, Gau and Chiang, *Sleep* 2009;**32**:671–9), antisocial behaviour and a fluctuating mood. Onset is before seven years of age. Symptoms can fade by puberty but inattention and antisocial behaviour may persist into adult life and may lead to poor achievement (see *1.7.2*). ADHD is one of the most inheritable of all mental health conditions (up to 85%) and so there is a major genetic component. Studies implicate dysregulation of frontal-subcortical-cerebellar catecholamine circuits, including abnormal dopamine transport and impaired neurotransmission (e.g. Kuntsi *et al*,

Neuromolecular Med 2006;**8**:461–84), especially in the nucleus accumbens and midbrain, areas that regulate reward and motivation (n=97, Volkow *et al*, *JAMA* 2009;**302**:1084–91), leading to a permanent state of dopamine deficiency.

Role of drugs *

As ADHD symptoms can lead to life-long impairment so drug treatment should be started early and combined with behavioural and environmental approaches. Pharmacotherapy is an essential component for the treatment package for ADHD and is effective in reducing core symptoms. Methylphenidate is the current first-line stimulant. There is a natural reluctance by many prescribers to use stimulants in younger children and so mild symptoms should be managed with environmental changes. Moderate-to-severe symptoms may require drug therapy as delayed starting of stimulants for ADHD results in a greater academic decline than starting earlier (n=11872, Zoëga et al, Pediatrics 2012;**130**:e53–62). The availability of licensed once-a-day formulations has increased retention in treatment over three months (66–75%), six months (50–65%) and at one year (40–55%) (n=13,489, van den Ban *et al*, *Atten Defic Hyperact Disord* 2010:**2**:213–20). Psychosocial interventions cannot be shown to be effective due to insufficient data (meta-analyses=8, Moriyama *et al*, *CNS Spectr* 2013;**18**:296–306).

Reviews: * general (Thapar and Cooper, *Lancet* 2015; in press; Sibley *et al*, *Clin Psychol Rev* 2014;**34**:218–32), stimulants in ADHD (Sinita and Coghill, *Neuropharmacology* 2014;**87**:271–81), pharmacotherapies (Santosh *et al*, *CNS Drugs* 2011;**25**:737–63), Canadian guidelines (Gorman *et al*, *Can J Psychiatry* 2015;**60**:62–76; FFT), ADHD plus comorbid tics (s=8, RCT, d/b, Pringsheim and Steeves, *Cochrane Database Syst Rev* 2011;**4**:CD007990), managing risks of ADHD medications (Manning, *J Clin Psychiatry* 2013;**74**:e19), overdose (Spiller *et al*, *CNS Drugs* 2013;**27**:531–43).

NB: Trials need to be interpreted carefully, as different diagnostic criteria may have been used.

BNF listed

Treatment with stimulants remains controversial in some quarters but the evidence points towards lack of negative effects:

- An early age of initiation of MTH does not increase the risk for negative outcomes (e.g. substance misuse) and probably has the opposite effect (n=354, >6 years, Mannuzza *et al*, *Am J Psychiatry* 2008;**165**:604–9)
- There is no statistically significant association between prescribed stimulants (6–17 years), and the degree of alcohol, drug or nicotine use in adult life (n=140[c=112], 10-year follow-up, Biederman *et al*, *Am J Psychiatry* 2008;**165**:597–603)
- There is no increased risk of sudden death with stimulants in ADHD (n=18637, McCarthy *et al*, *Drug Saf* 2009;**32**:1089–96)
- There are no changes in the trajectories of height over time cf controls, and that stimulants have no effect on growth (n=261, 10–11 years, Biederman *et al*, *J Pediatrics* 2010;**157**:635–40).

Atomoxetine *

Atomoxetine is a noradrenaline reuptake inhibitor with minimal effects on other transmitters. It is non-stimulant, with minimal abuse potential and no discontinuation syndrome. The usual dose is 0.5 mg/kg up to 40 mg/d for the first week, increased up to 100 mg/d (lower in 2D6 slow metabolisers). In adolescents, higher doses may be more effective than lower doses (1.4 vs 0.8 mg/kg/d; n=267, RCT, 40/52, Wietecha *et al*, *J Child Adolesc Psychopharmacol* 2009;**19**:719–30). Once-daily maintenance atomoxetine seems as effective and well tolerated as twice a day (e.g. n=218, RCT, d/b, Adler *et al*, *Ann Clin Psychiatry* 2006;**18**:107–13), and it may be effective throughout the day, including the next morning, unlike methylphenidate (n=197, RCT, d/b, p/c, 8/52, Kelsey *et al*, *Pediatrics* 2004;**114**:1–8, MS). The optimum effect is usually after 3/12 but with 50% in the first week (Bushe and Savill, *J Psychopharmacol* 2014;**28**:204–11;MI) so if switching from a stimulant continue the stimulant for several weeks before tapering down. Long-term treatment seems effective (s=13, n=714, open, 3–4 years, Donnelly *et al*, *J Am Acad Child Adolesc Psychiatry* 2009;**48**:176–85) and with only a minor effect on height, with none on those with the lowest height (n=412, >2

years, Spencer *et al*, *Pediatrics* 2005; **116**:74–80). A huge independent meta-analysis concluded short-term atomoxetine is safe and superior to placebo, although 40% still have significant symptoms (s=25, n=3928, d/b, Schwartz and Correll, *J Am Acad Child Adolesc Psychiatry* 2014;**53**:174–87). The UK SmPC states that people on atomoxetine should be monitored for signs of depression, suicidal thoughts or suicidal behaviour and referred for appropriate treatment if necessary, as increased suicidal thoughts or behaviour have been noted (s=12, n=1357), although the incidence was only 0.4% and with no completed suicides.
Reviews: * general (Garnock-Jones and Keating, *CNS Drugs* 2010;**24**:85–8), ADRs (s=22, Wietecha *et al*, *J Clin Psychiatry* 2013; **74**:1217–23).

Dexamfetamine

Amfetamine is clearly superior to placebo on a variety of key measures, remaining effective over 15 months (n=62, RCT, 15/12, Gillberg *et al*, *Arch Gen Psychiatry* 1997;**54**:857–64).
Review: * amfetamines (Mariotti *et al*, *Curr Clin Pharmacol* 2013;**8**:350–7).

Guanfacine *

Guanfacine is an alpha-2 antagonist licensed for treatment of ADHD in 6–17-year-olds where stimulants have not been suitable, tolerated or effective and has been available in USA since 2009. The starting dose is 1 mg/d for a week, then increased weekly to 4mg/d (ages 6–12) or up to 7 mg/d (ages 13–17; see SmPC for dose-weight titrations and monitoring requirements). Guanfacine can be taken in the morning or evening but, pragmatically, if somnolence is a problem it should be taken at night (n=333, RCT, d/b, p/c, 8/52, Newcorn *et al*, *J Am Acad Child Adolesc Psychiatry* 2013;**52**:921–30).
Efficacy: A systematic review and meta-analysis concluded that 59% benefitted on guanfacine monotherapy cf. 33% on placebo (s=7, n=1752, RCTs, p/c, 6-16/52, Ruggiero *et al*, *Eur Neuropsychopharmacol* 2014;**24**:1578–90). Another review concluded it is effective in 6–12-year-olds as monotherapy and as an adjunct to stimulants, but less so as monotherapy in adolescents (s=10, Elbe and Reddy, *J Can Acad Child Adolesc Psychiatry* 2014;**23**:48–60; FFT). Guanfacine is effective and tolerable over two years in completers (n=262[c=60], open, two years, Sallee *et al*, *J Child Adolesc Psychopharmacol* 2009;**19**:215–26). Guanfacine can help comorbid tics (n=34[c=33], RCT, d/b, p/c, 8/52, Scahill *et al*, *Am J Psychiatry* 2001;**158**;1067–74) and oppositional symptoms (n=217, RCT, d/b, p/c, 9/52, Connor *et al*, *CNS Drugs* 2010;**24**:755–68).
Adjunct: A review concludes adjunctive guanfacine monotherapy is superior to placebo, and especially effective for overall, hyperactivity and inattention symptoms (s=12, n=2276, RCT, p/c, Hirota *et al*, *J Am Acad Child Adolesc Psychiatry* 2014;**53**:153–73). Morning or evening guanfacine as an adjunct to stimulants is superior to placebo (n=461, RCT, d/b, p/c, 9/52, Wilens *et al*, *J Am Acad Child Adolesc Psychiatry* 2012;**51**:74–85). In sub-optimal response to methylphenidate/LDX, addition of guanfacine significantly reduced oppositional symptoms (n=455[c=378], RCT, d/b, p/c, Findling *et al*, *J Child Adolesc Psychopharmacol* 2014;**24**:245–52; FFT).
Reviews: * general (Bello, *Patient Prefer Adherence* 2015;**9**:877–85; FFT; Martinez-Raga *et al*, *Neuropsychiatr Dis Treat* 2015;**11**:1359–70; FFT).

Lisdexamfetamine (LDX) *

Lisdexamfetamine is licensed for ADHD in children aged six and over who have not responded to methylphenidate. LDX is a long-acting pro-drug from binding dexamfetamine to the amino acid l-lysine. It is inactive until metabolised, mostly in the red blood cells, releasing d-amphetamine. The onset of action is around 30–60 minutes after a dose, but having a consistent pharmacokinetic profile avoids the peak plasma levels associated with dexamfetamine, reducing the abuse potential. LDX has a subtly different mode of action to methylphenidate and so may have a significant role. The duration of action is at least 13 hours. The starting dose is 30 mg once a day, increased by 20 mg/d weekly. Doses can be taken before, with or after food. Once a day maintains the effect until at least 6.00PM, as does MTH-XL (n=317, RCT, d/b, p/c, a/c, Coghill *et al*, *Eur Child Adolesc Psychiatry* 2014;**23**:61–8). Short-term efficacy has been shown with a 78% response

Methylphenidate formulations: plasma profiles

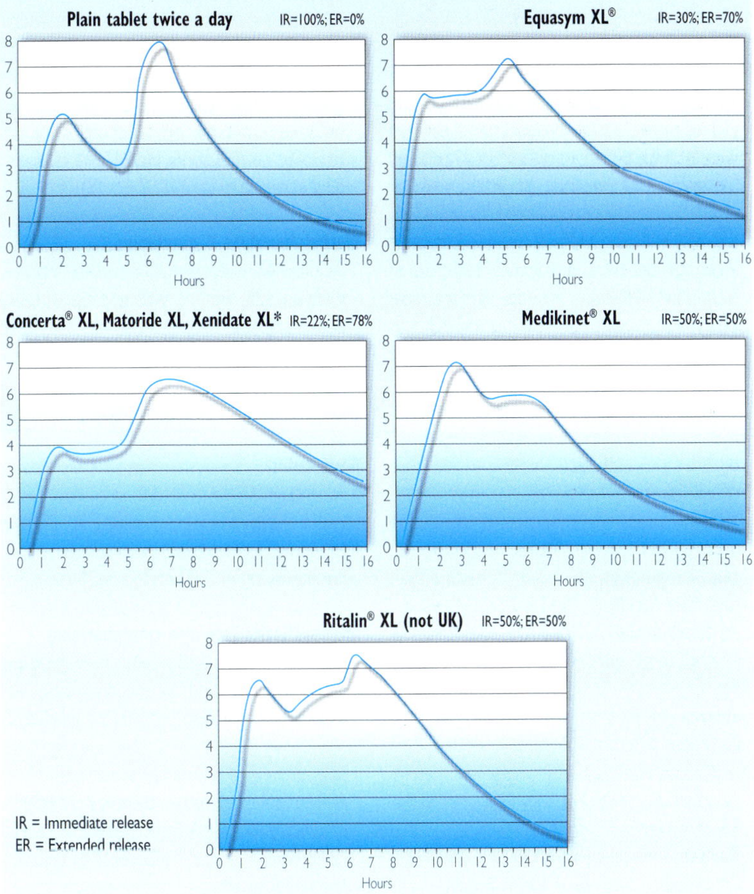

Note: Although Concerta XL , Matoride XL and Xenidate XL are classified as bioequivalent, there may be clinically significant differences in their release profiles, especially as they use different SR mechanisms. They may thus not be readily interchangeable. The BNF recommends prescribing by brand name.

(cf. 61% for OROS MTH and 14% placebo) while reasonably well tolerated (Study 325; n=336[c=196], RCT, d/b, p/c, 7/52, Coghill *et al, Eur Neuropsychopharmacol* 2013;**23**:1208–18). A network meta-analysis of short-term efficacy studies in ADHD without comorbidity concluded that the relative probability of treatment response for CGI-I was:

- Atomoxetine vs LDX=0.65
- Methylphenidate XL vs LDX=0.82
- Methylphenidate IR vs LDX=0.51
- Methylphenidate IR vs LDX=0.62

and that LDX was the most effective treatment, although these would not have been long enough for atomoxetine's full effect (s=32, Roskell *et al, Curr Med Res Opin* 2014;**30**:1673–85). Long-term use seems safe and effective (n=265, open, 48/52, Findling *et al, J Child Adolesc Psychopharmacol* 2013;**23**:11–21).

Reviews: * meta-analysis (s=5, n=1016, Maneeton *et al, Drug Des Devel Ther* 2015; **9**: 1927–36; FFT), general (Coghill *et al, CNS Drugs*

2014;**28**:497–511; Roncero and Alvarez, *Expert Rev Neurother* 2014;**14**:849–65; Madaan *et al*, *Neuropsychiatr Dis Treat* 2013;**9**:977–83).

Methylphenidate (see also introduction) *

At appropriate doses of methylphenidate (10–80 mg/d), a large proportion of children with ADHD obtain remission of symptoms. Methylphenidate's mode of action may be blockade of central dopamine transporters, and may enhance the motivation to complete a task by increasing dopamine. Predictors of a positive response include demonstrable inattention, normal or near normal IQ, low anxiety (Buitelaar *et al*, *J Am Acad Child Adolesc Psychiatry* 1995;**34**:1025–32), high levels of hyperactivity at school and relatively low age (n=36, RCT, Zeiner *et al*, *Acta Pediatr* 1999; **88**:298–303) and family history of response (n=19, Gazer-Snitovsky *et al*, *J Atten Disord* 2015; in press). A meta-analysis concluded methylphenidate is clearly superior to placebo, although effect size is smaller than might be expected (s=16, Koesters *et al*, *J Psychopharmacol* 2009;**23**:733–44). A review of the three established XL preparations (eg. Concerta® XL, Janssen, Equasym®, UCB Pharma, Medikinet®, Flynn) show they are genuinely different, no one is better than another overall, although may be for an individual (Coghill *et al*, *BMC Psychiatry* 2013; **13**:237).

Review: * kinetics (Frölich *et al*, *Expert Opin Drug Metab Toxicol* 2014;**10**:1169–83)

+ Combinations

Atomoxetine + methylphenidate

Adding methylphenidate to atomoxetine non-responders in previous stimulant non-responders seems pointless (n=25, RCT, p/c, d/b, Carlson *et al*, *Child Adolesc Psychiatry Mental Health* 2007;**1**:10), although there is a case of successful use in a 10-year-old boy (n=1, *J Child Adolesc Psychopharmacol* 2006;**16**:365–70).

Atomoxetine + olanzapine *

Olanzapine has helped reduce comorbid disruption and aggression as an adjunct for ADHD (n=11, open, 10/52, Holzer *et al*, *J Child Adolesc Psychopharmacol* 2013;**23**:415–8).

Methylphenidate + melatonin *

Long-term MTH may produce subtle changes in circulating serotonin and reduce melatonin levels (n=179, 4/52, Molina-Carballo *et al*, *J Psychiatr Res* 2013;**47**:377–83), so adjunctive melatonin can partly help improve sleep disturbance, but not core symptoms of ADHD (n=60[c=50], RCT, d/b, p/c, 8/52, Mohammadi *et al*, *Iran J Psychiatry* 2012;**7**:87–92).

Methylphenidate + quetiapine *

Adjunctively quetiapine can lead to improvement in 47% and be well tolerated (n=30, open, 3+9/52, Kronenberger *et al*, *J Child Adolesc Psychopharmacol* 2007;**17**:334–47).

• Unlicensed/some efficacy

Amantadine

Amantadine 100–150mg/d may have equivalent efficacy to methylphenidate 20–30 mg/d (n=40, RCT, d/b, 6/52, Mohammadi *et al*, *Hum Psychopharmacol* 2010;**25**:560–5).

Antipsychotics (see also combinations)

Although not recommended in ADHD, low doses can be used for uncontrollable and explosive behaviour. Long-term side-effects and worsening cognitive and learning functions may outweigh the potential advantages.

Aripiprazole was shown to have no evidence of efficacy in a systematic review in ADHD (s=2, RCT, d/b, p/c, Ghanizadeh, *Neurosciences (Riyadh)* 2013;**18**:323–9).

Risperidone may be as effective as methylphenidate in children and adolescents with moderate learning disabilities (n=45, s/b, 4/52, Filho *et al*, *J Am Acad Child Adolesc Psychiatry* 2005;**44**:748–55) and 1 mg/d can be useful for aggression in ADHD (n=25, RCT, p/c, 4/52, Armenteros *et al*, *J Am Acad Child Adolesc Psychiatry* 2007;**46**:558–65).

Bupropion *

Bupropion XL up to 450 mg/d may be effective and a systematic review of comparative studies suggests response rates and drop-outs are not significantly between bupropion and methylphenidate (s=4, n=146, RCTs, a/c, 6–16/52, Maneeton *et al*, *Neuropsychiatr Dis Treat* 2014;**10**:1439–49; FFT).

Buspirone

Buspirone (0.5 mg/kg/d) was equivalent to methylphenidate for symptoms of ADHD except inattention (n=34, RCT, d/b, 6/52, Davari-Ashtiani *et al*, *Child Psychiatry Hum Dev* 2010;**41**:641–8; see also n=17, open, 6/52, Mahmoudi-Gharaei *et al*, *Hum Psychopharmacol* 2011;**26**:155–60). An active comparison showed buspirone 20–30 mg/d to be less effective than methylphenidate 20–30 mg/d, albeit in only a short trial (n=40, RCT, d/b, 6/52, Mohammadi *et al*, *Acta Med Iran* 2012;**50**:723–8).

Clonidine

Clonidine (an alpha-2 agonist) can be used for treatment-resistant ADHD and an SR version (Kapvay®) is licensed in USA as add-on or monotherapy for ADHD in 6–17-year-olds, e.g. 0.1–0.3 mg/d may be effective (but less so than methylphenidate) in ADHD (e.g. n=122, RCT, d/b, p/c, 16/52, Palumbo *et al*, *J Am Acad Child Adolesc Psychiatry* 2008;**47**:180–8). It may be useful as an alternative to methylphenidate (n=50, RCT, d/b, Nair and Mahadevan, *J Trop Pediatr* 2009;**55**:116–21) and in stimulant-resistant ADHD (n=195, RCT, d/b, p/c, 8/52, Kollins *et al*, *Pediatrics* 2011:**127**:e1406–13). It may improve conduct, (e.g. n=198, RCT, d/b, p/c, Kollins *et al*, *Pediatrics* 2011;**127**:1406–13) and help reduce stimulant adverse effects (n=67, RCT, p/c, 6/52, Hazell and Stuart, *J Am Acad Child Adolesc Psychiatry* 2003;**42**:886–94).

Review: clonidine and alpha-2 adrenergic agonists (Sallee, *Postgrad Med* 2010;**122**:78–87).

Melatonin (see also combinations)

Melatonin advances circadian rhythms and enhances sleep time (review by Bendz and Scates, *Ann Pharmacother* 2010;**44**:185–91), but appears to have no effect on behaviour, cognition or QoL in ADHD (n=105, RCT, d/b, p/c, 4/52, Van der Heijden *et al*, *J Am Acad Child Adolesc Psychiatry* 2007;**46**:233–41).

Modafinil

Modafinil has some promise in ADHD, e.g. once-daily modafinil (170–425 mg/d) was superior to placebo, well tolerated and effective on all rating systems (n=46, RCT, d/b, p/c, 6/52, Kahbazi *et al*, *Psychiatry Res* 2009;**168**:234–7). The most recent review concludes that modafinil improves ADHD symptoms and behaviours compared to placebo (s=3, n=638, d/b, p/c, <9/52, Biederman and Pliszka, *J Pediatr* 2008;**152**:394–9), with no withdrawal symptoms on abrupt withdrawal (n=190, RCT, d/b, p/c, 9/52, Swanson *et al*, *J Clin Psychiatry* 2006;**67**:137–47).

Reboxetine

Reboxetine is a noradrenaline reuptake inhibitor, like atomoxetine, and so logically it could be useful in ADHD. Reboxetine 4–6 mg/d was as effective as methylphenidate 20–50 mg/d (n=33, d/b, 6/52, Arabgol *et al*, *Eur Child Adolesc Psychiatry* 2008;**18**:53–9), and 2–8 mg/d was almost as effective as methylphenidate 10–20 mg/d (n=27, open, 8/52, Cohen-Yavin *et al*, *Clin Neuropharmacol* 2009;**32**:179–82). It may have some efficacy in stimulant-resistant ADHD (eg. n=31, RCT, open, 6/52, Ratner *et al*, *J Am Acad Child Adolesc Psychiatry* 2005;**44**:428–33).

Selegiline

In an active comparison, selegiline and methylphenidate were equally effective for child and adolescent ADHD (n=40, RCT, 60/7, Mohammadi *et al*, *J Child Adolesc Psycho-pharmacol* 2004;**14**:418–25), but it has little effect on impulsivity (n=11, RCT, d/b, p/c, c/o, Rubenstein *et al*, *J Child Adolesc Psychopharmacol* 2006;**16**:404–15).

Tricyclics *

Cochrane concludes that most of the TCA evidence is for desipramine, which improves core symptoms in the short-term, but that its CV side-effects are an important restriction (s=6, n=216, RCT, p/c, Otasowie *et al*, *Cochrane Database Syst Rev* 2014;**9**:CD006997).

Valproate

In stimulant-resistant aggression in ADHD, 57% remitted on valproate compared with only 15% on placebo (n=27, RCT, d/b, p/c, 8/52, Blader *et al*, *Am J Psychiatry* 2009;**166**:1392–401).

Venlafaxine

A systematic review of venlafaxine in ADHD (two RCTs, three open) shows the data is poor and larger trials are needed (s=5, Ghanizadeh *et al, Rev Recent Clin Trials* 2013;**8**:2–8).

■ Unlicensed/possible efficacy

Agomelatine

Agomelatine might help ADHD by improving sleep patterns (n=10, p/c, Niederhofer, *J Atten Disord* 2012;**16**:346–8).

Ginkgo biloba

GB is less effective than methylphenidate (n=50, RCT, d/b, a/c, 6/52, Salehi *et al, Prog Neuropsychopharmacol Biol Psychiatry* 2010;**34**:76–80).

MAOIs

MAOIs are poorly effective but may be agents of last resort, although the dietary restrictions are difficult to manage.

Memantine

A pilot study suggested a dose-dependent improvement in ADHD-IV and CGI-S with memantine 10–20mg/d (n=16, open, 8/52, Findling *et al, J Acad Adolesc Psychopharmacol* 2007;**17**:19–33).

Nicotine

Daily transdermal nicotine has reduced hyperactivity and learning problems but was poorly tolerated (n=10, RCT, d/b, p/c, 2/52, Shytle *et al, World J Biol Psychiatry* 2002;**3**:150–5).

Omega-3 fatty acids + TAU *

Adjunctive omega-3 fatty acids seem to be only modestly effective in ADHD, but since they are relatively benign may be worth a try (s=10, n=699, RCT, p/c, Bloch and Qawasmi, *J Am Acad Child Adolesc Psychiatry* 2011:**50**:991–1000). Cochrane concludes that there is little evidence for PUFAs in ADHD, although there might be for a combination of omega-3 and omega-6-fatty acid supplementation (s=13, n=1011, Gillies *et al, Cochrane Database Syst Rev* 2012;**7**:CD007986) and a more recent study showed omega-3/6 had a clear positive effect on ADHD (n=75, RCT, p/c, 6/12, Johnson *et al, Atten Defic Hyperact Disord* 2012;**4**:199–204). Omega-3 supplements do not enhance the effects of methylphenidate in 7–15-year olds (n=69, RCT, d/b, p/c, 8/52, *J Res Med Sci* 2013;**18**:653–8).

SSRIs

Serotonin function may be abnormal in ADHD and fluoxetine 20–60mg/d has produced some statistical improvements in some rating scales (n=22, open, Barrickman *et al, J Am Acad Child Adolesc Psychiatry* 1991;**30**:762–7).

Zinc *

Zinc may have some efficacy, but only at 15mg twice a day, not once a day (n=52, RCT, d/b, p/c, 13/52, Arnold *et al, J Child Adolesc Psychopharmacol* 2011;**21**:1–19; review by Ghanizadeh and Berk, *Eur J Clin Nutr* 2013;**67**:122–4).

✱ Case reports

- **Duloxetine** (n=1, Niederhofer, *Eur Psychiatry* 2010;**25**:214–5)
- **Gabapentin** (e.g. n=1, Hamrin and Bailey, *J Child Adolesc Psychopharmacol* 2001;**11**: 301–9).

□ No efficacy

Benzodiazepines

These have been tried, but excitation and agitation may be counter-productive.

Caffeine

Caffeine is ineffective as a minor stimulant (Dulcan, *Pediatr Ann* 1985;**14**:383–400), as tolerance develops too rapidly.

Donepezil

Adjunctive donepezil is poorly tolerated and ineffectual for residual symptoms (n=13[c=7], open, 12/52, Wilens *et al, J Child Adolesc Psychopharmacol* 2005;**15**:947–55).

Folic acid *

Folic acid has no efficacy as an adjunct to MTH (n=49, RCT, d/b, p/c, 8/52, Ghanizadeh *et al, Iran J Psychiatry* 2013;**8**:108–12).

Homeopathy

There is no evidence for any efficacy in ADHD (s=4, n=168, Coulter and Dean, *Cochrane Database Syst Rev* 2007;**4**:CD005648).

St John's wort

SJW was ineffective in improving symptoms of ADHD (n=54, RCT, d/b, p/c, 8/52, Weber *et al*, *JAMA* 2008;**299**:2633–41).

1.7.2 ADHD IN ADULTS

Incidence and importance *

Adult ADHD is widely under-recognised. Up to 65% of adolescents with ADHD will have enduring symptoms, with around 3–4% adults affected, remarkably similar in different countries. Comorbidity is common, e.g. anxiety, BPD, SUD, depression, bipolar disorder, conduct disorders and eating disorders, thus making diagnosis tricky. Indeed, around 11–35% adults with SUD have ADHD (review Klassen *et al*, *Curr Drug Abuse Rev* 2012;**5**:190–8). Adults with ADHD may have lower educational achievement levels, but not because of low IQ (n=117, Antshel *et al*, *Psychol Med* 2009;**39**:1325–35).

Symptoms *

Adult ADHD may present as:

- Continuation of symptoms from adolescence
- Re-presentation after a treatment gap by young adults now realising they cannot cope
- First diagnosis, never diagnosed as children but with a history of symptoms
- Late-onset (as opposed to late diagnosis), which is controversial although a 40-year follow-up in Dunedin showed 6% incidence in children and 3% in adults BUT with virtually non-overlapping sets, with 90% adults lacking history as children (n=1037 [c=985], 38 years, Moffitt *et al*, *Am J Psychiatry* 2015;**172**:967–77).

Over 90% of adults with ADHD suffer from poor attention as the main symptoms (n=107, Wilens *et al*, *J Clin Psychiatry* 2009;**70**:1557–62), with work, family and social activities also affected. Other main symptoms in adults include driving problems (more accidents; Reimer *et al*, *Traffic Inj Prev* 2007;**8**:290–9), impulsivity and a lifetime history of sleep problems.

Role of drugs *

Prescribing of ADHD treatments drops significantly from the ages of 15–21 years, but at a greater rate than age-reported lessening of symptoms, suggesting premature stopping occurs in some people who need treatment (McCarthy *et al*, *Br J Psychiatry* 2009;**194**:273–7). Stimulants are as effective in adults as in younger people. LDX and atomoxetine are licensed for *de novo* treatment in adults.

A systematic review and meta-analysis has concluded that the main evidence in adults is for immediate release methylphenidate, rather than the XL preparations (s=22, n=2203, Peterson *et al*, *Psychopharmacology [Berl]* 2008;**197**:1–11). Self-reported compliance correlates well with actual compliance (Safren *et al*, *J Atten Disord* 2007;**10**:257–60) and many will self-medicate, e.g. with amphetamines if sub-optimally treated. Although diversion is possible (reportedly 16–29%), it is less likely with XL preps (s=21, n=113,104, Wilens *et al*, *J Am Acad Child Adolesc Psychiatry* 2008;**47**:21–31).

Reviews: * general (Volkow and Swanson, *N Engl J Med* 2013;**369**:1935–44), long-term efficacy and safety (Fredriksen *et al*, *Eur Neuropsychopharmacol* 2013:**23**:508–27), efficacy and tolerability of medicines in adult ADHD (Santosh *et al*, *CNS Drugs* 2011;**25**:737–63), BAP guidelines (Bolea-Alamañac *et al*, *J Psychopharmacol* 2014;**28**:179–203), treatment guidelines (Ramos-Quiroga *et al*, *Curr Med Res Opin* 2013;**29**:1093–104).

BNF listed

Atomoxetine *

Atomoxetine is licensed in UK for adult ADHD (including *de novo* treatment), where symptoms can be traced back to childhood and where there is some functional impairment. It has advantages in that the risk of diversion is minimal, it is not a controlled drug, and has no discontinuation or withdrawal symptoms (s=4, 9–10/52, Wernicke *et al*, *J Clin Psychopharmacol* 2004;**24**:30–5, MS). It can be given once-daily in adults for maintenance, with an effect lasting into the evening, and with continued efficacy for at least 6/12 (e.g. n=502, RCT, d/b, p/c, 24/52, Young *et al*, *Clin Neuropharmacol* 2011:**34**:51–60). It can help driving performance (n=18, p/c, c/o, 3/52, Barkley et al, *J Atten Disord* 2007;**10**:306–16) and comorbid social anxiety (n=442, RCT, d/b, p/c, 16/52, Adler et al, *Depress Anxiety* 2009;**26**:212–21). An integrated analysis concludes clear efficacy in adults in the short- and long-term (s=9, n=3374, RCTs, d/b, p/c, <6/12, Asherson et al, *J Psychopharmacol* 2014;**28**:837–46; FFT).

Reviews: * general (Durell et al, *J Atten Disord* 2010;**13**:401–6), side-effects (s=3, Wietecha et al, *J Clin Psychiatry* 2013;**74**:1217–23).

Lisdexamfetamine (Elvanse Adult®) *

Lisdexamfetamine (LDX) is licensed for adults with at least moderate severity. Efficacy has been shown (n=414, RCT, d/b, p/c, 4/52 +follow-on, Mattingly et al, *BMC Psychiatry* 2013;**13**;39; see Babcock et al, *BMC Pharmacol Toxicol* 2013;**13**:18), and an 86% symptom reduction in symptoms has been shown in college students (n=50, Dupaul et al, *J Atten Disord* 2012;**16**:202–20; n=36, Jasinski and Krishnan, *J Psychopharmacol* 2009;**23**:419–27). The Tmax in adults is 3.5–5.5 hours (n=47, RCT, d/b, p/c, Ermer et al, *Neuropsychiatr Dis Treat* 2013;**9**:219–29), likely to minimise its abuse potential.

Methylphenidate * (continuation only)

Methylphenidate is licensed for continuation treatment in adult ADHD but not for *de novo* treatment in the UK (although it is in USA, and Medikinet® is licensed for adults in Germany). There remains some controversy about dosing in adults but large studies show that 'robust' dosing (mean 1 mg/kg/d) may be highly effective (response 76% vs 19% placebo) compared to more traditional dosing (e.g. n=146, RCT, d/b, p/c, 6/52, Spencer et al, *Biol Psychiatry* 2005;**57**:456–63). Any lingering doubts about its efficacy should be dispelled by the study in 30 adult male prison inmates with ADHD/co-morbid disorders where the NNT for the primary outcome of improved ADHD symptoms after 5/52 was 1.1 (n=30, RCT, d/b, p/c, 5/52, Ginsberg and Lindefors, *Br J Psychiatry* 2012;**200**;68–73; 47/52 open extension, Ginsberg et al, *Eur Arch Psychiatry Clin Neurosci* 2012;**262**:705–24; FFT). Other efficacy studies show clear statistical efficacy, with a 50% response at 8/52 (cf 18% in placebo group) (eg. n=279, RCT, d/b, 13/52, Casas et al, *World J Biol Psychiatry* 2013;**14**:268–81), with a dose-dependent response, reduced with comorbid SUD (s=18, Castells et al, *CNS Drugs* 2011;**25**:157–69), low treatment failure over six months (21%) than placebo (50%) (n=725[c=584], RCT, d/b, p/c, 9/12, Huss et al, *Adv Ther* 2014;**31**:44–65), a low risk for diversion with XL preparations (n=50[c=39], RCT, d/b, p/c, c/o, 2x5/52, Jain et al, *J Clin Psychiatry* 2007;**68**:268–77) and improved driving performance (e.g. n=17, RCT, open, c/o, 6/12, Cox et al, *J Clin Psychopharmacol* 2012;**32**:225–30). There can be a modest rise in bp and heart rate (s=26, n=811, Godfrey, *J Psychopharmacol* 2009;**23**:194–205) and decrease in weight (n=550[c=275], open, one year, Adler et al, *J Clin Psychopharmacol* 2011;**31**:108–14). Cochrane concludes that methylphenidate IR is effective, with side-effects 'not of serious clinical significance' (s=11, n=474, RCT, d/b, p/c, Epstein et al, *Cochrane Database Syst Rev* 2014;**9**:CD005041).

Review: general (Nair and Moss, *Neuropsychiatr Dis Treat* 2009;**5**:421–32).

Unlicensed (but BNF listed for adolescents)

Dexamfetamine (licensed only 5-13years)

Cochrane concludes that amfetamines improve adult ADHD in the short-term but longer trials are needed (s=7, n=1091, p/c, Castells et al, *Cochrane Database Syst Rev* 2011;**6**:CD007813).

Guanfacine *

This alpha-2 noradrenergic agonist (similar to clonidine) is licensed for 6–17 year olds (n=17, d/b, p/c, c/o, Taylor and Russo, *J Clin Psychopharmacol* 2001;**21**:223–8).

+ Combinations

Atomoxetine + buspirone

The combination was not statistically superior to atomoxetine monotherapy but the trend was for a greater effect, and the trial was only 8/52, too short for atomoxetine (n=241, RCT, d/b, p/c, 8/52, Sutherland et al, *J Clin Psychiatry* 2012;**73**:445–50).

● Unlicensed/some efficacy

Bupropion *

A meta-analysis shows up to 400 mg/d to be well tolerated and clearly superior to placebo (s = 5, n = 349, RCT, p/c, Maneeton *et al*, *Psychiatry Clin Neurosci* 2011;**65**:611–7; see also n = 42, RCT, d/b, p/c, 6/52, Hamedi *et al*, *Acta Med Iran* 2014;**52**:675–80; FFT).

Clonidine

Clonidine ER is currently only licensed for 6–17-year-olds in the USA.

Duloxetine

Duloxetine may have a potential role (n = 30, RCT, d/b, p/c, 6/52, Bilodeau *et al*, *J Atten Disord* 2014;**18**:169–75).

■ Unlicensed/possible efficacy

Fish oils

High dose fish oil was better than flax oil or olive oil for correcting low serum phospholipid fatty acid levels in adults with ADHD (n = 30, RCT, 12/52, Young *et al*, *Reprod Nutr Dev* 2005;**45**:549–58).

Lamotrigine *

In adult ADHD and comorbid bipolar, a retrospective chart analysis showed 77% responded to lamotrigine at a mean dose of 125mg/d (n = 40, Öncü *et al*, *J Psychopharmacol* 2014;**28**:282–3).

Lithium

Lithium (≤1200 mg/d) was equivalent to methylphenidate (≤40 mg/d) on most outcome measures in one study (RCT, d/b, c/o, 2 x 8/52, Dorrego *et al*, *J Neuropsychiatry Clin Neurosci* 2002;**14**:289–95).

Memantine *

Memantine has been associated with improved ADHD symptoms and performance (n = 34[c = 28], open, 12/52, Surman *et al*, *World J Biol Psychiatry* 2012;**14**:291–8) and improved executive function (n = 26, RCT, d/b, p/c, 12/52, Biederman *et al*, *J Atten Disord* 2015; in press).

Modafinil

Modafinil was reasonably well tolerated but ineffectual in one trial (n = 338[c = 330], RCT, d/b, p/c, 9/52, Arnold *et al*, *J Atten Disord* 2014 **18**:133–44), unlike an earlier smaller trial (n = 22 [c = 21], RCT, p/c, c/o, 3 x 3/52, Taylor and Russo, *J Child Adolesc Psychopharmacol* 2000;**10**:311–20).

Nicotine

This indirect dopamine agonist (transdermal or smoked) improves concentration (s = 2, n = 17, d/b, c/o, Conners and Levin, *Psychopharmacol Bull* 1996;**32**:67–73), and is frequently used as self-medication by adults with ADHD.

Oxcarbazepine

Oxcarbazepine 300–1500 mg/d may be effective in some adults with ADHD (n = 9 [c = 8], open, 8/52, Davids *et al*, *Prog Neuropsychopharmacol Biol Psychiatry* 2006;**30**:1033–8).

Reboxetine

Reboxetine 8 mg BD seems to have some efficacy (n = 40, RCT, d/b, p/c, 6/52, Raihi *et al*, *Hum Psychopharmacol* 2010;**25**:570–6).

Venlafaxine

In treatment-naïve adults, venlafaxine 225 mg/d improved index ADHD symptoms, but did not separate from placebo (n=41, RCT, d/b, p/c, 6/52, Amiri *et al*, *Hum Psychopharmacol* 2012;**27**:76–81).

Vitamins

A micronutrient formula containing mainly vitamins and minerals, without omega fatty acids, seemed to work on self and observer but not clinician-rated rating scales (n = 80, RCT, d/b, p/c, 8/52, Rucklidge *et al*, *Br J Psychiatry* 2014;**204**;306–15).

✱ Case reports

- **Milnacipran** (n = 1, Kako *et al*, *Prog Neuropsychopharmacol Biol Psychiatry* 2007;**31**:772–5)
- **Moclobemide** (n = 1, Vaiva *et al*, *Prog Neuropsychopharmacol Biol Psychiatry* 2002; **26**:609–11)
- **Varenicline** (n = 1, 6/52, Cocores and Gold, *J Neuropsychiatry Clin Neurosci* 2008;**20**:494–5).

☐ No efficacy

Cholinesterase inhibitors

Adjunctive **donepezil** (n=6, open, 12/52, Wilens *et al*, *J Child Adolesc Psychopharmacol* 2005;**15**:947–55) and **galantamine** (n=36, RCT, d/b, p/c, 12/52, Biederman *et al*, *J Clin Psychopharmacol* 2006;**26**:163–6) are poorly tolerated and ineffective.

Homeopathy

There is no significant treatment effect (s=4, n=168, Coulter and Dean, *Cochrane Database Syst Rev* 2007;**17**:CD005648).

Selegiline

Selegiline was ineffective and had significant ADRs (n=24, RCT, d/b, p/c, 10/52, Ernst *et al*, *Psychopharmacol Bull* 1996;**32**:327–34).

1.8 AUTISTIC SPECTRUM DISORDERS (ASD)

Symptoms *

Autistic spectrum disorders (ASD) are neurodevelopmental in origin, characterised by an excessive or morbid dislike of others or society, not responding with normal human emotions towards other people, a morbid self-centred attitude and with major impairments or abnormalities in language, communication, reciprocity, social interactions, imagination and behaviour. The main features include 'autistic aloneness', poor speech and language development, an obsessive desire for sameness, bizarre behaviour or mannerisms, a restricted repertoire of activities and interests, rituals and compulsive behaviour. The incidence is 0.04%, (or 0.2% if including associated conditions), up to 25% develop seizures in adolescence, 75% have an IQ in the impaired range, and up to 60% need long-term residential care. There is some evidence that dietary gluten could be implicated in ASDs (Whiteley *et al*, *Front Hum Neurosci* 2012;**6**:344; Millward *et al*, *Cochrane Database Syst Rev* 2008;**2**:CD003498) but genetics seem to be the major origin (n=6243 pairs, Colvert *et al*, *JAMA Psychiatry* 2015;**72**:415–23).

Role of drugs

Drugs may be of limited use in treating some of the more severe behavioural symptoms. Self-injurious behaviour (SIB) is common (*see 1.23*) and may be helped by low dose antipsychotics, as autistic individuals seem very sensitive to moderate and higher doses. Only risperidone and methylphenidate have some efficacy for aggression (see 1.2) in ASD (s=21, Parikh *et al*, *J Child Adolesc Psychopharmacol* 2008;**18**:157–78). Again higher doses may be counter-productive. Family support, education, skills training, behavioural therapy and social support can be significant aspects of the overall management.

Reviews: * general (Kumar *et al*, *Pharmacol Rep* 2012;**64**:1291–304; Politte *et al*, *Harv Rev Psychiatry* 2014;**22**:76–92), pharmacotherapy (Young and Findling, *Curr Opin Psychiatry* 2015; **28**:91–101) efficacy (Kirino, *Clin Med Insights Pediatr* 2014;**8**:17–30), pharmacotherapy for young people (s=8, Dove *et al*, *Pediatrics* 2012;**130**:717–26; FFT), interventions for co-morbid catatonia (Dejong *et al*, *J Autism Dev Disord* 2014;**44**:2127–36), pharmacotherapy for irritability in ASD (s=23. RCTs, Elbe and Lalani, *J Can Acad Child Adolesc Psychiatry* 2012:**21**:130–46; FFT).

BNF listed

Risperidone *

Risperidone is licensed in the US for irritability associated with autistic disorder in children aged 5–16 years. Risperidone 0.5–3.5 mg/d does not affect core symptoms of ASDs but has moderate efficacy for irritable and aggressive behaviour (s=6, p/c; s=16 open; Sharma and Shaw, *J Pediatr Health Care* 2012; **26**:291–9), repetition and social withdrawal (s=3, Jesner *et al*, *Cochrane Database Syst Rev* 2007;**1**:CD005040). Long-term use seems safe and effective, e.g. for up to three years but response may disappear rapidly on discontinuation (n=32, 6/12, d/b, Autism Network, *Am J Psychiatry* 2005;**162**:1361–9). Raised prolactin and weight gain are risks so monitor carefully (n=20, 24/52, Gagliano *et al*, *J Child Adolesc Psychopharmacol* 2004;**14**:39–47). One review concludes it should be a drug of last resort (Dinnissen *et al*, *Expert Opin Drug Metab Toxicol* 2015;**11**:111–24).

• Unlicensed/some efficacy

Amantadine + risperidone

Adjunct: amantadine plus risperidone reduced hyperactivity and irritability in children with ASD (n=40, RCT, d/b, p/c, 10/52, Mohammadi *et al*, *Clin Neuropharmacol* 2013;**36**:179–84).

Antipsychotics * (see risperidone in BNF)

Low-dose antipsychotics have a role to play. As adverse reactions can be significant, a 'start low and go slow' mantra is recommended.

Aripiprazole is also licensed in USA for irritability associated with autism (n=244[c=199], open, one year, Marcus *et al*, *J Clin Psychiatry* 2011;**72**:1270–6) in 6–17-year-olds, including aggression, SIB, temper and mood lability. Doses of 5, 10 and 15mg/d all significantly improve aberrant or challenging behaviour and can be well tolerated (s=2, RCTs, n=316, Ching and Pringsheim, *Cochrane Database Syst Rev* 2012;**5**:CD009043). However, aripiprazole did not separate from placebo for preventing relapse to irritability symptoms in youngsters (6–17) with ASD (n=85, RCT, 26/52, p/c, Findling *et al*, *J Clin Psychiatry* 2014;**75**:22–30).

Paliperidone significantly improves irritability in ASD (n=25, open, 8/52, Stigler *et al*, *Psychopharmacology (Berl)* 2012;**223**:237–45).

Haloperidol 0.5–3mg/d can reduce behavioural symptoms (e.g. aggression and SIB).

Olanzapine (s=3, s=11; e.g. see n=12, RCT, open, 6/52, Malone *et al*, *J Am Acad Child Adolesc Psychiatry* 2001;**40**:887–94) and **clozapine** (open, n=3, Zuddas *et al*, *Am J Psychiatry* 1996;**153**:738) may also be effective, but there is little evidence that **amisulpride** (RCT, n=9) or **quetiapine** (open, n=6) are useful (s=13, n=133, Barnard *et al*, *J Psychopharmacol* 2002;**16**:93–101), although short-term quetiapine at low-dose may help reduce aggression and improve sleep (n=11, open, Golubchik *et al*, *Clin Neuropharmacol* 2011;**34**:216–9). **Ziprasidone** has been used (n=12, open, 6/52, Malone *et al*, *J Child Adolesc Psychopharmacol* 2007;**17**:779–90).

Reviews: * general (Politte *et al*, *Harv Rev Psychiatry* 2014;**22**:76–92), in children and adolescents (Young and Findling, *Curr Opin Psychiatry* 2015;**28**:91–101), irritability in ASD (Kirino, *Clin Med Insights Pediatr* 2014;**8**:17–30).

Celecoxib + risperidone

Adjunct: celecoxib 300mg/d to risperidone was superior to risperidone monotherapy for irritability, withdrawal and stereotypy, suggesting inflammation may be part of the process (n=40, RCT, d/b, p/c, 10/52, Asadabadi *et al*, *Psychopharmacol [Berl]* 2013;**225**:51–9).

Cyproheptadine + haloperidol

Adjunct: Cyproheptadine+haloperidol was superior to haloperidol alone for aberrant behaviour (RCT, d/b, p/c, 8/52, Akhondzadeh *et al*, *J Clin Pharm Ther* 2004;**29**:145–50).

Galantamine + risperidone

Adjunct: Galantamine up to 24mg/d improved irritability, lethargy and social withdrawal (n=40, RCT, d/b, p/c, 10/52, Ghaleiha *et al*, *J Psychopharmacol* 2014;**28**:677–85).

Memantine + risperidone *

Adjunct: Adjunctive memantine up to 20mg/d significantly improved irritability, stereotypy and hyperactivity (n=25, RCT, d/b, p/c, 10/52, Ghaleiha *et al*, *Int J Neuropsychopharmacol* 2013;**16**:783–9).

Methylphenidate

Monotherapy: Methylphenidate can have considerable negative effects on tantrums and moods but this may sometimes be outweighed by the positive effects on hyperactivity, attention and stereotypical behaviour (e.g. n=72[c=66], RCT, RUPPAN, *Arch Gen Psychiatry* 2005;**62**:1266–74).

N-acetylcysteine (NAC) + risperidone *

Adjunct: NAC decreased irritability in children and adolescents with ASD (n=40, RCT, d/b, p/c, 8/52, Ghanizadeh and Moghimi-Sarani, *BMC Psychiatry* 2013;**13**:196).

Pentoxifylline + risperidone

Adjunct: Pentoxifylline 600mg/d plus risperidone may have some effects on behaviour (n=40, RCT, d/b, p/c, 10/52, Akhondzadeh *et al*, *Prog Neuropsychopharmacol Biol Psychiatry* 2010;**34**:32–6).

Riluzole + risperidone *

Adjunct: Riluzole and risperidone reduced irritability in children with ASD, but caused weight gain (n=49[c=40], RCT, d/b, p/c, Ghaleiha *et al*, *Paediatr Drugs* 2013;**15**:505–14).

Topiramate + risperidone

Adjunct: Topiramate improved irritability, stereotypy and hyperactivity (n=40, RCT, d/b, p/c, 8/52, Rezaei *et al*, *Prog Neuropsychopharmacol Biol Psychiatry* 2010; **34**:1269–72).

■ Unlicensed/possible efficacy

Acamprosate *

Monotherapy: Acamprosate may help normalise the GABA: glutamate balance and two small trials have shown some efficacy (n=9, s/b, 12/52, Erickson *et al*, *J Autism Dev Disord* 2014;**44**:981–7; n=6, open, 10–30/52, Erickson *et al*, *J Child Adolesc Psychopharmacol* 2011:**21**:565–9).

Antidepressants *

SSRIs may have some role to play, particularly in adults with strong behavioural rigidity. Cochrane concludes that there is no evidence for SSRIs in children with ASD and some emerging evidence of harm, and only limited evidence for effectiveness in adults (s=9, n=320, RCT, Williams *et al*, *Cochrane Database Syst Rev* 2013;**8**:CD004677).

Agomelatine 25 mg/d has been tried (n=1, 10/52, Niederhofer, *Prim Care Companion CNS Disorders* 2011;**13**:101038).

Citalopram has no effect on repetitive behaviour (n=149, RCT, p/c, 12/52, King *et al*, *Arch Gen Psychiatry* 2009;**66**:583–90).

Duloxetine 40 mg/d had no advantage over other antidepressants for general ASD symptoms (n=2, 10/52, Niederhofer, *Prim Care Companion CNS Disorders* 2011;**13**:101038).

Fluoxetine (mean 10 mg/d) was superior to placebo for repetitive behaviours (n=45, RCT, d/b, p/c, c/o, 2x8/52, Hollander *et al*, *Neuropsychopharmacology* 2005;**30**:582–9) and up to 80 mg/d significantly improved repetitive behaviour, OCD and CGI scores in adults (n=37, RCT, d/b, p/c, Hollander *et al*, *Am J Psychiatry* 2012;**169**:292–9).

Mirtazapine 15–30 mg/d had some efficacy (50% were very much improved) in reducing inappropriate sexual behaviours in ASDs (n=10, open, 8/52, Coskun *et al*, *J Child Adolesc Psychopharmacol* 2009;**19**:203–6).

Tricyclics have limited and conflicting evidence that is insufficient to recommend TCA use in ASD (s=3, RCT, Hurwitz *et al*, *Cochrane Database Syst Rev* 2012;**3**:CD008372), although low dose amitriptyline may be useful for hyperactivity, impulsivity, aggression and SIB (n=50, Bhatti *et al*, *J Autism Dev Disord* 2013;**43**:1017–27).

Venlafaxine low dose (18.75 mg/d) has helped reduce SIB and ADHD-like symptoms in ASD (n=3, Carminati *et al*, *Prog Neuropsychopharmacol Biol Psychiatry* 2006;**30**:312–5).

Atomoxetine

Monotherapy: Atomoxetine is just about effective for ADHD symptoms in ASD (n=97, RCT, d/b, p/c, 8/52, Harfterkamp *et al*, *J Am Acad Child Adolesc Psychiatry* 2012:**51**:733–41).

Bumetanide *

Monotherapy: Bumetanide, which reduces intra-cellular chloride reinforcing GABA inhibition, can significantly improve autism rating scale (CARS) scores (n=60[c=54], RCT, d/b, p/c, 3/12, Lemonnier *et al*, *Transl Psychiatry* 2012; **2**:e202).

Buspirone + risperidone *

Adjunct: Buspirone (mean 6.7 mg/d) was more effective than risperidone monotherapy for irritability in ASD (n=40[c=34], RCT, d/b, p/c, 8/52, Ghanizadeh and Ayoobzadehshirazi, *Pediatr Neurol* 2015;**52**:77–81).

Cycloserine (D-cycloserine)

Monotherapy: Cycloserine was well tolerated and improved measures of social withdrawal (n=12, 6/52, Posey *et al*, *Am J Psychiatry* 2004; **161**:2115–7).

Donepezil

Monotherapy: A pilot study showed donepezil increases REM sleep time in ASD (n=5, Buckley *et al*, *J Child Adolesc Psychopharmacol* 2011;**21**:353–7 FFT).

Guanfacine *

Guanfacine can be effective for hyperactivity, impulsivity and distractibility in ASD (n=62[c=54], RCT, p/c, 8/52, Scahill *et al*, *Am J Psychiatry* 2015;**172:** 1197–206).

Melatonin ± TAU *

Monotherapy/adjunct: Melatonin may improve sleep latency (mean 47 minutes) and total sleep (mean 52 minutes), but not the number of night wakenings. An extensive review shows significant improvements in sleep latency, duration and better daytime behaviours (s=5, RCT, d/b, p/c, Rossignol *et al*, *Curr Clin Pharmacol* 2014;**9**:326–34). Long-term use may be needed as the effect may disappear on discontinuation (n=25, open, 7/12, Giannotti *et al*, *J Autism Dev Disord* 2006;**36**:741–52).

Review: practical advice on use (Doyen *et al*, *Eur Child Adolesc Psychiatry* 2011;**20**:231–9).

Memantine + TAU

Adjunct: Memantine may significantly improve disruptive behaviour, language and social behaviour, with no serious side-effects (n=151, open, 21/1, Chez *et al*, *J Child Neurol* 2007;**22**:574–9).

Naltrexone/opioid antagonists ± TAU *

Monotherapy/adjunct: A systematic review concludes that 77% who received naltrexone show statistically significant improvement in irritability and hyperactivity as was well tolerated (s=10, n=155, Roy *et al*, *J Intellect Disabil Res* 2014;**59**:293–306), but working out who would respond was the tricky bit.

Oxcarbazepine ± TAU *

Adjunct: For irritability/agitation in ASD 47% much improved on oxcarbazepine (n=30[c=23], RCS, open, Douglas *et al*, *J Autism Dev Disord* 2013;**43**:1243–7).

Oxytocin *

Monotherapy: Inhaled oxytocin may improve social behaviour and facial expression recognition (n=16, RCT, d/b, p/c. c/o, Guastella *et al*, *Biol Psychiatry* 2010;**67**:692–4; review by Cochran *et al*, *Harv Rev Psychiatry* 2013;**21**:219–47).

Propranolol ± TAU *

Monotherapy/adjunct: A single dose study showed propranolol significantly improved category fluency (n=28, d/b, p/c, c/o, Beversdorf *et al*, *Cogn Behav Neurol* 2011;**24**:11–7), and 20mg/d has been successful for hypersexual behaviours in adolescents with ASD (n=1, Deepmala and Agrawal, *Ann Pharmacother* 2014;**48**:1385–8).

Valproate ± TAU

Monotherapy/adjunct: There may be some improvement in behavioural symptoms associated with ASDs, e.g. aggression and impulsivity, particularly if an EEG abnormality or seizure history was present (n=14, open pilot, Hollander *et al*, *J Clin Psychiatry* 2001;**62**:530–4).

✹ Case reports

- Gabapentin (for disruptive and compulsive behaviours, Guglielmo *et al*, *J Clin Psychopharmacol* 2013;**33**:273–4).

☐ No efficacy

Ginkgo biloba + risperidone

Adjunctive GB has no apparent effect (n=47, RCT, d/b, p/c, Hasanzadeh *et al*, *Child Psychiatry Hum Dev* 2012;**43**:674–82).

Lamotrigine

Lamotrigine was ineffective on all measures (n=28, RCT, p/c, 18/52, Belsito *et al*, *J Autism Dev Disord* 2001;**31**:175–81).

Levetiracetam

Levetiracetam is ineffective (n=20, p/c, d/b, 10/52, Wasserman *et al*, *Int Clin Psychopharmacol* 2006;**21**:363–7), although some symptoms may improve (n=10, open, Rugino and Samsock, *J Dev Behav Pediatr* 2002; **23**:225–30).

Mecamylamine

Mecamylamine seems safe but ineffective (n=20, RCT, d/b, p/c, 14/52, Arnold *et al*, *J Child Adolesc Psychopharmacol* 2012:**22**:198–205).

Omega-3 fatty acids

Cochrane concludes a lack of evidence for efficacy (s=2, n=37, RCT. p/c, James *et al, Cochrane Database Syst Rev* 2011;**11**: CD007992).

Secretin

There is no evidence of any efficacy (s=16, RCT, p/c, Williams *et al, Cochrane Database Syst Rev* 2012;**4**:CD003495).

St. John's wort

SJW was ineffective for measures of autistic behaviour (n=3, Niederhofer, *Phytother Res* 2009;**23**:1521–3).

1.9 BENZODIAZEPINE DEPENDENCE and WITHDRAWAL

Although short-term benzodiazepine use at standard doses is usually without significant risk of toxicity and dependence, higher dose and longer-term use have potential risks. In BDZ withdrawal, minimal intervention (leaflet or group meeting) and clinician-led systematic discontinuation are both more effective than TAU (s=32, RCTs, Parr *et al, Addiction* 2009;**104**:13–24), but psychotherapy during BDZ tapering may actually be detrimental (n=180 [c=170], RCT, 15/12, Oude Voshaar *et al, Br J Psychiatry* 2006; **188**:188–9).

Reviews: withdrawing BDZs in primary care (Lader *et al, CNS Drugs* 2009;**23**:19–34), treatment (Heberlein *et al, Fortschr Neurol Psychiatr* 2009;**77**:7–15).

BNF listed

Antidepressants

Antidepressants may be useful for treating underlying anxiety and depression. **Mirtazapine** has been useful, particularly for sleep disturbance (n=1, Chandrasekaran, *Singapore Med J* 2008;**49**:166–7).

Characteristics of benzodiazepine users:

- Elderly maintained symptom-free by low and unchanging doses
- Chronic physical disorders controlled by BDZs (e.g. epilepsy)
- Where quality of life is so improved by BDZs that long-term use, preferably with intermittent/variable doses, is justified (e.g. chronic or severe anxiety or insomnia, people who relapse to alcohol and other more dangerous substances when BDZ-free).

Benzodiazepines *

A common strategy is to transfer from a current benzodiazepine to diazepam (if necessary), a longer-acting benzodiazepine, from which it may be easier to withdraw. Clonazepam has been used successfully for BDZ craving and withdrawal symptoms

How to minimise the risks of dependence:

- Carefully select patients (e.g. avoid in dependence-prone, lower education, multi-drug users, criminal backgrounds)
- Keep the dose low
- Use shorter courses or intermittent or variable doses
- Manage anxiety with other agents, e.g. SSRIs (Darke et al, *Addiction* 1994;**89**:1683–90).

Risk factors for poor withdrawal and abstinence (seek specialist advice): *

- Previously severe withdrawal reactions
- History of seizures
- Elderly or infirm
- History of abuse of alcohol/other drugs or continued alcohol intake
- Co-morbid severe medical or mental health (including personality) problems (n=180 [c=174], Voshaar et al, *Can J Psychiatry* 2006;**51**:445–52)
- High dose or longer-term use (e.g. >30 mg/d diazepam equivalent >1 year)
- Cluster B personality/Borderline PD (n=76, Vorma *et al, Subst Use Misuse* 2005;**40**:499–510)
- High neuroticism, higher behavioural inhibition and low social support (n=41, 28/52, O'Connor *et al, Addict Behav* 2004;**29**:583–93)
- Craving (n=124, Mol et al, *J Clin Psychiatry* 2007;**68**:1894–900).

Patients where withdrawal should not be attempted:

- *Older medically ill or with spasticity or epilepsy:* Benzodiazepine usually prescribed by a non-psychiatrist. Seldom abused, doses not escalated, effective long-term. Care with subtle cognitive changes that can occur
- *Psychiatric patients with panic or agoraphobic disorders:* Seldom abused, doses not escalated, necessary long-term
- *Psychiatric patients with recurrent dysphoria:* Long-term indications for use less clear. Abuse of other drugs often occurs
- *Chronic sleep-disordered problems:* Drug may be active or preventing a rebound syndrome.

Withdrawal symptoms in the dependent patient:

- *Psychological:* Tension (to above pre-treatment levels), restlessness, agitation, panic attacks
- *Physical:* Dry mouth, sweating, tremor, sleep disturbance, lethargy, headache, nausea, palpitations
- *Mental:* Impaired memory and concentration, confusion
- *Moderate:* Perceptual changes (i.e. hypersensitivity to light/sound), dysphoria, flu-like symptoms, anorexia, sore eyes, depersonalisation, depression, abnormal sensations of movement, rebound insomnia
- *Severe:* (rare) Convulsions, psychoses (e.g. visual hallucinations, paranoia), delusions.

(n=1, Maremmani *et al, Case Rep Psychiatry* 2013;**2013**:367594), a potential game-changer were it not also a benzodiazepine.

Pregabalin *

Another obvious option is to treat underlying anxiety with another anxiolytic, e.g. pregabalin. A Norwegian pharmacoepidemiological study suggested that 48% of people on BDZs were able to reduce their use when starting pregabalin (cf. only 14% on gabapentin: Bramness *et al, Basic Clin Pharmacol Toxicol* 2010;**107**:883–6) and 52.5% successfully withdrew from BDZ-hypnotics if pregabalin replaced it (n=40, open, Cho and Song, *J Clin Sleep Med* 2014;**10**:545–50). Starting pregabalin, then dropping the BDZ by 25% a week for four weeks was superior to placebo, albeit with a high drop-out rate (n=106[c=49], RCT, d/b, p/c, 12/52, Hadley *et al, J Psychopharmacol* 2012;**26**:461–70), although open trials may actually be more realistic (n=282, open, 12/52, Bobes *et al, Eur Psychiatry* 2012;**27**:301–7).

Review: review in BDZ dependence (Oulis and Kostantakopoulos, *Expert Opin Investig Drugs* 2012;**21**:1019–29).

● Unlicensed/some efficacy

Agomelatine

There are cases of agomelatine reducing the craving for BDZs (n=3, Müller *et al, Singapore Med J* 2012;**53**:e228–30).

Buspirone

Although buspirone may aggravate withdrawal symptoms, starting before a tapered discontinuation has been used successfully for stopping long-term BDZs (n=107, d/b, Rickels *et al, Am J Psychiatry* 2000;**157**:1973–9), even lorazepam (n=44, RCT, Delle Chiaie *et al, J Clin Psychopharmacol* 1995;**15**:12–9).

Carbamazepine

Carbamazepine 600–800 mg/d has been used and reduces the chance of withdrawal symptoms and relapse (n=40, RCT, 12/52, Schweizer *et al, Arch Gen Psychiatry* 1991;**48**:448–52).

■ Unlicensed/possible efficacy

Antihistamines

These may be useful as non-benzodiazepine hypnotics where insomnia is a problem.

Baclofen *

A study suggested that baclofen 20–40 mg/d can abolish BDZ-withdrawal symptoms (n=5,

Shukla *et al, J Neurosci Rural Pract* 2014; **5**[Suppl 1]: S53–4; FFT).

Clonidine

This may be a helpful adjunct in withdrawal, especially at relatively high dose.

Flumazenil

In high-dose BDZ dependence a flumazenil infusion and stabilisation with clonazepam led to over 50% abstinence (n=29, Quaglio *et al, Psychiatry Res* 2012;**198**:457–62). IV flumazenil has been used to reduce BDZ craving, lower relapse rates and improve outcomes (n=50, RCT, p/c, 6/52, Gerra *et al, Addict Biol* 2002;**7**:385–95).

Melatonin *

Melatonin CR has been successfully used to facilitate discontinuation of benzodiazepines (n=34, d/b, 6/52, Garfinkel *et al, Arch Intern Med* 1999;**159**:2456–60), although in older adults was ineffective as an adjunct to TAU (n=92[c=90], RCT, d/b, p/c, 4/52, Lähteenmäki *et al, Br J Clin Pharmacol* 2014; **77**:975–85).

Oxcarbazepine

Oxcarbazepine has facilitated rapid BDZ withdrawal in as little as 11 days (n=10, Croissant *et al, Am J Drug Alcohol Abuse* 2008; **34**:534–40).

Phenobarbital

A fixed-dose phenobarbital taper has been used successfully (n=310, 3/7, Kawasaki *et al, J Subst Abuse Treat* 2012;**43**:331–4).

Valproate

Valproate 150–1200mg/d may reduce the intensity of symptoms in protracted withdrawal (eg. n=4, Apelt and Emrich, *Am J Psychiatry* 1990;**147**:950–1), as well as acting as an anticonvulsant.

*** Case reports**

- **Topiramate** (n=1, Cheseaux *et al, Hum Psychopharmacol* 2003;**18**:375–7;n=1, Michopoulos *et al, World J Biol Psychiatry* 2006;**7**:265–7).

□ No efficacy

Antipsychotics

Low dose anxiolytic use may be useful, but may make withdrawal symptoms worse.

1.10 BIPOLAR MOOD DISORDER

1.10.1 PROPHYLAXIS AND MAINTENANCE
1.10.2 MANIA AND HYPOMANIA
1.10.3 BIPOLAR DEPRESSION
1.10.4 RAPID-CYCLING BIPOLAR DISORDER

Introduction

Bipolar mood disorder is a life-long illness with a variety of presentations, phases and sub-divisions. DSM-IV divides the condition into bipolar I (one or more manic or mixed episodes, wide mood swings), bipolar II (the most common form, one or more episodes of depression with at least one hypomanic but no manic episode), and bipolar III (pseudobipolar, often triggered by antidepressants, and which may present as a mixed state). There are many other classifications and sub-categories. Well-being and functioning are inversely proportional to the number of episodes, and so strategies to reduce relapse must be rigorously followed, especially minimising bipolar depression (see *1.10.3*).

Reviews: * meta-analysis of NNTs for bipolar drugs (Popovic *et al, Psychopharmacology [Berl]* 2011;**213**:657–67), general (Grande, *Lancet* 2015; in press).

1.10.1 PROPHYLAXIS AND MAINTENANCE

Role of drugs *

The optimum outcomes in bipolar occur with appropriate and consistent prescribing and adherence with mood stabilisers, training for the person to cope with stresses and risk factors, and family support. Lithium, valproate, olanzapine and quetiapine are widely used for the prophylaxis of bipolar disorder but must be used with care as rebound relapse on (rapid) discontinuation may occur (n=53, Franks *et al, J Psychopharmacol* 2008;**22**:452–6). A network meta-analysis concluded that all the main treatments for bipolar relapse prevention were superior to placebo, except aripiprazole, carbamazepine, imipramine and paliperidone, and that lithium should remain the first-line agent (s = 33, n = 4846, RCT, Miura *et al*, *Lancet Psychiatry* 2014;**1**:351–9). CBT does not appear to reduce overall episode recurrence in recurrent bipolar disorder (n = 253 [c = 200], RCT, s/b, 18/12, Scott *et al*, *Br J Psychiatry* 2006;**188**:313–20), except perhaps in people with fewer episodes, although NICE takes a different view.

Reviews: * general (Anderson *et al*, *Br Med J* 2012;**345**:e85; Geddes and Miklowitz, *Lancet* 2013;**381**:1672–82), nutrient therapies (Sylvia *et al*, *Psychother Psychosom* 2013;**82**:10–9).

BNF listed

Aripiprazole

Aripiprazole is licensed for prevention of recurrence of manic episodes in bipolar I, in people who have responded acutely. The maintenance dose is the same as the acute dose. In supporting studies, 15–30 mg/d was superior to placebo for reducing relapse in bipolar mania in those responding over 6/52 (e.g. n = 161, RCT, d/b, p/c, 6/12, Keck *et al*, *J Clin Psychiatry* 2006;**67**:626–37; two-year extension, n = 161, RCT, d/b, p/c, two years, Keck *et al*, *J Clin Psychiatry* 2007;**164**:1480–91). Relapse prevention has been shown, albeit with a high drop-out (n = 60[c = 20], RCT, d/b, 12+40/52, El-Mallakh *et al*, *J Affect Disord* 2012;**136**:258–66).

Reviews: meta-analysis with NNTs (Fountoulakis *et al*, *J Affect Disord* 2011;**133**:361–70), general (de Bartolomeis and Perugi, *Expert Opin Pharmacother* 2012;**13**:2027–36; Zupancic and Gonzalez, *Ther Clin Risk Manag* 2012;**8**:1–6; Fagiolini *et al*, *Expert Opin Pharmacother* 2011;**12**:473–88).

Carbamazepine

Carbamazepine is licensed as an alternative to lithium. Six studies of maintenance carbamazepine in bipolar disorder have shown equivocal results, e.g. incomplete protection (Post *et al*, *CNS Drugs* 2007;**21**:47–71). It has been suggested that the best thing you can do with carbamazepine in bipolar is to stop it and allow other drugs to reach therapeutic levels.

Review: * comparison of carbamazepine and lithium (RCTs, Ceron-Litvoc *et al*, *Hum Psychopharmacol* 2009;**24**:19–28).

Lamotrigine

Lamotrigine is licensed in UK for the maintenance treatment of bipolar I depression and relapse prevention (see *1.10.3*).

Lithium *

The use of lithium in bipolar was first published by Cade (*Med J Aust* 1949;**2**:349–52; discussion by Cole and Parker, *J Nerv Ment Dis* 2012; **200**:1101–4) and it is the gold standard for the treatment and prophylaxis of bipolar illnesses and, with care, can be safe and effective in bipolar I and II by reducing relapses and increasing inter-episodic intervals.

Efficacy: * Lithium clearly reduces the risk of relapse in bipolar disorder (61% with placebo, 33% with lithium), particularly for manic episodes and the latest systematic review and meta-analysis concludes the evidence for lithium prophylaxis has strengthened vs placebo (s = 7, n = 1580, RCT) and anticonvulsants (s = 7, n = 1305, RCT) and that it remains the most effective treatment option (Severus *et al*, *Int J Bipolar Disord* 2014;**2**:15; FFT). A 10-year study showed that excellent response occurs in about 9% of people on lithium over five years, but that response is 3% less for every admission pre-starting lithium, especially if manic (n = 3762, Kessing *et al*, *Int Clin Psychopharmacol* 2011;**26**: 323–8). Commencing lithium within the first ten years of onset (the sooner the better) predicts better outcomes compared to starting later on (n = 4714, Kessing *et al*, *Br J Psychiatry* 2014;**205**:214–20).

Lithium is most effective if monitored regularly, and the dose and therapy reviewed regularly to minimise side-effects (e.g. weight gain and cognitive dulling). The main problems appear to be when lithium is given to inappropriate people given insufficient support (see compliance), education and supervision, shown by naturalistic studies with poorer outcomes than controlled trials. Goodwin argues strongly that treatment with lithium should be for at least two years (and more probably three years at the minimum), and that up to two years it may have at best no beneficial effect (premature stopping resulting in premature recurrence of mania and suicidal activity).

Suicide reduction: * Lithium is more effective than placebo at reducing suicides (OR 0.13) and mortality from any cause (OR=0.38) (s=48, n=6674, Cipriani *et al, BMJ* 2013;**346**:f3646). Reduced suicide has been shown in Finland (n=826, Toffol *et al, J Affect Disord* 2015; **183**:159–65). Lithium associated in high-risk bipolar patients with reduced risk of suicidal attempts and significantly decreased suicide mortality (RR=0.39) and decreased all-cause mortality by 49%, not seen with valproate, antidepressants nor BDZs (n=826, mean 3.5 years, Toffol *et al, J Affect Disord* 2015;**183**:159–65). However, premature discontinuation can actually *increase* the risks, e.g. there was a sizeable reduction in mortality over all times studied (e.g. one year) but significantly increased risks shown if discontinuing lithium by 180 days (Smith *et al, Br J Psychiatry* 2015;**207**:55–63; see also n=21194, Smith *et al, BMC Psychiatry* 2014;**14**:357; FFT). Even higher lithium levels in drinking water may be associated with reduced suicide (Vita *et al, Int Clin Psychopharmacol* 2015;**30**:1–5) in e.g. Japan (n=18 municipalities in Oita, Ohgami *et al, B J Psychiatry* 2009;**194**:464–5), in women (Sugawara *et al, Int J Environ Res Public Health* 2013;**10**:6044–8), Austria (n=Austria, Kapusta *et al, Br J Psychiatry* 2011;**198**:346–50; unless you live at altitude, Helbich *et al, Geospat Health* 2013;**7**:209–18) and Texas (n=226 counties in Texas, Blüml *et al, J Psychiatry Res* 2013;**47**:407–11). The effect may be due to reduced dysphoria, anger, aggression and impulsivity (Müller-Oerlinghausen and Lewitzka, *Neuropsychobiology* 2010;**62**:43–9).

Mode of action: * Lithium may exert its effect via many mechanisms, e.g. inhibiting secondary messenger systems, or protein kinase C activity (an action shared with valproate and tamoxifen), neuroprotection by increasing hippocampal volume, regulating glycogen synthase kinase-3 (GSK-3) gene expression, up-regulation of Bcl-2 (major neuroprotective protein, with speculated rebound reduction in Bcl-2 production on withdrawal), protection from glutamate apoptosis and increased grey matter volume (review by Malhi *et al, CNS Drugs* 2013;**27**:135–53).

Dosing: * Once-daily lithium at night minimises renal damage cf. multiple daily doses (s=20, Carter *et al, Can J Psychiatry* 2013;**58**:595–600), reduces side-effects and simplifies dosage requirements (review Ljubicic *et al, Can J Psychiatry* 2008;**53**:323–31). There are several methods of predicting lithium dose and levels (e.g. n=60, Abou-Auda *et al, Bipolar Disord* 2008;**10**:369–76).

Plasma levels: Plasma levels of 0.4–0.8 mmol/L are generally considered safe and effective as prophylaxis, but below 0.4–0.6 mEq/L may be less protective against relapse. In the elderly, a third to half less lithium may be needed due to reduced clearance. Lower plasma levels of lithium may be better at preventing relapse of bipolar depression and higher levels better to prevent mania (n=64, 18/12, Severus *et al, J Affect Disord* 2009;**115**:466–70). Lithium is safe during Ramadan as long as the dose is taken at the same time every day (n=62, Farooq *et al, Int Clin Psychopharmacol* 2010;**25**:323–7).

Monitoring: * Plasma monitoring is variable, with many litigation cases for poor monitoring. Locally-run lithium databases and automated blood sample recall improves monitoring dramatically and almost abolishes non-accidental toxicity (n=1500, Kirkham *et al, Ther Adv Psychopharmacol* 2013;**3**:260–5).

Compliance or concordance: The main reason for lithium failure is non-compliance (either complete or erratic), and the patient (and any partner or caregiver) should be aware of the long-term commitment needed especially avoiding rapid discontinuation.

Discontinuation: Early (particularly manic) relapse following lithium discontinuation is now well recognised with numerous studies showing a significant risk from rapid discontinuation. If stopped in under 14 days, the risk of relapse is much higher (median 50% risk of relapse within four months, 100% over 3.5 years) than with slower (15–30 days) withdrawal, with a significant excess over the first six months (n=78, Baldessarini *et al, Am J Psychiatry* 1997; **154**:551–3) with excess morbidity being attributable to the first episode/relapse after discontinuation (n=42, 7 years, Cavanagh *et al, Acta Psychiatr Scand* 2004;**109**:91–5). Even controlled lithium discontinuation can lead to a high relapse in people who have had a good response for at least five years, so be careful (n=32, up to nine years, Yazici *et al*, *J Affect Disord* 2004;**80**:269–71). Decreasing lithium levels, (either through erratic compliance or major changes in dose) is also a powerful predictor of relapse (n=94, Perlis *et al*, *Am J Psychiatry* 2002;**159**:1155–9).

Lithium refractoriness: * The evidence is not robust that lithium is less effective on re-starting if treatment is interrupted but the trial score is currently only 3–2 (s=5, n=212, de Vries *et al*, *Bipolar Disord* 2013;**15**:645–9).

Reviews: * general (Licht, *CNS Neurosci Ther* 2012;**18**:219–26; Nivoli *et al*, *Neuropsychobiology* 2010;**62**:27–35), pharmacology, uses and toxicity (Oruch *et al*, *Eur J Pharmacol* 2014;**740**:464–73), meta-analysis of adverse effects (s=385, McKnight *et al*, *Lancet* 2012; **379**:721–8), intracellular pathways (Pasquali *et al*, *Behav Pharmacol* 2010;**21**:473–92), dosing equations (Nichols *et al*, *Ann Pharmacother* 2014;**48**:596–600).

Olanzapine *

Olanzapine is licensed for the prevention of manic relapse in people with bipolar disorder who have responded to it acutely. Two systematic reviews from Cipriani conclude that olanzapine helps prevent manic episodes, but only in people who respond in an acute or mixed episode and had not previously responded to lithium or valproate, (s=5, RCTs, Cipriani *et al*, *J Psychopharmacol* 2010;**24**:1729–38). So, the actual SmPC is precise and accurate but that data is limited and the evidence is stronger for lithium as a first-line maintenance treatment (s=5, n=1165, RCTs, Cipriani *et al*, *Cochrane Database Syst Rev* 2009;**1**:CD004367).

Review: use in adolescents with Bipolar I (McCormack, *CNS Drugs* 2010;**24**:443–52).

Quetiapine (see also combinations)

Quetiapine is licensed for the prevention of recurrence of mania, mixed states or depressive symptoms that responded to quetiapine in the acute state (review by Popovic *et al*, *Psychopharmacol [Berl]* 2011;**213**:657–67). Continuation therapy with quetiapine reduces relapse equivalent to lithium and significantly more than placebo (n=2438, <2 years, d/b, p/c, Weisler *et al*, *J Clin Psychiatry* 2011;**72**:1452–64), and it may also help comorbid panic and anxiety (n=149, RCT, d/b, p/c, 8/52, Sheehan *et al*, *J Affect Disord* 2013;**145**:83–94).

Review: use as bipolar maintenance (Janicak and Rado, *Expert Opin Pharmacother* 2012; **13**:1645–52).

Valproate/valproate semisodium/divalproex

Valproate is licensed for mania and relapse prevention (as Depakote® and Episenta®). Valproate was not quite superior to lithium or placebo in the time to any mood episode, but there was a noticeable trend for valproate over placebo and lithium, and was superior to placebo on nearly all secondary measures (n=372, RCT, d/b, p/c, one year, Bowden *et al*, *Arch Gen Psychiatry* 2000;**57**:481–9). Reduced suicide in bipolar has not been shown with valproate compared to lithium (n=20638, Goodwin *et al*, *JAMA* 2003;**290**:1467–73) or in high-risk patients (n=98, RCT, d/b, 30/12, Oquendo *et al*, *Am J Psychiatry* 2011;**168**:1050–6). See also entry under mania/hypomania (*1.10.2*).

+ Combinations (of drugs with some intrinsic mood stabilising activity)

Lithium + carbamazepine/oxcarbazepine

Lithium plus **carbamazepine** may help (e.g. n=33, Small *et al*, *Psychopharmacol Bull* 1995;**31**:265–72), but **oxcarbazepine** appeared more effective and better tolerated than carbamazepine as add-on to lithium for residual bipolar symptoms (n= 52[c=52], RCT, d/b, 8/52, Juruena *et al*, *Prog Neuropsychopharmacol Biol Psychiatry* 2009;**33**:94–9).

Lithium + quetiapine

In people stabilised on quetiapine plus lithium, continued treatment reduced the risk of relapse (20% vs 52%) compared to placebo (n=1953, open, <36/52; then n=628, RCT, d/b, p/c, <104/52, Suppes *et al*, *Am J Psychiatry* 2009;**166**:476–88). See 'some efficacy' section.

Quetiapine + valproate *

In people stable on quetiapine plus valproate, continued maintenance with both significantly increases the time to any mood event (s=2, n=1326, RCT, d/b, p/c, <2 years, Suppes *et al*, *Depress Anxiety* 2013;**30**:1089–98).

Valproate + carbamazepine

There have been several reports of efficacy, e.g. 69% responded when valproate was added to carbamazepine in non-responders (n=29, Schaff *et al*, *J Clin Psychiatry* 1993;**54**:380–4).

Valproate + lamotrigine

An open study has indicated some efficacy (reviewed by Freeman and Stoll, *Am J Psychiatry* 1998;**155**:12–21), although the combination requires great care to avoid lamotrigine-induced rash (see *4.4.2*).

Valproate + quetiapine

In people stabilised on quetiapine and valproate, continued treatment reduced the risk of relapse (20% vs 52%) compared to placebo (e.g. n=1953, open, <36/52; then n=628, RCT, d/b, p/c, <104/52, Suppes *et al*, *Am J Psychiatry* 2009;**166**:476–88). See also 'some efficacy'.

• Unlicensed/some efficacy

Antidepressants

Adjunct: A meta-analysis concludes that long-term adjunctive antidepressants are not superior to a mood stabiliser alone, and should further encourage reliance on MSs as the cornerstone of prophylaxis (s=12, n=350, RCT, >6/12, Ghaemi *et al*, *Acta Psychiatr Scand* 2008;**118**:347–56; comment by Young and Seim, *EBMH* 2009;**12**:49). See also bipolar depression (*1.10.3*).

Antipsychotics (see also aripiprazole, olanzapine and quetiapine in BNF listed)

The main roles of antipsychotics in bipolar disorder are:

1. Adjunctive to mood stabilisers for management of acute mania (see *1.10.2*) or psychotic depression.
2. Adjunctive maintenance in treatment-resistance.

Aripiprazole, quetiapine and olanzapine are licensed for relapse prevention of mania in responders (see BNF section). Many others are licensed for bipolar mania and might thus have some relapse prevention efficacy.

Asenapine is licensed in some non-EU countries for relapse prevention.

Clozapine may have some significant mood-stabilising effects in treatment-resistant bipolar or schizoaffective patients and a real-world naturalistic mirror-image study in TRBD showed clozapine (mean 307 mg/d) to produce a clinically significant reduction in bed-days (178 to 35), admissions (3.2 to 2) and co-medications (n=326, two years, Nielsen *et al*, *Bipolar Disord* 2012 ;**14**:863–9).

Paliperidone-stabilised acute manics remained well twice as long (588 days vs 283 days) with PPLAI than those switching to placebo (n=766, RCT, p/c, Berwaerts *et al*, *J Affect Disord* 2012;**138**:247–58, MS).

Risperidone LAI can help prevent relapse of mania but not depression (n=303, Quiroz *et al*, *Biol Psychiatry* 2010;**68**:156–62; review by Deeks, *Drugs* 2010;**70**:1001–12). In frequent relapsers, adjunctive risperidone LAI showed 23% relapses with RLAI + TAU vs 46% with placebo injection (n=124[c=64], RCT, d/b, p/c, one year, Macfadden *et al*, *Bipolar Disord* 2009;**11**:827–39).

Ziprasidone is licensed in US as an adjunct to lithium or valproate as maintenance in bipolar I (NNT=8, n=238, RCT, d/b, p/c, 24/52, Citrome, *Expert Rev Neurother* 2010;**10**:1031–7; see also Dubovsky and Dubovsky, *Expert Opin Pharmacother* 2011;**12**:817–24).

Reviews: * Bowden, *Neuropsychiatr Dis Treat* 2011;**7**:87–92; Sacchetti *et al*, *Expert Rev Clin Pharmacol* 2011;**4**:163–79), depot/LAI antipsychotics for maintenance (Gigante *et al*, *CNS Drugs* 2012;**26**:403–20), switching antipsychotics in bipolar (Grande *et al*, *Int J Neuropsychopharmacol* 2014;**17**:497–507), combinations (Buoli *et al*, *J Affect Disord* 2014;**152–4**:12–8).

Calcium-channel blockers + lithium *

Adjunct: This hazardous combination has not fulfilled early promise (review by Levy and Janicak, *Bipolar Disord* 2000;**2**:108–19), although **verapamil** 120–450 mg/d and **diltiazem** (n=8, open, 12/12, Silverstone and Birkett, *J Psychiatry Neurosci* 2000;**25**:276–80) may have some role as adjunct therapy in resistant cases.

Memantine + valproate/TAU *

Adjunct: Memantine was ineffective as an adjunct to valproate in Bipolar II (n=135, RCT, d/b, p/c, 12/52, Lee *et al, J Psychiatr Res* 2013;**47**:1343–8) but has been used long-term as an antimanic and mood stabiliser in Bipolar I (n=2, Serra *et al, J Clin Psychopharmacol* 2013;**33**:715–7), for managing post-lithium discontinuation with valproate (n=3, Serra *et al, Ther Adv Psychopharmacol* 2014;**4**:53–5; FFT) and at 10–30mg/d as an adjunct to TAU (n=40[c=35], 12/12, Koukopoulos *et al, J Affect Disord* 2011;**136**:163–6).

Spironolactone + TAU

Adjunct: Adjunctive spironolactone 50–100mg/d was effective for residual symptoms in some bipolar patients (n=4, Juruena *et al, J Psychopharmacol* 2009;**23**:985–7).

Tiagabine + TAU

Adjunct: Cochrane concludes that there is no robust evidence yet for an effect (s=0, n=0, Vasudev *et al, Cochrane Database Syst Rev* 2011;**12**:CD005173), although there are some case reports (e.g. n=13, open, Suppes *et al, Bipolar Disord* 2002;**4**:283–9).

Topiramate + TAU

Adjunct: Open studies suggest some efficacy, e.g. a mean dose of 180mg/d had a dose-related response and weight loss, as well as significant side-effects (n=76, open, Ghaemi *et al, Ann Clin Psychiatry* 2001;**13**:185–9) in TRBD (n=19, open, 12/52, Vieta *et al, World J Biol Psychiatry* 2003;**4**:172–6), and as maintenance, with low drop-outs and low relapses (n=56, open, 12/12, Lykouras and Hatzimanolis, *Curr Med Res Opin* 2004;**20**:843–7).

■ Unlicensed/possible efficacy

Cannabis + TAU

Adjunct: There are no published studies of efficacy but much anecdotal evidence (s=0, n=0, Ashton *et al, J Psychopharmacol* 2005;**19**:293–300).

Cholinesterase inhibitors + TAU

Adjunct: Adjunctive **galantamine** can improve episodic memory in cognitive dysfunction, but has little overall positive effect (n=30[c=16], RCT, d/b, p/c, 3/12, Ghaemi *et al, J Clin Psychopharmacol* 2009;**29**:291–5). **Donepezil** was not much use either (n=12, 3/12, Gildengers *et al, Int J Geriatr Psychiatry* 2008;**23**:704–11).

Gabapentin + TAU

Adjunct: See bipolar depression (*1.10.3*). Despite lacking efficacy in acute states, gabapentin added to a mood stabiliser (lithium, valproate or carbamazepine) may have some prophylactic effects (n=25, RCT, d/b, p/c, 12/12, Vieta *et al, J Clin Psychiatry* 2006;**67**:473–7).

Oxcarbazepine (see also combinations) **+ TAU**

Adjunct: There are case reports of success in bipolar II with comorbid substance abuse (n=4, Nasr, *Am J Psychiatry* 2002;**159**:1793).

Pramipexole + TAU

Adjunct: Pramipexole had no overall effect on improving cognition, one sub-group (n=50[c=45], RCT, d/b, p/c, 8/52, Burdick *et al, J Clin Psychiatry* 2012;**73**:103–12).

Tamoxifen + TAU (see also mania)

Adjunct: There is some interest in tamoxifen as a mood stabiliser in that it shares some intra-cellular properties with lithium, e.g. PKC inhibition (see review by Zarate and Manji, *CNS Drugs* 2009;**23**:569–82).

Vitamins and minerals + TAU *

Adjunct: An unrepeated trial of 36 dietary nutrients has produced a 55–66% reduction in symptoms and a reduction in medication levels, suggesting that bipolar disorder could be an error of metabolism, albeit of unknown mechanism (n=11, 6/12, open, Kaplan *et al, J Clin Psychiatry* 2001;**62**:936–44; review by Sarris *et al, Bipolar Disord* 2011;**13**:454–65).

□ No efficacy

Omega-3 fatty acids + TAU

Adjunctive O3FA, with or without cytidine, had no beneficial effects, with a non-significant statistical trend for worse outcomes (n=45, RCT, d/b, p/c, 4/12, Murphy *et al, J Clin Psychopharmacol* 2012;**32**:699–703).

1.10.2 MANIA AND HYPOMANIA

Symptoms

The main symptoms of hypomania, the more common and less severe form of mania, include an abnormal euphoric and labile mood (irritable, angry, grandiose), poor concentration, bright or untidy appearance, low sleep requirement, increased drive and energy, reduced insight, pressure of speech, flight of ideas, expansive thought and an overactive and intrusive manner. Effective treatment in acute phases is essential for long-term outcomes (review Tyrer, *J Psychopharmacol* 2006;**20**[suppl 2]:4–11).

Role of drugs

Hypomania or mania usually requires specific long-term mood-stabiliser treatment for the bipolar component (i.e. lithium, valproate, SGAs, carbamazepine, etc), and non-specific shorter-term treatments (e.g. antipsychotics, benzodiazepines) for the insomnia, agitation and hyperactivity to calm the person and prevent exhaustion and harm. Meta-analyses of antimanic agents' comparative efficacy and acceptability have concluded that:

- **Haloperidol** is superior to other treatments
- **Risperidone** and **olanzapine** are similar to each other and superior to all other agents except haloperidol
- **Lithium, quetiapine, valproate, ziprasidone, carbamazepine aripiprazole** and **asenapine** are of similar efficacy
- **Gabapentin, lamotrigine** and **topiramate** are no better than placebo

(s=68, n=16073, RCT, 3/52, Cipriani *et al, Lancet* 2011;**378**:1306–15; s=56, n=10,800, RCT, p/c, Yildiz *et al, Neuropsychopharmacology* 2011;**36**:375–89; FFT).

Treatment goals for mania should be:

1. Discontinue any manicogenic agents, including antidepressants and stimulants (see 5.7).
2. Stabilise any medical conditions.
3. Start non-specific calming medications, e.g. benzodiazepines, antipsychotics.
4. Start specific mood-stabilisers or relapse prevention agents (see *1.10.1*) preferably when the person is able to consent to longer-term therapy.
5. A night of sleep deprivation is likely to escalate any manic patient to a higher degree of mania and so hypnotic/sedative use should be considered appropriate.
6. Any comorbid substance misuse must also be tackled, as recovery is poorer in people with a history of substance abuse.

After recovery from a manic episode many people receive antipsychotics long-term. This may not always be the best thing to do, as one study showed that those continuing antipsychotics long-term had a quicker onset of depression, were more likely to discontinue, and have more EPS and dysphoria — a good collection of detrimental effects (n=27, RCT, p/c, d/b, 6/12, Zarate and Tohen, *Am J Psychiatry* 2004;**161**:169–71). See bipolar mood disorder (*1.10.1*) for maintenance strategies.

Reviews: * NNTs and response in acute bipolar (Tamayo *et al, Int J Neuropsychopharmacol* 2010; **13**:813–32), general (Pompili *et al, Neuropsychiatr Dis Treat* 2011;**7**:259–65; Chwieduk and Scott, *CNS Drugs* 2011;**25**:251–67), current acute bipolar guidelines (Nivoli *et al, J Affect Disord* 2012;**140**:125–41), nutritional therapies as adjuncts (Sylvia *et al, Psychother Psychosom* 2013; **82**:10–9).

BNF listed

Aripiprazole (see also combinations) *

Aripiprazole is licensed for prevention of recurrence of manic episodes in bipolar I, in people who have responded acutely, including in adolescents aged 13 years or older. The maintenance dose is the same as the acute dose. Successful use depends on appropriate initial dosing, titrating and adjusting as needed, plus appropriate adjunctive time-limited medicines, e.g. benzodiazepines, to minimise short-term ADRs (Goodwin *et al, Curr Med Res Opin* 2011;**27**:2285–99). It also seems to be effective for psychotic symptoms in mania and during maintenance, including monotherapy (s=4, RCT, Fountoulakis *et al, Ann Gen Psychiatry* 2009;**8**:27; FFT). In the main adjunctive study, aripiprazole plus lithium or valproate was superior to either as monotherapy (n=337[c=192], RCT, d/b, 12/12, Marcus *et al, Bipolar Disord* 2011;**13**:133–44, MS) except perhaps in mixed episodes (d/b, p/c, 52/52, Yatham *et al, J Affect Disord* 2013;**147**:365–72). In an open-label extension, aripiprazole seemed effective as an adjunct to lithium or valproate in the completers (n=283 [c=146], open, 6/12, Vieta *et al*, *Curr Med Res Opin* 2010;**26**:1485–96). Cochrane concludes that aripiprazole is effective for mania, albeit with GI disturbance and movement disorders (s=10, n=3340, p/c, a/c, RCTs, Brown *et al*, *Cochrane Database Syst Rev* 2013;**12**:CD005000).

Reviews: * general (McIntyre *et al*, *Neuropsychiatr Dis Treat* 2011;**7**:319–23; De Fazio *et al*, *Clin Drug Investig* 2010;**30**:827–41), use with mood stabilisers (de Bartolomeis and Perugi, *Expert Opin Pharmacother* 2012;**13**:2027–36).

Asenapine *

Asenapine is licensed for moderate-to-severe manic episodes associated with bipolar I disorder in adults. It has a high affinity for 5HT1A/ 1B/2A/2B/2C/5/6/7, D1/2/3/4, alpha 1 and 2, H1 and H2 but not cholinergic receptors. The sublingual tablet dissolves in seconds when placed *under* (not *on*) the tongue. It is 35% bio-available orally, but less than 2% if swallowed, so not drinking or eating for 10 minutes after a dose is recommended (Gerrits *et al*, *Biopharm Drug Dispos* 2010;**31**:351–7). In manic or mixed episodes in bipolar I, asenapine 5 mg BD was effective as 10 mg bd (n=367 [c=264], RCT, d/b, p/c, 3/52, Landbloom *et al*, *J Affect Disord* 2016;**190:** 103–10), superior to placebo at day 2 and with less weight gain than olanzapine (n=488, RCT, d/b, p/c, 3/52, McIntyre et al, J Affect Disord 2010;122:27–38), and as effective as olanzapine over 9/52 (n=504[c=308], RCT, b/d, p/c, 9/52, McIntyre *et al*, *Bipolar Disord* 2009;**11**:815 26). Asenapine may reduce depressive symptoms in bipolar I patients in manic or mixed states, although more data is needed (s=2, n=977, RCT, d/b, Szegedi *et al*, *BMC Psychiatry* 2011;**11**:101), and is effective as an adjunct to valproate or lithium, being significantly better at 3/52, and over 2–12/52 (n=324, RCT, d/b, p/c, 12/52, Szegedi *et al*, *J Clin Psychopharmacol* 2012;**32**:46–55).

Reviews: * in bipolar (s=5, n=1587, Gonzalez *et al*, *Patient Prefer Adherence* 2011;**5**:333–41; Samalin *et al*, *Ther Adv Chronic Dis* 2013;**4**:5–14; McIntyre, *CNS Neurosci Ther* 2011;**17**:645–8), general (Citrome, *Expert Opin Drug Saf* 2014;**13**:803–30; Young *et al*, *J Psychopharmacol* 2013;**27**[4 Suppl]:3–13; Cortese *et al*, *J Psychopharmacol* 2013;**27**[4 Suppl]:14–22), efficacy (McIntyre and Wong, *Clin Schizophr Relat Psychoses* 2012;**5**:217–20), meta-analysis and review of RCTs (Vita *et al*, *Int Clin Psychopharmacol* 2013;**28**:219–27).

Carbamazepine (see also combinations)

Carbamazepine MR up to 1600 mg/d was effective in 41% (cf. 22% for placebo) as monotherapy in acute bipolar mania (n=204 [c=96], RCT, d/b, p/c, 3/52, Weisler *et al*, *J Clin Psychiatry* 2004;**65**:478–84) as it was up to 1600 mg/d (pooled results analysis; s=2, n=443 [c=240], RCT, Weisler *et al*, *CNS Drugs* 2006;**20**:219–31).

Review: bipolar and mania (Stoner *et al*, *Pharmacotherapy* 2007;**27**:68–88).

Lithium (see also combinations)

Lithium can be effective in acute mania/ hypomania, although the onset of action may be delayed for five to seven days or longer (unless perhaps if loading doses are used). It is difficult to use in mania due to the need for loading doses (sparsely studied; n=15, open, Keck *et al*, *Bipolar Disord* 2001;**3**:68–72), monitoring blood levels, problems with stopping later or prematurely, and the need for two to three years minimum treatment duration. Serum levels of 0.9–1.4 mmol/L may be necessary in the *short-term* for a therapeutic effect but should be reduced once mood is normalised. Early improvement in the first week strongly predicts later response and remission (n=46, 4/52, open, Machado-Vieira *et al*, *J Affect Disord* 2013;**144**:160–4). At least four previous depressive or 10–12 previous manic episodes are associated with reduced antimanic response to lithium (Swann *et al*, *Acta Psychiatr Scand* 2000;**101**:444–51; n=40, RCT, d/b, p/c, 4/52, Kafantaris *et al*, *J Am Acad Child Adolesc Psychiatry* 2004;**43**:984–93).

Review: efficacy and side-effects in mania (Bowden, *J Clin Psychiatry* 2000;**61**[Suppl 9]:S35–S40).

Olanzapine (see also combinations) *

The starting dose for olanzapine in acute mania is 15 mg/d as monotherapy or 10 mg/d as an adjunct. Pooled data from three RCTs show olanzapine is effective in bipolar I mania, particularly when mixed features and more severe depressive symptoms (s=3, n=447, p/c, Tohen *et al, J Affect Disord* 2014;**168**:136–41). Olanzapine orodispersible tablets produce a plasma level profile similar to oral tablets but may be a suitable in some cases by assuring compliance. Cochrane concludes that olanzapine is effective in mania, possibly more so than valproate, but with more weight gain and somnolence (s=6, n=1422, Rendell *et al, Cochrane Database Syst Rev* 2003;**3**:CD004040), although the valproate was probably underdosed (Lu, *Evid Based Ment Health* 2003;**6**:28; FFT).

Quetiapine (see also combinations)
Quetiapine is licensed as monotherapy for acute manic episodes and relapse prevention in bipolar I disorder. Rapid dose with the XL formulation is 300mg on day one, 600mg on day two and then up to 800mg/d thereafter, and is effective at 400–800mg/d from day four (n=308, RCT, d/b, p/c, 3/52, Cutler *et al, Clin Ther* 2011;**33**:1643–58). Two RCTs have shown efficacy, e.g. quetiapine 400–800mg/d was as effective as haloperidol but better tolerated (n=302, RCT, d/b, p/c, 12/52, McIntyre *et al, Eur Neuropsychopharmacol* 2005;**15**:573–85), and up to 800mg/d was as effective as lithium and both were superior to placebo (n=302, RCT, d/b, p/c, 12/52, Bowden *et al, J Clin Psychiatry* 2005;**66**:111–21). An extension study in responders showed the time to recurrence was longer with lithium or quetiapine (cf placebo) for both mania and depression (n=1226, RCT, d/b, p/c, two years, Weisler *et al, J Clin Psychiatry* 2011;**72**:1452–64).

Risperidone (see also combinations)
Risperidone is licensed in the UK for monotherapy in bipolar mania. RCTs have shown efficacy, e.g. risperidone was more effective than placebo (42% vs 13% remission) (n=291, RCT, d/b, p/c, 3/52, Gopal *et al, J Clin Psychiatry* 2005;**66**:1016–20, MS; n=290, RCT, d/b, p/c, 3/52) and in mania (Khanna *et al, Br J Psychiatry* 2005;**187**:229–34 MS). Onset can be rapidly effective (within a week) as an adjunctive treatment to mood stabilisers, especially if carbamazepine-treated patients are excluded (n=151, RCT, d/b, p/c, 3/52, Yatham *et al, Br J Psychiatry* 2003;**182**:141–7; see *4.4.1* for reasons). It can be safely combined with valproate or lithium in acute mania (n=79, 12/52, Yatham *et al, Int Clin Psychopharmacol* 2004;**19**:103–9). Cochrane concludes that risperidone is effective in mania as both monotherapy and as an adjunct (s=6, n=1343, Rendell *et al, Cochrane Database Syst Rev* 2006;**1**:CD004043).
Review: general (Nguyen and Guthrie, *Ann Pharmacother* 2006;**40**:674–82).

Valproate semisodium (divalproex) *
Valproate semisodium (as Depakote®, Sanofi-Aventis, and Episenta®, Beacon) is licensed in the UK as monotherapy for acute mania and relapse prevention. There appears to be a linear relationship between valproate serum concentration and response in acute mania, best response being above 94mcg/mL presumably as trough levels, although this is unclear in the paper (n=374, s=3, RCT, Allen *et al, Am J Psychiatry* 2006;**163**:272–5), and so oral loading doses of valproate are probably more rapidly effective in mania, e.g. 20mg/kg/d may give a rapid response, often within three days (n=36, RCT, 6/7, McElroy *et al, J Clin Psychiatry* 1996;**57**:142–6). Even more aggressive dosing (30mg/kg/d on days 1–2, then 20mg/kg/d days 3–10) are as effective as quetiapine (200mg/d, 400mg/d, 600mg/d, up to 800mg/d), but works in three days (n=30, RCT, 21/7, Feifel *et al, Innov Clin Neurosci* 2011;**8**:29–35). In acute mania, oral or IV loading of valproate is quicker and more effective than a standard oral maintenance regimen (n=90, RCT, 7/7, Ghaleiha *et al, Neuropsychobiology* 2014;**70**:29–35). Prompt rapid stabilisation with valproate may allow transition to maintenance without antipsychotics (n=136, RCT, d/b, p/c, 21/7, Müller-Oerlinghausen *et al, J Clin Psychopharmacol* 2000;**20**:195–203). Cochrane concludes that there is consistent if limited evidence that valproate is effective in acute mania; it may be less effective than olanzapine but with less sedation and weight gain (s=10, Macritchie *et al, Cochrane Database Syst Rev* 2003;**1**:CD004052). The equivalent amount of valproic acid available from Depakote® 500mg (Sanofi-Aventis), Epilim EC® 500mg (Sanofi-

Aventis) and Epilim Chrono® 500mg (Sanofi-Aventis) are 500mg, 433mg and 433mg respectively.

Review: general (Bowden, *Bipolar Disord* 2003; **5**:189–202), loading dose strategies (Keck *et al*, *Bipolar Disord* 2000:**2**:42–6).

+ Combinations (by drugs with some possible intrinsic antimanic activity)

In acute mania, combinations are commonly used and a meta-analysis has concluded that adding an antipsychotic to an established mood stabliser is more effective than a mood stabliser alone (s=8, n=1124, RCT, Smith *et al*, *Acta Psychiatr Scand* 2007;**115**:12–20).

Review: * combinations in mania (Geoffroy *et al*, *CNS Neurosci Ther* 2012;**18**:957–64).

Aripiprazole + lamotrigine

The combination delayed the time to manic relapse in bipolar I cf. lamotrigine monotherapy, but not statistically significantly (NNT=9, n=351, RCT, p/c, 52/52, Carlson *et al*, *Bipolar Disorder* 2012;**14**:41–53).

Benzodiazepines + antipsychotics

Extensive clinical experience supports routine use of BDZs in mania, although there is remarkably little robust evidence. For acute mania they have a rapid onset, are highly sedative and are well tolerated, with no EPSEs but have little or no long-term role. Short-term medium or high doses of benzodiazepines can be used alone or as adjuncts to other therapies in acute phases of hypomania, e.g. **diazepam**, **lorazepam** or **clonazepam** (meta-analysis of clonazepam in mania, although there wasn't exactly a lot to meta-analyse; s=7, n=206, RCT, Curtin and Schulz, *J Affect Disord* 2004;**78**:201–8). See individual drugs or groups in this section (see also *Acute psychiatric emergency 1.1*).

Levetiracetam + TAU

Levetiracetam 500–2000mg/d showed some improvement in most manic patients, but was not wildly encouraging (n=34, open, 8/52, Post *et al*, *J Clin Psychiatry* 2005;**66**:370–4), although there are some cases of response (eg. n=10, open, 28/7, Grunze *et al*, *J Clin Psychiatry* 2003;**64**:781–4).

Lithium + antipsychotics

Olanzapine may enhance the antimanic response to lithium (n=2004, 12/52, Vieta *et al*, *J Affect Disord* 2008;**106**:63–72).

Quetiapine was effective and well tolerated as an adjunct (n=191 [c=105], RCT, 21/7, d/b, p/c, Sachs *et al*, *Bipolar Disord* 2004;**6**:213–23), and at 500mg/d (range 300–700mg/d), and was superior to placebo when combined with lithium (n=402, RCT, d/b, p/c, 6/52, Yatham *et al*, *J Clin Psychopharmacol* 2004;**24**:599–606).

Risperidone plus lithium was as effective as haloperidol plus a MS and more effective than an MS alone in acute mania (n=156, RCT, d/b, p/c, 3/52, Sachs *et al*, *Am J Psychiatry* 2002;**159**:1146–54).

Lithium + carbamazepine

The combination has been used in resistant cases. See *4.4.3* for neurotoxicity warning.

Olanzapine + carbamazepine

The combination had no advantage (and had more side-effects) over carbamazepine alone in mania (n=118, RCT, d/b, p/c, 6+20/52, Tohen *et al*, *Br J Psychiatry* 2008;**192**:135–43).

Valproate + antipsychotics

Amisulpride as valproate augmentation was as effective as haloperidol but better tolerated (n=123, RCT, open, 3/12, Thomas *et al*, *Neuropsychiatr Dis Treat* 2008;**4**:675–86).

Aripiprazole+valproate seems as effective as haloperidol plus valproate in acute mania, with less EPSE but more weight gain (n=42, RCT, s/b, 8/52, Jeong *et al*, *Clin Neuropharmacol* 2012;**35**:97–102).

Olanzapine adjunctively was superior to placebo in manic and mixed bipolar episodes, but with significant weight gain (n=344, RCT, d/b, 6/52, Tohen *et al*, *Arch Gen Psychiatry* 2002;**59**:62–9, MS; comment by Gardner, *Evid Based Ment Health* 2002;**5**:89; FFT).

Quetiapine augmentation was effective and well tolerated (eg. n=402, RCT, d/b, p/c, 6/52, Yatham *et al*, *J Clin Psychopharmacol* 2004;**24**:599–606).

Risperidone plus valproate was as effective as haloperidol plus MS and more effective than an MS alone in acute mania (n=156, RCT, d/b, p/c, 3/52, Sachs *et al*, *Am J Psychiatry*

2002;**159**:1146–54), and may be more effective more rapidly than haloperidol plus valproate in acute mania (n=41, RCT, s/b, 6/52, Ouyang *et al, Int J Psychiatry Clin Pract* 2012;**16**:178–88).

Phenytoin + haloperidol

Phenytoin augmentation of haloperidol in acute mania was more effective than haloperidol alone (n=39, RCT, 5/52, Mishory *et al, Am J Psychiatry* 2000;**157**:463–5).

Valproate + lithium

Valproate has been used to augment lithium in resistant rapid-cycling mania (e.g. n=12, open, Reischies *et al, Neuropsychobiology* 2002;**46**[Suppl 1]:S22–S27).

• Unlicensed/some efficacy

Allopurinol + lithium/valproate/haloperidol*

Adjunct: Allopurinol 600mg/d was significantly superior to placebo as an adjunct to lithium in mania and can be an alternative to antipsychotics (n=120, RCT, d/b, p/c, 4/52, Machado-Vieira *et al, J Clin Psychiatry* 2008;**69**:1237–45; FFT). As an adjunct to valproate, allopurinol increased the probability of remission 23-fold in one study (n=57[c=50], RCT, d/b, p/c, 4/52, Jahangard *et al, Eur Neuropsychopharmacol* 2014;**24**:1210–21), but another was unable to show any effect as an adjunct (n=180, RCT, p/c, 6/52, Weiser *et al, Bipolar Disord* 2014;**16**:441–7).

Antipsychotics *
(see also aripiprazole, asenapine, olanzapine, quetiapine and risperidone in BNF listed)

Hypomania has a hyperdopaminergic component (Cousins *et al, Bipolar Disord* 2009;**11**:787–806).

Amisulpride (about 700mg/d) was effective for mania in a pilot study (n=20[c=14], open, 6/52, Vieta *et al, J Clin Psychiatry* 2005;**66**:575–8).

Clozapine * is obviously problematic but may be effective in 72% treatment-resistant manics or schizoaffectives (e.g. n=38, RCT, one year, Suppes *et al, Am J Psychiatry* 1999;**156**:1164–9) with rapid titration in resistant episodes (up to 100mg on day 1) reducing the time to response and discharge compared to standard (n=23) titration (n=67[c=64], Ifteni *et al, J Affect Disord* 2014;**166**:168–72).

Haloperidol is probably superior to other antimanics (s=68, n=16073, RCT, 3/52, Cipriani *et al, Lancet* 2011;**378**:1306–15).

Paliperidone (review by Marino *et al, Neuropsychiatr Dis Treat* 2012;**8**:181–9) 12mg/d (but not lower) may be superior to placebo (n=469, RCT, d/b, p/c, 3/52, Berwaerts *et al, J Affect Disord* 2011;**129**:252–60), and as effective as quetiapine (n=493, RCT, d/b, 12/52, Vieta *et al, Bipolar Disord* 2010;**12**:230–43), but not effective as an adjunct to either lithium or valproate (n=300, RCT, d/b, p/c, 6/52, Berwaerts *et al, J Affect Disord* 2011;**129**:252–60).

Ziprasidone is licensed in the USA for acute mania, with a rapid response from 40–80mg BD (review by Cañas *et al, Expert Opin Pharmacother* 2011;**12**:2245–63).

Benzodiazepines (see combinations)

Donepezil + lithium *

Adjunct: There was some benefit from day one but no significant benefit after that (n=30[c=30], RCT, d/b, p/c, 4/52, Chen *et al, Neuropsychiatr Dis Treat* 2013;**9**:839–45).

Folic acid + valproate

Adjunct: Folic acid was superior to placebo as an adjuvant in acute mania, a fascinating finding (n=88, RCT, d/b, p/c, 3/52, Behzadi *et al, Acta Psychiatr Scand* 2009;**120**:441–5).

Medroxyprogesterone + TAU *

Adjunct: Adjunctive medroxyprogesterone acetate (a SERM) was superior to placebo for acute symptoms (n=51, d/b, p/c, RCT, 4/52, Kulkarni *et al, Psychoneuroendocrinology* 2014;**43**:52–61).

Tamoxifen

Monotherapy: Tamoxifen (a protein kinase C inhibitor) has a significant antimanic activity, with a response by day 5 at 20–140mg/d (n=16, d/b, p/c, 3/52, Zarate *et al, Bipolar Disorders* 2007;**9**:561–70), is remarkably well tolerated (n=66[c=50], RCT, d/b, p/c, 3/52, Yildiz *et al, Arch Gen Psychiatry* 2008;**65**:255–63) and effective as an adjunct to lithium (1–1.2mEq/L) in acute mania (n=40, RCT, d/b, p/c, 6/52, Amrollahi *et al, J Affect Disord* 2011;**129**:327–31).

Topiramate + lithium/valproate *

Adjunct: Topiramate appears to have no effect as an adjunct to lithium or valproate in bipolar I manic or mixed episodes (n=46, RCT, d/b, p/c, 8/52, Mirsepassi *et al, Iran J Psychiatry Behav Sci* 2013;**7**:11–5), but at least people can lose significant amounts of weight (n=287, RCT, d/b, p/c, 12/52, Chengappa *et al, J Clin Psychiatry* 2006;**67**:1698–1706). Cochrane has concluded that there is, as yet, insufficient evidence for use as monotherapy or adjunctive for acute mania (s=1, Vasu-dev *et al, Cochrane Database Syst Rev* 2006;1:CD003384).

Verapamil + lithium

Adjunct: Verapamil may be highly antimanic with lithium, possibly by enhancing pKC inhibition (n=50[c=50], RCT, d/b, 4/52, Singh, *Int J Psychiatr Clin Pract* 2008;**12**:303–8).

Zonisamide + TAU

Adjunct: Adjunctive zonisamide has improved mania in many patients but mood deteriorated in 32% patients, although nearly all lost weight (n=62[c=40], open, 8/52, McElroy *et al, J Clin Psychiatry* 2005;**66**:617–24).

■ Unlicensed/possible efficacy

Memantine

Memantine may have some efficacy and appears well tolerated (n=33, open, Keck *et al, Clin Neuropharmacol* 2009;**32**:199–204).

Tryptophan depletion

Acute tryptophan depletion may have an antimanic effect, albeit poorly tolerated (n=23[c=17],RCT,d/b,p/c,7/7,Applebaum *et al, Bipolar Disord* 2007;**9**:884–7).

✱ Case reports

- Eslicarbazepine * (n=1, treatment intolerant, Nath *et al, Clin Neuropharmacol* 2012;**35**:295)
- Propofol IV (n=1, Cluver and Hardesty, *J Clin Psychiatry* 2006;**67**:165–6).

□ No efficacy

Antidepressants

Antidepressants can precipitate, exacerbate or trigger mania (n=1864, Lim *et al, Bipolar Disord* 2001;**3**:165–73).

Caffeine

A high caffeine intake will risk disturbing sleep patterns and exacerbating mania (n=1, Caykoylu *et al, Prog Neuropsychopharmacol Biol Psychiatry* 2008;**32**:1349–50).

Calcitonin + TAU *

In refractory bipolar mania, intranasal calcitonin (200iu) was ineffective as an adjunct (n=46, RCT, d/b, p/c, 3/52, Vik *et al, Bipolar Disord* 2013;**15**:359–64).

Dipyridamole + lithium

Dipyridamole is ineffective as an adjunct to lithium (n=120, RCT, d/b, p/c, 4/52, Machado-Vieira *et al, J Clin Psychiatry* 2008;**69**:1237–45).

Fosphenytoin

IV fosphenytoin appears ineffective in acute mania (n=7, open, one hour, Applebaum *et al, J Clin Psychiatry* 2003;**64**:408–9).

Gabapentin ± TAU

Two studies failed to show any advantage as an adjunct or monotherapy (e.g. Pande *et al, J Clin Psychopharmacol* 1999;**19**:341–8).

Lamotrigine

Lamotrigine has no efficacy in acute mania and delays the time to manic relapse in pooled data.

Omega-3 fatty acids ± cytidine *

A meta-analysis showed no evidence for efficacy as an adjunct for mania (s=5, n=291, RCT, >4/52, Sarris *et al, J Clin Psychiatry* 2012;**73**:81–6). Both (individually or combined) were non-significantly worse than placebo in a small but adequately powered study (n=45, RCT, d/b, p/c, 4/12, Murphy *et al, J Clin Psychopharmacol* 2012;**32**:699–703).

Oxcarbazepine

Cochrane concludes that there is insufficient

evidence on the use for acute mania or rapid-cycling (s=7, n=368, RCT, Vasudev *et al, Cochrane Database Syst Rev* 2011;**12**:CD004857).

Tiagabine *

Cochrane concludes that there is no evidence for efficacy and highlights serious ADRs (s=0, n=0, RCTs, p/c, Vasudev *et al, Cochrane Database Syst Rev* 2013;**12**:CD004694).

Topiramate (see also adjuncts) *

An analysis concluded that there was no evidence to support routine use as monotherapy in mania (s=4, RCT, Kushner *et al, Bipolar Disord* 2006;**8**:15–27).

1.10.3 BIPOLAR DEPRESSION *

Bipolar depression is longer-lasting than unipolar depression, frequently misdiagnosed as unipolar depression, and is more likely to have psychosis, diurnal variation, and hypersomnia during depressive episodes, and a greater number of shorter episodes. It is clear that well-being and functioning are inversely proportional to the number of bipolar episodes and so strategies to reduce relapse must be rigorously followed. Bipolar depression can be potentiated by substance and alcohol misuse and is more difficult to treat.

Role of drugs *

For *acute* bipolar depression, a multiple treatments meta-analysis (s=29, n=8331, RCT, d/b, 4–16/52, Taylor *et al, Acta Psychiatr Scand* 2014;**130**:452–69) using effect sizes as the efficacy measure has concluded that:

- **Best performers**: olanzapine + fluoxetine, olanzapine, lurasidone
- **Also recommended**: quetiapine, valproate, SSRIs
- **Possible**: tricyclics, lithium
- **Little or no evidence**: lamotrigine (high switch risk, less robust acute efficacy), MAOIs, ziprasidone, aripiprazole and risperidone.

Although responding quickly is good news, it appears not to be a particularly good guide to how well someone will do long term. However, **not** improving at all in the first 14 days does seem to predict long-term poorer response (s=10, n=3369, RCT, d/b, p/c, Kemp *et al, J Affect Disord* 2011;**130**:171–9; see also systematic review and meta-analysis; s=7, de Fruyt *et al, J Psychopharmacol* 2012;**26**:603–17).

In *refractory* bipolar depression antidepressants *may* be effective if agitated people are excluded, and the risk of mania is only moderately greater than the risk of spontaneous mania; and bipolar TRD is not necessarily resistant to all treatments (s=15, Tondo *et al, Curr Psychiatry Rep* 2014;**16**:431).

The general principles of management include:

1. **Use mood stabilisers:** quetiapine, lurasidone and olanzapine/fluoxetine have good evidence for acute symptoms and relapse prevention.
2. **Optimise any antidepressants:** (see also antidepressants under unlicensed) The STEP-BD study concluded that longer-term adjunctive antidepressants have no therapeutic advantage, but at least they do not increase the risk of relapse, switches to mania or have greater ADRs (n=366, RCT, d/b, p/c, 26/52, STEP-BD, Sachs *et al, N Engl J Med* 2007;**356**:1711–22). Use with a MS and start with lowest switch risk drugs (see 5 below).
3. **Minimise any antidepressant exposure:** attempt gradual taper after a continuation phase if the person is genuinely euthymic, as premature discontinuing antidepressants within the first 3–6/12 of an episode has an up to three times higher relapse rate than those continuing for at least 8/12 (n=44, retrospective, one year, Altshuler *et al, J Clin Psychiatry* 2001;**62**:612–6).
4. **Avoid switching to manic or mixed states with antidepressants** — this usually occurs within the first 12 weeks (s=13[7 RCTs], Bond *et al, J Clin Psychiatry* 2008;**69**:1589–601), and is lower if antidepressants are used with a mood stabiliser. If mania develops, reduce the antidepressant dose immediately and allow the mood to settle for a month or so. Manic switch risk factors include past depressive episodes, history of rapid-cycling, alcohol misuse, previous suicide attempt and a history of switching, the majority of which are NOT antidepressant-related (n=2166, STEP-BD, Perlis *et al, Neuropsychopharmacology* 2010;**35**:2545–52).

5. **Avoid sudden dose changes** or switches.
6. **Offer ECT** for people at immediate risk of self-harm or unable to tolerate medication (n=6, Macedo-Soares *et al*, *J ECT* 2005;**21**:31–4), e.g. older people.
7. **Check thyroid function** — poor response in bipolar depression may be related to low FTI and high TSH levels, even if in the alleged therapeutic range (n=65, Cole *et al*, *Am J Psychiatry* 2002;**159**:116–21).

Reviews: * meta-analysis of monotherapy studies (s=24, p/c, mean 8/52, Selle *et al*, *Pharmacopsychiatry* 2014;**47**:43–52), pharmacotherapy for acute bipolar II depression (s=21, RCTs, Swartz and Thase, *J Clin Psychiatry* 2011;**72**:356–66) and bipolar I depression (Cerullo and Strakowski, *CNS Spectr* 2013;**18**:199–208), general (Vieta and Valenti, *CNS Drugs* 2013;**27**:515–29; Ketter *et al*, *J Clin Psychiatry* 2014;**75**:e10), stimulants, e.g. modafinil, armodafinil, lisdexamfetamine (Corp *et al*, *J Clin Psychiatry* 2014;**75**:1010–8), improving outcomes (Nierenberg *et al*, *J Clin Psychiatry* 2015;**76**:e10; FFT).

BNF listed

Lamotrigine

Lamotrigine is licensed in the UK for prevention of depressive episodes in people with bipolar I disorder (but *not* for *acute* episodes). Robust and independent meta-analysis of the five studies (three unpublished) show lamotrigine has a consistently beneficial, albeit modest, effect from 50–200mg/d, greater in more severe depression (s=5, n=1072, RCT, d/b, p/c, Geddes *et al*, *Br J Psychiatry* 2009;**194**:4–9), including in the elderly (n=57[c=38], open, 12/52, Sajatovic *et al*, *Bipolar Disord* 2011;**13**:294–302) but not in manic, mixed, rapid-cycling or unipolar depressive states (Amann *et al*, *J Psychopharmacol* 2011;**25**:1289–94). Addition of paroxetine helps, but not in people who have not responded to lithium and lamotrigine (n=124, RCT, d/b, p/c, 16/52, van der Loos *et al*, *Acta Psychiatr Scand* 2010;**122**:246–54) Increasing the dose slowly over 6/52 to 200mg/d minimises the incidence of serious rash, especially with valproate.

Reviews: * general (Tränkner *et al*, *Neuropsychiatr Dis Treat* 2013;**9**:101–11; Reid *et al*, *J Clin Psychiatry* 2013;**74**:675–84).

Quetiapine *

Quetiapine is licensed for the treatment of acute depressive episodes in bipolar disorder, and for prevention of recurrence if responding acutely. A slower dose increase is recommended (night-time, day 1 50mg; day 2 100mg; day 3 200mg; day 4 300mg) with an onset of action within one week (s=11, n=3488, RCTs, Suttajit *et al*, *Drug Des Devel Ther* 2014;**8**:827–38). Monotherapy efficacy has been proven in two robust RCTs showing response rates of 55% for 300mg/d and 600mg/d cf 36% with placebo (BOLDER I, n=542, RCT, d/b, p/c, 8/52, Calabrese *et al*, *Am J Psychiatry* 2005;**162**:1351–60; BOLDER II, n=509, RCT, d/b, p/c, 8/52, Thase *et al*, *J Clin Psychopharmacol* 2006;**26**:600–9), with no treatment-emergent mania and an NNT=5 for response and remission of bipolar depression (Cookson *et al*, *Int Clin Psychopharmacol* 2007;**22**:93–100). EMBOLDEN I (n=802, RCT, d/b, p/c, 8/52, Young *et al*, *J Clin Psychiatry* 2010;**71**:150–62), and EMBOLDEN II (n=740, RCT, d/b, p/c, 8/52, McElroy *et al*, *J Clin Psychiatry* 2010;**71**:163–74) showed 300–600mg/d was superior to placebo, paroxetine and lithium. Continuation treatment with quetiapine reduces relapse in bipolar I and II depression (n=584, RCT, d/b, p/c, <1 year, Young *et al*, *World J Biol Psychiatry* 2014;**15**:96–112).

Reviews: systematic review (Chiesa *et al*, *Int Clin Psychopharmacol* 2012;**27**:76–90), general (Sanford and Keating, *CNS Drugs* 2012;**26**:435–60).

+ Augmentation (by drugs with possible intrinsic activity)

Agomelatine + lithium/valproate *

Agomelatine was effective as an add-on to valproate or lithium, where 86% responded (n=28[c=26], open, 36/52, Fornaro *et al*, *Neuropsychiatr Dis Treat* 2013;**9**:243–51; FFT).

Aripiprazole + antidepressants

Adjunctive aripiprazole 20–30mg/d has been successful in TRBD (n=2, Karada *et al*, *Turk Psikiyatri Derg* 2011;**22**:269–72).

Lamotrigine + quetiapine

In quetiapine or lamotrigine monotherapy-resistant bipolar depression, adding the other increased the euthymia rate (0–46%) and decreased syndromal (80–30%) symptom rates (n=39[c=29], open, 12/52, Ahn *et al, Ann Clin Psychiatry* 2011;**23**:17–24).

Lamotrigine + valproate

The combination appeared superior to lamotrigine monotherapy on secondary measures, although primary measures were non-significant (n=86, RCT, d/b, p/c, 8/12, Bowden *et al, Acta Psychiatr Scand* 2012;**126**:342–50).

Lithium + fluoxetine

Fluoxetine augmentation of lithium in bipolar mood disorder can help prevent breakthrough depression (n=26, open, three-year, Tondo *et al, Int J Psychiatry Clin Pract* 1997;**1**:203–6).

Lithium + lamotrigine

The combination was significantly superior to lamotrigine monotherapy in acute bipolar depression (n=124, RCT, d/b, p/c, 8/52, van der Loos *et al, J Clin Psychiatry* 2009;**70**:223–31) and had an enduring effect (n=124, RCT, d/b, p/c, 76/52, van der Loos *et al, Bipolar Disord* 2011;**13**:111–7).

Lurasidone + lithium/valproate *

Adjunctive lurasidone significantly reduced MADRS scores compared to placebo, with lower discontinuations in a robust study (n=348, RCT, d/b, p/c, 6/52, Loebel *et al, Am J Psychiatry* 2014;**171**:169–77).

Olanzapine + fluoxetine (OFC)

The olanzapine-fluoxetine combination (OFC) is licensed for bipolar depression in the US as 'Symbyax' (6/25, 6/50, or 12/50 mg/day), and has been compared to olanzapine (5–20 mg/day), and placebo (n=833, RCT, d/b, p/c, 8/52, Tohen *et al, Arch Gen Psychiatry* 2003;**60**:1079–88), although there was no fluoxetine arm and so the combination's efficacy might be predominantly from fluoxetine (n=114 [c=83], RCT, open, 7+12/52, Tamayo *et al, J Clin Psychopharmacol* 2009;**29**:358–61). A systematic review and meta-analysis concludes that OFC improves response, remission and relapse but with a worse profile of ADRs (s=4, n=1330, RCTs, Silva *et al, J Affect Disord* 2013;**146**:310–8).

• Unlicensed/some efficacy

Antidepressants *

Monotherapy: A review noted that there is a 'striking incongruity between the wide use and weak evidence-base' for antidepressants in bipolar depression (Pacchiarotti *et al, Am J Psychiatry* 2013;**170**:1249–62). Numerous reviews come to many conclusions:

- Switching to mania occurs anyway but probably less common than widely believed (Vázquez *et al, Int J Neuro-psychopharmacol* 2013;**16**:1673–85)
- Antidepressants seem safe when combined with a mood stabiliser
- Antidepressant monotherapy cannot be recommended (especially in bipolar I) due to lack efficacy (s=15, n=2373, RCTs, <16/52, Sidor and Macqueen, *J Clin Psychiatry* 2011;**72**:156–67)
- Accelerated episode frequency is unproven but considered likely
- Apparent switching may be that anti depressants shorten depressed phases
- If mania develops, stopping or reducing the antidepressant dose is advisable
- A major predictor of mood instability is long-term exposure to antidepressants (n=53, 12/12, Strejilevich *et al, Ann Clin Psychiatry* 2011;**23**:186–92)
- Antidepressants used selectively with or without MS in non-agitated depressed bipolars may be effective for short periods, albeit with a moderate risk of manic elevations (n=1036, Tondo *et al, Acta Psychiatr Scand* 2013;**127**:355–64).

Reviews: * (McInerney and Kennedy, *Prim Care Companion CNS Disord* 2014;**16**; PCC.14r01653; FFT; Licht *et al, Acta Psychiatr Scand* 2008;**118**:337–46).

Bupropion has been used adjunctively in resistant bipolar depression (n=13, open, Erfurth *et al, Neuropsychobiol* 2001;**45**[Suppl 1]:S33–S36).

Citalopram may be a useful adjunct, with response rates rising past the first six weeks (n=20, RCT, d/b, 12/52, Schaffer *et al, J Affect Disord* 2006;**96**:95–9).

Escitalopram may have some efficacy (n=20, open, 12/52, Fonseca *et al*, *J Clin Psychiatry* 2006;**67**:81–6).

Fluoxetine * may have a low switch rate in bipolar I and II (s=8, Martinotti *et al*, *Expert Opin Pharmacother* 2013;**14**:1065–75).

Moclobemide 450–750mg/d may be effective, with less side-effects and fewer switches to mania (2 vs 6), indicating a useful potential role (n=156, RCT, 8/52, Silverstone *et al*, *Acta Psychiatr Scand* 2001;**104**:104–9).

Tricyclics should be avoided unless covered with mood stabilisers (n=136, Mundo *et al*, *J Affect Disord* 2006;**92**:227–30).

Tranylcypromine appeared effective (62.5% responded) in refractory bipolar depression in an incomplete study (n=19, RCT, open, Nolen *et al*, *Acta Psychiatr Scand* 2007;**115**:360–5).

Venlafaxine was effective in lithium non-responders, with no switches to mania (n=17, 12/52, Amsterdam *et al*, *Acta Psychiatr Scand* 2010;**121**:210–8), although response can reduce after repeated exposure (n=83, RCT, open, Amsterdam and Shults, *J Aff Disorders* 2009;**115**:234–40).

Antipsychotics (see also quetiapine & OFC)

Monotherapy: The main roles of antipsychotics in bipolar depression are as adjuncts to mood stabilisers and as adjuncts in maintenance.

Aripiprazole did not delay the time to relapse of depressive symptoms, although it did not increase it either (n=161[c=12], RCT, d/b, p/c, two years, Keck *et al*, *J Clin Psychiatry* 2007;**68**:1480–91).

Ziprasidone (mean 58mg/d) may have potential (n=30, Liebowitz *et al*, *J Affect Disord* 2009;**118**:205–8).

Olanzapine * monotherapy may be superior to placebo in bipolar depression, shown in a pooled analysis (s=2, n=1214, RCT, d/b, p/c, Tohen *et al*, *J Affect Disord* 2014;**164**:57-62) and a mean dose of 14mg/d produced response rates of 50% (cf. 21% with placebo) and remissions rates of 35% vs 12% (n=68[c=57], RCT, d/b, p/c, 8/52, Wang *et al*, *Psychopharmacology [Berl]* 2014;**231**:2811–8).

Inositol + TAU

Adjunct: Inositol may be useful in bipolar depression, e.g. 50% responded to 12g/d inositol cf. 30% on placebo (n=24, RCT, 6/52, Chengappa *et al*, *Bipolar Disord* 2000;**2**:47–55), and in TRBD where response was 17% (cf lamotrigine 24% and risperidone 5%; n=66, RCT, 16/52, open, Nierenberg *et al*, *Am J Psychiatry* 2006;**163**:210–6). However, it was not statistically or clinically superior to placebo as augmentation of lithium or valproate (n=17, RCT, d/b, p/c, 6/52, Eden Evins *et al*, *Bipolar Disord* 2006;**8**:168–74).

Ketoconazole + TAU

Adjunct: Ketoconazole, 400mg/d has been used as an adjunct in resistant bipolar depression, with no increase in manic symptoms (n=6, open, Brown *et al*, *Bipolar Disord* 2001;**3**:23–9).

Levothyroxine + TAU *

Adjunct: Adjunctive T4 to a MS has had no effect (n=20, RCT, d/b, p/c, 6/52, Uhl *et al*, *Pharmacopsychiatry* 2014;**47**:180–3), even high-dose levothyroxine 300mcg/d (n=62, RCT, d/b, p/c, 6/52, Stamm *et al*, *J Clin Psychiatry* 2014;**75**:162–8).

Lurasidone (license application due 2016) *

Adjunct/monotherapy: Lurasidone is licensed in US for bipolar depression as monotherapy or as an adjunct to valproate or lithium. The starting dose is 18.5mg/d, increasing up to a maximum of 111mg/d, which significantly reduces bipolar depression with discontinuations lower than placebo (n=505, RCT, d/b, p/c, 6/52, PREVAIL 2, Loebel *et al*, *Am J Psychiatry* 2014;**171**:160–8). See main entry under psychosis.

Memantine + lamotrigine/valproate *

Adjunct: A pilot study showed no statistically significant advantage of memantine (20mg/d) and lamotrigine (>100mg/d), but an early effect suggests that perhaps the dose was too high (n=29, RCT, d/b, p/c, 8/52, Anand *et al*, *Bipolar Disord* 2012;**14**:64–70). Adjunctive memantine 5mg/d to valproate had no apparent clinical effect, although TNFα-levels fell (n=214, RCT, d/b, p/c, 12/52, Lee *et al*, *J Clin Psychopharmacol* 2014;**34**:337–43).

Mifepristone + TAU

Adjunct: A one-week course of adjunctive mifepristone 600mg/d seems to produce a sustained improvement in spatial working memory enduring over 7/52, perhaps via a persistent improvement in hippocampal mineralo-corticoid receptor function (n=60, RCT, d/b, p/c, 8/52, Watson *et al*, *Biol Psychiatry* 2012:**72**:943–9).

Modafinil + TAU *

Adjunct: A meta-analysis showed adjunctive modafinil is effective for bipolar depression, including for symptoms of fatigue (s=4, n=568, RCTs, d/b, p/c, Goss *et al*, *J Clin Psychiatry* 2013;**74**:1101–7). Armodafinil 150mg appears to do the same (n=257, RCT, d/b, p/c, 8/52, Calabrese *et al*, *J Clin Psychiatry* 2010;**71**:1363–70).

N-acetylcysteine (NAC) + TAU

Adjunct: Bipolar disorder may be complicated by glutathione depletion and so adjunctive NAC may help to correct this, and is well tolerated (eg. n=149, RCT, open, 2/12, Berk *et al*, *J Affect Disord* 2011;**135**:389–94; n=17, RCT, p/c, 24/52, Maqalhães *et al*, *Rev Bras Psiquiatr* 2011;**33**:374–8).

Omega-3 fatty acids + TAU

Adjunct: A meta-analysis for use in bipolar depression shows strong evidence of moderate efficacy, for depression but not for mania (s=5, n=291, RCT, >4/52, Sarris *et al*, *J Clin Psychiatry* 2012;**73**:81–6), e.g. E-EPA was effective in bipolar depression, with 1–2g/d superior to placebo (n=75, RCT, d/b, p/c, 12/52, Frangou *et al*, *Br J Psychiatry* 2006;**188**:46–50). Dose may be important (n=12[c=8], open, 6/12, Osher *et al*, *J Clin Psychiatry* 2005;**66**:726–9).

Oxcarbazepine + lithium

Adjunct: The combination was effective in 60% and may have longer-term efficacy (n=17, open, 8/52+12/12, Benedetti *et al*, *J Affect Disord* 2004;**79**:273–7).

Pramipexole + lithium/valproate/MS *

Adjunct: Adjunctive pramipexole (a dopamine agonist) was clearly superior (60% response) to placebo (9%) in bipolar depression (n=21, RCT, d/b, p/c, 6/52, Zarate *et al*, *Biol Psychiatry* 2004;**56**:54–60) and a mean 1.7mg/d added to existing mood stabilisers led to a 67% response (cf. 20% with placebo) in bipolar depression (n=22, RCT, o/p, p/c, 6/52, Goldberg *et al*, *Am J Psychiatry* 2004;**161**:564–6).

Review: Dell'Osso and Ketter, *Int Clin Psychopharmacol* 2013;**28**:297–304.

Uridine + TAU

Adjunct: Uridine was well tolerated and reduced depressive symptoms in children (n=7, open, 6/52, Kondo *et al*, *J Child Adolesc Psychopharmacol* 2011:**21**:171–5; FFT).

Zonisamide + TAU

Adjunct: Adjunctive zonisamide (mean 236mg/d) may have modest effectiveness in bipolar depression (e.g. Wilson and Findling, *Expert Opin Pharmacother* 2007;**8**:111–3), but relatively poor tolerability (n=20[c=10], open, 8/52, Ghaemi *et al*, *J Clin Psychopharmacol* 2006;**26**:385–8), although up to 300mg/d as add-on had significant effects in 50% of completers (n=10[c=8], open, 8/52, Anand *et al*, *J Clin Psychiatry* 2005;**66**:195–8).

■ Unlicensed/possible efficacy

Gabapentin + TAU

Adjunct: Gabapentin has no antimanic activity (see *1.10.2*), although may have a role as an adjunct in refractory bipolar (review, s=40, Carta *et al*, *J Affect Disord* 2003;**75**:83–91).

Ketamine *

Adjunct: In TR-BPD, a single dose of ketamine followed by d-cycloserine 1000mg/d led to 50% remission (n=8[c=7], 4/52, Kantrowitz *et al*, *J Clin Psychiatry* 2015;**76**:737–8; FFT).

Monotherapy: Ketamine (an NMDA antagonist) IV infusion (0.5mg/kg) produces a robust, rapid and reliable improvement in bipolar depression symptoms (71% vs 6% with placebo), albeit short-lived (n=18, RCT, d/b, p/c, c/o, 28/7, Diazgranados *et al*, *Arch Gen Psychiatry* 2010;**67**:793–802; replicated: n=15, RCT, d/b, p/c, c/o, Zarate *et al*, *Biol Psychiatry* 2012;**71**:939–46).

Lisdexamfetamine *

A pilot study showed some potential efficacy

(n=25, RCT, d/b, p/c, 8/52, McElroy *et al*, *Int Clin Psychopharmacol* 2015;**30**:6–13).

Melatonin + TAU

Melatonin secretion is altered in bipolar disorder and so melatonin supplementation may have some role (review by Srinivasan *et al*, *World J Biol Psychiatry* 2006;**7**:138–51).

Methylphenidate + TAU

Small open studies have shown adjunctive methylphenidate effective and tolerable in 78% depressed bipolars (eg. n=14, open, 12/52, El-Mallakh, *Bipolar Disord* 2000;**2**:56–9), without apparent abuse or mood switching (n=16, Lydon and El-Mallakh, *J Clin Psychopharmacol* 2006;**26**:516–8).

Triiodothyronine (T3) + TAU

Triiodothyronine (mean 90mg/d) has been successful in treatment-resistant bipolar II (n=159, retrospective, Kelly and Lieberman, *J Affect Disord* 2009;**116**:222–6).

Valproate

A systematic review and meta-analysis has shown some evidence for some efficacy as monotherapy, with an NNT of 5.9 (41% response cf 24% response on placebo) (s=4, n=142, RCT, d/b, p/c, Smith *et al*, *J Affect Disord* 2010;**122**:1–9; bizarrely the same s=4, n=142, RCT, d/b, p/c, Bond *et al*, in the same *J Affect Disord* 2010;**124**:228–34).

✱ Case reports

- Oxycodone as an adjunct (Schiffman and Gitlin, *J Clin Psychiatry* 2012;**73**:992).

☐ No efficacy

Levetiracetam

Levetiracetam up to 2500mg/d was ineffective (n=42, RCT, d/b, p/c, 6/52, Saricicek *et al*, *J Clin Psychiatry* 2011;**72**:744–50).

Ziprasidone

Adjunctive ziprasidone (mean 90mg/d) shows no efficacy as an adjunct (n=298, RCT, d/b, p/c, 6/52, Sachs *et al*, *J Clin Psychiatry* 2011;**72**:1413–22).

1.10.4 RAPID-CYCLING BIPOLAR DISORDER

Introduction

Rapid-cycling bipolar disorder is a variant of bipolar mood disorder, where four or more mood episodes occur in one year. Although relatively uncommon and often transient (about 80% will resolve within a year), this sub-group accounts for up to 80% of lithium non-responders, antidepressant therapy of depressive phases can induce or worsen cycling, and that rapid-cycling is a risk factor for suicide and suicide attempts (n=345, mean 13 years, Coryell *et al*, *Arch Gen Psychiatry* 2003;**60**:914–20). Rapid-cyclers are more likely (cf. non-rapid-cycling) to have a younger age of onset, more enduring symptoms, more severe depression and impairment, more anxiety/mania (n=54257, Lee *et al*, *Br J Psychiatry* 2010;**196**:217–25), and be female and bipolar II (n=1742, STEP-BD, Schneck *et al*, *Am J Psychiatry* 2008;**165**:370–7). Risk factors include poor adherence (n=3640, Perlis *et al*, *J Clin Psychiatry* 2010;**71**:296–303), neurological damage, neuroendocrine factors (including hypothyroidism) and psychotropic drugs (e.g. alcohol, antidepressants, stimulants), as well as some genetic factors.

Role of drugs

There will probably always be a lack of robust data on the pharmacotherapy of rapid-cycling, due to the unpredictable and spontaneously remitting nature of the condition. The initial strategies must be:

1. Reduce or stop any potential cycle-promoters, e.g. antidepressants.
2. Add/optimise mood stabilisers (start with lithium for treatment-naïve patients). Lithium and anticonvulsants have equivalent effectiveness, and aripiprazole and olanzapine appear promising (s=25 [6 RCTs], Fountoulakis *et al*, *Bipolar Disord* 2013;**15**:115–37).
3. Add other drugs, e.g. antipsychotics, lamotrigine (especially for bipolar II), and perhaps valproate.
4. Levothyroxine and nimodipine may be effective in non-response to first-line agents and may be worth a therapeutic trial.
5. Minimise ADRs to enhance compliance.
6. Recognise that the full benefits may not be

apparent for several months so do not abandon treatment too early.

References: n=500, STEP-BD, Schneck *et al*, *J Clin Psychiatry* 2006;**67**[Suppl 11]:22–7.

Review: * systematic (Carvalho *et al*, *J Clin Psychiatry* 2014;**75**:e578–86).

BNF listed

Carbamazepine

The original carbamazepine study (n=32, open, Kishimoto *et al*, *Br J Psychiatry* 1983;**143**:327–31) showed a particular effect in rapid-cycling, and several studies (e.g. n=18, open, 6/12, Joyce, *Int Clin Psychopharmacol* 1988;**3**:123–9) have shown a long-term response rate ranging from 20–70%. Doubt has, however, been raised about long-term efficacy, as CBZ seems to lose efficacy over several years (e.g. n=24, open, four years, Post *et al*, *J Clin Psychopharmacol* 1990;**10**:318–27).

Lithium

Around 20% of rapid-cyclers are lithium responders, probably by reducing the intensity of relapses rather than the actual number. Lithium response may be better if the sequence of relapse is mania, depression and then remission, rather than depression, mania and remission. Poor compliance with lithium, particularly if intermittent (e.g. frequent abrupt stopping), may complicate treatment by inducing relapse.

Review: Muzina, *Bipolar Disord* 2009;**11**(Suppl 2):84–91.

+ Combinations

Lithium + carbamazepine

The combination can be useful in rapid-cyclers non-responsive to the individual drugs (e.g. n=16, retrospective, Di Costanzo and Schifano, *Acta Psychiatr Scand* 1991;**83**:456–9). See also interactions (*4.4.1*).

Lithium + valproate

Valproate seems as effective as lithium in preventing relapse in recently stabilised rapid-cyclers (n=60[n=254 in stabilisation phase], RCT, d/b, 20/12, Calabrese *et al*, *Am J Psychiatry* 2005;**162**:2152–61), although it has no additional efficacy with lithium (n=31, RCT, d/b, 6/12, Kemp *et al*, *J Clin Psychiatry* 2009;**70**:113–21).

Thyroid + antidepressants

Sub-therapeutic doses of T_3 tri-iodothyronine 25–50mcg/d or T_4 levothyroxine up to 100mcg/d have been used to augment tricyclics and phenelzine (although care is needed with any use of antidepressants in rapid-cycling). See levothyroxine/liothyronine.

• Unlicensed/some efficacy

Lamotrigine ± TAU

Adjunctive: Lamotrigine seems potentially useful as an adjunct in non-response to lithium plus valproate (n=36[c=16], d/b, p/c, 12/52, Wang *et al*, *Psychopharmacol Bull* 2010;**43**:5–21). The optimum dose appears to be 50–200mg/d, although doses as high as 600mg/d have been used.

Monotherapy: In the most robust study in rapid-cycling disorder, lamotrigine monotherapy was well tolerated and appeared useful in some (n=324, open+n=182, d/b maintenance phase, Calabrese *et al*, *J Clin Psychiatry* 2000; **61**:841–50), with survival rates favouring lamotrigine (significantly so in bipolar II patients), and 41% stable without relapse at 6/12 (cf. 26% placebo).

■ Unlicensed/possible efficacy

Calcium-channel blockers

Monotherapy: Old and unrepeated studies suggested a marked response in rapid-cycling in some people (e.g. n=12[c=9], RCT, d/b, p/c, Pazzaglia *et al*, *Psychiatry Res* 1993;**49**:257–72).

Clozapine

Clozapine may be effective in treatment-resistant rapid cycling (e.g. n=3, Suppes *et al*, *Biol Psychiatry* 1994;**36**:338–40).

Gabapentin

Some gabapentin monotherapy mania studies included some rapid-cyclers and moderate efficacy was reported (Shelton and Calabrese, *Curr Psychiatry Reports* 2000;**2**:310–15).

Olanzapine + TAU

Ten rapid-cyclers were classified as responding to adjunctive olanzapine during dysphoric mania (n=13, open, 4/52, Gonzalez-Pinto *et al*, *J Clin Psychopharmacol* 2002;**22**:450–4).

Quetiapine

Monotherapy: Quetiapine 300–600mg/d was effective for treating depressive episodes in rapid-cycling bipolar I and II (n=108, RCT, d/b, p/c, 8/52, Vieta *et al*, *Bipolar Disorder* 2007;**9**:413–25) and may be more effective than valproate, albeit with more side-effects (n=17, open, Langosch *et al*, *J Clin Psychopharmacol* 2008;**28**:555–60).

Risperidone LAI + TAU

Risperidone LAI was no more effective than TAU for preventing relapse, but may reduce the need for urgent care referrals (n=45, RCT, open, 12/12, Bobo *et al*, *Clin Neuropharmacol* 2011;**34**:224–33).

✹ Case reports

- **Clozapine + lamotrigine** (n=1, Bastiampillai *et al*, *J Psychopharmacol* 2010;**24**:1834–6)
- **Lamotrigine + valproate** (n=1, Woo *et al*, *Psychiatry Clin Neurosci* 2007;**61**:130–1)
- **Levetiracetam** (eg. n=1, Kaufman, *Epilepsy Behav* 2004;**5**:1017–20)
- **Topiramate + clozapine** (n=1, Chen *et al*, *Clin Neuropharmacol* 2005;**28**:136–8).

☐ No efficacy

Antidepressants + TAU *

TAU plus antidepressant continuation in rapid-cycling is associated with worsened maintenance outcomes cf. TAU plus discontinuation (n=68, El-Mallakh *et al*, *J Affect Disord* 2015;**184**:318–21), so antidepressant discontinuation has to be a first-line treatment. They should only be used in rapid-cyclers in low dose and only in acute severe depression.

1.11 BORDERLINE PERSONALITY DISORDER (BPD)

see also Aggression (*1.2*)

There are a large number of personality disorders, of which borderline personality disorder is but one. Treatment is usually directed towards managing symptom clusters, e.g. anxiety, aggression and impulsiveness, rather than the underlying personality disorder.

Symptoms

The main symptoms are a deeply ingrained maladaptive pattern of behaviour, recognisable from adolescence and continuing through adult life, continued boredom, anger, unstable relationships, impulsive self-harmful behaviour (e.g. gambling, stealing, binge-eating or drinking), fears of abandonment, variable moods, recurrent suicide threats or behaviour, and uncertainty about personal identity.

Role of drugs

People with BPD may account for up to 7.5% of psychiatric admissions, with a raised incidence of psychiatric morbidity and mortality, and use of a wide range of medication and services. Pharmacotherapy will not alter ingrained character traits or the effects of abuse, but they may produce modest benefits with the occasional striking result, and be more effective if combined with psychotherapy. Drug therapy, however, is fraught with problems, e.g. side-effects may be grossly exaggerated and people may be actively antimedication or continually demand more medication. Several meta-analyses of RCTs have concluded that the beneficial effects are as follows:

Aspect	Anti-psychotics	Anti-depressants	Mood stabilisers
Cognitive-perception	++	?	?
Anger	++/+++	+/++	++
Impulse-behaviour	+	o	++
Anxiety	?	+/++	+++
Depression	o	+	++
Global functioning	+	o	+

+++ Significant effect + Minor effect
++ Moderate effect o No effect

Cochrane concludes that the current data for pharmacotherapy in BPD is insufficient to make any recommendations (s=8, n=394, Khalifa *et al*, *Cochrane Database Syst Rev* 2010;**8**:CD007667; s=28, n=1742, Stoffers *et al*, *Cochrane Database Syst Rev* 2010;**6**:CD005653; comment by Lieb *et al*, *Br J Psychiatry* 2010;**196**:4–12; s=21, Ingenhoven *et al*, *J Clin Psychiatry* 2010;**71**:14–25; Mercer *et al*, *J Pers Disord* 2009;**23**:156–74).

Reviews: * general (Belli *et al*, *J Clin Med Res* 2012;**4**:301–8), psychopharmacology (Ripoll, *Curr Opin Psychiatry* 2012;**25**:52–8; Bateman *et al*, *Lancet* 2015;**385**:735–43), narcissistic personality disorder (Caligor *et al*, *Am J Psychiatry* 2015;**172**:415–22).

• Unlicensed/some efficacy

Antidepressants (see also no efficacy)

Some symptoms of BPD are shared with depression, e.g. self-condemnation, emptiness, hopelessness, boredom and somatic complaints, and so the use of antidepressants for some symptoms is logical. **SSRIs** may have a role, e.g. **sertraline** (n=16, 8/52, Kavoussi *et al*, *J Clin Psychiatry* 1994;**55**:137–41), **fluoxetine** (n=40, RCT, Coccaro and Kavoussi, *Arch Gen Psychiatry* 1997;**54**:1081–8) and **fluvoxamine** (n= 38, RCT, d/b, p/c, c/o, 24/52 total, Rinne *et al*, *Am J Psychiatry* 2002;**159**:2048–54). Careful dose titration is needed to minimise agitation. Generally tricyclics are considered ineffective (or even detrimental) in depression associated with BPD.

Antipsychotics *

It is generally accepted that people with borderline or schizotypical personality disorders may gain significant benefit from psychotherapy and small doses of antipsychotics.

Aripiprazole 15 mg/d (starting at a lower dose; n=3, Mobascher *et al*, *Pharmacopsychiatry* 2006;**39**:111–2) may improve many measures of BPD (n=52, RCT, d/b, p/c, 8/52, Nickel *et al*, *Am J Psychiatry* 2006;**163**:833–8).

Asenapine seems safe and effective for global BPD symptoms, especially where other treatments are not tolerated (n=12[c=8], open, 8/52, Martin-Blanco *et al*, *Int Clin Psychopharmacol* 2014;**29**:120–3).

Clozapine (25–100 mg/d) may significantly reduce aggressive incidents especially in the first 6/12 (eg. n=22, Frogley *et al*, *Ann Clin Psychiatry* 2013;**25**:125–34; n=7, Brown *et al*, *CNS Spectr* 2014;**19**:391–402) and significantly reduce SIB, seclusion and violence (n=7, Chengappa *et al*, *J Clin Psychiatry* 1999;**60**:477–84; n=1 Vohra, *Indian J Psychiatry* 2010;**52**:267–9).

Review: * use in BPD (Beri and Boydell, *Ann Clin Psychiatry* 2014;**26**:139–44).

Haloperidol and **trifluoperazine** have been used to reduce anger, hostility and behavioural symptoms, but are now obsolescent, as two studies show haloperidol to be poorly tolerated and no better than placebo (e.g. n=108, RCT, d/b, p/c, 6/52, Soloff *et al*, *Arch Gen Psychiatry* 1993;**150**:377–85).

Olanzapine may be effective for a range of symptoms, e.g. 5–10 mg/d showed a modest advantage over placebo for BPD, with predictable side-effects (eg. n=451 [c=294], RCT, d/b, p/c, Zanarini *et al*, *J Clin Psychiatry* 2011;**72**:1353–62) and if olanzapine helps in the short-term, then continued therapy will build upon that (s=2, n=472, d/b, p/c, Zanarini *et al*, *J Clin Psychopharmacol* 2012;**32**:398–402). A previous trial was negative (n=314, RCT, d/b, p/c, 12/52, Schulz *et al*, *Br J Psychiatry* 2008;**193**:485–92).

Paliperidone was effective and well tolerated for global BPD symptoms (n=18, open, 12/52, Bellino *et al*, *Depress Res Treat* 2011;**2011**:680194).

Quetiapine (range 175–400 mg/d) may be well tolerated and significantly improve impulsivity and other symptoms in severe BPD (n=23, open, 12/52, Villeneuve and Lemelin, *J Clin Psychiatry* 2005;**66**:1298–303). Higher doses may have an effect on hostility, suspiciousness and other rating scales (n=29 [c=23], open, Perrella *et al*, *Prog Neuropsychopharmacol Biol Psychiatry* 2007;**31**:158–63; n=16 [c=9], open, 8/52, Adityanjee *et al*, *Ann Clin Psychiatry* 2008;**20**:219–26). Lower doses, e.g. 150 mg/d may be as effective but better tolerated (n=95[c=64], RCT, d/b, p/c, 8/52, Black *et al*, *Am J Psychiatry* 2014;**171**;1174–82).

Risperidone * (mean 3.3 mg/d) can help adjunctively to TAU to improve BPD symptomatology, especially aggression and overall functioning (n = 15, open, 8/52, Rocca *et al*, *J Clin Psychiatry* 2002;**63**:241–4). RLAI has been used (Carrasco *et al*, *Psychopharmacology (Berl)* 2012;**224**:347–8).

Ziprasidone does not seem to have any significant effects (n = 60, RCT, d/b, p/c, 12/52, Pascual *et al*, *J Clin Psychiatry* 2008;**69**:603–8).

Lamotrigine

Lamotrigine was relatively well tolerated and highly significantly effective for anger in women with BPD (n = 27, RCT, d/b, p/c, 8/52, Tritt *et al*, *J Psychopharmacol* 2005;**9**:287–91).

Topiramate

Topiramate may help to reduce anger in men (n = 42, RCT, d/b, p/c, 8/52, Nickel *et al*, *Biol Psychiatry* 2005;**57**:495–9) and women (n = 29, RCT, d/b, p/c, 8/52, Nickel *et al*, *J Clin Psychiatry* 2004;**65**:1515–9). Up to 200 mg/d has reduced stress and some other symptoms in a relatively limited cohort (n = 56, RCT, d/b, 10/52, Loew *et al*, *J Clin Psychopharmacol* 2006;**26**:61–6).

Valproate

Valproate significantly reduced irritability, anger, impulsiveness and relationship tempestuousness in women with comorbid bipolar II and BPD and was well tolerated (n = 20, RCT, p/c, d/b, 6/12, Frankenburg and Zanarini, *J Clin Psychiatry* 2002;**63**:442–6).

■ Unlicensed/possible efficacy

Carbamazepine

Monotherapy: Carbamazepine may possibly be useful for aggression and episodic dyscontrol. Carbamazepine was suggested as superior to placebo for behaviour control (n = 16, d/b, p/c, c/o, 6/52, Cowdry and Gardner, *Arch Gen Psychiatry* 1988;**45**:111–9), but an RCT failed to show any effects (n = 20, RCT, 30/7, de la Fuente and Lotstra, *Eur Neuropsychopharmacol* 1994;**4**:479–86).

Duloxetine ± TAU

Duloxetine 60 mg/d had a positive effect on somatic and other symptoms in BPD (n = 18 [c = 14], open, 12/52, Bellino *et al*, *J Psychopharmacol* 2010;**24**:333–9).

Lithium ± TAU

Lithium has been reported to be useful for episodic dyscontrol and aggression in BPD, emotionally unstable adolescents and in alcoholics with a BPD, although the consequences of erratic compliance would be a significant disadvantage.

Omega-3 fatty acids + TAU *

O3FAs may improve function and psychotic symptoms in BPD and ultra-high risk for psychosis (n = 15, RCT, d/b, p/c, 12/12, Amminger *et al*, *Can J Psychiatry* 2013;**58**:402–8), and can be used with valproate (Bellino *et al*, *J Psychopharmacol* 2014;**28**:125–32).

Oxcarbazepine

Monotherapy: Oxcarbazepine up to 3 g may have a potential role (n = 17, open, Bellino *et al*, *J Clin Psychiatry* 2005;**66**:1111–5).

□ No efficacy

Amfetamines

Dexamfetamine appears ineffective, albeit with the occasional exception (reviewed by Stein in *Br J Psychiatry* 1992;**161**:167–84).

Benzodiazepines ± TAU

Adjunct: The occasional use of rapidly absorbed short-acting BDZs (e.g. **lorazepam**) may have a limited use in intermittent explosive disorders.

Monotherapy: Benzodiazepines are considered to be inappropriate in BPD due to their potential to disinhibit, induce rage reactions and lead to dependence, e.g. **alprazolam** was significantly worse than placebo for behavioural control (n = 16, d/b, p/c, c/o, 6/52, Cowdry and Gardner, *Arch Gen Psychiatry* 1988;**45**:111–9).

MAOIs

Phenelzine 60 mg/d appears no better than placebo (e.g. n = 108, RCT, d/b, p/c, 5/52, Soloff *et al*, *Arch Gen Psychiatry* 1993;**150**:377–85).

Reboxetine

There is a case of worsening symptoms (n = 1, Anghelescu *et al*, *J Neuropsychiatry Clin Neurosci* 2005;**17**:559–60).

1.12: CATATONIA

see also Psychosis and schizophrenia (*1.21*)

Symptoms

Catatonia is usually a rare and potentially lethal type of schizophrenia or mood disorder, (or even NMS; Vesperini *et al, Encephale* 2010;**36**:105–10) dominated by psychosis, catalepsy, stupor, extreme negativism, resistant rigidity, hyperpyrexia, excitement (purposeless motor activity not influenced by external stimuli), echopraxia, grimacing or posturing. It can be associated with mixed (rather than pure) manic episodes in bipolars, and so may be misdiagnosed and has been linked to ASDs (Takaoka and Takata, *Psychol Rep* 2007;**101**:961–9), or even be an ASD symptom (Dhossche *et al, Int Rev Neurobiol* 2006;**72**:151–64).

Role of drugs

ECT is generally considered the treatment of choice for various forms of catatonia, e.g. organic, lethal and schizophrenic (eg. n=50, Hatta *et al, J ECT* 2007;**23**:233–5). Benzodiazepines (usually high dose) are the first choice drug therapy. A careful history may elicit a drug-symptom association and the potentially offending drug(s) stopped. Antipsychotics are generally unhelpful.

Reviews: * general (Fink, *Acta Psychiatr Scand Suppl* 2013;**441**:1–47), clinical features, diagnosis, management and prognosis (Fink and Taylor, *Arch Gen Psychiatry* 2009;**66**:1173–7), interventions for catatonia in ASD (Dejong *et al, J Autism Dev Disord* 2014;**44**:2127–36).

+ Combinations

Asenapine + clozapine *

Catatonia resistant to ECT and clozapine responded when asenapine was added (n=1, Buoli *et al, Case Rep Psychiatry* 2013;**2013**:503601).

Lorazepam + amisulpride *

A 100% resolution rate over three days has been reported (n=15, Arora *et al, Am J Ther* 2015; in press).

Lorazepam + diazepam *

When used together for catatonia in schizophrenia, 86% responded within 24 hours (n=21, Lin and Huang, *Compr Psychiatry* 2013;**54**:1210–4).

Lorazepam + risperidone

Clonazepam-resistant catatonia has been treated with lorazepam plus risperidone (n=1, Grenier *et al, J Nerv Ment Dis* 2011;**199**:987–8; n=1, Prakash and Bagepally, *Gen Hosp Psychiatry* 2012;**34**:321.e5–6). See also separate drugs/groups.

Olanzapine + amantadine

A dramatic reduction of symptoms has been reported with memantine, a weak NMDA receptor antagonist (n=1, Babington and Spiegel, *Psychosomatics* 2007;**48**:534–6).

Zonisamide + aripiprazole *

This has been effective in ECT and BDZ-resistant periodic catatonia (n=1, Nakagawa *et al, J Neuropsychiatry Clin Neurosci* 2012;**24**:E9).

• Unlicensed/some efficacy

Amantadine See memantine.

Benzodiazepines

Despite many case series and reports, Cochrane concludes that the robust evidence base is lacking (s=0, n=0, RCT, Gibson and Walcott, *Cochrane Database Syst Rev* 2008;**4**:CD006570).

Lorazepam 3–6mg/d can produce complete response in 32% of people and improvement in 69% (n=107, Tibrewal *et al, Prog Neuropsychopharmacol Biol Psychiatry* 2010;**34**:1520–2), over 24 hours (many cases eg. n=2, Huang and Huang, *Chang Gung Med J* 2010;**33**:106–9) and can be given as IM (or diazepam IV if lorazepam fails; n=12, Huang et al, Biomed J 2013;36:35–9) and as an adjunct to ECT (Quinn *et al, J ECT* 2014;**30**:e13–15). Maintenance lorazepam has been effective long-term (eg. n=1, Grover and Aggarwal, *Gen Hosp Psychiatry* 2011;**33**:82.E1–3).

Clonazepam at 2.5mg/d orally or 1mg IV (e.g. n=1, Kumar, *Aust N Z J Psychiatry* 2001;**35**:391) and **midazolam** (n=1, Delise,

Am J Psychiatry 1991;**148**:809) have also been used.

Diazepam IV or lorazepam IM produced 100% resolution within a day in depressed people with catatonic features (n=7, Hung and Huang, *Clin Neuropharmacol* 2006;**29**:144–7) and when induced by haemodialysis (n=1, Tsai and Huang, *Prog Neuropsychopharmacol Biol Psychiatry* 2010;**34**:423–4).

Memantine

Amantadine and **memantine,** weak NMDA receptor antagonists, may have a role in improving symptoms of treatment-resistant catatonia (n=25, Carroll *et al, J Neuropsychiatry Clin Neurosci* 2007;**19**:406–12). There are reports of rapid, significant response of catatonic schizophrenia to memantine 10–20mg/d (e.g. n=1, Obregon *et al, J Psychiatr Pract* 2011;**17**:292–9) and amantadine (e.g. n=1, Muneoka *et al, Pharmacopsychiatry* 2010;**43**:151–2).

Zolpidem

There have been reports of dramatic improvement in catatonia with zolpidem (e.g. Mastain *et al, Rev Neurol* 1995;**151**:52–6), including a dramatic response when due to alcohol withdrawal (n=1, Cottencin *et al, Med Sci Monit* 2009;**15**;CS129–31), to the extent that it has been used as a diagnostic tool for catatonia, e.g. by inducing resolution in people thought to have schizophrenia and allowing interviews to take place (e.g. Thomas *et al, Lancet* 1997;**349**:702).

■ Unlicensed/possible efficacy

Antipsychotics *

Antipsychotics are generally considered unhelpful, but there are some cases of use.

Amisulpride has been effective (n=1, Cottencin *et al, Prim Care Companion J Clin Psychiatry* 2009;**11**:275–6), including multi-resistant chronic catatonia responding to amisulpride 1200mg/d over six months (n=1, Srikanth and Baxter, *Prog Neurol Psychiatry* 2007;**11**:13–6).

Aripiprazole has been used orally (n=1, Kirino, *Clin Schizophr Relat Psychoses* 2010;**4**:185–8; n=3, Vörös and Tényi, *Neuropsychopharmacol Hung* 2010;**12**:373–6) and IM (n=3, Vörös *et al, Pharmacopsychiatry* 2009;**42**:286–7).

Clozapine (n=2, Dursun *et al, J Psychopharmacol* 2005;**19**:432–3; n=1, Sixt *et al, Z Kinder Jugendosychiatr Psychother* 2009;**37**:209–14) has been successful.

Olanzapine has been successful in lethal catatonia (e.g. n=1, Ueda *et al, Psychiatry Clin Neurosci* 2012;**66**:465; n=1, Ueda et *al, Psychiatry Clin Neurosci* 2012;**66**:465), and encephalitis presenting as catatonia (n=1, Suzuki et *al, Rinsho Shinkeigaku* 2010; **50**:329–31).

Quetiapine may have more efficacy than other antipsychotics for catatonic schizophrenia (n=39, retrospective, Yoshimura *et al, Neuropsychiatr Dis Treat* 2013;**9**:1565–71).

Risperidone (n=2, Valevski *et al, Clin Neuropharmacol* 2001;**24**:228–31) has been used, including for periodic catatonia (Duggal and Gandotra, *Can J Psychiatry* 2005;**50**:241–2).

Carbamazepine

Carbamazepine has been used in lorazepam-resistant cases (n=9, Kritzinger and Jordaan, *Int J Neuropsychopharmacol* 2001;**4**:251–7; n=1, Padhy *et al, Prim Care Companion CNS Disord* 2011;**13**:PCC.10l00992).

Valproate

A very short review concluded the valproate was only mildly effective (Bowers and Ajit, *J Neuropsychiatry Clin Neurosci* 2007;**19**:197–8), although a prophylactic effect may occur (n=1, Yoshida *et al, J Clin Psychopharmacol* 2005;**25**:504–5).

■ Case reports

- **Lithium** (n=1, Padhy et *al, Prim Care Companion CNS Disord* 2011;**13**:PCC.10l00992)
- **Methylphenidate** (n=1, Prowler et *al, Psychosomatics* 2010;**51**:74–6)
- **Pregabalin** * (treatment resistant, n=1, Köhler et *al, J Clin Psychopharmacol* 2013;**33**:814–6)
- **Vitamin B12** (n=1, Berry et *al, Acta Psychiatr Scand* 2003;**108**:156–9).

1.13 DEMENTIA including:

1.13.1 Treatment of Alzheimer's disease
1.13.2 BPSD/BPSSD (behavioural and psychological [signs and] symptoms of dementia)
1.13.3 Vascular dementia
1.13.4 Dementia in Parkinson's disease
1.13.5 Prophylaxis and prevention

Symptoms

Dementia is a progressive and irreversible reduction in the level of previously attained intellect, memory and personality or emotional functioning. The main clinical features are:

- disturbed behaviour (disorganised, inappropriate, distracted, restless, antisocial)
- lack of insight
- impaired thinking (slow, impoverished, incoherent, rigid)
- poverty of speech and low mood
- poor cognitive function (forgetfulness, poor attention, disorientation in time and place)
- impaired memory.

Non-pharmacological interventions should include behavioural management, cognitive and multisensory stimulation, environmental design, physical activities, reality orientation and recreational activities.

Alzheimer's disease (AD) is characterised by amyloid beta accumulation and neuro-fibrillary tangles, with reduced levels of acetylcholine and other transmitters in the brain. The degree of dementia is associated more with the extent of neurofibrillary pathology than with the amyloid plaque burden. The symptoms of AD present with an insidious onset and steady deterioration, forgetfulness, lack of spontaneity, disorientation, depressed mood, decline in self-care, poor sleep (waking disorientated and perplexed), and intellectual impairment (dysphasia, dyspraxia, language decline). The incidence of comorbid cerebrovascular disease may be high, and ranges from 22% (n=548, Feldman *et al, Int J Geriatr Psychiatry* 2008;**24**:479–88) to 89% (n=232, Tabet *et al, Int J Clin Pract* 2009;**63**:338–45), depending on the threshold for identification.

Lewy body dementia is a variant of Alzheimer's disease and is more common in men. The key features include early onset, persistent and well-formed visual hallucinations and motor features of Parkinsonism. Patients may be extremely sensitive to antipsychotics and anticholinergics (Gold *et al, Front Neurol Neurosci* 2009;**24**:107–13), which may result in a sudden onset of EPSEs, profound confusion and deterioration, and can lead to premature death.

Vascular dementia is a variant of Alzheimer's disease (see separate section *1.13.3*).

Role of drugs

Currently, there are eight classes of agents for dementia (management and prevention, or delay):

- cholinesterase inhibitors (ChEIs)
- NMDA receptor blockers (e.g. memantine)
- antioxidants (including ginkgo biloba)
- anti-inflammatory agents
- neurotrophic factors (including HRT)
- antiamyloid agents (including cholesterol-lowering drugs)
- Tau protein inhibitors
- mitochondrial dysfunction regulators.

Several systematic reviews and meta-analyses show ChEIs and memantine to have a modest effect on neuropsychiatric and functional outcomes in Alzheimer's, e.g. they are able to stabilise or slow the decline in cognition, function, behaviour, and global change (Tan *et al, J Alzheimers Dis* 2014;**41**:615–31) and show a small but statistically significant effect on size in moderate-to-severe AD in combination (s=13, n=971, Muayqil and Camicioli, *Dement Geriatr Cogn Dis Extra* 2012;**2**:546–72; FFT).

Reviews: * general (Osborn and Saunders, *J Am Osteopath Assoc* 2010;**110**[9 Suppl 8]:S16–26), meta-analysis of anticholinesterases and memantine and severity of AD (Di Santo *et al, J Alzheimer's Dis* 2013;**35**:349–61), pharmacotherapy (Massoud and Léger, *Can J Psychiatry* 2011;**56**:579–88), dementia in Lewy body and Parkinson's (Ballard *et al, Drugs Aging* 2011;**28**:769–77), latest research (Herrmann *et al, Drugs* 2011;**71**:2031–65), phytochemicals for treatment and prevention (Howes and Perry, *Drugs Aging* 2011;**28**:439–68), BAP practice guidelines for anti-dementia drugs (O'Brien *et al, J Psychopharmacol* 2011;**25**:997–1019), pharmacotherapies for sleep disturbances in Alzheimer's disease (s=5, n=313, RCTs, p/c, Cleary *et al, Cochrane Database Syst Rev* 2014;**3**:CD009178).

1.13.1 TREATMENT OF ALZHEIMER'S DISEASE

BNF listed

CHOLINESTERASE INHIBITORS (ChEIs)

There are slight differences between the ChEIs. Donepezil inhibits AChE, rivastigmine inhibits AChE and BuChE, and galantamine both inhibits AChE and enhances ACh's action on nicotinic receptors. Outcomes appear better in males, people treated with NSAIDs and use of higher doses (n=843, open, three years, Wattamo *et al, Alzheimer's Res Ther* 2011;**3**:23). Cochrane concludes that all three are effective and that donepezil may be slightly better tolerated, although careful titration of galantamine and rivastigmine might overcome this (s=13, RCT, d/b, p/c, Birks, *Cochrane Database Syst Rev* 2006;**1**:CD005593).

Review: systematic review and meta-analysis comparing cholinesterase inhibitors (s=26, Hansen *et al, Clin Interv Aging* 2008;**3**:211–25; s=12, Lockhart *et al, Dement Geriatr Cogn Disord* 2009;**8**:389–403).

Donepezil

Donepezil is licensed for the symptomatic treatment of mild or moderate AD. The dose is 5mg/d for the first month, increasing to 10mg/d as tolerated. Efficacy has been shown in numerous studies, e.g. in the early stages (n=153, RCT, d/b, p/c, 24/52, Seltzer *et al, Arch Neurol* 2004;**61**:1852–6), in moderate AD (s=10, Whitehead *et al, Int J Geriatr Psychiatry* 2004;**19**:624–33), in severe AD (e.g. n=343, RCT, d/b, p/c, 24/52, Black *et al, Neurology* 2007;**69**:459–69) and in Lewy body dementia (n=140, RCT, d/b, p/c, 12/52, Mori *et al, Ann Neurol* 2012;**72**:41–52; FFT). Over the longer-term, it may slow progression to AD over the first year (n=769, three years, RCT, p/c, d/b, Petersen *et al, N Engl J Med* 2005;**352**:2379–88) and over two years, although the benefits are lost within six weeks of stopping (n=763, open, two years, Doody *et al, Arch Neurol* 2001;**58**:427–33). CYP2D6 ultra-rapid metabolisers may have lower steady-state plasma levels than normals, and show no improvement, a possible explanation of interindividual variation (n=42, Varsaldi *et al, Eur J Clin Pharmacol* 2006;**62**:721–6). Cochrane concludes that donepezil produces modest improvements in cognitive function, ADL, and behaviour over one year (s=23, n=5272, Birks *et al, Cochrane Database Syst Rev* 2006;**1**:CD001190).

Reviews: * general (Doody *et al, Curr Alzheimer Res* 2012;**9**:773–81), 10-year review (Cheewakriengkrai and Gauthier, *Expert Opin Pharmacother* 2013;**14**:331–8), different doses including 23mg/d (Tariot *et al, BMC Res Notes* 2012;**5**:283), kinetics and pharmacodynamics (Prvulovic and Schneider, *Expert Opin Drug Metab Toxicol* 2014;**10**:1039–50).

Galantamine *

Galantamine is a reversible competitive acetylcholinesterase inhibitor, but also stimulates pre- and post-synaptic nicotinic receptors and is indicated for mild-to-moderate AD. The optimum dose is 16mg/d for mild and 24mg/d for moderate AD (n=835, RCT, d/b, p/c, 5/12, Aronson *et al, Drugs Aging* 2009;**26**:231–9), and severe AD (n=407 [c=329], RCT, d/b, p/c, Burns *et al, Lancet Neurol* 2009;**8**:39–47). The effect is sustained, with significantly reduced mortality and decline in cognition and daily living activities compared to placebo over 2 years (n=2045[c=661], RCT, d/b, p/c, 24/12, Hager *et al, Neuropsychiatr Dis Treat* 2014;**10**:391–401). In co-morbid AD and cerebrovascular disease, galantamine showed improved cognitive function (n=285 [c=212], RCT, d/b, p/c, 6/12, Erkinjuntti *et al, J Psychopharmacol* 2008;**22**:761–8). Cochrane concludes that galantamine is effective at doses of 16–32mg/d, with a consistent effect at 3–6 months (s=10, n=6805, Loy and Schneider, *Cochrane Database Syst Rev* 2006;**1**:CD001747).

Review: general (Prvulovic *et al, Expert Opin Drug Metab Toxicol* 2010;**6**:345–54).

Rivastigmine *

Rivastigmine is licensed for the treatment of mild to moderately severe AD and for mild-to-moderate dementia in Parkinson's disease (see *1.13.4*). Efficacy has been shown in advanced moderate AD (e.g. n=44, RCT, p/c, 12/12, Karaman *et al, Dement Geriatr Cogn Disord* 2005;**19**:51–6), rapidly progressing AD (s=4, n=517, 26/52, Farlow *et al, Dement*

Geriatr Cogn Disord 2005;**20**:192–7) and in Lewy body dementia (n=49, RCT, d/b, Touchon *et al*, *Curr Med Res Opin* 2006;**22**:49–59) and in advanced dementia (Farlow *et al*, *Int J Geriatr Psychiatry* 2011;**26**:1236–43). Patches allow higher doses to be used with the same tolerability (Frampton, *Drugs Aging* 2014;**31**:639–49) and an observational study concluded that rivastigmine patches improve adherence, so presumably they work better if you stick to them (n=1104[c=928], 6/12, Adler *et al*, *Int J Clin Pract* 2014;**68**:465–70). And, vice versa. The manufacturer's advice about the application of patches must be followed carefully, e.g. site rotation, as 3.7% discontinue due to skin reactions (n=1195, RCT, p/c, 24/52, Cummings *et al*, *Clin Drug Invest* 2010;**30**:41–9). Cochrane concludes that rivastigmine is beneficial at 6–12mg/d in mild-to-moderate AD, with improvements in ADL and reduced rate of decline (s=13, RCT, d/b, >12/52, Birks and Grimley Evans, *Cochrane Database Syst Rev* 2015;**4**:CD001191).

Review: patches (Dhillon, *Drugs* 2011;**71**:1209–31).

NON-CHOLINESTERASE INHIBITORS

Memantine *

Memantine (an NMDA antagonist) is licensed in the UK and in some European countries for moderate-to-severe dementia (not just mild-to-moderately severe), a unique indication. It acts as a voltage-dependent, non-competitive NMDA-antagonist, blocking the effect of excess glutamate release, thought to be responsible for many symptoms and for disease progression. The dose is 5mg/d, adding 5mg/d each week, increased if needed up to the licensed maintenance dose of 20mg/d once a day. Efficacy has been shown in mild-to-moderate AD (n=470, RCT, d/b, p/c, 6/12, Bakchine and Loft, *J Alzheimer's Dis* 2007;**11**:471–9), for reducing deterioration in moderate-to-severe AD (n=2340, RCT, d/b, p/c, 16-28/52, Wilkinson *et al*, *Dement Geriatr Cogn Disord* 2013;**37**:71–85), and for global clinical and behavioural symptoms in Lewy body dementia (eg. n=199[c=159], RCT, d/b, p/c, 24/52, Emre *et al*, *Lancet Neurol* 2010;**9**:969–77) with a possible DLB disease-modifying effect (n=75[c=42], RCT, d/b, p/c, three years, Stubendorff *et al*, *Br Med J Open* 2014;**4**:e005158). Evidence is currently lacking for memantine in mild AD (s=3, n=1128, RCT, p/c, Schneider *et al*, *Arch Neurol* 2011;**68**:991–8) and dementia in Down's syndrome (n=173[c=148], RCT, d/b, p/c, 52/52, Hanney *et al*, *Lancet* 2012;**379**:528–36). Memantine may significantly delay clinical worsening of AD compared to placebo (s=9, n=2506, Hellweg *et al*, *Int J Geriatr Psychiatry* 2012;**27**:651–6), reducing the need for psychotropic drug use and nursing home burden (n=31 [c=24], open, 3/12, Herrmann *et al*, *CNS Drugs* 2011;**25**:425–33). A systematic review and meta-analysis concludes that memantine does not help cognition and motor function in LBD although it may be superior to placebo for the overall impression (Matsunga *et al*, *Am J Geriatr Psychiatry* 2014;**23**;373–83).

Reviews: * general (Herrmann and Lanctôt, *Expert Opin Pharmacother* 2011;**12**:787–800), safety (Yang *et al*, *J Alzheimer's Dis* 2013;**36**:445–58), long-term tolerability (n=702, up to nine years, Kitamura *et al*, *Nihon Ronen Igakkai Zasshi* 2014;**51**:74–84).

+ Combinations

Ginkgo biloba (GB) + ChEIs *

In people taking ChEIs, also taking GB showed a non-significant cognitive benefit (n=828, 12/12, Canevelli *et al*, *Phytomedicine* 2014;**21**:88–92).

Memantine + ChEIs

One meta-analysis and systematic review concluded that there is no benefit from the combination (s=3, n=1317, RCTs, 6/12, Farrimond *et al*, *Br Med J Open* 2012;**2**:e000917), but another (13 studies in all) suggested statistically significant improvements in moderate-to-severe AD, although the studies were heterogeneous (s=3, n=971, RCTs, Muayqil and Camicioli, *Dement Geriatr Cogn Dis Extra* 2012;**2**:546–72).

Rivastigmine + memantine may improve memory and executive function in mild-to-moderate AD and has a sustained effect on slowing cognitive and functional decline compared to an anticholinesterase or no treatment (n=382, 30/12, Atri *et al, Alzheimer Dis Assoc Disord* 2008;**22**:209–21). Rivastigmine patches can improve tolerability of the combination (n=117, open, 26/52, Olin *et al, Int J Geriatr Psychiatry* 2010;**25**:419–26), but probably only in specific cases (n=172[c=147], RCT, open, 24/52, Choi *et al, Curr Med Res Opin* 2011;**27**:1375–83).

Donepezil + memantine may be no better than either alone (n=295, 52/52, Howard *et al, N Engl J Med* 2012;**366**:893–903), although a post-hoc analysis suggested that adding memantine to donepezil significantly improved outcomes and reduced deterioration (s=2, n=510, RCT, d/b, p/c, 24/52, Atri *et al, Alzheimer's Res Ther* 2013;**5**:6).

Reviews: * general (Parsons *et al, Neurotox Res* 2013;**24**:358–69; Tan *et al, J Alzheimers Dis* 2014;**41**:615–31).

• Unlicensed/some efficacy

Cilostazol + donepezil *

Adjunct: Adjunctive cilostazol to donepezil reduced cognitive decline in mild (but not moderate/severe) dementia (n=70, 30/12, Ihara *et al, PLoS One* 2014;**9**:e89516).

Ginkgo biloba (GB)

The role of GB is still unclear. On the positive side, Ginkgo biloba extract (EGb 761®) was associated with a statistically significant improvement in cognitive symptoms (n=410, RCT, d/b, p/c, 24/52, Herrschraft *et al, J Psychiatr Res* 2012;**46**:716–23; although this data has been published three times, e.g. see also Bachinskaya *et al, Neuropsychiatr Dis Treat* 2011;**7**:209–15; Ihl *et al, Int J Geriatr Psychiatry* 2013;**26**:1186–94) and was equivalent to donepezil and superior to placebo on MMSE (e.g. n=96, RCT, d/b, 22/52, Yancheva *et al, Aging Ment Health* 2009;**13**:183–90). A systematic review concluded that GB is superior to placebo for improving cognitive function in dementia, although the differences were inconsistent (s=9, n=2372, 12–52/52, Weinmann *et al, BMC Geriatr* 2010;**10**:14). However, GB 120mg/d had no detectable effect on mild-to-moderate dementia (n=176, RCT, d/b, p/c, 6/12, McCarney *et al, Int J Geriatr Psychiatry* 2008;**23**:1222–30), and Cochrane concludes that there is no convincing evidence for its efficacy on cognition in dementia or in healthy adults (s=9, RCT, d/b, p/c, Geng *et al, Cochrane Database Syst Rev* 2010;**12**:CD007769).

Masitinib + TAU

Adjunct: Adjunctive masitinib (a mast cell stabiliser) to ChEIs/memantine slowed cognitive decline (n=34, RCT, p/c, 24/52, Piette *et al, Alzheimers Res Ther* 2011;**3**:16).

Nimodipine + galantamine *

Adjunct: Nimodipine did not add to galantamine's effect (n=21, RCT, d/b, p/c, 24/52, Caramelli *et al, Arq Neuropsiquiatr* 2014;**72**:411–7).

Sibutramine + TAU

Adjunct: Adjunctive sibutramine to donepezil had some efficacy in improving cognitive functioning in early and moderate AD (RCT, p/c, 3/12, Ollat *et al, Encephale* 2007;**33**:211–5).

SSRIs (see also sertraline in 'no efficacy') *

Some studies have shown a potential effect, e.g. **escitalopram** may be as effective as risperidone for BPSD (n=40, RCT, d/b, 6/52, Barak *et al, Int Psychogeriatr* 2013; **25**:1433-6), and **citalopram** was superior to placebo (n=85, RCT, d/b, 17/7, Pollock *et al, Am J Psychiatry* 2002;**159**:460–5).

Vitamin D + memantine *

Adjunct: In newly-diagnosed AD, adjunctive vitamin D statistically and clinically improved cognition cf memantine alone (n=43, open, 6/12, Annweiler *et al, Cogn Behav Neurol* 2012;**25**:121–7).

■ Unlicensed/possible efficacy

Antipsychotics *

A systematic review and meta-analysis concluded **aripiprazole** and **risperidone** can improve psychiatric symptoms and slow cognitive decline over 12/52 but with a high side effect burden (s=23, n=5819, RCTs, 12/52, Tan *et al, Alzheimer's Res Ther* 2015;**7**:20; FFT).

Doxycycline and rifampicin

Significantly reduced decline has been shown with doxycycline 200mg/d and rifampicin

300 mg/d for three months, which was well tolerated (n=101, RCT, t/b, p/c, 12/12, Loeb *et al*, *J Am Geriatr Soc* 2004;**52**:381–7).

Folic acid + TAU

Cochrane concludes that there is no consistent evidence either way for the use of folic acid (with or without B12) to treat or prevent AD (s=8, RCT, Malouf *et al*, *Cochrane Database Syst Rev* 2008;**4**:CD004514).

Ginseng

Cochrane concludes that the studies are only in healthy volunteers, so no conclusion is possible (s=5, RCT, d/b, p/c, Geng *et al*, *Cochrane Database Syst Rev* 2010;**12**:CD007769).

Insulin

Elevating insulin levels improves memory in people with AD (n=23+14 controls, Craft *et al*, *Arch Gen Psychiatry* 1999;**56**:1135–40).

Levodopa

Levodopa has produced 36% 'responders' for motor symptoms in DLB (n=14[c=10], Molloy *et al*, *J Neurol Neurosurg Psychiatry* 2005;**76**:1200–3).

Melatonin *

Poor sleep quality has been linked with Alzheimer's and melatonin shows significantly improved cognitive performance cf. placebo, the effect increasing with a longer treatment duration (n=80, RCT, d/b, p/c, 28/52, Wade *et al*, *Clin Interv Aging* 2014;**9**:947–61), and it can improve MCI and significantly reduce the need for benzodiazepines to manage behaviour (n=96, open, 15-60/12, Cardinali *et al*, *Am J Neurodegener Dis* 2012;**1**:280–91). Melatonin may not help cognitive or non-cognitive symptoms (s=3, Jansen *et al*, *Cochrane Database Syst Rev* 2006;**1**:CD003802).

Methylphenidate *

Methylphenidate 10–20 mg/d has been shown to be helpful for chronic apathy in dementia (eg. n=60, RCT, d/b, p/c, 6/52, Rosenberg *et al*, *J Clin Psychiatry* 2013;**74**:810–6).

Naftidrofuryl

Cochrane concludes that there is some low-level evidence that the cerebral vasodilator naftidrofuryl may have some positive effects on behaviour, cognition and mood (s=9, n=847, RCT, p/c, Lu *et al*, *Cochrane Database Syst Rev* 2011;**12**:CD002955).

Nutritional supplements *

There can be a significant positive effect on weight, BMI and cognition (s=12, n=1824, Allen *et al*, *Clin Nutr* 2013;**32**:950–7).

Omega-3 fatty acids *

Reduced levels of DHAs have been linked with dementia and so supplements may have some efficacy if started early (Cole *et al*, *Prostaglandins Leukot Essent Fatty Acids* 2009;**81**:213–21) and may help cognitive function in very mild AD (n=204[c=174], RCT, d/b, p/c, Freund-Levi *et al*, *Arch Neurol* 2006;**63**:1402–8; Calon, *Curr Alzheimer Res* 2011;**8**:470–8). Combined use with alpha lipoic acid has slowed cognitive and functional decline cf either or placebo (n=39[n=34], RCT, p/c, 12/12, Shinto *et al*, *J Alzheimers Dis* 2014;**38**:111–20).

Opioids *

Cochrane could find no firm evidence of efficacy for agitation in dementia (s=0, n=0, RCT, p/c, Brown *et al*, *Cochrane Database Syst Rev* 2015;**5**:CD009705).

Raloxifene

Raloxifene 60 mg/d significantly improves verbal memory in postmenopausal women over 69 years of age (n=213, RCT, d/b, p/c, 12/12, Jacobsen *et al*, *Menopause* 2010;**17**:309–14).

Testosterone

Men with AD receiving weekly testosterone enanthante 100 mg performed significantly better in spatial and memory tests, but with no change in aggression or unwanted behaviour (n=32, RCT, p/c, 6/52, Cherrier *et al*, *Neurology* 2005;**64**:2063–8).

Trazodone *

Trazodone 50 mg at night can cause no significant daytime sleepiness or naps, or effects on cognition or functionality in people with sleep problems in probable AD (n=30,

RCT, d/b, p/c, 3/52, Camargos *et al*, *Am J Geriatr Psychiatry* 2014;**22**:1565–74).

Valproate

Any improvement with valproate is associated with lower serum levels (40–60mcg/mL) and doses (7–12mg/kg/d) rather than higher doses, although the effect is modest anyway (s=20, Dolder *et al*, *J Pharm Pract* 2012;**25**:142–50) and it may double brain loss in mild-to-moderate AD (n=89, 12/12, Fleisher *et al*, *Neurology* 2011;**77**:1263–71).

Vinpocetine

Vinpocetine is well tolerated, but has only a minor effect (s=3, n=583, p/c, Szatmari and Whitehouse, *Cochrane Database Syst Rev* 2003;**1**:CD003119).

Vitamin E (alpha tocopherol) *

Vitamin E 2000iu/d slowed the progression of AD by 19% a year cf. placebo and decreased caregiver burden cf placebo and memantine (n=613[c=361], RCT, d/b, p/c, mean two years, Dysken *et al*, *JAMA* 2014;**311**:33–44), which means that Cochrane will need updating (s=3, RCTs, d/b, Farina *et al*, *Cochrane Database Syst Rev* 2012;**11**:CD002854).

✱ Case report

- **Lamotrigine** 100mg/d (n=1, 6/12, Devarajan *et al*, *Am J Psychiatry* 2000;**157**:1178).

☐ No efficacy

Cannabinoids

Cochrane concludes that there is no evidence that cannabinoids are effective for AD (s=1, Krishnan *et al*, *Cochrane Database Syst Rev* 2009;**2**:CD007204), so there goes my excuse.

Cycloserine (D-cycloserine)

Cycloserine (a partial agonist at NMDA receptors) may enhance implicit memory in Alzheimer's, but has no place in treatment (s=4, RCTs, d/b, Laake and Oeksengaard, *Cochrane Database Syst Rev* 2002;**2**:CD003153).

Nicotine

There is no reliable evidence for a beneficial effect (s=1, López-Arrieta *et al*, *Cochrane Database Syst Rev* 2001;**2**:CD001749).

NSAIDs (see also prevention, *1.13.5*)

Cochrane concludes an unproven efficacy of aspirin, steroidal and NSAIDs for AD (s=14, n=2235, RCTs, Jaturapatporn *et al*, *Cochrane Database Syst Rev* 2012;**2**:CD006378).

Pioglitazone

Pioglitazone is well tolerated but ineffective (n=29[c=25], RCT, d/b, p/c, 18/52, Geldmacher *et al*, *Arch Neurol* 2011;**68**:45–50).

Piracetam

Cochrane concludes that the evidence for this weak ACh release stimulator is too weak to prove an effect (Flicker and Grimley Evans, *Cochrane Database Syst Rev* 2001;**2**:CD001011).

Prednisone

Prednisone 10–20mg/d is ineffective (n=138, RCT, 56/52, Aisen *et al*, *Neurology* 2000;**54**:588–93).

Procaine

Procaine is probably detrimental (s=2, n=415, Szatmári and Bereczki, *Cochrane Database Syst Rev* 2008;**4**:CD005993).

Selegiline

Cochrane concludes that the evidence is poor, with no justification for use (s=17, RCTs, d/b, Birks and Flicker, *Cochrane Database Syst Rev* 2003;**1**:CD000442).

Sertraline *

Sertraline is ineffective for depression in AD, (HTA-SADD, n=326, RCT, p/c, Banerjee *et al*, *Health Technol Assess* 2013;**17**:1–166).

Statins *

Statins have no efficacy for treating Alzheimer's or vascular dementia (s=4, n=1154, RCT, d/b, >6/12, McGuinness *et al*, *Cochrane Database Syst Rev* 2014;**7**:CD007514).

Varenicline *

Varenicline is ineffective (n=66, RCT, d/b, p/c, c/o, 12/52, Kim *et al*, *Dement Geriatr Cogn*

Disord 2013;**37**:232–45).

Vitamins (see also Vitamin E)

Cochrane concludes that there is no evidence for pyridoxine 5mg, folic acid 1mg and iron (n=89, RCT, d/b, p/c, 26/52, Sun *et al, Clin Ther* 2007;**29**:2204–14).

1.13.2 BPSD/BPSSD (behavioural and psychological [signs and] symptoms of dementia)

BPSD has a cluster of cognitive and non-cognitive symptoms and occurs in up to 90% of people with dementia. BPSD is likely to be an imbalance in a range of transmitters rather than one neuro-transmitter abnormality. Symptoms include aggression, agitation, anxiety, wandering, hoarding, sexual disinhibition, apathy and disruptive vocal activity.

Role of drugs *

Symptoms of BPSD should be monitored for at least a month before treatment is considered, and non-drug approaches (e.g. environment, multisensory stimulation) used first. Anti-cholinesterases and memantine have modest efficacy and antidepressants may help depression (but more data is needed on agitation and aggression) but use of valproate is not supported by current data. Antipsychotics may be helpful for severe BPSD symptoms but use low doses, ensure adequate hydration and mobility, time limit and document fully.

Reviews: * general (Corbett *et al, Curr Treat Options Neurol* 2012;**14**:113–25), genetics (Borroni *et al, Curr Alzheimer Res* 2010;**7**:158–64), review of pharmacological treatments (s=29, Seitz *et al, Int Psychogeriatr* 2013;**25**:185–203).

BNF listed

Cholinesterase inhibitors *

Cholinesterase inhibitors may help BPSD by slowing disease progression in AD. A systematic review of all three in BPSD concluded the evidence was limited but they were certainly an option (s=14, median 24/52, Rodda *et al, Int Psychogeriatr* 2009;**21**:813–24).

Donepezil: a systematic review and meta-analysis indicated that it is effective for BPSD (s=4, RCTs, p/c, Lockhart *et al, Dement Geriatr Cogn Dis Extra* 2011;**1**:212–27;MS).

Galantamine: a pooled analysis suggested it might improve behavioural symptoms (s=3, n=2033, RCT, d/b, p/c, 3–6/12, Herrmann *et al, Am J Geriatr Psychiatry* 2005;**13**:527–34), but not as well as risperidone (n=100, RCT, 12/52, Freund-Levi *et al, Dement Geriatr Cogn Disord* 2014;**38**:234–44).

Rivastigmine: a meta-analysis showed 6–12 mg/d to be well tolerated and effective for BPSD (s=3, p/c, 6/12, Finkel *et al, Clin Ther* 2004;**26**:980–90).

Memantine *

A systematic review and meta-analysis suggested that memantine decreases NPI scores and may have a role in managing BPSD, although the effect size is relatively small (s=5, n=1750, RCT, d/b, p/c, Maidment *et al, Ann Pharmacother* 2008;**42**:32–8). In moderate-to-severe AD, a pooled analysis showed memantine to have a significant effect on neuropsychiatric symptoms and disease progression (s=3, RCT, p/c, 6/12, Wilcock *et al, J Clin Psychiatry* 2008;**69**:341–8), but did not improve agitation in moderate-to-severe AD (n=153, RCT, d/b, p/c, 12/52, Fox *et al, PloS One* 2012;**7**:e35185). It may help to reduce the need for antipsychotics (n=38, Suzuki *et al, Ther Adv Psychopharmacol* 2013;**3**:123–8).

Risperidone (see also antipsychotics)

Risperidone is licensed for the short-term treatment (up to 6/52) of persistent aggression in people with moderate-to-severe AD unresponsive to non-pharmacological approaches and when there is a risk of harm to self or others. A starting dose of 0.25mg BD is recommended, increased to an optimum of 0.5mg BD for most patients, although up to 1mg BD can be used. A mean dose of 1.5mg/d has been shown to be effective and well tolerated for BPSD, including sleep disturbances (n=338[c=321], open, 12/52, Durán *et al, Int Psychogeriatr* 2005;**17**:591–604), aggression, agitation and psychosis (n=337, RCT, p/c, 12/52, Brodaty *et al, J Clin Psychiatry* 2003;**64**:134–43). Additional care is needed in Lewy body dementia as, although psychotic and behavioural symptoms may respond well to low doses, severe EPSEs (especially rigidity) have occurred at 1 mg/d. Risperidone appears as effective as olanzapine (n=39, d/b, 14/7, Fontaine *et al*, *J Clin Psychiatry* 2003;**64**:726–30) and quetiapine (n=72[c=69], RCT, s/b, 8/52, Rainer *et al*, *Eur Psychiatry* 2007;**22**:395–403). Adequate hydration and movement is essential in the first four weeks of treatment.

+ Combinations

Memantine + donepezil

Adjunctive memantine may significantly improve BPSD in moderate-to-severe AD (n=404[c=322], RCT, d/b, p/c, Tariot *et al*, *JAMA* 2004:**291**:317–24) and significantly lower NPI scores by reducing agitation-related stress (d/b, p/c, 24/52, Cummings *et al*, *Neurology* 2006;**67**:57–63).

Dextromethorphan + quinidine *

A preliminary study showed a quinidine-dextromethorphan combination significantly reduced agitation and was generally well tolerated (n=220[c=194], RCT, d/b, p/c, 10/52, Cummings *et al*, *JAMA* 2015;**314**:1242–54).

■ Unlicensed/probable efficacy

Antipsychotics (see also risperidone) *

Cochrane concludes that antipsychotics can be withdrawn from people with BPSD without detrimental effects on behaviour, although two studies in people whose agitation or psychosis had previously responded well had more or quicker relapses so might not be candidates for discontinuation (s=9, n=606, RCTs, Declerq *et al*, *Cochrane Database Syst Rev* 2013: **3**:CD007726).

Aripiprazole 10 mg/d may be safe and effective for psychosis associated with AD, improving agitation and CGI (n=487, RCT, d/b, p/c, 10/52, Mintzer *et al*, *Am J Geriatr Psychiatry* 2007;**15**:918–31), but a mean 9 mg/d was ineffective in another trial (n=256, RCT, d/b, p/c, 10/52, Streim *et al*, *Am J Geriatr Psychiatry* 2008;**16**:537–50).

Haloperidol's SmPC now states that elderly people with dementia-related psychosis treated with antipsychotics are at a 1.6–1.7 times higher increased risk of death, most appearing to be either cardiovascular (e.g. heart failure, sudden death) or infections (e.g. pneumonia). If low dose haloperidol is effective for BPSD over 20/52, the effect is maintained over the next 24 weeks (n=44, RCT, d/b, p/c, 24/52, Devanand *et al*, *Int J Geriatr Psychiatry* 2011;**26**:937–43).

Olanzapine at low dose, e.g. 5–10 mg/d (but not 15 mg/d) may be superior to placebo in treating BPSD and psychosis (n=206, RCT, d/b, p/c, 6/52, Street *et al*, *Arch Gen Psychiatry* 2000;**57**:968–76), with 2.5 mg/d seems reasonable starting dose (n=652, RCT, 10/52, d/b, p/c, De Deyn *et al*, *Int J Geriatr Psychiatry* 2004;**19**:115–26).

Quetiapine is not approved for dementia-related psychosis due to a three-fold increased risk of CVA seen in RCTs with some SGAs. However, 25–150 mg/d has become a standard therapy for BPSD in dementia, e.g. quetiapine (50–400 mg/d) was as effective as risperidone (0.5–2 mg/d) for BPSD, with no cognitive impairment (n=72[c=69], RCT, s/b, 8/52, Rainer *et al*, *Eur Psychiatry* 2007;**22**:395–403), and 200 mg/d was superior to placebo, but 100 mg/d was not (n=333[c=63–65%], RCT, d/b, p/c, 10/52, Zhong *et al*, *Curr Alzheimer Res* 2007;**4**:81–93). It has, however, been associated with significant cognitive decline (e.g. n=40[c=27], RCT, d/b, p/c, 6/52, Paleacu *et al*, *Int J Geriatr Psychiatry* 2008;**23**:393–400).

Risperidone — see BNF Listed.

Ziprasidone IM may be useful for the short-term management of BPSD (n=14, open, 24/24, Rais *et al*, *Psychiatry (Edgmont)* 2010;**7**:17–24).

Cyproterone

Cyproterone 100 mg/d has shown significantly better efficacy and safety than haloperidol 2 mg/d in controlling mild aggression associated with AD (n=27, RCT, d/b, 3/12, Huertas *et al*, *J Clin Psychiatry* 2007;**68**:439–44; n=1, Bolea-Alamanac *et al*, *J Psychopharmacol* 2011; **25**:141–5).

Prazosin

Prazosin (mean 6 mg/d) was well tolerated and significantly useful for reducing BPSD (n=22, RCT, d/b, p/c, 8/52, Wang *et al*, *Am J Geriatr Psychiatry* 2009;**17**:744–51).

Table 1.13.1: The use of antipsychotics in elderly people with dementia *

Antipsychotics are widely used for symptomatic management of BPSD and can relieve psychotic symptoms. They must not be used as substitutes for poor care, and be monitored and reviewed regularly. Risperidone and olanzapine should not routinely be used for BPSD, as the risk of death (s=17, mean, 10/52, UK SmPC) is 1.6–1.7 times higher than with placebo (4.5% vs 2.6%), mostly CV (e.g. heart failure, sudden death) or infections (e.g. pneumonia).

Antipsychotic use in elderly people with BPSD *

Evidence for safety is limited:

- A prospective nursing home study did not show any increased mortality with antipsychotics (n=273, 12/12, Suh *et al, Int Psychogeriatr* 2005;**17**:429–41).
- A Medicaid analysis was unable to show that SGAs (including risperidone) were more likely to cause CVEs than haloperidol or benzodiazepines (n=8 million, Finkel *et al, Int Psychogeriatr* 2005;**17**;617–29).

The main risks are: *

- **Femur fracture**: increased risk (OR=1.3, n=7393, Liperoti *et al, J Clin Psychiatry* 2007;**68**:929–34).
- **Pneumonia**: 60% increased risk (n=22944, Knol *et al, J Am Geriatr Soc* 2008;**56**:661–6).
- **Decline and cerebrovascular events**:
  - → Carrying on with antipsychotics had a survival probability of 70% compared to 77% in a switch-to-placebo group at one-year, 46% vs 71% at two years, and 30% vs 59% at three years (n=128, RCT, p/c, Ballard *et al, Lancet Neurol* 2009;**8**:151–7)
  - → An increased risk of death at 30 days compared to non-users (n=27,259 pairs, Gill *et al, Ann Intern Med* 2007;**146**:775–86), but see below for interpretation of this
  - → All psychotropics are linked with more rapid cognitive and functional decline and not with improved BPSD, although it could be that they are prescribed to people with more risk of problems (n=230, mean 3.7 years, Rosenberg *et al, Int J Geriatr Psychiatry* 2012;**27**: 1248–57;FFT).
- **Increased risk of stroke**:
  - → The risk of stroke in people >65 years old prescribed antipsychotics (n=4223) is higher with SGAs (47 per 1000 pt years), butyrophenones (47), phenothiazines (72) and benzamides (25) than without (12; n=69939), but the risk was higher with FGAs than the SGAs (Sacchetti *et al, J Psychopharmacol* 2008;**22**:39–46).

The important case in the middle:

- Four large cohort studies show that the risk of CVAEs is higher in the first four weeks (OR 9.9) but falls to baseline after one month, and that chronic use is not associated with CVAEs (n=26157, Kleijer *et al, J Psychopharmacol* 2009;**23**:909–14; n=134,448, Sacchetti *et al, J Psychopharmacol* 2010;**24**:1131–32; n=37138, 10 years, Pariente *et al, Arch Intern Med* 2012;**172**:648–53).
- **The increased mortality occurs with higher doses**, e.g. haloperidol >1 mg/d, olanzapine >2.5 mg and risperidone >1 mg/d but not with quetiapine at any dose (n=18127, five years, Rossom *et al, J Am Geriatr Soc* 2010;**58**:1027–34). This may be due to dehydration and poor mobilisation.
- **The risk is highest in the first four week.**

Conclusion:

1. Use antipsychotics only as a last line of management:

- Nursing staff trained and supported to deliver enhanced psychosocial care can reduce antipsychotic use in nursing homes without an increase in agitation (n=349, RCT, s/b, 12/12, Fossey *et al, Br Med J* 2006;**332**:756–61; comment by Byrne, *EBMH* 2006; **9**:103).

- ADRs from the SGAs may be the limiting factor and the modest benefits may be outweighed by the risks (n=421, RCT, d/b, p/c, Schneider *et al, N Engl J Med* 2006;**355**: 1525–38).
- Although antipsychotics cause harm and the evidence is against them, use may be justified in a palliative care model, reducing stress to the person and relatives where life expectancy is short (Treloar *et al, Br J Psychiatry* 2010;**197**:88–90).
- Cochrane concludes that risperidone and olanzapine reduce aggression in dementia, but due to risk of severe CVA and EPSE they should not be used routinely unless there is marked distress (s=16, RCT, p/c, Ballard and Waite, *Cochrane Database Syst Rev* 2006; **1**:CD003476).

2. Ensure good fluid intake and mobility in the first four weeks:

- The main risk seems to be in the first four weeks (see 'The important case in the middle') and this may be due to dehydration and poor mobilisation (Ballard and Corbett, *CNS Drugs* 2010;**24**:729–39), rather than a platelet effect. So, ensuring adequate hydration and movement in the first month is **essential**.

3. Keep doses low and avoid haloperidol

- **Increased mortality occurs with higher doses,** e.g. haloperidol > 1 mg/d, olanzapine > 2.5 mg and risperidone > 1 mg/d, but not with quetiapine (n=18127, 5 years, Rossom *et al, J Am Geriatr Soc* 2010;**58**:1027–34; see also n=136393, 180/7, Gerhard *et al, Br J Psychiatry* 2014;**205**:44–51).
- The risk of mortality at 180 days (where RR=relative risk to risperidone) was highest with **haloperidol** (RR=1.5), **risperidone** (RR=1), **olanzapine** (RR=0.99), **valproate** (RR=0.91) and **quetiapine** (RR=0.73). The risk with haloperidol was highest in first 30 days, but decreased significantly and sharply after that (n=33604, 180/7, Kales *et al, Am J Psychiatry* 2012;**169**:71–9;FFT).
- In older people in nursing homes, the risk of mortality was highest with **haloperidol** (HR=2.07 cf. risperidone), none with **aripiprazole**, **olanzapine** and **ziprasidone**, and **quetiapine** had a decreased risk (HR 0.81) over the first 6/12, the effects strongest in the first 40/7, were dose-related (except for quetiapine), the same for any recorded diagnosis and seen for all causes in death, with no clinically meaningful differences (n=75445, 6/12, Huybrechts *et al, Br Med J* 2012;**344**:e977;FFT).

4. Discontinue where possible:

- **Most people with BPSD can have any antipsychotics withdrawn** except perhaps where agitation or psychosis had responded well, where relapse was quicker and more frequent (s=9, n=606, RCTs, p/c, Declercq *et al, Cochrane Database Syst Rev* 2013;**3**:CD007726; s=9, n=580, RCTs, Pan *et al, Dement Geriatr Cogn Disord* 2013;**37**:125–40).

5. Avoid absolutely in possible Lewy body dementia:

- Although psychotic and behavioural symptoms may respond well to low doses, severe EPSEs (especially rigidity) can occur at low doses, resulting in rapid deterioration and death unless discontinued quickly.

6. Review treatment effects regularly:

- Carry out a pre-treatment assessment, and repeat every 3–6 months to detect common ADRs such as postural hypotension, anticholinergic effects and EPSE.
- Single daily doses are usually appropriate once stable.
- Review doses regularly, and institute a periodic reduction in dose (e.g. by 10–25% every four weeks), and if no recurrence then continue the reduction every four weeks.

Topiramate

Topiramate 25–50mg/d may be as effective as risperidone 0.5–2mg/d for BPSD (n=48[n=41], RCT, d/b, 8/52, Mowla and Pani, *J Clin Psychopharmacol* 2010;**30**:40–3).

Yokukansan

Yokukansan, a traditional Japanese medicine, appears effective and well tolerated (eg. n=61, RCT, open, 4/52, Okahara *et al*, *Prog Neuropsychopharmacol Biol Psychiatry* 2010; **34**:532–6).

■ Unlicensed/possible efficacy

Analgesia

In moderate-to-severe dementia and BPSD, use of the analgesics paracetamol, morphine, buprenorphine patches or pregabalin all reduced agitation and improved behaviour (n=352, RCT, 8–12/52, Husebo *et al*, *Br Med J* 2011;**343**:d4065).

Antidepressants

Antidepressants may have some efficacy for comorbid depression. Cochrane concludes that SSRIs, mirtazapine and trazodone are relatively well tolerated (s=9, n76=692, Seitz *et al*, *Cochrane Database Syst Rev* 2011; **2**:CD008191) and can help with modest reductions of agitation in AD without significant ADRs or cognitive deterioration.

Aromatherapy

Melissa, an essential balm oil, has reduced agitation in severe dementia (n=71, d/b, p/c, Ballard *et al*, *J Clin Psychiatry* 2002;**63**:553–8). However, a comparison with donepezil (with raters wearing nose clips to ensure full blinding or whatever the word is for smelling) showed no evidence for Melissa's efficacy (n=114[c=84], RCT, d/b, p/c, 12/52, Burns *et al*, *Dement Geriatr Cogn Disord* 2011;**31**:158–64). Lavender oil produced a modest but significant reduction in agitation in a cunningly placebo-controlled trial (n=15, p/c, Holmes *et al*, *Int J Geriatr Psychiatry* 2002;**17**:305–8).

Benzodiazepines *

A systematic review concludes that there is no evidence to support routine use in BPSD, but there may be specific circumstances where use might be acceptable (s=5, Tampi and Tampi, *Am J Alzheimer's Dis Other Dement* 2014;**29**:565–74).

Carbamazepine

Carbamazepine may have some use for hostility and aggression in dementia not responding to antipsychotics (e.g. n=21, RCT, 6/52, Olin *et al*, *Am J Geriatr Psychiatry* 2001;**9**:400–5), but a literature review was less than enthusiastic (s=7, Konovalov *et al*, *Int Psychogeriatr* 2008;**20**:293–308).

Gabapentin *

Gabapentin has been used for BPSD and sexual disinhibition in dementia. In a review of 11 case reports, three case series and one chart review, gabapentin was in most cases well tolerated and effective, but the data is incomplete (Kim *et al*, *Drugs Aging* 2008;**25**:187–96). For aggression, 100% in a case series had 'impressive' responses (n=7, Cooney *et al*, *J Neuropsychiatry Clin Neurosci* 2013;**25**:120–5).

Melatonin

Melatonin (1.5–8.5mg/d) at night had no effect on sleep, circadian rhythms or agitation in Alzheimer's (n=41, RCT, p/c, d/b, 10/7, Gehrman *et al*, *Am J Geriatr Psychiatry* 2009; **17**;166–9), but is a low-risk option and may allow carers some respite too.

Yi-Gan San

Yi-Gan San (a traditional Chinese medicine) improved BPSD and ADL (n=52[c=52], RCT, open, 4/52, Iwasaki *et al*, *J Clin Psychiatry* 2005;**66**:248–52).

Zolpidem

Has been used for dementia-related insomnia and night-time wandering (Shelton and Hocking, *Ann Pharmacother* 1997;**31**:319–22).

✱ Case reports

- **Donepezil + gabapentin** (n=2, Dallocchio *et al*, *J Clin Psychiatry* 2000;**61**:64)
- **Propranolol** (n=1, Summers, *J Alzheimer's Dis* 2006;**9**:69–75).

☐ No efficacy

Cannabinoids

Cochrane concludes there is no evidence that cannabinoids improve BPSD or other symptoms of dementia (s=1, Krishnan *et al, Cochrane Database Syst Rev* 2009;**2**:CD007204).

Estrogen

Short-term estrogen may exacerbate BPSD (n=16, RCT, d/b, p/c, 4/52, Kyomen *et al, Am J Psychiatry* 2002;**159**:1225–7).

Oxcarbazepine

Oxcarbazepine has no significant effect (n=103, RCT, d/b, p/c, 8/52, Sommer *et al, Dement Geriatr Cogn Disord* 2009;**27**:155–63).

Valproate

Valproate appears ineffective for agitation in dementia, with unacceptable ADRs (s=3, Lonergan and Luxenberg, *Cochrane Database Syst Rev* 2009;**3**:CD003945), with 10–12mg/kg appearing not to delay emergence of agitation or slow cognitive decline in moderate Alzheimer's and had significant toxic effects (n=317[c=122], RCT, d/b, p/c, 24/12, Tariot *et al, Arch Gen Psychiatry* 2011;**68**:853–61).

1.13.3 VASCULAR DEMENTIA

Vascular dementia (VaD) is the second most common cause of dementia, affecting about 1–4% of people over 65. It can be comorbid with AD. VaD is characterised by impaired executive function rather than memory impairment, usually with an acute onset of disorientation. The other main symptoms are reading difficulties, loss of insight, apathy and gait apraxia.

Prevention of vascular dementia i.e. elimination of the main causes:

- hypertension significantly increases the risk of vascular dementia so rigorous treatment is a key measure to prevent progression (s=11, n=10625, Sharp *et al, Int J Geriatr Psychiatry* 2011;**26**:661–9)
- diabetes
- atherosclerosis
- CV disease (coronary artery disease, CHF, peripheral vascular disease)
- smoking
- atrial fibrillation
- lipid abnormalities
- hyperhomocystinemia
- sleep apnoea
- chronic infection.

(review by Baskys and Cheng, *Exp Gerontol* 2012;**47**:887–91).

Role of drugs

Cholinesterase inhibitors and memantine may produce small benefits but more data is needed (s=8, n=5183, RCT, 6/12, Kavirajan and Schneider, *Lancet Neurol* 2007;**6**:782–92), although another review concludes that there is insufficient evidence that cholinesterase inhibitors or memantine help (Zekry *et al, Front Neurol Neurosci* 2009;**24**:95–106).

Reviews: general (Rojas-Fernandez and Moorhouse, *Ann Pharmacother* 2009;**43**:1310–23), pharmacological treatment (Korczyn *et al, J Neurol Sci* 2012;**322**:2–10), role of herbal preps (Man *et al, Evid Based Complement Alternat Med* 2012;**2012**:426215).

BNF listed

Aripiprazole (see also antipsychotics)

Aripiprazole IM was well tolerated and superior to placebo for acute agitation in VaD (n=129, RCT, d/b, p/c, 24 hours, Rappaport *et al, J Am Med Dir Assoc* 2009;**10**:21–7).

Cholinesterase inhibitors (ChEIs) *

Donepezil can produce significant improvements in cognition and global functioning in VaD (s=2, n=1219, 24/52, Malouf and Birks, *Cochrane Database Syst Rev* 2004;**1**:CD004395), including over a year (s=2, n=885[c=707], RCT, 54/52, Wilkinson *et al, Int J Geriatr Psychiatry* 2009;**25**:305–13), but not global functioning (n=974, RCT, p/c, 24/52, Román *et al, Stroke* 2010;**41**:1213–21). **Galantamine** * may also be effective and Cochrane concludes that the data is limited but shows some advantage over placebo (s=2, n=1378, RCT, d/b, 6/12, Birks and Craig, *Cochrane Database Syst Rev* 2006;**4**:CD004746). **Rivastigmine** * may have some limited effect (s=3, n=800, RCTs, d/b, p/c, Birks *et al, Cochrane Database Syst Rev* 2013;**5**:CD004744).

Memantine

In mild-to-moderate VaD, memantine improves cognition and is well tolerated (n=579, RCT, d/b, p/c, 28/52, Wilcock *et al*, *Int Clin Psychopharmacol* 2002;**17**:297–305), and 20mg/d has improved ADAS-cog scores compared to placebo, where they declined (n=321 [c=288], RCT, p/c, 28/52, Orgogozo *et al*, *Stroke* 2002;**33**:1834–9). Cochrane, however, concludes that there is a small but beneficial effect at six months in AD, but no detectable effect in VaD (d/b, p/c, RCT, McShane *et al*, *Cochrane Database Syst Rev* 2005;**2**:CD003154).

■ Unlicensed/possible efficacy

Antihypertensives

Hypertension is a significant risk factor, and a persistent effect from calcium-channel blockers has been seen (review by Hanes and Weir, *Am J Geriatr Cardiol* 2007;**16**:175–82).

Antipsychotics * (see also aripiprazole)

In people with VaD, those exposed to olanzapine, risperidone or quetiapine (n=337) had no difference in mortality risk compared to non-exposed, suggesting that trials of antipsychotics for BPSD are justified (n=1531, Sultana *et al*, *Int J Geriatr Psychiatry* 2014;**29**:1249–54).

Huperzine A

Cochrane concludes that there is no evidence that Huperzine A (a herbal medicine) has any efficacy in VaD (s=1, n=14, Hao *et al*, *Cochrane Database Syst Rev* 2009;**2**:CD007365), but a more recent study suggests it may significantly improve cognitive function in mild-to-moderate VaD (n=78, RCT, d/b, p/c, 12/52, Xu *et al*, *Cell Biochem Biophys* 2012;**62**:55–8).

Statins *

For a review of possible efficacy see Giannopoulos *et al*, *J Alzheimer's Dis* 2014;**42** Suppl 3:S315–20.

● Case reports

- Finasteride (n=1, Na *et al*, *J Am Geriatr Soc* 2009;**57**:2161–2).

□ No efficacy

Cyproterone

Cyproterone was effective for aggression and impulsive behaviour but not aberrant motor behaviour in VaD (n=19, open, Caparros-Lefebvre and Dewailly, *Rev Neurol [Paris]* 2005;**161**:1071–8).

SSRIs

Citalopram appears to have no efficacy in VaD (n=98, RCT, d/b, 4/52, Nyth and Gottfries, *Br J Psychiatry* 1990;**157**:894–901).

1.13.4 PARKINSON'S DISEASE DEMENTIA (PDD)

Parkinson's disease dementia (PDD) and dementia with Lewy bodies (DLB) may overlap and have distinct cholinergic deficits.

Reviews: * general (Kurtz and Kaufer, *Curr Treat Options Neurol* 2011;**13**:242–54), drug treatments (Ballard *et al*, *Drugs Aging* 2011;**28**;769–77), treating psychosis and dementia in Parkinson's (Goldman and Holden, *Curr Treat Options Neurol* 2014;**16**:281).

BNF listed

Cholinesterase inhibitors (ChEIs)

Cholinesterase inhibitors are the primary treatment for PDD but need some extra care. Cholinesterase inhibitors may transiently worsen EPSE and tremor, and dystonias have been reported so care is needed. Rivastigmine is the only ChEI licensed for PDD. Modest improvements with ChEIs are possible and reduce the incidence of falls, albeit with higher rates of nausea and tremor (n=23, RCT, d/b, p/c, c/o, 15/52, Chung *et al*, *Neurology* 2010;**75**:1263–9), and not for visual hallucinations (Patel *et al*, *BMC Psychiatry* 2010;**10**:69). Cochrane concludes that cholinesterase inhibitors are effective, with a positive impact on global assessment, cognitive function, behavioural disturbance and ADL rating scales (s=6, n=1236, RCT, d/b, p/c, Rolinski *et al*, *Cochrane Database Syst Rev* 2012;**3**:CD006504).

Donepezil (not specifically licensed)

In PDD, donepezil 5–10mg/d appears well tolerated and does not worsen tremor but has shown no significant improvement, albeit with a definite trend towards improvement (n=550, RCT, p/c, 24/52, Dubois *et al, Mov Disord* 2012;**27**:1230–8), possibly due to poorer distribution across the brain (n=550, RCT, d/b, p/c, 24/52, Dubois *et al, Mov Disord* 2012;**27**:1230–8). Donepezil can also be poorly tolerated, and so a slow dose titration (e.g. starting at 2.5 mg) may optimise outcomes (n=24[c=14], Müller *et al, J Neural Transm Suppl* 2006;**71**:27–30). If 5mg/d begins to lose efficacy, increasing to 10mg/d may be effective (n=7, Ishikawa *et al, Psychogeriatrics* 2014;**14**:93–100).

Galantamine (not specifically licensed)

Galantamine for PDD seems effective and only 5% had minor increases in tremor (n=41, open, 24/52, Litvinenko *et al, Neurosci Behav Physiol* 2008;**38**:937–45). The authors were so pleased with the study because they managed to get it published twice (n=41, open, 24/52, Litvinenko *et al, Zh Nevrol Psikhiatr Im S S Korsakova* 2007;**107**:25–33). A smaller trial showed improvement in most people, although there was some mild worsening of tremor (3/13) and global symptoms (4/13) (n=16[c=13], open, 8/52, Aarsland *et al, Int J Geriatr Psychiatry* 2003;**18**:937–41).

Rivastigmine (licensed) *

Rivastigmine is licensed for dementia in PD but can increase nausea, vomiting and tremor (n=541 [c=410], RCT, d/b, 24/52, Emre *et al, N Engl J Med* 2004;**351**:2509–18; comment by Chow, *Evid Based Ment Health* 2005;**8**:41; FFT). In the longer term, rivastigmine does not exacerbate tremor or worsen other symptoms (n=334, open, 24/52, Oertel *et al, Drug Saf* 2008;**31**:79–94), improves executive function on a range of measures (n=541, RCT, d/b, p/c, 24/52, Schmitt *et al, CNS Neurosci Ther* 2010;**16**:330–6) and is well tolerated (n=583, RCT, 76/52, open, Emre *et al, Clin Neuropharmacol* 2014;**37**:9–16).

Review: general (Chitnis and Rao, *Expert Opin Drug Metab Toxicol* 2009;**5**:941–55).

Memantine (not specifically licensed) *

There is accumulating evidence for some efficacy at 10–20 mg/d:

On the positive side, memantine seemed effective for PDD with no apparent motor ADRs (e.g. n=72[c=56], RCT, d/b, p/c, 24/52, Aarsland *et al, Lancet Neurol* 2009;**8**:613–8), with 20 mg/d producing significant and substantial improvements in choice reaction time and word recognition (n=30, RCT, d/b, p/c, 24/52, Wesnes *et al, Int J Geriatr Psychiatry* 2015;**30**:46–54), but probably not gait (n=25, RCT, d/b, p/c, 90/7, Moreau *et al, J Neurol Neurosurg Psychiatry* 2013;**84**:552–5; FFT). It may reduce physical activity and sleep behaviour in PDD during sleep (n=42, RCT, p/c, 24/52, Larsson *et al, Int J Geriatr Psychiatry* 2010;**25**:1030–8). Longer treatment, e.g. up to a year at 20 mg/d (n=25, RCT, d/b, p/c, 22/52, Leroi *et al, Mov Disord* 2009;**24**:1217–21) may be essential to build on improved cognitive functions (one year, Litvinenko *et al, Neurosci Behav Physiol* 2010;**40**:149–55).

On the negative side, the largest studies show memantine does not appear to separate from placebo for global functioning, behaviour (n=120, RCT, d/b, p/c, Emre *et al, Lancet Neurol* 2010;**9**:969–77; n=199[c=159], RCT, d/b, p/c, 24/52, Emre *et al, Lancet Neurol* 2010;**9**:969–77), sleepiness, fatigue, depression and attention, although most elected to carry on after the trial so there may have been more subtle effects (n=40[c=36], RCT, d/b, p/c, 8/52, Ondo *et al, Parkinsonism Relat Disord* 2011;**17**:156–9).

Review: memantine and ChEIs (s=10, Wang *et al, J Neurol Neurosurg Psychiatry* 2015;**86**:135–43).

1.13.5 PROPHYLAXIS AND PREVENTION OF DEMENTIA

This section may be useful in helping advise patients, carers, friends and relatives about possible strategies for reducing the risk of dementia, especially where a family history exists. The genetic risk only accounts for 7% cases, but new cases could be reduced by:

- Eliminating depression, diabetes and eating more fruit and vegetable (21% reduction)
- Eliminating depression (10% reduction)
- Increasing education (18% reduction)

(n=1433, seven years, Ritchie *et al, Br Med J* 2010;**341**:c3885; FFT). The biggest avoidable causes of dementia seem to be, in descending order; low education, smoking, physical inactivity, depression, mid-life hypertension, diabetes and mid-life obesity (n = 3069, nine years, Yaffe *et al*, *Arch Neurol* 2012;**69**:1170–5).

General modifiable measures (see also vascular dementia) include:

- **Alcohol** — light to moderate alcohol consumption reduces the risk of Alzheimer's and VaD (n = 36746, Anstey *et al*, *Am J Geriatr Psychiatry* 2009;**17**:542–55)
- **Being overweight** in midlife increases the risk of dementia (n = 1152, 40 years, Hassing *et al*, *Int J Obes (Lond)* 2009;**33**:893–8; FFT) and those in the top third of weights are 2.5 times more likely to be cognitively impaired than those in the bottom third if aged 60–70 (n = 250, Yoon *et al*, *Age Aging* 2012;**41**:456–61; FFT)
- **Physical activity** and modest exercise improve cognition (n = 170 [c = 138], RCT, two years, Lauten-schlager *et al*, *JAMA* 2008;**300**:1027–37)
- **Hypertension** (see antihypertensives)
- **Lower cholesterol** (see statins)
- **Fruit and vegetables** — the risk of AD is lower with an increased intake of vegetables, but not fruit (s = 9, n = 44004, >6/12, Loef and Walach, *J Nutr Health Aging* 2012;**16**:626–30)
- **Not having diabetes** slows cognitive decline (n = 103, four years, Velayudhan *et al*, *Br J Psychiatry* 2010;**196**:36–40; FFT) and poor glucose control in diabetes is associated with worse cognitive function and greater decline (n = 3069, nine years, Yaffe *et al*, *Arch Neurol* 2012;**69**:1170–5; FFT)
- **Drinking 3–5 cups of tea or coffee a day** in midlife reduces the risk by 65%. The effect is most marked with tea but also occurs with coffee (s = 5, Eskelinen and Kivipelto, *J Alzheimers Dis* 2010;**20**(Suppl 1):167–74)
- **Having depression** is a risk factor for Alzheimer's (n = 357, Wilson *et al*, *Neurology* 2010;**75**:21–6; FFT)
- **Avoiding anticholinergics** (Jessen *et al*, *Eur Arch Psychiatry Clin Neurosci* 2010;**260** Suppl 2:S111–5; see also 'No efficacy').

Assessment of the risk of dementia:

Score	Risk factor
1–2	Older age
2–4	Poor cognitive performance
2	BMI < 18.5
1	> 1 apolipoprotein E epsilon 4 alleles
1	MRI shows white matter disease
1	Ventricular enlargement
1	Carotid artery thickening on ultrasound
1	History of bypass surgery
1	Slow physical performance
1	Lack of alcohol consumption

Over six years, the percentage of people developing dementia were:

- 4% with low scores (0-3)
- 23% with moderate scores (4-7)
- 56% with high scores (8-15).

(n = 3375, Barnes *et al*, *Neurology* 2009;**73**:173–9; FFT).

Reviews: * primary prevention strategies (Norton *et al*, *Lancet Neurol* 2014;**13**:788–94; Moretti *et al*, *CNS Neurol Disord Drug Targets* 2011;**10**:370–90), role of phytochemicals (Howes and Perry, *Drugs Aging* 2011;**28**:439–68), diet (Solfrizzi *et al*, *Expert Rev Neurother* 2011; **11**:677–708), recent advances (Solomon *et al*, *J Intern Med* 2014;**275**:229–50).

• Unlicensed/some efficacy

Cholinesterase inhibitors

A systematic review concludes that ChEIs do not delay the progression to AD or dementia when taken by people with MCI (s = 8, RCT, 24/52–3 years, Raschetti *et al*, *PLoS Medicine* 2007;**4**:e338; FFT). However, **donepezil** may delay progression in the presence of depression (n = 756, d/b, p/c, three years, Lu *et al*, *Neurology* 2009;**72**:2115–21; FFT).

NSAIDs *

The jury is still out on whether NSAIDs reduce the risk of AD.

The case for NSAIDs reducing the AD risk: *

- A significant effect, but with no advantage for SALAs (e.g. diclofenac, flurbiprofen, ibuprofen) over non-SALAs (e.g. celecoxib, etodolac, mefenamic acid, nabumetone, naproxen) (s=6, n=13499, Szekely *et al, Neurology* 2008;**70**:2291–8; FFT)
- Taking NSAIDs for more than five years, with the best evidence with ibuprofen (e.g. n=246199, Vlad *et al, Neurology* 2008;**70**:1672–7; FFT) and regular long-term low-dose aspirin (n=681 [c=489], five years, Kern *et al, Br Med J Open* 2012; **2**:e001288)
- Reduced cognitive decline, but only if started in midlife (<65 years) before the decline starts, for a minimum of two years and if the person has one or more predisposing APOE genotypes (n=3383, Hayden *et al, Neurology* 2007;**69**: 275–82)
- NSAIDs may have an adverse effect in the later stages of AD, but in asymptomatic people NSAIDs such as naproxen reduce the incidence of AD but only after 2–3 years, so the treatment effect varies according to the stage of the disease (n= 2528[c=2071], RCT, p/c, two years, Breitner *et al, Alzheimers Dement* 2011;**7**:402–11; FT).

The case against NSAIDs reducing AD risk:

- No effect on alleviating progression in people with mild-to-moderate AD (n=351, RCT, d/b, p/c, one year, Aisen *et al, JAMA* 2003;**289**:2819–26)
- No effect from low-dose aspirin 75 mg/d (n=310, RCT, open, mean three years, AD2000 Collaborative Group, *Lancet Neurol* 2008;**7**:41–9), ibuprofen 800 mg/d (n=132 [c=97], RCT, d/b, p/c, 12/12, Pasqualetti *et al, Aging Clin Exp Res* 2009;**21**:102–10), or celecoxib and naproxen (n=2528 [c=2117], RCT, d/b, p/c, mean two years, ADAPT Group, *Arch Neurol* 2008;**65**:896–905; FFT)
- Heavy NSAID users have a higher AD incidence than non-users, but this could be delayed onset (n=2736, 10 years, Breitner *et al, Neurology* 2009;**22**: 1899–905; FFT)
- Increased risk of intracerebral hemorrhages (HR=7.6) with longer-term use (s=2, n=433, RCT, Thoonsen *et al, Stroke* 2010;**41**:2690–2; FFT)
- Observational studies support NSAID use but RCTs do not (review by Wang *et al, J Alzheimer's Dis* 2015;**44**:385–96).

Review: * general (Gupta *et al, Am J Alzheimer's Dis Other Demen* 2014;**30**;178–82).

■ Unlicensed/possible efficacy

Antidepressants *

Depression is associated with an increased risk of dementia. Antidepressants may have neuroprotective effects and may cancel this out. A large retrospective study (1996–2005) in people with depression (n=37,658) showed a slightly reduced incidence of dementia in people taking longer-term tricyclics and MAOIs but the incidence with SSRIs was unchanged (n=37,658, Kessing *et al, Int Clin Psychopharmacol* 2011;**26**:316–22).

Antihypertensives (see also introduction) *

High and low bp is associated with faster cognitive decline in AD patients (s=11, n=10625, Sharp *et al, Int J Geriatr Psychiatry* 2011;**26**:661–9). A systematic review concluded that only ACE inhibitors and diuretics (n=1928+320, mean six years, Yasar *et al, Neurology* 2013;**81**:896–903) significantly reduce the risk for, and progression to, dementia (s=12, Shah *et al, Am J Geriatr Pharmacother* 2009;**7**:250 61). This was confirmed by a later study that ACE-Inhibitors are associated with slower rate of cognitive decline, independent of hypertension (n=616, Soto *et al, J Am Geriatr Soc* 2013;**61**:1482–8). A postmortem study showed less AD neuropathology in people treated with antihypertensives, even less than in non-hypertensive people (n=291, Hoffman *et al, Neurology* 2009;**72**:1720–6; FFT).

Review: * positive review of calcium-channel blockers positive review (Saravanaraman *et al, Rev Neurosci* 2014;**25**:231–46).

Beer

Beer contains silicone, which may reduce the bioavailability of aluminium (Gonzalez-Munoz *et al, Food Chem Toxicol* 2008;**46**:49–56). Well, it still seems to be working for my Dad.

Coffee/caffeine/tea (see also introduction) *

High blood caffeine levels (>1200ng/mL) are associated with no conversion to dementia over 2–4 years, whereas low caffeine levels were significantly associated with development of dementia, with increased levels being effective even after MCI has already appeared (n=124, <4 years, Cao *et al, J Alzheimers Dis* 2012;**30**:559–72). Higher intakes of caffeinated coffee (but not other sources of caffeine) was also related to better cognitive maintenance over five years in older women with vascular disorders (n=2475, Vercambre *et al, J Alzheimer's Dis* 2013;**35**:413–21). A pooled analysis shows a protective effect for coffee on developing AD (s=4, Barranco Quintana *et al, Neurol Res* 2007;**29**:91–5).

Review: * use to prevent dementia (Carman *et al, J Nutr Health Aging* 2014;**18**:383–92).

Estrogen (oestrogen)

Estrogen is a potent factor that prevents vascular disease and improves blood flow in diseased vessels in regions of the brain affected by AD, and also has an important role in the preservation and repair of neurons. Some trials have shown a potential effect in slowing decline or improving cognition, e.g. from long-term HRT in older women (n=2000, Carlson *et al, Neurology* 2001;**57**:2210–16), high-dose transdermal 17-beta-estradiol (n=20, RCT, p/c, 8/52, Asthana *et al, Neurology* 2001;**57**:605–12) and estrogen HRT, oral or transdermal (n=184, Maki *et al, Am J Psychiatry* 2001;**158**:227–33). It may only help if started before 49 years, and may possibly be detrimental after 60 (review by Craig and Murphy, *Ann N Y Acad Sci* 2010;**1205**:245–53). However, other trials have failed to show a protective effect from, e.g. conjugated estrogens (e.g. n=120, RCT, 12/12, Mulnard *et al, JAMA* 2000;**283**:1007–15), short-term estrogens (n=42 women, RCT, 16/52, Henderson *et al, Neurology* 2000;**54**:295–301), or estrogen replacement therapy (ERT) (n=2859, Alves de Moraes *et al, Am J Epidemiol* 2001;**154**:733–9; FFT) and it actually increased the risk in one study (n=4000, RCT, d/b, p/c, Shumaker *et al, JAMA* 2003;**289**:2651–62, 2663–72; comment by Sherwin and McGill, *EBMH* 2003;**6**:111; FFT). Cochrane concludes that HRT and ERT may have some effects, but there is insufficient evidence to indicate them for women with cognitive impairment (s=7, n=351, RCT, d/b, Hogervorst *et al, Cochrane Database Syst Rev* 2009;**1**:CD003799).

Reviews: general (Henderson, *Semin Reprod Med* 2009;**27**:283–93; FFT; Pike *et al, Front Neuroendocrinol* 2009;**30**:239–58; FFT).

Fish and n-3 fatty acids (see also omega-3 fatty acids)

People who eat fish at least once a week have 60% lower risk of developing AD compared with people who never, or seldom, eat fish (n=815, Morris *et al, Arch Neurol* 2003;**60**:940–6).

Folate

Cochrane concludes that there is no consistent evidence one way or the other for folic acid (with or without B12) to prevent AD (s=8, RCT, Malouf *et al, Cochrane Database Syst Rev* 2008;**4**:CD004514).

Insulin *

Insulin has been proposed (review by Rdzak and Abdelghany, *Pharmacotherapy* 2014;**34**:1317–23).

Interferon beta-1a *

Interferon beta-1a 22mcg s/c three times a week showed a non-significant reduction in disease progression (n=42, RCT, d/b, p/c, 1 year, Grimaldi *et al, J Neuroinflammation* 2014;**11**:30).

Lithium *

The case for lithium: *

- In bipolars, one year of continual lithium is associated with significantly reduced dementia risk in bipolars, but not with shorter durations of treatment (Gerhard *et al, Br J Psychiatry* 2015;**207**:46–51)
- Bipolars have an increased risk of dementia compared to the general population (19% vs 7%), but this is reduced in lithium takers (n=1423, Terao *et al, Prog Neuropsychopharmacol Biol Psychiatry* 2006;**30**:1125–8; n=114, Nunes *et al, Br J Psychiatry* 2007;**190**:359–60; FFT)
- Lithium can reduce CSF concentrations of P-tau and improve performance (n=45,

RCT, d/b, p/c, 12/12, Forlenza *et al, Br J Psychiatry* 2011;**198**:351–6; FFT)

- Lithium may produce a sustained increase in grey matter volume within 10–12 weeks (n=36, Lyoo *et al, Neuropsychopharmacology* 2010;**35**:1743–50; FFT), and block the accumulation of amyloid-beta peptides
- Standard and trace doses of lithium reduce dementia (s=18, Mauer *et al, Aust N Z J Psychiatry* 2014;**48**:809–18).

The case against lithium:

- A study failed to show lithium protects against the onset of dementia (Dunn *et al, Alzheimer Dis Assoc Disord* 2005;**19**:20–2)
- There appears no effect on GSK-3, which regulates tau protein (n=71, 10/52, Hampel *et al, J Clin Psychiatry* 2009;**70**:922–31)
- Lithium had no effect on MMSE in mild-to-moderate Alzheimer's disease (n=22 [c=8], open, < 12/12, *Int J Geriatr Psychiatry* 2008;**23**:704–11).

Reviews: * possible mechanisms (might be neuroprotection [Diniz *et al, Neuropsychiatr Dis Treat* 2013;**9**:493–500]) increased expression of anti-apoptotic genes, increased grey matter, and hippocampal volume: Forlenza *et al, Drugs Aging* 2012;**29**:335–42).

Melatonin

Melatonin and its analogues have been proposed as potentially having some value (Srinivasan *et al, Int J Alzheimers Dis* 2010,**2011**; 741974; FFT).

Memantine

Memantine may improve cognitive function in some populations of postmenopausal women at risk of dementia (n=22, open, 6/12, Wroolie *et al, Acta Neurol Scand* 2008;**119**:172–9).

Raloxifene

Raloxifene, a selective estrogen receptor modulator, 120mg/d (but not 60mg/d) may reduce the risk of cognitive impairment in postmenopausal women by 33% (n=5386, three years, Yaffe *et al, Am J Psychiatry* 2005;**162**:683–90).

Red wine

Moderate consumption could help reduce or slow AD due to its phenolic content (Anon, *Duke Med Health News* 2007;**13**:7–8). It's such a pity I can't tolerate red wine.

Rifampicin

A comparison of doxycycline and rifampicin seemed to show both had an effect in people with mild-to-moderate AD (n=101, RCT, t/b, p/c, 12/12, Loeb *et al, J Am Geriatr Soc* 2004;**52**:381–7).

Statins

Even moderately raised midlife serum total cholesterol is associated with an increased risk of AD (n=9844, 43 years, Solomon *et al, Dement Geriatr Cogn Disord* 2009;**28**:75–80; FFT), but it is unclear if statins help reverse this.

The case for statins:

- Lovastatin, pravastatin and atorvastatin substantially lower the risk of developing dementias (eg. n=60,000, Josefson, *Br Med J* 2000;**321**:1040; FT)
- Statin users are about half as likely to develop dementia as those not taking them (n=1674, five years, Cramer *et al, Neurology* 2008;**71**:344–50; FFT)
- In AD, use of statins is associated with a delay in functional decline (n=216, three years, Rosenberg *et al, Am J Geriatr Psychiatry* 2008;**16**:883–92; FFT)
- In cognitively normal people, statin therapy has been associated at autopsy with reduced neurofibrillary tangle burden, so starting statins before the onset of AD could be important (n=110, Li *et al, Neurology* 2007;**69**:878–85)
- Non-statin cholesterol-lowering drugs do not show this effect (n=6992, 15 years, Haag *et al, J Neurol Neurosurg Psych* 2009;**80**:13–7)
- Short-term studies show no effect but if taken for more than a year (n=23443, 3–25 years) the risk of dementia is 29% lower (s=16, Swiger *et al, Mayo Clin Proc* 2013;**88**:1213–21).

The case against statins:

- Use over 4–5 years had no association with a lower incidence of dementia (eg. n=2798, Rea *et al, Arch Neurol* 2005;**62**:1047–51).

Conclusion: * Cochrane concludes that statins have no benefit (s=4, n= 1154, McGuinness *et al, Cochrane Database Syst Rev* 2014;**7**:CD007514), but probably do little harm (s=2, McGuinness and Passmore, *J Alzheimer's Dis* 2010;**20**:925–33).

Reviews: * meta-analysis concluding a slight benefit (Wong *et al, Pharmacoepidemiol Drug Saf* 2013;**22**:345–58), general (Sánchez-Ferro *et al, Neuropsychiatr Dis Treat* 2013;**9**:55–63).

Vitamins *

High homocysteine levels have been shown to increase the risk of AD. B vitamins lower homocysteine and might slow the rate of atrophy in older people with MCI. However, brain shrinkage is not the same as dementia, although there might be some relationship (n=271 [c=168], RCT, d/b, p/c, 24/12, Smith *et al, PLoS One* 2010;**5**:12244; FFT).

The case for vitamins:

- Common antioxidants (vitamins C, E and beta-carotene) all decrease the risk of AD, especially vitamin E (s=7, Li *et al, J Alzheimers Dis* 2012;**31**:253–8)
- B12 or folate deficiency doubles the risk of AD (n = 370, Wang *et al, Neurology* 2001;**56**:1188–94)
- Vitamin E and C supplements may protect against VaD and improve cognitive function in later life in men (n=3385, Masaki *et al, Neurology* 2000;**54**:1265–72)
- Vitamin C may have a protective effect but avoiding deficiency is likely to be the most beneficial action (Harrison, *J Alzheimers Dis* 2012;**29**:711–26; FFT)
- Severe vitamin D deficiency increases the risk of AD 2.25-fold, simple deficiency reduces this to 1.69-fold (n= 1658, mean 5.6 years, Littlejohns *et al, Neurology* 2014;**83**:920–8), but it is still unclear if supplementation will slow this (n=382, four years, Miller *et al, JAMA Neurol* 2015; **72**: 1295–303).

The case against vitamins:

- In MCI, vitamin E 2000 IU had no effect on impairment and did not slow progression to AD (n=769, three years, RCT, p/c, d/b, Petersen *et al, N Engl J Med* 2005;**352**:2379–88; FFT)
- B6, B12 and folate supplementation was ineffective in reducing cognitive decline (n=409 [c=340], RCT, d/b, p/c, 18/12, Aisen *et al, JAMA* 2008;**300**:1774–83; FFT)
- An independent analysis concluded that B12 does not improve brain function (s= 18, *Ont Health Technol Assess Ser* 2013;**13**:1–45).

□ No efficacy

Anticholinergics

People taking a drug with an anticholinergic effect have an increased risk of cognitive decline, dementia (HR=1.65) (n=6912, four years, Carrière *et al, Arch Intern Med* 2009;**169**:1317–24; FFT) and death, but discontinuing decreases the risk.

Ginkgo biloba *

GB clearly has no effect on reducing the rates of dementia and this has been shown in numerous hopeful studies, e.g. over 5–6 years (n=3069, RCT, d/b, p/c, median six years, DeKosky *et al, JAMA* 2008;**300**:2253–62; FFT; n=2820, RCT, d/b, p/c, five years, Vellas *et al, Lancet Neurol* 2012:**11**:851–9; n=2820, RCT, d/b, p/c, five years, Vellas *et al, Lancet Neurol* 2012;**11**:851–9), in people with early memory problems (n=2854[c=2426], two years, Hirsch, *Ann Intern Med* 2013;**158**:JC7). A meta-analysis concludes GB does not prevent the progression of neurodegeneration (Yang *et al, Am J Clin Med* 2014;**42**:505–21). However, a longer but less robust study showed less decline with GB (EGb761) than placebo (n=3612, 20 years, Amieva *et al, PLoS One* 2013;**8**:e52755).

Omega-3 fatty acids

Cochrane concludes that O3FAs do not prevent deterioration of cognitive function, although trials may need to be much longer to detect an effect (s=3, n=4080[c=3536], <40/12, Sydenham *et al, Cochrane Database Syst Rev* 2012;**6**:CD005379).

Reviews: general (Huang, *J Alzheimer's Dis* 2010;**21**:673–90; Jicha and Markesbery, *Clin Interv Aging* 2010;**5**:45–61; FFT).

Piracetam *

Piracetam showed worsening cognitive decline

than GB (n=3612, 20 years, Amieva *et al*, *PLoS One* 2013;**8**:e52755).

Zinc

A systematic review showed no evidence that zinc deficiency is a risk factor (s=55, Loef *et al*, *Nutr Neurosci* 2012;**15**:2–12).

1.14 DEPRESSION

1.14.1 UNIPOLAR DEPRESSION

see also Postpartum depression (*1.14.2*), Bipolar depression (*1.10.3*), Rapid-cycling bipolar disorder (*1.10.4*), Depression in Parkinson's disease (*1.14.3*), Dysthymia (*1.14.4*), Mania and hypomania (*1.10.2*)

Depression is a common condition, affecting up to 3% of the population per year, but it remains underdiagnosed and undertreated (especially in men and in the under 30s). The overall cost of depression (e.g. work, family, other illnesses) is high for this eminently treatable condition, although the UK press still seems to have generally archaic views on this, with an apparent strong anti-pharmacotherapy bias.

Symptoms

Depression presents with a mixture of biological symptoms (insomnia or hypersomnia, diurnal variation in mood, low appetite, fatigue or loss of energy, constipation, loss of libido, weight loss or gain) and psychiatric symptoms (depressed mood, loss of interest or pleasure, poor memory, psychomotor agitation or retardation, recurrent thoughts of death or suicide, anxiety, feelings of worthlessness or guilt, including delusions). Atypical depression includes the symptoms of depression, plus two from hypersomnia, hyperphagia, rejection sensitivity and severe lethargy.

Role of drugs *

Antidepressants have a major role in acute depression (hastening recovery, reducing suffering) and minimising relapse (their most potent effect), are not addictive, and do not generally lose efficacy with prolonged use. Adequate doses are needed for a clinical effect.

Antidepressants may enhance the effectiveness of psychotherapy (NNT=7, s=16, n=852, Cuijpers *et al*, *Acta Psychiatr Scand* 2010;**121**:415–23), but most CBT trials use waiting list controls, which is actually worse than nothing (n=368, RCT, p/c, 10/52, Hegerl *et al*, *Int J Neuropsychopharmacol* 2010;**13**:31–44) and the most recent meta-analysis for CBT shows a lower effect size with higher quality studies and strong indications of publication bias, but no evidence CBT was better or worse than other treatments, but combined CBT and antidepressants was superior (s=115, Cuijpers *et al*, *Can J Psychiatry* 2013;**58**:376–85).

Treatment of depression

The general principles of the medicines treatment of depression (with antidepressants) can be summed up by the six Ds:

- Diagnosis
- Drug-induced
- Drug
- Dose
- Duration
- Discontinuation

1. **Diagnosis:** Making, or being able to make, a diagnosis helps. An obvious statement, but diagnosis does start with a D.
2. **Drug-induced causes eliminated:** See list in Chapter 5.5, as well as physical (e.g. low folate levels) and environmental causes.
3. **Drug:** * The main antidepressants appear to have broadly similar efficacy, although there are some subtle differences in efficacy and acceptability (see comparative section). As non-compliance or inadequate dosage are the main causes of drug failure, the choice of drug should consider this. The Cipriani network meta-analysis compared bupropion, citalopram, duloxetine, escitalopram, fluoxetine, fluvoxamine, milnacipran, mirtazapine, paroxetine, reboxetine, sertraline, and venlafaxine for the acute treatment of unipolar major depression in adults (s=117, n=25,928, RCT, Cipriani *et al*, *Lancet* 2009;**373**:746–58) and concluded that:
   - Escitalopram, mirtazapine, venlafaxine and sertraline were significantly more effective than duloxetine, fluoxetine, fluvoxamine, paroxetine and reboxetine (the least efficacious antidepressant)
   - Escitalopram and sertraline showed the best profile of acceptability, with significantly fewer discontinuations than duloxetine,

fluvoxamine, paroxetine, reboxetine, and venlafaxine
- Sertraline and escitalopram (now available as a generic) were first choices due to the most favourable balance between benefits, acceptability and acquisition costs
- A more recent network meta-analysis concluded that agomelatine, escitalopram and mirtazapine had the best efficacy-tolerability balance (s = 76, Khoo *et al*, *CNS Drugs* 2015;**29**:695–712).

4. **Dose:** The therapeutic range of newer anti-depressants is well-established, but seems less well-known for the tricyclics, e.g. the need for tricyclic doses of 125–150 mg/d in 95% adults. Once-daily dosing is as effective as multiple daily doses, regardless of drug half-life.

5. **Duration:**

5a. Acute therapy — SSRIs can be started at half the standard dose for a few days to improve tolerability. The person must be monitored for akathisia, anxiety, agitation and suicidal ideation early in treatment.

Onset of action: It is a common misperception that antidepressants take four weeks to work. It is more accurate to say that the 'time to substantial remission' (full statistical separation from placebo) may take four weeks in clinical trials (rarely powered to detect an earlier onset), but the onset of action may in fact be much quicker because:
- There are detectable positive effects after three hours (eg. n = 21 [c = 16], RCT, c/o, s/b, Bruhl *et al*, *Neuropsychopharmacology* 2010;**35**:521–33; FFT)
- There is symptomatic improvement in a week (s = 28, n = 5872, RCT, Taylor *et al*, *Arch Gen Psychiatry* 2006;**63**:1217–23; FFT) and 57% of differences are apparent by week two (s = 47, n = 8500, d/b, p/c, Pasternak and Zimmerman, *J Clin Psychiatry* 2005;**66**:148–58)
- Early improvement (> 50% reduction in HAM-D) at 2/52 predicted response at 6/52 in 59% people (n = 149, RCT, d/b, a/c, Vermeiden *et al*, *Psychopharmacology [Berl]* 2015;**232**:1347–56).

There is, however, a small cohort where response is delayed and can take ≤12/52 (n = 811, Uher *et al*, *J Clin Psychiatry* 2011; **72**:1478–84). Improvement within two weeks strongly predicts later outcomes, lower anxiety, and higher function (eg. n = 568, 12/52, Kim *et al*, *J Affect Disord* 2011;**129**:183–90; s = 41, n = 6562, p/c, 4–8/52, Szegedi *et al*, *J Clin Psychiatry* 2009;**70**:344–53) and leads to better long-term compliance, as the recovery is associated with starting antidepressants. Telling people antidepressants take four weeks to work will of course mean any rapid improvement will be attributed to other reasons. Higher starting doses speed response, but lead to increased drop-outs and ADRs (s = 9, n = 2340, RCT, d/b, p/c, Papakostas *et al*, *World J Biol Psychiatry* 2010;**11**:300–7), although spreading out the first doses across a day reduces the ADRs from peak plasma levels and can improve tolerability.

If unimproved at:	The chances of eventually converting to a responder are:		
Week 1	36% (n = 302)		
Week 2	29% (n = 208)		
Week 3	18% (n=151)		
Week 4	17% (n = 120)	23% (n = 118)	50% (n = 117)
Week 5	9% (n = 91)		
Week 6		10% (n=61)	33% (n = 60)
Week 12			30% (n = 46)

(n = 627, open, 12/52 + 52/52 continuation, Posternak *et al*, *J Clin Psychiatry* 2011;**72**:949–54). If depression remains completely unchanged after four weeks of therapeutic dosing, an alternate should be tried (n = 840, 12/52, open, Quitkin *et al*, *Am J Psychiatry* 2003;**160**:734–40), with these times probably doubled in the elderly and in chronic depression (review by Gelenberg and Chesen, *J Clin Psychiatry* 2000;**61**:712–21).

5b. Continuation therapy — effective treatment of depression requires continuation while the person remains vulnerable, with doses the **same or close to the therapeutic dose**. If a first episode of depression remits in 12 weeks, continued treatment for six months minimises the risk of relapse, but longer may give little additional benefit, except in people with additional relapse risk factors (n=395, RCT, 52/52, Reimherr *et al, Am J Psychiatry* 1998;**155**:1247–53). Relapse has been significantly lower with antidepressants in every study over the last 25 years, with an average relapse reduction of 52% cf. placebo, and not due to antidepressant withdrawal in the placebo group (s=15, RCTs, d/b, Borges *et al, J Clin Psychiatry* 2014;**75**:205–14). A large US study showed that older people (≥60 years) with untreated depression had a death rate twice as high over an average of eight years than people without depression, and that the rate for treated depression (combination of therapies, including antidepressants) was the same as people without depression (n=1226, Gallo *et al, Br Med J* 2013;**346**:f2570).

5c. Maintenance or relapse prevention — Maintenance therapy is appropriate for people with chronic depression, three or more episodes, or two episodes with risk factors (late or early onset, short interval between episodes, rapid onset, dysthymia, positive family history, comorbidity, incomplete response and low work adjustment). In recurrent MDD, the risk of relapse increases by 16% with each successive episode, but the risk of recurrence progressively decreases as duration of recovery increases (n=318, open, 10 years, Solomon *et al, Am J Psychiatry* 2000;**157**:229–33), so keeping people well pays dividends.

General minimum treatment duration recommendations:

- First episode — six months post-recovery
- Second episode — 1–3 years
- Third episode — five years or longer (n=128, RCT, d/b, p/c, three years, Frank *et al, Arch Gen Psychiatry* 1990;**47**:1093–9; two-year follow-up, Kupfer *et al, Arch Gen Psychiatry* 1992;**49**:769–73)
- Fourth episode — the person should have a very good reason to stop.

6. **Discontinuation:** Slowly reduce doses over a minimum of four weeks, as stopping rapidly (1–7 days) leads to a shorter time to relapse compared to slower (14/7 or more) discontinuation (n=224, open, Baldessarini *et al, Am J Psychiatry* 2010;**167**:934–41). Discontinuation syndromes have been reported for nearly all antidepressants (particularly paroxetine and venlafaxine), usually appear within 1–3 days of stopping and can improve within a week (although they can last much longer). See switching antidepressants in *2.2.7* for a further review.

Treatment-resistant depression (TRD) *

TRD is defined (after STAR*D) as failure of two treatment trials and is more likely where treatment was started after 6/12 of symptoms (n=270, Bukh *et al, J Affect Disord* 2013;**145**:42–8). Options include:

1. Exclude bipolar depression (see *1.10.3*): 16% people with TRD met the full DSM-IV-R criteria for bipolar, a further 31% met bipolarity specific criteria (n=5635, BRIDGE study, Angst *et al, Arch Gen Psychiatry* 2011;**68**:791–8) and a third eventually convert to bipolar (n=122, Dudek *et al, J Affect Disord* 2013;**144**:112–5). A follow-up of people being treated for unipolar MDD for up to eight years showed that 7.6–12.1% were subsequently diagnosed as bipolar, and that this was more likely in people poorly responding to antidepressants, a useful predictor (n=3944, Li *et al, Br J Psychiatry* 2012;**200**:45–51).

2. Escalate antidepressant doses for an adequate duration: This is appropriate for drugs with a dose-response curve or to tolerance. Push SSRI doses to the BNF maximum.

3. Check plasma levels: to detect non-concordance or possible 2D6 ultrarapid metabolisers who may rapidly metabolise tricyclics.

4. Switch antidepressants: The pros and cons (Shelton *et al, CNS Drugs* 2010;**24**:131–61) are:

- **Pros**: avoidance of polypharmacy; lower TEAEs; lower costs
- **Cons**: cannot build on a partial response; monotherapy switches after two treatments have only a limited effect (see STAR*D).

Ensure all drug classes have been tried optimally, e.g. SSRIs, tricyclics, SNRIs, mirtazapine, agomelatine, moclobemide (adequate doses e.g. over 600mg/d) and MAOIs (see *C2.2.6*).

5. Augment or combine: The pros and cons (Shelton *et al, CNS Drugs* 2010;**24**:131–61) are:

- **Pros:** can build on improvements achieved so far; especially with partial response
- **Cons:** results in multiple medicines; higher costs; more ADRs.

Use logical combinations of antidepressants, (see later in this section), e.g. mirtazapine, lithium, carbamazepine (but not with tricyclics, see *4.3.1*), valproate, or lithium/SSRI/tryptophan.

6. Assure compliance: Around 42% people stop antidepressants within the first 30 days, 30% in the next 60 days (mostly due to lack of efficacy), and only 28% carry on beyond three months (n=829, Olfson *et al, Am J Psychiatry* 2006;**163**:101–8).
7. Manage ADRs: If response occurs but ADRs are limiting, see *Chapter 6* for strategies to manage, e.g. sexual dysfunction, sedation, etc.
8. Check folate levels: See adjunctive therapy.
9. Consider individual CBT: In TRD combining antidepressants and psychotherapy has the best outcomes (s=10, Spijker *et al, Can J Psychiatry* 2013;**58**:386–92).

Reviews: * general (Vieta and Colom, *Ann Med* 2011;**43**:512–30), drug treatments (Schlaepfer *et al, J Psychopharmacol* 2012;**26**:587–602), refractory depression in older people (s=14, Cooper *et al, Am J Psychiatry* 2011;**168**:681–8), inflammatory cytokines (Makhija and Karunakaran, *Aust N Z J Psychiatry* 2013;**47**:828–39), glutamatergic approaches to MDD (ketamine, memantine and riluzole; Owen, *Drugs Today* 2012;**48**:469–78), psychotic depression (Nelson, *Curr Psychiatry Rep* 2012;**14**:619–23).

Loss of antidepressant effect *

Loss of efficacy (operational tolerance, tachyphylaxis, or 'poop-out') has been reported during long-term maintenance therapy. Possible causes include non-compliance, loss of initial placebo response, loss of true drug effect, pharmacological tolerance, accumulation of detrimental metabolites, change in illness pathology, unrecognised rapid-cycling, switching and cycle acceleration in bipolars, antidepressant-induced paradoxical effects and a genuine lack of prophylactic efficacy (review, Targum, *Innov Clin Neurosci* 2014;**11**:24–8; FFT).

Strategies to overcome loss of efficacy include:

1. **Increase** the dose.
2. **Decrease** the dose (especially if there is a 'therapeutic window') or have a **drug holiday** (≥3–4 weeks), although both of these are poorly supported by the literature.
3. **Switch** to a different drug or class.
4. **Ensure compliance**.
5. **Augment** with, e.g. mood stabilisers, anticonvulsants, thyroid, another antidepressant or dopamine agonists.

Suicidality *

The relationship between antidepressants and suicide (see *C5.15*) seems much clearer, with a pan-Europe study showing a clear inverse correlation between Standardised Death Rate for suicide and Defined Daily Dose antidepressant usage (29 years, 29 countries, Gusmão *et al, PLoS One* 2013;**8**:e66455). There may be a slight rise in the under 25s, probably undiagnosed bipolar depression. In young Swedish people, a comparison of all suicides in the 10–19 age group in 1992–2003 and 2004–2010 (post-EMA warning), suicide in the latter years increased for five consecutive years (60.5% total) and the increase was in individuals not treated with antidepressants (n=845, Isacsson and Ahlner, *Acta Psychiatr Scand* 2013;**129**:296–302; FFT).

Reviews: complementary and alternative medicines (s=185, RCTs, Freeman *et al, J Clin Psychiatry* 2010;**71**:682–8), adolescent depression (Thapar *et al, Br Med J* 2010;**340**:c209).

BNF listed

SELECTIVE SEROTONIN REUPTAKE INHIBITORS (SSRIs) *

SSRIs are first choice antidepressants due to their efficacy, overdose safety and side-effect profile, although their ADR profiles and interaction potential may show clinical differences, as well as efficacy and tolerability differences.

Citalopram

Citalopram is well tolerated from 20–40mg/d but not recommended above 40mg/d due to the alleged QTc prolongation. Cochrane (s=37, RCTs, Cipriani *et al, Cochrane Database Syst Rev* 2012;**7**:CD006534; FFT) concludes that citalopram is more effective than paroxetine and reboxetine, more acceptable than tricyclics, reboxetine and venlafaxine, but less effective than escitalopram (e.g. n=240[c=203], RCT, d/b, 6/52, Ou *et al, Psychopharmacology (Berl)* 2011;**213**:639–46). Relapse prevention has been shown in adults (n=427, RCT, 44–77/52, Hochstrasser *et al, Br J Psychiatry* 2001;**178**:304–10; FFT) and the elderly (n=121, RCT, 48/52, Klysner *et al, Br J Psychiatry* 2002;**181**:29–35).

Reviews: systematic review and meta-analysis (s=8, n=2025, Apler, *Br Med J Open*

2011;1:e000106; FFT), in later life depression (Seitz *et al*, *Int J Geriatr Psychiatry* 2010; **25**:1296–305).

Escitalopram

Escitalopram, the pharmacologically active enantiomer of citalopram (a mix of R- and S-citalopram), is at least twice as potent as citalopram on a mg for mg basis. It binds to the primary serotonin binding site **and** the allosteric site, whereas R-citalopram blocks the allosteric site in a dose-dependent manner, reducing the antidepressant effect on the primary site. The maximum UK dose is 20mg/d (adults) and 10mg (over 65s). The optimal dose in moderate MDD seems to be 10mg/d with 20mg/d the optimum in severe depression (p/c, 8/52, Bech *et al*, *Pharmacopsychiatry* 2006;**39**:128–34). Numerous meta-analyses have shown escitalopram superior to other antidepressants (eg. s=117, n=25,928, RCT, Cipriani *et al*, *Lancet* 2009;**373**:746–58; s=14, Cipriani *et al*, *Cochrane Database Syst Rev* 2009;**2**:CD006532; FFT). Relapse prevention has been shown (n=590[c=437], open, 12/12, Wade *et al*, *Ann Clin Psychiatry* 2006;**18**:83–9; n=139, RCT, d/b, p/c, 52/52, Kornstein *et al*, *J Clin Psychiatry* 2006;**67**:1767–75; MS).

Reviews: * general (Kirino, *Patient Prefer Adherence* 2012;**6**:853–61), enantiomer advantages (Leonard and Taylor, *J Psychopharmacol* 2010;**24**:1143–52; FFT), pharmacogenetics (Blazquez *et al*, *Eur Child Adolesc Psychiatry* 2012;**21**:599–610), comparative review (Sanchez *et al*, *Int Clin Psychopharmacol* 2014;**29**:185–96; MS).

Fluoxetine *

Fluoxetine is licensed for depression, with or without anxiety. Although 20mg/d is the standard dose, some resistant depressions may respond to 60–80mg/d. It is clearly superior to placebo and slightly superior to tricyclics with significantly fewer drop-outs (rigorous meta-analysis, s=30, n=4120, Bech *et al*, *Br J Psychiatry* 2000;**176**:421–8; FFT) with relapse prevention efficacy (n=140, RCT, 48/52, Gilaberte *et al*, *J Clin Psychopharmacol* 2001;**21**:417–24), although an independent review suggested inferior efficacy to other antidepressants (s=131, Cipriani *et al*, *J Clin Psychiatry* 2006;**67**:850–64). Cochrane concludes that the data is uncertain and draws no conclusions (s=171, n=24868, RCTs, Magni *et al*, *Cochrane Database Syst Rev* 2013;**7**:CD004185; FFT).

> **Switching or discontinuing antidepressants**
>
> For a table on switching antidepressants and the gaps needed, or advice on the problems of discontinuing, see *Chapter 2.2.7.*

Fluvoxamine

Recent meta-analyses conclude that there are no significant differences between fluvoxamine and other antidepressants (s=54, n=5122, RCT, Omori *et al*, *Cochrane Database Syst Rev* 2010;**3**:CD006114; FFT), but that it has more G/I ADRs.

Paroxetine *

Paroxetine is licensed for depression, including with comorbid anxiety, with 20mg/d being the optimum dose. Optimum plasma levels of 20–60ng/ml have been suggested (Tomita *et al*, *Ther Drug Monit* 2014;**36**:480–5). Relapse prevention has been shown (n=116, RCT, d/b, p/c, two years, Reynolds *et al*, *N Engl J Med* 2006;**354**:1130–8; FFT). Two meta-analyses are less than enthusiastic, noting only a modest advantage over placebo (s=11, n=unclear, Sugarman *et al*, *PLoS One* 2014;**9**:e106337) and inferior to citalopram and that the studies were at risk of bias (s=115, n=26134, RCTs, a/c, Purgato *et al*, *Cochrane Database Syst Rev* 2014;**4**:CD006531). Paroxetine's half-life increases from 10 to 21 hours on chronic dosing, but reduces when this is stopped, which may in part explain the many reports of discontinuation effects (see 2.2.2).

Review: general (Gibiino and Serretti, *Expert Opin Pharmacother* 2012;**13**:421–31).

Sertraline

Sertraline is similar to fluoxetine but with

TABLE 1.1: THE RATIONALE AND RISKS FOR COMBINATIONS OF ANTIDEPRESSANTS

SS	serotonin syndrome very possible
(SS)	serotonin syndrome possible or rarely reported
SSU	serotonin syndrome unlikely
LR	low rationale
SR	some rationale
HR	high rationale
UR	unknown rationale
LH	relatively low hazard or risk
MH	medium hazard or risk either known or predicted
HH	high hazard or risk of problems known or predicted so specialist monitoring required
UH	unknown or undocumented hazard
SM-LDT	specialist monitoring required and limit dose of tricyclic
VM	consider venlafaxine (>200 mg/d) or mirtazapine instead for combined 5-HT and NA/NE reuptake blockade
CI	see *Chapter 1* for data on positive use of combination
C4/5	see *Chapters 4* or *5* for data on risk of interaction or adverse consequences

	Citalopram/ escitalopram	Fluoxetine	Fluvoxamine	Paroxetine	Sertraline	Tricyclics	MAOIs	Venlafaxine	Mirtazapine	Reboxetine	Trazodone	Duloxetine	Moclobemide	Agomelatine
Fluoxetine	SS LR-HH													
Fluvoxamine	SS LR-HH	SS LR-HH												
Paroxetine	SS LR-HH	SS LR-HH	SS LR-HR											
Sertraline	SS LR-HH	SS-C4/5/5 LR-HH	SS LR-HH	SS LR-HH										
Tricyclics	SS-C4/5 LR-HH-CI	SS-C4/5 LR-HH-CI SM-LDT	SS-C4/5 LR-HH-CI SM-LDT	SS-C4/5 LR-HH-CI SM-LDT	SS-C4/5 LR-HH-CI									
MAOIs	(SS)-C4/5 SR-HH	(SS)-C4/5 SR-HH	(SS)-C4/5 SR-HH	(SS)-C4/5 SR-HH	(SS)-C4/5 SR-HH	(SS) SR-HH-CI								
Venlafaxine	SS LR-HH	SS-C4/5 LR-HH	SS LR-HH	SS MR-HH-CI	SS-C4/5 LR-HH	SS LR-HH	SS-C4/5 SR-HH							
Mirtazapine	SSU LR-UH	(SS) LR-UH	SSU LR-UH	SSU C4/5 LR/LH	SSU C4/5 LR-LH	SSU C4/5 LR-LH	SSU C4/5 SR-MH	SSU HR-LH						
Reboxetine	SSU SR-UH VM	SSU SR-UH VM	SSU SR-UH VM	SSU SR-UH VM	SSU SR-UH VM	SSU C4/5 LR-MH	SSU C4/5 LR-HH	SSU LR-UH	SSU MR-UH					
Trazodone	SS LR-UH	SS-C4/5 LR-MH	SS- C4/5 LR-UH	SS LR-UH	SS LR-UH	(SS) SR-MH	(SS)-C4/5 SR-HH	SS LR-HH	SSU SR-UH	SSU SR-UH VM				
Duloxetine	SS LR-HH	SS LR-MH	SS LR-HH	SS LR-HH	(SS) LR-HH	(SS)-C4 SR-LH	(SS)-C4 SR-HH	SS LR-HH	SSU SR-UH	SSU SR-UH VM	SS LR-HH			
Moclobemide	(SS)-C4/5 SR-MH	(SS)-C4/5 SR-LH	(SS)-C4/5 SR-MH	(SS)-C4/5 SR-MH	(SS) SR-MH	(SS0-C4/5 SR-HH	(SS) LR-HH	(SS)-C4/5 SR-HH	SSU SR-UH	SSU SR-UH	(SS) SR-UH	(SS) SR-UH		
Agomelatine	SSU HR-LH	SSU HR-LH	SSU HR-MH	SSU HR-LH	SSU HR-LH	SSU HR-LH	SSU HR-LH	SSU HR-LH	SSU HR-LH	SSU HR-LH	SSU HR-LH	SSU HR-LH	SSU HR-LH	
Tryptophan	(SS)-C4/5 UR-MH	(SS)-C4/5 UR-MH	(SS)-C4/5 UR-MH	(SS)-C4/5 UR-MH	(SS)-C4/5 UR-MH	(SS)-C4/5 UR-MH	(SS)-C4/5 UR-MH	(SS) UR-MH	SSU UR-LH	SSU UR-LH	(SS) UR-MH	(SS) UR-MH	SSU UR-MH	SSU UR-LH

a shorter half-life. In recurrent depression (≥3 episodes of MDD in four years), sertraline 50 mg/d and 100 mg/d have shown relapse prevention efficacy (n = 371, RCT, p/c, d/b, 18/12, Lépine *et al*, *Am J Psychiatry* 2004;**161**:836–42), but not in the elderly (n = 113[c = 31], RCT, d/b, p/c, two years, Wilson *et al*, *Br J Psychiatry* 2003;**182**:492–7; MS;FFT). The Cipriani meta-analysis concludes sertraline is the best antidepressant due to the most favourable balance between benefits, acceptability and acquisition costs (s = 117, n = 25,928, RCT, Cipriani *et al*, *Lancet* 2009;**373**:746–58).

Review: pharmacokinetic profile (DeVane *et al*, *Clin Pharmacokinet* 2002;**41**:1247–66).

TRICYCLICS

Doses of 125–150 mg/d of tricyclics are effective in depression and clearly superior to placebo but due to cardiac and overdose toxicity, sedation and anticholinergic effects, are not recommended first-line. In the UK, NICE recommends an ECG before prescribing tricyclics in people at significant risk of cardiovascular disease. If using tricyclics, a therapeutic dose must be used before assessing the response.

Review: toxicity (Nutt, *J Psychopharmacol* 2005;**19**:123–4).

Amitriptyline *

Cochrane concludes that amitriptyline is at least as effective as other antidepressants, but with a higher side-effect burden (s = 39, n = 3509, < 12/52, Leucht *et al*, *Cochrane Database Syst Rev* 2013;**12**:CD009138).

Clomipramine

Clomipramine is a predominantly serotonergic tricyclic with an active metabolite, often used for depression with an obsessional component.

Dosulepin (dothiepin)

Dosulepin is toxic in overdose and NICE recommends it is not prescribed. Although often used to aid sleep, dosulepin disrupts REM sleep with no sleep-promoting effects (n = 12, RCT, 5/52, d/b, p/c, Wilson *et al*, *J Psychopharmacol* 2002;**16**:321–31).

Doxepin

Doxepin is a standard tricyclic with moderate sedation, with fewer anticholinergic and cardiac effects than older tricyclics.

Imipramine

Imipramine is a standard tricyclic. It may provoke fragmentation of motor activity during sleep (n = 52, Volkers *et al*, *Eur Neuropsychopharm* 2002;**12**:273–8).

Lofepramine

Lofepramine is NICE's tricyclic of choice, and may have slightly less ADRs than other tricyclics. It is surprisingly safe in overdose, appearing to block the cardiotoxic effects of the main metabolite desipramine (Lancaster and Gonzalez, *Drugs* 1989;**37**:123–40).

Nortriptyline

Nortriptyline has low cardiotoxic side-effects. In TRD (failing 1–5 adequate trials), 40% may respond (12% remission), although 35% may not tolerate it (n = 116, RCT, 12/52, Mulsant *et al*, *Am J Geriatr Psychiatry* 2001;**9**:406–14).

Trimipramine

Trimipramine is structurally related to levomepromazine and has significant sedative properties. High doses (up to 400 mg/d) may be effective for delusional depression (n = 94[c = 57], RCT, d/b, p/c, 6/52, Künzel *et al*, *J Psychiatr Res* 2009;**43**:702–10).

OTHER ANTIDEPRESSANTS

Agomelatine *

Agomelatine is a 5HT2C and 5HT2B antagonist and a melatonin M1 and M2 agonist. The effective dose is 25–50 mg/d (10 mg/d is the minimum: n = 549, RCT, p/c, 6/52, Kennedy *et al*, *Eur Neuropsychopharmacol* 2014;**24**:553–63), with 80% of responders taking 25 mg/d (n = 21, RCT, d/b, p/c, 6/52, Kennedy and Emsley, *Eur Neuropsychopharmacol* 2006;**16**:93–100). Meta-analysis of published and unpublished studies shows agomelatine has similar efficacy to standard antidepressants, but did not analyse for ADRs (s = 20, n = 7460, RCT, d/b, p/c or a/c, Taylor *et al*, *Br Med J* 2014;**348**:g1888). However, a pooled analysis of all the head-to-head studies of agomelatine (vs. venlafaxine, sertraline, fluoxetine, paroxetine or escitalopram) showed agomelatine significantly superior to SSRIs/SNRI on HAM-D and CGI, including in severe depression (s=6, RCT, d/b, Kasper *et al, Int Clin Psychopharmacol* 2013;**28**:12–9) and with fewer drop-outs due to ADRs (s=13, n=4495, RCT, Guaiana *et al, Cochrane Database Syst Rev* 2013;**12**:CD008851; s=6, n=1871, RCT, Huang *et al, Aust N Z J Psychiatry* 2014;**48**:663–71), with no sexual side-effects, improved sleep (n=303, RCT, d/b, 6/52, Kasper *et al, J Clin Psychiatry* 2010;**71**:109–20), and with no withdrawal or rebound effects. It appears to be effective also in realistic naturalistic studies in TRD (n=110, Sparshatt *et al, Acta Psychiatr Scand* 2013;**128**:203–11) and the elderly and severely depressed (n=3317, open, 12/52, Laux *et al, Pharmacopsychiatry* 2013;**45**:284–91). Transient aminotransferase elevations can be seen at the higher dose (n=511, RCT, d/b, p/c, 8/52, Zajecka *et al, J Clin Psychopharmacol* 2010;**30**:135–44) and so precautionary LFTs are required at 0, 3, 6, 12 and 24 weeks.

Reviews: * general (Smeraldi and Delmonte, *Expert Opin Drug Saf* 2013;**12**:873–80; MacIsaac *et al, Expert Opin Pharmacother* 2014; **15**:259–74 Pae, *Expert Opin Pharmacother* 2014;**15**:443–7), meta-analysis (s=9, n= 3943, Singh *et al, Int J Neuropsychopharmacol* 2012; **15**:417–28), mode of action (Stahl, *CNS Spectr* 2014;**19**:207–12; Guardiola-Lemaitre *et al, Br J Pharmacol* 2014;**171**:3604–19), efficacy and tolerability (Plesnicar, *Patient Prefer Adherence* 2014;**8**:603–12).

Duloxetine

Duloxetine is an SNRI that also weakly inhibits dopamine reuptake, but with no histamine, dopamine, cholinergic or adrenergic receptor affinity. The standard dose is 60mg/d (but starting at a lower dose may improve tolerability; s=6, n=1619, d/b, p/c, Pritchett *et al, J Psychiatr Res* 2007;**41**:311–8). Follow-on studies show relapse prevention efficacy (e.g. n=288, RCT, d/b, p/c, <52/52, Perahia *et al, J Clin Psychiatry* 2009;**70**:706–16). Cochrane concludes that duloxetine has no advantages over other antidepressants and was less effective and tolerable than most SSRIs and venlafaxine, albeit with insufficient studies (s=16, n=5735, RCTs, Cipriani *et al, Cochrane Database Syst Rev* 2012;**10**:CD006533).

Reviews: general (Bochsler *et al, Expert Rev Neurother* 2011;**11**:1525–39), in MDD (Monteleone *et al, Cent Nerv Syst Agents Med Chem* 2011;**11**:174–83), kinetics and interactions (Knadler *et al, Clin Pharmacokinet* 2011;**50**:281–94).

> **Switching or discontinuing antidepressants**
>
> For a table on switching antidepressants and the gaps needed, or advice on the problems of discontinuing, see *Chapter 2.2.7*.

Flupentixol

The standard initial dosage is 1mg as a single morning dose, which can be increased to 2mg/d (maximum 3mg/d) if there is inadequate clinical response. The effect is probably mainly as an anxiolytic.

Mianserin

Mianserin is a tetracyclic with marked $5HT_{2A}$ and $5HT_{2C}$ antagonism, safety in overdose, low cardiotoxicity and marked sedation.

Mirtazapine

Mirtazapine blocks presynaptic alpha-2 adreno-receptors (increasing noradrenaline transmission) and indirectly enhances serotonergic transmission, with additional $5\text{-}HT_2$ and $5\text{-}HT_3$ receptor blockade minimising the incidence of serotoninergic side-effects, e.g. nausea, headache and sexual dysfunction. The optimum starting dose of 30mg/d is well tolerated and less sedating than 15mg/d. Cochrane concludes that it may be clinically superior to SSRIs and venlafaxine in terms of onset of action at two weeks and after six weeks, albeit with a unique ADR profile (eg. s=29, n=4974, RCTs, Watanabe *et al, Cochrane Database Syst Rev* 2011;**12**:CD006528; FFT). Relapse prevention is significantly superior to placebo (n=156, RCT, d/b, 40/52, Thase *et al, J Clin Psychiatry* 2001;**62**:782–8).

Reviews: * general (Alam *et al, Prim Care Companion CNS Disord* 2013;**15**:13r01525; Benjamin and Doraiswamy, *Expert Opin Pharmacother* 2011;**12**:1623–32), ADRs (Watanabe *et al, CNS Drugs* 2010;**24**:35–53).

Moclobemide

Moclobemide (a Reversible Inhibitor of Monoamine oxidase-A) inhibits only MAO-A (not MAO-B), so an excess of tyramine in the body will displace moclobemide from MAO-A, allowing tyramine metabolism to occur, MAO-B remaining free. This results in a 'cheese-reaction' usually only at amounts above 100–150mg of tyramine (see *4.3.4*), unlikely under normal conditions. A meta-analysis showed it to be about equipotent with reference antidepressants in agitated-anxious depressive patients, and superior to placebo (s=38, n=2416, d/b, Delini-Stula *et al, J Affect Disord* 1995;**35**:21–30). Moclobemide appears to be benign even in massive overdose (n=106, Isbister *et al, Br J Clin Pharmacol* 2003;**56**:441–50; FFT).

Reboxetine

Reboxetine is a selective noradrenaline re-uptake inhibitor with no other significant effects at 8mg/d. Efficacy has been shown vs. placebo in severe depression (s=4, RCT, d/b, p/c, 8/52, Montgomery *et al, J Clin Psychopharmacol* 2003;**23**:45–50), but a more recent scathing report suggested that as 74% of patient data was not published, the studies *en masse* do not show reboxetine to be effective, rather that it is inferior to SSRIs and possibly harmful cf. placebo. While early dose-finding studies are often inconclusive, this does lend credence to the clinical impression, i.e. 'it isn't much cop' (s=13, n=4098, p/c, Eyding *et al, Br Med J* 2010;**341**:c4737; FFT).

Selegiline transdermal *

Emsam® transdermal patches are licensed in the UK for use in TRD on a named-patient basis. Efficacy has been shown in acute depression (response NNT=11, remission NNT=9; s=5, 6-8/52, Citrome *et al, J Affect Disord* 2013;**151**:409–17) and relapse prevention (n=322, RCT, d/b, p/c, 52/52, Jang *et al, J Affect Disord* 2013;**151**:854–9), but a high placebo response confused the adolescent study (n=308[c=205], d/b, p/c, RCT, DelBello *et al, J Child Adolesc Psychopharmacol* 2014;**24**:311–7). The transdermal route allows higher doses than possible orally, with no need for dietary restrictions (eg. n=289, d/b, p/c, 8/52, Amsterdam, *J Clin Psychiatry* 2003;**64**:208–14).

Trazodone *

Trazodone (enthusiastic review, Fagiolini *et al, CNS Drugs* 2012;**26**:1033–49) increases NA and 5-HT turnover with low cardiotoxicity and anticholinergic side-effects, but a higher risk of drowsiness and nausea. Trazodone 300–350mg/d is more effective than placebo (n=412, RCT, d/b, p/c, 8/52, Sheehan *et al, Psychiatry (Edgmont)* 2009;**6**:20–33; FFT). It is best taken with food to reduce peak blood levels (review of off-licensed use, Bossini *et al, Expert Opin Pharmacother* 2012;**13**:1707–17).

Venlafaxine

Venlafaxine is an SNRI with 5-HT reuptake inhibition across the dosage range, NA reuptake inhibition becoming significant from 150mg/d and dopamine reuptake inhibition above 225mg/d. This may lead to a dose-response relationship with greater efficacy at higher doses (e.g. s=32, Smith *et al, Br J Psychiatry* 2002;**180**:396–404; FFT), including up to 375mg/d (n=96, retrospective, Vanoli *et al, J Psychopharmacol* 2008;**22**:434–40). A meta-analysis of all data (including unpublished) concludes that venlafaxine is a valid alternative for SSRI/TCA non-responders, rather than a first-line choice (s=56, n=13652, RCTs, Schueler *et al, Acta Psychiatr Scand* 2011;**123**:247–65), with a greater effect on remission in more severe depression (s=31, n=6492, Schmitt *et al, Eur Arch Psychiatry Clin Neurosci* 2009;**259**:329–39). In head-to-head studies, venlafaxine was superior to SSRIs for response and remission, but had higher drop-outs (s=26, n=5858, RCT, d/b, de Silva and Hanwella, *Int Clin Psychopharmacol* 2012;**27**:8–16). Relapse prevention has been shown in prior responders to venlafaxine over two years in the PREVENT studies (review, s=2, n=1354, by Kornsten, *Expert Rev Neurother* 2008;**8**:737–42).

The UK MHRA recommendations on venlafaxine are that it is:

- still to be reserved as second-line treatment
- only contraindicated in people with an identified high risk of a serious cardiac ventricular arrhythmia or with uncontrolled hypertension. No baseline ECG is needed, but regular bp is recommended.

The higher overdose toxicity with venlafaxine may be due to increased use in people at higher risk of suicide (including TRD), e.g. venlafaxine (n=27096) patients were 4–6 times more likely to have been previously hospitalised for depression than patients on fluoxetine (n=134996) or citalopram (n=52035) (n=214127, Mines *et al*, *Pharmacoepidemiol Drug Saf* 2005;**14**:367–72, MS). Discontinuation effects may be significant (*2.2.6*).

Reviews: venlafaxine vs. duloxetine (s=54, n=18180, Schueler *et al*, *Acta Psychiatr Scand* 2011;**123**:247–65).

Vortioxetine *

Vortioxetine is a new antidepressant with potent serotonin reuptake inhibition plus 5-HT3, 5-HT7 and 5-HT1D antagonism, 5-HT 1B partial agonism and 5-HT 1A agonism. In a unique Single Technology Appraisal, NICE approved its use as a third-line antidepressant in the UK. The standard starting dose is 10mg/d in the under 65s (5mg/d in the over 65s), which can then go to 5–20mg/d.

Efficacy: Two meta-analyses show vortioxetine is significantly more effective than placebo, with low drop-outs due to ADRs or lack of efficacy (s=12, RCT, d/b, p/c, 6–12/52, Pae *et al*, *J Psychiatry Neurosci* 2014;**39**:140129; FFT; s=11, n=6145, RCTs, <8/52, Meeker *et al*, *Syst Rev* 2015;**4**:21; FFT). It is at least as effective as venlafaxine (n=424, RCT, d/b, a/c, Wang *et al*, *Curr Med Res Opin* 2015;**31**:785–94). More recent studies show efficacy vs. placebo in duloxetine-validated studies (n=604, RCT, d/b, p/c-a/c, 8/52, Boulenger *et al*, *Int Clin Psychopharmacol* 2014;**29**:138–49; FFT; n=614, RCT, d/b, p/c-a/c, 8/52, Mahableshwarkar *et al*, *Psychopharmacology [Berl]* 2015;**232**:2061–70; FFT). Lack of weight gain, metabolic, cardiac and sexual effects and meaningfully improved cognitive functioning (at 5–15mg) give vortioxetine a significant potential role (Al-Sukhni *et al*, *Expert Opin Drug Saf* 2015;**14**:1291–304; Alvarez *et al*, *Neuropsychiatr Dis Treat* 2014;**10**:1297–307; FFT).

Cognition: Vortioxetine significantly improves cognitive functioning (RCT, d/b, p/c-a/c, 8/52, Mahableshwarkar *et al*, *Neuropsychopharmacology* 2015;**40**:2025–37), with a beneficial objective and subjective effect on cognition that is statistically significant and a direct effect of the molecule as it is largely independent of the antidepressant effect (n=602, RCT, d/b, p/c, 8/52, McIntyre *et al*, *Int J Neuropsychopharmacol* 2014;**17**:1557–67; FFT). There are no negative effects on driving or cognitive functioning (n=24, d/b, p/c-a/c, c/o, 3x15/7, Theunissen *et al*, *Clin Pharmacol Ther* 2013;**93**:493–501). Efficacy over one year has been shown (n=1073[c=538], open, 12/52, Jacobsen *et al*, *Int Clin Psychopharmacol* 2015;**30**:255–64; FFT).

Reviews * general (Kelliny *et al*, *Ther Clin Risk Manag* 2015;**11**:1193–212; FFT; Schatzberg *et al*, *J Clin Psychiatry* 2014;**75**:1411–8; FFT), cognitive symptoms (Al-Sukhni *et al*, *Expert Opin Drug Saf* 2015;**14**:1291–304), Acute treatment (systematic review and meta-analysis, Meeker *et al*, *Syst Rev* 2015;**4**:21; FFT), FDA review (Thase, *J Clin Psychiatry* 2015;**76**:e120–1; FFT).

MONOAMINE OXIDASE INHIBITORS (MAOIs)

Reviews: * use in primary care (Culpepper, *J Clin Psychiatry* 2012;**73**[Suppl 1]:37–41), general (Shulman *et al*, *CNS Drugs* 2013;**27**;789–97), efficacy in TRD (n=150, Fekadu *et al*, *Br J Psychiatry* 2012;**201**:369–75).

Isocarboxazid

Isocarboxazid is a hydrazine derivative that irreversibly blocks the MAO enzyme (editorial by Shader and Greenblatt, *J Clin Psychopharmacol* 1999;**19**:105–6).

Phenelzine

Phenelzine is a hydrazine derivative that irreversibly blocks the MAO enzyme, and is NICE's MAOI of choice, although they recommend that it is only initiated by specialist mental health professionals (including GPs with a special interest in mental health). A comparison of tranylcypromine and phenelzine showed no significant difference between them, with a 52% response rate in severe TRD (n=77[c=67], d/b, 5/52, Birkenhäger *et al*, *J Clin Psychiatry* 2004;**65**:1505–10).

Tranylcypromine

Tranylcypromine is a non-hydrazine amfetamine-related MAOI with stimulant effects and a greater incidence of adverse drug interactions. Tranylcypromine did poorly in TRD in the STAR*D study (n=109, open, McGrath *et al, Am J Psychiatry* 2006;**163**:1531–41), although the mean dose was only 37 mg/d (doses towards 100 mg/d or more may be much more effective, and a mean 52 mg/d produced a 59% remission rate in TRD; n=32, Adli *et al, Pharmacopsychiatry* 2008;**41**:252–7), more patients were switched because of previous medication intolerance and the 2/52 washout/lead-in would have led to shorter treatment duration.

OTHER ANTIDEPRESSANTS

Lithium (see also combinations) *

Lithium monotherapy in the treatment and prophylaxis of unipolar (as well as bipolar) depression is well-established and associated with lower mortality, e.g. in unipolar depression lithium reduces suicides (OR 0.36) and deaths from any cause (OR=0.13) (s=48, n=6674, Cipriani *et al, Br Med J* 2013;**346**:f3646), with an 88% risk reduction (s=8, n=329, 4–5 years, Guzzetta *et al, J Clin Psychiatry* 2007;**68**:380–3). Some antidepressant response to lithium is probably mood stabilisation in undiagnosed bipolar depression (Faedda *et al, Am J Psychiatry* 2001;**158**:1337–9). Cochrane concludes that lithium is effective for relapse-prevention of long-term unipolar depression (s=8, n=475, Cipriani *et al, Cochrane Database Syst Rev* 2006;**4**:CD003492).

Reviews: lithium augmentation and bipolarity (Inoue *et al, J Affect Disord* 2011;**129**:64–7), in depression (Bschor, *Drugs* 2014;**74**:855-62), predictors of efficacy (Sugawara *et al, J Affect Disord* 2010;**125**:165–8), long-term outcomes (Adli *et al, Neuropsychobiology* 2009;**60**:23–30). See main entry under bipolar mood disorder (*1.10*) and bipolar depression (*1.10.3*).

Tryptophan (discontinued in UK) *

Tryptophan is a naturally occurring amino acid and precursor to serotonin and has been used in combination with other antidepressants. Meta-analysis has shown good evidence for reduced plasma tryptophan levels in people with MDD, particularly so if untreated (s=25, n=1716, Ogawa *et al, J Clin Psychiatry* 2014;**75**:e906–15) and Cochrane concludes that the trial data is limited and unreliable, but suggests tryptophan may be superior to placebo (s=2, n=64, Shaw *et al, Cochrane Database Syst Rev* 2002;**1**:CD003198) and may be as effective as fluoxetine (n=70[c=60], RCT, a/c, 8/52, Jangid *et al, Asian J Psychiatr* 2013;**6**:29–34).

+ Combinations (of drugs with some intrinsic antidepressant activity)

Adding a second antidepressant to an ineffective first has little evidence to support it (s=5, n=483, d/b, p/c, Lopes Rocha *et al, J Affect Disord* 2013;**144**:1–6), but in partial response there may be some advantage for combined NA and 5-HT reuptake blocking drugs, which can produce a quicker effect. It could, however, be that this produces higher success rates by treating different depressive subgroups. It might even be better to start with combined antidepressants from the start, e.g. remission rates were higher with mirtazapine + venlafaxine (58%), mirtazapine + fluoxetine (52%) and mirtazapine + bupropion 150 mg/d than fluoxetine (25%) (n=105, RCT, d/b, 6/52, Blier *et al, Am J Psychiatry* 2010;**167**:281–8).

Reviews: general (Connolly and Thase, *Drugs* 2011;**71**:43–64) strategies for combination and augmentation for depression (Carvalho *et al, Curr Opin Psychiatry* 2009;**22**:7–12).

Agomelatine + bupropion *

A 60% remission rate in TRD with the combination compared favourably to a 40% response with monotherapy, an impressive NNT of 4 (n=30, open, Sühs *et al, Brain Behav* 2015;**5**:e00318; FFT).

Bupropion + SSRIs/SNRIs/MAOIs *

Bupropion 200–300 mg/d may be very effective as augmentation in partial response to SSRIs (n=60, RCT, s/b, p/c, 4/52, Gulrez *et al, Basic Clin Pharmacol Toxicol* 2012;**110**:227–30). Addition of bupropion 150–300mg/d in **escitalopram** non-responders improved response cf bupropion monotherapy (n=135, open, 18/52, Maron *et al, J Clin Psychiatry* 2009;**70**:1054–6). In TRD with atypical features, **duloxetine** plus bupropion had no advantage over bupropion monotherapy (n=46, RCT, d/b, p/c, 6/52, Fornaro *et al, Eur Neuropsychopharmacol* 2014;**24**:1269-78). Bupropion and **tranylcypromine** has been successful for TRD (eg. n=2, Quante and Zeugmann, *J Clin Psychopharmacol* 2012; **32**:572–4).

Lithium + antidepressants *

In TRD, the best evidence is for augmentation with lithium, e.g. there is an NNT of 5 for response (s=30, n>500, open; s=10, n=269, RCT, d/b, p/c, Bauer *et al, Neuropsychobiology* 2010;**62**:36–42; FFT), a substantial effect with SSRIs, mostly within 1–2 weeks (review by Zullino and Baumann, *Pharmacopsychiatry* 2001;**34**:119–27), maintained for 6/12 (n=30, RCT, d/b, p/c, 6/52, open 4/12 extension, Bauer *et al, Am J Psychiatry* 2000;**157**:1429–35), as well as having an anti-suicidal effect in MDD (n=167, Lauterbach *et al, Acta Psychiatr Scand* 2008;**118**:469–79). Predictors of efficacy include being bipolar, >3 previous MDDs and a family history of MDD/bipolar in a first-degree relative (n=79, 8/52, Sugawara *J Affect Disord* 2010;**125**:165–8). So, lithium works in bipolar depression, even if it has not been diagnosed.

Review: * review (s=10, RCT, p/c, Bauer *et al, CNS Drugs* 2014;**28**:331–42).

Lithium + tryptophan + antidepressants (eg. clomipramine, SSRI or phenelzine)

There have been reports of 55% remission rates in severe depression, eg. from:

- clomipramine (150–300mg/d) or an SSRI to tolerance *plus*
- tryptophan (2–4g/d) *plus*
- lithium (standard levels).

Alternatives to clomipramine include phenelzine and the SSRIs. Tryptophan enhances the action of SSRIs on 5-HT sites and improves 5-HT absorption. Lithium also affects 5-HT and is effective in bipolar depression.

Mirtazapine + venlafaxine/SSRIs

In persistent MDD, addition of mirtazapine to existing therapy produced a response rate of 64% cf. 20% with placebo (n=26, RCT, d/b, p/c, 4/52, Carpenter *et al, Biol Psychiatry* 2002; **51**:183–88). Mirtazapine has also been used with high-dose venlafaxine to block 5HT2 and 5HT3 receptors, reducing sexual and anxiety side-effects from venlafaxine, and allowing higher doses to be tolerated. The combination might have been under-rated in STAR*D phase 4 because the QIDS score was actually 23.5% vs only 12.1% for tranylcypromine. A retrospective study showed response rates of 50% at 8/52, and 56% at 6/12, with mirtazapine ADRs predominant (n=32, Hannan *et al, J Psychopharmacol* 2007;**21**:161–4).

Reboxetine + duloxetine

In duloxetine-resistant depression, addition of reboxetine produced an impressive 70% remission rate (n=79[c=71], open, 12/52, Seguí *et al, J Psychopharmacol* 2010;**24**:1201–7).

Reboxetine + mirtazapine

Addition of reboxetine in mirtazapine-resistant depression may be an effective strategy (n=14, 12/52, Lopez-Munoz *et al, Clin Neuropharmacol* 2006;**29**:192–6).

Reboxetine + SSRIs

This logical combination has been used successfully, e.g. reboxetine added to SSRI/mirtazapine/venlafaxine partial or non-responders has produced a well-tolerated improvement (n=61, open, 6/52, Rubio *et al, J Affect Disord* 2004;**81**:67–72), escitalopram and reboxetine may provide a rapid response (n=3, Camarasa *et al, Prog Neuropsychopharmacol Biol Psychiatry* 2005; **29**:165–8), and addition of reboxetine in SSRI-resistant depression has produced 50% response and 34% remission rates, but we still await RCTs to confirm this effect (n=141, open, 12/52, López-Muñoz *et al, Pharmacopsychiatry* 2007;**40**:14–9).

SSRIs + SSRIs

Although there are anecdotal reports of success, the combination cannot be recommended and risks serotonin syndrome.

Tricyclics + MAOIs

Although **extreme** caution is advised, the combination has been effective in some TRDs, e.g. isocarboxazid plus amitriptyline (n=25, open, Berlanga and Ortega-Soto, *J Affect Disord* 1995;**34**:187–92). Tranylcypromine plus clomipramine is known to be dangerous (at least two deaths). Most problems occur when a tricyclic is added to an MAOI rather than vice versa. Separate doses (e.g. MAOI in the morning, tricyclic in the evening), add one to the other in low dose and build up slowly, or stop all antidepressants, wait a week, and start both together at low dose and build up again.

Tricyclics + SSRIs

High dose fluoxetine (60 mg/d) appears more effective in partial or non-responders to 20 mg/d than a fluoxetine/desipramine combination (n=41, RCT, d/b, 4/52, Fava *et al*, *Am J Psychiatry* 1994;**151**:1372–4). Avoid the combination due to the high risk of an adverse interaction (*4.3.2*).

Venlafaxine + agomelatine *

The combination has been successfully used (n=1, DaHale *et al*, *Gen Hosp Psychiatry* 2014;**36**:e3).

Venlafaxine + SSRIs

SSRIs have been used successfully to augment venlafaxine (n=4, Gonul *et al*, *Prog Neuro-psychopharmacol Biol Psychiatry* 2003;**27**:889–91), but the combination is not recommended.

• Adjuncts/unlicensed/some efficacy

A systematic review and meta-analysis concludes that adjunctive quetiapine (OR=1.92), aripiprazole (OR=1.85), thyroid (OR=1.84) or lithium (OR=1.56) are significantly more effective than placebo (s=48, n=6654, RCTs, p/c, Zhou *et al*, *J Clin Psychiatry* 2015;**76**:e487–98).

Antiglucocorticoids eg. metyrapone + TAU*

Adjunct: Cochrane concludes there is no advantage for antiglucocorticoids over placebo (s=9, RCTs, Gallagher *et al*, *Cochrane Database Syst Rev* 2008;**1**:CD005168). Metyrapone has been used (review by Sigalas *et al*, *Ther Adv Psychopharmacol* 2012;**2**:139–49; FFT).

Antipsychotics ± antidepressants *

Aripiprazole (OR=2.01), quetiapine (OR=1.79) and risperidone (OR=2.37) seem to be effective in psychotic depression (s=14, RCT, Spielmans *et al*, *PLoS Med* 2013;**10**:e1001403, with olanzapine and risperidone showing some promise (s=28, n=8487, RCT, d/b, Komossa *et al*, *Cochrane Database Syst Rev* 2010;**12**:CD008121).

Aripiprazole:

Adjunct: Aripiprazole is approved in US as add-on to antidepressants for adults with MDD, but a monotherapy license would require longer-term studies. There are many RCTs showing a modest effect as an adjunct to SSRIs or venlafaxine at 2.5–5 mg/d with a quicker and clinically meaningful response in TRD with NNT=6 for response and NNT=8 for remission (s=3, n=1038, RCT, d/b, p/c, 6/52, Nelson *et al*, *Int Clin Psychopharmacol* 2012;**27**:125–33), especially if symptoms worsened during antidepressant monotherapy (s=3, n=1065, RCT, d/b, p/c, 6/52, Nelson *et al*, *CNS Spectr* 2014;**19**:528–34; FFT; same data Stewart *et al*, *J Affect Disord* 2014;**162**:20–5). Lack of improvement at two weeks significantly predicts lack of remission (s=3, RCT, d/b, 8/52, Muzina *et al*, *Am J Manag Care* 2011;**17**:793–801;FFT), and a clinically meaningful response at two weeks predicts response at 6/52 (s=3, n=1064, RCT, n=4, d/b, p/c, 6/52, Casey *et al*, *Prim Care Companion CNS Disord* 2012;**13**:11m01251) In a huge trial of TRD with high drop-outs, adjunctive aripiprazole mean 10 mg/d produced 70% remission in the completers (n=1002[c=323], open, <52/52, Berman *et al*, *Neuropsychiatr Dis Treat* 2011;**7**:303–12; FFT; n=225, RCT, 8/52, Fava *et al*, *Psychother Psychosom* 2012;**81**:87–97)

Amisulpride:

Monotherapy: 50 mg/d may have antidepressant activity comparable with fluoxetine 20 mg/d, (n=281, d/b, Smeraldi, *J Affect Disord* 1998;**48**:47–56), paroxetine 20 mg/d (n=272, RCT, d/b, 56/7, Cassano *et al*, *Int Clin Psychopharmacol* 2002;**17**:27–32) and for psychotic depression in the elderly (n=11, Politis *et al*, *Prog Neuropsychopharmacol Biol Psychiatry* 2008;**32**:1227–30).

Clozapine has been used as an adjunct in

refractory psychotic depression (n=1, Dassa *et al, Br J Psychiatry* 1993;**163**:822–4).

Olanzapine-fluoxetine * **(OFC):**
This is licensed in US for treatment-resistant unipolar and bipolar depression. A pooled analysis showed OFC superior to fluoxetine or olanzapine individually, and that absence of early improvement is highly predictive of overall response failure (s=5, Tohen *et al, J Clin Psychiatry* 2010;**71**:451–62). Olanzapine plus sertraline improved psychotic depression better than olanzapine alone, suggesting that olanzapine monotherapy may not be a potent antidepressant (n=259, RCT, d/b, p/c, 12/52, Meyers *et al, Arch Gen Psychiatry* 2009;**66**:838–47; FFT). In TRD, OFC-responders increased the time to relapse over 27/52 compared to fluoxetine monotherapy, at the cost of weight gain and metabolic changes (n=444, RCT, 47/52, 27/52, Brunner *et al, Neuropsychopharmacology* 2014;**39**:2549–59; MS; FFT). Adjunctive olanzapine does not improve slow-wave sleep but may improve sleep continuity and depression (n=25, RCT, d/b, p/c, 35/7, Lazowski *et al, BMC Psychiatry* 2014;**14**:202).

Review: * safety of OFC (Cristancho and Thase, *Expert Opin Drug Saf* 2014;**13**:1133–41).

Perphenazine added to a tricyclic did not improve efficacy in psychotic depression (n=36, RCT, d/b, 4/52, Mulsant *et al, J Clin Psychiatry* 2001;**62**:597–604).

Quetiapine:
Adjunct: Quetiapine XL is licensed in US and Europe (review by Connolly and Thase, *Drugs* 2011;**71**:43–64) for adjunctive treatment in sub-optimal response to antidepressant monotherapy. Adding quetiapine to citalopram was almost statistically significant superior to placebo (n=41, RCT, d/b, p/c, 6/52, Quante *et al, Psychiatr Danub* 2013;**25**:214–20) and improved sleep disturbance and quality cf. placebo in TRD (s=2, n=919, RCT, d/b, p/c, 6/52, Bauer *et al, Int J Neuropsychopharmacol* 2013;**16**:1755–65).
Monotherapy: A meta-analysis of quetiapine monotherapy in depression concludes that quetiapine XL 300mg/d (but not 150mg/d; s=2, RCT, d/b, p/c, 6/52, Sanford, *CNS Drugs* 2011;**25**:803–13) is effective in 4/7 (s=3, n=1497, RCTs, p/c, Maneeton *et al, BMC Psychiatry* 2012;**12**:160; FFT). Quetiapine monotherapy improves sleep disturbance cf. placebo in MDD (s=4, n=1379, RCTs, 6–8/52, Trivedi *et al, Int J Neuropsychopharmacol* 2013;**16**:1733–44). Maintenance monotherapy reduces relapse by 66% (n=776, RCT, d/b, p/c, 12/12, Liebowitz *et al, Depress Anxiety* 2010;**27**:964–76).

Risperidone:
Adjunct: 1–2mg/d augmentation of sub-optimally effective antidepressants has increased response and remission (n=274, RCT, d/b, p/c, 6/52, Mahmoud *et al, Ann Intern Med* 2007;**147**:593–602; comment by Barbee, EBMH 2008;**11**:77). In non-psychotic, unipolar TRD, add-on risperidone 0.5–3mg/d produced more rapid response and higher remission rates (n=97, RCT, d/b, p/c, 4/52, Keitner *et al, J Psychiatr Res* 2009;**43**:205–14; FFT).

Sulpiride 100mg/d may accelerate the antidepressant effect of paroxetine 10–40mg/d (n=41 [c=33], RCT, open, 12/52, Uchida *et al, J Clin Psychopharmacol* 2005;**25**:545–51).

Ziprasidone has been used as augmentation in SSRI-resistance (n=64, RCT, open, 6/52, Dunner *et al, J Clin Psychiatry* 2007;**68**:1071–7).

Reviews: * in TRD (Kato and Chang, *CNS Drugs* 2013;**27**[Suppl 1];S11–9), general (Han *et al, Expert Rev Neurother* 2013;**13**:851–70).

Benzodiazepines ± TAU *

Adjunct: Cochrane concludes that BDZ augmentation of antidepressants, e.g. **clonazepam** (optimum dose 2.5–6mg/d, response takes 2–4 weeks; Morishita, *Hum Psychopharmacol* 2009;**24**:191–8) leads to fewer drop-outs and less depression severity at 1–4 weeks, but the effect disappears at 6–8 weeks. Thus, short-term use may be successful, possibly by minimising initial SSRI side-effects (e.g. anxiety), improving sleep, or a direct action (s=9, n=679, Furukawa *et al, Cochrane Database Syst Rev* 2002;**1**:CD001026). Predictors of response include negative family history of psychiatric illness, and doses of 2.5–4mg/d (n=120, Morishita and Arita, *Hum Psychopharmacol* 2007;**22**:27–31).

Botulinum toxin injections ± TAU *

Monotherapy: A single botulinum toxin injection in the forehead produced a rapid, strong and sustained alleviation of depression with

MDD, leading the authors to conclude that facial muscles not only express mood states, but may regulate them as well (n=30, RCT, d/b, p/c, 16/52, Wollmer *et al*, *J Psychiatr Res* 2012:**46**:574–81), the effect lasting six months even though the cosmetic effects only lasted 12–16 weeks (n=30, RCT, d/b, p/c, c/o, 24/52, Magid *et al*, *J Clin Psychiatry* 2014;**75**:837–44).

Bupropion ± TAU *

Adjunct: See combinations.

Monotherapy: Bupropion, a dopamine and noradrenaline reuptake inhibitor, is licensed in many countries for the treatment of depression, as well as for smoking cessation. A meta-analysis of bupropion studies shows 300mg/d (max 450mg/d) is as effective and tolerable as venlafaxine (s=3, n=1117, RCTs, Maneeton *et al*, *Drug Des Devel Ther* 2013;**7**:1053–62) for MDD and for co-morbid anxiety (s=10, n=2890, RCT, d/b, p/c, Papakostas *et al*, *J Psychiatr Res* 2008;**42**:134–40), but with no more sexual dysfunction than placebo (s=7, RCT, d/b, Thase *et al*, *J Clin Psychiatry* 2005;**66**:974–81), less nausea, diarrhoea and somnolence, but higher cardiovascular, proconvulsive (at doses up to 450mg/d; Pesola and Avasarala, *J Emerg Med* 2002;**22**:235–9) and overdose toxicity. The maximum dosage of 450mg/d should be adhered to since the risk of seizures is dose related (see *3.4*).

Review: general (Moreira, *Clin Drug Investig* 2011;**31**[Suppl 1]:5–17).

Buspirone ± TAU

Adjunct: Buspirone shares some pharmacodynamic properties with pindolol, augmentation of SSRIs may produce marked improvement in TRD, e.g. adding 20–60mg/d buspirone to SSRI non-responders significantly reduced MADRS scores at the end of week one compared to placebo, but both groups were equivalent at six weeks (n=102, RCT, p/c, d/b, 6/52, Appelberg *et al*, *J Clin Psychiatry* 2001;**62**:448–52). However, another trial suggested that buspirone actually slowed the onset of action of fluoxetine (n=120, RCT, open, 12/52, Onder and Tural, *J Affect Disord* 2003;**76**:223–7), so care is needed.

Monotherapy: Buspirone may be superior to placebo, but less effective than imipramine in MDD in old age (n=177, RCT, Schweizer *et al*, *J Clin Psychiatry* 1998;**59**:175–83).

Carbamazepine ± TAU

Adjunct: Carbamazepine augmentation may be useful in SSRI non-responders (n=6, Steinacher *et al*, *Eur Neuropsychopharmacol* 2002;**12**:255–60), but beware of potential interactions, e.g. carbamazepine does not augment mirtazapine and reduces its plasma levels (n=46, 5/52, open, Schüle *et al*, *World J Biol Psychiatry* 2009;**10**:390–9).

Monotherapy: Evidence for use as a pure anti-depressant is poor. See main entry under *1.10*.

Cholinesterase inhibitors ± TAU *

Adjunct: **Donepezil** augmentation of sertraline may improve cognition in older people with depression and MCI (n=23, RCT, d/b, p/c, 8/52, Pelton *et al*, *Int J Geriatr Psychiatry* 2008;**23**:670–6; FFT) and may reduce REM latency (n=16, c/o, Perlis *et al*, *Biol Psychiatry* 2002;**51**:457–62) but does not reduce the risk of relapse or prevent progression to MCI or dementia (n=130, RCT, d/b, p/c, two years, Reynolds *et al*, *Arch Gen Psychiatry* 2011;**68**:51–60). Adding **galantamine** to venlafaxine or citalopram had no effect in MDD in 'older' (>50) adults and with increased drop-outs (n=38, RCT, d/b, p/c, 24/52, Holtzheimer *et al*, *Int J Geriatr Psychiatry* 2008;**23**:625–31).

Creatine monohydrate + SSRIs

Adjunct: In women with MDD, creatine 5g/d was rapidly effective as an add-on to an SSRI (n=52[c=40], RCT, d/b, p/c, 8/52, Lyoo *et al*, *Am J Psychiatry* 2012 **169**:937–45).

Curcumin + antidepressants *

Adjunct: Curcumin was not different to placebo as an adjunct to escitalopram or venlafaxine (n=40, RCT, d/b, p/c, 5/52, Bergman *et al*, *Clin Neuropharmacol* 2013;**36**:73–7). The trial may have been too short as it appears to be superior to placebo in weeks 4–8, but not in the first four weeks (n=56, RCT, d/b, p/c, 8/52, Lopresti *et al*, *J Affect Disord* 2014;**167**:368–75).

Dexamfetamine

Monotherapy: Dexamfetamine may be effective

for depression and fatigue, with one successful trial in men with HIV (n=23, RCT, 2/52, Wagner and Rabkin, *J Clin Psychiatry* 2000;**61**:436–40).

DHEA (dehydroepiandrosterone)

Monotherapy: DHEA (an adrenal androgen and neurosteroid) 90–450mg/d was effective for mid-life depression (n=18/52, RCT, d/b, p/c, c/o, 18/52, Schmidt *et al*, *Arch Gen Psychiatry* 2005;**62**:154–62), and in non-major depression in HIV/AIDS (n=145 [c=133], RCT, p/c, d/b, 8/52, Rabkin *et al*, *Am J Psychiatry* 2006;**163**:59–66), possibly by reducing the vulnerability to stress.

Estradiol/estrogens ± TAU

(see also combinations) *

Adjunct: Estrogen supplementation of SSRIs may enhance their effectiveness in, e.g. postnatal depression (see *1.14.2*) and the menopause (n=145, Miller *et al*, *J Am Geriatr Soc* 2002;**50**:1826–30). Low-dose estrogen 0.625mg/d augmentation of partially effective SSRIs in perimenopausal depression significantly improved mood, but not memory (n=17, RCT, d/b, p/c, 6/52, Morgan *et al*, *J Clin Psychiatry* 2005;**66**:774–80), but it did not enhance the effectiveness of sertraline in postmenopausal women with MDD, although it might have speeded the onset of response (n=22, RCT, p/c, 10/52, Rasgon *et al*, *J Psychiatr Res* 2007;**41**:338–43).

Monotherapy: Estrogen receptors occur in the CNS and loss of estrogen reduces serotonergic and other functioning, and so estrogen supplements may improve depressive (but not cognitive) symptoms in post-menopausal women (n=19, RCT, p/c, c/o, 24/52, Schiff *et al*, *Psychoneuroendocrinology* 2005;**30**:309–15), e.g. a progesterone derivative (chlormadinone) plus ethinylestradiol improved mood in women (n=50000, open, <12/12, Huber *et al*, *Clin Drug Invest* 2008;**28**;783–91). However, an earlier study showed transdermal estradiol did not improve depressive symptoms in postmenopausal women (n=57, RCT, d/b, p/c, 8/52, Morrison *et al*, *Biol Psychiatry* 2004;**55**:406–12).

Reviews: depression in women (Studd, *Climacteric* 2011;**14**:637–42) general (Estrada-Camarena *et al*, *Behav Pharmacol* 2010;**21**:451–64), mechanisms of action (Osterlund, *Biochim Biophys Acta* 2010;**1800**:1136–44), transdermal estradiol (Moses-Kolko *et al*, *Clin Obstet Gynecol* 2009;**52**;516–29; FFT).

Glucocorticoid antagonists

See dexamethasone, hydrocortisone, ketoconazole and mifepristone.

Fludrocortisone + SSRIs

Adjunct: Fludrocortisone (a mineralocorticoid receptor agonist) did not improve the efficacy of escitalopram, but speeded up the response (n=64, RCT, d/b, p/c, 5/52, Otte *et al*, *J Psychiatr Res* 2010:**44**:339–46).

Folate and methylfolate *

Folate is a naturally occurring B vitamin necessary for the synthesis of norepinephrine, serotonin and dopamine (Fava and Mischoulon, *J Clin Psychiatry* 2009;**70**[Suppl 5]:12–7), and low RBC folate levels have been linked to persistent depression and a poor response to antidepressants, an easily rectified problem (e.g. n=2948, Morris *et al*, *Psychother Psychosom* 2003;**72**:80–7).

Adjunct: In females, augmentation of fluoxetine with folic acid 5mg/d was more effective than 1.5mg/d (n=42, RCT, d/b, 6/52, Venkatasubramanian *et al*, *J Affect Disord* 2013; **150**:644–8). In TRD methylfolate 15mg/d (but not 7.5mg/d) was a safe and effective adjunct to SSRIs (s=2, n=223, RCT, d/b, p/c, 60/7, Papakostas *et al*, *Am J Psychiatry* 2012;**169**:1267–74; n=75, RCT, d/b, p/c, 60/7, Papakostas *et al*, *J Clin Psychiatry* 2014;**75**:855–63; review by Papakostas *et al*, *Can J Psychiatry* 2012;**57**:406–13).

Monotherapy: People on methylfolate monotherapy (n=52) self-reported 68% response and 46% remission, after a mean 95 days therapy, suggesting a slow-onset effect (n=554, open, Shelton *et al*, *Prim Care Companion CNS Disord* 2013;**15**:13m01520; FFT).

Hydrocortisone

IV hydrocortisone produced a significantly greater and robust improvement in HAM-D scores than ovine CRH or placebo (n=22, RCT, d/b, p/c, 2/7, DeBattista *et al*, *Am J Psychiatry* 2000;**157**:1334–7; comment by Watson and Young, *Am J Psychiatry* 2001;**158**:1536–7).

Hyoscine

Monotherapy: A robust and rapid response occurred during short-term treatment with IV scopolamine in TRD (n=39[c=18], RCT, d/b, p/c, c/o, 5/7, Furey and Drevets, *Arch Gen Psychiatry* 2006;**63**:1121–9;FFT).

Infliximab ± TAU

Adjunct and monotherapy: Infliximab, a tumour necrosis factor antagonist, infusion does not have general antidepressant activity, but may improve symptoms in someone with high baseline inflammatory markers (n=60, RCT, d/b, p/c, 12/52, Raison *et al, JAMA Psychiatry* 2013;**70**:31–41; FFT).

Ketamine ± TAU *

The anaesthetic ketamine appears to be an extremely rapid-acting antidepressant. It has no effect on monoamines, possibly acting by blocking glutamatergic NMDA receptors, increasing BDNF (n=22, Haile *et al, Int J Neuropsychopharmacol* 2014;**17**:331–6; FFT) or many other candidate modes of action.

Route: IV infusion is known to be very effective and robust and shows a rapid effect maintained for 2/52 (n=42, Permoda-Osip *et al, Psychiatr Pol* 2014;**48**:35–47). Rapid IV infusion over two minutes may be poorly tolerated (n=4, d/b, p/c, c/o, Lai *et al, World J Biol Psychiatry* 2014;**15**:579–84). Other possible routes include IM (n=2, Harihar *et al, Indian J Psychiatry* 2013;**55**:186–8), intranasal (where 50mg produced 40% responders in 48 hours; n=20[c=18], RCT, d/b, p/c, c/o, Lapidus *et al, Biol Psychiatry* 2014;**76**:970–6) and sublingual (where dosing every 2–7 days gave a 77% response in TRD) (n=26, open, Lara *et al, Int J Neuropsychopharmacol* 2013;**16**:2111–7).

Efficacy: Systematic reviews and meta-analyses conclude that ketamine as a single dose for unipolar and bipolar depression produces its highest clinical remission (OR=7) at 24 hours, with three days (OR=4), and 7 days (OR=4) also superior to placebo (s=7, n=183, RCT, d/b, p/c, McGirr *et al, Psychol Med* 2015;**45**: 693–704) and that the effect size is bigger for repeat infusions but seems to wear off by 12–14 days (s=21, n=437, Coyle and Laws, *Hum Psychopharmacol* 2015;**30**:152–63). Ketamine infusion can also have a rapid and practical, albeit short-lived, effect on suicidal ideation in TRD (s=9, n=137, Reinstatler and Yussef, *Drugs R D* 2015;**15**:37–43) with no effect on the BSI (Beck Scale of Suicidal Ideation) over 24 hours but a significant effect at 48 hours, albeit no longer significant at seven days (n=24[c=24], RCT, a/c, Murrough *et al, Psychol Med* 2015;45:3571–80). Predictors of response over a week include higher BMI, a family history of alcohol dependence (n=42, Permoda-Osip *et al, Psychiatr Pol* 2014;**48**:35–47) and a lack of suicide attempts (s=4, Niciu *et al, J Clin Psychiatry* 2014;**75**:e417–23).

Efficacy vs ECT: In a comparison, IV ketamine was as effective as ECT in MDD but with a more rapid onset (n=18, RCT, 1/52, Ghasemi *et al, Psychiatry Res* 2014;**215**:355–61). Higher B12 levels may facilitate response (n=20, Permoda-Osip *et al, Pharmacopsychiatry* 2013;**46**:227–8).

Long-term: Ketamine may be effective with repeated doses (n=3, 12/12, open, Szymkowicz *et al, J Affect Disord* 2013;**147**:416–20).

Practicalities: An NHS environment can be used (n=28, 6/12 follow-up, Diamond *et al, J Psychopharmacol* 2014;**28**:536–44). The effect may be reduced by benzodiazepines (Ford *et al, Aust N Z J Psychiatry* 2015;49:1227).

Reviews: * systematic review and meta-analysis (Lee *et al, Gen Hosp Psychiatry* 2015;**37**:178-84), general (Iadarola *et al, Ther Adv Chronic Dis* 2015;**6**:97–114; FFT; Hasselmann *et al, Curr Neuropharmacol* 2014;**12**:57–70), mode of action (Kavalali and Monteggia, *Am J Psychiatry* 2012;**169**:1150–6), systematic review and meta-analysis (Caddy *et al, Ther Adv Psychopharmacol* 2014;**4**:75–99).

Ketoconazole + antidepressants

Adjunct: Ketoconazole inhibits cortisol secretion, lowering levels and may have a slow-onset antidepressant effect, particularly in hypercortisolemic (but not normal) patients (n=20, RCT, d/b, p/c, 4/52, Wolkowitz *et al, Biol Psychiatry* 1999;**45**:1070–74), but probably not in TRD (n=16, RCT, Malison *et al, J Clin Psychopharmacol* 1999;**19**:466–70).

Lamotrigine ± TAU *

One review concludes there is little data on lamotrigine in TRD (s=1, RCT, d/b, Thomas *et al, J Ment Health* 2010;**19**:168–75; FFT). Remember that even missing two days' doses means retitrating.

Adjunct: Lamotrigine (see *1.10.3*) may have a role as an adjunct at 200mg/d for refractory unipolar depression, enhancing the onset of paroxetine (n=40, p/c, d/b, 9/52, Normann *et al, J Clin Psychiatry* 2002;**63**:337–44), albeit with a modest (n=23, RCT, d/b, p/c, 6/52, Barbosa *et al, J Clin Psychiatry* 2003;**64**:403–7) at best effect (e.g. n=96[c=65], RCT, d/b, p/c, 10/52, Barbee *et al, J Clin Psychiatry* 2011;**72**:1405–12). Response to adjunctive lamotrigine in TRD may have a plasma-level relationship (above 12.7micromol/L or 3.3mcg/ml) (n=34, open, 8/52, Kagawa *et al, Ther Drug Monit* 2014;**36**:730–3), or with a therapeutic window of 5–11 mcg/mL (n=25, open, Katayama *et al, Pharmacopsychiatry* 2014;**47**:111–4).

Levothyroxine (synthetic T4) + TAU

Adjunct: Low TSH and higher T4 levels are associated with depressive syndrome in young adults (n=6869, Forman-Hoffman *et al, Acta Psychiatr Scand* 2006;**114**:132–9). Thyroid supplementation, e.g. levothyroxine 150–300mcg/d may accelerate the onset of tricyclic response in non-refractory depression (5/6 studies found T3 significantly superior to placebo, especially in women: meta-analysis, Altshuler *et al, Am J Psychiatry* 2001;**158**:1617–22). The combination of T3+T4 may be no better than T4 monotherapy (n=40, RCT, d/b, p/c, 15/52, Sawka *et al, J Clin Endocrinol Metab* 2003;**88**:4551–5).

Liothyronine + TAU
(L-isomer of triiodothyronine, T3) *

Free thyroid hormone concentrations are associated with depression severity, and treatment with triiodothyronine is likely to be better then levothyroxine because of individual differences in hormone metabolism (Berent *et al, Mol Biol Rep* 2014;**41**:2419–25).

Adjunct: A meta-analysis showed liothyronine 50mcg augmentation produces twice as many responses in refractory depression compared to controls, with moderately large improvements (s=5, RCTs, Cooper-Kazaz and Lerer, *Int J Neuropsychopharmacol* 2008;**11**:685–99). T3 mean 90mg/d was effective in TRD with 33% achieving full remission after failing an average of 14 antidepressants (n=159, retrospective, Kelly and Lieberman, *J Affect Disord* 2009;**116**:222–6), although T3 25mcg/d had no additional benefit over placebo on any measures as an adjunct to sertraline (n=153, RCT, d/b, p/c, 8/52, Garlow *et al, J Psychiatry Res* 2012;**46**:1406–13).

Review: HUNT study (Panicker *et al, Clin Endocrinol [Oxf]* 2009;**71**:574–80).

Lisdexamfetamine + TAU *

Adjunct: In escitalopram non-remitters, augmentation by LDX 20–50mg/d reduced depressive symptoms with an NNT=6.7 (n=173, RCT, p/c, d/b, 6/52, Trivedi *et al, J Clin Psychiatry* 2013;**74**:802–9) and 20–70mg/d improved response rates and cognitive functioning in mild MDD (n=143[c=119], RCT, d/b, p/c, 9/52, Madhoo *et al, Neuropsychopharmacology* 2014;**39**:1388–98).

Monotherapy: LDX will not be licensed as monotherapy after two negative phase III trials.

Memantine + TAU *

Adjunct: No changes in MADRAS scores were seen with memantine 20mg/d as an adjunct in TRD (n=31[c=26], RCT, d/b, p/c, 8/52, Smith *et al, J Clin Psychiatry* 2013;**74**:966–73).

Monotherapy: Memantine 5–20mg/d is ineffective for MDD (n=32, RCT, d/b, p/c, Zarate *et al, Am J Psychiatry* 2006;**163**:153–5).

Methylphenidate ± TAU

Cochrane concluded that there is reasonable evidence for short-term psychostimulants (methylphenidate, dexamfetamine, modafinil) to reduce the symptoms of depression (s=24, RCT, Candy *et al, Cochrane Database Syst Rev* 2008;**2**:CD006722).

Adjunct: Methylphenidate may be effective as augmentation where incomplete response has occurred with antidepressants, including the elderly, where apathy and withdrawal (but not hopelessness) are prominent features. Methylphenidate 10–40mg/d may improve apathy and fatigue (n=145, RCT, d/b, p/c, 5/52, Ravindran *et al, J Clin Psychiatry* 2008;**69**:87–94; n=30, RCT, d/b, p/c, 14/7, Kerr *et al, J Pain Symptom Manage* 2012;**43**:68–77).

Monotherapy: Methylphenidate can be used

as monotherapy in acute depression as it has the major advantage of a rapid action (often within 48 hours), although the effect tends to be transient and it may worsen anxiety and insomnia and be poorly tolerated in people with age-related cognitive decline (n=60, RCT, p/c, d/b, Turner *et al*, *Psychopharmacol [Berl]* 2003;**168**:455–64).

Modafinil + SSRIs

Cochrane concluded that there is reasonable evidence for short-term modafinil and other stimulants to reduce the symptoms of depression (s=24, RCT, Candy *et al*, *Cochrane Database Syst Rev* 2008;**2**:CD006722).

Adjunct: Modafinil 200 mg BD plus fluoxetine 40 mg/d was significantly superior to fluoxetine plus placebo for MDD (n=46[c=44], RCT, d/b, p/c, 6/52, Abolfazli *et al*, *Depress Anxiety* 2011;**28**:297–302) and may help in people with fatigue and sleepiness in MDD over the short-term.

N-acetylcysteine (NAC) + TAU *

Adjunct: The anti-inflammatory NAC had little effect as an adjunct in MDD (n=252, RCT, d/b, p/c, 28/52, Berk *et al*, *J Clin Psychiatry* 2014;**75**:628–36).

Nimodipine + SSRIs

Adjunct: Nimodipine augmentation of fluoxetine has been successful for 'vascular depression' (n=101, RCT, d/b, p/c, 8/52, Taragano *et al*, *Int Psychogeriatr* 2005;**17**:487–98).

NSAIDs/COX-2 inhibitors + TAU *

Depression may be a failure in the stress system, inflammation may be a precipitating and perpetuating factor, and glucocorticoid receptor resistance may occur (Krishnadas and Cavanagh, *J Neurol Neurosurg Psychiatry* 2012;**83**:495–502), e.g:

- A third of people with MDD show elevated peripheral inflammatory markers
- Having an inflammatory illness increases the rate of MDD
- Raised cytokines increase the risk of MDD.

Adjunct: Meta-analysis shows anti-inflammatories, especially **celecoxib** (n=40, RCT, d/b, p/c, 6/52, Abbasi *et al*, *J Affect Disord* 2012:**141**:308–14; n=40, RCT, p/c, 6/52, Akhondzadeh *et al*, *Depress Anxiety* 2009;**26**:607–11), decrease depressive symptoms without significant ADRs, although the studies showed a high risk of bias (s=14, n=6262, RCT, p/c, Köhler *et al*, *JAMA Psychiatry* 2014;**71**:1381–91). However, aspirin or statin use did not reduce depression incidence in people aged 35–66 in the community (n=1631, mean five years, Glaus *et al*, *J Affect Disord* 2015;**182**:126–31).

Review: general (Andrade, *J Clin Psychiatry* 2014;**75**:975–7).

Omega-3 fatty acids ± TAU

The variable results from PUFA (omega-3 fatty acids) studies may be due to differential effects between eicosapentaenoic acid (EPA) and docosahexaenoic acid (DHA). A meta-analysis suggests that PUFA supplements containing >60% of total EPA+DHA in a dose range of 200–2200 mg/d of EPA in excess of DHA were effective (s=15, n=916, RCT, d/b, p/c, Sublette *et al*, *J Clin Psychiatry* 2011;**72**:1577–84; FFT; s=28, RCTs, Martins, *J Am Coll Nutr* 2009;**28**:525–42). A later systematic review and meta-analysis concludes that there is a small, non-significant benefit from omega-3 fatty acids as adjunct or monotherapy in MDD, with a probably high publication bias (s=13, n=731, RCT, p/c, Bloch and Hannestad, *Mol Psychiatry* 2012;**17**:1272–82; FFT). Intakes of fish and omega-3 fatty acids may be inversely associated with chronic depression, so supplementation may be helpful in people for whom fish is not an acceptable source (n=3317, 20 years, Colangelo *et al*, *Nutrition* 2009;**25**:1011–9; FFT).

Adjunct: There seems more evidence for adjunctive therapy. In TRD, augmentation with omega-3 fatty acids improved symptoms (Krawczyk and Rybakowski, *Psychiatr Pol* 2012;**46**:585–98), increased total response with citalopram (n=42, RCT, p/c, 9/52, Gertsik *et al*, *J Clin Psychopharmacol* 2012;**32**:61–4) and was a safe adjunct to SSRIs (n=80, Safa *et al*, *Ther Adv Psychopharmacol* 2013;**3**:186–90) but not for depression in diabetics (n=25, RCT, d/b, p/c, 12/52, Bot *et al*, *J Affect Disord* 2010;**126**:282–6), or as augmentation of sertraline 50 mg/d (n=122, RCT, d/b, 10/52, Carney *et al*, *JAMA* 2009;**302**:1651–7; FFT). A recent meta-analysis claims a significant benefit for omega-3 fatty acids as adjuncts in depression cf placebo (s=19, RCTs, Grosso *et al*, *PLoS One* 2014;**9**:e96905; FFT).

Monotherapy: There appears little evidence for efficacy as monotherapy. EPA-E 1g/d was ineffective for MDD, albeit well tolerated (n=57 [c=35], RCT, d/b, p/c, 8/52, Mischoulon *et al*, *J Clin Psychiatry* 2009;**70**:1636–44; FFT), eicosapentaenoic acid (EPA) and docosahexaenoic acid (DHA) were ineffective (n=196[c=154], RCT, d/b, p/c, 8/52, Mischoulon *et al*, *J Clin Psychiatry* 2015;**76**:54–61), there was no effect in perinatal depression (n=26, RCT, d/b, p/c, 6/52, Rees *et al*, *Aust N Z J Psychiatry* 2008;**42**:199–205) and a meta-analysis identified a lack of benefit for omega-3 fatty acids monotherapy in MDD (s=19, RCTs, Grosso *et al*, *PLoS One* 2014;**9**:e96905; FFT).

Review: general (Su *et al*, *Expert Opin Investig Drugs* 2013;**22**:1519–34).

Phenytoin

Monotherapy: Phenytoin (up to 400 mg/d) was as effective as fluoxetine (up to 21 mg/d) for MDD (n=33 [c=28], RCT, d/b, Nemets *et al*, *J Clin Psychiatry* 2005;**66**:586–90).

Pindolol + SSRIs

Adjunct: Antidepressants, e.g. SSRIs may act by inhibiting the 5-HT reuptake pump, increasing 5-HT but this also enhances 5-HT at 5-HT1A receptors situated on the cell body that operate a feedback loop, thus cancelling each other out. Over a period of weeks, however, the pre-synaptic 5-HT1A receptors become desensitised. Pindolol selectively blocks 5-HT1A receptors, and inhibits this initial feedback loop to increase the speed of onset of action. An eloquent systematic review concluded that pindolol is clearly effective to enhance the onset of action of SSRIs, most clearly up to four weeks (s=11, Whale *et al*, *J Psychopharmacol* 2010;**24**:513–20; n=30, RCT, d/b, p/c, 6/52, Portella *et al*, *J Clin Psychiatry* 2011;**72**:962–9). Pindolol may improve response (70% vs 40%) and speed of response (53 days vs 19 days) only in first episode depression but not in recurrent depression (Portella *et al*, *Eur Neuropsychopharmacol* 2009;**19**:516–9).

Pioglitazone + SSRIs

Adjunct: Pioglitazone 30 mg/d was highly effective as an adjunct to citalopram, with a well tolerated, earlier and more robust improvement (n=40, RCT, d/b, p/c, 6/52, Sepanjnia *et al*, *Neuropsychopharmacology* 2012;**37**:2093–100).

Pramipexole ± TAU *

Monotherapy: Pramipexole (a dopamine D2/D3 agonist licensed for Parkinson's disease) has been used with some success (n=22, case series, Ostow, *Am J Psychiatry* 2002;**159**:320–1; n=174, RCT, p/c, 8/52, Corrigan *et al*, *Depress Anxiety* 2000;**11**:58–65).

Adjunct: In TRD, pramipexole was safe and potentially effective (n=60, RCT, d/b, p/c, 8/52, Cusin *et al*, *J Clin Psychiatry* 2013;**74**:636–41).

SAM-e (S-adenosyl-L-methionine) ± SSRIs *

Adjunct: SAMe (a naturally occurring cellular molecule) was effective and well tolerated as an adjunct to SSRIs in TRD (n=73, RCT, d/b, p/c, 6/52, Papakostas *et al*, *Am J Psychiatry* 2010;**167**:942–8), with IM or IV use well supported, but less so for oral use (Papakostas, *J Clin Psychiatry* 2009;**70** [Suppl 5]:18–22).

Monotherapy: SAMe has failed to statistically beat placebo, although neither did escitalopram (n=189, RCT, d/b, p/c, 12/52, Mischoulon *et al*, *J Clin Psychiatry* 2014;**75**:370–6).

Review: general (Papakostas *et al*, *Can J Psychiatry* 2012;**57**:406–13).

Statins + SSRIs *

Adjunct: Lovastatin 30 mg/d was superior to placebo as an adjunct to fluoxetine (n=68, RCT, d/b, p/c, 6/52, Ghanizadeh and Hedayati, *Depress Anxiety* 2013;**30**:1084–8).

St John's wort (SJW) ± TAU *

Adjuncts: Care is needed in adjunctive therapy (particularly if purchased OTC — see *4.3.3.10*).

Monotherapy: SJW is available over-the-counter in most European countries in a variety of preparations. The mode of action is uncertain but may include serotonin and/or norepinephrine reuptake inhibition, MAO-A and B inhibition and sigma receptor activity. A variety of systematic reviews and meta-analyses conclude SJW has modest effects in MDD (e.g.

s = 13, Rahimi *et al*, *Prog Neuropsychopharmacol Biol Psychiatry* 2009;**33**:118–27) with relapse prevention over 6/12 (n = 426, RCT, d/b, p/c, 26/52, Kasper *et al*, *Eur Neuropsychopharmacol* 2008;**18**:803–13). Cochrane concludes that SJW is superior to placebo in MDD, equivalent to standard antidepressants and with fewer side-effects, although the source of SJW may be relevant (s = 29, n = 5489, Linde *et al*, *Cochrane Database Syst Rev* 2008;**4**:CD000448). Most studies are short-term (up to 6/52), and many have high (up to 50%) drop-out rates, indicating that transient mild depression may be common in participants.

Review: ADRs (s = 35, Knüppel and Linde, *J Clin Psychiatry* 2004;**5**:1470–9).

Testosterone ± TAU *

Low free testosterone levels are associated with a higher prevalence of depression, e.g. older men with low total or free testosterone levels are 1.5–2.7 times more likely to develop depression (n = 3987, Almeida *et al*, *Arch Gen Psychiatry* 2008;**65**:283–9). A review concluded that men with depressive symptoms and testosterone deficiency should have a 3/12 trial of testosterone (Khera, *Arch Esp Urol* 2013;**66**:729–36).

Adjunct: Weekly testosterone cypionate 100–200 mg/d has helped some men with late-onset (but not early onset) depression (n = 15, RCT, 6/52, Perry *et al*, *J Clin Psychiatry* 2002;**63**:1096–101). Testosterone gel may be an effective non-parenteral route (n = 22, RCT, p/c, 8/52, Pope *et al*, *Am J Psychiatry* 2003;**160**:105–11), although it was ineffective for TRD with plasma testosterone < 350 ng/mL (n = 100, RCT, p/c, d/b, 6/52, Pope *et al*, *J Clin Psychopharmacol* 2010;**30**:126–34).

Monotherapy: In men with metabolic syndrome, low testosterone, erectile dysfunction and depression, depot testosterone undecanoate significantly im-proved mood, most markedly in men with low baseline total testosterone (n = 184, RCT, d/b, p/c, 30/52, Giltay *et al*, *J Sex Med* 2010;**7**:2572–82).

Review: in depression (Amore *et al*, *Int J Endocrinol* 2012;**2012**:280724).

Topiramate + TAU

Adjunct: In TRD topiramate 100–200 mg/d can augment SSRIs, with a 32% reduction in HAM-D cf 6% with placebo (n = 53[c = 42], RCT, d/b, p/c, 8/52, Mowla and Kardeh, *Prog Neuropsychopharmacol Biol Psychiatry* 2011;**35**:970–3).

Vardenafil

Monotherapy: Vardenafil is effective for erectile dysfunction in milder MDD, and depressive symptoms may improve with treatment of a contributory symptom (n = 280, RCT, d/b, p/c, Rosen *et al*, *Am J Psychiatry* 2006;**163**:79–87).

Vitamin D + TAU *

Adjunct: Low serum levels of vitamin D are associated with depressive symptoms, but it is unclear if supplementation has any effect (s = 14, n = 31424, Anglin *et al*, *Br J Psychiatry* 2013;**202**:100–7), e.g. folic acid 2.5mg/d, B6 (50mg/d) and B12 (1mg/d) had no effect on reducing depression in mid-life and older women over seven years (n = 4331, RCT, p/c, seven years, Okereke *et al*, *Br J Psychiatry* 2015;**206**:324–31). A once-yearly (autumn) dose of vitamin D3 500,000iu for 3–5 years had no effect on mood in women over the age of 70 (n = 2317, RCT, d/b, p/c, 3–5 years, Sanders *et al*, *Br J Psychiatry* 2011;**198**:357–64; FFT). However, vitamin D3 1500u plus fluoxetine 20 mg/d was significantly more effective from week 4 than fluoxetine monotherapy for MDD (n = 42[c = 40], RCT, d/b, p/c, 8/52, Khoraminya *et al Aust N Z J Psychiatry* 2013;**47**:271–5).

Ziprasidone *

Monotherapy: Ziprasidone was ineffective for MDD in one study (n = 120, RCT, d/b, p/c, 12/52, Papakostas *et al*, *J Clin Psychiatry* 2012;**73**:1541–7), although 40–160 mg/d may help MDD in people with psychomotor symptoms (n = 106, RCT, d/b, p/c, 12/52, Jeon *et al*, *Int Clin Psychopharmacol* 2014;**29**:332–8).

■ Unlicensed/possible efficacy

Beta-blockers (see also pindolol)

Monotherapy: Although beta-blockers can induce depression, continuous use post percutaneous coronary intervention (PCI) reduces the risk of depression by 49%, ranging between 36% for low dose and 58% for high dose (n=685, one year, Battes *et al, J Affect Disord* 2012;**136**:751–7: FFT).

Chromium

Monotherapy: Chromium picolinate may be an option in atypical depression, with a potential effect within two weeks (n=15, 8/52, p/c, Davidson *et al, Biol Psychiatry* 2003;**53**:261–4).

Dexamethasone + TAU

Adjunct: This synthetic glucocorticoid can show a rapid and marked improvement given IV or orally (e.g. n=10, 6/52, Dinan *et al, Acta Psychiatr Scand* 1997;**95**:58–61), although probably only in a minority. This interesting effect may be via upregulation of glucocorticoid receptors, an effect shared with the SSRIs.

Review: glucocorticoids (Kling *et al, Depress Anxiety* 2009;**26**:641–9; FFT).

Magnesium + TAU

Adjunct: Inadequate dietary magnesium intake may be a cause of TRD (Eby and Eby, *Med Hypotheses* 2010;**74**:649–60).

Mifepristone

Monotherapy: Mifepristone 600–1200mg/d (a glucocorticoid antagonist) may be an option, the theory being that 'the psychosis in MDD is caused by excessive activation of the HPA axis' (n=30, open, 7/7, Belanoff *et al, Biol Psychiatry* 2002;**52**:386–92).

Minocycline + TAU

Adjunct: Minocycline 150mg/d seemed effective in psychotic depression (n=25, open, Miyaoka *et al, Prog Neuropsychopharmacol Biol Psychiatry* 2012;**37**:222–6).

Opiates + TAU

Adjunct: Some anecdotal cases suggest that oxycodone, buprenorphine (Callaway, *Biol Psychiatry* 1996;**39**:989–90), or oxymorphone may produce a sustained effect in refractory and chronic depression, as well as reducing psychogenic pain and distress (review by Berrocoso *et al, Curr Pharm Des* 2009;**15**:1612–22). The potential for abuse limits their use.

Pergolide + TAU

Adjunct: The dopamine agonist pergolide has been moderately successful in open trials as an adjunct (e.g. n=20, open, Izumi *et al, J Affect Disord* 2000;**61**:127–32).

Pregabalin + TAU

Adjunct: In older people pregabalin is useful for augmenting antidepressants in comorbid depression (n=94, open, 12/52, Karaiskos *et al, Int J Ger Psychiatry* 2013;**28**:100–5).

Riluzole + TAU

Adjunct: Riluzole (mean 75mg/d), a dopamine agonist, may be useful as an adjunct to antidepressants, with a significant effect within the first week (n=10, open, 12/52, Sanacora *et al, Biol Psychiatry* 2007;**61**:822–5; FFT).

Valproate + TAU *

Adjunct: There are some reports of efficacy as augmentation of paroxetine in TRD with a 49% remission rate (n=39, RCT, 8/52, a/c, Fang *et al, J Clin Psychopharmacol* 2011;**31**: 638–42).

Vitamins + TAU *

Adjunct: Although vitamin B supplements (B12 500mcg; B6 25mg; folic acid 2mg) had no effect on enhancing citalopram's effect at 12 weeks, they enhanced and sustained the effect at one year (n=153, RCT, d/b, p/c, 52/52, Almeida *et al, Br J Psychiatry* 2014;**205**:450–7).

Zinc + TAU

Adjunct: An extraordinary study (n=75, d/b, p/c, 12/52, Siwek *et al, J Affect Disord* 2010; **126**:447–52), that urgently needs replicating, suggested that:

- Serum zinc is significantly lower (by 22%) in depressed cf non-depressed people
- Zinc levels increase with response to a tricyclic regardless of zinc supplementation
- People with TRD have 14% lower zinc levels than people with non-resistant depression
- Oral zinc increases serum zinc levels
- There is an inverse relationship between serum zinc and response.

Zonisamide + duloxetine

Adjunct: In people not responding to duloxetine 60mg/d, addition of zonisamide 75mg/d may enhance the response rates (n=40, open, 24/52, Fornaro *et al*, *Ann Gen Psychiatry* 2011;**10**:23; FFT).

✱ Case reports ✱

- **Oxytocin**, as adjunct to escitalopram (Scantamburlo *et al*, *J Neuropsychiatry Clin Neurosci* 2011;**23**:E5)
- **Tramadol** (review by Barber, *Exp Clin Psychopharmacol* 2011;**19**:123–30)
- **Varenicline** (n=1, Grosshans *et al*, *Addiction* 2009;**104**:859–61).

☐ No efficacy

Atomoxetine + TAU

Atomoxetine augmentation is of no benefit (n=276, RCT, d/b, p/c, 8/52, Michelson *et al*, *J Clin Psychiatry* 2007;**68**:582–7) and it is in fact a failed antidepressant (n=15[c=11], open, 8/52, Carpenter *et al*, *J Clin Psychiatry* 2005;**66**:1234–8).

Benzodiazepines (monotherapy)

Benzodiazepines have no antidepressant activity but can help reduce anxiety symptoms.

Caffeine

Some depressed people may have increased sensitivity to caffeine (Lee *et al*, *Am J Psychiatry* 1988;**145**:632–5).

Inositol + SSRIs

Inositol is not effective as augmentation of SSRIs (n=27, RCT, p/c, Levine *et al*, *Biol Psychiatry* 1999;**45**:270–3).

Spironolactone + SSRIs

Adjunct: Spironolactone (a mineralocorticoid receptor antagonist) did not improve the efficacy of escitalopram, even in responders (n=64, RCT, d/b, p/c, 5/52, Otte *et al*, *J Psychiatr Res* 2010:**44**:339–46).

1.14.2 POSTPARTUM DEPRESSION (PPD) see also Unipolar depression (*1.14.1*)

Symptoms:

PPD is defined as MDD with an onset within one month of childbirth, although it can pre-date childbirth. The incidence ranges from 6–14% (e.g. (n=865, Miyake *et al*, *J Affect Disord* 2006;**96**:133–8), peaking in the third month, and with a second peak at nine months (n=506, Gjerdingen *et al*, *J Womens Health (Larchmt)* 2011;**20**:381–6; FFT). The recurrence rate may be as high as 25% (Wisner *et al*, *J Clin Psychiatry* 2001;**62**:82–6). The Edinburgh Postnatal Depression Scale (Cox *et al*, *Br J Psychiatry* 1987;**150**:782–6) is the most widely used assessment tool. There is a well-established relationship between maternal depression and impaired childhood development, e.g. poor cognitive function, behavioural inhibition, emotional maladjustment, poor bonding, slowed development, and child neglect (e.g. Carter *et al*, *J Am Acad Child Adolesc Psychiatry* 2001;**40**:18–26), and the quicker the mother gets better, the better the child does (n=80, 1–2 years, Wickramaratne *et al*, *Am J Psychiatry* 2011;**168**:593–602). So, there is huge risk in not treating, especially as PPD carries an increased risk of suicide.

Causes:

There are numerous and dramatic changes in hormones in the postnatal period and estrogen, progesterone and other hormonal fluctuations may be the main culprits, although rapid changes in estrogen and progesterone may not be a cause (n=192, 7/12, Klier *et al*, *J Psychiatr Res* 2007;**41**:273–9).

Risk factors for PPD: ✱

- Postpartum blues (Reck *et al*, *J Affect Disord* 2009;**113**:77–87)
- MDD or anxiety in pregnancy
- Previous depression (n=588, McCoy *et al*, *J Reprod Med* 2008;**53**:166–70)
- Stopping antidepressants during pregnancy
- Cigarette smoking (n=588, McCoy *et al*, *J Reprod Med* 2008;**53**:166–70)
- Low partner support
- Epilepsy, especially with polypharmacy and multiparity (n=56, Galanti *et al*, *Epilepsy Behave* 2009;**16**:426–30; FFT)
- Low serum zinc (n=66[c=58], 30/7, Wójcik *et al*, *Pharmacol Rep* 2006;**58**:571–6; FFT)
- Vitamin D deficiency in mid-pregnancy (n=796, Robinson *et al*, *Arch Women's Ment Health* 2014;**17**:213–9).

Not risk factors for PPD:

- Low serum magnesium (n=66, 30/7, Wójcik

et al, Pharmacol Rep 2006;**58**:571–6; FFT)
- Low folate, pyridoxine or cobalamin (n=865, Miyake *et al, J Affect Disord* 2006;**96**:133–8)
- Medroxyprogesterone acetate depot — use immediately postpartum does not seem to predispose to PPD (n=247, Tsai and Schaffir, *Contraception* 2010;**82**:174–7).

Role of drugs: *

There are some concerns regarding infant exposure to antidepressants, but the multiple adverse effects of untreated PPD are outweighed by this risk if drugs and doses are chosen carefully. The potential effects of antidepressants in breast-feeding must be considered (see *C3.9*; Fortinguerra *et al, Pediatrics* 2009;**124**:547–56; FFT). Antidepressants show larger effect sizes than non-pharmacological treatments (Cuijpers *et al, J Clin Psychol* 2008;**64**:103–18) and IPT is unproven (s=11, Miniati *et al, Arch Women's Ment Health* 2014;**17**:257–69). ECT may be an option in an emergency (n=5, Forray and Ostroff, *J ECT* 2007;**23**:188–93). Adding antidepressants to supportive care in PPD can bring forward response (n=254, RCT, 18/52, Sharp *et al, Health Technol Assess* 2010;**14**:1–153; FFT). SSRIs can delay secretory activation by around 15 hours immediately postpartum, so might delay the onset of breast-feeding (n=431, Marshall *et al, J Clin Endocrin Metabol* 2010;**95**:837–46; FFT).

Prevention:

A protective effect has been shown by nortriptyline (n=51, RCT, d/b, p/c, 20/52, Wisner *et al, J Clin Psychiatry* 2001;**62**:82–6) and sertraline (n=22, RCT, d/b, p/c, 20/52, Wisner *et al, Am J Psychiatry* 2004;**161**:1290–2), although the effect seemed to go if stopped at 20 weeks.

Reviews: * meta-analysis of treatments (s=21, McDonagh *et al, Obstet Gynecol* 2014;**124**:526–34; Sockol *et al, Clin Psychol Rev* 2011;**31**:839–49; FFT), general (Guille *et al, J Midwifery Womens Health* 2013;**58**:643–53; Stuart-Parrigon and Stuart, *Curr Psychiatry Rep* 2014;**16**:468), pharmacotherapy (Kim *et al, Expert Opin Pharmacother* 2014;**15**:1223–34), complementary and alternative medicines (Deligiannidis and Freeman, *Best Pract Res Clin Obstet Gynaecol* 2014;**28**:85–95).

BNF listed *

PPD is not a specific indication so technically all antidepressants are licensed (see *1.14.1*). Cochrane concludes that SSRIs are effective but that the evidence base for PPD is of low quality due to the small sample sizes (s=6, n=596, RCT, p/c, Molyneaux *et al, Cochrane Database Syst Rev* 2014;**9**:CD002018). Another systematic review concluded that SSRIs were effective, well tolerated and consistently (but not clearly) superior to other treatments (s=6, n=595, De Crescenzo *et al, J Affect Disord* 2014;**152–4**:39–44). Specific PPD studies are listed below.

Citalopram

Citalopram and reboxetine significantly improved the mother's perception of the baby's facial expressions to be more positive, thereby possibly mitigating the negative effects of depression in infant development, a subtle effect (n=39, RCT, d/b, p/c, 7/7, Stein *et al, J Psychopharmacol* 2012;**26**:670–6; FFT).

Fluoxetine

Fluoxetine 20mg/d and CBT both improved depressive symptoms more than placebo, but the combination had no advantage over monotherapy (n=87, RCT, d/b, p/c, 12/52, Appleby *et al, Br Med J* 1997;**314**:932–6; FFT).

Fluvoxamine

Fluvoxamine (mean 150mg/d) showed a 67% remission rate in a small study (n=6, open, 8/52, Suri *et al, Am J Psychiatry* 2001;**158**:1739–40).

Paroxetine

Paroxetine (max 40mg/d) has produced greater remission (37%) vs placebo (14%) at week 8, but this was not statistically significant (n=70, RCT, d/b, p/c, 8/52, Yonkers *et al, J Clin Psychiatry* 2008;**69**:659–65; FFT). Paroxetine (max 50mg/d, 87.5% response) and CBT (79% response) were both effective in another study (n=35, RCT, 12/52, Misri *et al, J Clin Psychiatry* 2004;**65**:1236–41).

Reboxetine See citalopram.

Sertraline *

Sertraline (up to 200mg/d) was as effective as

nortriptyline (up to 150mg/d) (n=109, RCT, 24/52, Wisner *et al, J Clin Psychopharmacol* 2006;**26**:353–60) and 50–200mg/d increased response over placebo from 26% to 59% (remission from 21% to 53%), especially if the depression started within 4/52 of childbirth (n=38, RCT, d/b, p/c, 6/52, Hantsoo *et al, Psychopharmacol [Berl]* 2014;**231**:939–48).

Venlafaxine

A small study showed possible efficacy, including perhaps with comorbid anxiety (n=15, open, 8/52, Cohen *et al, J Clin Psychiatry* 2001;**62**:592–6).

• Unlicensed/some efficacy

Aripiprazole + TAU *

Aripiprazole 2–10mg/d appeared safe and effective as an adjunct to antidepressants (n=10[c=8], open, Sharma and Sommerdyk, *Arch Women's Ment Health* 2015;**18**:131–4).

Benzodiazepines + TAU

Adjunct: Benzodiazepines may be useful for short-term anxiety and insomnia, but nothing specific has been published.

Bupropion

Monotherapy: Bupropion 150–400mg/d has produced 37.5% remission and 37.5% response, but with no effect on comorbid anxiety (n=8, open, 8/52, Nonacs *et al, Int J Neuropsychopharmacol* 2005;**8**:445–9).

Calcium + TAU

Calcium has been mentioned in one review (s=7, Dennis *et al, Can J Psychiatry* 2004;**49**:467–75).

Estrogens

Monotherapy: Cochrane concludes that estrogen (eg. sublingual beta-estradiol) is associated with greater improvement in severe PPD than placebo, and may be of modest value (s=2, n=229, Dennis *et al, Cochrane Database Syst Rev* 2008;**4**:CD001690). Women on transdermal 17-beta-estradiol may have a greater remission rate (review by Moses-Kolko *et al, Clin Obstet* 2009;**52**:516–29; FFT).

Riboflavin

Moderate consumption of riboflavin (vitamin B2) may be protective (n=865, Miyake *et al, J Affect Disord* 2006;**96**:133–8).

Selenium

Monotherapy: Prenatal selenium 100mcg/d significantly reduced postnatal depression scores (EPDS) and might have a role in prevention of PPD (n=166[c=85], RCT, d/b, p/c, 8/12, Mokhber *et al, J Matern Fetal Neonatal Med* 2011;**24**:104–8).

St. John's wort

St John's wort might be considered by some people as 'natural' and hence safe, but that is unproven and there is no published data on use in PPD (short review by Goldman *et al, Can Fam Physician* 2003;**49**:29–30; FFT).

□ No efficacy

Levothyroxine

Women with high antenatal thyroid antibody levels may be at greater risk of developing PPD (e.g. n=57, Lambrinoudaki *et al, J Affect Disord* 2010;**121**:278–82), but this is not corrected by daily thyroxine (n=446, RCT, d/b, p/c, 5/12, Harris *et al, Br J Psychiatry* 2002;**180**:327–30; FFT).

Omega-3 fatty acids *

Reviews of omega-3 fatty acids conclude that current trials show no evidence of effectiveness, are not robust and are too small (s=8, Ramakrishnan, *Matern Child Nutr* 2011;**7** Suppl 2:99–111). Docosahexanoic acid (DHA) showed no effect in PPD, cognitive skills or language development in children if taken from before 21 weeks to term (Wojcicki and Heyman, *J Matern Fetal Neonatal Med* 2010;**24**:680–6; FFT). Cochrane concludes there is insufficient evidence that DHA or EPA prevent PPD (s=2, n=305[c=203], RCTs, Miller *et al, Cochrane Database Syst Rev* 2013;**10**:CD009104).

Reviews: general (Levant, *Depress Res Treat* 2011;**2011**:467349; FFT; Jans *et al, Br J Nutr* 2010;**104**:1577–85).

Progesterones

Cochrane concludes norethisterone enthanate significantly increased the risk of postpartum depression (s=2, n=229, Dennis *et al*, *Cochrane Database Syst Rev* 2008;**4**:CD001690).

Vitamin D *

There appears no association between PPD and vitamin D levels during pregnancy, and there may be a higher risk of PPD in women with the highest vitamin D levels (n=1480, Nielsen *et al*, *PLoS One* 2013;**8**:e80686).

1.14.3 DEPRESSION IN PARKINSON'S DISEASE (DPD)

see also Unipolar depression (*1.14.1*)

Introduction

The prevalence of MDD in people with PD is around 45% (Lemke, *Eur J Neurol* 2008;**15** Suppl 1:21–5) and the incidence over 10 years is 70% (n=122, Piccinni *et al*, *Compr Psychiatry* 2012;**53**:727–31; n=685, Jasinska-Myga *et al*, *Can J Neurol Sci* 2010;**37**:61–6; FFT), and another 25% will have milder depression. After withdrawal of dopamine agonists, up to 20% may suffer central effects, e.g. depression and anxiety (n=26, Rabinak *et al*, *Arch Neurol* 2010;**67**:58–63).

Role of drugs

DPD may be secondary to an underlying neuroanatomic degeneration and so standard antidepressants may be less than usually effective and this may be why depression may be an early symptom of PD (n=7270, Alonso *et al*, *J Neurol Neurosurg Psychiatry* 2009;**80**:671–4; FFT). Standard antidepressants do not generally seem to make Parkinsonian symptoms worse (n=76640, Gony *et al*, *Clin Neuropharmacol* 2003;**26**:142–5; n=62 [c=52], Dell'Agnello *et al*, *Clin Neuropharmacol* 2001;**24**:221–7).

Treatment strategies include:

1. **Exclude/treat any organic causes,** e.g. hypothyroidism (more prevalent in PD, McDonald *et al*, *Biol Psychiatry* 2003;**54**: 363–75).
2. **Use of antidepressants:**
   - SSRIs — care is needed if co-prescribing with selegiline as this can precipitate serotonin syndrome (*C5.13*)
   - Tricyclics may be poorly tolerated. Low-dose TCAs may be more effective than SSRIs (see amitriptyline; n=77, RCT, 12/12, Serrano-Dueñas, *Rev Neurol* 2002;**35**:1010–41; FFT), although a noradrenergic drug such as desipramine may have a quicker effect (n=48, RCT, d/b, p/c, 30/7, Devos *et al*, *Mov Disord* 2008;**23**:850–7).
3. **Augment with dopamine agonists**, e.g. pramipexole (but this can cause impulse dyscontrol and psychosis), as can rotigitine (n=6/28, Schreglmann *et al*, *Parkinsonism Relat Disord* 2012;**18**:207–9).
4. **Consider ECT**, although the incidence of delirium is high.

Reviews: diagnosis and treatment (Costa *et al*, *Arq Neuropsiquiatr* 2012;**70**:617–20; FFT), general (Barone, *Eur J Neurol* 2011;**18**[Suppl 1]:11–5).

BNF listed

No antidepressants are specifically licensed for depression in PD (DPD), and there seems to be some significant differences in efficacy and tolerability.

SSRIs

A systematic review and meta-analysis of RCTs was unable to prove conclusively that SSRIs are effective for DPD and suggested that higher doses may be needed, or that they may only help with more severe depression (s=10, n=430, RCT, 4–52/52, Skapinakis *et al*, *BMC Neurol* 2010;**10**:49; FFT).

Citalopram

A pilot study suggested a significant effect on depression and anxiety with no motor ADRs (n=10, open, 8/52, Menza *et al*, *J Neuropsychiatry Clin Neurosci* 2004;**16**:315–9), and improved bradykinesia in people also taking levodopa (n=46, open, 4/12, Rampello *et al*, *Clin Neuropharmacol* 2002; **25**:21–4).

Escitalopram

Escitalopram has a low effect on remission (n=14, Weintraub *et al*, *J Neuropsychiatry Clin Neurosci* 2006;**18**:377–83; FFT).

Fluoxetine *

Fluoxetine can be effective for DPD without impairing motor performance (n = 18, open, 80/7, Kostic *et al*, *Vojnosanit Pregl* 2012;**69**:1067–75), although marked worsening of motor symptoms has occurred (n=4, Steur, *Neurology* 2003;**43**:211–3).

Paroxetine

A large and robust RCT over 12/52 has shown that paroxetine (40 mg/d; n=42) significantly improved DPD and did not worsen motor functions (n = 115, RCT, d/b, p/c, 12/52, Richard *et al*, *Neurology* 2012;**78**:1229–36), although there may be slight worsening of motor symptoms (n = 14, 2/52, Chung *et al*, *Neurology* 2005;**64**:1797–8) and older studies were less positive (n=52, RCT, p/c, 8/52, Menza *et al*, *Neurology* 2009;**72**:886–92; FFT).

Sertraline

A naturalistic study showed sertraline (mean dose 66 mg/d) was effective in DPD and also had a positive impact on PD symptoms, albeit with worsening symptoms a few cases (n = 373[c = 310], Kulisevsky *et al*, *Eur J Neurol* 2008;**15**:953–9).

OTHERS ANTIDEPRESSANTS

Duloxetine

Duloxetine had no adverse effects in DPD and 65% reported varying degrees of pain relief (n = 23 [c = 20], open, 6/52, Djaldetti *et al*, *Clin Neuropharmacol* 2007;**30**:201–5).

MAOIs (see also selegiline)

Non-selective MAOIs, e.g. tranylcypromine have limited use but the MAO-A inhibitor moclobemide may be better. An open study with tranylcypromine showed slight improve-ment in motor symptoms and no unexpected ADRs (n = 37 [c = 27], 33/52, Fahn and Chouinard, *J Neural Transm Suppl* 1998;**52**:49–61).

Moclobemide

Moclobemide 300–600 mg/d was effective in 90% patients, although worsening or onset of tremor occurred in 50% (n = 12 [c = 10], open, 12/52, Giménez-Roldán *et al*, *Parkinsonism Relat Disord* 1997;**3**:219–25).

Reboxetine

Reboxetine seems effective, with an increasing effect over at least 4/12, and no increased motor symptoms (n = 17, 4/12, Pintor *et al*, *Gen Hosp Psychiatry* 2006;**28**:59–64).

Tricyclics

A meta-analysis suggests that tricyclics may be associated with a delay in starting dopaminergic therapy cf. no antidepressants (s = 6, n = 2064, Paumier *et al*, *Mov Disord* 2012;**27**:880–7).

Venlafaxine

A large and robust RCT over 12/52 has shown that venlafaxine XL (up to 225 mg/d; n = 34) significantly improved DPD and did not worsen motor functions (n = 115, RCT, d/b, p/c, 12/52, Richard *et al*, *Neurology* 2012; **78**:1229–36).

• Unlicensed/some efficacy

Bupropion

Successful use with motor symptom improvement has been reported (n = 1, Zaluska and Dyduch, *Int Psychogeriatr* 2011;**23**:325–7), as has improved comorbid panic and depression (n = 1, Gebhardt *et al*, *J Clin Pharm Ther* 2008; **33**:575–7).

Dopamine antagonists

See **pergolide** and **pramipexole** and review (Leentjens, *Drugs* 2011;**71**:273–86).

Omega-3 fatty acids ± TAU

Fish oils seem to improve DPD, either as monotherapy or as an adjunct (n = 31 [c = 29], RCT, d/b, p/c, 12/52, da Silva *et al*, *J Affect Disord* 2008;**111**:351–9).

Pergolide + levodopa

Pergolide as add-on to levodopa was not effective for self-reported depression, although lower levodopa doses were needed (n = 41, RCT, 8/12, Rektorová *et al* *Eur J Neurol* 2003;**10**:399–406).

Pramipexole

A meta-analysis has shown pramipexole improves mood and motivational symptoms, even in people without DPD (s= 14, RCT, d/b, p/c, Leentjens *et al*, *Clin Ther* 2009;**31**:89–98), e.g. 0.375–2 mg/d was clearly superior to placebo in a large trial (n=296[c=287], RCT, d/b, p/c, Barone *et al*, *Lancet Neurol* 2010;**9**:573–80) and 1.5–4.5 mg/d was as effective as sertraline 50 mg/d, with a significantly greater number of remissions, and no motor ADRs (n=67[c=62], Barone *et al*, *J Neurol* 2006;**253**:601–7). Pramipexole can also lower levodopa dose requirements (n=41, RCT, 8/12, Rektorová *et al Eur J Neurol* 2003;**10**:399–406).

Quetiapine

Psychotic anxious depression in PD has remitted with quetiapine (n= 1, Link *et al*, *Mov Disord* 2009;**24**:2431–2).

Selegiline

The MAO-B irreversible inhibitor selegiline is available transdermally in US for depression (review by Riederer and Laux, *Exp Neurobiol* 2011;**20**:1–17). Low oral doses are used for PD but high oral doses are needed (requiring MAOI diet) for DPD. Transdermal selegiline allows low doses to be absorbed, so is probably the only practical route for use (review by Frampton and Plosker, *Drugs* 2007;**67**:257–65).

Tianeptine

Tianeptine seems safe and effective, with no motor ADRs (n= 18, 3/12, Levin, *Zh Nevrol Psikhiatr Im S S Korsakova* 2006;**106**:20–5).

Trazodone

Trazodone seems to improve DPD (n=20, RCT, p/c, Werneck *et al*, *Arq Neuropsiquiatr* 2009;**67**:407–12; FFT).

□ No efficacy

Atomoxetine

Atomoxetine appears ineffective for DPD, although it improves cognitive performance and wakefulness (n=55, RCT, p/c, 8/52, Weintraub *et al*, *Neurology* 2010;**75**:448–55; FFT).

1.14.4 DYSTHYMIA (OR PERSISTENT DEPRESSIVE DISORDER)

see also Depression (*1.14*)

Symptoms

Dysthymia or persistent depressive disorder (DSM-5) is a low-grade chronic depression (often with anxiety) of insidious onset, chronic course (lasting at least two years with permanent or intermittent symptoms) and a high risk of relapse. It has few of the physical symptoms of depression and is compatible with stable social functioning. Almost all sufferers eventually develop super-imposed major depression (n=86, three-year follow-up, Klein *et al*, *Am J Psychiatry* 2000;**157**:931–9). The life-time prevalence rate may be around 3–6%, and higher in the elderly. It has been considered by some to be similar to depressive personality disorder or anxiety.

Role of drugs

Antidepressants are effective in dysthymia, and a meta-analysis showed antidepressants to actually have a wider margin of efficacy than in MDD, partly due to a lower placebo response rate in dysthymia (s= 17, Levkovitz *et al*, *J Clin Psychiatry* 2011;**72**:509–14). There is no proven significant differences between classes, but they should form part of an overall treatment strategy including, e.g. psychological therapies. A greater sensitivity to side-effects has been noted in dysthymics. SSRIs and moclobemide appear favoured. Cochrane concludes that drug therapy might as well be chosen on the basis of potential side-effects (s= 14, de Lima and Hotopf, *Cochrane Database Syst Rev* 2003;**3**:CD004047).

Reviews: diagnosis and treatment (de Lima and Hotopf, *Drug Saf* 2003;**26**:55–64), SSRIs and TCAs (s=20, von Wolff *et al*, *J Affect Disord* 2013;**144**:7–15; FFT).

• Unlicensed/some efficacy

ALCAR (acetyl-l-carnitine)

ALCAR may be as effective and tolerable as amisulpride (n=204, RCT, d/b, 12/52, Zanardi and Smeraldi, *Eur Neuropsychopharmacol* 2006;**16**:281–7).

Antipsychotics ± TAU

Cochrane concludes that for SGAs in dysthymia, **quetiapine** monotherapy is more effective than placebo, and that augmentation with **aripiprazole** or quetiapine (and possibly **olanzapine** or **risperidone**) may be superior to placebo (s=28, n=8487, Komossa et al, *Cochrane Database Syst Rev* 2010;**12**:CD008121). There is some evidence for low-dose **amisulpride** (e.g. n=313, RCT, d/b, 12/52, Amore *et al, Int Clin Psychopharmacol* 2001;**16**:317–24).

Review: substituted benzamides in dysthymia (Pani and Gessa, *Mol Psychiatry* 2002;**7**:247–53; FFT).

Bupropion

Bupropion SR up to 400mg/d was effective in 71% patients in one trial, with those having a history of substance misuse less likely to respond (n=21, open, 8/52, Hellerstein *et al, J Clin Psychopharmacol* 2001;**21**:325–9).

L-acetylcarnitine (LAC) *

LAC, the acetyl ester of naturally occurring carnitine, was as effective as fluoxetine but with a quicker onset (n=80, RCT, d/b, p/c, 7/52, Bersani *et al, Eur Neuropsychopharmacol* 2013;**23**:1219–25).

Moclobemide

Moclobemide (mean 675mg/d) appears to be significantly more effective for dysthymia than imipramine (mean 220mg/d), with less side-effects (n=315, RCT, Versiani *et al, Int Clin Psychopharmacol* 1997;**12**:183–93).

SSRIs *

SSRIs are probably the treatment of choice for dysthymia.

Citalopram (mean 39mg/d) appeared effective in 73% of 'pure' dysthymics in a small study (n=21, open, 12/52, Hellerstein *et al, Int Clin Psychopharmacol* 2004;**19**:143–8).

Fluoxetine 20mg/d may be more effective than placebo, with 50% of the non-responders at three months improving with a dose increase to 40mg/d (n=140, RCT, Vanelle *et al, Br J Psychiatry* 1997;**170**:345–50), but may have limited efficacy in elderly people (n=90[c=71], RCT, d/b, p/c, 12/52, Devanand *et al, Am J Geriatr Psychiatry* 2005;**13**:59–68).

Paroxetine was superior to placebo in two RCTs (e.g. n=40, RCT, d/b, p/c, 12/52, Ravindran *et al, Asian J Psychiatr* 2013;**6**:157–61).

Sertraline, up to 200mg/d, may be effective in dysthymia without major depression (n=310, RCT, p/c, 12/52, Ravindran *et al, J Clin Psychiatry* 2000;**61**:821–7; n=410, RCT, d/b, p/c, Hellerstein *et al, Am J Psychiatry* 2000;**157**:1436–44).

Testosterone

In hypogonadal older men, testosterone gel may be effective for subsyndromal depression (n=33, RCT, d/b, p/c, 24/52, Shores *et al, J Clin Psychiatry* 2009;**70**:1009–16) with IM injections as an alternative (n=23, RCT, d/b, p/c, Seidman *et al, J Clin Psychopharmacol* 2009;**29**:216–21).

Tricyclics

Tricyclics at robust doses, e.g. imipramine 50–300mg/d may be effective but with high drop-outs in long-standing dysthymia (n=416, RCT, 12/52, p/c, Kocsis *et al, Am J Psychiatry* 1997;**154**:390).

■ Unlicensed/possible efficacy

Duloxetine

A small study has suggested some efficacy for duloxetine in dysthymia (n=24[c=19], open, Koran *et al, J Clin Psychiatry* 2007;**68**:761–5).

Mirtazapine

Mirtazapine 15–45mg/d was effective in 73% in a small trial (n=15[c=11], open, 10/52, Dunner et al, *Depress Anxiety* 1999;**10**:68–72).

Sildenafil

Sildenafil has produced improvement, not related to erectile function, in middle-aged depressed men (n=20, open, 6/52, Orr *et al, J Nerv Ment Dis* 2008;**196**:496–500).

Venlafaxine

Several open studies suggest some efficacy, e.g. up to 225–300mg/d was effective in 71% of completers (eg. n=23[c=18], open, 12/52, Devanand *et al, J Geriatr Psychiatr Neurol* 2004;**17**:219–24).

✱ Case reports

- **Chromium** (n=5, s/b, McLeod *et al, J Clin Psychiatry* 1999;**60**:237).

□ No efficacy

St John's wort

Dysthymia is unresponsive to SJW (n=150, RCT, d/b, p/c, 6/52, Randlov *et al*, *Phytomedicine* 2006;**13**:215–21).

1.15 EATING DISORDERS

1.15.1 Anorexia nervosa
1.15.2 Bulimia nervosa
1.15.3 Binge-eating disorder

DSM-5 includes three eating disorders; anorexia nervosa (AN), bulimia nervosa (BN), binge-eating disorder (BAD) and eating disorders not otherwise specified (EDNOS). Although sociocultural explanations are important anorexia, bulimia and obesity may be heterogeneous disorders with a complex aetiology, including genetic factors and the environment.

Reviews: AFSBP Guidelines (Aigner *et al*, *World J Biol Psychiatry* 2011;**12**:400–43), general (Treasure *et al*, *Lancet* 2010;**375**:583–93), anticonvulsants for eating disorders (McElroy *et al*, *CNS Drugs* 2009;**23**:139–56), pharmacotherapy (Flament *et al*, *Int J Neuropsychopharmacol* 2012; **15**:189–207).

1.15.1 ANOREXIA NERVOSA (AN)

Symptoms:

The main diagnostic symptoms are:

- Amenorrhoea in females (absence of three consecutive menstrual cycles)
- Refusal to maintain body weight over the minimum normal for age and height
- Intense fear of gaining weight or being fat
- Disturbance in body perception, e.g. feeling fat even when emaciated.

Anorexia usually starts in the late teens, with distorted body image and relentless dieting. People with AN may avoid carbohydrates, induce vomiting, abuse laxatives, take excess exercise, binge eat and suffer depression and social withdrawal. It may occur in up to 8–13 per 100000 population, and 90% are female.

Role of drugs

Drug therapy is generally most useful as a supportive measure to treat any concurrent conditions. In severely emaciated patients, enteral feeding or even TPN may be necessary.

Reviews: * overall management (Milano *et al*, *ISRN Pharmacol* 2013;**2013**:352865; Watson and Bulik, *Psychol Med* 2013;**43**:2477–500), adolescent eating disorders: definitions, symptomatology, epidemiology and comorbidity (Herpertz-Dahlmann, *Child Adolesc Psychiatr Clin N Am* 2009;**18**:31–47), use of SGAs (McKnight and Park, *Eur Eat Disord Rev* 2010;**18**:10–21), severe and enduring AN (Hay *et al*, *Aust N Z J Psychiatry* 2012;**46**:1136–44).

• Unlicensed/some efficacy

Nutritional feeding

TPN may be necessary in severe anorexia where life-threatening weight loss has occurred, particularly if accompanied by low potassium levels and where conventional therapies have failed. Osteoporosis (Misra and Klibanski, *Rev Endocr Metab Disord* 2006; **7**:91–9) and osteopenia can be frequent and severe complications (Golden, *Adolesc Med* 2003;**14**:97–108). Vitamin D and calcium supplements are essential.

Reviews: medical complications (Gentile, *Nutrients* 2012;**4**:1293–303), tube feeding and nutrition (Gentile *et al*, *Clin Nutr* 2010;**29**:627–32).

Treatment of any PMS

This may help any premenstrual exacerbations.

■ Unlicensed/possible efficacy

Antidepressants (see also fluoxetine)

Citalopram 20mg/d has been used successfully (e.g. n=52, RCT, Fassino *et al*, *Eur Neuropsychopharmacol* 2002;**12**:453–9).

Dronabinol *

Dronabinol 5mg/d for 4/52 produced a small but significant weight gain (n=25[c=24], RCT, d/b, p/c, c/o, 12/52, Andries *et al*, *Int J Eat Disord* 2014;**47**:18–23).

Oxytocin *

There may be a deranged oxytocin system in AN that may normalise on recovery (Maquire *et al*, *Eur Eat Disord Rev* 2013;**21**:475–8). Intranasal oxytocin has attenuated the attentional bias for eating and fat shape stimuli in patients with AN (n=64, d/b, p/c, c/o, Kim *et al, Psychoneuroendocrinology* 2014;**44**:133–42).

Zinc

Zinc 100mg/d produced an increase in BMI twice that of placebo (n=35, RCT, d/b, p/c, Birmingham *et al, Int J Eat Disord* 1994;**15**:251–5) and 14mg/d for two months has been advocated as routine in all people with AN (RCT, Birmingham and Gritzner, *Eat Weight Disord* 2006;**11**:109–11).

✱ Case reports

- **Mirtazapine** (n=1, Safer *et al, Int J Eat Disord* 2011;**44**:178–81; n=1, Jaafar *et al, Aust N Z J Psychiatry* 2007;**41**:768–9)
- **Mirtazapine + olanzapine** (n=1, 6/12, Wang *et al, Prog Neuropsychopharmacol Biol Psychiatry* 2006;**30**:306–9)
- **Tramadol** 225mg/d (n=1, Mendelson, *Am J Psychiatry* 2001;**158**:963–94).

□ No efficacy

Antipsychotics *

Although there has been much enthusiasm for antipsychotics in AN, a meta-analysis of SGAs concludes that olanzapine, quetiapine and risperidone are not superior to placebo but some people do benefit (s=7, n=201, RCTs, Dold *et al, Psychother Psychosom* 2015;**84**:110–6).

Aripiprazole has shown efficacy in reducing eating-related pre-occupations and rituals (n=75, open, Marzole *et al, PLoS One* 2015;**10**:e0125569; FFT).

Haloperidol * low-dose has been suggested as an adjunct in severe AN (n=13, open, 6/12, Cassano *et al, Int J Eat Disord* 2003;**33**:172–7; n=9, RCR, Mauri *et al, Eat Weight Disord* 2013;**18**:329–32).

Olanzapine 5mg/d may help OCD and AN, with reduced fixed body perceptions and improved insight. Two RCTs showed only a trend for benefit but no statistical difference (eg. n=23[c=17], RCT, d/b, p/c, 8/52, Attia *et al, Psychol Med* 2011;**41**:2177–82), and it was ineffectual for under-weight adolescent females with AN (n=20[c=15], RCT, d/b, p/c, 10/52, Kafantaris *et al, J Child Adolesc Psychopharmacol* 2011;**21**:207–12).

Quetiapine 150–300mg/d has improved some general psychiatric symptoms in anorexia (n=19[c=14], open, 10/52, Powers *et al, Int J Eat Disord* 2007;**40**:21–6) and quetiapine 100–400mg/d plus TAU was superior to TAU for a range of key symptoms (n=33, RCT, open, 12/52–1 year, Court *et al, J Psychiatr Res* 2010;**44**:1027–34), but there was no apparent effect in the only RCT (n=15[c=10], RCT, d/b, p/c, 8/52, Powers *et al, Eur Eat Disord Rev* 2012;**20**:331–4; FFT).

Risperidone was ineffective for adolescents and young adults with AN, although there was a transient improvement at initiation (n=40, RCT, d/b, p/c, 9/52, Hagman *et al, J Am Acad Child Adolesc Psychiatry* 2011;**50**:915–24; FFT) and an effect maintained over 17/12 (n=1, Kracke and Tosh, *Springerplus* 2014;**3**:706; FFT).

Review: in children and adolescents (Mehler-Wex *et al, Eur Eat Disord Rev* 2008; **16**:100–8).

Fluoxetine

Fluoxetine had no advantage over placebo in anorexia following weight restoration (n=93, RCT, d/b, p/c, <1 year, Walsh *et al, JAMA* 2006;**295**:2605–12).

Topiramate

Topiramate caused relapse of AN in a patient when used for epilepsy (n=1, Rosenow *et al, Am J Psychiatry* 2002;**159**:2112–3).

1.15.2 BULIMIA NERVOSA (BN)

Symptoms

The main diagnostic symptoms are:

- Recurrent binge eating and lack of control
- An urge to overeat (including lack of control of eating during binges)
- Regular self-induced vomiting, laxative abuse, strict dieting or fasting
- Persistent over-concern with body shape and weight.

There must be a minimum of two binge episodes per week for at least three months. Weight and menses are normal. Prevalence rates are about 1% for young women and 0.1% for young men.

Role of drugs

Cochrane concludes that all antidepressants appear equally effective, but with a high drop-out rate (Bacaltchuk and Hay, *Cochrane Database Syst Rev* 2003;**4**:CD003391) and do not work purely as antidepressants. Side-effects (especially anticholinergic) can be severe and result in non-compliance. Drugs should be part of an individualised programme with nutrition and CBT the most effective interventions, although Cochrane concludes that the evidence for the efficacy of CBT in bulimia is small and of variable quality (s=48, n=3054, Hay *et al*, *Cochrane Database Syst Rev* 2009;**4**:CD000562). **Review:** general (Hay and Claudino, *Clin Evid [Online]* 2010;**2010**:1009; FFT).

BNF listed

Fluoxetine (see also other SSRIs)

Fluoxetine 60mg/d has a significant effect on binge-eating and purging, eating attitudes, behaviour and food craving, e.g. it was superior to placebo as maintenance therapy (eg. n=150, RCT, 12/12, Romano *et al*, *Am J Psychiatry* 2002;**159**:96–102) and in adolescent bulimia (n=10, open, 8/52, Kotler *et al*, *J Child Adolesc Psychopharmacol* 2003;**13**:329–35), but may have no benefit over a year once weight has been restored (n=93, RCT, d/b, p/c, 12/12, Walsh *et al*, *JAMA* 2006;**295**:2605–12). Bulimics who fail to report at least a 60% decrease in binge-eating or vomiting by week 3 are unlikely to respond (s=2, n=785, Sysko *et al*, *Psychol Med* 2010;**40**:999–1005; FFT). Improvement is independent of depression scores. Its long half-life may help with missed doses.

• Unlicensed/some efficacy

SSRIs (see also fluoxetine above)

Citalopram may be useful for depressed people with bulimia (n=37, RCT, s/b, Leombruni *et al*, *Adv Ther* 2006;**23**:481–94).

Fluvoxamine 200mg/d may reduce binge-eating and purging and may be well tolerated (e.g. n=12, RCT, p/c, 12/52, Milano *et al*, *Adv Ther* 2005;**22**:278–83).

Paroxetine was reported to have no beneficial effect in an unpublished study.

Sertraline was significantly effective in most measures in two short studies (n=34, RCT, d/b, 6/52, McElroy *et al*, *Am J Psychiatry* 2000;**157**:1004–6; n=18, open, 8/52, Sloan *et al*, *Int J Eat Dis* 2004;**36**:48–54).

Topiramate

A systematic analysis suggested topiramate is effective for the short-term treatment of BN but long-term use is unproven (s=5, n=655, RCTs, Arbaizar *et al*, *Gen Hosp Psych* 2008;**30**:471–5). There have been some case reports of success (n=5, Barbee, *Int J Eat Disord* 2003;**33**:468–72).

■ Unlicensed/possible efficacy

Buspirone

Buspirone may have similar efficacy to fluoxetine in short-term management of bulimic symptoms (n=57, open, 12/52, Rajewski and Rybakowski, *Psychiatr Pol* 2006; **40**:75–82).

Lamotrigine

Lamotrigine has been used to treat bulimia with comorbid bipolar (Rybakowski and Kaminska, *Prog Neuropsychopharmacol* 2008; **32**:2004–5).

MAOIs

MAOIs can be effective if dietary restrictions can be overcome.

Ondansetron

Ondansetron was reported to be effective in three small, short-term trials and may be an option after failure of conventional therapies (reviews by Fung and Ferrill, *Ann Pharmacother* 2001;**35**:1270–3). Decreased binge-eating and vomiting has been shown with ondansetron 24mg/d, possibly due to a pharmacological decrease in vagal neuro-transmission (n=28, RCT, Faris *et al*, *Lancet* 2000;**355**:792–7; editorial by Kiss, *Lancet* 2000;**355**:769–70).

Oxcarbazepine

Oxcarbazepine has been used for self-mutilating bulimic patients (Cordas *et al*, *Int J Neuropsychopharmacol* 2006;**9**:769–71).

PMS treatments

Pyridoxine and progesterones may help to minimise the effects of premenstrual relapses.

Reboxetine

Reboxetine 4mg/d has produced a rapid response (50% decrease in bulimic behaviour) in 60% patients (n=28, RCT, 3/12, Fassino *et al, J Psychopharmacol* 2004;**18**:423–8).

Stimulants

In women with comorbid ADHD and bulimia, complete response in binge eating has been reported with stimulants (n=6, Dukarm, *J Women's Health [Larchmt]* 2005;**14**:345–50).

Tricyclics

Tricyclics have been used but high relapse rates suggest serious limitations with long-term efficacy (n=80, RCT, d/b, p/c, 6/12, Walsh *et al, Am J Psychiatry* 1991;**148**:1206–12).

Zonisamide

Zonisamide (up to 300mg/d) reduced SIB and other impulsive behaviours in bulimia nervosa (n=17[c=10], open, one year, Idini *et al, Rev Bras Psiquiatr* 2011;**33**:418–9; FFT).

✱ Case reports

- Aripiprazole (n=3, Trunko *et al, Int J Eat Disord* 2010;**44**:269–75)
- Duloxetine 120mg/d (e.g. n=1, Christensen and Averbuch, *Psychiatry (Edgmont)* 2009;**6**:27–8; FFT).

□ No efficacy

Carbamazepine

No effect was seen in one study (n=6, Safai-Kutti and Kutti, *Am J Psychiatry* 1986;**143**:1059).

Clozapine

Bulimia has acutely worsened with clozapine 350mg/d (n=1, Brewerton and Shannon, *Am J Psychiatry* 1992;**149**:1408).

Cyproheptadine

Cyproheptadine appears to be detrimental in bulimia (n=72, RCT, d/b, Halmi *et al, Arch Gen Psychiatry* 1986;**43**:177–81).

Lithium

Despite early enthusiasm, lithium appears no more effective than placebo (n=91, Hsu *et al, J Nerv Mental Dis* 1991;**179**:351–5).

Mianserin

No effect was seen at 60mg/d (n=50, 8/52, Sabine *et al, Br J Clin Pharmacol* 1983;**15**:195S–202S; FFT).

1.15.3 BINGE-EATING DISORDER (BED)

Symptoms

BED is characterised by binge-eating large amounts of food in discrete time periods, which is not then followed by compensatory behaviours such as purging or vomiting. BED is a chronic condition (mean duration 14 years, n=888, Pope *et al, Am J Psychiatry* 2006;**163**:2181–3), with a longer duration than bulimia or anorexia. Many (but not all) patients are obese and may seek treatment for this. CBT is effective for behavioural and psychological features of BED, but not for the obesity (n=108[c=86], RCT, 16/52, d/b, p/c, Grilo *et al, Biol Psychiatry* 2005;**57**:301–9). Higher rates of comorbid psychiatric conditions, especially depression, are seen.

Role of drugs

A meta-analysis of p/c trials concluded that pharmacotherapy had a clinical advantage over placebo for achieving short-term remission and weight-loss from BED, but there was no data for a long-term effect. Combining with psychotherapy does not enhance the effect (s=33, p/c, Reas and Grilo, *Obesity (Silver Spring)* 2008;**16**:2024–38; FFT). Studies on fluvoxamine, fluoxetine, sertraline, citalopram, sibutramine and topiramate have shown some efficacy.

Reviews: * general (Marazziti *et al, Eur Rev Med Pharmacol Sci* 2012;**16**:2102–7; McElroy *et al, Expert Opin Pharmacother* 2012;**13**:2015–26), novel treatments (Marazziti *et al, Curr Med Chem* 2011;**18**:5159–64), therapeutics options (Ramacciotti *et al, Eat Weight Disord* 2013;**18**:3–9).

● Unlicensed/some efficacy

Atomoxetine

Atomoxetine 40–120mg/d was fairly well

tolerated and significantly reduced binge-eating ratings (n=40[c=36], RCT, d/b, p/c, 10/52, McElroy *et al*, *J Clin Psychiatry* 2007;**68**:390–8).

Bupropion

Weight gain was significantly greater with bupropion 300mg/d than placebo, but there were no other significant differences (n=61[c=54], RCT, d/b, p/c, 8/52, White and Grilo, *J Clin Psychiatry* 2013;**74**:400–6).

Duloxetine

The only study showed duloxetine (mean 79mg/d) was effective in BED with comorbid MDD (n=40, d/b, p/c, 12/52, Guerdjikova *et al*, *Int J Eat Disord* 2012;**45**:281–9).

Lamotrigine *

Lamotrigine had a significant effect on all measures of BED in one study but, unfortunately, so did placebo, which may have disguised any effect, or not, as the case may be (n=51, RCT, d/b, p/c, 16/52, Guerdjikova *et al*, *Int Clin Psychopharmacol* 2009;**24**:150–8). There is a case series suggesting a possible positive effect (n=5, Trunko *et al*, *Int J Eat Disord* 2014;**47**:329–34).

Lisdexamfetamine *

LDX is licensed for moderate-to-severe BED in USA, but is not for weight loss (Reas and Grilo, *Expert Opin Pharmacother* 2015; **16**:1463–78) and is on its way to a European license. The only published trial showed that 50–70mg/d decreased BE days, BE cessation and global improvement, and was well tolerated (n=259, RCT, d/b, p/c, 11/52, McElroy *et al*, *JAMA Psychiatry* 2015;72:235–46; systematic review by Citrome, *Int J Clin Pract* 2015;**69**:410–21).

Sibutramine

Two RCTs have shown sibutramine 15mg/d to reduce binge episodes, weight and mental state but with significant ADRs (e.g. n=304, RCT, d/b, p/c, 24/52, Wilfley *et al*, *Am J Psychiatry* 2008; **165**:51–8).

SSRIs (see also 'no efficacy')

The SSRIs seem to have some efficacy. **Citalopram** may be effective in reducing binge-eating frequency, weight and severity (n=38, RCT, d/b, p/c, 6/52, McElroy *et al*, *J Clin Psychiatry* 2003;**64**:807–13). **Sertraline** 100–200mg/d and **fluoxetine** 40–80mg/d were equally effective for measures of BED (n=42, RCT, d/b, 6/12, Leombruni *et al*, *Prog Neuropsychopharmacol Biol Psychiatry* 2008; **32**:1599–605). **Fluoxetine** (mean dose 71mg/d) was well tolerated and effective in reducing binge-eating frequency, weight and illness severity (n=60, RCT, d/b, 6/52, Arnold *et al*, *J Clin Psychiatry* 2002;**63**:1028–33), but was less effective than individualised CBT (n=116, >2 years, Devlin *et al*, *Obesity [Silver Spring]* 2007;**15**:1702–9).

Topiramate ± TAU

Adjunct: Topiramate 200mg/d improved the short-term efficacy of CBT (n=73, RCT, d/b, p/c, 21/52, Claudino *et al*, *J Clin Psychiatry* 2007;**68**:1324–32). There may be a dose-response as up to 600mg/d produced an enduring improvement in some people with BED, albeit poorly tolerated (e.g. n=61, 14+42/52, RCT, d/b, p/c, McElroy *et al*, *J Clin Psychiatry* 2004;**65**:1463–9).

Monotherapy: A systematic analysis has suggested that topiramate is effective for the short-term treatment of BED, but long-term use is unproven (s=5, n=655, RCTs, Arbaizar *et al*, *Gen Hosp Psych* 2008;**30**:471–5).

Review: general (Leombruni *et al*, *Neuropsychiatr Dis Treat* 2009;**5**:385–92; FFT).

■ Unlicensed/possible efficacy

Acamprosate

Acamprosate was not statistically different to placebo, although all measures improved (n=40, RCT, d/b, p/c, 10/52, McElroy *et al*, *Int J Eat Disord* 2011;**44**:81–90).

Lithium + topiramate

Lithium has augmented topiramate in comorbid bipolar and BED, (n=12, open, Kotwal *et al*, *Hum Psychopharmacol* 2006; **21**:425–31).

Memantine

Memantine 5–20mg/d may reduce binge-eating in BED but has little effect on BMI (n=19[c=9], open, 12/52, Brennan *et al*, *Int J Eat Disord* 2008;**41**:520–6).

Reboxetine

Reboxetine 8 mg/d produced a remarkable reduction in binge days per week, decreased BMI and improved other measures (n=9[c=5], open, 12/52, Silveira *et al*, *Eat Weight Disorder* 2005;**10**:93–6).

Sodium oxybate

Oxybate (mean 7 g/d) appeared very effective for BED but with a high drop-out rate (n=12[c=5], open, 16/52, McElroy *et al*, *Int J Eat Disord* 2011;**44**:262–8).

Zonisamide

Zonisamide 100–600 mg/d may significantly reduce binge-eating frequency and other measures (n=15[c=8], open, 12/52, McElroy *et al*, *J Clin Psychiatry* 2004;**65**:50–6).

□ No efficacy

Fluvoxamine (see also SSRIs)

Fluvoxamine was no better than placebo in BED (n=20, RCT, d/b, p/c, Pearlstein *et al*, *Arch Women Ment Health* 2003;**6**:147–51).

1.16 INSOMNIA

Insomnia, the difficulty in initiating or maintaining sleep, is generally a symptom of an underlying problem, not an illness itself and should be treated as such. Insomnia can be caused by a variety of external (e.g. environment) and internal stimuli (e.g. mental health problems, e.g. ADHD, stress, emotional conflict, physical illness and drugs, see *5.14*), and can be transient, chronic, initial or with early morning wakening. The causes, where possible, should be determined and treated, as well as placing emphasis on sleep hygiene.

Principles of sleep hygiene:*

Although widely used and logical, there is actually no evidence base for sleep hygiene, although *not* doing any of these will not help sleep.

1. Avoid excessive use of caffeine (particularly within 3–6 hours of going to bed), alcohol or nicotine. A hot milky drink may help.
2. Do not stay in bed for prolonged periods if not asleep. Go to another dimly lit room — watching TV can have an alerting effect.
3. Avoid back-lit screens (e.g. TV, PC, iPad) for an hour before going to bed, as the blue light emitted inhibits the release of melatonin.
4. Avoid daytime naps or long periods of inactivity.
5. A warm bath or exercise a few hours before bedtime may promote sleep.
6. Avoid engaging in strenuous exercise or mental activity near bedtime (although sex can aid sleep).
7. Make sure that the bed and bedroom are comfortable and avoid extremes of noise, light, temperature and humidity.
8. Establish a regular bedtime routine, e.g. going to bed and rising at the same time, regardless of sleep duration.
9. Diet — carbohydrate (e.g. pasta) can help sleep, but not eating a big meal within about two hours of going to bed. Sugar may inhibit sleep, as may some vitamin supplements.

Role of drugs

Assuming sleep hygiene is good, any hypnotics should always be used on a 'when required' basis, as tolerance may develop to the sedative effects within 2–3 weeks. Short-term use for short-term reasons is usually without problem and can be useful and comforting for the patient. Longer-term use needs the risk:benefit analysis considered. About 30% of older people prescribed BDZs or Zs may still be taking them two months later, but since they seem to be effective it may be that effort should go into avoiding long-term use, rather than stopping short-term use for treatment of some symptoms of mania, anxiety and depression (n=129, Simon and Ludman, *Gen Hosp Psychiatry* 2006;**28**:374–8; FFT). In a much-disputed study, the risks of mortality or cancer over 2.5 years appeared significantly higher with hypnotics, even with less than 18 pills per year, suggesting that there must be some other explanations, or the world's premature death rates ought to be much higher (n=10529+23676, Kripke *et al*, *Br Med J Open* 2012;**2**:e000850).

Reviews: * BAP Guidelines for treatment of insomnia, parasomnias and circadian rhythm disorders (Wilson *et al*, *J Psychopharmacol* 2010;**24**:1577–1600), general (Ioachimescu and El-Solh, *Expert Opin Pharmacother* 2012;**13**:1243–60), sleep disturbances in Alzheimer's (s=5, n=313, RCTs, p/c, McCleery *et al*, *Cochrane Database Syst Rev* 2014;**3**:CD009178).

BNF listed

BENZODIAZEPINES

Benzodiazepines may be extremely useful in the short-term management of insomnia, helping to facilitate or initiate essential high-quality sleep. A meta-analysis has indicated benzodiazepines are effective in improving sleep latency and duration, but ADRs (e.g. drowsiness and dizziness) are common, although methodologically these studies are flawed. Users of benzodiazepines are at greater risk of road-traffic accidents, especially if combined with alcohol (s=27, Rapoport *et al*, *J Clin Psychiatry* 2009;**70**:663–73). Although relatively safe in overdose, BDZs (especially flunitrazepam and nitrazepam) have been implicated in 39% of drug poisoning suicides in Sweden from 1992–1996, so care is needed (Carlsten *et al*, *Scand J Public Health* 2003;**31**:224–28).

Flunitrazepam

This longer-acting benzodiazepine may have an abuse potential and its misuse may be underrated as a trigger for admission to forensic settings (n=60, Dåderman and Edman, *Psychiatry Res* 2001;**103**:27–42).

Flurazepam

Flurazepam has a short half-life but with longer-acting metabolites that can cause a hangover in older people (n=25, RCT, d/b, p/c, c/o, Boyle *et al*, *Hum Psychopharmacol* 2009;**24**:61–71).

Loprazolam

Loprazolam is an intermediate-acting benzodiazepine with a half-life of 7–15 hours.

Lormetazepam

Lormetazepam is an intermediate-acting benzodiazepine. Short-term use has no effect on daytime vigilance or motor task performance, with only minimal psychomotor impairment in younger adults (n=18, RCT, d/b, p/c, Fabbrini *et al*, *Clin Ther* 2005;**27**:78–83).

Nitrazepam

Nitrazepam is a longer-acting benzodiazepine similar to diazepam, and has active metabolites. Stable plasma levels can be attained in five days, so avoid use in the elderly.

Predicting hypnotic dependence risk
(Tyrer, *Br Med J* 1993;**306**:706–8;FFT)

Factor	Score
Benzodiazepine hypnotic used	3
Dose higher than BNF mean	2
Duration of treatment >3 months	2
Dependent personality	2
Short elimination half-life drug	2
Tolerance or dose escalation	2
Total	
No dependence, abrupt withdrawal	=0
Some dependence risk, withdraw over two weeks recommended	=1–4
Strong dependence risk, withdraw over 4–12 weeks	=5–8
High risk of dependence, withdraw gradually plus support programme	=8–13

Temazepam

Temazepam is a shorter-acting benzodiazepine, whose abuse potential has been well recognised. 7.5mg and 15mg appear equally effective (n=131, RCT, d/b, Erman *et al*, *Curr Med Res Opin* 2004;**20**:441–9).

'Z' HYPNOTICS

The 'Z' hypnotics are now widely used and offer many benefits over the benzodiazepines. **Zolpidem** is potent and quick-acting (often within 15 minutes) and ideal for initiating sleep and has many fans in the pharmaceutical and medical worlds. **Zopiclone** has a slower onset but longer action. The incidence of dependence with zopiclone and zolpidem is remarkably lower than hypnotic BDZs, and they are relatively safe (n=58, Hajak *et al*, *Addiction* 2003;**98**:1371–8).
Review: * cognitive effects (Stranks and Crowe, *J Clin Exp Neuropsychol* 2014;**36**:691–700).

Zaleplon

Zaleplon is a pyrazolopyrimidine hypnotic, a selective full agonist at the omega-1 benzodiazepine receptor (Noguchi *et al*, *Eur J Pharmacol* 2002;**434**:21–8).

Zolpidem *

Zolpidem is a imidazopyridine that binds preferentially to the omega-1 benzodiazepine receptor. It has a rapid onset and a short duration of action but does not affect sleep architecture. Zolpidem 10mg taken at night up to 3–5 times a week significantly improved overall sleep, which was sustained, with no evidence of rebound, dose escalation or withdrawal, showing that true PRN hypnotic use may be highly effective and safe (n=199, RCT, p/c, 12/52, Perlis *et al*, *J Clin Psychiatry* 2004;**65**:1128–37). Zolpidem does not lose its efficacy after 8/12 continuous therapy (n=91, RCT, d/b, p/c, 8/12, Randall *et al*, *Sleep* 2012;**35**:1551–7) and even after a year there were no withdrawal symptoms or rebound insomnia when stopped or, to be precise, 30–40% *did* suffer rebound insomnia, but this did not differ between zolpidem and placebo (n=33, RCT, d/b, p/c, 12/12, Roehrs *et al*, *J Psychopharmacol* 2012;**26**:1088–95). Although zolpidem causes minimal cognitive, memory and equilibrium adverse effects (n=48, RCT, d/b, p/c, c/o, Allain *et al*, *Eur J Clin Pharmacol* 2003;**59**:179–88), it is apparently a strong and independent risk factor for falls in in-patient units (n=4962+11358, Kolla *et al*, *J Hosp Med* 2013;**8**:1–6) and the FDA in USA have reduced the maximum nightly dose of zolpidem to 5mg due to concerns about a hangover effect.

Reviews: general (Greenblatt and Roth, *Expert Opin Pharmacother* 2012;**13**:879–93; Dang *et al*, *CNS Neurosci Ther* 2011;**17**:387–97), kinetics (de Haas *et al*, *J Psychopharmacol* 2010;**24**:1619–29).

Zopiclone *

Zopiclone is an established non-benzodiazepine hypnotic, albeit only licensed in the UK for up to 7.5mg/d for up to four weeks. Zopiclone is equivalent, but not superior, to BDZs (s=45, n=2672, meta-analysis, Holbrook *et al*, *CMAJ* 2000;**162**:225–33; FFT). Impaired driving effects can be seen up to 11 hours after a 7.5mg dose (s=4, n=101, d/b, c/o, Leufkens and Vermeeren, *Clin Ther* 2014;**36**:141–50). Eszopiclone and SSRIs improve sleep and depression and anxiety (s=2, n=347, RCT, d/b, p/c, 8/52, Fava *et al*, *J Clin Psychiatry* 2011;**72**:473–9.

OTHER HYPNOTICS

Antihistamines

Antihistamines may be effective and are often used as OTC sleep aids. **Promethazine** has a relatively long half-life and a low abuse potential. **Diphenhydramine** may have an abuse potential and has been strongly linked to cognitive impairment and decline in older people (n=426, Agoustini *et al*, *Arch Intern Med* 2001;**161**:2091–7). However, while causing drowsiness they do not actually lead to a quality or refreshing sleep.

Barbiturates

Barbiturates should only be used for severe, intractable insomnia where there are compelling reasons, and only in people already taking barbiturates. Toxicity in overdose can be high.

Chloral hydrate

Chloral hydrate has properties similar to the barbiturates and is relatively safe in the elderly, as the half-life is not significantly lengthened. An abuse potential exists and it can be toxic in overdose.

Clomethiazole (chlormethiazole)

Clomethiazole is a thiamine derivative with sedative-hypnotic and anticonvulsant properties. It has a rapid onset of action and short half-life even in the elderly, although they may be more sensitive to it. Dependence and abuse have been reported, generally in people who are dependence prone (n=5, Hession *et al*, *Lancet* 1979;**ii**:953–4). It is unsafe in overdose.

Melatonin (Circadin®) *

Circadin® is the only melatonin product licensed in the UK as a monotherapy course up to 13 weeks for primary insomnia in people aged 55 and over. Melatonin is an agonist at M1, M2 and M3 receptors. The dose is 2mg 1–2 hours before bedtime and after food (which slows absorption). The Circadin® tablets contain a synthetic melatonin, which is released over several hours to match the normal human melatonin profile (increasing after dark, peaking at 2–4 AM, then diminishing), as older people with primary insomnia secrete significantly lower levels of melatonin than healthy elderly people with good sleep quality. A meta-analysis concludes melatonin produces a modest reduction in sleep latency and increased sleep time, with a longer duration and higher doses being more effective and with no reduction in effect over time (s=19, n=1683, RCT, p/c, Ferracioli-Oda *et al, PLoS One* 2013;**8**:e63773). Melatonin is also effective in under-55s (n=791 [c=746], RCT, d/b, p/c, 7/12, Wade *et al, Curr Med Res Opin* 2011;**27**:87–98) and in shift workers (n=86, RCT, d/b, p/c, c/o, Sadeghniiat-Haghighi *et al, J Circadian Rhythms* 2008;**6**:10; FFT). There are no withdrawal symptoms on discontinuation (n=170[c=164], RCT, d/b, p/c, 7/52, Lemoine *et al, J Sleep Res* 2007;**16**:372–80; FFT). Adjunctive melatonin can help older people discontinue conventional hypnotics (n=22, RCT, d/b, c/o, 4/12, Garzón *et al, Aging Clin Exp Res* 2009;**21**:38–42), although a larger study suggested lack of effect over placebo for sedative withdrawal in older people with primary insomnia (n=92[c=89], RCT, d/b, p/c, 8/52, Lähteenmäki *et al, Br J Clin Pharmacol* 2014;**77**:975–85). Any loss in efficacy over time may be due to slower 1A2 metabolism and subsequent accumulation and toxicity, so it can help to lower the dose (n=3, Braam *et al, J Intellect Disabil Res* 2010;**54**:547–55).

Reviews: * general (Lyseng-Williamson, *Drugs Aging* 2012;**29**:911–23; Lemoine and Zisapel, *Expert Opin Pharmacother* 2012;**13**:895–905), use for insomnia in over 55s (s=16, Vural *et al, Drugs Aging* 2014;**31**:441–51).

• Unlicensed/some efficacy

Other sedative drugs the person may already be taking, especially antipsychotics and antidepressants, may be prescribed as a single dose at night (but not SSRIs). In longer-term therapy most can be given this way, although again these are only causing sedation, not aiding quality or refreshing sleep, e.g. they may disrupt REM sleep. If using antidepressants, a review suggests choosing sedating ones over activating ones, low anticholinergic effects, 5HT2A or 2C blockers over pure histamine blockers and using the lowest dose possible (e.g. doxepin 1–3 mg, mirtazapine 15 mg, trazodone 50 mg, trimipramine 25 mg; Wiegand, *Drugs* 2008;**68**:2411–7).

Agomelatine

Agomelatine can help poor sleep if related to MDD (reviewed by Quera-Salva *et al, Hum Psychopharmacol* 2010;**25**:222–9).

Doxepin *

Doxepin at low dose is one of the most potent antihistamines known and 1 mg, 3 mg and 6 mg are superior to placebo for improving objective and subjective sleep measures in primary insomnia, with no apparent ADRs or residual effects (n=67, RCT, d/b, c/o, Roth *et al, Sleep* 2007;**30**:1555–61; FFT), with significant and sustained improvements over five weeks, with no rebound or residual effects (n=221, RCT, d/b, p/c, 37/7, Krystal *et al, Sleep* 2011;**34**:1433–42; FFT), even in elderly adults with chronic primary insomnia at 3–6 mg/d (n=254, RCT, d/b, p/c, 4/52, Lankford *et al, Sleep* Med 2012;**13**:133–8) and 3 mg/d (n=240, RCT, d/b, p/c, 12/52, Krystal *et al, Sleep* 2010;**33**:1553–61; FFT). In transient insomnia, doxepin 6 mg shows significant benefits on sleep onset, maintenance, duration and quality (n=565, RCT, d/b, p/c, Roth *et al, Sleep Med* 2010;**11**:843–7). It was ineffective for sleep in people with MDD (n=17, open, Mews *et al, Prim Care Companion CNS Disord* 2014;**16**:13m01567).

Reviews: general (Goforth, *Expert Opin Pharmacother* 2009;**10**:1649–55; Weber *et al, CNS Drugs* 2010;**24**:713–20).

Mirtazapine

Insomnia is reported by 90% of depressed people, and stimulation of 5-HT2 receptors is thought to underlie the insomnia and adverse changes in sleep architecture seen with SSRIs/SNRIs. Mirtazapine blocks 5-HT2 receptors and may improve sleep, e.g. 30 mg increased sleep efficiency and decreased wakenings (and their duration), but with no effect on REM. A thorough review (including 12 RCTs) showed a consistent improvement in sleep efficiency, sleep time and sleep quality (s=23, Dolder *et al, Ann Clin Psychiatry* 2012;**24**:215–

24). Mirtazapine may in fact help normalise abnormal REM sleep (n=32, Schittecatte *et al*, *Psychiatry Res* 2002;**109**:1–8), unlike SSRIs.

Quetiapine *

Quetiapine 25–100mg is sedative, probably at least partly through its antihistaminic effects (s=4, Coe and Hong, *Ann Pharmacother* 2012;**46**:718–22). It improves sleep architecture in 2–4 days in unipolar or bipolar depression and self-reported sleep quality, but the effects wear off with continued treatment (n=15[c=11], s/b, 28/7, Gedge *et al*, *Neuropsychiatr Dis Treat* 2010;**6**:501–8; FFT). Quetiapine may be a useful non-addictive hypnotic in recovering alcohols (n=20, p/c, 8/52, Chakravorty *et al*, *J Clin Psychopharmacol* 2014;**34**:350–4).

Reviews: * general (Anderson and Vande Griend, *Am J Health Syst Pharm* 2014;**71**:394-402), use in addictive conditions (Terán *et al*, *Subst Use Misuse* 2008;**43**:2169–71).

■ Unlicensed/possible efficacy

Anticonvulsants

A review of AED effects on sleep concludes that **gabapentin**, **pregabalin** (Holsboer-Trachsler and Prieto, *Int J Neuropsychopharmacol* 2013;**16**:925–36; review by Roth *et al*, *Sleep Med Rev* 2014;**18**:241–51), **clobazam** and **carbamazepine** reduce sleep latency and/or increase sleep efficiency; **phenobarbital, valproate** and **levetiracetam** (higher dose) aggravate daytime sleepiness; whereas **tiagabine** (n=207, RCT, d/b, p/c, Roth *et al*, *Sleep* 2006;**29**:335–41), **topiramate** and **zonisamide** don't (Jain and Glauser, *Epilepsia* 2014;**55**:26–37).

Alcohol

Alcohol is not recommended for routine use as a hypnotic because, although it causes sedation, it increases slow-wave sleep, reduces and disrupts REM sleep, the diuretic effect may be counter-productive and overdose can have serious consequences. Rebound arousal can occur with higher doses when blood concentrations reach zero, leading to awakening. It is, however, widely used as self-medication and is available in a number of highly palatable formulations, e.g. Farmer's and anything sold at the Ivy House, Stradbroke. Interestingly, ageing Scotch whisky upregulates GABA receptors more than younger or blended Scotch (regardless of ethanol concentration), and is better at calming and inducing sleep (Koda *et al*, *J Agriculture Food Chem* 2003;**51**:5238–44). Reasonable quantities of Spanish beer can also provide sufficient melatonin (and the higher the alcohol content, the more the melatonin) to increase the human body's antioxidant capacity (n=1, b=18, Maldonado *et al*, *Clin Nutr* 2009;**28**:188–91).

Cherry Tart juice beverage

Chronic insomnia in older people can respond to Cherry Tart juice beverage, albeit with a modest effect (n=15, RCT, d/b, p/c, 2x2/52, Pigeon *et al*, *J Med Food* 2010;**13**:579–83; FFT).

Donepezil

Cholinesterase inhibitors have been shown to improve REM sleep in younger and elderly healthy adults (n=42, d/b, p/c, Schredl *et al*, *Pharmacopsychiatry* 2006;**39**:205–8).

Gabapentin

In alcoholics with persistent insomnia, gabapentin may improve sleep (n=55, open, 6/52, Karam-Hage and Brower, *Psych Clin Neurosci* 2003;**57**:542–4; FFT), perhaps by enhancing slow-wave sleep and improving sleep quality (n=18, open, 4/52, Lo *et al*, *Clin Neuropharmacol* 2010;**33**:84–90). Intractable insomnia in bipolar has responded markedly to gabapentin, which then also improved mood (n=1, Egashira *et al*, *Clin Neuropharmacol* 2011;**34**:129–30).

Herbal and OTC preparations

There is an extensive review (Meolie *et al*, *J Clin Sleep Med* 2005;**1**:173–87) of oral, non-prescription treatments for insomnia, e.g. herbals and others, including passionflower, valerian, Jamaican dogwood, hops, Californian poppy, chamomile, lemon balm, St John's wort, kava kava, wild lettuce, skullcap, Patrina root, older histamine-1-receptor antagonists, calcium, vitamin A, nicotinamide, magnesium, vitamin B12, tryptophan, 5-hydroxytryptophan, dietary changes, Natrum muriaticum and Yoku-kan-san-ka-chimpi-hange. It concluded that the studies were small, of inadequate design and lacked statistical analysis. There was insufficient data to recommend any, except preliminary but conflicting data on valerian and H1-antagonists. There are significant potential risks for Jamaican dogwood, kava kava and tryptophan.

Nicotine

Low concentrations of nicotine can cause mild sedation and relaxation but higher levels cause arousal and agitation.

Trazodone

There is little or no data (except perhaps in depressed people) on trazodone's efficacy or tolerability (s=18, Mendelson, *J Clin Psychiatry* 2005;**66**:469–76). It appears ineffective for sleep in people on methadone maintenance (n=137[c=121], d/b, p/c, 1/12, Stein *et al, Drug Alcohol Depend* 2012;**120**:65–73).

☐ No efficacy

Caffeine *

Caffeine competes with the inhibitory neurotransmitter adenosine, causing cortical arousal and decreased sleep and 150mg before retiring has a marked effect on sleep latency, reduces sleep efficacy and REM periods. Its half-life of five hours means any ingested near bedtime will affect sleep latency. It can reduce total sleep time even if taken six hours before bedtime, so avoid substantial use for a minimum of six hours pre-bedtime (Drake *et al, J Clin Sleep Med* 2013;**9**:1195–200). If only I could. See caffeinism (*1.28*).

SSRIs *

SSRIs can obviously help insomnia caused by depression by treating the root cause but should not be taken at night When entering REM sleep 5HT, NA and H1 levels drop to zero, so any drug enhancing serotonin will affect this and disrupt REM sleep.

MANIA AND HYPOMANIA

see Bipolar – Mania and hypomania (*1.10.2*)

1.17 NARCOLEPSY

Symptoms

Narcolepsy is a rare and often misdiagnosed disabling neurological disorder of excessive daytime sleepiness, sleep paralysis, hypnagogic hallucinations, cataplexy (sudden loss of muscle tone provoked by strong emotions, e.g. laughter) and abnormalities in REM sleep. Other specific symptoms include catalepsy (an abrupt, bilateral loss of skeletal muscle tone), hypnagogic hallucinations (vivid dreams while falling asleep or waking), sleep paralysis and automatic behaviour (unconscious functioning while asleep). There is a strong genetic linkage, and normally starts in the 20s or 30s. The incidence ranges from 0.01-0.1% of the population. Narcolepsy is probably caused by the loss of some of the 10–20K neurons responsible for producing the neuropeptide hypocretin/orexin, the role of which is to keep us awake.

Role of drugs

The use of stimulants or modafinil is considered first-line treatment. The risks of pharmacotherapy are usually outweighed by the risks to the person of driving, work-place and other mishaps. The role of oxybate is as yet unclear. Some antidepressants may be useful in resistant cases (s=5, n=246, Vignatelli *et al, Cochrane Database Syst Rev* 2008;1:CD003724).

BNF listed

Dexamfetamine

Dexamfetamine acts by enhancing the release of noradrenaline, dopamine and serotonin, but the stimulant effect appears to be mainly via dopamine. Dexamfetamine 5–50mg/d can be highly effective, although doses of 40–60mg/d appear more effective. Although dexamfetamine may have problems from chronic stimulant ingestion, many can take it for decades without apparent adverse consequences.

Methylphenidate (unlicensed but BNF listed)

Methylphenidate 5–10mg/d (up to 60mg/d) can be used. Tolerance can be a problem, with drug holidays helpful. It has been considered as good as dexamfetamine and may have a better side-effect profile (reviewed by Challman and Lipsky, *Mayo Clin Proc* 2000;**75**:711–21).

Modafinil

Modafinil is licensed in UK for symptomatic relief of excessive sleepiness associated with narcolepsy. Its precise mechanism of action is unclear, but may activate the hippocampus which receives afferents from the hypothalamus, the centre of the sleep–wake rhythm, promoting wakefulness. It significantly increases daytime sleep latency but does not suppress cataplexy. Modafinil 600 mg/d appears the maximum tolerated dose and splitting the doses, e.g. 200 mg BD/TDS may help promote wakefulness throughout a day compared to once-daily (s=2, n=56, RCT, d/b, Schwartz *et al*, *J Neuropsychiatry Clin Neurosci* 2005;**17**:405–12), with no tolerance or withdrawal in a 40-week follow-on (n=271, RCT, 9/52, Modafinil study group, *Neurology* 2000;**54**:1166–75). A review and meta-analysis concludes that modafinil is effective for excessive daytime sleepiness but not cataplexy (s=9, n=1054, RCTs, Golicki *et al*, *Med Sci Monit* 2010;**16**:RA177–86).

Reviews: mode of action (Ballon and Feifel, *J Clin Psychiatry* 2006;**67**:554–66), pharmacokinetics (Robertson and Hellriegel, *Clin Pharmacokinet* 2003;**42**:123–37).

Sodium oxybate

Sodium oxybate (the sodium salt of gamma-hydroxybutyrate [GHB]), is licensed for cataplexy in adults with narcolepsy. Oxybate probably promotes slow (delta) wave sleep consolidating night-time sleep, increasing stage 3 and 4 sleep, reducing the onset of REM sleep.

Abuse potential: GHB can be abused for its euphoric and weight loss effects, and its amnesic effect has led to it being used as a date-rape drug (Gonzalez and Nutt, *J Psychopharmacol* 2005;**19**:195–204), although the risk of abuse/misuse may have been over-rated and may actually be very low (n=26000, Wang *et al*, *J Clin Sleep Med* 2009;**5**:365–71; FFT).

Dose: The starting dose is 4.5 g/d (2x2.25 g), titrated slowly every two weeks (or longer) up to 9 g/d as a BD dose (bedtime and 2.5–4 hours later, due to its short half-life). If oxybate is stopped for more than 14 days it should be retitrated, although withdrawal symptoms with therapeutic doses are minimal (n=55, Anon, *J Toxicol Clin Toxicol* 2003;**41**:131–5).

Efficacy: A systematic review and meta-analysis showed 9 g/d at night significantly reduces cataplexy and daytime sleepiness in narcolepsy for up to at least 21/12 (s=6, RCT, Alshaikh *et al*, *J Clin Sleep Med* 2012;**8**:451–8).

Switching: When switching to oxybate, gradual withdrawal of antidepressants can lead to a short-term increase in cataplexy, especially with TCAs (n=57, Ristanovic *et al*, *Sleep Med* 2009;**10**:416–21).

Reviews: general (Mayer, *Expert Rev Neurother* 2012;**12**:519–29; Ahmed and Thorpy, *Clin Chest Med* 2010;**31**:371–81).

● Unlicensed/some efficacy

Selegiline

Two old trials showed a potent and dose-related effect, at doses of at least 20 mg/d (e.g. n=30, RCT, d/b, p/c, 4/52, Mayer *et al*, *Clin Neuropharmacol* 1995;**18**:306–19).

■ Unlicensed/possible efficacy

SSRIs

These are generally considered less effective than tricyclics but some rare positive results have appeared with, e.g. fluoxetine (Langdon *et al*, *Sleep* 1986;**9**:371–2).

Tricyclics

Clomipramine and imipramine have been used for cataplexy and sleep paralysis, particularly in stimulant-resistant or intolerant patients. Tricyclic ADRs can be significant and rebound cataplexy can occur with abrupt withdrawal (n=57, 7/52, Ristanovic *et al*, *Sleep Med* 2009;**10**:416–21).

Venlafaxine

Venlafaxine has been used for narcolepsy with cataplexy at 37.5–112.5 mg/d in children (n=6, Møller and Østergaard, *J Child Adolesc Psychopharmacol* 2009;**19**:197–201).

✱ Case reports ✱

- **Donepezil** 10 mg/d (n=1, 3/12, Niederhofer,

J Clin Sleep Med 2006;**2**:71–2)
- **Temazepam** (n=1, Kansagra *et al, J Clin Sleep Med* 2013;**9**:499–500).
- **Tranylcypromine + modafinil** (n=1, Clemons *et al, Sleep Med* 2004;**5**:509–11).

1.18 OBSESSIVE-COMPULSIVE DISORDERS (OCD)

OCD is a serious and potentially life-destroying condition. It is not to be confused with OCB (obsessive-compulsive behaviour) where the person enjoys doing the various OCD traits (e.g. tidying, being a pharmacist), a stark comparison with true OCD where the sufferer hates the OCD actions and cannot control them.

1.18.1 OBSESSIVE-COMPULSIVE DISORDER (OCD)

Symptoms

OCD has a lifetime prevalence of around 2–3%, an early onset (childhood or adolescence), and frequently becomes chronic and disabling if untreated. It is characterised by recurrent and intrusive thoughts of compulsive, stereotyped, repetitive behaviour, e.g. recurrent checking, hand-washing. Functioning is impaired by obsessive thoughts and rituals. Resisting these compulsions causes heightened anxiety and distress.

Role of drugs *

There is much evidence that the cause of OCD is related to a dysfunctional serotonin system, and SSRIs and clomipramine have been shown to be effective (e.g. s=17, n=3097, RCTs, p/c, Soomro *et al, Cochrane Database Syst Rev* 2008; **23**:CD001765). Overall:

1. Drug: Only antidepressants affecting the serotonin system are effective:
   - the SSRIs and clomipramine are effective (but with different side-effects) and both are superior to non-serotonergic drugs
   - clomipramine is perhaps slightly more effective than the SSRIs
   - tricyclics (other than clomipramine) and mirtazapine seem ineffective
   - comorbid depression does not seem necessary for improvement in obsessive-compulsive symptoms.
2. Dose: The daily dose usually needs to be high, e.g. 250–300 mg clomipramine, or 60–80 mg fluoxetine or paroxetine which, although not well tolerated, are clearly associated with improved efficacy (s=9, n=2268, RCT, d/b, p/c, Bloch *et al, Mol Psychiatry* 2010;**15**: 850–5; FFT). In resistant OCD, even higher doses may be needed, e.g. citalopram up to 120 mg/d, escitalopram up to 50 mg/d, fluoxetine 100 mg/d, paroxetine up to 80 mg/d, sertraline 250–300 mg/d over at least a year (n=26, retrospective, Pampaloni *et al, J Psychopharmacol* 2010;**24**:1439–45).
3. a. Duration for response: Response is slow so continue with the maximum tolerated dose of an SSRI for **three months** (25% respond given adequate dose and duration).
   b. Duration for relapse prevention: A minimum of 1–2 years is recommended as relapse is common on discontinuation. The risks of long-term therapy may be outweighed by the risks of relapse. If someone is on an SSRI and in partial or complete remission then the risk of relapsing is about 33% (1 in 3) if stopping. The median time to worsening was 39 weeks. If on an SSRI but still symptomatic, the risk of becoming more unwell is about 10%. In other words, if the SSRI is working, stopping it means you may well get unwell, but if it isn't, things can't get much worse (n=252, five years, Grant *et al, Int Clin Psychopharmacol* 2013;**28**:200–5; FFT).
4. Treatment resistance: Switching from an SSRI (e.g. paroxetine) to venlafaxine or vice versa may be an effective strategy if there is lack of response (n=150, RCT, d/b, Denys *et al, J Clin Psychiatry* 2004;**65**:37–43; review by Bhui, *EBMH* 2004;**7**:114; FFT). Failing that, add an antipsychotic (see separate entry), although only 30% will show a meaningful response.
5. Discontinuation: Gradual discontinuation over several months is widely recommended.

In the UK, NICE's guidance on OCD uses a stepped care approach. However, this does not fully emphasise the need to use higher doses for prolonged periods of time. Drugs may only reduce symptomatology by 30–60%, but this is a significant benefit for many people and facilitate engagement with psychological therapies (n=100[c=86, RCT, p/c, 8/52, Simpson *et al,*

JAMA Psychiatry 2013;**70**:1190–9), especially if immediately after drug response (n=96[c=59], RCT, s/b, 12/52, Tenneij *et al*, *J Clin Psychiatry* 2005;**66**:1169–75; comment by Cottraux, *EBMH* 2006;**9**:53). If ERP (exposure response therapy) is not effective, switching to an SSRI (e.g. fluvoxamine) is more effective than CBT (n=48[c=45], RCT, 12/52, van Balkom *et al*, *Psychother Psychosom* 2012; **81**:366–74).

Reviews: * general (Franklin and Foa, *Annu Rev Clin Psychol* 2011;**7**:229–43; Marazziti and Consoli, *Expert Opin Pharmacother* 2010;**11**:331–43), pharmacotherapy (Fineberg *et al*, *Aust N Z J Psychiatry* 2013;**47**:121–41), BAP Guidelines (Baldwin *et al*, *J Psychopharmacol* 2014;**28**:403–439), non-antidepressants for OCD (Abdel-Ahad and Kazour, *Curr Clin Pharmacol* 2015; in press), serotonergics drugs (Pizarro *et al*, *Expert Opin Pharmacother* 2014;**15**:1391–401) BDNF in OCD (Maina *et al*, *J Affect Disord* 2010;**122**:174–8), IV routes of treatment (Ravindran *et al*, *J Psychopharmacol* 2010;**24**:287–96), pharmacogenomics (Brandl *et al*, *Pharmacogenomics* 2012;**13**:71–81).

BNF listed

Clomipramine

Clomipramine up to 250mg/d is superior to placebo and non-serotonergic drugs (e.g. n=122, RCT, d/b, p/c, 12/52, Foa *et al*, *Am J Psychiatry* 2005;**162**:151–61; see also review of meta-analyses in introduction).

Escitalopram

Escitalopram is licensed for OCD at a dose of 10–20mg/d, with 10mg/d as effective as (and better tolerated than) paroxetine 40mg/d. Escitalopram 20mg/d was effective as early as six weeks (n=466, RCT, d/b, p/c, 24/52, Stein *et al*, *Curr Med Res Opin* 2007;**23**:701–11). High-dose escitalopram (up to 50mg/d, mean 34mg/d) may be needed in resistant OCD (n=67[c=64], open, 16/52, Rabinowitz *et al*, *Int Clin Psychopharmacol* 2008;**23**:49–53) and some may need up to 60mg/d (n=246, open, Shim *et al*, *Int Clin Psychopharmacol* 2011;**26**:284–90). Relapse prevention is well-established, with an NNT for prevention of relapse of 3.3 (s=4, RCT, d/b, 24/52, Bech *et al*, *J Clin Psychiatry* 2010;**71**:121–9).

Fluoxetine

Fluoxetine has a significant clinical effect at 20–60mg/d, developing over 13 weeks, and continuing to be effective for at least nine months with few side-effects (e.g. n=130, RCT, p/c, 12/12, Romano *et al*, *J Clin Psychopharmacol* 2001;**21**:46–52). It may be more effective in washers and with obsessive thoughts rather than checkers (n=265, Farnam *et al*, *Arch Iran Med* 2008;**11**:522–5; FFT).

Fluvoxamine

Fluvoxamine has been shown to be partially or very effective in several trials and it may be equivalent to clomipramine but better tolerated (n=227, RCT, d/b, 10/52, Mundo *et al*, *Hum Psychopharmacol* 2001;**16**:461–8).

Paroxetine

Paroxetine is licensed for OCD and for relapse prevention at doses of 40–60mg (reviews by Owen, *Drugs Today (Barc)* 2008;**44**:887–93). Higher doses are necessary, particularly in acute OCD, as 20mg/d is not effective (n=348, RCT, d/b, p/c, 12/52, Hollander *et al*, *J Clin Psychiatry* 2003;**64**:1113–21).

Sertraline

Sertraline is licensed for OCD in adults and in children and adolescents (dose: 6–12 years, 25–50mg/d; for 13–17 years, use the adult dose but with at least a week between dose increases, and a lower body weight may require lower doses). Sertraline is slightly more effective than fluoxetine and as well tolerated (n=150, RCT, d/b, 6/12, Bergeron *et al*, *J Clin Psychopharmacol* 2002;**22**:148–54). Rapid titration to 150mg/d over five days may give a faster onset of action in acute OCD, with similar tolerability to slower (15 days) titration (n=32, s/b, 12/52, Bogetto *et al*, *Eur Neuropsychopharm* 2002;**12**:181–6). High-dose sertraline (up to 400mg/d) may be effective in TR-OCD (n=66, RCT, d/b, 12/52, Ninan *et al*, *J Clin Psychiatry* 2006;**67**:15–22). Relapse prevention has been shown, with lack of prominent discontinuation symptoms (n=649[c=223], RCT, 6/12, Koran *et al*, *Am J Psychiatry* 2002;**159**:88–95; review by Soomro, *EBMH* 2002;**5**:115; FFT).

+ Combinations with SSRIs/clomipramine*

Reviews: * rationale and use of adjunctive dopamine antagonists for TR-OCD (Koo et al, *Expert Rev Neurother* 2010;**10**:275–90), augmentation strategies (Arumugham and Reddy, *Expert Rev Neurother* 2013;**13**:187–203).

Antipsychotics + SSRIs/clomipramine *

Meta-analysis shows antipsychotics are clearly superior to placebo as adjuncts to SSRIs in TR-OCD (s=14, n=491, RCT, d/b, p/c, Dold et al, *Int J Neuropsychopharmacol* 2015;**18**: pyv047; FFT). If successful, they should probably continue for at least several months, as relapse on discontinuation is high.

Risperidone has the most evidence and is effective as SSRI augmentation at 0.5 mg/d (n=45, RCT, d/b, p/c, 6/52, Erzeovesi et al, *Eur Neuropsychopharmacol* 2005;**15**:69–74) to 3 mg/d (e.g. n=70, RCT, 12/52, McDougle et al, *Arch Gen Psychiatry* 2000;**57**:794–801; comment by Ramasubbu, *Arch Gen Psychiatry* 2002;**59**:472–3), and more effective than aripiprazole as an adjunct (n=41, RCT, s/b, 8/52, Selvi et al, *Hum Psychopharmacol* 2011;**26**:51–7).

Aripiprazole may have some efficacy as augmentation of SSRIs, e.g. in TR-OCD (c=30, RCT, d/b, p/c, 16/52, Muscatello et al, *J Clin Psychopharmacol* 2011;**31**:174–9), with doses of 10 mg significantly reducing Y-BOCS scores (n=39, RCT, d/b, p/c, 12/52, Sayyah et al, *Depress Anxiety* 2012;**29**:850–4), albeit with a risk of EPSEs at 2–12 mg/d (e.g. n=13, >7/52, open, Higuma et al, *World J Biol Psychiatry* 2012;**13**:14–21).

Olanzapine is less effective and the only RCT showed no efficacy in fluoxetine-refractory OCD (n=44, RCT, p/c, 6/52, Shapira et al, *Biol Psychiatry* 2004;**55**:553–5).

Quetiapine 400–600 mg/d has been ineffective as an adjunct to an SSRI in TR-OCD (n=40, RCT, d/b, p/c, 12/52, Kordon et al, *J Clin Psychopharmacol* 2008;**28**:550–4), but up to 400 mg/d may have some efficacy in TR-OCD (s=3, n=102, RCT, d/b, p/c, Fineberg et al, *Int Clin Psychopharmacol* 2006;**21**:337–43) and in another trial more people with TR-OCD responded to adjunctive quetiapine (54%) than aripiprazole (27%) (n=44, RCT, d/b, 12/52, Shoja Shafti and Kaviani, *Ther Adv Psychopharmacol* 2015;**5**:32–7; FFT). Starting quetiapine 300–450 mg/d *with* an SSRI may significantly enhance the number of responses (n=76 [c=66], RCT, d/b, p/c, 10/52, Vulink et al, *J Clin Psychiatry* 2009;**70**:1001–8).

Paliperidone 9 mg/d showed some efficacy as an adjunct to SSRIs in TR-OCD (n=34, d/b, p/c, 8/52, Storch et al, *J Clin Psychiatry* 2013;**74**:e527–32).

Celecoxib + SSRIs

Adjunct: Celecoxib 400 mg/d was significantly more effective as an adjunct to fluoxetine than fluoxetine monotherapy (n=50, RCT, d/b, p/c, 8/52, Sayyah et al, *Psychiatry Res* 2011; **189**:403–6).

Clomipramine + SSRIs

Citalopram plus clomipramine has been useful in TR-OCD (n=16, open, 3/12, Pallanti et al, *Eur Psychiatry* 1999;**14**:101–6), and around 50% of people taking clomipramine (after failing at least two SSRIs previously) responded after addition of citalopram up to 60 mg/d (n=20, 11/12, Marazziti et al, *CNS Spectr* 2008;**13**:971–6). An unusual study in TR-OCD showed that clomipramine+fluoxetine was superior to fluoxetine+quetiapine or fluoxetine+placebo and was well tolerated, but concluded that higher doses of fluoxetine should be used for longer before any combination therapy (n=54 [c=40], RCT, d/b, p/c, 12/52, Diniz et al, *J Clin Psychopharmacol* 2011;**31**:763–8).

Dexamfetamine and caffeine + SSRIs

In partial response to SNRIs or SSRIs, augmentation with dexamfetamine (30 mg/d) or caffeine (300 mg/d) were equally effective in improving residual symptoms, although this book's author thinks there must be many people who already take at least 300 mg/d caffeine without any need for an augmentation strategy (s=2, n=24, RCT, d/b, 5/52, Koran et al, *J Clin Psychiatry* 2009;**70**:1530–5).

Gabapentin + SSRIs

Gabapentin up to 3600 mg/d has been used in people only partially responsive to fluoxetine 30–100 mg/d (n=5, open, 6/52, Cora-Locatelli et al, *J Clin Psychiatry* 1998;**59**:480–1).

Granisetron + SSRIs

Granisetron 2mg/d as an adjunct to fluvoxamine, led to response and remission rates of 100% and 90% respectively, cf. 35% with placebo, and with good tolerability, an extraordinary outcome (n=42[c=39], RCT, d/b, p/c, 8/52, Askari *et al*, *CNS Drugs* 2012;**26**:883–92).

Lamotrigine + SSRIs *

Lamotrigine 100mg/d added to a stable SSRI is well tolerated and improves response in TR-OCD (n=40 [c=33], RCT, d/b, p/c, 16/52, Bruno *et al*, *J Psychopharmacol* 2012:**26**:1456–62; cases in n=2, Arrojo-Romero *et al*, *Case Rep Psychiatry* 2013;**2013**:612459).

Memantine + SSRIs/clomipramine *

Two RCTs have shown adjunctive memantine to have significant efficacy in TR-OCD (n=40[c=29], RCT, d/b, p/c, 12/52, Haghighi *et al*, *Psychopharmacol [Berl]* 2013;**228**:633–40), with 20mg/d well tolerated and producing 89% remission cf. 32% with placebo, a major finding (n=42[c=38], RCT, d/b, p/c, 8/52, Ghaleiha *et al*, *J Psychiatr Res* 2013;**47**:175–80). This is supported by many earlier reports (n=44, s/b, Stewart *et al*, *J Clin Psychopharmacol* 2010;**30**:34–9; n=12, open, 12/52, Bakhla *et al*, *Ind Psychiatry J* 2013;**22**:149–52).

Mirtazapine + citalopram

Mirtazapine 15–30mg/d may accelerate the response to citalopram at four weeks, but with similar response rates from week 8, which could be significant in severe OCD, although a robust study would be needed to confirm this (n=49, s/b, 12/52, Pallanti *et al*, *J Clin Psychiatry* 2004;**65**:1394–9; comment by Schüle and Laakmann, *EBMH* 2005;**8**:42; FFT). In mirtazapine-responders, discontinuation has led to relapse, suggesting a prophylactic effect (n=30, d/b, p/c, 8/52, Koran *et al*, *J Clin Psychiatry* 2005;**66**:515–20).

Ondansetron + SSRIs *

Adjunct: Although ondansetron is 'strikingly effective' in some controlled trials, at best ondansetron 1–8mg/d is an experimental adjunct (s=6, n=142, Andrade, *J Clin Psychiatry* 2015;**76**:e72–5).

Pindolol + SSRIs

Pindolol 7.5mg/d may enhance the response to paroxetine in multiple SSRI-resistant OCD (n=14, d/b, p/c, 6/52, Dannon *et al*, *Eur Neuropsychopharmacol* 2000;**10**:165–9).

Pregabalin + SSRIs

Adjunctive pregabalin 225–675mg/d improved OCD symptoms in a small pilot trial (n=10, open, 12/52, Oulis *et al*, *Int Clin Psychopharmacol* 2011;**26**:221–4).

Topiramate + SSRIs

Topiramate 100–200mg/d as augmentation in SSRI-resistant OCD can lead to a good response, e.g. a mean 32% reduction in Y-BOCS, with no placebo response (n=49[c=41], RCT, d/b, p/c, 12/52, Mowla *et al*, *CNS Spectr* 2010;**15**:613–7). It may be better for compulsions, but not obsessions (n=36, RCT, d/b, p/c, 12/52, Berlin *et al*, *J Clin Psychiatry* 2011;**72**:716–21).

Tricyclics + clomipramine

Addition of nortriptyline 50mg/d to clomipramine 150mg/d produced a more rapid onset of action than clomipramine alone (n=30, d/b, p/c, RCT, Noorbala *et al*, *J Clin Pharm Ther* 1998;**23**:155–9).

• Unlicensed/some efficacy

Citalopram

Citalopram has been shown to be as effective as fluvoxamine and paroxetine. Predictors of response include a longer duration of more severe illness, no previous SSRI and an adequate dose for adequate duration (RCT, Stein *et al*, *Int Clin Psychopharmacol* 2001;**16**:357–61). Very high dose citalopram (160mg/d) may be effective in severe, resistant OCD (n=1, Bejerot and Bodlund, *Acta Psychiatr Scand* 1998;**98**:423–4).

Venlafaxine

Venlafaxine has been shown to be as effective as paroxetine but not superior (n=150, RCT, d/b, Denys *et al*, *J Clin Psychopharmacol* 2003;**23**:568–757), and almost as effective as clomipramine (n=47; 150–225mg/d) but better tolerated (n=73, RCT, s/b, 12/52, Albert

et al, *J Clin Psychiatry* 2002;**63**:1004–9).
Review: SNRIs in OCD (Dell'Osso et al, *J Clin Psychiatry* 2006;**67**:600–10).

■ Unlicensed/possible efficacy

Agomelatine ± TAU *

Monotherapy: In partial/non-responders to SSRIs, switching to agomelatine 50mg/d has had some efficacy (n=6, Fornaro, *Ann Gen Psychiatry* 2011;**10**:5; FFT), and there are other case reports of success (n=1, da Rocha and Correa, *Clin Neuropharmacol* 2011;**34**:139–40; n=1, De Berardia et al, *J Clin Psychopharmacol* 2012;**32**:289–90).
Adjunct: Complete response of TR-OCD has been reported with agomelatine augmentation of escitalopram (n=1, De Berardis et al, *Case Rep Psychiatry* 2012;**2012**:642752).

Buprenorphine + TAU *

A small pilot study showed that adjunctive buprenorphine (400–600mcg/d) gave 30% improvement in Y-BOCS in 57% patients (n=7, Liddell et al, *Ther Adv Psychopharmacol* 2013;**3**:15–9).

Cycloserine (D-cycloserine) + CBT

Cycloserine 100mg given before CBT improves OCD and depressive symptoms (n=23, RCT, d/b, p/c, 5/52, Wilhelm et al, *Am J Psychiatry* 2008;**165**:335–41), and when used before exposure therapy (d/b, p/c, Kushner et al, *Biol Psychiatry* 2007;**62**:835–8).

Glycine + TAU

Glycine 60g/d was poorly tolerated but had some significant sustained responses in a pilot study (n=24[c=14], RCT, d/b, p/c, 12/52, Greenberg et al, *J Psychiatr Res* 2009;**43**:664–70).

Mirtazapine

Monotherapy: Mirtazapine 60mg/d has shown advantage over placebo (n=30[c=26], open, 12/52 followed by d/b, p/c discontinuation, 8/52, Koran et al, *J Clin Psychiatry* 2005;**66**:515–20).

Morphine + TAU

Rather puzzlingly, once-weekly oral morphine was effective in some people with TR-OCD, unlike lorazepam or placebo (n=23, RCT, d/b, p/c, c/o, 6/52, Koran et al, *J Clin Psychiatry* 2005;**66**:353–9).

Phenelzine

Monotherapy: Phenelzine 60mg/d is inferior to fluoxetine (80mg/d) except in people with asymmetry or other atypical obsessive symptoms (n=60, RCT, Jenike et al, *Am J Psychiatry* 1997;**154**:1261–4).

Riluzole + TAU

Adjunct: Riluzole 100mg/d appears to have some efficacy in TR-OCD (n=13, open, Coric et al, *Biol Psychiatry* 2005;**58**:424–8).

✸ Case reports *

- **Amantadine** augmentation (n=1, Pasquini et al, *J Clin Psychopharmacol* 2010;**30**:85–6)
- **Carbamazepine** 1200mg/d (n=1, Aggarwal et al, *Indian J Med Sci* 2009;**63**:468–9; FFT)
- **Carbamazepine + clomipramine** (n=1, Iwata et al, *J Clin Psychiatry* 2000;**61**:528–9)
- **Lamotrigine** 150mg/d (n=1, Uzun et al, *J Psychopharmacol* 2010;**24**:425–7)
- **Nicotine chewing gum** (n=1, Pasquini et al, *Prog Neuropsychopharmacol Biol Psychiatry* 2005;**29**:157–9)
- **Oxcarbazepine** (n=1, McMeekin, *J S C Med Assoc* 2002;**98**:316–20)
- **Paliperidone** (n=1, Angelucci et al, *Prog Neuropsychopharmacol Biol Psychiatry* 2009;**33**:1277–8)
- **Psilocybin** (n=9, Moreno et al, *J Clin Psychiatry* 2006;**67**:1735–40)
- **Risperidone** monotherapy (n=1, Chiou et al, *Clin Neuropharmacol* 2015;**38**:114–6).

□ No efficacy

Benzodiazepines ± TAU

Adjunct: Augmentation of sertraline was ineffective (n=37, RCT, d/b, p/c, 12/52, Crockett et al, *Ann Clin Psychiatry* 2004;**16**:127–32).
Monotherapy: BDZs seem ineffective in treating OCD, although clonazepam may be helpful for specific sub-groups with comorbid anxiety (n=27, d/b, p/c, 10/52, Hollander et al, *World J Biol Psychiatry* 2003;**4**:30–4).

Bupropion

Bupropion had no significant effect as monotherapy in OCD (n=12, open, 8/52, Vulink *et al*, *J Clin Psychiatry* 2005;**66**:228–30).

Clozapine

Clozapine has been used for OCD symptoms in schizophrenia (n=15, open, Reznik *et al*, *Pharmacopsychiatry* 2004;**37**:52–6), but is usually ineffective (n=10, McDougle *et al*, *Am J Psychiatry* 1995;**152**:1812–4), or even detrimental (e.g. Baker *et al*, *J Clin Psychiatry* 1992;**53**:439–42).

Flutamide

The anti-androgen flutamide was ineffective in one trial (n=8, Altemus *et al*, *J Clin Psychiatry* 1999;**60**:442–5).

Ketamine *

Ketamine infusion does not seem effective for TR-OCD (n=10, 3/7, open, Bloch *et al*, *Biol Psychiatry* 2012;**72**:964–70).

Inositol + SSRIs

The only RCT has shown inositol to have no effect on symptoms (n=10, RCT, d/b, p/c, c/o, 6/52, Fux *et al*, *Int J Neuropsychopharmacol* 1999;**2**:193–5).

Lithium + SSRIs

Lithium augmentation of fluvoxamine in OCD was ineffective (n=30, d/b, p/c, McDougle *et al*, *J Clin Psychopharmacol* 1991;**11**:175–84).

Minocycline + TAU

Minocycline is not effective as an adjunct in OCD, except perhaps in early onset and in hoarders (n=9, 12/52, open, Rodriguez *et al*, *J Clin Psychiatry* 2010;**71**:1247–9; FFT).

Naltrexone + SSRIs/clomipramine

Naltrexone augmentation in SSRI-resistant OCD is ineffective (n=10, RCT, d/b, p/c, c/o, 5/52, Amiaz *et al*, *Eur Neuropsychopharmacol* 2008;**18**:455–61).

Oxytocin

Initial enthusiasm was not confirmed in a study of intranasal administration (n=3, Salzberg and Swedo, *Am J Psychiatry* 1992;**149**:713–4).

Trazodone

Trazodone up to 300mg/d appears to be ineffective (n=21, d/b, c/o, 10/52, Pigott *et al*, *J Clin Psychopharmacol* 1992;**12**:156–62).

Tricyclics (except clomipramine)

Imipramine (Volavka *et al*, *Psychiatry Res* 1985;**14**:85–93), amitriptyline and nortriptyline have been shown to be ineffective.

1.18.2 BODY DYSMORPHIC DISORDER (BDD)

Symptoms

BDD is characterised by a disabling preoccupation with an imagined or minor defect in appearance (especially skin, hair and nose), with time-consuming behaviours such as mirror gazing, excessive camouflaging and the need for reassurance. The adult incidence is thought to be around 0.5–1% (Bohne *et al*, *Psychosomatics* 2002;**43**:486–90), although it may be as high as 2.4% (Koran *et al*, *CNS Spectr* 2008;**13**:316–22). It has a fluctuating or episodic course, often life-long, with a higher risk/comorbidity in people with depression, social phobia, SUDs, OCD and eating disorders. There is a high risk of suicide, e.g. around a quarter may have attempted suicide sometime during their life, 2.6% per year and 0.3% succeed (Phillips and Menard, *Am J Psychiatry* 2006;**163**:1280–2; FFT), which is 45 times higher than the general population and 2–3 times more than depression and bipolar.

Role of drugs

There are few trials or RCTs in BDD. NICE recommends using either an SSRI or more intensive targeted CBT for moderate BDD. The onset of action of SSRIs (as in OCD) may be delayed for up to 12/52. The best evidence is available for fluoxetine; clomipramine monotherapy is a second line; with buspirone as an adjunct in resistant cases. Treatment duration should be 12 months if effective to prevent relapse and allow further improvement. TCAs (other than clomipramine), SNRIs, MAOIs, anxiolytics (except short-term) or antipsychotic monotherapy are not recommended. Cochrane concludes that SSRIs/clomipramine are superior to placebo and to desipramine (s=2, n=96) and CBT may be effective (s=3, n=83), mostly in women (s=5, n=179, Ipser *et al*, *Cochrane Syst Database Rev* 2009; **1**:CD005332).

Reviews: * general (Gupta *et al*, *Semin Cutan Med Surg* 2013;**32**:78–82; Fang *et al*, *Psychiatr Clin North Am* 2014;**37**:287–300; Mufaddel *et al*, *Prim Care Companion CNS Disord* 2014;**15**:12r01464; Veale and Bewley, *BMJ* 2015; **350**:h2278).

● Unlicensed/some efficacy

Clomipramine

Clomipramine was clearly superior to desipramine in BDD, even if delusions were prominent (n=29, RCT, d/b, c/o, 16/52, Hollander *et al*, *Arch Gen Psychiatry* 1999;**56**:1033–9).

Fluoxetine

A 53% response rate (cf. 18% with placebo) has been seen (NNT=2.7, n=67, RCT, d/b, p/c, 12/52, Phillips *et al*, *Arch Gen Psychiatry* 2002;**59**:381–8) and may have a protective effect against suicide (n=67, RCT, d/b, p/c, 12/52, Phillips and Kelly, *Int Clin Psychopharmacol* 2009;**24**:26–8; FFT).

■ Unlicensed/possible efficacy

Buspirone + SSRIs

A small open study showed a 46% response with buspirone as augmentation of SSRIs (n=13, open, Phillips, *Psychopharmacol Bull* 1996;**32**:175–80).

Citalopram

An open study showed a 73% response rate in BDD (n=15, open, 12/52, Phillips and Najjar, *J Clin Psychiatry* 2003;**64**:715–20).

Escitalopram

A small study showed some well tolerated efficacy (47% were much improved) in BDD (n=15 [c=11], open, Phillips, *Int Clin Psychopharmacol* 2006;**21**:177–9; FFT).

Fluvoxamine

Fluvoxamine has had a 63% response rate using BDD-YBOCS (review by Irons, *Neuropsychiatr Dis Treat* 2005;**1**:289–99; FFT).

Levetiracetam

Levetiracetam (mean 2000 mg/d) has improved many measures of BDD (n=17, open, 12/52, Phillips and Menard, *CNS Spectr* 2009;**14**:252–60; FFT).

Olanzapine + SSRIs

Olanzapine (up to 15 mg/d) augmentation of fluoxetine was effective in 33%, but 67% remained unchanged (n=6, d/b, p/c, 8/52, Phillips, *Am J Psychiatry* 2005;**162**:1022–3; FFT).

Venlafaxine

Venlafaxine (minimum 150 mg/d) may improve global severity and specific symptoms (n=17 [c=11], open, 12–16/52, Allen *et al*, *CNS Spectr* 2008;**13**:138–44).

✱ Case reports

- **Aripiprazole + fluvoxamine** (n=1, Uzun and Ozdemir, *Clin Drug Investig* 2010;**30**:707–10)
- **Bupropion** (n=1, Nardi *et al*, *Aust N Z J Psychiatry* 2005;**39**:112; Canan *et al*, *J Clin Psychopharmacol* 2013;**33**:133–4)
- **Glycine** (n=1, Cleveland *et al*, *Neural Plast* 2009;**2009**:768398; FFT).

□ No efficacy

Pimozide + fluoxetine

Pimozide was ineffective as an adjunct to fluoxetine (n=28, d/b, p/c, 8/52, Phillips, *Am J Psychiatry* 2005;**162**:377–9; FFT).

1.19 PANIC DISORDER

see also Anxiety disorder (*1.6*)

Symptoms

Panic disorder is characterised by sudden attacks of anxiety, where physical symptoms predominate, peaking within 10 minutes and with an associated fear of serious consequences, e.g. heart attack. These attacks need to include four of the following: palpitations, abdominal distress/nausea, numbness/tingling, inability to breathe or shortness of breath, choking, sweating, chest pains, dizziness, depersonalisation (common), flushes/chills, fear of dying and trembling/shaking. The lifetime prevalence of panic disorder is about 5% in the USA (Grant *et al*, *J Clin Psychiatry*

2006;**67**:363–74), with a point prevalence of 1.5% (males) and 2.8% (females). There is frequently a family history and it can also be a presenting feature of depression.

Role of drugs *

In general, short-term benefits may be gained with drug therapy. The main principle is to start low and go slow (to minimise initial jitteriness), and accept that response may take some time to occur. A meta-analysis of drugs concludes that the most effective is venlafaxine; then fluoxetine, paroxetine, sertraline to citalopram, with reboxetine and fluvoxamine least effective (s=50, n=5236, Andrisano *et al, Int Clin Psychopharmacol* 2013;**28**;33–45). After a standard dose SSRI for 6/52, there is little evidence for increasing the dose (n=39, Simon *et al, J Clin Psychiatry* 2009;**70**:1563–70; FFT). Benzodiazepines have a quicker onset of action but obvious potential problems, e.g. dependence and tolerance, and NICE concludes that they have a poor long-term outcome. Placebo responders tend to show an early and temporary remission. Relapse rates at 6–12 months can be as high as 75% and stopping antidepressants suddenly (over 1–7 days) leads to an increased relapse rate, occurring more rapidly (half the time it would take otherwise) than stopping over 14 days or longer (n=398, mean three-year follow-up, Baldessarini *et al, Am J Psychiatry* 2010;**167**:934–41). Cochrane concludes that there is no evidence for psychotherapy as an adjunct for BDZs in panic disorder (s=3, n=243, Watanabe *et al, Cochrane Database Syst Rev* 2009;**2**:CD005335).

Reviews: * SSRIs (Mochcovitch and Nardi, *Expert Rev Neurother* 2010;**10**:1285–93), general (Freire *et al, CNS Neurol Disord Drug Targets* 2014;**13**:1057–65), review and meta-analysis (s=234, n=37333, Bandelow *et al, Int Clin Psychopharmacol* 2015;**30**:183–92).

BNF listed

Benzodiazepines ± TAU

Benzodiazepines are rapidly effective and useful in people needing immediate relief. Many benzodiazepines have been studied, e.g. **alprazolam** (s=8, n=631, RCTs, Moylan *et al, J Clin Psychopharmacol* 2011;**31**:647–52) and **clonazepam**, which is longer-acting, with 1–2 mg/d the best balance between benefit and tolerability and it may have a sustained effect (n=67, open, three years, Nardi *et al, Psychiatry Res* 2005;**137**:61–70). Use of clonazepam, slowly tapered after four weeks, as an initial adjunct to paroxetine can facilitate longer-term monotherapy (n=60, RCT, p/c, 12/52, Pollack *et al, J Psychopharmacol* 2003;**17**:276–82). The main problem is discontinuation, where relapse may be more common with shorter-acting benzodiazepines, so transferring to an SSRI is advisable. In people asymptomatic for at least a year, tapering clonazepam at 0.25 mg/week can be successful, without major withdrawal symptoms or relapse (n=73, open, Nardi *et al, J Clin Psychopharmacol* 2010;**30**:290–3).

Citalopram

Citalopram is licensed in the UK for panic disorder, with or without agoraphobia. The starting dose in panic disorder is 10 mg/d for one week, increasing to 20–30 mg/d as the optimum dose, to a maximum of 60 mg/d, with 20–60 mg/d appearing effective and well tolerated over one year.

Escitalopram

Escitalopram is licensed in the UK for panic disorder, with or without agoraphobia. The initial dose is 5 mg/d for the first week, then 10 mg/d, increasing to a maximum of 20 mg/d. Escitalopram and citalopram appear equally effective in panic disorder (n=366, RCT, d/b, p/c, 10/52, Stahl *et al, J Clin Psychiatry* 2003;**64**:1322–7).

Paroxetine

Paroxetine is licensed for panic and agoraphobia. A 10 mg/d starting dose is recommended. Several studies have shown a significant effect, e.g. as effective as citalopram (n=58, RCT, s/b, 60/7, Perna *et al, Pharmacopsychiatry* 2001;**34**:85–90). The optimum effective dose is 40 mg/d. After 12 months' treatment, a further year of paroxetine did not reduce relapse rates compared to discontinuation (with or without agoraphobia) (n=143, open, three years, Dannon *et al, BMC Psychiatry* 2004;**11**:16; FFT).

Tricyclics

Tricyclics are effective in panic disorder. They may take four weeks to start to work and 12 weeks for maximal effect. Start at a low dose (10–25 mg/d) to avoid the common initial jitteriness. **Clomipramine** is as effective as paroxetine, but with a slower onset of action and more side-effects, and may have a biphasic response, symptoms worsening over 12 weeks before improving. **Imipramine** is effective (vs placebo) in all studies using doses above 150 mg/d and with a substantial prophylactic efficacy (n = 18, RCT, Mavissakalian and Perel, *Ann Clin Psychiatry* 2001;**13**:63–7). Although long-term maintenance is needed for most people, early detection of relapse may be a viable alternative (n = 51, RCT, d/b, 12/12, Mavissakalian and Perel, *J Clin Psychopharmacol* 2002;**22**:294–9).

• Unlicensed/some efficacy

Fluoxetine

Monotherapy: Fluoxetine 20 mg/d is superior to placebo when initial doses are kept very low (2.5–5 mg/d) then increased, as higher doses produce side-effects such as anxiety and over-stimulation, possibly due to serotonergic supersensitivity. If there is no response by 6/52, an increase up to 60 mg/d may help (n = 180 [c = 153], 12/52, RCT, Michelson *et al*, *Br J Psychiatry* 2001;**179**:514–8; FFT).

Fluvoxamine

Monotherapy: Fluvoxamine has been compared favourably with placebo and cognitive therapy (n = 55, RCT, p/c, 8/52, Black *et al*, *Arch Gen Psychiatry* 1993;**50**:44–50), but not all placebo controlled trials have shown efficacy.

Gabapentin

Monotherapy: Gabapentin 600–3600 mg/d may have anxiolytic effects in severe panic disorder (n = 103, RCT, d/b, p/c, 8/52, Pande *et al*, *J Clin Psychopharmacol* 2000;**20**:467–71).

Mirtazapine

Monotherapy: Mirtazapine may be a rapidly effective alternative to SSRIs (n = 28, RCT, open, 12/52, Boshuisen *et al*, *Int Clin Psychopharmacol* 2001;**16**:363–8) and of similar efficacy and tolerability to fluoxetine (n = 27, RCT, 8/52, Ribeiro *et al*, *Braz J Med Biol Res* 2001;**34**:1303–7; FFT).

Sertraline

Monotherapy: Pooled data indicates that sertraline is an effective treatment for panic disorder, even in people with risk factors for poor response (s = 4, n = 664, d/b, Pollack *et al*, *J Clin Psychiatry* 2000;**61**:922–7) and prevents relapse (n = 240, RCT, d/b, p/c, 8/52, Kamijima *et al*, *Int Clin Psychopharmacol* 2005;**20**:265–73). Early response predicts final remission, a useful aid to decision-making (n = 544, p/c, Pollack *et al*, *J Psychiatr Res* 2002;**36**:229–36). Sertraline is enhanced by self-administered CBT (n = 251, RCT, p/c, 12/52, Koszycki *et al*, *Psychol Med* 2011;**41**:373–83).

Review: Hobgood and Clayton, *Drugs Today (Barc)* 2009;**45**:351–61.

■ Unlicensed/possible efficacy

Aripiprazole + TAU

A pilot study suggested aripiprazole may be useful as an adjunct in resistant panic disorder (e.g. n = 10, open, 8/52, Hoge *et al*, *CNS Spectr* 2008;**13**:522–7).

Cycloserine (D-cycloserine) + CBT

D-cycloserine may enhance the response to CBT in panic (n = 31, RCT, d/b, p/c, Otto *et al*, *Biol Psychiatry* 2010;**67**:365–70).

Duloxetine

Duloxetine 60–120 mg/d may have some efficacy (n = 15, open, 6/52, Simon *et al*, *CNS Neurosci Ther* 2009;**15**:19–23).

Inositol

Inositol 12 g/d may improve panic symptoms, and was superior to fluvoxamine 150 mg/d in one study (n = 20, RCT, c/o, 8/52, Palatnik *et al*, *J Clin Psychopharmacol* 2001;**21**:335–9).

Lamotrigine + TAU

Some success has been reported in chronic panic (n = 4, 14/12, Masdrakis *et al*, *Clin Neuropharmacol* 2010;**33**:126–8).

Levetiracetam

Levetiracetam was effective in 84% completers in a pilot study (n=18[c=13], open, 12/52, Papp, *J Clin Psychiatry* 2006;**67**:1573–6).

MAOIs

Tranylcypromine 60mg/d appears to be effective for comorbid panic and social anxiety, but not 30mg/d, or the panic symptoms alone (n=36, d/b, 12/52, Nardi *et al, Psychiatry Res* 2010;**175**:260–5). **Phenelzine** 45–90mg/d may be effective (n=1, Buch and Wagner, *J Clin Psychiatry* 2007;**68**:335–6).

Moclobemide

Moclobemide was ineffective in one study (n=55, RCT, p/c, 8/52, Loerch *et al, Br J Psychiatry* 1999;**174**:205–12), but comparisons with clomipramine (n=135, RCT, 8/52, Kruger and Dahl, *Eur Arch Psych Clin Neurosci* 1999;**249**[Suppl 1]:S19–S24) and fluoxetine (RCT, d/b, 8/52, Tiller *et al, Eur Arch Psych Clin Neurosci* 1999;**249**[Suppl 1]:S7–S10) show similar efficacy, albeit with sub-therapeutic doses of the comparator drugs.

Olanzapine

Olanzapine (mean 12.3mg/d) was remarkably effective in reducing refractory panic attacks, with 50% even being panic-free at the trial end (n=10, open, 8/52, Hollifield *et al, Depress Anxiety* 2005;**21**:33–40).

Reboxetine

Reboxetine is less effective than citalopram (n=19, RCT, s/b, c/o, 18/52, Seedat *et al, Int Clin Psychopharmacol* 2003;**18**:279–84) and paroxetine (n=68, RCT, s/b, Bertani *et al, Pharmacopsychiatry* 2004;**37**:206–10).

Valproate

Valproate 300–1500mg/d may be useful for resistant panic disorder (e.g. n=13[c=10], open, 8/52, Baetz and Bowen, *Can J Psychiatry* 1998;**43**:73–7).

Venlafaxine

Monotherapy: Venlafaxine (75–225mg/d) was superior to placebo for panic disorder, higher doses being most effective (n=624, RCT, p/c, 12/52, Pollack *et al, Psychopharmacol [Berl]* 2007;**194**:233–42), although a previous study was negative (n=361, RCT, d/b, p/c, 10/52, Bradwejn *et al, Br J Psychiatry* 2005;**187**:352–9; FFT). Very low doses are sometimes effective (n=2, Orenstein and Raskind, *J Clin Psychiatry* 2010;**71**:89–91).

✸ Case reports

- **Bupropion** (n=1, Gebhardt *et al, J Clin Pharm Ther* 2008;**33**:575–7)
- **Hydroxyzine** 25mg TDS (n=1, Iskandar *et al, Prim Care Companion CNS Disord* 2011;**13**:PCC10l01126; FFT)
- **Olanzapine + paroxetine** (n=1, Chao, *Pharmacopsychiatry* 2004;**37**:239–40)
- **Pramipexole + SSRIs** (n=2, Marazziti *et al, Am J Psychiatry* 2001;**158**:498–9)
- **Quetiapine** (n=1, Pitchot and Ansseau, *Asian J Psychiatr* 2012;**5**:204–5).

◆ Others

Other drugs tried include **pindolol** (see Mathew *et al, Psychopharmacol Bull* 2001;**35**:97–110).

☐ No efficacy

Buspirone *

Cochrane concludes that there is too little data and what is available isn't encouraging (s=3, n=170, RCT, p/c, Imai *et al, Cochrane Database Syst Rev* 2014;**9**:CD010828).

Caffeine

Caffeine is anxiogenic, particularly in panic disorder, and challenge doses of 480mg can provoke panic attacks (n=98, RCT, d/b, 1/52, Nardi *et al, Psychiatry Res* 2009;**169**:149–53).

1.20 POST-TRAUMATIC STRESS DISORDER (PTSD)

Symptoms *

PTSD is an anxiety disorder resulting from an extreme stressful event, e.g. serious threat to life or involvement of a loved one in a catastrophic event, and where a personal vulnerability exists. The person then re-experiences the event recurrently through dreams and feelings. The four core symptoms are re-experiencing, avoidance, negative cognition/mood and hyperarousal. PTSD may be a quite common yet unrecognised cause of significant morbidity and mortality. The lifetime prevalence may be 1–9%. Only drugs with a significant effect on the serotonin system seem to be effective.

Role of drugs *

Current data suggest that 'positive' symptoms (e.g. nightmares, etc) respond better to drugs, whereas 'negative' symptoms of avoidance (e.g. social withdrawal) are less responsive. SSRIs (e.g. sertraline and paroxetine) are effective in the short term (6–12/52), and for relapse prevention over 6–12/12. Higher doses of serotonergic drugs for longer periods (at least 5–12 weeks) seem necessary. Extended treatment is needed, as there is a great risk of relapse and symptom recurrence if discontinued. BDZs are probably ineffective (review by Asnis *et al*, *Drugs* 2004;**64**:383–404). One meta-analysis concludes CBT, exposure therapy and EMDR (eye movement desensitisation and reprocessing) are effective, as are paroxetine, sertraline, fluoxetine, risperidone, topiramate and venlafaxine, but queries the validity of psychotherapy studies that use waiting-list controls (s=137, Watts *et al*, *J Clin Psychiatry* 2013;**74**:541–50). Another systematic review and meta-analysis showed fluoxetine, paroxetine and venlafaxine have the best evidence (s=51, RCTs, Hoskins *et al*, *Br J Psychiatry* 2015;**206**:93–100). Cochrane concludes that there is moderate evidence for hydrocortisone for the prevention of PTSD but not any others drugs, albeit with small sample sizes (s=9, n=345, <12/52, Amos *et al*, *Cochrane Database Syst Rev* 2014;**7**:CD006239).

Reviews: * BAP Guidelines (Baldwin *et al*, *J Psychopharmacol* 2014;**28**:403–39) pharmacotherapy (Jeffreys *et al*, *J Rehab Res Dev* 2012;**49**:703–15), non-antidepressant long-term treatments (Kerbage and Richa, *Curr Clin Pharmacol* 2014; in press), new directions in pharmacotherapy (Green, *Adv Psychiatr Treat* 2013;**19**:181–90), changes in brain structure (s=15, Thomaes *et al*, *J Psychiatry Res* 2014;**50**:1–15), alpha-2 receptor agonists (clonidine and guanfacine: Belkin and Schwartz, *Drugs Context* 2015;**4**:212286; FFT).

BNF listed

Paroxetine

Paroxetine at standard doses of 20–40mg/d (maximum 50mg/d) has been shown to be effective and well tolerated in adults (both male and female) with chronic PTSD (n=551, RCT, p/c, 12/52, Marshall *et al*, *Am J Psychiatry* 2001;**158**:1982–8), for dissociation in chronic PTSD in adults (n=52, RCT, d/b, p/c, 10/52, Marshall *et al*, *Depress Anxiety* 2007;**24**:77–84) and possibly for chronic PTSD (n=52[c=25], 12/12, open, Kim *et al*, *Psychiatry Clin Neurosci* 2008;**62**:646–52).

Sertraline

Sertraline is licensed for PTSD in women, but may not be effective in men. Two RCTs have shown sertraline 50–200mg/d (mean 150mg/d) to be effective for global and functional outcomes and symptom severity (n=187, RCT, 12/52, Brady *et al*, *JAMA* 2000;**283**:1837–44; critical review by Bisson, *EBMH* 2000;**3**:110; FFT; n=208, RCT, p/c, 12/52, Davidson *et al*, *Arch Gen Psychiatry* 2001;**58**:485–92). Sertraline seems particularly effective in treating psychological symptoms of PTSD, e.g. anger, anhedonia, detachment and numbing as opposed to somatic symptoms, e.g. insomnia and exaggerated startle response (n=400, 12/52, Davidson *et al*, *Psychol Med* 2002;**32**:661–70). It was effective in Iranian war veterans (n=70[c=64], RCT, d/b, p/c, 10/52, Panahi *et al*, *Psychol Med* 2011;**41**:2159–66) and may be effective for acute PTSD in children (n=26, RCT, d/b, p/c, 24/52, Stoddard *et al*, *J Child Adolesc Psychopharmacol* 2011:**21**:469–77) and for relapse prevention (n=26 [c=26], d/b, p/c, 24/52, Stoddard *et al*, *J Child Adolesc Psychopharmacol* 2011:**21**:469–77).

• Unlicensed/some efficacy

Hydrocortisone *

There are five studies (n=164) which show a large effect size for reducing the risk of PTSD (mentioned in Sijbrandij *et al*, *Lancet Psychiatry* 2015;**2**:413–21). A 10-day course of hydrocortisone 20mg bd (started within 12 hours of the trauma) can reduce PTSD in acutely injured trauma patients, and 30mg oral

hydrocortisone prior to prolonged exposure for US Veterans improved retention in treatment (n=24, RCT, p/c, Yehuda *et al*, *Psychoneuroendocrinology* 2015;**51**:589–97). Cochrane concludes that there is moderate evidence for hydrocortisone for the prevention of PTSD (s=9, n=345, <12/52, Amos *et al*, *Cochrane Database Syst Rev* 2014;**7**:CD006239).
Review: * De Kleine *et al*, *Eur J Psychotraumatol* 2013;**4**:21626; FFT).

Prazosin *

Prazosin may have a significant role for some PTSD symptoms, such as for recurrent nightmares (s=21, Kung *et al*, *Mayo Clin Proc* 2012;**87**:890–900; FFT; n=100, RCT, p/c, 8/52, Ahmadpanah *et al*, *Neuropsychobiology* 2014;**69**:235–42). The initiation dose is 1 mg/d, maintenance is usually 2–6 mg/d at night (military studies have used 10–16 mg at night), with a relatively rapid response in weeks (really good review by Green, *J Psychiatr Pract* 2014;**20**:253–9). Higher doses, e.g. 30–45 mg/d at night may be needed in resistant cases (n=2, Koola *et al*, *Ther Adv Psychopharmacol* 2014;**4**:43–7). In soldiers with PTSD prazosin 25 mg/d in men (2–5 mg mid-morning and 10–20 mg at night), and 12 mg/d in women was effective for trauma nightmares, sleep quality and hyperarousal (n=67, RCT, p/c, 15/52, Raskind *et al*, *Am J Psychiatry* 2013;**170**:1003–10). The effect can be maintained over the long term (n=324[c=237], open, >6/12, Byers *et al*, *J Clin Psychopharmacol* 2010;**30**:225–9). A US Veterans study suggested that suboptimal dosing in 80% (mean 3.6mg/d cf. recommended 6mg/d) and early discontinuation in 60% (less than a year) are the major causes of undertreatment and poor response (n=12844, Alexander *et al*, *J Clin Psychiatry* 2015;**76**:e639–44).
Reviews: * general (Berardis *et al*, *Curr Drug Targets* 2015;**16**:1094–106; s=11, Hudson *et al*, *Prim Care Companion CNS Disord* 2012;**14**:11r01222), in combat-related PTSD nightmares (Writer *et al*, *J Neuropsychiatry Clin Neurosci* 2014;**26**:24–33).

SSRIs (paroxetine and sertraline are licensed)

Citalopram may be partly effective (n=2, Khouzam *et al*, *Mil Med* 2001;**166**:921–3).
Escitalopram (up to 20 mg/d) was effective in 45% people (n=25[c=24], open, 12/52, Robert *et al*, *J Clin Psychiatry* 2006;**67**:1522–6).
Fluvoxamine 100–300 mg/d (mean 150 mg) appeared to improve combat-related PTSD but not depressive symptoms (n=15, open, 14/52, Escalona *et al*, *Depress Anxiety* 2002;**15**:29–33).
Fluoxetine appears to be effective and well tolerated for PTSD (s=7, RCT, Xu *et al*, *Neurosciences [Riyadh]* 2011;**16**:257–62). Care is needed initially in people with comorbid panic attacks, as fluoxetine may increase panic and anxiety so start low and go slow.

Topiramate

Topiramate (up to 400 mg/d) may have significant effects on re-experiencing symptoms and treatment outcome scales in civilian PTSD (e.g. n=38, RCT, d/b, p/c, Tucker *et al*, *J Clin Psychiatry* 2007;**68**:201–6). Topiramate (mean 100 mg/d) significantly improved reexperiencing and avoidance PTSD symptoms in 82% people in a more recent trial (n=35, RCT, d/b, p/c, 12/52, Yeh *et al*, *CNS Neurosci Ther* 2011;**17**:305–10).

Venlafaxine

Venlafaxine 37.5–300 mg/d (mean 222 mg/d) may be significantly more effective than placebo for enduring PTSD (n=329, RCT, d/b, p/c, 6/12, Davidson *et al*, *Arch Gen Psychiatry* 2006;**63**:1158–65; review, Pae *et al*, *Expert Rev Neurosci* 2007;**7**:603–15).

■ Unlicensed/possible efficacy

Agomelatine

There is one case of response (n=1, De Berardis *et al*, *Ann Clin Psychiatry* 2012;**24**:241–2; duplicate case by De Berardis *et al*, *Case Rep Psychiatry* 2012;**2012**:642752).

Antipsychotics ± TAU *

Meta-analysis shows that **olanzapine** and **risperidone** are superior to placebo as adjuncts for PTSD symptoms, particularly intrusion' symptoms (s=7, n=192, RCT, d/b, p/c, Pae *et al*, *Int Clin Psychopharmacol* 2008;**23**:1–8).
Aripiprazole should be started at a low dose, i.e. 5 mg/d rather than 10 mg/d, with a slower

titration, to aid tolerability (eg. n=32 [c=23], open, 16/52, Mello *et al, Rev Bras Psiquiatr* 2008;**30**:358–61; FFT) and a mean 13 mg/d produced a 53% response rate with PTSD (e.g. n=10 [c=8], open, 12/52, Youssef *et al, Int Clin Psychopharmacol* 2012;**27**:191–6).

Clozapine has been used successfully in comorbid psychosis and PTSD (n=1, Hamner, *Am J Psychiatry* 1996;**153**:841) and in abused adolescents with psychosis and TR-PTSD (n=6, Wheatley *et al, J Clin Psychopharmacol* 2004;**24**:167–73).

Levomepromazine may help reduce sleep problems in PTSD (Aukst-Margetic *et al, Eur Psychiatry* 2004;**19**:235–6).

Olanzapine augmentation of SSRIs may be useful (e.g. n=19, d/b, p/c, 8/52, Stein *et al, Am J Psychiatry* 2002;**159**:1777–9) and it has shown efficacy in non-combat related chronic PTSD (n=28 [c=28], RCT, d/b, p/c, 8/52, Carey *et al, Hum Psychopharmacol* 2012;**27**:386–91).

Quetiapine * (mean 200–250 mg/d) augmentation of SSRIs may be helpful in TR-PTSD (eg. n=15, open, 8/52, Ahearn *et al, Int Clin Psychopharmacol* 2006;**21**:29–33). Quetiapine 25–400 mg/d monotherapy may reduce psychotic and PTSD symptoms (e.g. n=53, open, 8/52, Kozaric-Kovacic and Pivac, *Int J Neuropsychopharmacol* 2007;**10**:253–61).

Risperidone has been used as an adjunct in resistant combat PTSD, was well tolerated and produced a modest improvement (n=40, RCT, d/b, p/c, 5/52, Hamner *et al, Int Clin Psychopharmacol* 2003;**18**:1–8) at 2–4 mg/d (n=26, open, 6/52, Kozaric-Kovacic *et al, J Clin Psychiatry* 2005;**66**:922–7). Lower dose risperidone 1–3 mg at night can help combat nightmares (n=4, Detweiler *et al, Consult Pharm* 2011;**26**:920–8), although less so as an adjunct to sertraline (n=45 [c=34], Rothbaum *et al, J Clin Psychiatry* 2008;**69**:520–5).

Ziprasidone has been used successfully (n=2, Siddiqui *et al, J Psychiatry Neurosci* 2005;**30**:430–1; FFT).

Benzodiazepines

Although generally considered ineffective, potential anti-arousal effects can be useful and beneficial effects have been seen with **clonazepam** at 4–5 mg/d, although it was largely ineffective in improving sleep disturbances and nightmares in combat-related PTSD (n=6, 2+2/52, p/c, c/o, s/b, Cates *et al, Ann Pharmacother* 2004:**38**:1395–9). Care is needed with possible abuse, induction of depression, the potential for the release of impulsive or antisocial behaviour and severe withdrawal reactions (review by Nardi *et al, Curr Drug Targets* 2013;**14**:353–64).

Beta-blockers *

Early data suggested that propranolol might reduce the consolidation of emotional memory in PTSD (eg. Rosenberg, *Am J Bioeth* 2007;**7**:27–8), e.g. propranolol 40 mg TDS (n=19, open, Vaiva *et al, Biol Psychiatry* 2003;**54**:947–9). A meta-analysis of memory consolidation and reconsolidation studies suggested propranolol reduced recalled emotional materials in healthy adults, but was unsure if this applies to more traumatic memories (s=18, n=567, RCT, d/b, p/c, Lonergan *et al, J Psychiatry Neurosci* 2013;**38**:222–31).

Duloxetine

In men with PTSD, duloxetine 60–120 mg/d showed promise (n=21 [c=20], open, 8/52, Walderhaug *et al, Pharmacopsychiatry* 2010; **43**:45–9).

Gabapentin

Successful use has been reported (e.g. n=30, Hamner *et al, Ann Clin Psychiatry* 2001;**13**:141–6; n=1, Malek-Ahmadi, *Ann Pharmacother* 2003;**37**:664–6).

Hydroxyzine *

Hydroxyzine may improve sleep and reduce nightmares but is not as effective as prazosin (n=100, RCT, p/c, 8/52, Ahmadpanah *et al, Neuropsychobiology* 2014;**69**:235–42).

Ketamine *

IV ketamine was significantly and rapidly effective for chronic PTSD after 24 hours (n=41, RCT, d/b, c/o, a/c, Feder *et al, JAMA Psychiatry* 2014;**71**:681–8), although it has made PTSD worse (n=50, Schonenberg *et al, J Psychopharmacol* 2008;**22**:493–7).

Lamotrigine *

Lamotrigine can decrease aggression in TR-PTSD (Kozaric-Kovacic and Eterovic, *Clin Neuropharmacol* 2013;**36:**94–5).

Levetiracetam + TAU

Levetiracetam (mean 2000mg/d) may be useful as augmentation in refractory PTSD (n=23, retrospective, mean 10/52, Kinrys *et al, J Clin Psychiatry* 2006;**67**:211–4).

Liothyronine/triiodothyronine + SSRIs

Triiodothyronine 25mcg/d has been used successfully to augment ineffective SSRI monotherapy (n=5, 8/52, Agid *et al, J Clin Psychiatry* 2001;**62**:169–73).

MAOIs

Phenelzine may exert a notable effect on intrusive and avoidance symptoms (n=60, RCT, d/b, 8/52, Kosten *et al, J Nerv Ment Dis* 1991;**179**:366–70), possibly via a strong inhibitory effect on REM sleep.

MDMA (Ecstasy) *

MDMA did not seem to help psychotherapy in PTSD (n=12, RCT, d/b, p/c, 1 year, Ochen *et al, J Psychopharmacol* 2013;**27**:40–52), although it might do (Chabrol, *J Psychopharmacol* 2013;**27**:865) by helping relax the person as an adjunct (n=20, Mithoefer *et al, J Psychopharmacol* 2011;**25**:439–52).

Mirtazapine

Studies have suggested an effect on symptoms at 45mg/d (64% response vs 20% for placebo; n=29, RCT, d/b, p/c, 8/52, Davidson *et al, Biol Psychiatry* 2003;**53**:188–91). For PTSD nightmares, mirtazapine may have some significant effects, perhaps on sleep (n=>300, open, Lewis, *Am J Psychiatry* 2002;**159**:1948–9). A continuation study showed a modest enduring effect for six months (n=15[c=12], 24/52, Kim *et al, Psychiatry Clin Neurosci* 2005;**59**:743–7).

Phenytoin

Phenytoin may have some efficacy and may be associated with changes in brain structure (n=9, open, 3/12, Bremner *et al, J Clin Psychiatry* 2004;**65**:1559–64; Bremner *et al, J Psychopharmacol* 2005;**19**:159–65).

Pregabalin ± TAU *

A small pilot study suggested pregabalin may be useful for accident-related PTSD (e.g. n=9, 6/52, Pae *et al, Int Clin Psychopharmacol* 2009; **24**:29–33; n=1, Paslakis *et al, Prog Neuropsychopharmacol Biol Psychiatry* 2011;**35**:1160–1). *Adjunct:* A pilot study showed adjunctive use was just about statistically effective for severity of PTSD but not depression, anxiety or QoL (n=37, RCT, d/b, p/c, 6/52, Baniasadi *et al, J Psychiatr Pract* 2014;**20**:419–27).

Tiagabine *

Tiagabine 8mg/d (range 4–12mg/d) may have some acute (n=7, open, 8/52, Taylor, *J Clin Psychiatry* 2003;**64**:1421–5) and relapse prevention efficacy (n=29[c=19], open, 12/52, Connor *et al, Psychopharmacol (Berl)* 2006;**184**:21–5). Tiagabine 2–12mg has helped improve sleep and a good response on the first night predicts subsequent PTSD response (n=20, Krystal *et al, J Psychopharmacol* 2014;**28**:457–65).

Tricyclics

Amitriptyline (n=46, p/c, 8/52, Davidson *et al, Arch Gen Psychiatry* 1990;**4**:259–69) and **imipramine** (n=60, RCT, p/c, 8/52, Kosten *et al, J Nerv Ment Dis* 1991;**179**:366–70) have been shown to produce a modest but clinically meaningful effect with doses of 300mg/d needed for at least eight weeks.

Valproate

Intrusion, hyperarousal and depressive symptoms and non-combat-related PTSD may respond to valproate (see systematic review and meta-analysis, although data was limited; s=8, Adamou *et al, Curr Med Res Opin* 2007;**23**:1285–91).

• Case reports *

- DHEA (dehydroepiandrosterone) (n=5, Sageman and Brown, *J Clin Psychiatry* 2006;**67**:493–6)
- Memantine (n=4, 12/52, Battista *et al, Psychiatry* 2007;**70**:167–74; n=1, Chopra *et al, J Clin Psychopharmacol* 2011;**31**:787–8)
- Oxcarbazepine (n=1, Berigan, *Can J Psychiatry* 2002;**7**:973–4)

- **Rivastigmine** in TR-PTSD (n = 3, 6/12, Fayyazi *et al*, *J Clin Psychopharmacol* 2013;**33**:706–9)
- **Terazosin** (n = 1, Salviati *et al*, *Clin Ter* 2013;**164**:133–7).

□ No efficacy

Bupropion

Bupropion may improve depression but not PTSD (n = 30, d/b, p/c, 8/52, Becker *et al*, *J Clin Psychopharmacol* 2007;**27**:193–7).

Flumazenil

Two studies have shown no effects (e.g. Coupland *et al*, *Biol Psychiatry* 1997;**41**:988–90).

Guanfacine *

Two studies have shown no detectable effect on any PTSD symptoms (n = 63, RCT, d/b, p/c, 8/52, Neylan *et al*, *Am J Psychiatry* 2006;**163**:2186–8; RCT, d/b, p/c, 8/52+8/52 open extension, Davis *et al*, *Psychopharmacol Bull* 2008;**41**:8–18).

Naltrexone

Only non-significant improvements were seen in a small, short trial (n = 8, open, 2/52, Lubin *et al*, *Hum Psychopharmacol* 2002;**17**:181–5).

PSYCHIATRIC EMERGENCY, ACUTE

see Acute psychiatric emergency (*1.1*)

1.21 PSYCHOSIS AND SCHIZOPHRENIA

1.21.1. Psychosis and schizophrenia
1.21.2. First episode (early intervention)
1.21.3. Cognitive impairment
1.21.4. Negative symptoms *
1.21.5. Psychosis in Parkinson's disease

Symptoms

Schizophrenia is an enduring and fluctuating mental health problem with a high risk of relapse. Schneider's 'First rank symptoms' are often used as the main diagnostic features. They include hearing thoughts spoken aloud, hallucinations ('third person', running commentary and somatic), thought withdrawal or insertion, thought broadcasting, delusional perceptions and feelings, or actions experienced as being made or influenced by external agents. Japan has dropped schizophrenia as a term and 'salience syndrome' has been suggested (van Os, *Acta Psychiatr Scand* 2009;**120**:363–72).

Possible causes of schizophrenia *

The dopamine hypothesis, i.e. excess dopamine activity in the mesolimbic remains the most enduring explanation for the main symptoms but there are many other theories, e.g. hypofunction of the glutamate systems, particularly at the NMDA sub-type of glutamate receptor, combined dopamine hyperfunction, glutamate hypofunction, 5-HT_2 hyperfunction and part of an inflammatory process. There are currently 22 locations on the human genome linked to schizophrenia (Ripke *et al*, *Nature Genetics* 2013;**45**:1150–9).

Role of drugs in schizophrenia

Antipsychotics have a major role in the management of the symptoms of schizophrenia, but there is no clear choice of first-line antipsychotic. This is complicated further because the placebo response (1960 to 2013) in antipsychotic trials has significantly increased, possibly due to inflation of baseline scores, less severe illness, and higher expectations as a result of more effective treatments, because placebo only works if you think it might do (s = 105, RCTs, 4–24/52, Rutherford *et al*, *JAMA Psychiatry* 2014;**71**:1409–21). The terms 'atypical' and 'typical' have no real meaning but until a better classification term is agreed upon, the abbreviations SGA (second generation antipsychotic) and FGA (first generation antipsychotic) will be used here.

1. Choice of antipsychotic *

There have only been two major independent direct comparisons between antipsychotics.

(i) **CATIE** (n = 1493, RCT, < 18/12, Lieberman *et al*, *N Engl J Med* 2005;**353**:1209–23; FFT) compared olanzapine, risperidone, perphenazine, quetiapine and ziprasidone. Among the many findings were:

- 74% people discontinued their first antipsychotic within 18 months
- Olanzapine (7.5–30 mg/d) had the lowest drop-out rate (but with known side-effects)
- Perphenazine (8–32 mg/d) was as effective as the SGAs
- In those who did not respond to a SGA, clozapine was more effective than switching

to another SGA (n=99, CATIE, McEvoy *et al*, *Am J Psychiatry* 2006;**163**:600–10).

(ii) CUtLASS compared switching to either an FGA or SGA in people who needed a change and showed striking consistency over all studied drugs for quality of life scores (n=227, RCT, open-s/b, 12/12, Jones *et al*, *Arch Gen Psychiatry* 2006;**63**:1079–87). The antipsychotic choice in the acute phase thus remains an individual decision.

2. Early-onset and limitation of progression

Evidence is accumulating that antipsychotics started after symptoms first appear, or even in a prodromal stage, may prevent or delay the progression of schizophrenia. See *1.21.2*.

3. Acute phase *

Many antipsychotics have an immediate calming effect (relieving distress in the acute stage) and then reduce the intensity of psychotic symptoms. Higher doses are no more effective than lower doses and potentially give the recipient an adversive experience.

Onset of action: analyses have shown that:

- Only minimal improvement (<20% reduction in PANSS or BPRS) predicts non-response at six weeks or later with an 86–90% accuracy
- Significant symptom reduction occurs in up to week 4, with smaller reductions after that
- Improvement with clozapine was significant every week over a year
- There is no evidence (except for lurasidone) that, if there is lack of improvement after two weeks, increasing the dose then converts people to responders
- See also first episode/EIS, which may be subtly different.

(s=34, n=9460, Samara *et al*, *Am J Psychiatry* 2015;**172**:617–29; s=19, up to one year, Suzuki *et al*, *Br J Psychiatry* 2011;**199**:275–80; FFT; s=5, p/c, RCTs, O'Gorman *et al*, *Hum Psychopharmacol* 2011;**26**:282–90).

4. Relapse prevention *

Relapse occurs in around 80% of untreated schizophrenics and so maintenance therapy, which reduces relapse rates significantly, is usually an important component of management, although it can be difficult to motivate people to continue while relatively asymptomatic but experiencing side-effects. A systematic review and meta-analysis including two-year follow-ups has shown that antipsychotics reduce relapse but have side-effects (s=65, n=6493, RCT, p/c, Leucht *et al*, *Lancet* 2012;**379**:2063–71; see also Leucht *et al*, *Cochrane Database Syst Rev* 2012;**5**:CD008016).

Two-year outcomes	Antipsychotics	Placebos
Relapses	27% NNT=3	64%
Readmitted	10% NNT=5	26%
Side-effects	16%	9%
Sedation	13%	9%
Weight gain	10%	6%

Many people will need to balance the positive effects of the drug (e.g. symptom suppression) and the negative effects (e.g. side-effects), and finding a good reason not to relapse, e.g. family, friends or job, may aid effective maintenance therapy. Long-term side-effects, particularly the under-rated akathisia, weight gain and dysphoria, tend to reduce compliance and so efforts to reduce and manage ADRs are vital.

Mortality: An 11-year study of mortality in people with schizophrenia concluded that there is no evidence of an increase in deaths with antipsychotics and that the gap in life expectancy between people with schizophrenia and the general population is reducing, e.g. there was a lower mortality in people with schizophrenia taking antipsychotics (for 7–11 years during the study period) than not, (n=66881 schizophrenics from national register cf. 5.2 million in general population, 11 years, Tiihonen *et al*, *Lancet* 2009;**374**:620–7; critical appraisal De Hert *et al*, *Schizophr Res* 2010;**117**:68–74).

Intermittent therapy ('use of medication only during periods of incipient relapse or symptom exacerbation rather than continuously') is superior to placebo, but less effective than continuous treatment (s=17, n=2252, RCTs, 6/52–2 years, Sampson *et al*, *Cochrane Database Syst Rev* 2013;**7**:CD006196) and risks sudden relapse.

Dose: Many people with schizophrenia are on long-term antipsychotics (depot/LAI or oral) at the dose they received when acutely ill and there is abundant evidence that this may not be applicable in schizophrenia, as continuous antipsychotic intake is 'topping-up' D2 blockade as significant D2 blockade can persist for 16 weeks after discontinuing depots (Pani *et al*, *Eur Psychiatry* 2007;**22**:267–75). Reducing doses from their acute levels may actually improve outcomes and symptoms, but (and it is a big but) some people appear to need higher doses long-term. This does not mean not trying to reduce doses, but that care is needed to prevent unnecessary and potentially catastrophic relapses.

The use of high dose antipsychotic medication (Thompson, *Br J Psychiatry* 1994;**164**:448–58; revised by Royal College of Psychiatrists, 2006)

The upper end of the dose ranges of older antipsychotics is often not clearly established and usually defined by limits of safety and the SPCs. Doses above these limits should only be used 'with caution and under specialist supervision'. 'Chlorpromazine equivalents' have been used to compare drugs or calculate total doses of multiple drugs, but maximum doses vary between drugs, and dosage equivalents are of only limited use (see *2.2.1*). The evidence and scientific rationale for the effectiveness of high doses is very limited.

Main dangers of high dose antipsychotics:

1. Sudden cardiac-related death, e.g. QT prolongation, torsades de pointes.
2. CNS toxicity, e.g. CNS and respiratory depression, hypoxia, seizures.

Main uses of antipsychotics above BNF limits:

1. **Psychiatric emergency:** see 'Acute psychiatric emergency' (*Chapter 1.1*).
2. **Acute treatment**: i.e. after the emergency, but before the antipsychotic takes full effect. Doses should be reduced as soon as possible once the patient has responded.
3. **Long-term treatment**: e.g. in TRS where residual symptoms impair living or rehabilitation:
   - **as polypharmacy**: not recommended unless with a carefully arrived at rationale
   - **poor resources**: inappropriate if to compensate for inadequate resources/environment

Factors to be considered before prescribing high-dose antipsychotics:

- The diagnosis is fully confirmed and documented
- Plasma levels are therapeutic and compliance with the regimen is assured
- Treatment duration has been fully adequate
- Reduced doses for a trial period have been tried to rule out, e.g. akathisia
- Adverse social and psychological factors have been minimised
- Alternative antipsychotic therapies tried.

If exceeding standard BNF doses, the following should be routine and documented:

- Multidisciplinary team and patient (or advocate) discussion, obtaining valid consent if possible, thoroughly recording the decision and reasoning, including target signs and symptoms, and outcome evaluation
- Consideration of any contraindications, e.g. cardiac, age, renal, hepatic, weight, and smoking, and any interactions, e.g. with tricyclics, carbamazepine, etc
- ECG pre-treatment to exclude QTc prolongation, repeated every 1–3 months, especially with haloperidol
- Doses increased only slowly
- Regular checks carried out on pulse, bp temperature and hydration
- Prescription reviewed regularly and reduced after three months if no improvement.

5. Discontinuation *

If antipsychotics are stopped, relapse may be delayed for 2–6 months, with the individual often feeling better (due to a reduced side-effect burden) before the relapse.

Reducing doses or stopping antipsychotics in someone on a high dose long-term:

- Check the history carefully to confirm that there is clear evidence of previous illness
- If so, proceed only with great caution (especially if any evidence of a forensic history or potential) and document carefully
- A history of non-compliance without relapse is good, but do not taken as confirmation that antipsychotics are not needed
- Make only small changes each time
- Relapse peaks at about 2–6 months post-dose reduction or discontinuation so allow 6/12 to assess the outcome of each change
- Have a robust system in place for detecting early signs of relapse, e.g. increasing or reintroducing doses to restabilise the person
- Consider the consequences of relapse, damage to the individual and others, and previous events
- Remember that some people need higher doses and there is much to gain by reducing doses, but more to lose should the person relapse and not be able to return to their previous levels of functioning.

Medication risk factors for relapse:

- Antipsychotic used: e.g. some SGAs may be linked to lower rehospitalisation rates (n=1039, 2 years, Rabinowitz *et al*, *Am J Psychiatry* 2001;**158**:266–9)
- Doses: These may need to be lower in some ethnic groups (n=192, 6/52, Emsley *et al*, *J Clin Psychiatry* 2002;**63**:9–14). Higher long-term doses lead to extra ADRs and a higher risk of non-compliance
- Duration of untreated psychosis (DUP): longer DUP is a good predictor of poor outcomes
- Unmanaged substance misuse: reduces antipsychotic effects in dual diagnosis, with sooner and longer readmissions, especially if non-compliant (n=99, four years, Hunt *et al*, *Schizophr Res* 2002;**54**:253–64)
- Non-compliance/concordance/adherence.

Suicide prevention *

Up to 5–10% of people with schizophrenia will commit suicide, usually near symptom onset (n=22598, Palmer *et al*, *Arch Gen Psychiatry* 2005;**62**:247–53). Clozapine has a clear anti-suicide effect and is licensed in the US for reduction in recurrent suicidal behaviour in schizophrenia and schizoaffective disorder, if taken for a minimum of two years. Risperidone and olanzapine may give some protection compared to other (excluding clozapine) antipsychotics (n=756, five years Barak *et al*, *Psychopharmacol [Berl]* 2004;**175**:215–9).

Reviews: * general (Leucht *et al*, *Int J Neuropsychopharmacol* 2011;**14**:269–84), systematic review of published meta-analyses of oral antipsychotics (n=91, Citrome, *Expert Opin Pharmacother* 2012:**13**:1545–73), antipsychotics for TRS (Van Sant and Buckley, *Expert Opin Pharmacother* 2011;**12**:411–34), BAP Guidelines for pharmacological treatment of schizophrenia (Barnes *et al*, *J Psychopharmacol* 2011;**25**:567–620), modes of action (Correll, *J Clin Psychiatry* 2014;**75**:e23), mid-term and long-term effectiveness in schizophrenia, suggesting clozapine is most effective, followed by olanzapine, then risperidone, and then the rest (Glick *et al*, *J Clin Psychiatry* 2011;**72**:1616–27).

1.21.1 PSYCHOSIS AND SCHIZOPHRENIA

BNF listed

FIRST GENERATION (OR TYPICAL) ANTIPSYCHOTICS (FGAs)

PHENOTHIAZINES

Chlorpromazine *

Cochrane concludes that chlorpromazine remains a global benchmark for schizophrenia, as a well-established, effective but imperfect treatment (s=55, Adams *et al*, *Cochrane Database Syst Rev* 2014;**1**:CD000284), with relapse prevention efficacy (s=10, n=1042, Almerie *et al*, *Cochrane Database Syst Rev* 2007; **1**:CD006329). The optimum dose is in the 400–800 mg/d range, with no advantages for lower or higher doses (s=4, n=1012, RCT, Liu and De Haan, *Cochrane Syst Database Rev* 2009; **2**:CD007778). IV use is not recommended unless the injection is diluted and the patient is in a supine position.

Levomepromazine (methotrimeprazine) *

Cochrane concludes there is little information on levomepromazine for schizophrenia (s=4, n=192, RCTs, Sivaraman *et al, Schizophr Bull* 2012;**38**:219–20; FFT), but that it causes less EPSE than haloperidol and more hypotension than risperidone, not really ground-breaking conclusions.

Pericyazine *

Pericyazine is a piperidine phenothiazine, with marked sedative and hypotensive side-effects. Use as a low-dose anxiolytic-sedative has increased since the fall of thioridazine. The little that has been published is not of any quality (s=5, RCT, Matar *et al, Cochrane Database Syst Rev* 2014;**5**:CD007479).

Perphenazine *

Perphenazine is a piperazine phenothiazine with a relatively short half-life (8–12 hours). Thanks to CATIE, perphenazine has been shown to be non-inferior to olanzapine, risperidone and quetiapine at 18 months (n=1049, Rosenheck and Lin, *J Nerv Ment Dis* 2014;**202**:18–24) but Cochrane concludes that there is poor and incomplete reporting (s=31, n=4662, RCT, a/c, Hartung *et al, Cochrane Database Syst Rev* 2015;**3**:CD003443).

Prochlorperazine

Prochlorperazine is a piperazine phenothiazine better known for its use as an antiemetic and in Ménières disease, but is also licensed for schizophrenia and acute mania.

Promazine

Promazine is similar to chlorpromazine and has a minor role as a non-dependence-prone hypnotic.

Trifluoperazine *

Trifluoperazine is a piperazine phenothiazine, sometimes claimed to have 'activating' effects at low doses. Cochrane concludes that trifluoperazine is superior to placebo (s=10, n=686, RCT, p/c, Koch *et al, Cochrane Database Syst Rev* 2014;**1**:CD010226) and of similar efficacy to other antipsychotics (s=13, n=1162, Marques *et al, Cochrane Database Syst Rev* 2004;**1**:CD003545), but that the data is inconclusive and of poor quality (s=7, n=422, RCT, 4–52/52, Tardy *et al, Cochrane Database Syst Rev* 2014;**7**:CD009396).

BUTYROPHENONES

Benperidol

Benperidol is a potent D2 blocker originally marketed as specific for antisocial sexual behaviour. Cochrane concludes that there is insufficient evidence to assess its effectiveness and it is inferior to perphenazine (s=1, n=40, RCT, Leucht and Hartung, *Cochrane Database Syst Rev* 2005;**2**:CD003083). See *1.24*.

Haloperidol (see also LAIs/depots) *

Haloperidol is the standard reference butyrophenone used for the treatment of acute and chronic psychosis, both orally and as an injection (aqueous and depot), although in the CUtLASS study few people remained on haloperidol long-term. The new BNF oral limit is 20 mg/d, but Cochrane concludes doses in the range 3–7.5 mg have optimum efficacy in uncomplicated acute schizophrenia and that people should be reluctant to prescribe or take more than 7.5 mg/d (s=19, Donnelly *et al, Cochrane Database Syst Rev* 2013;**8**:CD001951). Improvement in the first two weeks is predictive of response, but increasing the dose above 6.6 mg/d (±2 mg) in non-responders does not improve response (n=101, Giegling *et al, J Psychiatr Res* 2010;**44**:487–92). Cochrane concludes that haloperidol is of similar efficacy to low-potency FGAs (s=17, n=877, RCT, 2–12/52, Tardy *et al, Cochrane Database Syst Rev* 2014;**7**:CD009268), but that its ADRs are such that alternative antipsychotics should be prescribed (s=25, n=4651, RCTs, Adams *et al, Cochrane Database Syst Rev* 2014;**11**:CD003082). The UK SmPC recommends an ECG before treatment due to the risk of a dose-related increase in QT-interval, especially if given by the IV, rather than IM, route.

THIOXANTHENES

Flupentixol (see also LAIs/depots) *

Cochrane concludes that the data on flupentixol is almost entirely lacking (s=1, n=45, Shen *et al, Cochrane Database Syst Rev* 2013;**11**:CD009777; see also; Grohmann *et al, Eur Arch Psychiatry Clin Neurosci* 2014;**264**:131–41). It has also been compared with olanzapine (n=28, RCT, d/b, 4/52, Gattaz *et al, Pharmacopsychiatry* 2004;**37**:279–85) and risperidone (n= 144, RCT, d/b, 25/52, Ruhrmann *et al, Prog Neuropsychopharmacol Biol Psychiatry* 2007;**31**:1012–22). Oral flupentixol is occasionally used in low dose for anxiety and depression.

Zuclopenthixol (see also LAIs/depots)

Zuclopenthixol is a relatively long-acting oral antipsychotic, and in a trial of oral vs depot zuclopenthixol in people with violence and schizophrenia, violence was inversely proportional to compliance, and much lower in the depot group (n=46, RCT, s/b, 12/12, Arango *et al, Eur Psychiatry* 2006;**21**:34–40). Cochrane concludes that oral zuclopenthixol is a viable option but needs routine anticholinergics (s=18, n=1578, Kumar and Strech, *Cochrane Database Syst Rev* 2005;**4**:CD005474).

DIPHENYLBUTYLPIPERIDINES

Pimozide *

Pimozide is licensed for chronic schizophrenia and other psychoses, especially paranoid and monosymptomatic hypochondriacal psychoses, e.g. parasitosis. Cochrane concludes it is effective but there is no data to support or refute its use in delusional disorders (s=32, Mothi and Sampson, *Cochrane Database Syst Rev* 2013;**11**:CD001949), which is based almost entirely on case reports (Generali and Cada, *Hosp Pharm* 2014;**49**:134–5).

BENZAMIDES, substituted

Amisulpride

Amisulpride blocks pre-synaptic D2 and D3 autoreceptors at lower doses, and higher doses blocks post-synaptic receptors, with little effect on other receptors albeit with dose-dependent hyperprolactinaemia (RCT, d/b, 6/12, Mortimer *et al, Int Clin Psychopharmacol* 2004;**19**:63–9). Two meta-analyses show some effect at 50–100mg/d for predominantly negative symptoms and lower use of anticholinergic drugs (e.g. s=18, n=2214, RCT, Leucht *et al, Am J Psychiatry* 2002;**159**:180–90). Cochrane concludes that studies vs SGAs are short, but that it is more effective than ziprasidone with less weight gain than risperidone or olanzapine (s=10, n=1549, Komossa *et al, Cochrane Database Syst Rev* 2010;**1**:CD006624; FFT).

Reviews: general (Nuss and Tessier, *Curr Med Res Opin* 2010;**26**:787–801), TDM (Sparshatt *et al, Acta Psychiatr Scand* 2009;**120**:416–28).

Sulpiride *

Sulpiride is a specific dopamine (D2, plus some D3 and D4) receptor blocker. Cochrane concludes that sulpiride may be effective but the evidence is extremely limited (s=2, n=113, Wang and Sampson, *Cochrane Database Syst Rev* 2014;**4**:CD007811). It was the most commonly chosen FGA in the CUtLASS study (n=227, RCT, open-s/b, 12/12, Jones *et al, Arch Gen Psychiatry* 2006;**63**:1079–87).

SECOND GENERATION (OR ATYPICAL) ANTIPSYCHOTICS (SGAs)

'Atypical' has been a widely-used term to describe a diverse group of antipsychotics with individual characteristics, e.g. minimal EPS, lack of sedation or a fast dissociation from D2 receptors. The CATIE, CUtLASS and the Leucht meta-analysis (s=150, n=21533, d/b, Leucht *et al Lancet* 2009;**373**:31–41; FFT) have shown similar efficacy between SGAs but different ADRs.

Aripiprazole (see also LAIs/depots and APE) *

Aripiprazole is a dopamine D2 and $5HT_{1A}$ receptor partial agonist, and a $5HT_{2A}$ receptor antagonist. Its dopamine receptor agonism is at a lower level than dopamine, while blocking endogenous dopamine (100% D2 occupancy by aripiprazole reduces dopaminergic activity to about 30%). The starting dose should be 5mg/d if the person is switching from another antipsychotic, increasing to 10mg/d, and then 15mg/d as tolerated. The time to steady state can take up to four weeks so rapid dose escalation is not advisable (Uzun *et al*, *Psychiatr Danub* 2005;**17**:67–75). Plasma levels may be helpful in optimising doses (n=45, Lin *et al*, *J Clin Psychopharmacol* 2011;**31**:758–62).

The optimum dose of aripiprazole appears to be 10–25mg/d, with up to 10mg/d for agitation and hostility (s=22, RCT, d/b, p/c, <1 year, Charpeaud *et al*, *Encephale* 2014;**40**:62–73), with doses above 20mg/d providing no additional benefit (s=5, Mace and Taylor, *CNS Drugs* 2009;**23**:773–80). Cochrane concludes that aripiprazole may be effective for schizophrenia, with efficacy similar to FGAs (s=9, n=3122, Bhattacharjee and El-Sayeh, *Cochrane Database Syst Rev* 2008;**3**:CD006617), with low prolactin and QTc effects (noting very high drop-out rates and lack of much usable data; s=9, n=2585, RCT, Belgemwar and El-Sayeh, *Cochrane Database Syst Rev* 2011;**8**:CD006622), and that comparisons with other SGAs are of limited quality and incomplete, with a drop-out rate of 30–40% (s=174, n=17244, RCTs, Khanna *et al*, *Cochrane Database Syst Rev* 2014;**1**:CD006569). Long-term efficacy has been shown (n=214, one year, Chrzanowski *et al*, *Psychopharmacology (Berl)* 2006;**189**:259–66), where 15mg/d seemed well tolerated and effective (n=310, RCT, p/c, d/b, 6/12, Pigott *et al*, *J Clin Psychiatry* 2003;**64**:1048–56; comment by Mortimer, *EBMH* 2004;**7**:41; FFT; noting placebo level side-effects, no dose titration, simple dosing, that 30% of stable people relapsed over 6/12 when switched, and a lack of symptom reduction in more severely ill people).

Reviews: extensive (Croxtall, *CNS Drugs* 2012;**26**:155–83; Sparshatt *et al*, *J Clin Psychiatry* 2010;**71**:1447–56), general (Park *et al*, *Expert Rev Neurother* 2011;**11**:1541–52), use in TRS (Mossaheb and Kaufmann, *Neuropsychiatr Dis Treat* 2012;**8**:235–44).

Clozapine (see also *Tables 1.2–1.6*) *

Clozapine is indicated for treatment-resistant schizophrenia (TRS) and unresponsive psychotic disorders in Parkinson's disease. Before starting, patients should have a physical examination and any cardiac disease excluded.

Efficacy: * Clozapine is probably effective in up to 30–50% of people with TRS (n=268, RCT, d/b, p/c, 6/52, Kane *et al*, *Arch Gen Psychiatry* 1988;**45**:789–96), with an early response possible after 4–6 weeks of treatment (s=19, n=1745, RCT, d/b, Sherwood *et al*, *J Psychopharmacol* 2012;**26**:1175–84). Response may rise to 60% if adequate doses are given for up to 12 months, e.g. 50–76% responded, the peak response occurring at 12–24 weeks (n=84, open, 52/52, Lieberman *et al*, *Am J Psychiatry* 1994;**151**:1744–52), but with little to gain beyond eight weeks at any particular dose if no response is seen (n=50, open, Conley *et al*, *Am J Psychiatry* 1997;**154**:1243–7). Cochrane concludes that clozapine is clearly superior and has a differential efficacy (s=42, n=3950, Essali *et al*, *Cochrane Database Syst Rev* 2009;**1**:CD000059), including compared to olanzapine (s=7, n=648, RCTs, Souza *et al*, *CNS Spectr* 2012;**18**:82–9).

Blood levels: * Plasma levels are best taken 10–12 hours post-dose (Flanaghan, *Br J Clin Pharmacy* 2011;**3**:18–20) and may be useful in optimising therapy or if a poor response occurs. ADRs can be far higher than spontaneously reported, and plasma level-related, especially in the under 18s (n=545, Couchman *et al*, *Early Interven Psychiatry* 2013;**7**:122–30). See *Table 1.6*.

Review: * predictors of plasma levels (Rajkumar *et al*, *Int Clin Psychopharmacol* 2013;**28**:50–6).

Blood dyscrasias: Clozapine can cause a usually reversible neutropenia in 3–4% of people, which may lead on to agranulocytosis in 0.8% over one year, with a non-dose-related higher risk in older people and those with lower base-line wbc counts. The onset peaks at around 8–10 weeks (range 0.5–24+ weeks), lasts for between 12 and 20 days (see *Table 1.2*). The incidence after three years is lower than with carbimazole (where blood monitoring is not considered necessary). The UK CPMS database indicates that agranulocytosis is 2.4-fold higher in Asians compared to Caucasians, and there is an age-related increase in risk of 53% per decade, but no dose-relationship (n=12760, Munro *et al*, *Br J Psychiatry* 1999;**175**:576–80). Clozapine can induce transient granulocytopenia without a rise in granulocyte colony stimulating factor (G-CSF) levels. Use in people with benign ethnic neutropenia (BEN) may be allowed with haematologist advice. See 6.2 for dyscrasia management advice.

Rechallenge: Of 53 patients rechallenged after clozapine-induced leucopenia or neutropenia, 38% had a further dyscrasia and, in most of these, it was more severe, longer-lasting and of a quicker onset than the original episode, but 55% were rechallenged successfully and remained in treatment (n=53, Dunk *et al, Br J Psychiatry* 2006;**188**:255–63; FFT). If stopping clozapine due to serious ADRs, careful rechallenge can be considered after neutropenia and NMS, but not after agranulocytosis or myocarditis (n=138, Manu *et al, Schizophr Res* 2012;**134**:180–6; FFT):

Adverse reaction as the reason to stop clozapine	n=	Rechallenge success rate over 16–96/52
Neutropenia	112	70%
Agranulocytosis	15	20%
NMS	5	100%
Myocarditis	4	75%
Pericarditis	1	100%

Review: review of plasma levels (McKee *et al, Clin Schizophr Relat Psychoses* 2011;**5**:26–32).

Suicide reduction: Clozapine is licensed for suicide reduction in schizophrenia in the US. The incidence can be as high as 5–10%, a startling comparison with the 2% risk reversible agranulocytosis. The InterSePT study (n=980, RCT, d/b, two years, Meltzer *et al, Arch Gen Psychiatry* 2003;**60**:82–91) showed a 25% reduction in suicide events cf. olanzapine and a Swedish study (2006–9) showed lower suicide rates (OR=0.45) and attempted suicide (OR=0.44) with clozapine than haloperidol, with reduced rehospitalisations (n=26046, Ringbäck Weitoft *et al, Pharmacoepidemiol Drug Saf* 2014;**23**:290–8). Not all data is consistent (n=1514 plus 2830 matched-controls, four years, Sernyak *et al, Am J Psychiatry* 2001;**158**:931–7; disputed by Ertugrul and Meltzer, *Am J Psychiatry* 2002;**159**:323–5).

Reviews: * general (Hill and Freudenreich, *Clin Schizophr Relat Psychoses* 2013;**6**:177–85 Fakra and Azorin, *Expert Opin Pharmacother* 2012;**13**:1923–35), predictors of response in TRS (n=633, mirror-image, Nielsen *et al, J Clin Psychopharmacol* 2012;**32**:678–83), pharmacogenetics (s=124, Kohlrausch, *Rev Bras Psiquiatr* 2013;**35**:305–17), guidelines for use (Warnez and Alessi-Severini, *BMC Psychiatry* 2014;**14**:102).

Lurasidone *

Lurasidone is licensed for schizophrenia and has a high D2 and 5HT2A and 5HT7 antagonism, some alpha-2c affinity, alpha-2A antagonism and 5-HT1A partial agonism, but no relevant H1 or M1 activity (Ichikawa *et al, Neurochem Int* 2012;**61**:1133–43). The starting dose is 37mg/d (US 40mg/d) up to a maximum of 148mg/d (US 160mg/d). Efficacy vs placebo has been shown in three key studies: PEARL 1 for acute exacerbations (n=500, RCT, d/b, p/c, 6/52, Nasrallah *et al, J Psychiatr Res* 2013;**47**:670–7); PEARL 2 with the active non-comparator olanzapine (n=478, RCT, d/b, p/c, a/c, 6/52, Meltzer *et al, Am J Psychiatry* 2011;**168**:957–67); and PEARL 3 (with the active non-comparator quetiapine; n=488, RCT, d/b, p/c, a/c Loebel *et al, Schizophr Res* 2013;**145**:101–9). In a pooled analysis of short-term trials, lurasidone also significantly improved depressive symptoms in people with schizophrenia (s=4, n=1330, RCT, d/b, p/c, 6/52, Nasrallah *et al, CNS Spectr* 2014;**20**:140–7). Two studies have shown relapse prevention over at least 6/12 (n=148[c=98], open, 6/12, Citrome *et al, CNS Spectr* 2014;**19**:330; n=254[c=113], open, 6/12, Stahl *et al, J Clin Psychiatry* 2013;**74**:507–15). Lurasidone and quetiapine were both equivalent for relapse prevention, BUT there were lower relapses vs quetiapine over 12/12 (24% vs 34%) and readmissions (n=292[c=140], d/b, 12/12, Loebel *et al, Schizophr Res* 2013;**147**:95–102). Lurasidone causes less daytime drowsiness than quetiapine XR when both are taken at night (n=486, RCT, d/b, p/c, 6/52, Loebel *et al, CNS Spectr* 2014;**19**:197–205). It appears weight, glucose, lipid and prolactin neutral. It is best taken at night with a snack of food (>350 calories, independent of fat content) to enhance absorption 2–3-fold (s=2, n=42, open, c/o, Preskorn *et al, Hum Psychopharmacol* 2013;**28**:495–505). The main side-effects are somnolence, akathisia, EPS and nausea.

Clozapine UK prescribing and monitoring summary

Clozapine is indicated in the UK for treatment-resistant schizophrenia and psychosis in Parkinson's disease, ie. patients 'non-responsive' or 'intolerant' of conventional antipsychotics (*Table 1.2*). It can be dispensed on a weekly, fortnightly or four-weekly basis (*Table 1.3*), but only following a satisfactory blood result (*Table 1.4*).

Table 1.2: Summary of UK clozapine prescribing restrictions

'Non-responsive'	Lack of satisfactory clinical improvements despite the use of at least two marketed antipsychotics prescribed at adequate dose for an adequate duration
'Intolerant'	The impossibility of achieving clinical benefit with conventional antipsychotics because of severe or untreatable neurological or other adverse reactions, eg. extrapyramidal or tardive dyskinesia
Patient requirements	Hospital-based originally. Normal white blood cell and differential blood counts. Enrolled with clozapine non-rechallenge database (CNRD)
Prescriber and dispensing requirements	Consultant must be registered with CNRD (clozapine non-rechallenge database). Hospital or nominated community pharmacy must be registered with CNRD

Table 1.3: Summary of UK clozapine minimum blood test requirements *

Blood tests	Required frequency	Validity
Pre-treatment	Single blood screen	10 days, if satisfactory (green)
First 18 weeks of treatment First sample at three days	Weekly (usually Monday or Tuesday)	11 days (not including day of sample) if satisfactory (green)
Weeks 19–52	Every two weeks if blood results have been satisfactory	21 days (not including day of sample) if satisfactory (green)
Weeks 53 onwards	Every four weeks, if 'stable haematological profile'	42 days (not including day of sample) if satisfactory (green)
Discontinuation (temporary or permanent)	Weekly (up to 18 weeks), or fortnightly (19 weeks onwards) for four weeks after completely stopping clozapine	In total one month's follow-up is required at previous monitoring frequency e.g. 4x1/52, 2x2/52 or 1x4/52.. If test result has not been, or does not go red, clozapine may be restarted. See *Table 1.5*

Table 1.4: Summary of UK test results

Results	Meaning	Action
Green	Satisfactory	Routine tests
Amber	wbc or neutrophil counts below accepted levels	Repeat test twice a week until either red or green
Red	wbc below $3000/mm^3$ and/or absolute neutrophils below $1500/mm^3$	Immediate cessation of therapy. Sample blood daily until patient recovered. No further prescribing allowed unless an error has occurred or Consultant takes full responsibility.

Table 1.5: Summary of temporary breaks in clozapine therapy advice *

1. Dose		
Dose on discontinuation	Break	Dose on restart (contact supplying pharmacy for advice)
Any	<48 hours	Restart on previous dose
Any	>48 hours	Restart at 12.5–25mg and build up gradually to previous dose to minimise dose-related side-effects
2. Sampling frequency		
Previous monitoring frequency	Break	Monitoring on restart
Weekly	< 1 week	Weekly, no need to restart 18-week period
Weekly	> 1 week	Weekly, **must** restart 18-week period
After 18 weeks *		
Fortnightly	3 days	Fortnightly
Fortnightly	≥3 days	Weekly for six weeks, then fortnightly
Four-weekly	≤3 days	Four-weekly
Four-weekly	>3 days	Weekly for six weeks, then four-weekly
Fortnightly or four-weekly	>4 weeks	Requires full re-registration and monitoring again fully as if commencing for the first time.

Table 1.6: Summary of clozapine plasma level interpretation *

Trough clozapine	Clinical response	Advice
<0.01 ('not detected')	Any	Clozapine unlikely to have been taken for at least a week pre-sample unless early in initiation phase and the dose with dose under 100mg/d. Low plasma levels may occur in CYP1A2 ultra-rapid metabolisers (review by Greenwood-Smith *et al*, *J Psychopharmacol* 2003;**17**:234–8) and may account for some non-responders.
<0.35mg/l	Good	Repeat at six months, then annually unless response deteriorates or ADRs become troublesome.
	Poor or incomplete	If poor adherence possible, consider psychoeducation or supervised administration. A suspension is available, which **MUST** be shaken for a **full 90 seconds** before administering. Repeat assay after adherence intervention. If no improvement, consider cautious dose increase (extra care above 450mg/d because of the increased risk of ADRs, particularly seizures.) Monitor mental state and side-effects. Review patient again and repeat the assay after at least one week on the new dose. Low plasma levels may occur in CYP1A2 ultra-rapid metabolisers (see above).
0.35–0.60mg/l	Good	Repeat at six months, then annually unless response deteriorates or ADRs become troublesome. If ADRs persist or are serious, consider cautious dose reduction (e.g. 25mg/d in week 1, and a further 25mg/d in week 2, etc.), but bear in mind the possible loss of response.
	Poor or incomplete	If clozapine has continued for at least 3–6 months at the current dose, consider psychosocial intervention. Augmentation with other psychoactive drugs can be considered (see separate section). Any such attempts should be carefully considered with respect to side-effects (including the risk of neutropenia) and possible interactions. Avoid drugs with known potential for causing agranulocytosis.
0.61–0.99mg/l	Good, with no clinical features of toxicity	Review treatment. Consider a cautious dose reduction (e.g. 25mg/d in week 1 and a further 25mg/d in week 2, etc.), but balance this reduction against the risk of diminishing the response to clozapine. Consider an anticonvulsant (not carbamazepine) as prophylaxis against seizures as 0.61–0.99mg/l increases the risk of seizures (Flanagan, *CPD Clin Biochem* 2006;**7**:3–18), if dose reduction is thought inadvisable. Monitor the patient's mental state. Repeat assay after at least one week on a new dose, otherwise repeat three-monthly.
	Poor, incomplete or reduced and/or clinical features of toxicity	Consider a cautious dose reduction (see above) to bring plasma clozapine to below 0.6mg/L. Monitor the patient's mental state. Repeat assay after at least one week on a new dose.
1.0–1.9mg/l	Good — no clinical features of toxicity	Review treatment. Consider cautious dose reduction (as above) to bring plasma level below 1.0 and possibly below 0.6mg/L, but balance this against risk of reduced response to clozapine. Consider using valproate as prophylaxis against seizures. Monitor the patient's mental state. Repeat the assay after at least one week on a new dose, otherwise three-monthly. Remember that plasma levels may continue to rise in the short term, even after dose reduction.
	Poor, incomplete or reduced and/or with clinical features of toxicity	Consider a cautious dose reduction (see above) to bring plasma levels to below 1.0 and possibly below 0.6mg/L. Monitor the patient's mental state. Repeat the assay after at least one week on a new dose. Remember that plasma levels may continue to rise in the short term, even after dose reduction.
>2mg/l	Good, with no clinical features of toxicity	Review urgently. Consider a cautious dose reduction (see above) to bring plasma level to below 1.0mg/L, and possibly below 0.6mg/L. Seriously consider an anticonvulsant (not carbamazepine) as prophylaxis against seizures. Monitor the patient's mental state. Repeat the assay after at least one week on a new dose. Plasma clozapine may continue to rise in the short term, even after the dose has been reduced.
	Poor, incomplete or reduced and/or with clinical features of toxicity	Review urgently. If the patient is being treated in the community, consider admitting for observation. Consider withholding clozapine for 24 hours and re-starting at 75% of the last dose, and thereafter reducing the dose cautiously (see above) to bring plasma clozapine to below 1.0mg/L, and possibly below 0.6mg/L. Seriously consider using an anticonvulsant (not carbamazepine) prophylaxis against seizures. Monitor the patient's mental state. Repeat the assay after at least one week on a new dose. Plasma clozapine may continue to rise in the short term, even after the dose has been reduced.
Others*	Plasma clozapine: norclozapine ratios	The usual ratio of clozapine:norclozapine is about 1.25:1 and should stay the same for any individual. A ratio of >2 suggests clozapine N-demethylation has become saturated (n=26796, Couchman *et al*, *Ther Drug Monit* 2010;**32**:438–47, often at high doses), smoking ceased, enzyme inhibitor drug started, recent missed doses or a non-trough sample. Ratio <1 suggests last dose missed, rapid metabolism (1A2 ultra-rapid metabolism), smoking started or starting an enzyme-inducing drug. Anecdotally, a sample at 4–6 hours, that is closer to 1:1 suggests ultra-rapid metabolism.

Reference: by kind permission Bob Flanaghan, CMHP Bulletin 2011; Carol Paton and Hannah Macfarlane

NB: EU dosing is slightly different to US, as the EU just includes the active moiety whereas US includes the HCl salt, so EU to US dose equivalents are 18.5 mg = 20 mg; 37 mg = 40 mg and 74 mg = 80 mg.

Reviews: * meta-analysis (s = 212, n = 43049, Leucht *et al*, *Lancet* 2013;**382**:951–62), general (Bruijnzeel *et al*, *Expert Opin Pharmacother* 2015;**16**:1559–65; Sanford, *CNS Drugs* 2013;**27**:67–80; Tarazi and Riva, *Expert Opin Drug Discov* 2013;**8**:1297–307).

Olanzapine (see also LAIs/depots) *

Olanzapine is licensed for the treatment of schizophrenia and for relapse prevention. It blocks a wide variety of receptors, e.g. 5HT2A/C, 5HT3, 5HT6, D1–5, M1–5, alpha-1 and H1, with some mesolimbic dopamine selectivity. The starting dose is 10 mg/d (range 5–20 mg/d, mean 15–18 mg/d), with a systematic review and meta-regression concluding the optimum dose is 10–15 mg/d, perhaps lower in smoking females (s = 15, Bishara *et al*, *J Clin Psychopharmacol* 2013;**33**:329–35). It appears effective for relapse prevention (n = 583, RCT, d/b, one year, Beasley *et al*, *J Clin Psychopharmacol* 2003;**23**:582–94, MS). Cochrane concludes olanzapine may be slightly more effective than other antipsychotics but that unfamiliar rating scales make firm conclusions difficult to draw (s = 55, n > 10000, Duggan *et al*, *Cochrane Database Syst Rev* 2005;**2**:CD001359) and its known metabolic and weight ADRs, and 49% drop-out rate from trials, make any conclusions 'tentative' (s = 50, n = 9476, Komossa *et al*, *Cochrane Database Syst Rev* 2010;**3**:CD006654; FFT).

High dose olanzapine: * This may be more effective than other antipsychotics except clozapine (s = 60 RCTs, n = 33360; s = 27 observational studies, n = 202591, Soares-Weiser *et al*, *Eur Neuropsychopharmacol* 2013;**23**:118–25; review by Batail *et al*, *Schizophr Res* 2014;**159**:411–4), but 45–160 mg/d has been linked with significant EPS and sedation and, in this study, with 2–5 deaths (n = 91, Petersen *et al*, *Clin Toxicol [Phila]* 2014;**52**:39–43).

Review: TDM/plasma levels, dosing and interactions (Patel *et al*, *J Clin Psychopharmacol* 2011;**31**:411–7).

Paliperidone (see also LAIs/depots) *

Paliperidone is the 9-hydroxy metabolite of risperidone and is an antagonist at alpha-1, alpha-2 adrenergic, and H1 receptors, with no affinity for cholinergic, muscarinic or beta-1 or beta-2 adrenergic receptors. It licensed in UK for schizophrenia from age 15 and schizoaffective disorder (12 mg/d the optimum dose; n = 316, RCT, p/c, 6/52, Canuso *et al*, *J Clin Psychiatry* 2010;**71**:587–98). The starting and standard dose for schizophrenia is 6 mg once a day (using the OROS sustained release system), with placebo level EPS and no dose titration needed. Administration with a high fat, high caloric meal increases peak concentration by 60% and the AUC by 54% compared with fasting conditions. Paliperidone is effective at 6–12 mg/d in acute schizophrenia (s = 3, n = 1326, RCT, d/b, p/c, 6/52, Meltzer *et al*, *J Clin Psychiatry* 2008;**69**:817–29), quicker-acting and more effective than quetiapine in acute schizophrenia (n = 397 [c = 281], RCT, d/b, p/c, 6/52, Canuso *et al*, *Am J Psychiatry* 2009;**166**:691–701) and for relapse prevention (s = 3, n = 1083, 52/52, open extension, Emsley *et al*, *Int Clin Psychopharmacol* 2008;**23**:343–56). Cochrane concludes paliperidone is effective (s = 5, n = 3067, RCT, p/c, Nussbaum and Stroup, *Cochrane Database Syst Rev* 2008;**2**:CD006369).

Reviews: general (Wang *et al*, *Clin Drug Investig* 2012;**32**:497–512), plasma levels (Nazirizadeh *et al*, *Eur J Clin Pharmacol* 2010;**66**:797–803; de Leon *et al*, *Psychosomatics* 2010;**51**:80–8).

Quetiapine *

Quetiapine is an established antipsychotic with characteristic transiently high D2 occupancy which drops rapidly over 12–14 hours and may explain the low EPS and low prolactin elevation (s = 20, review by Sparshatt *et al*, *J Clin Psychiatry* 2011;**72**:1108–23). The target dose of 600 mg/d (range 150–750 mg/d) is probably the most effective. Doses need to be titrated up gradually over several days, to reduce the incidence of postural hypotension. Quetiapine's onset of action is significant by the end of week one (SANS and BPRS), sooner than usually expected (s = 3, n = 620, RCT, d/b, Small *et al*, *Curr Med Res Opin* 2004;**20**:1017–23).

High-dose quetiapine: In TRS, quetiapine continued at 800mg/d was not inferior to a trial of higher doses (mean 1144mg/d) (n=131, RCT, d/b. p/c, 8/52, Honer *et al*, *J Clin Psychiatry* 2011;**73**:13–20) and in people not responding to 600mg for 4/52, there was no advantage of increasing the dose to 1200mg/d for 8/52 and added tolerability issues (n=60, RCT, d/b, 8/52, Lindenmayer *et al*, *J Clin Psychopharmacol* 2011;**31**:160–8). There has been response to high dose (1200mg/d and 1400mg/d) post-clozapine (Chandrappa and Ho, *Ther Adv Psychopharmacol* 2012;**2**:207–9). Cochrane concludes that quetiapine is more effective than placebo but no difference could be detected against FGAs (s=12, n=3443, RCT, Srisurapanont *et al*, *Cochrane Database Syst Rev* 2004;**2**:CD000967), albeit with less weight gain, ECG abnormalities, EPSE, prolactin (s=43, n=7217[c=4547], RCTs, Suttajit *et al*, *Cochrane Database Syst Rev* 2013;**5**:CD007815). The drop-out rate from quetiapine is relatively high, with most stopping it within a few weeks (s=25, RCT, Asmal *et al*, *Cochrane Database Syst Rev* 2013;**11**:CD006625; FFT).

Reviews: TDM (n=487, Handley *et al*, *Ther Adv Psychopharmacol* 2013;**3**:129–37; Wittman *et al*, *Neuro Endocrinol Lett* 2010;**31**:203–7).

Risperidone (see also LAIs/depots) *

Risperidone is licensed for acute and chronic psychosis and is a D2 and 5HT2 blocker.

Efficacy: Risperidone has shown efficacy across a wide range of symptoms of psychosis and schizophrenia. Relapse prevention has been shown over one year (eg. n=404,[c=374], RCT, one year, Wang *et al*, *Am J Psychiatry* 2010;**167**:676–85).

Dose: Risperidone's optimum dose in schizophrenia is 4–6mg/d, lower doses being consistently less effective and >6mg/d having more side-effects, and with less efficacy at >10mg/d (Ezewuzie and Taylor, *J Psychopharmacol* 2006;**20**:86–90), but with 1–4mg/d of value in first episodes (Li *et al*, *Cochrane Database Syst Rev* 2009;**4**:CD007474). Titration to 6mg/d over three days is standard practice, but a slower titration has been recommended (over weeks rather than days, stabilising on 2–4mg/d initially before proceeding to higher doses), particularly in the drug-naïve and elderly, as this markedly reduces the final doses needed, reduces EPS and improves compliance. Even very low dose (1–2mg/d) can lead to dramatic improvements in the prodromal phase or first episode schizophrenia (see *1.21.2*).

Cochrane concludes risperidone is effective but that the data is incomplete and it has more EPSE and prolactin increases cf other SGAs (s=45, n=7760, RCT, d/b, Komossa *et al*, *Cochrane Database Syst Rev* 2011;**1**:CD006626; FFT).

Reviews: TDM (Nazirizadeh *et al*, *Eur J Clin Pharmacol* 2010;**66**:797–803), plasma levels (n=51, Yasui-Furukori *et al*, *J Psychopharmacol* 2010;**24**:987–94), pharmacokinetics (n=50 and review, Uchida *et al*, *Ther Drug Monit* 2012; **34**:182–7).

Ziprasidone (not licensed in the UK)

Ziprasidone is licensed in many countries for schizophrenia and schizoaffective disorder and 5–20mg/d is effective for acute psychosis and effective for relapse prevention (e.g. n=168, d/b, 196/52, Potkin *et al*, *Int J Neuropsychopharmacol* 2009;**12**:1233–48). It may have some efficacy in TRS (n=147, RCT, d/b, p/c, 18/52, Sacchetti *et al*, *Schizophr Res* 2009;**110**:80–9). Cochrane concludes that ziprasidone is slightly less effective than amisulpride, olanzapine and risperidone but with a low weight gain (s=9, n=3361, Komossa *et al*, *Cochrane Database Syst Rev* 2009;**4**:CD006627; FFT).

Reviews: general (Fagiolini *et al*, *Expert Opin Pharmacother* 2010;**11**:2199–220), kinetics (s=31, Stip *et al*, *Clin Ther* 2011;**33**:1853–67).

LONG-ACTING AND DEPOT INJECTIONS *

The major advantages for depots/LAIs is assured compliance and steady plasma levels, with associated and proven reduction in relapses, rehospitalisation and severity of relapse. There may also be some reduction in bioavailability problems (a few people metabolise antipsychotics extensively via the first-pass effect). LAIs/depots can lead to reduced relapses, stable therapeutic effects and better downward titration of doses to reduce the incidence of side-effects, especially as low treatment retention rates are well recorded (Nasrallah, *Acta Psychiatr Scand* 2007;**115**:260–7).

The major disadvantages include the impossibility of altering a dose quickly if side-effects develop (e.g. dystonia, NMS), patients having no control over or involvement in their treatment or, worse still, being seen as a punishment. Depot injections are also painful, with the pain declining over 10 days, and may lead to a negative patient attitude towards medication (n=34, Bloch *et al*, *J Clin Psychiatry* 2001;**62**:855–9), although there is some evidence to the contrary (Walburn *et al*, *Br J Psychiatry* 2001;**179**:300–7; FFT). Meticulous (Z-tracking) injection technique is essential (Cocoman and Murray, *J Psychiatr Ment Health Nurs* 2008;**15**:424–34).

Meta-analysis suggests that, over two years, depots are equivalent to oral antipsychotics for relapse prevention (s=21, n=5176, RCT, 24/12, Kishimoto *et al*, *Schizophr Bull* 2014;**40**:192–213), but only provided oral antipsychotics are actually taken. Study design is important (s=13, Kirson *et al*, *J Clin Psychiatry* 2013;**74**:568–75).

Reviews: * general (Manchanda *et al*, *Can J Psychiatry* 2013;**58**(5 Suppl 1):5S–13S; s=3, n=1182, Peuskens *et al*, *BMC Psychiatry* 2012;**12**:130; FFT), SGA LAIs (Rauch and Fleischhacker, *CNS Drugs* 2013;**27**:637–52), formulations (Park *et al*, *Arch Pharm Res* 2013;**36**:651–9), LAI pharmacokinetics (Spanarello and La Ferla, *Curr Clin Pharmacol* 2014;**9**:310–7).

Licensed UK depot/LAI sites *

Depot/LAI	Licensed IM routes
Aripiprazole	Gluteal, deltoid
Flupentixol decanoate	Gluteal, lateral thigh
Fluphenazine decanoate	Gluteal
(Fluspirilene)	Gluteal, lateral thigh
Haloperidol decanoate	Gluteal
Olanzapine pamoate	Gluteal
Paliperidone palmitate	Gluteal, deltoid
(Pipothiazine palmitate)	Gluteal
Risperidone	Gluteal, deltoid
Zuclopentixol decanoate	Gluteal, lateral thigh

Pharmacokinetics

The tables on *pages 156–159* show plasma levels for each depot as single doses (although these have been difficult to obtain and are not reliable), and as computer-generated profiles for multiple doses (based on single-dose profiles). Half-life is often longer on chronic administration.

Aripiprazole (Abilify Maintena®, Lundbeck)*

- Duration of action=6–8 weeks
- Tmax/peak=7–24 days (5–7 days with continuous treatment)
- Elimination half-life=30 days (300mg) and 47 days (400mg)
- Time to steady state=8–10 weeks

Aripiprazole LAI is a once-monthly suspension injection. The starting dose is 400mg monthly, with 10–20mg/d oral aripiprazole continued for 14/7. If the person has not had aripiprazole before they must have tolerability and potential efficacy assessed first, and the trials used 10–30mg/d for 4–12/52, with the person stable for 4/52. After reaching steady state with the LAI (2/12 inc. 2/52 oral supplement) the plasma levels are the following approximate equivalents:

- 200mg/month=c7.5mg/d (sub-therapeutic)
- 300mg/month=c20mg/d orally
- 400mg/month=c25mg/d orally

(n=41[c=22], open, 24/52, Mallikaarjun *et al*, *Schizophr Res* 2013;**150**:281–8; FFT)

The dose can be reduced to 300mg/month if ADRs occur or if taking concomitant strong 3A4 or 2D6 inhibitors for more than 14 days.

Efficacy: In people stable on oral aripiprazole, switching to ALAI produced a significantly longer time to impending relapse cf. placebo (10% vs 40% respectively) with fewer drop-outs from ADRs cf. placebo (e.g. n=403, RCT, d/b, p/c, one year, Kane et al, *J Clin Psychiatry* 2012;**73**:617–24), with relapse rates at 26/52 being 7% (ALAI 400mg/m), 8% (10-30mg/d oral) and sub-therapeutic ALAI 22% (50mg/m) (n=662, RCT, d/b, a/c, Fleischhacker *et al*, *Br J Psychiatry* 2014;**205**:13-44; FFT). Relapse prevention has been shown (n=710, RCT, d/b, two years, Fleischhacker *et al*, *Int Clin Psychopharmacol* 2013;**28**:171–8; n=183, mirror-image, Kane *et al*, *J Med Econ* 2013;**16**:917–25). Clinical profile same in obese and non-obese patients (n=662, RCT, d/b, a/c, De Hert *et al*, *Neuropsychiatr Dis Treat* 2015;**11**:1299–306; FFT). QoL, effectiveness and acceptability for ALAI seems greater overall than PPLAI (n=295[c=183], RCT, s/b,

28/52, Naber *et al, Schizophr Res* 2015;**168**:498-502; FFT). The most common ADR is pain at the site of injection (n=710, Kane et al, *J Clin Psychiatry* 2012;**73**:617–24).

Reviews: * general (Potkin *et al, Curr Med Res Opin* 2013;**29**:1241–51; Motiwala *et al, Patient Prefer Adherence* 2013;**7**:1181–7).

Flupentixol decanoate *
(e.g. Depixol®, Lundbeck)

- Duration of action = 3–4 weeks
- Peak = 7–10 days
- Rate limiting half-life = 8 days (single dose), 17 days (multiple doses)
- Time to steady state = 10–12 weeks.

Flupentixol decanoate is a thioxanthene licensed in people stabilised on oral therapy first (SmPC). Cochrane recommends using standard doses as higher doses (100–200 mg) have no advantage in relapse prevention (s=15, n=626, Mahapatra *et al, Cochrane Database Syst Rev* 2014;**6**:CD001470).

Fluphenazine decanoate
(e.g. Modecate®, Sanofi) *

- Duration of action = 1–3 weeks
- Peak = 6–48 hours
- Rate-limiting half-life = 6–10 days (single doses), 14–100 days (multiple doses)
- Time to steady state = 6–12 weeks.

Fluphenazine decanoate is a phenothiazine and a four-week interval between injections is possible. Efficacy data is limited, showing little difference between depots and orals (s=73, n=4870, RCT, Maayan *et al, Cochrane Database Syst Rev* 2015;**2**:CD000307). 25 mg every 2–6 weeks produces similar side-effects, efficacy and relapse rates, but with reduced drug exposure using the longer dosage interval.

Fluspirilene (Redeptin®, Imap®)

- Duration of action = 1.5 weeks
- Peak = within two days
- Rate limiting half-life = 7–9 days
- Time to steady state = 5–6 weeks.

Fluspirilene is a water-based weekly micro-crystalline injection, is only available in the UK as an import. Cochrane concludes it has no advantage over orals or other depots, albeit (s=12, n=525, RCT, Abhijnhan *et al, Cochrane Database Syst Rev* 2007;**1**:CD001718).

Haloperidol decanoate
(Haldol Decanoate®, Janssen)

- Duration of action = six weeks
- Peak = 3–9 days
- Rate limiting half-life = 18–21 days (single + chronic)
- Time to steady state = 10–12 weeks at monthly dosing.

Haloperidol decanoate is a butyrophenone and a four-week interval between injections is possible. An analysis suggests a maximal effect at 50 mg/4 weeks, with no evidence that doses above 100 mg/4 weeks have any additional effects (s=13, Taylor, *Psychiatr Bull* 2005;**29**:104–7), e.g. rates of deterioration with 50–100 mg/month were not significantly different to 25 mg/month, and ADRs were higher (n=105, RCT, d/b, Kane *et al, Am J Psychiatry* 2002;**4**:554–60; review by Marois and Roy, *EBMH* 2002;**5**:113; FFT). It is best reserved for chronic relapsing schizophrenics only responsive to haloperidol.

Olanzapine pamoate *
(Zypadhera®, Zyprexa Relprevv®, Lilly)

- Duration of action = about 6 weeks
- Tmax/peak = 2–4 days
- Half-life = 30 days
- Time to steady state = 12 weeks.

Olanzapine pamoate is licensed for patients who have previously received oral doses. It releases olanzapine slowly over at least 6–8 weeks post-injection, so care is needed after discontinuation. Oral supplementation is not recommended, e.g. in acute TRS, olanzapine pamoate every two or four weeks was more effective than placebo, despite no use of oral doses (RCT, d/b, p/c, 8/52, Lauriello *et al, J Clin Psychiatry* 2008;**69**:790–9).

Efficacy: Olanzapine LAI appears as effective and well tolerated as oral olanzapine, apart from injection-related adverse events (n=1065, RCT, d/b, 24/52, Kane *et al, Am J Psychiatry* 2010;**167**:181–9). After two years out-patients on olanzapine LAI maintained and improved over baseline functioning, albeit not differently from oral olanzapine (n=524, RCT, open, two years, Ascher-Svanum *et al, Neuropsychiatr Dis Treat* 2014;**10**:1125–31; apparent duplicate publication: Detke *et al, J Clin Psychopharmacol* 2014;**34**:426–34). There is no evidence of accumulation, even after six years (Heres *et al*, *Int Clin Psychopharmacol* 2014;**29**:299–312).

Doses: These should be as per this chart for the first two months, then reduced.

Dose conversion:

Oral dose	Starting dose (initial 2/12)	Maintenance dose (after 2/12)
10 mg/d	210 mg 2/52 or 405 mg 4/52	150 mg 2/52 or 300 mg 4/52
15 mg/d	300 mg 2/52	210 mg 2/52 or 405 mg 4/52
20 mg/d	300 mg 2/52	300 mg 2/52

The two-month loading dose is due to a significant (but not enormous) difference between steady state and initiation levels. A US registry shows that most prescribers continue with the same initial dose instead of switching to a lower maintenance dose, showing lack of reassessment of doses, ignorance or laziness (n=1694, Case *et al*, *Curr Med Res Opin* 2013;**29**:1533–7).

Post-injection delirium/sedation syndrome (PDSS): * Unpredictable (in 1.4% patients; 0.07% injections, n=2054, injections=45000; Detke *et al*, *BMC Psychiatry* 2010;**10**:43) and idiosyncratic excessive sedation, resembling olanzapine overdose (Citrome, *Int J Clin Pract* 2009;**63**:140–50), can occur 1–6 hours post-injection, with full recovery within 24–72 hours. The manufacturer's data (n=338, Bushe *et al*, *BMC Psychiatry* 2015;**15**:65; FFT) shows:

- Only 20% get impaired consciousness
- 50% PDSS events occur within 15 minutes
- 66% PDSS events occur within 30 minutes
- 86% PDSS events occur within 1 hour
- 50% of all PDSS occur in the first three injections of a course
- PDSS occurs when an IM injection goes through a vein (the bond splits when exposed to large amounts of water, e.g. blood). It is not an injection technique issue but probably a genetic variation in venous distribution
- All cases resolve within 72 hours (s=3, n=931 [c=393], <6 years [mean 3], McDonnell *et al*, *Int Clin Psychopharmacol* 2014;**29**:322–31; FFT)
- The most common symptoms are sedation (61%), confusion (56%), dysarthria (54%), somnolence (46%), dizziness (45%).

A review of PDSS shows it is only associated with olanzapine, although one case was reported on placebo in a paliperidone trial (s=33, Novakovic *et al*, *Clin Neuropharmacol* 2013;**36**:59–62). The patient must be observed in a healthcare facility by appropriately qualified personnel for at least three hours post-injection for signs and symptoms of apparent overdose.

Reviews: * general (Schöttle *et al*, *Expert Opin Drug Saf* 2013;**12**:897–903), pooled analysis of injection site ADRs with olanzapine (Atkins *et al*, *BMC Psychiatry* 2014;**14**:7).

Paliperidone palmitate *
(Xeplion®, Invega Sustenna®, Janssen)

- Duration of action=up to about 4/12
- Tmax/peak=median 13 days
- Rate limiting half-life=25–49 days
- Time to steady state=2/52 with titration as SmPC
- Cmax is 28% higher with deltoid over gluteal injection.

Paliperidone palmitate LAI (PPLAI) is licensed for maintenance treatment of schizophrenia in people previously responsive to paliperidone (the major metabolite of risperidone) or risperidone without prior stabilisation on the oral preparation. It uses a nanocrystal technology formulation, allowing both an early and a sustained release.

PPLAI has a specific dose schedule:

- Initial dose is 150 mg in the deltoid muscle. No oral supplementation is needed
- 100 mg should be given on day 8, again in the deltoid muscle (if switching directly from risperidone LAI these two starting doses do not have to be in the deltoid)
- Then as per dose equivalent or schedule, which can be in the gluteal or deltoid sites
- Under exceptional circumstances the day 8 dose can be ±2 days, and monthly doses ±7 days without a clinically significant effect on plasma concentrations. The second dose window was increased to ±4/7 in US in 2013 (Samanti *et al*, *Neuropsychiatr Dis Treat* 2013;**6**:721–30; FFT).

Efficacy: This has been show in a large

number of studies in acute schizophrenia (e.g. n=514, RCT, d/b, p/c, 13/52, Nasrallah *et al*, *Neuropsychopharmacology* 2010;**35**:2072–82; FFT; n=652, RCT, d/b, p/c, 13/52, Pandina et al, *J Clin Psychopharmacol* 2010;**30**:235–44), where 150mg separates from placebo after four days in acute schizophrenia (n=312, RCT, d/b, p/c, 13/52, Alphs *et al*, *Ann Gen Psychiatry* 2011;**11**:12; MS; FFT). It has equivalent efficacy to haloperidol decanoate with more weight gain and raised prolactin but less akathisia (n=311, RCT, d/b, a/c, <24/12, McEvoy *et al*, *JAMA* 2014;**311**:1978–87). A naturalistic study showed 65% retention at one year, higher with people started as out-patients, switching from risperidone and if using the correct dose initiation (n=210[c=200], one year, Attard *et al*, *Acta Psychiatr Scand* 2014;**130**:46–51).

PPLAI vs risperidone LAI: PPLAI was not quite as effective as risperidone LAI over one year (n=749, RCT, d/b, one year, Fleischhacker et al, *Int J Neuropsychopharmacol* 2012;**15**:107–18), close in another (n=452, RCT, open, Li *et al*, *Prog Neuropsychopharmacol Biol Psychiatry* 2011;**35**:1002–8), and probably non-inferior in a third (n=1220, RCT, d/b, 13/52, Pandina *et al*, *Prog Neuropsychopharmacol Biol Psychiatry* 2011;**35**:218–26).

PPLAI vs oral risperidone: In the first month PPLAI was as effective as oral risperidone (n=913, RCT, d/b, 13/52, Gopal *et al*, *Innov Clin Neurosci* 2011;**8**:26–33; MS; FFT) and sub optimal responders to risperidone orally may significantly improve on PPLAI (n=216, d/b, p/c, 13/52, Sliwa *et al*, *Schizophr Res* 2011;**132**:28–34; MS).

Relapse prevention is clear, with an NNT=2 for prevention of relapse (eg. s=8, Gopal *et al*, *Neuropsychiatr Dis Treat* 2011;**7**:93–101; MS; FFT; n=212[c=113], one year, Coppola *et al*, *BMC Psychiatry* 2012;**12**:26, FFT).

Cochrane concludes that PPLAI is safe and effective cf. placebo, but is associated with substantial increases in prolactin (s=5, n=2215, RCT, Nussbaum and Stroup, *Cochrane Database Syst Rev* 2012;**6**:CD008296).

Reviews: * general (Chue and Chue, *Expert Rev Neurother* 2012;**12**:1383–97; Kim *et al*, *Patient Prefer Adherence* 2012;**6**:533–45), guidelines for practical use (Newton *et al*, *Curr Med Res Opin* 2012;**28**:559–67), dosing and switching (Samtani *et al*, *CNS Drugs* 2011;**25**:829–45), use in schizophrenia (Carter, *Drugs* 2012;**72**:1137–60), comparison of pharmacology with risperidone (Corena-McLeod, *Drugs R D* 2015;**15**:163–74; FFT).

1

Pipothiazine palmitate (discontinued) *

- Duration of action = 4–6 weeks
- Peak = 9–10 days
- Rate limiting half-life = 14–21 days
- Time to steady state = 8–12 weeks.

Pipothiazine is an obsolete piperidine phenothiazine (Dinesh *et al*, *Cochrane Database Syst Rev* 2004;**4**:CD001720).

Risperidone (RLAI) *

(Risperdal Consta®, Janssen)

- Duration of action = 4–6 weeks
- Peak = 5–6 weeks
- Rate limiting half-life = 14–21 days
- Time to steady state = 6–8 weeks.

RLAI is licensed for schizophrenia and other psychoses and uses risperidone molecules in a synthetic and absorbable polymer microsphere base suspended in water.

Dose and release: * The initial dose is 25–37.5mg fortnightly, with a maximum of 50mg every two weeks, with no statistical advantage for 100mg/fortnight over 50mg/fortnight (n=160, RCT, d/b, a/c, 6/12, Meltzer *et al*, *Schizophr Res* 2014;**154**:14–22). Plasma levels are stable after 3–4 injections and maintained for 4–5 weeks after the last injection. Elimination is complete 7–8 weeks after the last injection. The deltoid and gluteal injection routes have the same release, Cmax and AUC (s=2, Thyssen *et al*, *J Clin Pharmacol* 2010;**50**:1011–21).

Switching from oral: * See *C2.2.1.2*.

A careful switching study (n=50[c=45], RCT, s/b, 48/52, Bai *et al*, *J Clin Psychiatry* 2007;**68**:1218–25) concluded:

- oral dose <3mg/d = RLAI 25mg 2/52
- oral 3–5mg/d = RLAI 37.5mg 2/52
- oral >5mg/d = RLAI 50mg 2/52.

Where possible, people should be pre-treated with risperidone orally before RLAI is started to rule out any severe EPS, hypotensive or other idiosyncratic reactions. Oral cover may be needed for the first 3–4 weeks, then tapered during weeks

Depot and longer-acting injection pharmacokinetics

These graphs show the known plasma levels of the available longer-acting antipsychotic injections in the UK. The single dose kinetics are reasonably well-established for many of these preparations. The multiple-dose graphs are computer-generated as little or no data exists on long-term kinetics, with downward arrows indicating when injections are given. These graphs will, however, give *some* indication of the time to steady state, and the length of time before plasma levels fall to zero after a depot has been stopped, although half-lives tend to lengthen with chronic use. The 'y' axis units are not established for any of the multiple dose graphs, and there will of course be inter-individual variation.

Flupentixol decanoate single dose

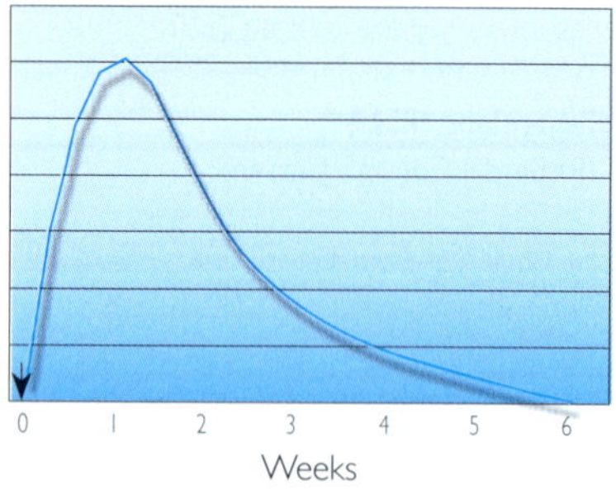

Flupentixol decanoate 1/52

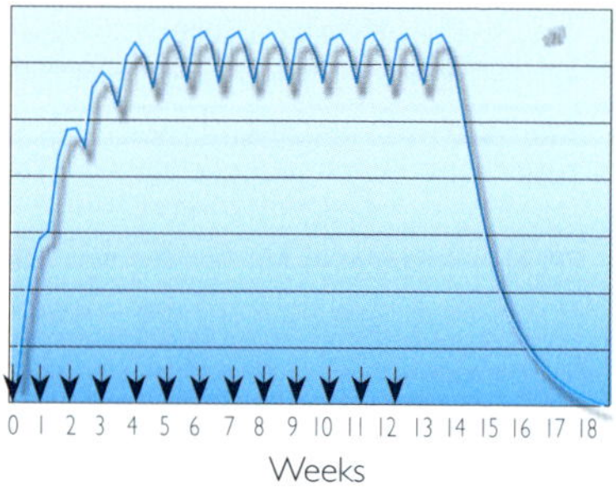

Flupentixol decanoate 2/52

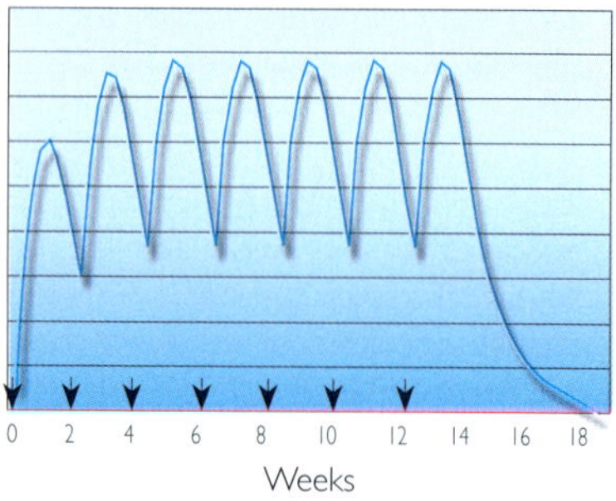

Fluphenazine decanoate single dose

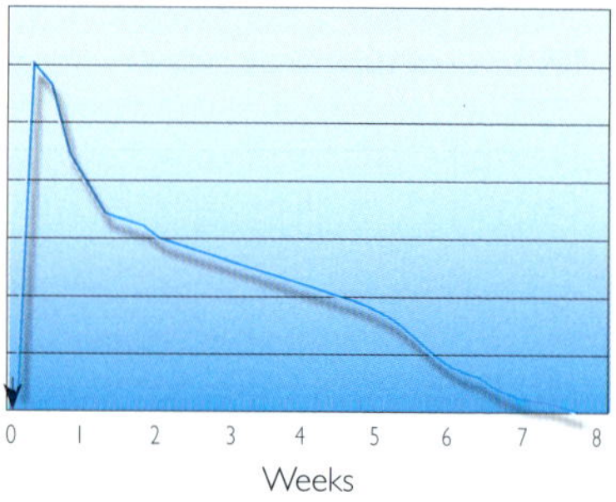

Fluphenazine decanoate 2/52

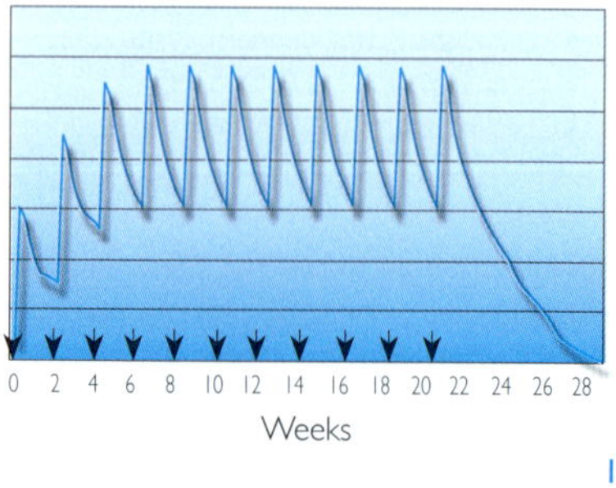

Fluphenazine decanoate 4/52

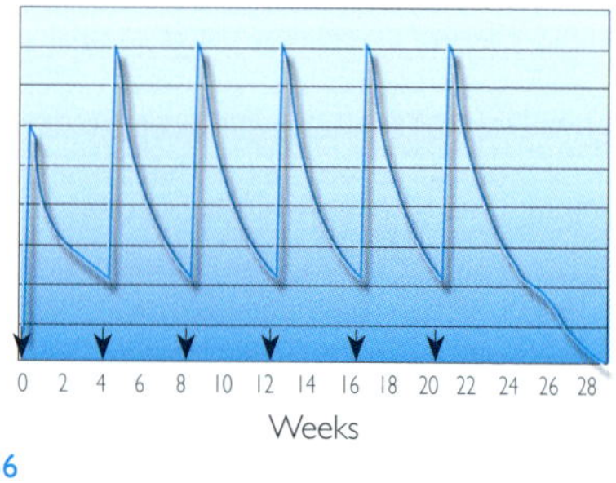

Fluspirilene

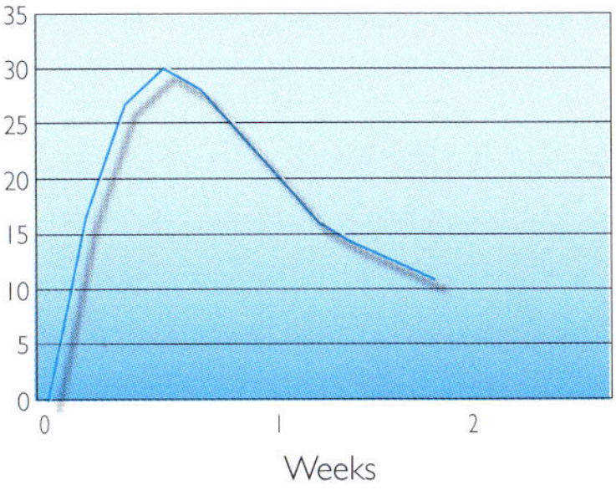

Haloperidol decanoate single dose

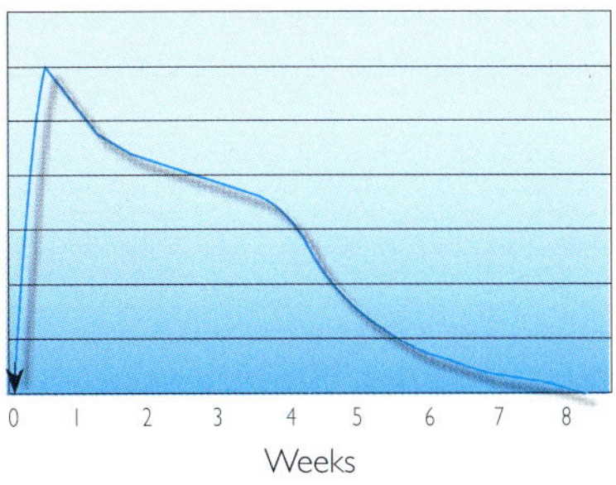

Haloperidol decanoate 2/52

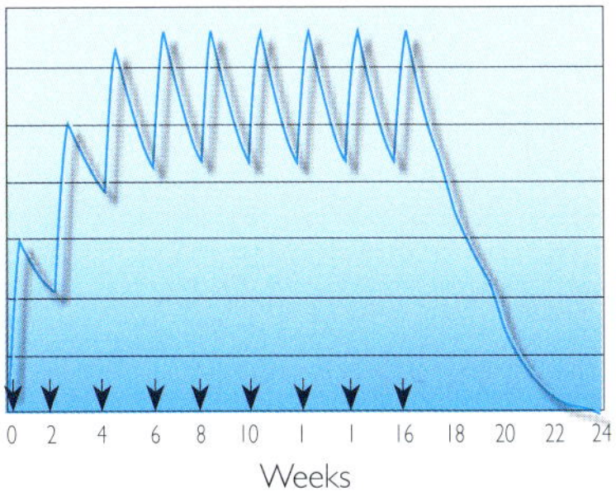

Haloperidol decanoate 4/52

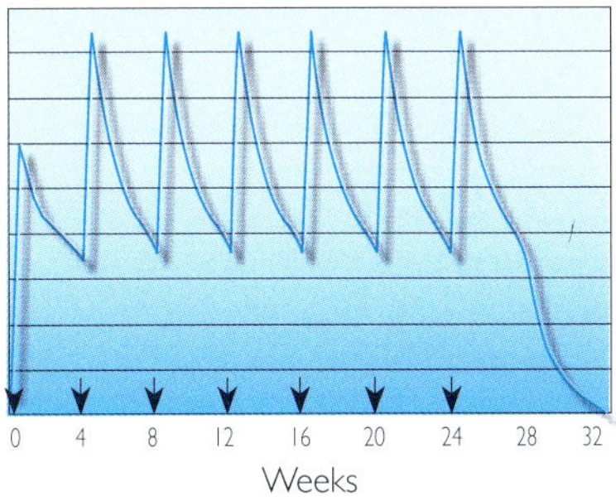

Olanzapine pamoate single dose (based on 405mg)

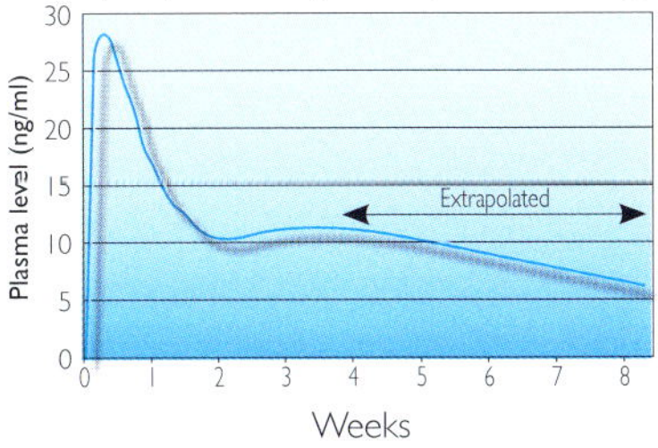

Olanzapine pamoate 200mg every 2/52

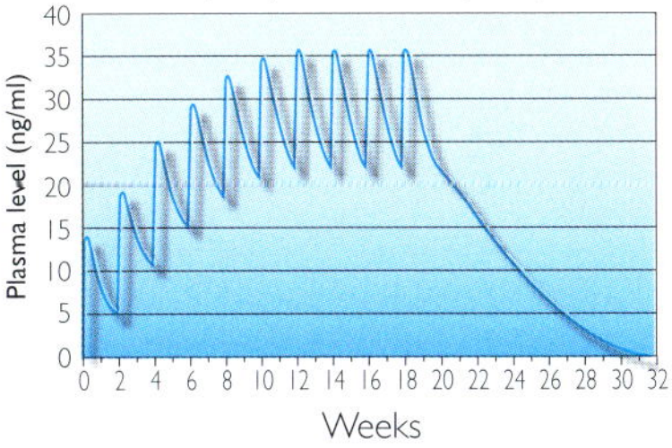

Olanzapine pamoate 405mg every 4/52

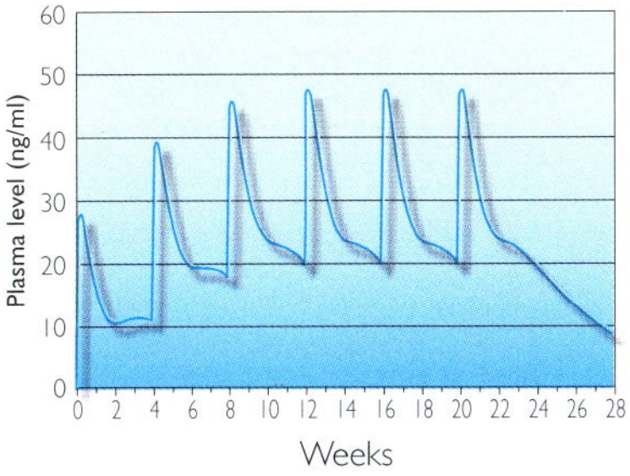

Pipotiazine palmitate single dose

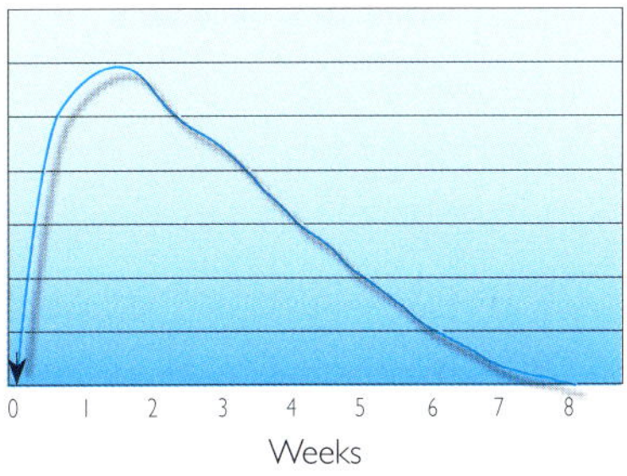

Risperidone Consta single dose

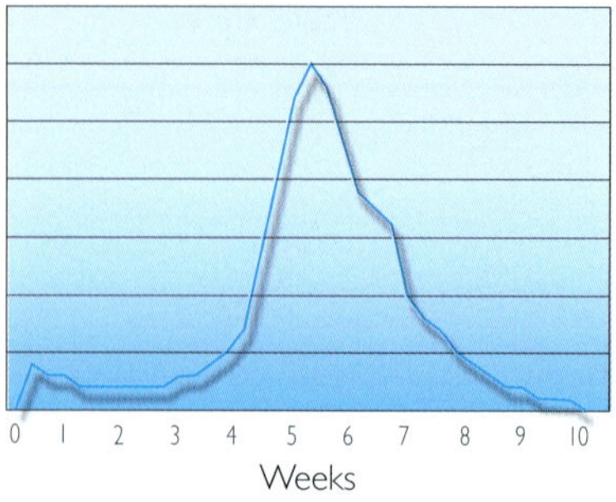

Risperdal Consta 2/52

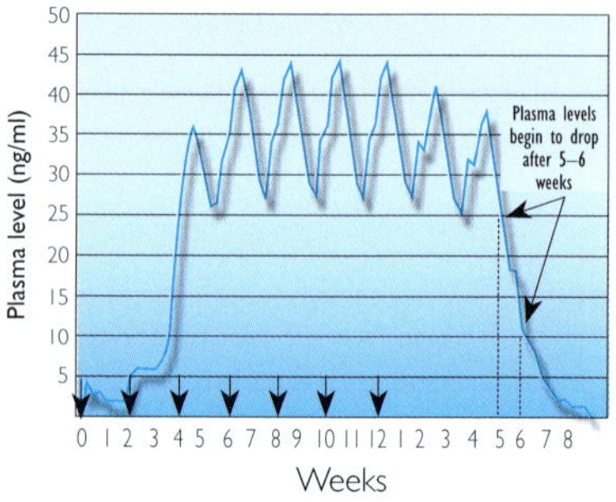

Zuclopenthixol decanoate single dose

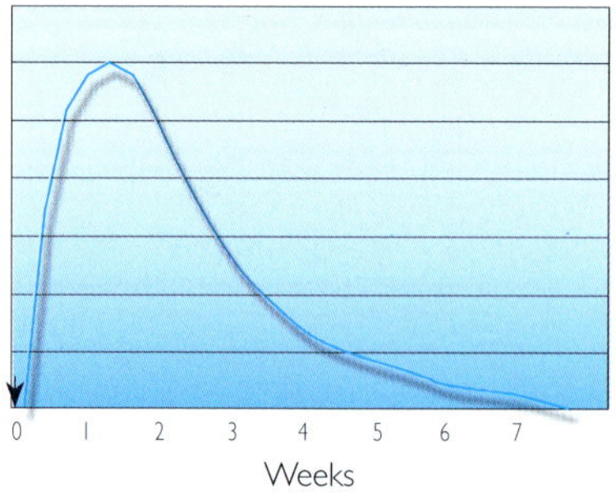

Zuclopenthixol decanoate 1/52

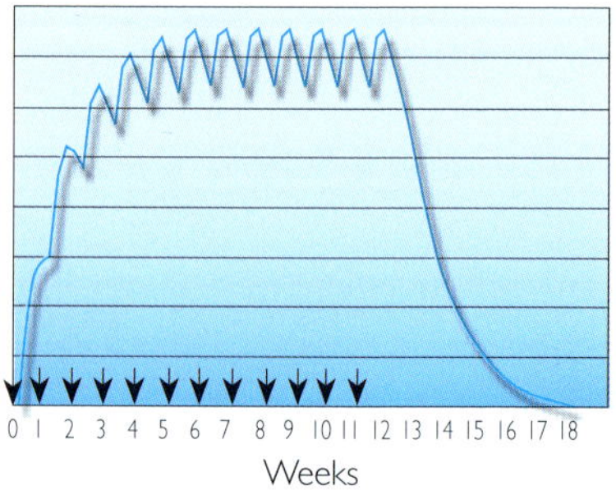

Zuclopenthixol decanoate 2/52

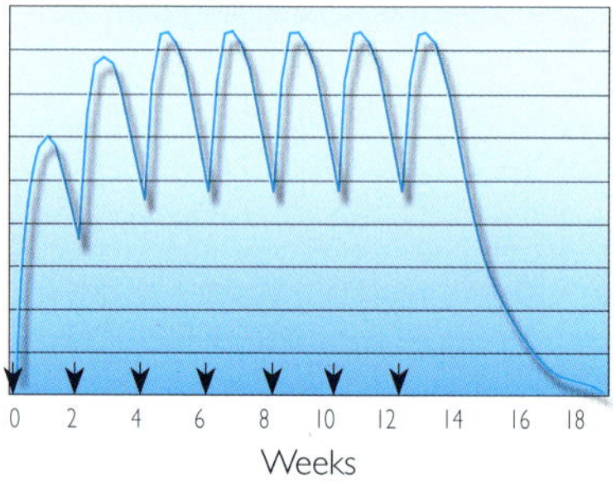

Zuclopenthixol acetate single dose

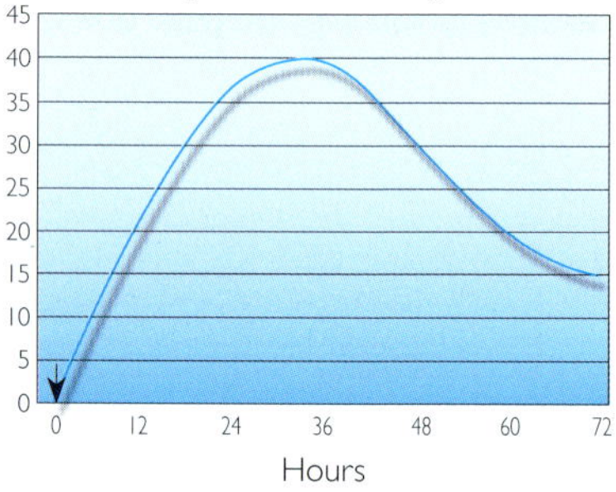

Paliperidone palmitate initiation: 150mg day 1, 100mg day 8

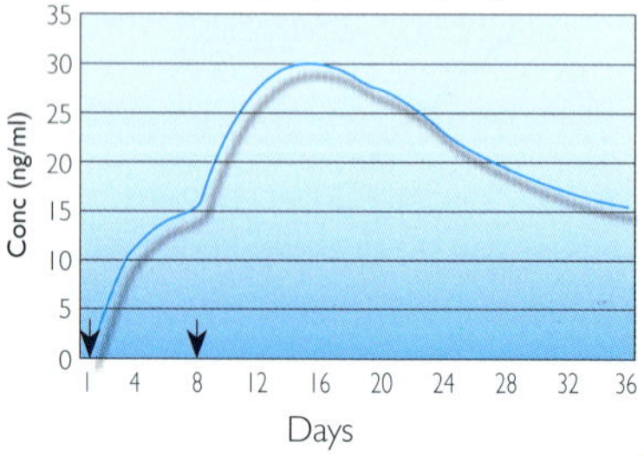

Paliperidone palmitate 50mg monthly then stopping

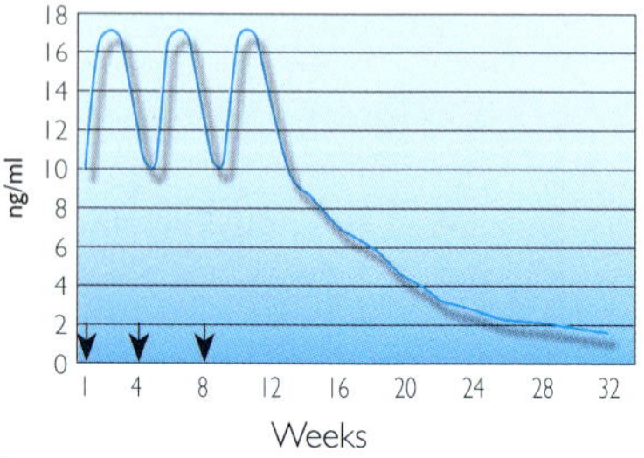

Paliperidone palmitate 100mg monthly then stopping

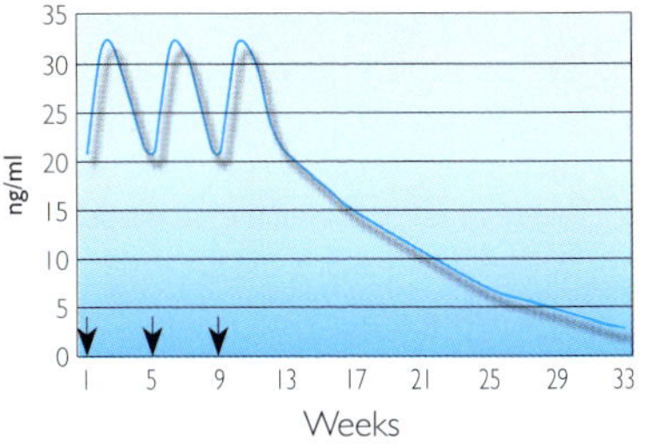

Paliperidone palmitate 150mg monthly then stopping

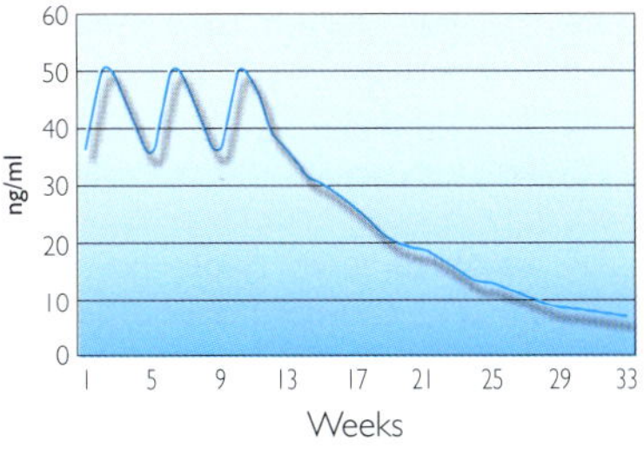

Aripiprazole Maintena single 400 mg dose

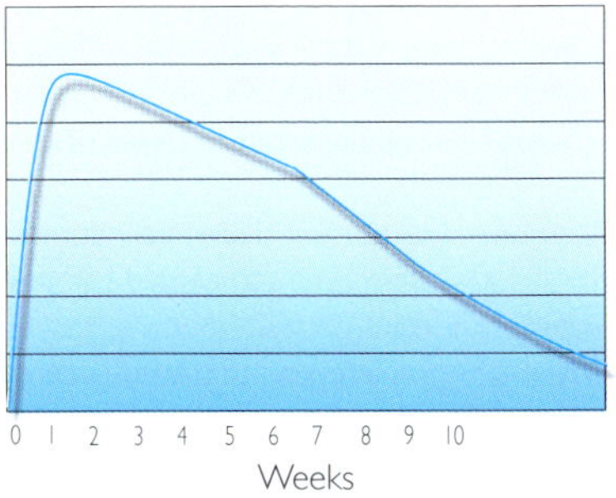

Aripiprazole Maintena

Oral for 2/52 with 400 mg dose, then 4x400 mg doses, then stopped

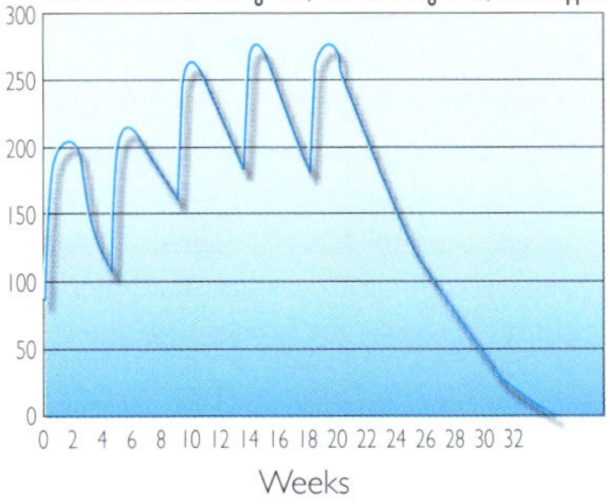

4–5. Steady state occurs about 6–8 weeks after each dose change, and some have recommended dose increases only every eight weeks (Knox and Stimmel, *Clin Ther* 2004;**26**:1994–2002).

Efficacy: This has been shown against oral olanzapine (n = 377, RCT, open, one year, Keks *et al*, *Br J Psychiatry* 2007;**191**:131–9; MS; FFT) and zuclopenthixol depot (n = 115, RCT, open, 6/12, Rubio *et al*, *Can J Psychiatry* 2006;**51**:531–9). Optimum efficacy may take many months, e.g. half of those with a good outcome at 6/12 had not yet improved by 3/12, with a 34% reduction in the readmission rate cf. non-use, and a 50% reduction when used as monotherapy (n = 1859, 12/12, Grimaldi-Bensouda *et al*, *Schizophr Res* 2012;**134**:187–94), with a similar reduction shown in a mirror-image study at one year (n = 67, three years, Niaz and Haddad, *Acta Psychiatr Scand* 2007;**116**:36–46). There may be a significant effect on negative symptoms when used for a prolonged period of time (n = 842 [c = 631], 6/12, Curtis *et al*, *J Psychopharmacol* 2008;**22**:254–61). However, in other news, RLAI was no better at preventing relapse and rehospitalisation in at-risk people with schizophrenia cf. any oral antipsychotic (n = 369, RCT, Rosenheck *et al*, *N Engl J Med* 2011;**364**:842–51; FFT) and was not superior to FGA-LAIs (n = 4532, 2700 patient years, Nielsen *et al*, *Schizophr Bull* 2014;**41**:627–36).

Factors predicting response: RLAI seems to produce more favourable outcomes in previous poor concordance and older people (n = 250, 6/12, Taylor *et al*, *Int J Neuropsychopharmacol* 2006;**9**:685–94), out-patients and those not previously treated with clozapine (n = 211, six years, Taylor and Cornelius, *J Psychopharmacol* 2010;**24**:995–9).

Review: general (Bobo and Shelton, *Expert Rev Neurother* 2010;**10**:1637–58).

Zuclopenthixol acetate *

(Clopixol Acuphase®, Lundbeck)

- Duration of action = 2–3 days
- Peak = 24–40 hours
- Rate limiting half-life = 32 hours ± 7.

Zuclopenthixol acetate's initial dose is

50–150mg and provides a reduction in psychotic symptoms over about 78 hours. The maximum licensed cumulative dose is 400mg over two weeks, with no more than four injections. Cochrane concludes that there is inadequate data on Acuphase® and no convincing evidence either way in APE compared to IM haloperidol (s=9, Jayakody *et al, Cochrane Database Syst Rev* 2012;**4**:CD000525; FFT). See also *1.1*.

Zuclopenthixol decanoate
(Clopixol®, Lundbeck)

- Duration of action=2–4 weeks
- Peak=4–9 days
- Rate limiting half-life=17–21 days (multiple doses)
- Time to steady state=10–12 weeks.

Zuclopenthixol decanoate is a thioxanthene that has also been used in high dose for aggression and, although not indicated, particularly in learning disabilities and forensic patients.

+ Combinations of antipsychotics

Polypharmacy with antipsychotics falls into three main categories:

- Two or more drugs of the same class
- Multiclass (two or more drugs of different classes at full dose)
- Adjunctive and augmentation (low doses of one with a standard dose of another).

Appropriate reasons for the use of antipsychotic combinations include:

- Failure to respond to clozapine
- Poor tolerance to clozapine, with a second antipsychotic as augmentation of a low clozapine dose
- As augmentation in clozapine partial response
- People unwilling to stop an existing antipsychotic or choosing not to try clozapine
- During a switch from one to another
- When discontinuing a depot poses an unacceptable risk, e.g. forensic patients
- As a temporary measure during an acute exacerbation of illness.

Inappropriate reasons for the use of antipsychotic combinations include:

- Confusing a sedative effect with an antipsychotic effect
- Not waiting sufficient time for an antipsychotic to work before making a switch
- Failing to plan and communicate a switch, which is then never fully completed
- Where clinical improvement occurs before completion of a switch, and the clinician 'quits while ahead'
- Using higher dose combinations to make up for inadequate resources and environment.

Despite widespread use of combinations, and few RCTs, use of multiple antipsychotics is associated with a major increase in drug exposure, adverse events and time in hospital, but with no apparent clinical gain compared to monotherapy (n=70 pairs, Centorrino *et al, Am J Psychiatry* 2004;**161**:700–6). Combinations should only be used if standard monotherapy is ineffective, and then only with carefully monitored outcomes (clinical and adverse) and discontinued if no clear advantage is seen.

Reviews:* editorial review of the lack of evidence and trials of combinations (Zink *et al, Curr Opin Psychiatry* 2010;**23**:103–11), meta-analysis of use with glutamate modulators (s=13, Veerman *et al, Pharmacopsychiatry* 2014;**47**:185–94).

Clozapine combinations & augmentation

Two meta-analyses suggest that a second antipsychotic can be modestly beneficial in partial response to clozapine and that tolerability does not seem to be adversely affected (s=14, n=735, RCT, d/b, p/c, Taylor *et al, Acta Psychiatr Scand* 2012;**125**:15–24). There is some evidence for augmentation with amisulpride, aripiprazole and mirtazapine (s=62, n=1556, Porcelli *et al, Eur Neuropsychopharmacol* 2012;**22**:165–82).

Reviews: general (Mossaheb *et al, World J Biol Psychiatry* 2010;**11**:502–5), augmentation in TRS unresponsive to clozapine (Sommer *et al, Schizophr Bull* 2012;**38**:1003–11; FFT).

Amisulpride+clozapine (see also sulpiride)*

Combining a specific D2-blocker with clozapine is a well-known strategy. There are some studies, albeit no RCTs, e.g. amisulpride may significantly improve the response to clozapine (eg. n=56[c=50], s/b, 8/52, Genç *et al, Adv Ther* 2007;**24**:1–13) and may have a significant anti-aggressive action (n=6, Hotham *et al, CNS Spectr* 2014;**19**:403–10).

Aripiprazole + clozapine *

A systematic review and meta-analysis recently concluded that the data is limited but suggests aripiprazole augmentation minimises cardiac and metabolic risks, and improves symptoms, but causes agitation and akathisia (s=4, n=347, p/c, RCTs, 8–24/52, Srisurapanont *et al, J Psychiatr Res* 2015:**62**:38–47).

Cholinesterase inhibitors + clozapine

See *1.21.3* for the effect on cognition.

Clonidine + clozapine

Adjunctive clonidine has been used (n=1, Dardennes *et al, Prog Neuropsychopharmacol Biol Psychiatry* 2010;**30**:724–5).

Duloxetine + clozapine

Duloxetine 60mg/d improved negative and other symptoms in TRS, but had no effect on cognitive functioning (n=40 [c=33], RCT, d/b, p/c, 16/52, Mico' *et al, Int Clin Psychopharmacol* 2011;**26**:303–10).

Ginkgo biloba + clozapine

Adjunctive ginkgo biloba had some beneficial effects on negative symptoms, but not positive or overall symptoms (n=42, p/c, 12/52, Doruk *et al, Int Clin Psychopharmacol* 2008;**23**:223–7).

Lamotrigine + clozapine

A meta-analysis concluded that lamotrigine augmentation of clozapine was superior to placebo, with a clinically meaningful benefit (s=5, n=161, RCT, p/c, 10–24/52, Tiihonen *et al, Schizophr Res* 2009;**109**:10–4).

Levothyroxine + clozapine *

There is a single case of clear response of psychosis with combination (n=1, Seddigh *et al, Case Rep Psychiatry* 2015; **2015**:678040; FFT).

Lithium + clozapine

Lithium augmentation may provide additional clinical benefit in schizoaffective but not schizophrenic patients (n=20, p/c, 4/52, Small *et al, J Clin Psychopharmacol* 2003;**23**:223–8).

Memantine + clozapine

Memantine 20mg/d augmentation has been associated with improvement in positive and negative symptoms in TRS (n=21 [c=21], RCT, d/b, p/c, 12/52, de Lucena *et al, J Clin Psychiatry* 2009;**70**:1416–23).

Minocycline + clozapine *

In TRS, adjunctive minocycline 200mg/d had no effect on overall BPRS scores but significant improvements were seen in working memory, avolition and anxiety/depression (n=52, RCT, d/b, p/c, 10/52, Kelly *et al, J Clin Psychopharmacol* 2015;**35**:374–81).

Mirtazapine + clozapine

Mirtazapine augmentation has improved negative symptoms (especially apathy and anhedonia) and BPRS scores (n= 24, RCT, d/b, p/c, 8/52, Zoccali *et al, Int Clin Psychopharmacol* 2004;**19**:71–6).

Olanzapine + clozapine

There is a case report of use (n=1, Rhoads, *J Clin Psychiatry* 2000;**61**:678–80).

Pimozide + clozapine *

This combination was no more effective than clozapine monotherapy (eg. n=32[c=28], RCT, d/b, p/c, 12/52, Gunduz-Bruce *et al, Schizophr Res* 2013;**143**:344–7).

Quetiapine + clozapine

Quetiapine has some effect as augmentation, albeit less than amisulpride (n=56 [c=50], s/b, 8/52, Genç *et al, Adv Ther* 2007;**24**:1–13).

Raloxifene + clozapine *

Raloxifene 60–120mg/d has successfully augmented clozapine in TRS (n=1, Shivakumar and Venkatasubramanian, *Indian J Psychiatry* 2012;**54**:394).

Reboxetine + clozapine *

An uncontrolled study concluded reboxetine had no discernible positive effects and a trend for worsening of cognitive functioning (n=15, open, 12/52, Bruno *et al, J Clin Psychopharmacol* 2014;**34**:620–3).

Risperidone + clozapine

Risperidone has improved sub-optimal clozapine response, reduced relapses and improved social functioning, as oral (n=40, RCT, d/b, p/c, 12/52, Josiassen *et al*, *Am J Psychiatry* 2005;**162**:130–6) and as RLAI (n=4, one year, Kim *et al*, *J Psychopharmacol* 2010;**24**:981–6), although prolactin levels can rise four-fold (n=40, open, Henderson *et al*, *J Clin Psychiatry* 2001;**62**:605–8). Earlier studies were negative and the optimum response may be with lower risperidone doses for a longer duration (s=15[2=RCT], n=86, Kontaxakis *et al*, *Eur Arch Psychiatry Clin Neurosci* 2006;**256**:350–5).

Ropinirole + clozapine

This may help TRS negative symptoms (Michaelopoulou *et al*, *J Clin Psychopharmacol* 2012;**32**:719–20).

Sulpiride + clozapine

Cochrane concludes that the combination is probably more effective than clozapine alone (s=4, n=221, Wang *et al*, *Cochrane Database Syst Rev* 2010;**1**:CD008125).

Topiramate + clozapine

Three RCTs now show adjunctive topiramate to be ineffective in TRS and may even be detrimental (eg. n=80[c=63], RCT, d/b, p/c, 17/52, Behdani *et al*, *Arch Iran Med* 2011;**14**:270–5; FFT). Topiramate should not be used as anticonvulsant cover for clozapine (e.g. n=1, Hofer *et al*, *J Clin Psychiatry* 2003;**64**:1267–8).

Ziprasidone + clozapine *

In TRS, ziprasidone augmentation was effective (n=40, RCT, d/b, p/c, 16/52, Muscatello *et al*, *J Clin Psychopharmacol* 2014;**34**:129–33) including compared with risperidone (n=24, open, RCT, 6/52, Zink *et al*, *J Psychopharmacol* 2009;**23**:305–14).

Other antipsychotic combinations

Amisulpride + aripiprazole

Worsening psychosis has occurred when aripiprazole was added to amisulpride (n=1, Adan-Manes and Garcia-Parajua, *J Clin Pharm Ther* 2009;**34**:245–6).

Amisulpride + risperidone or ziprasidone

Adjunctive amisulpride (mean 693 mg/d) led to 80% improving (n=15, open, Lerner *et al*, *Clin Neuropharmacol* 2005;**28**:66–71).

Aripiprazole + quetiapine or risperidone

Adjunctive aripiprazole 2–15 mg/d added to partially effective risperidone or quetiapine had no effect on TRS symptoms, but helped reduce prolactin levels (n=323[c=225], RCT, d/b, p/c, 16/52, Kane *et al*, *J Clin Psychiatry* 2009;**70**:1348–57).

Olanzapine + amisulpride

Amisulpride augmentation may have some benefit, although this study was not particularly robust (n=49, open, 3/12, Molina *et al*, *Pharmacopsychiatry* 2011;**44**:142–7).

Olanzapine + quetiapine

There is a case report of use (n=1, Dunkley and Reveley, *J Psychopharmacol* 2005;**19**:97–101).

Olanzapine + risperidone

The combination was successful in TRS resistant to sequential olanzapine, quetiapine and risperidone monotherapy (e.g. n=17[c=17], open, 8/52, Suzuki *et al*, *Hum Psychopharmacol* 2008;**23**:455–63).

Olanzapine + sulpiride

Sulpiride 600 mg/d augmentation of partially effective olanzapine had no effect on PANSS, but significantly improved depressive symptoms (n=17, RCT, 8/52, Kotler *et al*, *Int Clin Psychopharmacol* 2004;**19**:23–6).

Quetiapine + amisulpride

In quetiapine partial response, addition of amisulpride had some beneficial effects but significantly increased weight and prolactin (n=6, open, 8/52, Englisch *et al*, *Clin Neuropharmacol* 2010;**33**:227–9).

• Unlicensed/some efficacy

Allopurinol + TAU *

Adjunct: Allopurinol is an adenosine agonist that may reduce dopamine receptors' affinity for dopamine, which may then have antipsychotic and anxiolytic effects. The main RCT showed no effect on PANSS (n=248, p/c, 8/52, Weiser *et al, Schizophr Res* 2012;**138**:35–8), but three single centre studies suggested some effect (n=59[c=51], RCT, d/b, p/c, 8/52, Dickerson *et al, Schizophr Res* 2009;**109**:66–9), with haloperidol (n=46, RCT, d/b, p/c, 8/52, Akhondzadeh *et al, Prog Neuropsychopharmacol Biol Psychiatry* 2005;**29**:253–9) and 300–600mg/d in TRS (n=35[c=22], d/b, p/c, c/o, 12/52, Brunstein *et al, J Clin Psychiatry* 2005;**66**:213–9).

Amantadine (see memantine)

Antidepressants (see negative symptoms)

Asenapine * (see also bipolar mania)

Monotherapy: Asenapine is licensed in some non-EU countries for acute schizophrenia (e.g. US) and relapse prevention. It has a high affinity for 5HT1A/1B/2A/2B/2C/5/6/7, D1/2/3/4, alpha 1 and 2, H1 and H2 receptors but not cholinergic receptors. A meta-analysis of asenapine for acute schizophrenia concludes that it is effective and superior to placebo and comparable to risperidone and olanzapine (s=4, Szegedi *et al, J Clin Psychiatry* 2012;**73**:1533–40; FFT), including adolescents (n=306, RCT, d/b, p/c, 8/52+26/52 open, Findling *et al, J Child Adolesc Psychopharmacol* 2015;**25**:384–96; FFT). Lack of improvement within two weeks predicts lack of subsequent response (s=3, n=1008, RCT, 6/52, Leucht and Zhao, *J Psychopharmacol* 2014;**28**:387–94). There is robust long-term relapse prevention efficacy compared to placebo (12% vs 47%; n=386[c=207], RCT, d/b, p/c, 26/52, Kane *et al, J Clin Psychiatry* 2011;**72**:349–55) and for up to two years in total, with no extra TEAEs (n=400, Schoemaker *et al, Pharmacopsychiatry* 2012;**45**:196–203). See main entry under bipolar mania *1.10.2*).

Reviews: overview (Potkin, *J Clin Psychiatry* 2011;**72**[Suppl 1]:14–18), efficacy data (McIntyre and Wong, *Clin Schizophr Relat Psychoses* 2012;**5**:217–20), general (Citrome, *Neuropsychiatr Dis Treat* 2011;**7**:325–39; FFT).

Aspirin + TAU

Adjunct: Aspirin 1000mg/d as an adjunct to regular antipsychotics may have a significant effect on PANSS scores, with speculation that inflammation may be a new target for treatment (n=70, RCT, d/b, p/c, 3/12, Laan *et al, J Clin Psychiatry* 2010;**71**:520–7).

Benzodiazepines ± TAU *

Adjunct: Short-term use may reduce anxiety, tension and insomnia and high doses may have some tranquillising effects but may increase the suicide risk by 91% (n=2588, four years, Tiihonen *et al, Arch Gen Psychiatry* 2012;**69**:476–83). Cochrane concludes that there is little or no evidence that BDZs are useful as adjunctive therapy in schizophrenia, although widely used to augment antipsychotics in acute states (s=34, n=2657, Dold *et al, Cochrane Database Syst Rev* 2012:**11**:CD006391).

Monotherapy: Cochrane concludes that there is little or no evidence that BDZs are useful as monotherapy in schizophrenia (s=34, n=2657, Dold *et al, Cochrane Database Syst Rev* 2012:**11**:CD006391). See also 'Acute psychiatric emergency' (*1.1*).

Buspirone + TAU

Adjunct: Buspirone as an adjunct to risperidone significantly improved PANSS scores and was surprisingly well tolerated (n=46, RCT, d/b, p/c, 8/52, Ghaleiha *et al, J Clin Psychopharmacol* 2010;**30**:678–82).

Chinese herbal medicines + TAU

Adjunct: A systematic review and meta-analysis suggested that use might help some outcomes (s=7, RCTs, Rathbone *et al, Br J Psychiatry* 2007;**190**:379–84; FFT; disputed by Werneke, *EBMH* 2008;**11**:19).

Cholinesterase inhibitors See *1.21.3*.

Cox-2 inhibitors + risperidone

Adjunct: Celecoxib 400mg/d may produce a significant reduction in PANSS compared to risperidone monotherapy (n=50, RCT, d/b, p/c, 5/52, Muller *et al, Eur Arch Psychiatry Clin Neurosci* 2004;**254**:14–22) and reduce EPSEs (n=60, RCT, d/b, p/c, 8/52, Akhondzadeh *et al, Schizophr Res* 2007;**90**:179–85).

D-serine (see also sarcosine) **+ TAU**

Adjunct: D-serine (a full NMDA receptor agonist)

plus olanzapine or risperidone, significantly improved PANSS and was well tolerated (n=39, RCT, d/b, p/c, c/o, 6/52, Heresco-Levy *et al, Biol Psychiatry* 2005;**15**:577–85).

Dipyridamole + haloperidol

Adjunct: Adjunctive dipyridamole was superior to haloperidol monotherapy, possibly via an effect on the interaction between the adenosine and dopamine systems (n=30, RCT, Akhondzadeh *et al, J Clin Pharm Ther* 2000; **25**:131–8).

Estradiol/estrogens ± TAU *

Adjunct: **Estrogen** as an adjunct to haloperidol significantly reduced positive and general symptoms in women (n=32, RCT, d/b, p/c, 8/52, Akhondzadeh *et al, Prog Neuropsychopharmacol Biol Psychiatry* 2003;**27**:1007–12), including those of child-bearing age with chronic schizophrenia (n=32, RCT, p/c, d/b, 4/52, Ghafari *et al, Clin Schizophr Relat Psychoses* 2013;**6**:172–6). There may be specific antipsychotic-like effects in women (n=125, Bergemann *et al, Psychol Med* 2007;**37**:1427–36), e.g. 100 mcg **estradiol** significantly reduced positive and general psychopathology (n=102, RCT, p/c, 28/7, Kulkarni *et al, Arch Gen Psychiatry* 2008;**65**:955–60; generally positive comment by Crespo-Focorro *et al, EBMH* 2009;**12**:55). **Raloxifene** (an estrogen modulator) 120 mg/d led to a significantly quicker recovery cf. 60 mg/d and placebo, suggesting a potential role in postmenopausal women with schizophrenia (n=33, RCT, d/b, p/c, 12/52, Usall *et al, J Clin Psychiatry* 2011;**72**:1552–7).

Monotherapy: Transdermal estrogen did not prevent relapse of postnatal affective psychosis if started within 48 hours of delivery (n=29, open, 12/7, Kumar *et al, J Clin Psychiatry* 2003;**64**:112–8).

Famotidine + TAU *

Adjunct: Famotidine has improved PANSS scores cf. placebo (n=30, RCT, p/c, 4/52, Meskanen *et al, J Clin Psychopharmacol* 2013;**33**:472–8).

Ginkgo biloba + TAU (see also GB + clozapine)

Adjunct: Ginkgo biloba has enhanced the effectiveness of haloperidol and reduced EPS (n=109, RCT, d/b, p/c, 12/52, Zhang *et al, J Clin Psychiatry* 2001;**62**:878–83; comment by Knable, *EBMH* 2002;**5**:90; FFT).

Lamotrigine + TAU (see also lamotrigine + clozapine)

Adjunct: In comorbid schizophrenia/schizo-affective disorder and OCD, lamotrigine 200 mg/d (plus olanzapine or quetiapine, plus SSRI or BDZ) gave a significant 83% response (n=9, open, 8/52, Poyurovsky *et al, J Psychopharmacol* 2010;**24**:861–6; review by Tiihonen *et al, Schizophr Res* 2009;**109**:10–4).

L-theanine + TAU

Adjunct: L-theanine, an amino acid found virtually only in tea, may have psychoactive properties. Augmentation of antipsychotics in schizophrenia or schizoaffective disorders has improved positive activation and anxiety symptoms, so more studies may be worth it (n=60[c=40], RCT, d/b, p/c, 8/52, Ritsner *et al, J Clin Psychiatry* 2011;**72**:34–42).

L-lysine + risperidone *

L-lysine 6 g/d as an adjunct to risperidone was tolerable and improved negative and general symptoms of chronic schizophrenia (n=72, RCT, d/b, p/c, 8/52, Zeinoddini *et al, J Psychiatr Res* 2014;**59**:125–31).

Memantine + TAU (see also clozapine) *

Adjunct: A meta-analysis concluded that adjunctive use of the NMDA receptor antagonists amantadine (s=5, n=220) and memantine (s=3, n=186) may improve cognitive function, although the trials were small (s=8, n=406, RCT, p/c, Kishi and Iwata, *J Psychiatr Res* 2013;**47**:1143–9).

Minocycline + TAU *

Adjunct: Risperidone plus minocycline 200 mg/d improved PANSS negative scores cf. risperidone, albeit not quite statistically significantly (n=43[c=35], RCT, p/c, 8/52, Ghanizadeh *et al, Recent Pat Inflamm Allergy Drug Discov* 2014;**8**:211–5). Acute catatonic symptoms have responded to minocycline (n=2, Miyaoka *et al, Prog Neuropsychopharmacol Biol Psychiatry* 2007;**31**:304–7).

Mirtazapine + TAU
(see also mirtazapine + clozapine)

Adjunct: Adjunctive mirtazapine has improved depressive symptoms with no increased psychosis (n=41, RCT, d/b, p/c, 12/52, Terevnikov *et al*, *Hum Psychopharmacol* 2011;**26**:188–93).

Penfluridol

Monotherapy: Penfluridol is a butyrophenone licensed in some countries (e.g. India) for psychosis. Its main advantage is that it is an oral antipsychotic that can be taken once a week at around 20mg (e.g. Khorana and Patel, *Indian J Physiol Pharmacol* 1988;**32**:293–8; n=30, 12/52, Vaidyalingam, *J Postgrad Med* 1990;**36**:100–3). A slightly obscure additional advantage is that in *Plasmodium falciparum* (malaria) penfluridol may reverse mefloquine resistance (Oduola *et al*, *Trans R Soc Trop Med Hyg* 1993;**87**:81–3). Cochrane concludes it to be a viable option especially in people with antipsychotic needs and poor adherence, but who do not like depots (s=25, n=1024, Soares and Lima, *Cochrane Database Syst Rev* 2006;**2**:CD002923).

Sarcosine (N-methylglycine) + TAU

Adjunct: Sarcosine was superior to placebo as add-on to TAU for TRS, unlike d-serine, which was not (n=60, RCT, d/b, p/c, 6/52, Lane *et al*, *Int J Neuropsychopharmacol* 2010;**13**.451–60).

Topiramate + TAU (see also clozapine)

Adjunct: Adjunctive topiramate in TRS has reduced PANSS scores in some (n=26, RCT, d/b, p/c, c/o, 2x12/52, Tiihonen *et al*, *J Clin Psychiatry* 2005;**66**:1012–5;IS) and reduced weight gain (n=32, RCT, d/b, p/c, Afshar *et al*, *J Psychopharmacol* 2009;**23**:157–62).

Valproate ± TAU *

Adjunct: Valproate may be useful as an adjunct to risperidone or olanzapine for acute exacerbations of schizophrenia (n=249, RCT, d/b, 4/52, Casey *et al*, *Neuropsychopharmacol* 2003;**28**:182–92; FFT), for functional hallucinations (n=1, Rajkumar, *Indian J Psychol Med* 2012;**34**:76–8; FFT) and in very severe schizophrenia (n=28, open, Suzuki *et al*, *Hum Psychopharmacol* 2009;**24**:628–38).

Monotherapy: Cochrane concludes that there is no data to support or refute its use as monotherapy in schizophrenia (s=7, n=519, Schwarz *et al*, *Cochrane Database Syst Rev* 2008;**3**:CD004028).

Review: * off-license use in schizophrenia (Horowitz *et al*, *PLoS One* 2014;**9**:e92573).

■ Unlicensed/possible efficacy

Betel nut

Males with schizophrenia chewing large quantities of betel nut (an anti-muscarinic) have significantly milder positive symptoms than low users (n=65, Sullivan *et al*, *Am J Psychiatry* 2007;**164**:670).

Flunarizine (not licensed in UK)

Flunarizine has some dopamine-blocking properties, and may be as effective as haloperidol and, with a half-life of 2–7 weeks, could have a potential role as a long-acting oral antipsychotic (n=70, RCT, d/b, 12/52, Bisol *et al*, *J Clin Psychiatry* 2008;**69**:1572–9).

Gabapentin + TAU

Adjunct: Gabapentin was well tolerated and significantly improved PANSS and CDSS with risperidone or olanzapine, but sadly so did placebo (n=10, open, p/c, 8/52, Gabriel, *Neuropsychiatr Dis Treat* 2010;**6**:711–7).

Lithium * (see also lithium + clozapine)

Lithium-responsive psychosis may be familial and perhaps genetically distinct from the majority of schizophrenias.

Monotherapy: Cochrane concludes that lithium is ineffective as a sole agent, but may potentially be useful in a few people (s=20, n=611, Leucht *et al*, *Cochrane Database Syst Rev* 2007;**3**:CD003834).

Melatonin + TAU

Melatonin 3mg/d may be useful as a hypnotic in schizophrenia (see insomnia, n=40, RCT, d/b, p/c, 15/7, Kumar *et al*, *J Clin Psychiatry* 2007;**68**:237–41), but not in those with better sleep efficiency (n=19, RCT, c/o, p/c, Shamir *et al*, *J Clin Psychiatry* 2000;**61**:373–7).

Review: * in schizophrenia (Morera-Fumero

and Abreu-Gonzalez, *Int J Mol Sci* 2013; **14**:9037–50).

Nifedipine + TAU

Adjunct: Adjunctive nifedipine is of low efficacy (n=62, open, 10/52, Dzhuga and Kozlovskii, *Zh Nevrol Psikhiatr Im S S Korsakova* 2009;**109**:32–5).

Omega-3 fatty acids * + TAU

There is some evidence for abnormal phospholipid metabolism in schizophrenia, and trials with PUVAs have produced inconsistent but usually favourable findings. Long-chain omega-3 fatty acid (E-EPA and DHA) deficiency has been implicated in CV disease, a primary cause of excess mortality and the majority of people with schizophrenia may have very low in long-chain omega-3 fatty acids, a risk for CV mortality and morbidity (n=44, McNamara *et al, Cardiovasc Psychiatry Neurol* 2013;**2013**:796462).

Adjunct: E-EPA was not shown to be effective (n=53, RCT, d/b, p/c, 12/52, Berger *et al*, J Clin Psychiatry 2007;**68**:1867–75), although a small open study of adjunctive omega-3 fatty acids and vitamins E and C to haloperidol suggested significantly improved symptoms on all rating scales, particularly on reduced akathisia (n=17, open, Sivrioglu *et al, Prog Neuropsychopharmacol Biol Psychiatry* 2007;**31**:1493–9). Cochrane concludes the evidence is still inconclusive (s=8, n=517, Joy *et al, Cochrane Database Syst Rev* 2006;**3**:CD001257).

Review: * Marano *et al, Clin Ter* 2013;**164**:e529–37.

Ondansetron + TAU

Adjunct: Ondansetron may be an effective adjunct to risperidone or haloperidol, especially for negative symptoms, but a large RCT is needed (s=6, Bennett and Vila, *Ann Pharmacother* 2010;**44**:1301–6).

Oxcarbazepine + TAU

Adjunct: Oxcarbazepine has been used in acute schizophrenia (n=6, open, Leweke *et al, Am J Psychiatry* 2004;**161**:1130–1).

Pregabalin + TAU

Adjunct: Pregabalin may be effective for comorbid anxiety in schizophrenia (n=11, open, Englisch *et al, J Clin Psychopharmacol* 2010;**30**:437–40).

Raloxifene (see estradiol/estrogens) *

Sodium nitroprusside *

A single four-hour infusion of sodium nitroprusside showed a rapid improvement in all symptoms (n=20, RCT, d/b, p/c, 1/7, Hallak *et al, JAMA Psychiatry* 2013;**70**:668–76).

Tetrabenazine

Tetrabenazine has been used for the treatment of psychoses but the high incidence of side-effects makes this a relatively unsuitable drug.

● Case reports *

- **Dronabinol** (n=4, Schwarcz and Karajgi, *J Clin Psychiatry* 2010;**71**:1552–3)
- **Pergolide + amisulpride** (n=1, Roesch-Ely *et al, Pharmacopsychiatry* 2006;**39**:115–6)
- **Rivastigmine** (hallucinations, n=1, Abad *et al, Iran J Psychiatry* 2011;**6**:161–3).

□ No efficacy

Ayurvedic medicine

Ayurvedic medicine may have some effects, but the data is inadequate (s=3, n=250, Agarwal *et al, Cochrane Database Syst Rev* 2007;**4**:CD006867).

Buspirone

Buspirone has various receptor activities, e.g. dopamine antagonism but exacerbation of psychosis has been reported.

Caffeine

Excess caffeine consumption can present as psychosis and increase arousal, but moderate use probably has little effect on anxiety, depression and psychosis (e.g. n=26, RCT, d/b, c/o, Mayo *et al, Br J Psychiatry* 1993;**162**:543–5).

Cannabidiol

In TRS, only one patient showed mild improvement with cannabidiol (n=3, 35/7, Zuardi *et al, J Psychopharmacol* 2006;**20**:683–6).

Cannabis *

Cochrane concludes that there is insufficient evidence to support or refute the use of cannabis to treat schizophrenia (s=8, n=530, RCT, McLoughlin *et al*, *Cochrane Database Syst Rev* 2014;**10**:CD004837; FFT).

Carbamazepine ± TAU *

Cochrane could not recommend carbamazepine for routine use, either as monotherapy, augmentation or maintenance (s=10, n=258, RCT, Leucht *et al*, *Cochrane Database Syst Rev* 2014;**5**:CD001258). Carbamazepine also induces CYP3A4 and reduces the plasma levels of many antipsychotics.

Creatine + TAU

Adjunctive creatine 5g/d had no effect on cognitive function or symptoms (n=12, RCT, d/b, p/c, c/o, 3/12, Kaptsan *et al*, *J Clin Psychiatry* 2007;**68**:881–4).

Methylphenidate + TAU

Bolus IV methylphenidate has been used to exacerbate symptoms in an attempt to predict those people likely to relapse if antipsychotics are discontinued (mentioned in Klein and Wender, *Arch Gen Psychiatry* 1995;**52**:429–33).

Statins + risperidone *

Lovastatin had no effect as an adjunct to risperidone (RCT, d/b, p/c, 8/52, Ghanizadeh *et al*, *Psychiatry Res* 2014;**219**:431–5).

Varenicline *

There is naturally concern about the use of varenicline for smoking cessation in people with schizophrenia, but a systematic review and meta-analysis concludes that varenicline is not superior to placebo for smoking cessation, in schizophrenia anyway (s=7, n=439, RCT, d/b, p/c, Kishi and Iwata, *Eur Arch Psychiatry Clin Neurosci* 2014;**265**:259–68).

Vitamin B6

No difference in PANSS scores was detectable with B6 supplementation in stable chronic schizophrenia (n=15, d/b, p/c, c/o, 9/52, Lerner *et al*, *J Clin Psychiatry* 2002;**63**:54–8).

1.21.2 FIRST EPISODE (EARLY INTERVENTION) *

1

Early intervention can include both treating a first episode or prodromal symptoms quickly, and treating people at high risk before symptoms actually appear. Social decline, associated with neurocognitive deficits, often occurs in the prodromal phase, or in the early course of schizophrenia, thus management is vital.

Duration of Untreated Psychosis (DUP)

A meta-analysis and systematic review (s=33, Penttilä *et al*, *Br J Psychiatry* 2014;**205**:88–94) found that a longer DUP (mean is 49 months, range 1–312/12; n=80, Primavera *et al*, *Ann Gen Psychiatry* 2012;**11**:21; FFT) shows a modest but consistent relationship with:

- worse symptoms (n=80, Fraguas *et al*, *Schizophr Res* 2014;**152**:130–8) and poor social functioning independent of symptoms
- less chance of remission and reduced improvement after one year (e.g. a DUP longer than 30 days adversely impacted on long-term outcome in Hong Kong; n=153[c=112], 13 years, Tang *et al*, *Schizophr Res* 2014;**153**;1–8)
- impaired verbal IQ, verbal learning and working memory
- greater transition to schizophrenia (systematic review and meta-analysis; s=11 n=1246, RCTs, Stafford *et al*, *BMJ* 2013; **346**:f185; n=2923, Queirazza et al, *Br J Psychiatr* 2014;**204**:299–305).

Role of antipsychotics in first episodes

- Minimise deterioration (or even perhaps prevent the illness developing, s=11 n=1246, RCTs, Stafford *et al*, *BMJ* 2013;**346**:f185)
- Reduce stigma from symptoms, aiming for complete, not incomplete, remission
- Increase engagement by minimising adverse experience with medication through use of minimum effective doses.

Antipsychotic therapy is usually considered as essential treatment, and is definitely more effective if taken regularly.

Response to antipsychotics in first episodes

Response at six months in drug-naïve schizophrenia shows five distinct trajectories:

- rapid response 10%
- gradual response 44%
- remaining mildly ill 28%
- unsustained clinical response 13%
- remain very unwell 5%.

The only predictor of rapid response was employment (OR 2.5) (n=467, Nordon *et al, Acta Psychiatr Scand* 2013;**28**:200–5). Factors predicting lack of remission at one year are:

- longer DUP
- worse negative symptoms
- only completing primary education.

(n=174, RCT, open, one year, Diaz *et al, Psychiatry Res* 2013;**206**:181–7).

Optimum use of antipsychotics in first episodes

1. Initiate antipsychotics carefully:

- Slow titration is needed, both starting and stopping, to minimise side-effects
- The cumulative response rate is about 40% at 8/52 (see n=522, RCT, median 30/52, Emsley *et al, Am J Psychiatry* 2006;**163**:743–45), but 65% at 16/52, showing many first-episodes respond between weeks 8 and 16 and that limited early improvement does not help identify eventual non-responders (n=112, RCT, open, Gallego *et al, J Clin Psychiatry* 2011;**72**:1691–6; FFT).

2. Choice of antipsychotic:

- Systematic reviews conclude that the SGAs are not superior to FGAs, although may be more acceptable to younger people (s=13, n=1112, RCT, Kumar *et al, Cochrane Database Syst Rev* 2013;**10**:CD009582; s=15, n=2522, RCT, Crossley *et al, Br J Psychiatry* 2010;**196**:434–9; FFT) which seems a good enough reason to choose SGAs.

3. Optimise doses:

- Relatively low doses e.g. risperidone 4mg/d, olanzapine 15.3mg/d, haloperidol 5.4mg/d may be equally effective for first episode psychosis, with haloperidol worst for EPSE and olanzapine worst for weight gain (n=172, RCT, open, 6/52, Crespo-Facorro *et al, J Clin Psychiatry* 2006;**67**:1511–21)
- The best outcomes with antipsychotics in EIS seem to be to get the best out of the first drug, as response to subsequent antipsychotics (except clozapine) seems to diminish (n=244, Agid *et al, Eur Neuropsychopharmacol* 2013;**23**:1017–22). Response rates are:
  - 1st drug, mean 75% response (olanzapine 82%, risperidone 64%)
  - 2nd drug, if first didn't work, mean 20% response (olanzapine 25%, risperidone 4%)
  - 3rd drug: clozapine can be as high as 75%
  - High doses seem to be of low efficacy or detrimental to outcomes.

4. Patient choice considered a high priority:

- Consider what the patient prefers. Weight gain is the most unpopular side-effect and its impact on the user must not be trivialised. It is 3–4 times more common in younger, first-episode patients compared to older, chronic patients. The increase is consistent by drug (olanzapine, risperidone, haloperidol) but idiosyncratic by individual (s=51, n=14769, Alvarez-Jiménez *et al, CNS Drugs* 2008;**22**:547–62)
- Minimise 'obvious' ADRs that might make the person appear abnormal, e.g. EPSE, which can also reduce compliance and engagement (n=42, Amminger *et al, Schizophr Res* 2002;**54**:223–30)
- Explain that there is no clear way of treating prodromal symptoms without the high risk of treating 'false positives' (review by Larsen *et al, Acta Psychiatr Scand* 2001;**103**:323–4).

5. Adequate duration of treatment:

- Long-term treatment retention is low — as few as 12% of youths are still on the same treatment at one year (n=54, Findling *et al, J Am Acad Child Adolesc Psychiatry* 2010;**49**:583–94; FFT). The risk of relapse in people treated for EIS is increased by:
  - Medicine non-adherence (4-fold increase)
  - Persistent SUDs (3-fold increase)
  - Carers' critical comments (2.3-fold increase) (s=29, n=3978, Alvarez-Jimenez *et al, Schizophr Res* 2012;**139**:116–28)
- On discontinuation, up to 78% may experience an exacerbation or relapse within one year, and 96% may do so within two years (n=53, RCT, open, 18/12, Gitlin *et al, Am J Psychiatry* 2001;**158**:1835–42)
- There are high discontinuation rates from

antipsychotics over the first 24 months, which do not seem to vary between drugs (n=110[c=32], 24/12, Noguera *et al*, *J Clin Psychopharmacol* 2013;**33**:463–71)

- Advise person that not taking antipsychotics for several years may almost inevitably lead to relapse and rehospitalisation (n=104, Robinson *et al*, *Arch Gen Psychiatry* 1999;**56**:241–7). The optimum duration of therapy is as yet unclear.

6. Optimise long-term dosing:

- The risk from low doses appears low compared to the risk of relapse and subsequent potential deterioration, e.g. the risk of relapse in stable first-episode psychosis is twice as high if discontinuing an antipsychotic compared to maintenance with a low-dose antipsychotic (43% vs 21%), with 30% requiring restarting antipsychotics and only 20% successfully discontinuing (n=131, RCT, open, 18/12, Wunderink *et al*, *J Clin Psychiatry* 2007;**68**:654–61)
- After 6/12 of remission from a first episode with an antipsychotic, dose reduction or gradual discontinuation had a better outcome at seven years than continued treatment or placebo (n=128[c=103], open, RCT, seven years, Wunderink *et al*, *JAMA Psychiatry* 2013;**70**;913–20).

7. Treatment is monitored:

- Many antipsychotics have a high incidence of EPS (even low dose haloperidol), raised prolactin and adverse cognitive effects. Others have higher incidence of weight gain (which should be dealt with early) and diabetes, which needs to be screened for, monitored and managed.

Reviews: * antipsychotic use in children and adolescents (Schneider *et al*, *J Psychopharmacol* 2014;**28**:615–623), management (Taylor *et al*, *J Psychopharmacol* 2012;**26**[5 Suppl]:3–5), general (Mattai *et al*, *Curr Opin Psychiatry* 2010;**23**:304–10), EPSE in EIS (Haddad et *al*, *J Psychopharmacol* 2012;**26**[Suppl]:15–26), LAIs in EIS (Emsley *et al*, *Early Interv Psychiatry* 2013;**7**:247–54).

BNF listed

Amisulpride

Amisulpride (mean 250 mg/d) is licensed from age 15 years upwards (n=14[c=12], open, 6/52, Murphy *et al*, *Hum Psychopharmacol* 2006; **21**:511–7).

Aripiprazole *

Aripiprazole is licensed in the UK for schizophrenia in adolescents aged 15 years or older (US 13–17 years). Nearly 50% of the PANSS decrease is in the first two weeks and 75% by week three, so week 3 is a better prediction of response than earlier (n=294, RCT, d/b, p/c, 6/52, Correll *et al*, *J Am Acad Adolesc Psychiatry* 2013;**52**:689–98; n=59[c=38], 6/52, open, Park *et al*, *Int Clin Psychopharmacol* 2014;**29**:77–85). Response can be 79% by week 12 (n=45[c=42], open, 12/52, Takahashi *et al*, *Clin Neuropharmacol* 2009;**32**:149–50; n=21, open, 8/52, Lee *et al*, *Psychiatry Clin Neurosci* 2010;**64**:38–43). In drug-naïve people with an ultra-high risk or already in a first episode, aripiprazole up to 7.5 mg/d seems effective for less severe positive (but not negative) symptoms, albeit with adverse effects (n=31[c=29], open, 4/52, Liu *et al*, *J Clin Psychopharmacol* 2013;**33**:18–23). Aripiprazole was equivalent to risperidone for positive symptom response, superior for negative symptoms but produced more akathisia (n=198, RCT, d/b, a/c, 12/52, Robinson *et al*, *Schizophr Bull* 2015;**41**:1227–36). Beware of hyperprolactinaemia as 60% may get subnormal prolactin levels cf. 8% with placebo (Safer *et al*, *J Child Adolesc Psychopharmacol* 2013;**23**:282–9; FFT).

Clozapine *

Clozapine is licensed from age 16 upwards. Early use of clozapine (after as few as 25 weeks in people failing two other antipsychotics) has been associated with significant and meaningful reductions in symptoms (n=54, d/b or open, Sporn *et al*, *J Am Acad Child Adolesc Psychiatry* 2007;**46**:1349–56), but it has more ADRs and toxicity (n=25, RCT, d/b, 8/52+open two-year follow-up, Shaw *et al*, *Arch Gen Psychiatry* 2006;**63**:721–30).

Reviews: * clozapine's role (Remington *et al*, *Am J Psychiatry* 2013;**170**:146–51), in refractory early-onset schizophrenia (Schneider *et al*, *Eur Psychiatry* 2014;**29**:1–10).

Haloperidol

Haloperidol is licensed for childhood behavioural disorders and schizophrenia, with no age limit. There is a sad irony that the only antipsychotic licensed in this age group is probably the one you would least want to use. Haloperidol 2 mg/d is much better tolerated than 8 mg/d and as effective, shown by PANSS scores (n=40, RCT, d/b, 6/52, Oosthuizen *et al, Int J Neuropsychopharmacol* 2004;**7**:125–31), has equivalent efficacy to olanzapine, although drop-out rates were high and this trial excluded more severely ill people (n=263[c=83], RCT, d/b, one year, Strakowski *et al, Schizophr Res* 2005;**78**:161–9) and equivalent to risperidone (both 2–4 mg/d) for first-episode schizophrenia, with similar ADRs and drop-outs (n=151, RCT, d/b, one year, Gaebel *et al, J Clin Psychiatry* 2007;**68**:1763–74). Unlike olanzapine, haloperidol is associated with reduced grey matter volume in a first episode, either due to haloperidol-induced toxicity or differential olanzapine efficacy (n=263, RCT, d/b, volunteer controlled, 24/12, Lieberman *et al, Arch Gen Psychiatry* 2005;**62**:361–70).

Olanzapine *

Olanzapine is only licensed in the UK from age 18 years upwards. Low dose olanzapine has superior efficacy, lower discontinuations, greater retention in treatment and reduced side-effects compared to haloperidol (e.g. n=107, RCT, d/b, p/c, 6/52, Kryzhanovskaya *et al, J Am Acad Child Adolesc Psychiatry* 2009;**48**:60–70), although weight gain (mean 15.4 kg) is a significant adverse effect (n=263, open, two years, Zipursky *et al, Br J Psychiatry* 2005;**187**:537–43; FFT). Response or non-response (>20% improvement) at weeks 2 and 3 were most robust predictors of response or non-response outcome at 6/52 with olanzapine (n>69, 6/52, p/c, Stentebjerg-Olesen *et al, Eur Child Adolesc Psychiatry* 2015;24:1485–96). Olanzapine (2.5–20 mg/d) and risperidone (1–6 mg/d) have been shown to be equipotent in first-episode schizophrenia (e.g. n=100[c=77], RCT, open, 6/12, Cuesta *et al, Br J Psychiatry* 2009;**194**:439–45; FFT), but the FDA have warned about the increased risk of weight gain and hyperlipidemia with long-term olanzapine in the 13–17 age group.

Review: use in adolescents (McCormack, *CNS Drugs* 2010;**24**:443–52).

Paliperidone

The dose for a first episode is 1.5–12 mg/d, and it does not need to be weight-related (n=201, RCT, d/b, p/c, 6/52, Singh *et al, Biol Psychiatry* 2011;**70**:1179–87).

Quetiapine *

Quetiapine is licensed for schizophrenia in adults but not recommended for under 18s due to lack of data. Low EPS, weight gain and prolactin effects make quetiapine a suitable antipsychotic in EIS. Doses of 200–800 mg/d can be used (n= 156 O/Ps, RCT, 12/52, Amr *et al, Int Arch Med* 2013;**6**:47; FFT; n=220, RCT, d/b, p/c, 6/52, Findling *et al, J Child Adolesc Psychopharmacol* 2012;**22**:327–42), but with a high drop-out due to lack of efficacy (n=202, RCT, open, one year, Crespo-Facorro *et al, Psychopharmacology [Berl]* 2014;**231**:357–66). After a first episode of psychosis, 41% of people who said they took quetiapine for the next year had relapsed, whereas 79% of those who stopped had relapsed, a difference of 38% (n=178, RCT, d/b, 12/12, Hui *et al, Schizophr Res* 2013;**150**:297–302). Long-term efficacy has been shown in people stable after one year, where a further year showed relapse of 41% cf. 79% placebo (n=178, RCT, d/b, p/c, 12/12, Chen *et al, Br Med J* 2010;**341**:c4024; FFT).

Risperidone *

Risperidone is licensed from age 15 years upwards and is a standard first choice. It needs a low but adequate dose, e.g. 1–3 mg/d seems optimum, and as effective as 4–6 mg/d but with less ADRs (n=160, RCT, d/b, p/c, 6/52, Haas *et al, J Child Adolesc Psychopharmacol* 2009;**19**:611–21), so it makes little pharmacological sense escalating doses at an early stage in a first episode (n=49, d/b, 8/52, Merlo *et al, J Clin Psychiatry* 2002;**63**:885–91). In the 75% who initially clinically improve, relapses are delayed longer with risperidone (mean 3.3 mg/d; median 466 days) than haloperidol (mean 2.9 mg/d; median 205 days) (n=555, RCT, d/b, <5 years, median 30/52, Schooler *et al, Am J Psychiatry* 2005;**162**:947–53). Risperidone 1–6 mg/d was equipotent with olanzapine (2.5–20 mg/d) in first-episode schizophrenia, but patients may be more stable with risperidone (eg. n=112, RCT, open, 4/12, Robinson *et al*, *Am J Psychiatry* 2006;**163**:2096–102). Use of RLAI improves compliance and reduces relapse rate (n=50[c=32], open, two years, Emsley *et al*, *Int Clin Psychopharmacol* 2008;**23**:325–31) in first episode schizophrenia compared to oral risperidone (n=50, Kim *et al*, *Prog Neuropsychopharmacol Biol Psychiatry* 2008; **32**:1231–5). Although 81% of patients discontinue treatment over the first two years, the LAI allows this to be more easily detected (n=37, Weiden *et al*, *J Clin Psychiatry* 2012;**73**:1224–33).

• Unlicensed/some efficacy

Celecoxib + TAU

Adjunct: Adding further weight to the hypothesis of inflammation as a contributor to schizophrenia, amisulpride 200–1000 mg/d plus celecoxib 400 mg or placebo showed a significantly better outcome in first episodes with celecoxib, including improved negative symptoms (n=49, RCT, d/b, p/c, 6/52, Müller *et al*, *Schizophr Res* 2010;**121**:118–24).

Minocycline + TAU

Adjunct: Minocycline, which modulates the glutamatergic system, has improved general outcome in first-episode patients as an add-on to SGAs (n=54, RCT, d/b, p/c, 6/12, Levkovitz *et al*, *J Clin Psychiatry* 2010;**71**:138–49)

Omega-3 fatty acids *

Monotherapy: In an extraordinary study of young people at ultra-high risk of developing psychotic disorders, a 3/12 course of omega-3 fatty acids 1.2 g/d (PUFAs) reduced transition to psychotic disorder from 27.5% (placebo) to 4.9% (PUFA) over one year, an NNT of 4 (n=81[c=76], RCT, d/b, p/c, 12/12, Amminger *et al*, *Arch Gen Psychiatry* 2010;**67**:146–54). Beat that if you can, and it certainly trumps the previous negative study (n=69, RCT, d/b, p/c, 12/52, Berger *et al*, *J Clin Psychiatry* 2007;**68**:1867–75). However, two reviews were luke-warm, noting a limited evidence base in treatment or prevention of schizophrenia, but, as it has a low risk of harm, adjunctive use may be of some assistance (Akter *et al*, *J Clin Pharm Ther* 2012;**37**:132–9) and so might be an alternative in some people (Mees *et al*, *Psychiatr Danub* 2011;**23** Suppl 1:S118–22). After 2–3 years stability and antipsychotic tapering, replacement with omega-3 fatty acids plus the metabolic antioxidant alphalipoic acid had no effect on relapse, showing that antipsychotic discontinuation even after 2–3 years carries a very high risk of relapse (n=33, RCT, d/b, p/c, Emsley *et al*, *Schizophr Res* 2014;**158**:230–5).

1.21.3 COGNITIVE IMPAIRMENT

Cognitive impairment is a known complication of schizophrenia and of antipsychotics, and so methods to improve cognitive function are needed. In overall neurocognitive scores, quetiapine and olanzapine performed best, then risperidone, ziprasidone, amisulpride and haloperidol, in that order, but with significant differences in specific cognitive tasks (s=9, RCTs, >6/12, Désaméricq *et al*, *Eur J Clin Pharmacol* 2014;**70**:127–34).

Reviews: general (Galletly, *Psychopharmacol [Berl]* 2009;**202**:259–73), pharmacological treatment of cognition in schizophrenia (Barch, *Curr Top Behav Neuosci* 2010;**4**:43–96).

Combinations and adjuncts

Antidepressants + TAU *

A systematic review and meta-analysis concluded that there was no evidence of a clinically significant effect on cognitive function, but some statistical advantages (s=11, n=568, RCTs, d/b, p/c, Vernon *et al*, *Schizophr Res* 2014; **159**:385–94).

Aripiprazole + TAU *

Adjunct: Adjunctive aripiprazole to olanzapine or risperidone improved motor speed but some cognitive functions deteriorated (n=36, RCT, d/b, p/c, 12/52, Yasui-Furukori *et al*, *J Psychopharmacol* 2012;**26**:806–12). As an adjunct to risperidone it had no effect on cognitive function but did reduce prolactin (n=35, RCT, d/b, p/c, 24/52, Lee *et al*, *Clin Psychopharmacol Neurosci* 2013;**11**:60–6).

Buspirone + TAU

Adjunct: Buspirone may improve attention, but not statistically (n=73, RCT, d/b, p/c, 6/12, Sumiyoshi *et al*, *Schizophr Res* 2007;**95**:158–68).

Cholinesterase inhibitor + antipsychotic *

Adjunct: A meta-analysis concludes that cholinesterase inhibitors may produce modest improvements but that other strategies are unproven (s=26, d/b, p/c, n=1104, Choi *et al*, *Br J Psychiatry* 2013;**203**:172–8) and Cochrane concords with that conclusion (Singh *et al*, *Cochrane Database Syst Rev* 2012;**1**:CD007967). **Donepezil** 5–10mg/d appeared to have little effect on cognitive deficits in schizophrenia (e.g. n=26, RCT, d/b, p/c, 16/52, Kohler *et al*, *Cognit Neuropsychiatry* 2007;**12**:412–21), but 10mg/d as an adjunct to risperidone significantly improved negative symptoms in chronic schizophrenia with cognitive impairments (n=30, RCT, d/b, p/c, 12/52, Akhondzadeh *et al*, *Prog Neuropsychopharmacol Biol Psychiatry* 2008;**32**:1810–5).
Galantamine adjunctively may improve refractory cognition, e.g. improved processing speed, WAIS-III and verbal memory (n=86, RCT, d/b, p/c, 12/52, Buchanan *et al*, *Am J Psychiatry* 2008;**165**:82–9), but 24mg/d had no apparent effect on cognitive function in stable schizophrenia with low baseline functioning (n=83[c=73], RCT, d/b, p/c, 12/52, Conley *et al*, *Clin Neuropharmacol* 2009;**32**:69–74; FFT).
Rivastigmine up to 9mg/d as an adjunct had no effect on cognitive function in schizophrenia with significant impairment (n=20, RCT, c/o, 6/12, Chouinard *et al*, *Curr Med Res Opin* 2007;**23**:575–83; n=40[c=21], RCT, d/b, p/c, 24/52, Sharma *et al*, *Schizophr Res* 2006;**85**:73–83), although up to 16mg BD may be more effective (n=16, 12/12, Lenzi *et al*, *Clin Neuropharmacol* 2003;**26**:317–21).
Review: * use to improve cognition in schizophrenia, individually or combined (Koola *et al*, *Schizophr Res* 2014;**157**:84–9).

Clozapine + risperidone

These did not significantly improve cognitive function cf. clozapine alone (n=30, RCT, d/b, p/c, 6/52, Akdede *et al*, *J Clin Psychiatry* 2006;**67**:1912–9).

Ginseng + antipsychotics

Adjunct: HT1001 (a commercial Ginseng prep) has improved working memory in schizophrenia (n=64, d/b, p/c, 4/52, Chen and Hui, *Phytother* 2012;**26**:1166–72).

Lurasidone *

Improved cognitive performance was shown with lurasidone 40–160mg/d cf. quetiapine 200–800mg/d (n=236, d/b, 6/12, Harvey *et al*, *Schizophr Res* 2015;**166**:334–8; FFT).

Minocycline + antipsychotic *

Adjunct: Minocycline 200mg/d, a glutamate system modulator, improved cognitive functioning in first-episode patients as an add-on to SGAs (n=54, RCT, d/b, p/c, 6/12, Levkovitz *et al*, *J Clin Psychiatry* 2010;**71**:138–49).

Mirtazapine + risperidone

Adjunct: Augmentation of risperidone significantly improved cognitive symptoms, but at the cost of weight gain (n=21, RCT, d/b, p/c, 8/52, Cho *et al*, *Prog Neuropsychopharmacol Biol Psychiatry* 2011;**35**:208–11), and improved a range of cognitive functions (n=37, RCT, d/b, p/c, 6/52, Stenberg *et al*, *Int J Neuropsychopharmacol* 2010;**13**:433–41).

Modafinil + antipsychotic

Adjunct: Modafinil 200mg/d has produced improvements in cognitive functioning in schizophrenia (n=20, RCT, d/b, p/c, c/o, Turner *et al*, *Neuropsychopharmacol* 2004;**29**:1363–73; FFT), but 300mg/d added to clozapine had no effect on impaired cognition (n=35, RCT, d/b, p/c, 8/52, Freudenreich *et al*, *J Clin Psychiatry* 2009;**70**:1674–80).

Oxytocin + antipsychotic *

Adjunct: Intranasal oxytocin can improve verbal memory in schizophrenia (n=15, 3/52, Feifel *et al*, *Schizophr Res* 2012;**139**:207–10), reduce psychotic symptoms (n=20, RCT, p/c, 14/7, Pedersen *et al*, *Schizophr Res* 2011;**132**:50–3; n=40[c=37], RCT, d/b, p/c, 8/52, Modabbernia *et al*, *CNS Drugs* 2013;**27**;57–65), improve olfactory identification (n=28[c=28], RCT, d/b, p/c, 3/52, Lee *et al*, *Schizophr Res* 2013;**145**:110–5), improve social perception (n=81, p/c, c/o, Fischer-Shofty *et al*, *Schizophr Res* 2013;**146**:357–62), and improve higher level social cognitive tasks (n = 23, RCT, p/c, Davis *et al*, *Schizophr Res* 2013;**147**:393–7) and social cognition (n = 60, RCT, d/b, p/c, c/o, Woolley *et al*, *Psychoneuroendocrinology* 2014;**47**:116–25). **Reviews:** * general (De Berardis *et al*, *CNS Neurol Disord Drug Targets* 2013;**12**:252–64; Macdonald and Feifel, *Acta Neuropsychiatr* 2012;**24**:130–46; FFT).

Pregnenolone + antipsychotic

Adjunct: Pregnenolone (a neurosteroid that may enhance cognition and modulates NMDA receptors) 30 mg/d was superior to placebo and pregnenolone 200 mg/d for positive symptoms and EPS in schizophrenia (n = 58 [c = 44], RCT, d/b, p/c, 8/52, Ritsner *et al*, *J Clin Psychiatry* 2010;**71**:1351–62; n = 21 [c = 18], RCT, d/b, p/c, 8/52, Marx *et al*, *Neuropsychopharmacology* 2009;**34**:1885–903; FFT).

Tropisetron + risperidone

Adjunct: Tropisetron (an alpha-7 nicotinic acetylcholine receptor agonist) appears well tolerated and significantly improved cognitive deficits (but not PANSS) in schizophrenia (n = 40 [c = 33], RCT, d/b, p/c, 8/52, Shiina *et al*, *Ann Gen Psychiatry* 2010;**9**:27; FFT).

Varenicline + TAU

Adjunct: Varenicline (≤2 mg/d) may improve cognition in some people with schizophrenia (n = 120, RCT, d/b, p/c, 8/52, Shim *et al*, *Neuropsychopharmacology* 2012;**37**:660–8; FFT).

□ No efficacy

Acamprosate

Acamprosate has no positive or negative effects on cognitive functioning in schizophrenia, so can safely be used for alcohol dependence (n = 23, RCT, d/b, p/c, 12/52, Ralevski *et al*, *J Nerv Ment Dis* 2011;**199**:499–505).

Atomoxetine + antipsychotic

Adjunctive atomoxetine was ineffective for improving cognitive impairment (n = 32, RCT, d/b, p/c, 8/52, Kelly *et al*, *J Clin Psychiatry* 2009;**70**:518–25).

Cycloserine (D-cycloserine) + antipsychotic

In severe negative symptoms and cognitive impairment (without marked positive, depressive or EPSE) there was no improvement when either glycine or cycloserine were added (n = 157, RCT, d/b, p/c, 12/52, Buchanan *et al*, *Am J Psychiatry* 2007;**164**:1593–602).

D-serine + antipsychotic

Adjunct: D-serine 2 g/d did not appear to improve cognition, although the placebo response was relatively high (n = 195, RCT, d/b, p/c, 16/52, Weiser *et al*, *J Clin Psychiatry* 2012;**73**:e728–34).

Dehydroepiandrosterone (DHEA) + TAU

Adjunct: DHEA 400 mg/d had little effect on positive symptoms and EPS in schizophrenia (n = 58 [c = 44], RCT, d/b, p/c, 8/52, Ritsner *et al*, *J Clin Psychiatry* 2010;**71**:1351–62).

Fluvoxamine + antipsychotic

Adjunct: Fluvoxamine was ineffective for cognition (n = 48, RCT, d/b, p/c, 12/52, Niitsu *et al*, *J Clin Psychopharmacol* 2012;**32**:593–601).

Glycine + antipsychotic

See cycloserine above.

Guanfacine *

One study showed no significant effect although some trends for improvements (n = 40 [c = 38], RCT, d/b, p/c, 4/52, Friedman *et al*, *Neuropsychopharmacology* 2001;**25**:402–9; FFT)

Memantine + antipsychotic

Although adjunctive memantine did not improve cognitive functioning in schizophrenia, it did not exacerbate positive symptoms (n = 26, p/c, 12/52, Lee *et al*, *Psychiatry Investig* 2012;**9**:166–73; FFT).

Reboxetine + olanzapine

Adjunctive reboxetine 4 mg/d to olanzapine 10 mg/d has no effect on cognitive function (p/c, d/b, Poyurovsky *et al*, *Isr J Psychiatry Relat Sci* 2009;**46**:213–20; FFT).

Rosiglitazone + clozapine

Rosiglitazone had no effect on cognition as an

adjunct to clozapine (n=19, RCT, d/b, p/c, 8/52, Yi *et al, Psychiatry Res* 2012;**200**:79–82).

1.21.4 NEGATIVE SYMPTOMS *

Symptoms and incidence:
Negative symptoms of schizophrenia may be linked to untreated positive symptoms or antipsychotic side-effects but remain difficult to manage. They lead to functional impairment of, e.g. normal emotional responses, thought processes, blunting or flattening of affect, apathy, anhedonia, and asociality. They reduce QoL, increase disability and burden, and lead to poorer long-term outcomes. Primary negative symptoms are prominent and persistent in up to 26% of people with schizophrenia, and may occur in up to 58% out-patients at any given time.

Role of drugs
Negative symptoms respond less well to medicines than positive symptoms and drug options are very limited. SGAs and adjunctive antidepressants may have modest efficacy.
Reviews: * general (Foussias *et al, J Psychopharmacol* 2015;**29**:116–126; Chue and Lalonde, *Neuropsychiatr Dis Treat* 2014:**10**;777–89; FFT).

Combinations and adjuncts

5HT3 antagonists * (ondansetron, granisetron, tropisetron)
Meta-analysis suggests 5HT3-ANTs are more effective for negative symptoms than placebo (s=6, n=311, RCTs, p/c, Kishi *et al, Neuromolecular Med* 2014;**16**:61–9).

Antidepressants + antipsychotics *
Adjunct: A systematic review and meta-analysis concluded that antidepressants have modest effects on negative symptoms, statistically significant for fluoxetine and trazodone but not for other antidepressants, e.g. mirtazapine, reboxetine, mianserin, fluvoxamine, sertraline, paroxetine and citalopram (s=23, n=819, Singh *et al, Br J Psychiatry* 2010;**197**:174–9; FFT). They may also reduce the risk of suicide, e.g. in Finns developing schizophrenia:
- Antidepressants reduced the risk by 85%
- Benzodiazepines increased the risk by 91%
- Two or more antipsychotics were not associated with increased all-cause mortality cf. monotherapy.

(n=2588, 35 suicides, four years, Tiihonen *et al, Arch Gen Psychiatry* 2012;**69**:476–83).
Citalopram added to SGAs had no effect on any clinical or cognition measures (n=19, RCT, p/c, c/o, 24/52, Friedman *et al, J Clin Psychopharmacol* 2005;**25**:237–42; n=58, RCT, d/b, p/c, 4/52, Hinklemann *et al, J Clin Psychopharmacol* 2013;**33**:686–90).
Escitalopram was well tolerated but ineffective for negative symptoms in chronic schizophrenia (n=40 [c=34], RCT, d/b, p/c, 10/52, Iancu *et al, Psychiatry Res* 2010;**179**:19–23), but significant improvement has been reported with escitalopram and aripiprazole (n=1, Tsai *et al, Psychiatry Clin Neurol* 2014;**68**:582–3).
Fluoxetine significantly improved PANSS in small open studies of TRS (e.g. n=9, open, 6/52, Goff *et al, Am J Psychiatry* 1990;**147**:492–4).
Fluvoxamine is ineffective as augmentation (n=30, open, 12/52, Takashi *et al, Hum Psychopharmacol* 2002;**17**:95–8). Only use with clozapine with extreme care.
Mirtazapine appears clearly and robustly superior to placebo despite the Singh meta-analysis, mirtazapine on almost all measures of improvement as an adjunct in TRS (n=39, RCT, d/b, 6/52, Joffe *et al, Schizophr Res* 2009;**108**:245–51), including risperidone (significantly improved PANSS total scores cf placebo: n=40, RCT, d/b, p/c, 8/52, Abbasi *et al, Schizophr Res* 2010;**116**:101–6), although not all studies are positive (n=40, RCT, d/b, p/c, 6/52, Berk *et al, Hum Psychopharmacol* 2009;**24**:233–8).
Paroxetine has been used successfully (n=8, open, 30/12, Jockers-Scherübl *et al, J Clin Psychiatry* 2001;**62**:573).
Reboxetine was ineffective (n=58, RCT, d/b, p/c, 4/52, Hinklemann *et al, J Clin Psychopharmacol* 2013;**33**:686–90).
Sertraline may improve negative or depressive symptoms (n=26, d/b, p/c, 8/52, Mulholland *et al, J Psychopharmacol* 2003;**17**:107–12).
Tricyclics are at best ineffective as adjuncts (n=58, RCT, d/b, p/c, 4/52, Kramer *et al, Arch Gen Psychiatry* 1989;**46**:922–8).

Asenapine *
Asenapine has had an effect on persistent

negative symptoms over 6/12 and might even be better over the next 6/12 (n=502, 12/12, Potkin *et al*, *Schizophr Res* 2013;**150**:442–9).

Cholinesterase inhibitors + TAU

Adjunct: Galantamine may improve refractory negative symptoms (n=86, RCT, d/b, p/c, 12/52, Buchanan *et al*, *Am J Psychiatry* 2008;**165**:82–9), but not in every study (n=83 [c=73], RCT, d/b, p/c, 12/52, Conley *et al*, *Clin Neuropharmacol* 2009;**32**:69–74; FFT).

Cycloserine (D-cycloserine) + TAU

Adjunct: Cycloserine, a partial agonist of NMDA glutamate receptors, has significantly reduced negative symptoms as an adjunct to risperidone and olanzapine (n=24, d/b, p/c, c/o, 6/52, Heresco-Levy *et al*, *Am J Psychiatry* 2002;**159**:480–2).

Cyproheptadine + haloperidol

Adjunct: Adding cyproheptadine 24mg/d to haloperidol 30mg/d has significantly reduced negative symptoms (n=30, RCT, Akhondzadeh *et al*, *J Clin Pharm Ther* 1999;**24**:49).

Desmopressin + risperidone *

Adjunct: DDAVP spray 20mcg/d as an adjunct has shown significant improvement in negative symptoms in chronic schizophrenia (n=40, RCT, d/b, p/c, 8/52, Hosseini *et al*, *Eur Neuropsychopharmacol* 2014;**24**:846–55).

DHEA (dehydroepiandrosterone) + TAU

Adjunct: DHEA 100mg/d might improve negative symptoms, although Cochrane concludes that the studies are short, inconclusive and unconvincing (s=3, n=126, Elias and Kumar, *Cochrane Database Syst Rev* 2007;**3**:CD006197).

Folate + TAU

Adjunct: Folate supplements did not improve negative symptoms except in people with at least one copy of the MTHFRT allele (n=32 [c=28], RCT, d/b, p/c, 12/52, Hill *et al*, *Schizophr Res* 2011:**127**:41–5). An earlier review concluded that the data was inadequate, inconsistent and unconvincing (s=7, n=885, Muntjewerff and Blom, *Prog Neuropsychopharmacol Biol Psychiatry* 2005;**29**:1133–9).

Folate + vitamin B12 *

Adjunct: Folate and vitamin B12 supplements can improve negative symptoms of schizophrenia but only in people with genetic variants of the 484T gene (n=140[c=121], RCT, d/b, p/c, 16/52, Roffman *et al*, *JAMA Psychiatry* 2013;**70**:481–9).

Glycine + TAU

Adjunct: High-dose glycine (0.8g/kg/d) added to olanzapine or risperidone significantly reduced negative symptoms by 23% and improved cognitive function (e.g. n=17, RCT, d/b, p/c, c/o, 6/52, Heresco-Levy *et al*, *Biol Psychiatry* 2004;**15**:165–71), although some studies are negative (n=30, d/b, p/c, Evins *et al*, *Am J Psychiatry* 2000;**157**:826–8).

Granisetron + risperidone *

Adjunct: Granisetron (2mg/d) as an adjunct to risperidone (up to 6mg/d) showed significantly greater improvement on negative subscales, albeit not for positive/general symptoms (n=40[c=38], RCT, d/b, p/c, 8/52, Khodaie-Ardakani *et al*, *J Psychiatr Res* 2013;**47**:472–8).

Memantine + risperidone *

Adjunct: Memantine is tolerable and significantly improves primary negative symptoms (n=40[c=38], RCT, d/b, p/c, 8/52, Rezaei *et al*, *J Clin Psychopharmacol* 2013;**33**:336–42).

Minocycline + risperidone *

Minocycline 200mg/d can improve negative symptoms, particularly in early-phase schizophrenia (n=92, RCT, d/b, p/c, 16/52, Liu *et al*, *Schizophr Res* 2014;**153**:169–76; n=144[c=94], Chaudhry *et al*, *J Psychopharmacol* 2012;**26**:1185–93).

Mirtazapine + risperidone *

Adjunct: A meta-analysis showed adjunctive mirtazapine can improve negative symptoms (s=5, RCT, d/b, Vidal *et al*, *Clin Schizophr Relat Psychoses* 2014;**9**: 88–95).

Modafinil + antipsychotic

Adjunct: A systematic review and meta-analysis concluded that (ar)modafinil 200mg/d significantly reduced negative symptoms with no effects on other symptoms (s=8, n=372,

RCT, Andrade *et al*, *J Psychiatr Res* 2015;**60**:14–21).

N-acetylcysteine (NAC) + risperidone *

As an adjunct to risperidone, NAC (<2g/d) reduced negative and total PANSS symptoms, but not positive or general symptoms (n=42, RCT, d/b, p/c, 8/52, Farokhnia *et al*, *Clin Neuropharmacol* 2013;**36**:185–92).

Oxytocin + antipsychotics *

Adjunct: Oxytocin intranasal spray with risperidone improved positive symptoms by week 8, and improved negative and total symptoms, but probably not clinically significantly (n=40[c=37], RCT, d/b, p/c, 8/52, Modabbernia *et al*, *CNS Drugs* 2013;**27**:57–65) and can improve negative symptoms (n=14, RCT, d/b, p/c, 6/52, Gibson *et al*, *Schizophr Res* 2014;**156**:261–5).

Riluzole + risperidone *

Adjunct: Riluzole can improve negative symptoms cf. placebo (n=50, RCT, d/b, p/c, 8/52, Farokhnia *et al*, *Psychopharmacology [Berl]* 2014;**231**:533–42).

Selegiline + TAU

Adjunct: Low-dose oral selegiline may improve negative symptoms of schizophrenia (n=67, d/b, p/c, 12/52, Bodkin *et al*, *Am J Psychiatry* 2005;**162**:388–90).

Sildenafil + risperidone

Adjunct: Sildenafil added to risperidone significantly improved negative symptoms of schizophrenia (n=40, RCT, d/b, p/c, 8/52, Akhondzadeh *et al*, *Psychopharmacol (Berl)* 2011;**213**:809–15).

1.21.5 PSYCHOSIS IN PARKINSON'S DISEASE (PPD)

Symptoms and incidence:

Up to 20% of people with Parkinson's disease (PD) and on drug treatment are actively psychotic at any one time and up to 50% have psychosis at some point. Psychotic symptoms are most commonly visual hallucinations (14%), auditory hallucinations (7%), illusions or misidentifications (7%) and paranoia (5%). These are five times more likely with comorbid depression and sleep-wakefulness (n=191, Lee and Weintraub, *Mov Disord* 2012;**27**:858–63; FFT). Symptoms are generally persistent and difficult to treat.

Causes:

Psychosis can occur as part of the PD process or, more often, as an ADR of dopamine agonists (see C5). The psychosis needs managing fully as it causes distress to the person and carers and leads to the need for early residential care and early death, whereas effective treatment reduces premature mortality (n=59, 26/12, open, Factor *et al*, *Neurology* 2003;**60**:1756–61).

Management:

1. Optimise any dopamine agonists, as early management reduces the risk of deterioration (Zahodne and Fernandez, *Curr Treat Options Neurol* 2010;**12**:200–11; FFT).
2. Exclude organic causes, e.g. infection or electrolyte imbalances.
3. If not too distressing, consider not treating but monitoring carefully.
4. Adjust or stop anticholinergics or dopamine agonists; the order of discontinuing should be anticholinergics, amantadine, MAO-B inhibitors, dopamine agonists and then COMT inhibitors (Fernandez, *Cleve Clin J Med* 2012;**79**:28–35). Levodopa should be reduced to the minimum effective and tolerable doses.
5. Clozapine is the first (and probably only) antipsychotic choice. Start at 6.25mg/d and keep doses below 50mg/d. Quetiapine can be tried, but has failed major controlled trials. Olanzapine, aripiprazole, ziprasidone and others are likely to have greater motor ADRs than acceptable; straight dopamine blockers such as risperidone and haloperidol should be avoided (review, Eng and Welty, *Am J Geriatr Pharmacother* 2010;**8**:316–30).
6. Consider a cholinesterase inhibitor, as they can sometimes help people with PD not on dopamine agonists (review by Friedman, *Parkinsonism Relat Disord* 2010;**16**:553–60).
7. ECT can be used for refractory psychosis (e.g. Ueda *et al*, *J ECT* 2010;**26**:111–5), including combined with clozapine (n=2, Factor *et al*, *J Neuropsychiatry Clin Neurosci*

1995;**7**:304–7; n=1, Muralidharan *et al, Indian J Psychiatry* 2011;**53**:156–8; FFT).

Reviews: * general (Herrmann *et al, Drugs Aging* 2013;**30**:19–22; Goldman and Holden, *Curr Treat Options Neurol* 2014;**16**:281).

BNF listed

Clozapine

Clozapine is the only antipsychotic licensed in the UK for PPD and also the only one where there is good evidence for efficacy. Two RCTs show a low dose (mean 25–35 mg/d) significantly improves drug-induced psychosis without significant motor deterioration (n=60, RCT, d/b, p/c, 20/52, Pollak *et al, J Neurol Neurosurg Psychiatry* 2004;**75**:689–95; FFT; n=60, RCT, d/b, p/c, 14/12, PSG, *N Engl J Med* 1999;**340**:757–63; FFT). Follow-up studies have shown continued efficacy (n=39, >2 years, Fernandez *et al, Mov Disord* 2004;**19**:831–3) even up to five years (n=32, Klein *et al, Clin Neuropharmacol* 2003;**26**:8–11). Higher doses (e.g. 70 mg/d) may be poorly tolerated (n=43 [c=23], Gomide *et al, Arq Neuropsiquiatr* 2008;**66**:611–4; FFT). A retrospective chart review showed that *all* patients who were admitted to nursing homes in US stopped clozapine (even if effective) due to logistical issues, so this needs to be resolved (n=38, Hack *et al, PLoS One* 2014;**9**:e91545).

• Unlicensed/some efficacy

Aripiprazole

Although aripiprazole 1–5 mg/d can be successful (n=3, Lopez-Meza *et al, J Neuropsychiatry Clin Neurosci* 2005;**17**:421–2), many have exacerbation of motor symptoms (n=14 [c=8], open, Friedman *et al, Mov Disord* 2006;**21**:2078–81).

Clomipramine

Psychosis with comorbid depression both improved with clomipramine (n=1, Meco and Bernardi, *Prog Neuropsychopharmacol Biol Psychiatry* 2007;**31**:311–3).

Mirtazapine *

There are many cases of reduced auditory hallucinations in PPD with mirtazapine (e.g. n=1, Tagai *et al, Psychogeriatrics* 2013;**13**:103–7; n=1, Godschalx-Dekker and Siegers, *Pharmacopsychiatry* 2014;**47**:81–3).

Olanzapine

Olanzapine has relatively low EPSEs and might be thought of as a viable option but two studies failed to show olanzapine efficacy for dopamimetic-induced psychosis (s=2, p/c, 4/52, Breier *et al, Biol Psychiatry* 2002;**52**:438–45;MS), and most studies show worsening of motor symptoms (e.g. n=30[c=27], RCT, d/b, p/c, 9/52, Ondo *et al, Mov Disord* 2002;**17**;1031–5).

Pimavanserin * (not licensed in UK)

Pimavanserin is a 5-HT2A inverse agonist, effective for PPD (n=199[c=185], RCT, d/b, p/c, 6/52, Cummings *et al, Lancet* 2014;**383**:533–40) by potentiating the antipsychotic effects of very low dose risperidone and reducing haloperidol's EPSEs, allowing low doses to be used. It has been granted Breakthrough Therapy status in USA.

Reviews: * general (Hacksell *et al, Neurochem Res* 2014;**39**:2008–17; FFT; Friedman, *Expert Opin Pharmacother* 2013;**14**;1969–75).

Quetiapine *

Quetiapine has relatively low EPSEs and might be thought of as another viable option, but all the RCTs (s=5, n=138, 8–12/52) are negative, except the one that excluded delusions (n=58 [c=32], RCT, d/b, p/c, 3/12, Rabey *et al, Mov Disord* 2007;**22**:313–8; review by Shotbolt *et al, Ther Adv Neurol Disord* 2010;**3**:339–50). Quetiapine may be worth a cautious trial but do not expect too much.

Risperidone

Low dose risperidone (mean 1.1 mg/d) can improve PPD without motor ADRs in some people (n=17[c=15], open, 12/52, Mohr *et al, Mov Disord* 2000;**15**:1230–7).

Ziprasidone

Ziprasidone (mean 35 mg/d) was as effective and well tolerated as clozapine (mean 32 mg/d) for PPD (n=16[c=14], RCT, s/b, 4/52, Pintor *et al, Clin Neuropharmacol* 2012;**35**:61–6).

RAPID-CYCLING BIPOLAR DISORDER

see Bipolar disorder, rapid-cycling (*1.10.4*)

1.22 SEASONAL AFFECTIVE DISORDER (SAD)

see Depression (*1.14*), Mania and hypomania (*1.10.2*) and Bipolar mood disorders (*1.10*)

SAD is a recurrent affective disorder, predominantly major depression, but it can include mania or hypomania. It has a characteristic seasonal relationship, usually autumn or winter for at least two or three years, with full remission at a characteristic time of the year and outnumbering any non-seasonal episodes. The incidence may be around 1–10% (e.g. 2.4% in North Wales) and peaks in winter. Atypical depressive features include hypersomnia, increased appetite and weight and carbohydrate cravings. It may be caused by excess melatonin secretion, delayed or reduced amplitude circadian rhythms, or serotonergic dysfunction. It is often undiagnosed and half of sufferers are given other depressive diagnoses and antidepressants (n = 1999, Michalak *et al*, *Br J Psychiatry* 2001;**179**:31–4; FFT). Light therapy is first choice for SAD (n=96, RCT, Lam *et al*, *Am J Psychiatry* 2006;**163**:805–12) and, although better tolerated than fluoxetine, it is not without risk, with side-effects including jumpiness (9%), headache (8%), and nausea (16%).

Role of drugs

While phototherapy is well established, drug treatment, e.g. bupropion and sertraline may also be effective. The risk of seasonal major depression can be minimised by starting an antidepressant early in the season while the person is still well (e.g. with bupropion 150–300mg/d; s=3, n=1042, RCT, p/c, Modell *et al*, *Biol Psychiatry* 2005;**58**:658–67). Cochrane concludes that there is weak evidence for fluoxetine as superior to placebo and equivalent to light therapy, but that's about all (s=3, n=204, 5–8/52, RCT, Thaler *et al*, *Cochrane Database Syst Rev* 2011;**12**:CD008591).

Reviews: * general (Kurlansik and Ibay, *Am Fam Physician* 2012;**86**:1037–41; FFT), long-term treatment (Westrin and Lam, *CNS Drugs* 2007;**21**:901–9).

● Unlicensed/some efficacy

Bupropion *

Bupropion XL is licensed in the USA for SAD, using 150–300mg/d and where treatment is started in the autumn while the person is still well (s=3, n=1042, RCT, p/c, d/b, Modell *et al*, *Biol Psychiatry* 2005;**58**:658–67; review by Niemegeers *et al*, *Expert Opin Drug Metab Toxicol* 2013;**9**:1229–40).

Sertraline

Sertraline (50–200mg/d) was significantly superior to placebo in winter pattern SAD in one study (n=187, RCT, d/b, p/c, O/P, 8/52, Moscovitch *et al*, *Psychopharmacol (Berl)* 2004;**171**:390–7).

■ Unlicensed/possible efficacy

Agomelatine

Seasonal depression may respond to agomelatine (n=37, open, 14/52, Pjrek *et al*, *Psychopharmacology [Berl]* 2007;**190**:575–9).

Beta-blockers

Early enthusiasm for pre-sunrise **propranolol** 60mg/d (n=33, d/b, p/c, Schlager, *Am J Psychiatry* 1994;**151**:1383–5) has waned. **Atenolol** appears even less effective (n=19, d/b, p/c, c/o, Rosenthal *et al*, *Am J Psychiatry* 1988;**145**:52–6).

Duloxetine

Duloxetine may be useful for SAD (n=26, open, 8/52, Pjrek *et al*, *Pharmacopsychiatry* 2008;**41**:100–5).

Melatonin

Melatonin secretion is altered in SAD and exogenous melatonin may have some role (review, Srinivasan *et al*, *World J Biol Psychiatry* 2006;**7**:138–51).

Modafinil

Modafinil may significantly reduce fatigue and sleepiness in SAD (n=13 [c=9], open, 8/52, Lundt, *J Affect Disord* 2004;**81**:173–8).

Reboxetine

A pilot study indicated a rapid and significant

effect, including for atypical symptoms in the first week (n=16, open, 6/52, Hilger *et al*, *Eur Neuropsychopharmacol* 2001;**11**:1–5).

SSRIs (see also sertraline)

Light therapy has an early onset of action and, in responders, **citalopram** significantly reduces relapse in the continuation phase (n=282, p/c, 15/52, Martiny *et al*, *Acta Psychiatr Scand* 2004;**109**:230–4). **Escitalopram** 10–20mg/d appears effective and very well tolerated (n=20, open, 8/52, Pjrek *et al*, *Pharmacopsychiatry* 2007;**40**:20–4) and **fluoxetine** 20mg/d was superior to placebo (59–34%), but was not quite statistically significant (n=68, p/c, 5/52, Lam *et al*, *Am J Psychiatry* 1995;**152**:1765–70).

□ No efficacy

Ginkgo biloba

'Bio-Biloba' was ineffective for preventing winter depression (n=27, RCT, 10/52, Lingaerde *et al*, *Acta Psychiatr Scand* 1999;**100**:62–6).

1.23 SELF-INJURIOUS BEHAVIOUR (SIB)

SIB is a self-destructive behaviour resulting in significant tissue damage, but without lethal intent. It can occur in learning disabilities (e.g. Lesch-Nyhan syndrome), as well as in OCD, sadomasochism, schizophrenia and personality disorders. There seems to be a variety of causes, e.g. relief of dysphoria, poor impulse control and dissociation.

Role of drugs *

Opiate antagonists may be useful where a reward mechanism seems to exist. There is some evidence of a serotonergic involvement. Antipsychotics seem to work mainly via a non-specific sedating mechanism. Cochrane concludes that there is no evidence for antidepressants, antipsychotics or natural products reducing repetitive self-harm (except a small unpublished trial of flupentixol (s=7, n=546, RCT, p/c or a/c, Hawton *et al*, *Cochrane Database Syst Rev* 2015;**7**:CD011777) and that there is no robust evidence for any drug therapy in learning disabilities (s=5, n=50, RCTs, d/b, p/c, Rana *et al*, *Cochrane Database Syst Rev* 2013;**4**:CD009084).

Review: * pharmacological interventions (Gormez *et al*, *J Psychopharmacol* 2014;**28**:624–32).

● Unlicensed/some efficacy

Antipsychotics *

Antipsychotics are frequently prescribed but evidence for their efficacy is suggestive rather than conclusive. **Risperidone** was effective for up to 52 months in 75% of developmentally disabled in-patients (n=31, Ruedrich *et al*, *J Intellect Disabil Res* 2008;**52**:132–40). Low-dose **olanzapine** (5mg/d) has been used successfully for SIB (n=2, Hough, *J Clin Psychiatry* 2001;**62**:296–7). **Clozapine** 150–400mg/d has been effective for SIB in people with a BPD (n=4, Zarzar and McEvoy, *Ther Adv Psychopharmacol* 2013;**3**:272–4) or learning disabilities (n=2, Hammock *et al*, *J Autism Dev Disord* 2001;**31**:109–13).

Naltrexone/naloxone

There is conflicting data about the efficacy of naltrexone in SIB. Some studies show some effects when used in adequate dose for an adequate duration, e.g. 25–100mg/d orally (n=4, Sandman *et al*, *Am J Ment Retard* 1990;**95**:93–102), although lower doses (e.g. 10–50mg/d) may also be effective and it undoubtedly helps some people (e.g. n=1, 32/52, Griengl *et al*, *Acta Psychiatr Scand* 2001;**103**:234–6; n=1 plus review, White and Schultz, *Am J Psychiatry* 2000;**157**:1574–82). Some trials have shown a lack of efficacy (e.g. n=33, d/b, p/c, c/o, Willemsen-Swinkels *et al*, *Arch Gen Psychiatry* 1995;**52**:766–73). SIB may get worse over the first few weeks of naltrexone, but then improve and so short studies could miss the effect. There is some evidence of raised opioid peptide activity in autism, Fragile-X syndrome and other mental handicaps.

Review: Symons *et al*, *Ment Retard Dev Disabil Res Rev* 2004;**10**:193–200.

■ Unlicensed/possible efficacy

Buspirone

In people with LD, SIB and anxiety, 64%

responded to doses of 20–45 mg/d, with a maximal response at three weeks (n=14, open, Ratey *et al*, *J Clin Psychiatry* 1989;**50**:382).

Lithium

Some old studies have suggested that lithium is effective in aggression and SIB with lithium levels of 0.7–1.0 mEq/L (n=42, d/b, p/c, 4/12, Craft *et al*, *Br J Psychiatry* 1987;**150**:685–9).

Omega-3 fatty acids

Omega-3 fatty acids may reduce suicidal markers and improve well-being in recurrent self-harmers, but have no effect on impulsivity, aggression and hostility (n=49, RCT, d/b, p/c, 12/52, Hallahan *et al*, *Br J Psychiatry* 2007;**190**:118–22; FFT).

Oxcarbazepine

Oxcarbazepine has been used for SIB in bulimia (Cordas *et al*, *Int J Neuropsychopharmacol* 2006;**9**:769–71).

*** Case reports**

- **Cholinesterase inhibitors** (n=1, Alagiakrishnan *et al*, *J Am Geriatr Soc* 2003;**51**:1326)
- **Lamotrigine + fluoxetine** (n=1, Schupak, *Prog Neuropsychopharmacol Biol Psychiatry* 2007;**31**:1337–8)
- **Pregabalin** (n=1, Fornaro *et al*, *Gen Hosp Psychiatry* 2012;**34**:321.e1–4)
- **Topiramate** (n=1, Cassano *et al*, *Bipolar Disorders* 2001;**3**:161).

1.24 SEXUAL DEVIANCY DISORDERS

Sexual deviancy disorders are abnormalities of a basic biological drive and are recognised as psychiatric syndromes. They include exhibitionism, fetishism, sexual masochism or sadism, paedophilia and voyeurism, but not rape (considered a sexual expression of aggression rather than an aggressive expression of sexuality). The main characteristic is of intense, recurrent sexual arousal and fantasies, particularly connected with inanimate objects, children, non-consenting adults or the self.

Role of drugs *

Pharmacotherapy is controversial but may sometimes be a useful adjunct to other therapies, due to the chronic nature of the disease and its high and unpredictable relapse rates. Combining pharmacology with psychotherapy is associated with better outcomes, e.g. antiandrogens plus CBT seems most effective for severe paraphilias and SSRIs for milder paraphilias and sexual compulsions. LHRH antagonists work similarly to physical castration but are reversible. Deviant sexual behaviour is rare in women and so drug therapy is usually aimed at reducing sexual drive in men.

Reviews: * drug treatment of paraphilic and non-paraphilic sexual disorders (Assumpção *et al*, *Psychiatr Clin North Am* 2014;**37**:173–181; Garcia and Thibaut, *Drugs* 2011;**71**:771–90).

BNF listed

Benperidol

Benperidol is a butyrophenone which, although touted for the control of deviant antisocial sexual behaviour, has no proven use other than as an antipsychotic (*Drug Ther Bull* 1974;**12**:12).

Cyproterone (acetate)

Cyproterone is licensed to treat severe hypersexuality and sexual deviation in men. It has both antiandrogenic and antigonadotropic actions and disrupts the receptors' response to androgens. It can reduce sexual interest, drive and arousal, as well as deviant fantasies and behaviour, and significantly reduces some sexual behaviours in paraphilias and paedophilia (n=19, RCT, d/b, p/c, c/o, Bradford *et al*, *Arch Sex Behav* 1993;**22**:383–402). The onset of action may be delayed for 2–3 weeks and is reversible within 3–6 weeks of stopping. An adequate trial of four months is usually recommended. A depot injection is available on a named patient basis and a syrup can be made.

Triptorelin pamoate *

Triptorelin pamoate is an LHRH antagonist presented as a 3-monthly injection and is licensed for testosterone reduction in adult men with severe sexual deviation. The published evidence is sparse (n=6, Thibaut *et al*, *Acta Psychiatr Scand* 1993;**87**:445–50).

• Unlicensed/some efficacy

LHRH antagonists

Luteinising hormone-releasing hormone (LHRH, gonadorelin) antagonists can produce reversible chemical castration and have a potent effect on sexual deviancy. A thorough but dated review concluded that LHRH antagonists offer a treatment option for severe paraphilia, with little or no relapse if the patient remains under treatment (s=13, n=118, Briken *et al*, *J Clin Psychiatry* 2003;**64**:890–7). **Nafarelin** and **flutamide** (a pure antiandrogen similar to cyproterone) have been used. **Leuprolide** acetate is an alternative and a depot leuprolide significantly suppressed self-reported deviant sexual interests and behaviour and was well tolerated, although bone demineralisation occurred in 25% (n=12, open, Krueger and Kaplan, *Arch Sex Behav* 2001;**30**:409–22).

SSRIs

Reduced daily frequency and duration of paraphilia and related disorders has been shown (n=26, open, case series, Kafka and Hennen, *J Clin Psychiatry* 2000;**61**:664–70; n=1, Mania *et al*, *Prim Care Companion J Clin Psychiatry* 2006;**8**:106; FFT). **Citalopram** has been effective for hypersexuality in early Alzheimer's disease (n=1, Tosto *et al*, *Neurol Sci* 2008;**29**:269–70). SSRI-induced anorgasmia may be a contributory factor to this effect.

■ Unlicensed/possible efficacy

Medroxyprogesterone (acetate)

Medroxyprogesterone has indirect anti-androgenic activity by inhibiting testosterone release from the testes and increasing its clearance, resulting in suppression of sexual arousal and libido. It was successful in a case series for inappropriate sexual behaviour in elderly men with dementia (n=5, case series, Light and Holroyd, *J Psychiatry Neurosci* 2006;**31**:132–4; FFT).

Methylphenidate

Methylphenidate has been used cautiously to augment the effect of SSRIs in paraphilias and related disorders (n=26, Kafka and Hennen, *J Clin Psychiatry* 2000;**61**:664–70).

Mirtazapine

Mirtazapine 15–30mg/d had some efficacy (50% were very much improved) in reducing inappropriate sexual behaviours in people with ASD (n=10, open, 8/52, Coskun *et al*, *J Child Adolesc Psychopharmacol* 2009;**19**:203–6).

Naltrexone *

Naltrexone had a positive response in 15 adolescent sexual offenders, with a therapeutic window of 50–200mg/d. Of the six non-responders, five responded to leuprolide (n=21, open, Ryback, *J Clin Psychiatry* 2004;**65**:982–6; see also n=1, effective over 11/12, Firoz *et al*, *Asian J Psychiatr* 2014;**8**:67–8). Compulsive sexual behaviour has been treated with naltrexone and SSRIs (n=2, Raymond *et al*, *Int Clin Psychopharmacol* 2002;**17**:201–5).

✱ Case reports *

- **Aripiprazole** (Reeves and Perry, *J Clin Psychopharmacol* 2013;**33**:145–6)
- **Carbamazepine** (n=1, Freymann *et al*, *Pharmacopsychiatry* 2005;**38**:144–5; n=1, Bach *et al*, *Mov Disord* 2009;**24**:1241–2)
- **Gabapentin** (n=3, Alkhalil *et al*, *Am J Ther* 2004;**11**:231–5)
- **Lithium** for sexual obsessions in Asperger's Syndrome (n=1, Shahani, *J Neuropsychiatry Clin Neurosci* 2012;**24**:E17)
- **Oxcarbazepine** (n=1, Corretti and Baldi, *Arch Sex Behav* 2010;**39**:1025–6)
- **Propranolol** 10mg BD (n=1, Deepmala and Agrawal, *Ann Pharmacother* 2014;**48**:1385–8)
- **Quetiapine** (n=1, Prakash *et al*, *Am J Alzheimer's Dis Other Demen* 2009;**24**:136–40)
- **Rivastigmine** (n=1, Canavelli *et al*, *Alzheimer Dis Assoc Disord* 2013;**27**:287–8)
- **Topiramate** (n=1, Khazaal and Zullion, *BMC Psychiatry* 2006;**6**:22; FFT).

1.25 SOCIAL ANXIETY DISORDER (SOCIAL PHOBIA DISORDER)

see also Anxiety disorder (*1.6*)

Social anxiety is the second most common phobia (incidence in USA is 5%; n=43093, Grant *et al*, *J Clin Psychiatry* 2005;**66**:1351–61) where the person fears public ridicule, scrutiny and negative evaluation, with fear of embarrassment, criticism or making a public mistake. Feared situations include public speaking, social gatherings, writing under supervision or eating and drinking in public. Anticipatory anxiety leads to impaired performance. This is a serious and disabling anxiety disorder, associated with reduction in quality of life (s=3, n=829, RCTs, p/c, Stein and Kean, *Am J Psychiatry* 2000;**157**:1606–13) and a high risk of alcohol dependence and abuse, but is underdiagnosed with less than 5% of sufferers receiving a diagnosis (n=3862, Katzelnick *et al*, *Am J Psychiatry* 2001;**158**:1999–2007). Early diagnosis and treatment may be vital (Kahalid-Khan *et al*, *Paediatr Drugs* 2007;**9**:227–37).

Role of drugs

Meta-analyses of the effect sizes (including all six UK SSRIs) conclude that SSRIs are more effective than placebo, with improvements also in social and occupational functioning (e.g. s=15, n=3527, RCT, d/b, p/c, 10–24/52, Hansen *et al*, *Int Clin Psychopharmacol* 2008;**23**:170–9; FFT). Effect sizes are highest with phenelzine, then paroxetine, venlafaxine and moclobemide (s=39, p/c, RCT, Davis *et al*, *Expert Opin Pharmacother* 2014;**15**:2281–91). The only predictor of response is length of treatment, which should be at least 12 weeks (Stein *et al*, *J Clin Psychiatry* 2002;**63**:152–5).

Reviews: * meta-analysis (s=234, n=37333, Bandelow *et al*, *Int Clin Psychopharmacol* 2015;**30**:183–92), evidence-based pharmacotherapy (Blanco *et al*, *Int J Neuropsychopharmacol* 2013;**16**:235–49), general (Canton *et al*, *Neuropsychiatr Dis Treat* 2012;**8**:203–15; FFT).

BNF listed

Escitalopram *

Escitalopram should be started at 10mg/d, increased to a maximum of 20mg/d or reduced to 5mg/d, depending upon response. Any trial should last at least four weeks before further intervention is considered (s=40, Baldwin *et al*, *Hum Psychopharmacol* 2009;**24**:269–75). Efficacy has been shown, e.g. 10–20mg/d is superior to placebo (54% vs 39% response) using the LSAS total score (n=358, RCT, p/c, d/b, 12/52, Kasper *et al*, *Br J Psychiatry* 2005;**186**:222–6; FFT). It is effective for relapse prevention (placebo=50%, escitalopram 20%) with an NNT of 3.3 (s=4, RCT, d/b, 24/52, Bech *et al*, *J Clin Psychiatry* 2010;**71**:121–9) and to help the fear of blushing (n=39[c=28], open, 12/52, Pelissolo and Moukheiber, *J Clin Psychopharmacol* 2013;**33**:695–8).

Paroxetine

Paroxetine is superior to placebo, e.g. at 20–50mg/d reducing symptoms and avoidance, with 40mg/d the optimum dose (n=384, d/b, 12/52, Liebowitz *et al*, *J Clin Psychiatry* 2002;**63**:66–74). Lack of response at eight weeks does not necessarily predict long-term lack of response and so a minimum of 12 weeks' treatment is necessary (review, s=3, Stein *et al*, *J Clin Psychiatry* 2002;**63**:152–5). It may be effective for relapse prevention (n=323[c=257], RCT, p/c, 36/52, Stein *et al*, *Arch Gen Psychiatry* 2002;**59**:1111–8).

Venlafaxine

Venlafaxine XL is licensed for moderate-to-severe generalised social anxiety disorder (n=279[c=173], RCT, d/b, p/c, 12/52, Liebowitz *et al*, *J Clin Psychiatry* 2005;**66**:238–47). The standard dose of 75mg/d is as effective and well tolerated as paroxetine 20–50mg/d (n=413[c=318], RCT, p/c, d/b, 12/52, Liebowitz *et al*, *Arch Gen Psychiatry* 2005;**62**:190–8), although 150–225mg/d has been used (n=386, d/b, p/c, 6/12, Stein *et al*, *Psychopharmacol (Berl)* 2005;**177**:280–8), with lower doses in children and adolescents (n=293, RCT, p/c, 16/52, March *et al*, *Biol Psychiatry* 2007;**62**:1149–54).

Combinations

Paroxetine + clonazepam

Unlike panic disorder, combining a BDZ with paroxetine did not lead to a quicker response (n=28[c=19], RCT, d/b, p/c, 10/52, Seedat and Stein, *J Clin Psychiatry* 2004;**65**:244–8).

• Unlicensed/some efficacy

Benzodiazepines

Benzodiazepines have a rapid onset, good tolerability and flexible dosing, but cause sedation, lack of coordination and long-term use has potential risks. **Diazepam** may be ineffective but **clonazepam** has been widely studied (Jefferson, *J Clin Psychiatry* 2001;**62**[Suppl 1]:S50–S53).

Botulinum toxin

Severe axillary hyperhydrosis has been treated with botulinum toxin, significantly improving overall disability (n=40, RCT, p/c, 8/52, Connor *et al*, *J Clin Psychiatry* 2006;**67**:30–6).

Gabapentin

Gabapentin (900–3600 mg/d) may be well tolerated and significantly reduce symptoms (n=69, RCT, d/b, p/c, 14/52, Pande *et al*, *J Clin Psychopharmacol* 1999;**19**:341–8), and 1800 mg/d was as effective as tiagabine for symptom reduction (n=8, RCT, d/b, c/o, 2x4/52, Urbano *et al*, *Prim Care Companion J Clin Psychiatry* 2009;**11**:123; FFT).

MAOIs

Response rates with **phenelzine** are 54% (at 12/52) and 48% (at 24/52) but 72% and 78% respectively if combined with cognitive behavioural group therapy (n=128, Blanco *et al*, *Arch Gen Psychiatry* 2010;**67**:286–95; FFT). MAOIs may need robust dosing, e.g. mean dose of phenelzine of 66 mg/d (n=7, open, Aarre, *Nord J Psychiatry* 2003;**57**:313–5) and tranylcypromine 60 mg/d (n=36, d/b, 12/52, Nardi *et al*, *Psychiatry Res* 2010;**175**:260–5).

Moclobemide

Moclobemide was more effective for subjective general anxiety, CBT for avoidant behaviour and the combination most rapidly effective (n=81 [c=66], RCT, p/c, 6/12+24/12, Prasko *et al*, *Neuro Endocrinol Lett* 2006;**27**:473–81).

Pregabalin

Two studies have shown that 600 mg/d is the minimum effective dose (e.g. n=329, RCT, d/b, p/c, 11/52, Feltner *et al*, *Int Clin Psychopharmacol* 2011;**26**:213–20). Relapse prevention efficacy has been shown over six months at 450 mg/d (n=153, RCT, d/b, p/c, 26/52, Greist *et al*, *Int Clin Psychopharmacol* 2011;**26**:243–51).

SSRIs (paroxetine, escitalopram and venlafaxine are licensed)

Improvement in social anxiety symptoms may lag behind depression resolution, and may need more than 12 weeks for full response (n=21, open, 12/52, Schneier *et al*, *Depress Anxiety* 2003;**17**:191–6).

Citalopram 40 mg/d appears well tolerated and as effective (75% response) as moclobemide (n=71, RCT, s/b, 8/52, Atmaca *et al*, *Hum Psychopharmacol* 2002;**17**:401–5).

Fluvoxamine may have some role (e.g. n=279, RCT, p/c, 12/52, Davidson *et al*, *J Clin Psychopharmacol* 2004;**24**:118–25; n=112, 24/52 extension, Stein *et al*, *Int J Neuropsychopharmacol* 2003;**6**:317–23).

Fluoxetine up to 60 mg/d was not superior to placebo, although placebo had a high response rate (n=60, RCT, d/b, 14/52, Kobak *et al*, *J Clin Psychopharmacol* 2002;**22**:257–62).

Sertraline is licensed in some countries for social anxiety. Up to 200 mg/d is more effective than placebo (e.g. n=415, RCT, d/b, p/c, 12/52, Liebowitz *et al*, *J Clin Psychiatry* 2003;**64**:785–92) and effective as relapse prevention, but relapse may occur on discontinuation (n=375, RCT, p/c, d/b, one year, Haug *et al*, *Br J Psychiatry* 2003;**182**:312–8; FFT).

Tiagabine (see gabapentin)

■ Unlicensed/possible efficacy

Cannabidiol

A report suggests cannabidiol reduces social anxiety symptoms (n=10, d/b, p/c, c/o, Crippa *et al*, *J Psychopharmacol* 2011;**25**:121–30).

Oxytocin

Intranasal oxytocin reduces anticipatory anxiety before public speaking, but not the fear of speaking itself (n=14, p/c, de Oliveira *et al*, *J Psychopharmacol* 2012;**26**:497–504).

Quetiapine

One study showed a slight positive effect as monotherapy (n=15, RCT, p/c, Vaishnavi *et al*, *Prog Neuropsychopharmacol Biol Psychiatry* 2007;**31**:1464–9), but single doses of 25 mg were ineffective for social anxiety, and caused drowsiness (n=20, RCT, d/b, p/c, c/o, Donahue *et al*, *J Anxiety Disord* 2008;**23**:362–8).

☐ No efficacy

Atomoxetine

Atomoxetine was ineffective for social anxiety (n=27, RCT, d/b, p/c, 10/52, Ravindran *et al*, *J Clin Psychopharmacol* 2009;**29**:561–4).

Beta-blockers

There is no evidence for efficacy, except perhaps where management of tremor is essential, e.g. musicians (e.g. nadolol; n=31, d/b, c/o, s/b, James and Savage, *Am Heart J* 1984;**108**:1150–5). Pindolol 15mg/d was no more effective than placebo in augmenting SSRIs (n=14, d/b, p/c, c/o, 4/52, Stein *et al*, *Am J Psychiatry* 2001;**158**:1725–7), but illicit self-medication with propranolol (up to 320mg/d) has been reported (n=1, Fontanella, *Rev Bras Psiquiatr* 2003;**25**:228–30; FFT), with symptoms manageable with adjunctive paroxetine, so maybe it does work, but at higher doses.

Caffeine

Caffeine induces more severe performance anxiety suggesting a hyperreactivity to caffeine (n=28+26, RCT, d/b, c/o, Nardi *et al*, *Psychiatry Res* 2009;**169**:149–53).

Levetiracetam

Levetiracetam was well tolerated but slightly inferior to placebo for social anxiety (e.g. n=217, RCT, d/b, p/c, 12/52, Stein *et al*, *J Clin Psychiatry* 2010;**71**:627–31).

Mirtazapine

Mirtazapine 30–45mg/d was ineffective in the major trial (n=60, RCT, d/b, p/c, 12/52, Schutters *et al*, *Int Clin Psychopharmacol* 2010;**25**:302–4), but seemed effective in women with social anxiety without comorbid psychiatric illness (n=66[c=60], RCT, d/b, p/c, 10/52, Muehlbacher *et al*, *J Clin Psychopharmacol* 2005;**25**:580–3).

St John's wort

SJW was not superior to placebo in one trial (n=40, RCT, p/c, 12/52, Kobak *et al*, *J Clin Psychopharmacol* 2005;**25**:51–8).

Sulpiride

Sulpiride has no detectable effect (n=23, RCT d/b, p/c, c/o, Bell *et al*, *J Psychopharmacol* 2013;**27**:146–51).

Valproate

A small study showed valproate completely ineffective at up to 1500mg/d (n=16, mentioned by Jefferson, *J Clin Psychiatry* 2001;**62**[Suppl 1]:S50–S53).

1.26 TOURETTE'S SYNDROME (GILLES DE LA TOURETTE)

see also OCD (*1.18*) and SIB (*1.23*)

The main diagnostic symptoms of this hereditary disorder include multiple tics, vocal tics (grunts, snarls, throat clearing and obscenities), stereotyped movements (jumping and dancing), overactivity, learning difficulties and emotional problems. The incidence is 1–5 per 10000 and is more common in males. It has an onset at 5–6 years, beginning with respiratory or vocal tics with grunting or barking noises. Psychiatric comorbidity is common, e.g. OCD, anxiety, depression and ADHD.

Role of drugs

If the condition is affecting the person's abilities to function, drug therapy may be useful. Low starting doses, gradual increases and adequate therapeutic trials are necessary.

Reviews: * general (Cavanna and Seri, *BMJ* 2013;**347**:f4964; Kurlan, *New Engl J Med* 2010;**363**:2332–8), emerging treatments (Termine *et al*, *Int Rev Neurobiol* 2013;**112**:445–80); pharmacotherapies (Egolf and Coffey, *Drugs Today [Barc]* 2014;**50**:159–79; Roessner *et al*, *Neuropharmacology* 2013;**68**:143–9).

BNF listed

Haloperidol

Haloperidol 0.5–40mg/d was the licensed drug of choice and remains a treatment option. Side-effects may be limiting and its efficacy has been questioned (n=22, p/c, d/b, Sallee *et al*, *Am J Psychiatry* 1997;**154**:1057–62). See also pimozide and nicotine chewing gum.

Pimozide

Cochrane concludes that pimozide is effective (s=6, n=162, RCT, Pringsheim and Marras,

Cochrane Database Syst Rev 2009;**2**:CD006996). ECG is essential monitoring (see *3.2.1*).

• Unlicensed/some efficacy

Antipsychotics (see also BNF Listed) *

Aripiprazole response rates have been 66% (vs. 45% for placebo; n=61[c=54], RCT, d/b, p/c, 10/52, Yoo *et al*, *J Clin Psychiatry* 2013;**74**:772–80). The optimum dose is around 12mg (range 5–45mg) and, although around 33% do not tolerate or respond, aripiprazole can be very effective for the rest (eg. n=100, retrospective, Wenzel *et al*, *J Clin Psychopharmacol* 2012;**32**:548–50).

Fluphenazine can be effective over 26 years, with no cases of TD (n=268, Wijemanne *et al*, *Mov Disord* 2014;**29**:126–30).

Olanzapine (mean 14.5mg/d) has improved aggression and tics, albeit with significant weight gain (n=10, RCT, s/b, 10/52, Stephens *et al*, *J Child Adolesc Psychopharmacol* 2004;**14**:255–66; n=12, open, 6/12, McCracken *et al*, *J Child Adolesc Psychopharmacol* 2008;**18**:501–8; FFT) and response has been maintained at eight years despite a reduction to 2.5mg/d (n=1, Hwang, *Acta Neurol Taiwan* 2012;**21**:165–8).

Quetiapine (mean 175mg/d) may have some efficacy (n=12, retrospective, 8/52, Copur *et al*, *Clin Drug Invest* 2007;**27**:123–30), albeit poorly tolerated (n=12[c=9], open, 8–12/52, de Jonge *et al*, *J Clin Psychiatry* 2007;**68**:1148–50).

Risperidone (mean 2.5mg/d) was clearly superior to placebo on global assessment of Tourette symptoms (n=48, RCT, d/b, p/c, Dion *et al*, *J Clin Psychopharmacol* 2002;**22**:31–9), and a mean dose of 3.8mg/d was at least as effective as pimozide but much better tolerated (n=50, d/b, 12/52, Bruggeman *et al*, *J Clin Psychiatry* 2001;**62**:50–6).

Sulpiride 200–400mg/d has been used, as has **amisulpride** (n=1, Fountoulakis *et al*, *Ann Pharmacother* 2004;**38**:901).

Review: antipsychotics in Tourette's (Cath *et al*, *Tijdschr Psychiatr* 2008;**50**:593–602; FFT).

Clonidine ± TAU

Clonidine 0.1–0.6mg/d may be as effective as haloperidol. Clonidine or methylphenidate alone, or in combination are effective for ADHD with comorbid tics (n=16, RCT, p/c, 16/52, TSSG, *Neurology* 2002;**58**:527–36; review by Goldberg, *EBMH* 2002;**5**:122; FFT), and clonidine 0.1mg/d has been effective (n=12[c=10], RCT, d/b, c/o, 15/52, Hedderick *et al*, *Pediatr Neurol* 2009;**40**:420–5).

Lorazepam ± TAU

Lorazepam 1.5–10mg/d has been useful as adjuvant therapy.

Pergolide

Pergolide (up to 300mcg/d) monotherapy may be safe and effective in children with Tourette's disorder, chronic motor or vocal tic disorder (n=245, RCT, 6/52, Gilbert *et al*, *Neurology* 2000;**54**:1310–6).

Topiramate *

The evidence for topiramate monotherapy in Tourette's is promising, but not conclusive (s=14, n=1003, RCTs, Yang *et al*, *Pediatr Neurol* 2013;**49**:344–550).

■ Unlicensed/possible efficacy

Cannabinoids

THC doses of up to 10mg/d show significant trends in favour of THC on a variety of measures, with no reported adverse effects (n=24, RCT, d/b, 6/52, Muller-Vahl *et al*, *J Clin Psychiatry* 2003;**64**:459–65). In a survey of people with Tourette's who had tried marijuana, 82% reported reduced or remitted motor and vocal tics, urges and OCD symptoms (n=17, Muller-Vahl *et al*, *Acta Psychiatr Scand* 1998;**98**:502–6).

Fluoxetine

Fluoxetine has improved Tourette's symptoms (n=32, open, Como and Kurlan, *Neurology* 1991;**41**:872–4).

Methylphenidate

Methylphenidate can precipitate or aggravate tics (Klein, *Arch Gen Psychiatry* 1995;**52**:429–33), but generally not enough to contraindicate a trial for ADHD with Tourette's (Gadow *et al*, *Arch Gen Psychiatry* 1995;**52**:444–55).

Nicotine + haloperidol

Transdermal nicotine (7mg/d) appears superior

to placebo as an adjunct to haloperidol (eg. n=70 [c=56], d/b, p/c, Silver *et al*, *J Clin Psychiatry* 2001;**62**:707–14). Nicotine chewing gum is an alternative and PRN usage may have a low risk.

Ondansetron

In haloperidol-resistant Tourette's, ondansetron 24mg/d significantly improved tic severity on one rating scale but not on others (n=30, RCT, d/b, p/c, 3/52, Toren *et al*, *J Clin Psychiatry* 2005;**66**:499–503).

Tetrabenazine

For a review of use see Porta *et al*, *Clin Drug Investig* 2008;**28**:443–59.

Valproate *

A systematic review and meta-analysis concluded valproate should not be routinely used for Tourette's in children (s=5, n=247, RCT, Yang *et al*, *Psychiatry Res* 2015;**226**:411–7), although there are cases of response (n=1, Ye and Lippmann, *Clin Neuropharmacol* 2014;**37**;36–7).

● Case reports *

- **Duloxetine** 40mg/d (n=1, Niederhofer, *Prim Care Companion J Clin Psychiatry* 2010;**12**:PCC.09l00889; FFT)
- **Finasteride** 5mg/d (n=1, Bortolato *et al*, *Am J Psychiatry* 2007;**164**:1914–5)
- **Paliperidone** (n=1, Guan and Tsai, *Psychiatry Clin Neurosci* 2013;**67**:128)
- **Quetiapine + clozapine** (n=1, Lan *et al*, *J Child Adolesc Psychopharmacol* 2015;**25**:188–90).

□ No efficacy

Levetiracetam

In a small, but perfectly formed trial, levetiracetam (10mg/kg/d) was completely ineffective (n=12 [c=10], RCT, d/b, c/o, 15/52, Hedderick *et al*, *Pediatr Neurol* 2009;**40**:420–5).

Omega-3 fatty acids

O3FAs had no effect on reducing tics in Tourette's (n=33, RCT, d/b, p/c, 20/52, Gabbay *et al*, *Pediatrics* 2012;**129**:1493–500; FFT).

Pramipexole

Pramipexole seems ineffective for tics, although it may decrease some comorbid ADHD symptoms (n= 63, RCT, d/b, p/c, 6/52, Kurlan *et al*, *Mov Disord* 2012;**27**:775–8).

1.27 TRICHOTILLOMANIA

see also OCD (*1.18*)

Symptoms

Trichotillomania presents as impulsive pulling out of a person's own hair (e.g. scalp, eyebrows, eyelashes, pubic, chest), resulting in relief of tension and hair loss. It is associated with OCD, and can occur in the presence of learning disability, anxiety, depression, schizophrenia and borderline personality disorder. It can be episodic or chronic, and is more common in females.

Role of drugs *

A range of psychological and behaviour therapies can be used and may be most effective when combined with pharmacotherapy. A review has concluded that clomipramine is effective, but that SSRIs are not (s=7, Bloch *et al*, *Biol Psychiatry* 2007;**62**:839–46), and trials need to be at least 8–10 weeks' duration to prove or disprove an effect in an individual case. HRT (habit reversal training) combined with sertraline is more effective than either approach alone (n=24, RCT, d/b, Dougherty *et al*, *J Clin Psychiatry* 2006;**67**:1086–92). Dermatological help is beneficial. Cochrane concludes that the data on pharmacotherapy is small and insufficient to recommend any treatment as yet (s=8, n=204, RCT, 6-12/52, Rothbart *et al*, *Cochrane Database Syst Rev* 2013;**11**:CD007662).

Reviews: * general (Rothbart and Stein, *Expert Opin Pharmacother* 2014;**15**:2709–19; Duke *et al*, *Clin Psychol Rev* 2010;**30**:181–93; Huynh *et al*, *Semin Cutan Med Surg* 2013;**32**:88–94).

+ Combinations

Antipsychotics + SSRI

There have been reports of symptom improvement when **olanzapine** 10mg/d was added to **fluoxetine** 40mg/d (n=2, Srivastava *et al*, *Aust NZ J Psychiatry* 2005;**39**:112–3) or **citalopram** (n=4, Ashton, *Am J Psychiatry* 2001;**158**:1929–30). Resistant trichotillomania has responded to **risperidone** augmentation of **fluvoxamine** (n=1, Gabriel, *Can J Psychiatry* 2001;**46**:285–6).

● Unlicensed/some efficacy

Clomipramine
Several studies (s=7, Bloch *et al*, *Biol Psychiatry* 2007;**62**:839–46) have shown clomipramine at around 180mg/d to be effective in some people with trichotillomania.

Olanzapine (see also combinations)
Olanzapine monotherapy has shown robust efficacy (85% vs 17%) for a wide range of symptoms (n=25[c=25], RCT, d/b, p/c, 12/52, Van Ameringen *et al*, *J Clin Psychiatry* 2010;**71**:1336–43). Up to 10mg/d has produced a significant reduction in hair pulling and anxiety, with 22% achieving full remission (n=18, open, 3/12, Stewart and Nejtek, *J Clin Psychiatry* 2003;**64**:49–52).

■ Unlicensed/possible efficacy

Aripiprazole
A small pilot study suggested aripiprazole (mean 7.5mg/d) might have some efficacy (n=12[c=11], open, 8/52, White and Koran, *J Clin Psychopharmacol* 2011;**31**:503–6), and 1.5–3mg/d has been completely effective (n=1, Yasui-Furukori and Kaneko, *Clin Neuropharmacol* 2011;**34**:258–9).

Bupropion
Bupropion 300–450mg/d has improved SSRI-resistant trichotillomania (n=1, Bipeta and Yerramilli, *J Med Case Rep* 2011;**5**:557; FFT; n=1, Bhanji and Margolese, *J Clin Psychiatry* 2004;**65**:1283) and has been used for relapse prevention (Klipstein and Berman, *J Clin Psychopharmacol* 2012;**32**:298–9).

Lithium
80% patients tried on lithium showed reduced hair pulling and some hair regrowth, possibly via an effect on aggressive behaviour in bipolar disorder (n=10, open, 14/12, Christenson *et al*, *J Clin Psychiatry* 1991;**52**:116–20; Sharma and Corpse, *Arch Women's Ment Health* 2008;**11**:305–6).

N-acetylcysteine (NAC) *
NAC (a glutamate modulator) was ineffective in the only RCT (n=39, RCT, d/b, p/c, Bloch *et al*, *J Am Acad Child Adolesc Psychiatry* 2013;**52**:231–40). Earlier studies had been more promising (eg. n=50, d/b, p/c, 12/52, Grant *et al*, *Arch Gen Psychiatry* 2009;**66**:756–63).

Naltrexone *
Naltrexone has produced a numerical but non-statistically significant reduction in hair-pulling (n=51, RCT, d/b, p/c, 8/52, Grant *et al*, *J Clin Psychopharmacol* 2014;**34**:134–8).

SSRIs (see also combinations)
A major review concluded that SSRIs lack significant clinical effect (s=7, Bloch *et al*, *Biol Psychiatry* 2007;**62**:839–46), although there have been some positive reports, e.g. **citalopram** (a modest but significant effect; n=14, open, 12/52, Stein *et al*, *Eur Arch Psychiatry Clin Neurosci* 1997;**247**:234–6), **escitalopram** (n=1, Bhatia and Sapra, *Eur Psychiatry* 2004;**19**:239–40) and **fluoxetine** (e.g. Winchel *et al*, *J Clin Psychiatry* 1992;**53**:304–8), where the dose needs to be high (up to 80mg/d).

✱ Case reports

- **Aripiprazole + clonazepam** (n=1, Virit *et al*, *J Clin Pharm Ther* 2009;**34**:723–5)
- **Inositol** (n=3, Seedat *et al*, *J Clin Psychiatry* 2001;**62**:60–1)
- **Oxcarbazepine** 1200mg/d (n=1, Leombruni and Gastaldi, *Clin Neuropharmacol* 2010;**33**:107–8)
- **Quetiapine** (n=1, Khouzam *et al*, *Psychiatry* 2002;**65**:261–70)
- **Risperidone + naltrexone** (n=1, Oravecz and Štuhec, *J Am Med Dir Assoc* 2014;**15**:301–2)
- **Valproate** (n=1, Adewuya *et al*, *J Child Adolesc Psychopharmacol* 2008;**18**:533–6).

1.28 CAFFEINISM

Caffeine is an antagonist at adenosine receptors, which increases dopamine activity. Caffeine consumption is classed as follows:

- 250–500mg/d=moderate use

- 600–900 mg/d = caffeinism
- 1000 mg/d and above = toxic range.

Caffeine dependence has features of a typical psychoactive substance dependence, i.e. withdrawal, continued use despite drug-induced problems, tolerance and persistent desire or unsuccessful attempts to cut down or control use. Tolerance develops very quickly to the stimulant effect, e.g. complete tolerance to sleep disruption from 400 mg/d occurs in seven days.

Caffeine withdrawal *

Caffeine withdrawal is a DSM-5 diagnosis and the 14 main withdrawal symptoms fall into three groups (Ozsungur *et al*, *Psychopharmacology [Berl]* 2009;**201**:541–8):

1. Fatigue and headache (52%) — more likely with high habitual use.
2. Dysphoric mood, rebound drowsiness — more likely with high habitual use.
3. Flu-like, somatic — no more likely with high habitual use than low use.

Symptoms of caffeinism (acute or chronic)

Adverse effects of low-to-moderate doses: Diuresis, increased gastric secretion, fine tremor, increased skeletal muscle stamina, mild anxiety, negative mood, palpitations and nervousness.

Adverse effects of high doses: Chronic insomnia, persistent anxiety, restlessness, tension, irritability, tremulousness, panic, poor concentration, confusion, disorientation, paranoia, delirium, tremor, muscle twitching, convulsions, vertigo, dizziness, tinnitus, auditory and visual hallucinations, facial flushing, hyperthermia, nausea, vomiting, abdominal discomfort and tachypnoea. High caffeine use is also associated with high daily cigarette use, aggression, conduct disorder, ADHD and social problems in adolescents (n = 132, Martin *et al*, *Scientific World Journal* 2008;**8**:512–6; FFT).

Adverse consequences: There is some contradictory evidence about the effect of caffeine on people with mental health problems. Clearly, high doses can cause significant effects. Acute high doses (10 mg/kg) significantly increase arousal and have a psychotogenic effect in schizophrenics and make it more resistant to antipsychotics, as well as exacerbate GAD and insomnia. There are reports of lack of correlation between caffeine consumption and anxiety and depression.

Methods of caffeine reduction

1. Recognition of the problems of excess caffeine consumption (>750 mg/d) and the likely benefits of reduction.
2. Identification of all current caffeine sources and the pattern of consumption.
3. Implementation of a planned gradual reduction, e.g. weaker drinks, taken less often, increasing use of caffeine-free equivalent drinks (particularly at 'usual' drinking times of the day) or mixing caffeine and decaffeinated coffee to give a lower strength.
4. Use of analgesia (caffeine-free, of course) for withdrawal headaches.
5. Setting a target for consumption, which does not need to be complete abstinence, e.g. caffeine drinks only at set times in the day, e.g. on rising, etc.

Caffeine content *

Commercial US tea or coffee samples (Chin *et al*, *J Anal Toxicol* 2008;**32**:702–4; FFT) suggest:

- Ordinary teas (green or black) range between 14–61 mg/serving (defined as 6–8oz), with no observable trend by variety
- Herbal teas have no caffeine detectable
- Decaffeinated teas all contain less than 12 mg/serving
- All contained more caffeine the longer they were brewed
- For American specialty coffees, the mean caffeine content ranges from 5.2–12.2 mg/g for powder and 0.23–0.49 mg/g for decaffeinated coffee (Hackett *et al*, *J Anal Toxicol* 2008;**32**:695–701; FFT), so the content of a cup is thus 36–85 mg.

Calculating caffeine intake:

Source	Caffeine content per 100 mL	Caffeine content per container
Brewed coffee	55–85 mg	140–210 mg/cup
Instant coffee	35–45 mg	85–110 mg/cup
Decaf. coffee	2 mg	5 mg/cup
Cocoa	3 mg	7 mg/cup
Brewed tea	25–55 mg	55–140 mg/cup
Coca-cola	11 mg	36 mg/can
Pepsi cola	7 mg	22 mg/can
Milk chocolate		22 mg/100 g
Alka-Seltzer XS		40 mg/tablet
Red Bull (varies by country)		80 mg/250 mL
Relentless		160 mg/500 mL
Lucozade alert		120 mg/60 mL
Lucozade Energy		80mg/500 mL

A cup is taken as being 250 mL

Positive consequences: It has to be mentioned that regular coffee drinkers are less likely to get type 2 diabetes, stroke, depression, early death from any cause, Parkinson's and Alzheimer's (Patil *et al, Mo Med* 2011;**108**:431–8), and rates of depression are lower in women who have four cups of coffee a day or more and were inversely proportional to total intake. Decaffeinated coffee had no associated additional risk (n=50739, 10-year follow-up, Lucas *et al, Arch Intern Med* 2011;**171**:1571–8; FFT). So, caffeine isn't all bad.

Reviews: caffeine and mental health (Lara, *J Alzheimer's Dis* 2010;**20**(Suppl 1):S239–48), caffeine craving questionnaire (West and Roderique-Davies, *J Psychopharmacol* 2008; **22**: 80–91).

1.29 ELECTROCONVULSIVE THERAPY (ECT)

ECT was first used in its current form in 1938 (Linington and Harris, *Br Med J* 1988;**297**:1354–5; FFT). It is effective for rapid and short-term improvement in severe unipolar and bipolar depression (n=220, Bailine *et al, Acta Psychiatr Scand* 2010;**121**:431–6), where other treatments have proven ineffective or life is threatened. It can also be used in mania (especially manic delirium), in TRS where it has helped 54% of people, particularly for positive symptoms (n=253, open, Chanpattana and Sackeim, *J ECT* 2010;**26**:289–98), and more rarely catatonia and drug-resistant Parkinsonism. ECT is probably superior to, or at least as effective as, antidepressants and tends to be quicker-acting in severely depressed people. ECT may be better than antidepressants for the short-term treatment of acute depression (s=6, n=256, UK ECT Group, *Lancet* 2003;**361**:799–808; comment by Bauer, *EBMH* 2003;**6**:83; FFT), although combining maintenance ECT with antidepressants may improve outcomes (n=58, retrospective chart review, Gagné *et al, Am J Psychiatry* 2000;**157**:1960–5).

Induction agents: * **Propofol** (review in ECT, Rasmussen, *J ECT* 2014;**30**:210–5) is widely used as it is well tolerated and short-acting with a quick recovery, although it shortens seizure length by up to 30%, but without significant effect on clinical outcomes (n=62, RCT, Bauer *et al, J ECT* 2009;**25**:85–90). Inhaled **sevoflurane** can be used (n=31, RCT, d/b, Rasmussen *et al, J ECT* 2007;**23**:236–8). **Ketamine** has its own antidepressant effect (see C1) and might enhance ECT (e.g. n=1, Niemegeers *et al, J ECT* 2014;**30**:e31–2) although the only RCT was negative (n=18, RCT, Abdallah *et al, J ECT* 2012;**28**:157–61; systematic review and meta-analysis; McGirr *et al, J Psychiatr Res* 2015;**62**:23-30). A systematic review and meta-analysis of **etomidate** showed EEG seizure duration was longer than methohexital by 2.23s, thiopental by 11.81s and propofol by 17.65sec and that etomidate produced better seizure duration, with myoclonus and painful injection most common ADRs (s=17, Singh *et al, J ECT* 2015;**31**:213–25).

Post-ECT memory loss and agitation: *

Thiamine 50–200mg/d may lead to a rapid resolution (3–5 days) of post-ECT confusion and memory loss, and so thiamine deficiency is implicated in post-ECT confusional state (n=3, Linton *et al, Int J Geriatr Psychiatry* 2002;**7**:189–92).

Promethazine 25–50mg orally 1–2 hours before ECT has been used successfully for severe post-ECT agitation (n=8, Vishne *et al, J ECT* 2005;**21**:118–21).

Cholinesterase inhibitors e.g. **donepezil** can been used successfully for post-ECT memory loss and cognitive deficits (n=45, RCT, t/b, p/c, Prakash *et al, J ECT* 2006;**22**:163–8), as can **rivastigmine** 3–4.5mg (n=30, RCT, d/b, p/c, <4/52, Stryjer *et al, Clin Neuropharmacol* 2012;**35**:161–4) and **galantamine** (n=39, RCT, d/b, p/c, 2/7, Matthews *et al, J ECT* 2013;**29**;170–8).

Dexmedetomidine is an anaesthetic effective for post-ECT agitation (n=1, Cohen and Stewart, *J ECT* 2013;**29**:e23–4).

Liothyronine may abolish post-ECT memory-loss (n=60, d/b, Ghafur *et al, Indian J Psychiatry* 2012;**54**:154–8), unlike piracetam, which doesn't (n=18, d/b, c/o, 3/7, Mindus *et al, Acta Psychiatr Scand* 1975;**51**:319–26), although it might slightly enhance ECT's clinical effect (n=38, RCT, d/b, p/c, >2/52, Tang *et al, J ECT* 2002;**18**:130–7).

Reviews: * comprehensive reviews (Lisanby, *N Engl J Med* 2007;**357**:1939–45), propofol, etomidate and thiopental (Canbek *et al, J ECT* 2014;**31**:91–7), in adolescents (s=39, Lima *et al, Ann Gen Psychiatry* 2013;**12**:17) and in TRD (Kellner *et al, Am J Psychiatry* 2012;**169**:1238–44).

Post-ECT headache: *

Ibuprofen 600mg/d 90 minutes before ECT may reduce the frequency and severity of post-ECT headache (n=34, RCT, p/c, d/b, Leung *et al*, *J Clin Psychiatry* 2003;**64**:551–3).

Mirtazapine may relieve post-ECT headaches and nausea, possibly by 5HT2 and 5HT3 antagonism (case series, Li *et al*, *J ECT* 2011;**27**:165–7).

Topiramate has been used where the headache does not respond to typical pain medicines (e.g. Ye *et al*, *J ECT* 2013;**29**:e49), and where the best reference is also the shortest in this whole book.

5HT$_1$-receptor antagonists such as **eletriptan** (n=72, Kertesz *et al*, *J ECT* 2014;31:105–9), or **sumatriptan** (White *et al*, *Headache* 2006; **46**:692) may help post-ECT headache.

Drug considerations

There are no RCTs of ECT given with concurrent anticonvulsants and one thorough review suggests that there is no evidence that ECT and anticonvulsants cannot be used together (Sienaert and Peuskens, *J ECT* 2007;**23**:120–3).

Agomelatine

There is no published experience on the use of agomelatine with ECT, but no pro- or anticonvulsant effects have been shown (MI).

Amisulpride *

Amisulpride appears safe with ECT, with no significant differences between amisulpride and control groups (n=20+20 controls, Takács *et al*, *Psychiatr Danub* 2013;**25**:76–9; FFT).

Antipsychotics (see also clozapine)

Antipsychotics lower the seizure threshold and would be expected to lead to seizures at lower ECT doses. A review concluded that the combination was safe and effective (Braga and Petrides, *J ECT* 2005;**21**:75–83).

Aripiprazole: no problems reported (n=4, Masdrakis *et al*, *J ECT* 2008;**24**:236–8).

Paliperidone: no problems (n=9, 83 ECTs, Masdrakis *et al*, *Gen Hosp Psychiatry* 2011;**33**: 9–10).

Risperidone LAI: no problems (n=1, Sengul *et al*, *J ECT* 2009;**25**:282–3).

Weekly ECT followed by maintenance as an adjunct to **sulpiride** (n=17), **risperidone** (n=26) and **olanzapine** (n=27) showed long-term safety and some efficacy (especially with olanzapine), albeit with a high drop-out rate (n=70 [c=32], two years, Ravani *et al*, *Psychiatr Danub* 2009;**21**:179–86; FFT).

Benzodiazepines

Benzodiazepines may lessen the improvement with unilateral ECT (n=124, Jha and Stein, *Acta Psychiatr Scand* 1996;**94**:101–4), even several months after stopping, probably by raising the seizure threshold, reducing seizure duration, increasing sub-maximal seizures or by increasing the number of treatments needed.

Bupropion

Use with ECT has been reported (n=2, Kellner *et al*, *J Clin Psychopharmacol* 1994;**14**:215–6), as have prolonged seizures (n=1, Conway and Nelson, *J ECT* 2001;**17**:216–8) and a case of status epilepticus lasting for 12 days after the fourth ECT (n=1, Dersch *et al*, *Pharmacopsychiatry* 2011;**44**:344–6).

Caffeine

Caffeine 125–240mg IV has been used to augment seizure duration (reported by the ideally named Coffey *et al*, *Am J Psychiatry* 1990;**147**:579–85; Jaffe and Dubin, *Am J Psychiatry* 1992;**149**:1610).

Carbamazepine

Seizure durations were slightly shorter with carbamazepine, but this appeared to have no dramatic effect on either the efficacy or side-effects of ECT (n=7, Zarate *et al*, *Ann Clin Psychiatry* 1997;**9**:19–25).

Ciprofloxacin

There is a case of prolonged ECT seizures related to concurrent ciprofloxacin 1g/d (n=1, Kisa *et al*, *J ECT* 2005;**21**:43–4).

Clozapine *

The UK SmPCs recommend suspending clozapine for 24 hours pre-ECT to reduce risk of unwanted or prolonged seizures, protracted delirium or serious hypersalivation (eg. n=2, Manjunatha *et al*, *Indian J Psychol Med* 2011;**33**:80–2; FFT). There have, however, been some case series suggesting clozapine and ECT can be an effective and safe combination provided care is taken, e.g.

even from 24 ECTs with clozapine 1600mg/d (n=1, Keller *et al*, *J ECT* 2009;**25**:280–1). ECT and clozapine improved TRS more than either alone (PANSS score reductions 71% combination, 46% clozapine and 40% placebo) with no significant adverse effects (n=18, p/c, Masoudzadeh and Khalilian, *Pak J Biol Sci* 2007;**10**:4287–90). Clozapine (mean 518mg/d, range 200–900mg/d) and 2–20 sessions of ECT were probably safe and with short-term efficacy (72% showing marked initial improvement but only in 23% beyond 4/12) and in resistant cases (n=22, Havaki-Kontaxaki *et al*, *Clin Neuropharmacol* 2006;**29**:52–6). In adolescents, response to ECT when taking clozapine is similar when taking other antipsychotics or BDZs, charges needed were the same and surprisingly rehospitalisation was lower with the clozapine group cf. non-clozapine group over one year follow-up (n=28, Flamarique *et al*, *J Clin Psychopharmacol* 2012;**32**:756–66). There may be greater efficacy in schizoaffective patients (n=43, Gazdag *et al*, *Ideggyogy Sz* 2006;**59**:261–7). However, not omitting doses is a risky strategy, especially with higher doses of clozapine where the seizure threshold may be significantly lower.

Duloxetine *

Duloxetine has been used successfully (n=1, Hanretta and Malek-Ahmadi, *J ECT* 2006;**22**:139–41), but tachycardia has been reported (n=1, Heinz *et al*, *J ECT* 2013;**29**:e33–5; see short review; Eraslan *et al*, *J ECT* 2011;**27**:51–2).

Escitalopram

There is a report of ECT being well tolerated with escitalopram 20mg/d (n=3, Masdrakis *et al*, *J ECT* 2008;**24**:289–).

Flumazenil

Effective ECT was only possible in a benzodiazepine-dependent depressed woman when the anticonvulsant effect of clonazepam was reversed by flumazenil 0.1mg (n=1, Berigan *et al*, *Am J Psychiatry* 1995;**152**:957).

Ibuprofen (see also headache)

Ibuprofen might increase seizure duration (Kessler, *J Clin Psychiatry* 2004;**65**:442).

Lamotrigine

A retrospective study suggested ECT is well tolerated and effective with lamotrigine, albeit with the occasional missed seizure (n=19, Sienaert *et al*, *J ECT* 2011;**27**:148–52).

Lithium

A prospective study concluded that lithium 'is by and large safe' with ECT provided serum that levels are kept at the lower end of the range. But, maximum heart rate and maximum systolic bp are lower with lithium and post-ECT recovery time is directly correlated with serum lithium levels (n=55, Thirthalli *et al*, *World J Biol Psychiatry* 2011;**12**:149–55). There are some cases of, e.g. prolonged seizure, serotonin syndrome, focal seizures (n=3, Sartorius *et al*, *World J Biol Psychiatry* 2005;**6**:121–4) and delirium (n=1, Sadananda *et al*, *Gen Hosp Psychiatry* 2013;**35**:678.e1–2). Elderly people may be more susceptible to this combination. Some sources recommend discontinuing lithium 48 hours before ECT to prevent this neurotoxicity and not re-starting for several days after the last treatment (Ferrier *et al*, *Adv Psychiatr Treat* 1995;**1**:102–10), although discontinuing lithium would risk discontinuation effects and be potentially dangerous (see lithium in *1.10*).

Review: * general (Rasmussen. *J ECT* 2015;**31**:87–90), safety issues (n=90, Volpe and Tavares, *J Neuropsychiatry Clin Neurosci* 2012;**24**:E33).

MAOIs

A review has concluded that there is no dangerous interaction between MAOIs and ECT (n=4, Dolenc *et al*, *J ECT* 2004;**20**:258–61).

Mirtazapine (see also headache)

There are cases of successful and uneventful use (n=2, Farah, *Convul Ther* 1997;**13**:116–7).

Moclobemide

The SmPC recommends suspending moclobemide for 24 hours pre-ECT, although there are no data to support this.

Moxifloxacin

Moxifloxacin has been associated with prolonged seizures (n=1, Reti and Davydow, *J ECT* 2007;**23**:289–90).

Naloxone
Naloxone has no detectable effect (Rasmussen *et al*, *Convuls Ther* 1997;**13**:44–6).

Rivastigmine (see also memory loss)
There is a case of eight ECTs being successful in a person taking rivastigmine throughout (n=1, Zink *et al*, *J ECT* 2002;**18**:162–4).

Selegiline
There appears no problems with transdermal selegiline and ECT (n=2, Horn *et al*, *Psychosomatics* 2010;**51**:176–8).

SSRIs *
A small study showed a significantly longer seizure duration in people taking SSRIs cf. other antidepressants (n=13, Potokar *et al*, *Int J Psychiatr Clin Pract* 1997;**1**:277–80):
Citalopram: caution advised (SmPC).
Fluoxetine appears not to cause prolonged seizures (n=12, Gutierrez-Esteinou and Pope, *Convul Ther* 1989;**5**:344–8).
Fluvoxamine's SmPC recommends a four-day gap between stopping fluvoxamine and ECT due to reports of prolonged seizures.
Paroxetine seizure length may be twice as long after ECT (n=14, Curran, *Acta Psychiatr Scand* 1995;**92**:239–40).
Sertraline: caution advised (SmPC).

Steroids
In chronic steroid users, additional 'stress doses' are sometimes given before general anaesthesia, but this appears unnecessary for prednisolone (n=27, Rasmussen *et al*, *J ECT* 2008;**24**:128–30).

Theophylline
Theophylline 100–400mg IV has facilitated ECT seizures in previous ECT-resistance (n=7, Leentjens *et al*, *Convuls Ther* 1996;**12**:232–7), although status epilepticus and increased seizure duration have been reported.

Trazodone
Low-dose use does not seem to produce any problems (n=100, Krahn *et al*, *J Clin Psychiatry* 2001;**62**:108–10), although a prolonged seizure has been reported (n=1, Lanes and Ravaris, *Am J Psychiatry* 1993;**150**:525).

Tricyclics
There appear to be no routine problems and nortriptyline might even enhance ECT and reduce cognitive adverse effects (n<319, RCT, Sackeim *et al*, *Arch Gen Psychiatry* 2009;**66**:729–37). The use of anaesthetics could enhance the risk of cardiac arrhythmias and hypotension.

Valproate
Seizure durations may be slightly shorter with valproate but with no effect on the efficacy or side-effects (n=42, RCT, d/b, Jahangard *et al*, *J ECT* 2012;**28**:118–23) and may help ECT-induced migraine (n=1, Rovrs and Roks, *J ECT* 2012;**28**:64–5).

Venlafaxine
Venlafaxine may reduce ECT's efficacy and worsen cognitive adverse effects (n<319, RCT, Sackeim *et al*, *Arch Gen Psychiatry* 2009;**66**:729–37). Venlafaxine seems safe if propofol is the anaesthetic, although asystole has been reported (n=13, Gonzalez-Pinto *et al*, *J Neuropsychiatry Clin Neurosci* 2002; **14**:206–9).

Vortioxetine *
There is no experience as yet, and so caution is recommended (SmPC).

Zopiclone
Reduced seizure length has been reported with zopiclone the previous night (n=2, Tobiansky, *J Psychopharmacol* 1991;**5**:268–9), and so is best avoided.

Ziprasidone
There are cases of safe and well tolerated use (n=8, Masdrakis *et al*, *J ECT* 2010;**26**:139–42).

2 SELECTING DRUGS, DOSES AND PREPARATIONS

Contents

2.1	**Relative side-effects of:**	
2.1.1	Hypnotics	194
2.1.2	Antidepressants	195
2.1.3	Antidepressants pharmacokinetics and receptor effects	197
2.1.4	Antipsychotics	199
2.1.5	Antipsychotics — pharmacokinetics and receptor effects	201
2.1.6	Anxiolytics	203
2.2	**Switching or discontinuing psychotropics**	**204**
2.2.1	Antipsychotics	205
2.2.1.1	General advice	205
2.2.1.2	Specific drug switches	206
2.2.1.3	Antipsychotic dose equivalents	213
2.2.1.4	Post-switching antipsychotic issues	214
2.2.1.5	Depot and LAI injections	216
2.2.2	Benzodiazepines	216
2.2.3	Anticholinergics	216
2.2.4	Drugs of abuse	216
2.2.5	ADHD treatments	226
2.2.6	Anticholinesterase inhibitors	226
2.2.7	Antidepressants	228

TABLE 2.1.1: HYPNOTICS — RELATIVE SIDE-EFFECTS *

Class	Drug	Usual night dose mg/d	Adult max dose mg/d	Elderly max dose mg/d	Elimination half-life (hours) adult	Elimination half-life (hours) elderly	G/I upset	Hang-over	Dependence potential
Shorter-acting benzodiazepines									
1a	Loprazolam	1	2	7	10	24	❍	●	●
1a	Lormetazepam	1	1.5+	<Ad	10	14	❍	●	●
1a	Temazepam	10–20	40	20	5–11	14+	❍	●	●●
Longer-acting benzodiazepines									
1b	Flunitrazepam (U)	1	2	1	35	35	❍	●●	●
1b	Flurazepam	15	30	15+	47–95	?	❍	●●●	●●
1b	Nitrazepam	5	10	5	18–36	40+	❍	●●●	●
Chloral and derivatives									
2	Chloral betane	707	5 tabs	<Ad?	7–10	Same	●●●	●	●
Other hypnotics									
3	Clomethiazole#	N/A#	2 caps#	Same	4–5	Same	❍	●	●●
4	Promethazine	25	50	–	10–19	10–19	❍	●●	❍
5	Zaleplon	10	10	5	2	3	❍	❍	❍
6	Zopiclone	7.5	7.5	<Ad	3.5–6	8	●	●	●
7	Zolpidem	5	(10)	10	2(2–3)	Longer	❍	❍	❍
8	Melatonin	2	2	2	3.5–4	3.5–4	❍	❍	❍

Classes

1a = Shorter-acting or minimally-accumulating benzodiazepines
1b = Longer-acting or accumulating benzodiazepines
2 = Chloral and derivative
3 = Clomethiazole (chlormethiazole)
4 = Antihistamine
5 = Pyrazolopyrimidine
6 = Imidazopyridine
7 = Cyclopyrrone
8 = Melatonin

Side-effects frequency (severity will be dose-related)

●●● = Marked effect
●● = Moderate effect
● = Mild effect
❍ = Little or nothing reported
? = No information available

Other abbreviations

Usual night dose = suggested usual dose for an adult in the UK SmPC
Adult max dose = suggested maximum adult hypnotic dose in the UK SmPC
Elderly max dose = suggested maximum elderly hypnotic dose in the UK SmPC
# = 1 capsule is therapeutically equivalent to 5 mL syrup. Indicated for severe insomnia in the elderly only
U = unlicensed in UK

TABLE 2.1.2: ANTIDEPRESSANTS — RELATIVE SIDE-EFFECTS *

Drug	Adult max dose mg/d	Elderly max dose mg/d	Relative side-effects (most will be dose-related): Anti-cholinergic	Cardiac	Nausea ‡	Sedation	Overdose §	Pro-convulsant potential	Sexual dysfunction
Tricyclics									
Amitriptyline	200	75	●●●	●●●	●●	●●●	●●●	●●	●●
Clomipramine	250	75	●●●	●●	●●	●●	●	●●	●●●
Dosulepin (dothiepin)	150	75	●●	●●	○	●●●	●●●	●●	●●
Doxepin	300	<Adult	●	●●	●	●●	●●	●●	●●
Imipramine	300	50	●●	●●	●●	●	●●●	●●	●●
Lofepramine	210	<Adult	●●	●	●	●	○	○	●●
Nortriptyline	150	50	●●	●	●●	●	●●	●	●●
Trimipramine	300	<Adult	●●●	●●	●	●●	●●	●	●●
SSRIs									
Citalopram	60	40	○	○	●●●	○	●	○	●●
Escitalopram	20	<20	○	○	●●	○	○	○	●●
Fluoxetine	(20)	(60)	○	○	●●	○	○	○	●●
Fluvoxamine	300	300	●	○	●●●	●	○	○	●
Paroxetine	50	40	○	○	●●	○	○	○	●●●
Sertraline	200	200	○	○	●●	○	○	○	●●
MAOIs									
Isocarboxazid	60	<Adult	●●	●●	●●	○	●●	○	●
Phenelzine	90	(90)	●	●	●●	●	●●●	○	●
Tranylcypromine	CA30	(30)	●	●	●●	●	●●●	○	●

TABLE 2.1.2: ANTIDEPRESSANTS — RELATIVE SIDE-EFFECTS (CONT) *

Drug	Adult max dose mg/d	Elderly max dose mg/d	Relative side-effects (most will be dose-related)						
			Anti-cholinergic	Cardiac	Nausea ‡	Sedation	Overdose §	Pro-convulsant potential	Sexual dysfunction
Others									
Agomelatine	50	50	❍	❍	❍	❍	❍	❍	❍
Bupropion/amfebutamone (U)	(450)	(450)	●	❍	●	❍	●●	●●●	❍
Duloxetine	120	120	❍	❍	●●	●	?	?	●●
Flupentixol	3	2	●●	❍	❍	●	●	?	●
Mianserin	90+	<Adult	●	❍	❍	●●●	❍	❍	●
Mirtazapine	45	45	❍	❍	❍	●●	❍	●●	❍
Moclobemide	600	600?	●	❍	●	❍	❍	?	●
Reboxetine	12	Not recommended	●	●	●	❍	❍	❍	❍
Trazodone	600	Care above 300	●	●	●●●	●●	●	❍	●●
Tryptophan	6g	6g	❍	❍	●	●●	●	❍	❍
Venlafaxine	375	375	❍	❍	●●	❍	●	❍?	❍
Vortioxetine	20	Care above 10	❍	❍	●●	❍	●	❍	❍

Side-effects frequency (severity will be dose-related)

●●● = Marked effect
●● = Moderate effect
● = Mild effect
❍ = Little or minimal effect
? = No information or little reported
U = Unlicensed in UK for depression

Other abbreviations

‡ = Typical serotonergic side-effect
Adult max dose = Maximum adult oral antidepressant dose in UK SmPC
Elderly max dose = Maximum elderly oral antidepressant dose as stated in UK SmPC. Most state that half the adult dose may be sufficient
Overdose § = Based on UK Fatal Toxicity Index (Henry *et al*, *BMJ* 1995;**310**:221–4; FFT). For review of epidemiology and relative toxicity of antidepressant drugs in overdose see Henry (*Drug Saf* 1997;**16**:374–90)

TABLE 2.1.3: ANTIDEPRESSANTS — PHARMACOKINETICS AND RECEPTOR EFFECTS *

Drug	Major active metabolites	Half-life (t½ in hours)	Peak plasma conc (Tmax in hours)	Reuptake inhibition			Receptor affinity										
				5-HT SERT	NA/NE NET	DA DAT	5HT1A	5HT1D	5HT2A	5HT2B	5HT2C	5HT3	5HT7	Melatonin	Histamine-1	Aplha-1	Muscarinic
Tricyclics																	
Amitriptyline		8–24	6	+++	++	O	+		+++		+++		+	O	+++	++	++
	Nortriptyline	See below															
Clomipramine		17–28	2.5	+++	++	O	+		+		++	++	+	O	++	++	++
	Desmethylclomipramine	>36	4–24	+++	++	O	O		+		++	++	+	O	++	++	
Dosulepin		14–40	3	+++	++	O	O		+					O	+++	+	++
(dothiepin)	Desmethyldothiepin	22–60	2														
Doxepin		8–24	4	++	++	O	+		++		+++			O	+++	++	++
	Desmethyldoxepin	30–72	–														
Imipramine		4–18	2	++	++	O	O		+		+		O	O	++	++	++
	Desipramine	12–24	(4–5)	+	+++	O	+				+		O	O	++	+	+
Lofepramine		1.6	1–2	++	+++	O								O			++
	Desipramine	As above		+	++++	O											
Nortriptyline		18–96	(4–5)	++	+++	O	+		+++		+++			O	++	++	++
Trimipramine	(Desmethyltrimipramine)	7–23	3	++	O	O			++		++	O		O	++	++	+
Selective serotonin reuptake inhibitors (SSRIs)																	
Citalopram		33	2–4	+++	O	O	O		O	O	O			O	O	O	O
Escitalopram		30	2–4	+++	O	O	O		O	O	O			O	O	O	O
Fluoxetine		24–140	6–8	+++	+	O			+	O	+			O	O	O	O/+
	Norfluoxetine	168–216	–	+	–	–											
Fluvoxamine	None	13–22	2–8	+++	+	O								O	O	O/+?	O
Paroxetine	None	24	6	+++	+	O								O	O		+
Sertraline		25–36	4–10	+++	+	+								O	O	+	O
	Desmethylsertraline	66–109	8–12	+	–	–											

TABLE 2.1.3: ANTIDEPRESSANTS — PHARMACOKINETICS AND RECEPTOR EFFECTS (CONT) *

Drug	Major active metabolites	Half-life (t½ in hours)	Peak plasma conc (Tmax in hours)	Reuptake inhibition			Receptor affinity										
				5HT SERT	NA/NE NET	DA DAT	5HT1A	5HT1D	5HT2A	5HT2B	5HT2C	5HT3	5HT7	Melatonin	Histamine-1	Alpha-1	Muscarinic
Monoamine oxidase inhibitors																	
Isocarboxazid	Not known	N/K	2–3	↑	↑	↑											
Phenelzine	Not known	1.5	2–3	↑	↑	↑											
Tranylcypromine	Not known	2.5	2–3	↑	↑	↑											
Others																	
Agomelatine	None	1–2	1–2	❍	❍	❍	❍	❍	❍	+	+			++	❍	❍	❍
Bupropion		3–16 (variable)	4	❍	❍	+	❍		❍	❍	❍			❍	❍	❍	❍
	Hydroxybupropion	12–38															
Duloxetine	Not known	8–17	6	+++	+++	+	❍	❍	+	❍	+		❍	❍	❍	❍	❍
Flupentixol	Not known	35	3–8	–	–	–											
Mianserin		12–29	1–3	❍	++	❍			++						+++	++	+
	Desmethyl-8-hydroxy																
Mirtazapine	None	20–40	1–3	↑	↑	❍			++	❍	++	❍	+	❍	+++	+	+
Moclobemide	None	1–2	1	↑	↑	↑											
Reboxetine	Not known	13	2	❍	+++	❍											
Trazodone		3–7	½–2	++#	❍	❍	+	+	++	++	+	❍	+	❍	+	❍	❍
	mCPP			+	❍	❍	++	+	++	++	++	+	+	❍	+	❍	❍
Venlafaxine §		1–2	5(2–7)	++§	+§	+§	❍	❍	❍	❍	❍	❍	❍	❍	❍	❍	❍
	Desmethylvenlafaxine		10(8–13)														
Vortioxetine	None	66	7–11	+++	(↑)	❍	++‡	+				++	+		❍	❍	❍

Abbreviations

+++ = Potent reuptake inhibitor or receptor affinity
++ = Moderate reuptake inhibitor or receptor affinity
+ = Minor reuptake inhibitor or receptor affinity
❍ = Minimal/no reuptake inhibitor or receptor
§ = Dose-dependent reuptake inhibition
↑ = Cytoplasm levels increase
‡ = Partial Agonism
SERT = Serotonin Transporter
NET = Noradrenaline/norepinephrine Transporter
DAT = Dopamine (Active) Transporter

Receptor functions and associations

5HT1A = Memory, learning, anxiety, mood
5HT1D = Vasoconstriction
5HT2A = Mood and anxiety
5HT2B = Empathy
5HT2C = Appetite, mood
5HT3 = Anxiety, emesis
5HT7 = Cognition, mood
Melatonin = Sleep-wake
Histamine = Wakefulness, appetite
Alpha-1 = Smooth muscles, bp
Muscarinic = Cognition

TABLE 2.1.4: ANTIPSYCHOTICS — RELATIVE SIDE-EFFECTS *

Drug	Adult max dose mg/d	Elderly max dose mg/d	Relative side-effects (most will be dose-related)								
			Anti-cholinergic	Cardiac	EPSE	Hypo-tension	Sedation	Minor O/D	Weight gain	Prolactin	Procon-vulsant
Phenothiazines											
Chlorpromazine	1000	<Adult	●●	●●	●●	●●●	●●●	●●●	●●●	●●●?	●●●
Levomepromazine (methotrimeprazine)	1000	NR	●●●	●●	●●?	●●●	●●●	●●●	?	●●●?	●●?
Promazine	800	<Adult	●●	●●	●	●●	●●	●●	?	●●●?	●●?
Pericyazine	(300)	<Adult	●	●●	●	●●	●●●	●●	?	●●●?	●●?
Perphenazine	24	<Adult	○	●●	●●	●	●●	●●	●●●	●●●?	●●?
Trifluoperazine	–	<Adult	●●●	●●	●●	●	●	●●	?	●●●?	●
Other first generation											
Benperidol	1.5	<Adult	?	?	?	●	●●	?	?	●●●?	●?
Haloperidol	30	30	●●	●●	●●●	●	●	●	●	●●●	●?
Flupentixol	18	<Adult	●●	○	●●	○	●	●	●	●●?	●?
Zuclopenthixol	150	<Adult	●●	●	●●●	●	●●	●●	?	●●?	○?
Pimozide	20	<Adult	●●●	●●●	●●	●●	●	●	○	●●●?	●
Amisulpride	1200	1200	●●	○	●	○	○	○	●	●●	●?
Sulpiride	2400	2400	●	○	●	○	●	●	●	●●	○?
Depot and long-acting injections (continued on the next page) ♦											
Flupentixol decanoate	400–1/52	<Adult	●●	○	●●	○	●	●	?	●●?	●?
Fluphenazine decanoate	100–2/52	<Adult	●●	●●	●●●	●	●●	●	●	●●●?	●
Fluspirilene *(discontinued in UK)*	20–1/52	<Adult	●●	●	●●	●●	●●	?	?	●●●?	●
Haloperidol decanoate	300–4/52	<Adult	●	●●	●●●	●	●	●	●	●●●	●
Pipotiazine palmitate *(discontinued)*	200–4/52	<Adult	○	●●	●●	●	●	?	?	●●●?	●●?
Zuclopenthixol decanoate	600–1/52	<Adult	●●●	●	●●●	●	●●	●●	?	●●?	○?

TABLE 2.1.4: ANTIPSYCHOTICS — RELATIVE SIDE-EFFECTS (CONT) *

Drug	Adult max dose mg/d	Elderly max dose mg/d	Relative side-effects (most will be dose-related)								
			Anti-cholinergic	Cardiac	EPSE	Hypo-tension	Sedation	Minor O/D	Weight gain	Prolactin	Procon-vulsant
Depot and long-acting injections (continued) †											
Aripiprazole LAI	400-month	See SmPC	❍	●	●	❍	❍	?	●	❍	❍
Risperidone LAI	50–2/52	25–2/52	❍	❍	●	●	●?	❍	●	●●	❍
Olanzapine pamoate	300–2/52	See SmPC	●	❍	❍	❍	●●	❍	●●●	●	●●
Paliperidone palmitate	150–month	See SmPC	❍	❍	●	●	●	❍	●	●●	❍
Second generation/atypicals											
Aripiprazole	30	30	❍	●	●	❍	❍	?	●	❍	❍
Asenapine *(Unlicensed use in UK)*	(10)	(20)	❍	❍	●	●	●●	?	●	❍	❍
Clozapine	900	(900)	●●	●●●	❍	●	●●●	?	●●●	❍	●●●
Lurasidone	148 (=160)‡	≤Adult	❍	❍	●	❍	●	?	❍	❍	❍
Olanzapine	20	20	●	❍	❍	❍	●●	❍	●●●	●	●●
Paliperidone	12	12	❍	❍	●	●	●	❍	●	●●	❍
Quetiapine	800	<Adult	●	●	❍	●	●●	●	●	●	●
Risperidone	(16)	4	●	❍	●	●	●?	❍	●	●●	❍
Ziprasidone *(Unlicensed in UK)*	–	–	❍	●●	❍	❍	❍	?	❍	❍	❍

Side-effects frequency (severity will be dose-related)

●●● = Marked effect
●● = Moderate effect
● = Mild/transient effect
❍ = Little or minimal effect
? = No information or little reported
‡ = Europe 148mg = 160mg USA dose

Other abbreviations

Adult max dose = Maximum adult oral antipsychotic dose as stated in UK SmPC or BNF. May be different for other indications

Elderly max dose = Maximum oral antipsychotic dose in the elderly as stated in UK SmPC or BNF. Most state that a starting dose of half to a quarter of the adult dose should be adequate, with smaller dose increments

† = 100–2/52 means 100mg every two weeks; 400–1/52 means 400mg every week, etc

TABLE 2.1.5: ANTIPSYCHOTICS — PHARMACOKINETICS AND RECEPTOR EFFECTS

Drug/group	Receptor affinity										$5HT_{2a}:D_2$ affinity ratio	Half-life (t½ in hours)	Time to peak (oral) (2) hours	Main active metabolite(s)
	D_1	D_2	D_3	D_4	$5HT_{1A}$	$5HT_{2A}$	M_1	α-1	α-2	H_1				
Phenothiazines														
Chlorpromazine	++	+	++	+		+++	++	+++	+	+++	10:1	6(2–119)	3(IM 1–4, IV 2–4)	Many
Fluphenazine HCl Fluphenazine decanoate	++	+++	+++	++		++	+	++	❍	?	1:2	FHCl 33 FD 14–27/7	FHCl 3	Some, unclear if active
Levomepromazine	++	++	+++	?		+++	+++	+++	❍	+++	5:1	15–30	1–3	Some, unclear if active
Pericyazine[3]	++?	+?	++?	+?		+++?	+++?			++?		NK	NK	NK
Perphenazine	++	++	NK	?		+++	+	++	++	+++	2:1	10(8–12)	4–8	Some, unclear if active
Trifluoperazine	++	++	NK	+		+++	+	+++	+	+	2:1	24	2–4	Several
Other first generations														
Benperidol	+?	+++	+?	+?		+?	❍?	+?	+?	++?	NK	8	2	1% unchanged in urine
Haloperidol HCl Haloperidol decanoate	++	+++	+++	+++	+	++	+	++	+	+	1:25	HHCl 21 (9–38) HD 21/7	2–6	Hydroxy-haloperidol
Flupentixol HCl Flupentixol decanoate												FHCl 22–36 FD 3–7/7(1)	FHCl 3–6 FD 3–10/7	Inactive
Zuclopenthixol HCl Zuclopenthixol decanoate Zuclopenthixol acetate	++	+++	+	NK		+++	++	++	NK	+	1:3	20	ZHCl 3–4 ZD 5–7 days ZA 24–48	Inactive
Sulpiride	❍	+++	+	❍		❍	❍	❍	❍	❍	1:50	6–8	2–6	Nil
Amisulpride	❍	+++	+++	❍		❍	❍	❍	❍	❍		12–17	1–4	Nil
Pimozide	+	+++	+++	+		+++	+	+++	+	❍	1:5	53–55	6–8	Some, unclear if active
Fluspirilene	NK	NK	NK	NK	NK	NK	NK	NK	NK	NK	NK	32–300	1–48	Inactive

TABLE 2.1.5: ANTIPSYCHOTICS — PHARMACOKINETICS AND RECEPTOR EFFECTS (CONT) *

Drug/group	Receptor affinity[5] D_1	D_2	D_3	D_4	$5HT_{1A}$	$5HT_{2A}$	M_1	α-1	α-2	H_1	$5HT_{2a}$:D_2 affinity ratio	Half-life (t½)	Tmax (time to peak, oral)[2]	Main active metabolite(s)
Second generation/Atypicals														
Aripiprazole Aripiprazole LAI	❍	++++	❍	❍	PAg	AAnt	❍	❍	❍	❍	N/A	75(31–146) 30–46 days	3–7 hours 3 days (deltoid) 7 days (gluteal)	Dehydroaripiprazole
Asenapine	++	+++	++	++	+++	+++	❍	++	++	+	20:1?	6–23 hours[8]	0.5–1.5 hours	Minor
Clozapine	++	++[4]	++	++	++	+++	+++	+++	++	+++	20–30:1	4–12 hours	2–3 hours	Norclozapine
Lurasidone	❍?	+++	❍?	❍?	PAg	+++	❍	++	++	❍		18 hours	1–3 hours	ID-14283
Olanzapine Olanzapine pamoate	++	++[4]	++	++	+	+++	++	++	+	+++	50:1	30(21–54) hours 30(13–42)/7	3–6 hours 2–4 days	Inactive
Paliperidone Paliperidone palmitate	+	+++	+++	++	+	+++	❍	+++	++	+++		23 hours 29–45 days	23–29 hours 13 days	None known
Quetiapine	❍	++	+	+	++	++	❍	++	❍	+++	1:1	7 hours	1.5, XL 5–6 hours	N-desalkylquetiapine (t½ 12 hours)
Risperidone Risperidone LAI	+	+++	++	++	++	+++	❍	+++	+++	++	8–11:1	20–30 hours 21–28 days?	1–2 (7) hours 35 days	Hydroxyrisperidone
Ziprasidone	+	+++	++	+	+++	+++	❍	++	+	❍	3:1	7	4–5 hours	Many

Receptor binding: +++ = High affinity; ++ = Moderate; + = Low; ❍ =Very low; NK = Not known; ? = Possible; PAg = Partial agonist with very high affinity; AAnt = Antagonist

1. Flupentixol decanoate's half-life is longer (up to 17 days) on continuous administration
2. Time to oral peak may vary if taken with food or the site of LAI injection
3. Receptor-binding studies for pericyazine have not been published, but it has been reported to have some differences to chlorpromazine
4. Olanzapine and clozapine appear to have some D2 limbic selectivity
5. Inclusion of a receptor may give some guide to therapeutic action and adverse effects
6. There is a considerable degree of variation between published sources, depending upon how the results are presented, whether they are single studies or averages, the receptor sources, assay type, etc. These figures should be taken only as a guide, eg. there is little, or nothing published about fluspirilene or pericyazine
7. All oral preparations, including tablets, orodispersible and liquid
8. Biphasic half-life: 6 hours for the first 18 hours, then terminal half-life is 23 hours.

TABLE 2.1.6: ANXIOLYTICS — RELATIVE SIDE-EFFECTS *

Class	Drug	Usual dose mg/d	Adult max dose mg/d	Elderly max dose mg/d	Half-life (hours) Adult (+ range)	Half-life (hours) Elderly	Hang-over	Dependence potential
Shorter-acting benzodiazepines								
Ia	Lorazepam	4	4	<Ad	12 (8–25)	Same	●●●	●●●
Ia	Oxazepam	30	120	80	8 (5–15)	Same	●●	●●
Longer-acting benzodiazepines								
Ib	Chlordiazepoxide	30	100	<50	12 (6–30)	L	●●●	●●
Ib	Clobazam	30	60	20	18 (9–77)	L	●	●●
Ib	Diazepam	6	30	15	32 (21–50)	L	●●●	●●
Beta-blockers								
2	Oxprenolol	80	80	80	4# (3–6)	Same	❍	❍
2	Propranolol	80	120	–	2# (1–2)	Same	❍	❍
Other anxiolytics								
3	Buspirone	30	45	45	7 (2–11)	Same	❍	❍
4	Pregabalin	300	600	<600	6	L	❍	❍
5	Duloxetine	30	120	120	8–17	Same?	❍	❍
5	Venlafaxine	75	75	75	1–2	Same	❍	❍
6	Escitalopram	10	20	<Ad	30	L	❍	❍
6	Paroxetine	20	50	40	c24	c24	❍	❍

Classes:
Ia = Shorter-acting or minimally-accumulating benzodiazepines
Ib = Longer-acting or accumulating benzodiazepines. These also have metabolites that enhance their length of action
2 = Beta-blockers
3 = Azapirone (azaspirodecanedione)
4 = Anticonvulsant
5 = SNRI
6 = SSRI

Side-effects frequency (severity will be dose-related)
●●● = Marked effect ❍ = Little or nothing reported
●● = Moderate effect
● = Mild effect

Other abbreviations
Adult max dose = Suggested maximum oral dose in the UK SmPC. Most recommend treatment for up to four weeks
Elderly max dose = Suggested maximum oral dose in the elderly in the UK SmPC. Most state that half the adult dose should be adequate
# = Pharmacological action longer than half-life suggests
L = Longer in elderly than younger adults

The data on this and the previous pages is based on a large number of papers. Note was taken of presentation of data, equivalence of dose used, etc. When non-comparable papers are excluded, there is a surprisingly high level of consistency on reported relative side-effects. Individual's response may, of course, vary widely. Many effects may be dose-related.

2.2 SWITCHING OR DISCONTINUING PSYCHOTROPICS

Switching psychotropics can be achieved using a variety of methods, varying in rate, overlap, gap and complexity. The main types are summarised in the graphs and comments. The remarks below specifically relating to antipsychotics are marked with †.

Switch 1: Drug-free interval
(Discontinue first drug, leave drug-free interval, introduce second drug)

Advantages:

1. Minimises combined ADRs.
2. Relapse risk is not too high if the person is relatively stable and the gap is not prolonged.
3. Minimal interaction potential.
4. Side-effects from the second drug are less likely to be confused with discontinuation effects from the first drug.
5. Anticholinergic doses can be titrated as needed. †
6. Ideal (but often impractical) for switches to clozapine to reduce the additive myelosuppressive potential. †
7. Lowest medication error potential.

Disadvantages:

1. Takes time, which delays the desired relief of symptoms or side-effects.
2. Potential for relapse or deterioration during the gap and changeover.
3. Early relapse before reaching a therapeutic dose of the second drug might be interpreted as its lack of efficacy.

Switch 2: No interval
(Stop first drug, start second immediately)

Advantages:

1. Straightforward.
2. Low medication error potential.
3. Can be used for inpatient settings with better supervision.
4. Appropriate where an acute severe ADR has occurred, e.g. statutory abrupt withdrawal of clozapine due to a blood dyscrasia. †
5. May be acceptable for high-risk switches to clozapine to reduce additive myelosuppressive potential, but retaining antipsychotic cover. †

TABLE 2.2.1: SWITCHING PSYCHOTROPICS

Switch 1: Drug-free interval (safest)

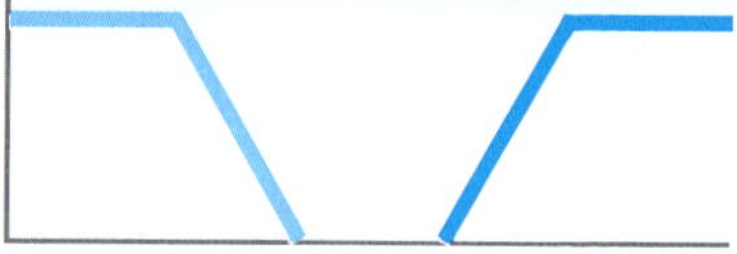

Switch 2a: No interval (generally preferred)

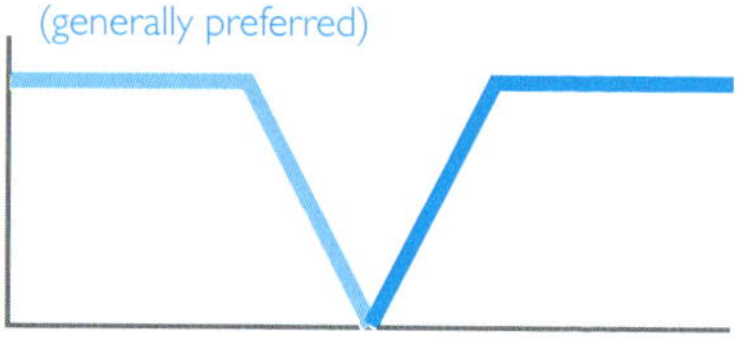

Switch 2b: Abrupt switch (risks discontinuation symptoms)

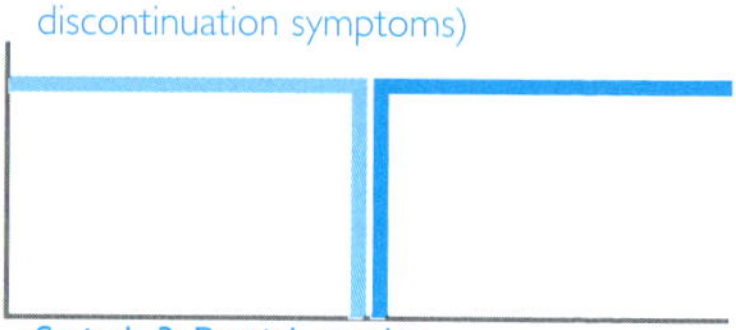

Switch 3: Partial overlap (usually acceptable)

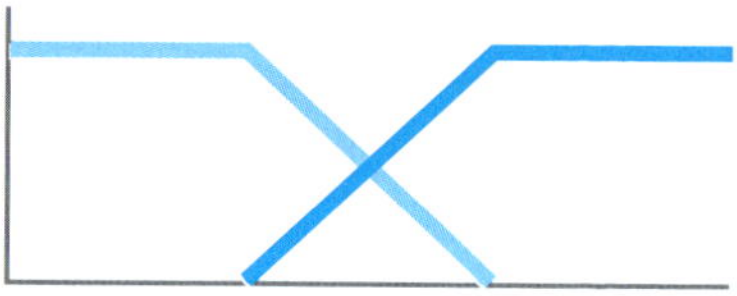

Switch 4a: Overlap (risks NMS, serotonin syndrome and combined ADRs)

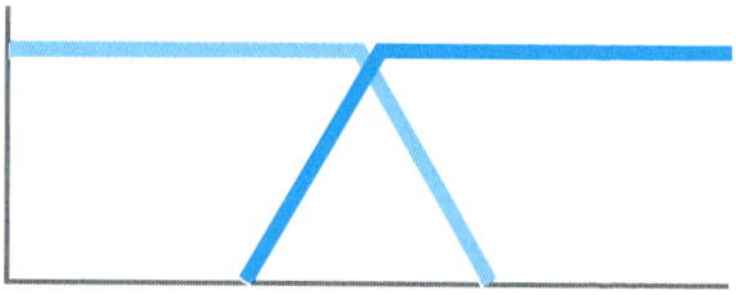

Switch 4b: Full overlap (same risks as 4a)

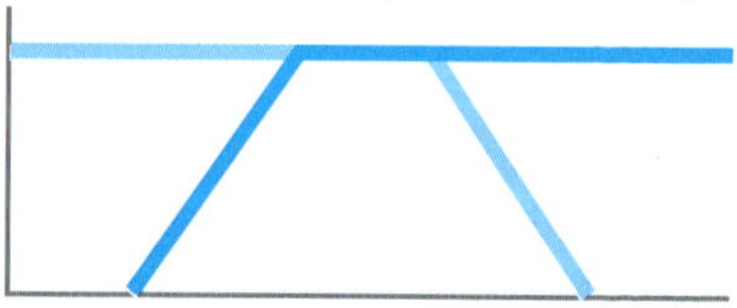

Switch 5: Incomplete (switch never finished, default polypharmacy, avoid)

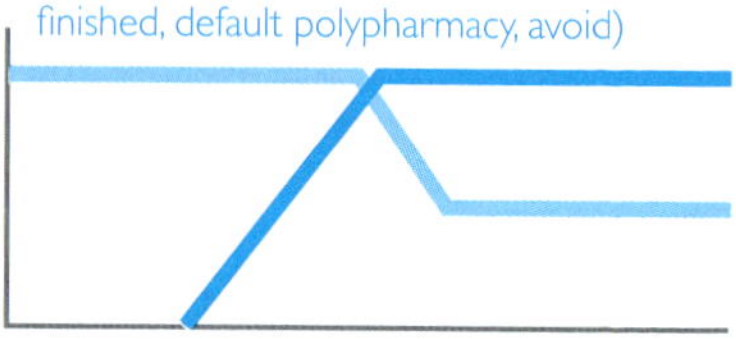

Disadvantages:*
1. May raise unrealistic expectations of a rapid improvement on the second drug.
2. Combined ADRs, usually short-lived.
3. Potential for drug interactions if the first drug has a long half-life, e.g. fluoxetine.
4. Rapid discontinuation of the first drug may produce higher relapse rates, e.g. antipsychotics.
5. Discontinuation effects from the first drug may be interpreted as ADRs of the second.
6. Can be destabilising for patient if abrupt.

Switch 3: Partial overlap

(Add new drug, either at standard dose or titrated upwards, while slowly tapering the first drug down)

Advantages:
1. Appropriate when symptom control is needed but there is a high risk of relapse or deterioration.
2. No abrupt potentially destabilising changes
3. May be unavoidable for LAI/depot to oral switches, where plasma levels will decline slowly. †
4. Useful where cholinergic rebound may occur. Anticholinergic cover can be retained for several weeks. †

Disadvantages:
1. Two drugs may be given at sub-therapeutic doses.
2. Combined ADRs may occur.
3. Potential for drug interactions, especially with antidepressants.
4. Potential for medication errors if not planned fully in advance — involve patient and carers if the patient is at home.
5. High potential for polypharmacy if the switch is never completed (see Switch 5). †

Switch 4: Full overlap

(Add new drug to therapeutic dose and then slowly taper previous drug)

Advantages:
1. Safest if relapse prevention is of the greatest concern.
2. Most appropriate if the person has recently (e.g. < 3 months) recovered from an acute relapse with the first drug.
3. Low risk of discontinuation effects from the first drug.
4. If a depot to oral antipsychotic switch, this may be a low risk opportunity to assess compliance with oral drugs. †
5. Slow taper is possible and is better for drugs with a high anticholinergic activity.
6. 4b is probably the safest for aripiprazole.

Disadvantages:
1. Combined ADRs may occur.
2. Potential for severe reactions, e.g. NMS or serotonin syndrome.
3. Potential for other drug interactions.
4. Potential for medication errors if not planned and completed fully.
5. High potential for polypharmacy if switch never completed (see switch 5 below).

Switch 5: Incomplete

(Add new drug to therapeutic dose and then never stop previous drug)

This can occur if the switch is started but the treatment plan is not passed on, or the person improves and there is a reluctance to discontinue the first drug. Default polypharmacy should be avoided. Long-term monotherapy is beneficial, as it is easier to judge accurately the effectiveness of any given drug, and medication regimens are simple and not confused by polypharmacy (extensive review, Weiden *et al*, *J Clin Psychiatry* 1998;**59**[Suppl 19]:36–49). Monotherapy should thus always be tried first and if, at some time later, a rational, planned and assessed polypharmacy is tried, that is reasonable.

2.2.1 SWITCHING AND DISCONTINUING ANTIPSYCHOTICS

2.2.1.1 GENERAL ADVICE ON SWITCHING ANTIPSYCHOTICS

Reasons for switching antipsychotics include:
1. Persistent positive (distressing and disruptive) symptoms.
2. Persistent negative (restrictive and burdening) symptoms.
3. Relapse despite compliance.
4. Persistent distressing adverse effects e.g. EPS, akathisia, hyperprolactinaemia, weight gain, sedation and sexual dysfunction.
5. Oral to LAI or other formulation change.

Main risks of discontinuing (or switching) antipsychotics:

1. Cholinergic rebound (e.g. nausea, vomiting, restlessness, see 18a), if a second drug has less anticholinergic effect or anticholinergics are withdrawn too soon. It can be brief and predictable, but severe.
2. Withdrawal dyskinesias, e.g. rebound akathisia (may be confused with anxiety), dystonia and worsening tardive dyskinesia. These may be partly cholinergic rebound, and can be minimised by slow tapering.
3. Relapse or destabilisation — rates of up to 50% at six months after abrupt discontinuation have been reported (n = 1,210, Viguera *et al*, *Arch Gen Psychiatry* 1997;**54**:49–55), particularly in schizophrenia, with increased use of in-patient and crisis services (n=651, open, 12/12, Faries *et al*, *BMC Psychiatry* 2009;**9**:54; FFT). Gradual discontinuation reduces this risk (review by Tranter and Healy, *J Psychopharmacol* 1998;**12**:401–6). True relapses tend to occur from 1–6 months after abrupt withdrawal of oral drugs and 3–6 months with depots, due to the persistence of the drug at receptor level (see also *2.2.1.4*).
4. Anxiety or stress from the switch causing symptom flare-up.
5. Medication errors during the switch.
6. The second antipsychotic may be less effective than the first, or have different but still unacceptable side-effects, with premature abandonment and an inadequate trial.

General principles for switching antipsychotics:

1. Ensure the optimum effect is obtained from the first drug
2. Set a treatment target and measure. Make sure the key aims are not easier and less risky to achieve by, e.g. dose or timing adjustment of the current antipsychotic.
3. Avoid switches:
    - coinciding with major life stress events
    - after a change in treatment team — allow full assimilation first
    - from a drug that was successfully used to treat a major relapse in the last 3–6/12
    - in people previously non-compliant with oral drugs now stable for under a year on a depot (Weiden *et al*, *J Clin Psychiatry* 1997;**58**[Suppl 10]:63–72).
4. Slowly taper any anticholinergic and reintroduce if necessary for any emergent symptoms.
5. Monitor mental and physical state regularly (particularly during the first month).

Before switching an antipsychotic:

1. Warn about possible ADRs (e.g. weight, sedation, change in prolactin).
2. Discuss the need for an adequate trial and the need to complete the switch.
3. Agree how to define success or failure, and the chances thereof.
4. Warn that the new antipsychotic is not perfect, and that the process is swapping one set of side-effects for another.

Reviews: * switching due to side-effects (Mukundan *et al*, *Cochrane Database Syst Rev* 2010;**12**;CD006629), Newcomer *et al*, *J Clin Psychiatry* 2013;**74**:1108–20), chlorpromazine equivalents (s = 11, Patel *et al*, *Schizophr Res* 2013; **149**:141–8).

2.2.1.2 SPECIFIC DRUG SWITCHES

1. Phenothiazine to phenothiazine

Switches 2 or 3 are probably reasonable where equivalent doses are used.

2. Phenothiazine to D2-blocker

As 1 above, but beware of cholinergic rebound (see 18a) and stronger D2-blockade leading to additional EPSE.

3. Switching to a FGA depot (Table 2.2.4)

Remember that FGA depot peak plasma levels may vary (see *Table 2.2.2*), and so reduce doses accordingly. Beware of additive EPSEs.

3a. Oral antipsychotic to FGA depot/LAI: See *Table 2.2.5* (*p.217*). For **aripiprazole** to haloperidol decanoate start haloperidol decanoate as per SmPC and taper down aripiprazole after six weeks.

3b. Switching from one FGA depot to another FGA depot: See 2.2.5.

3c. Combined oral antipsychotic plus depot/

LAI to depot/LAI monotherapy:

This can be a difficult procedure and relapses may occur more frequently, particularly in the first 3–4 months when antipsychotic levels might be inadvertently sub-therapeutic (Soni *et al*, *Acta Psychiatr Scand* 1992;**85**:354–9). If the risk of relapse is high, any change should probably be done verging on the side of caution, e.g. increasing the depot dose, then reducing oral doses later.

3d. FGA depots to others:

Stop the depot and introduce the next antipsychotic when the next depot dose would have been due, remembering that a slow decay in depot plasma levels may occur so beware of adding the new drug too quickly, e.g. 33% of people stopping fluphenazine decanoate had notable plasma levels 12/52 after the last dose (Gitlin *et al*, *J Clin Psychopharmacol* 1988;**8**:53–6). Depots are occasionally given more often than strictly necessary.

2

TABLE 2.2.2: SWITCHING ANTIPSYCHOTICS *

From \ To	Pheno-thia-zines	D2 blockers	FGA depots	Aripip-razole[15]	Asena-pine[15]	Cloza-pine[15]	Lurasi-done	Olanza-pine[15]	Olanza-pine[15] pamoate	Paliperi-done palm	Risperi-done	Risperi-done consta	Quetia-pine[15]
Pheno-thiazines	RT (1)	RT (2)	RT (3)	RT (4)	RT (12)	Care (5,)	NOP (16)	NOP (6)	NOP (13)	RT (15)	RT (7)	RT (8a)	RT (9a)
D2 blockers	RT (10)	RT (11)	RT (3)	RT (4)	RT (12)	Care (5)	NOP (16)	NOP (6)	NOP (13)	RT (15)	RT (7)	RT (8a)	RT (9b)
FGA depots	RT (3)	RT (3)	RT (3)	RT (3,4)	RT (3,12)	Care (3,5)	NOP (16)	RT (3,6)	NOP (3,13)	RT (15)	RT (3,7)	RT (3,8c)	RT (3,9c)
Aripiprazole[15]	RT (4)	RT (4)	RT (3,4)	-	RT (12)	Care (4,5)	NOP (16)	RT (4,6)	NOP (13)	RT (15)	RT (4,7)	RT (4,8a)	NOP (4,9d)
Asenapine[15]	RT (12)	RT (12)	RT (3,12)	RT (4,12)	-	NOP (5,12)	NOP (16)	RT (6,12)	NOP (12,13)	RT (15)	RT (7,12)	RT (8a,12)	RT (9,12)
Clozapine[15]	Care (5)	Care (5)	Care (3,5)	RT (4,5)	NOP (5,12)	-	NOP (16)	Care (5,6c)	NOP (5,13)	RT (15)	RT (5,7)	RT (5,8a)	RT (5,9e)
Lurasidone[16]	NOP (16)	NOP (16)	NOP (16)	NOP (16)	NOP (16)	NOP (16)	-	NOP (16)	NOP (16)	NOP (16)	NOP (16)	NOP (16)	NOP (16)
Olanzapine[15]	NOP (6)	NOP (6)	NOP (3,13)	RT (1,6)	RT (6,12)	Care (5,6)	NOP (16)	-	NOP (6,13)	RT (15)	RT (6,7)	RT (6,8a)	NOP (6,9f)
Olanzapine pamoate[15]	RT (13)	RT (13)	RT (3,13e)	RT (4,13)	RT (13,12)	RT (5,13)	NOP (16)	RT (6,13)	-	RT (15)	RT (7,13)	RT (8,13)	RT (9,13)
Paliperidone palmitate	RT (15)	RT (15)	RT (15)	RT (15)	RT (15)	RT (15)	NOP (16)	RT (15)	RT (15)	-	RT (15)	RT (15)	RT (15)
Risperidone	RT (14)	RT (14)	RT (3,14)	RT (4, 14)	RT (14,12)	Care (5, 14)	NOP (16)	NOP (6a, 14)	NOP (13,14)	RT (15)	-	RT (8d, 14)	NOP (9g, 14)
Risperidone Consta	RT (8e)	RT (8e)	RT (3,8)	RT (4,8e, 17)	RT (8e,12)	Care (5, 8e)	NOP (16)	RT (6,8, 15)	NOP (8a,13)	RT (15)	RT (7,8e)	-	RT (8e,9)
Quetiapine[15]	NOP (9,14)	NOP (9,14)	NOP (3,14)	RT (4,9, 14)	RT (9,12, 14)	Care (5, 9,14)	NOP (16)	NOP (6, 9,14)	NOP (9,13,14)	RT (15)	RT (7, 9,14)	RT (8a,9, 14)	-
Stopping	RT (18)	RT (18)	RT (18)	RT (18)	RT (18)	RT (18)	RT (18)	RT (18)	RT (18)	RT (18)	RT (18)	RT (18)	RT (18)

NOP = No obvious problems, although there is the definite risk of NMS with **all** switches
RT = Read text
Care = Great care needed, also read text
D2 blockers = sulpiride, amisulpride, haloperidol, flupentixol and zuclopenthixol

4. Switching to aripiprazole oral or LAI*

4a. Any to oral aripiprazole:

Abrupt switching to oral aripiprazole can often be poorly tolerated, especially in people with milder rather than more severe symptoms (n=77, RCT, open, 12/52, Pae *et al*, *Clin Drug Invest* 2010;**30**:187–93). Aripiprazole strongly binds to dopamine receptors, with a long half-life, displacing almost every other antipsychotic, and stimulating receptors to about 30% activity. This abrupt change from minimal dopamine activity to 30% within hours can lead to abrupt worsening, be acutely distressing and adversive, possibly via a dopamine supersensitivity and particularly after high doses of other antipsychotics (n=264, Takase *et al*, *J Psychopharmacol* 2015;**29**:383–9). A cross-taper is most likely to be successful, starting aripiprazole at 5mg/d (SmPC mentions 10mg/d), then increasing stepwise to 15mg/d and then reducing the previous antipsychotic by 25% twice a week (n=53[c=48], RCT, open, 14/52, Takeuchi *et al*, *J Clin Psychopharmacol* 2008;**28**:540–3; n=77, RCT, open, 12/52, Pae *et al*, *Eur Neuropsychopharmacol* 2009;**19**:562–70). Although three switches (abrupt; immediate aripiprazole start with tapered reduction of first drug; or a 14-day cross-taper) from risperidone or olanzapine were reportedly well tolerated (n=269, 8/52, Byerly *et al*, *Schizophr Res* 2009;**107**:218–22), the data is inconsistent (e.g. 12/52, Ryckmans *et al*, *Pharmacopsychiatry* 2009;**42**:114–21) and olanzapine and quetiapine may need a smoother switching process with a longer cross-taper (n=45[c=31], 12/52, Lin *et al*, *Chang Gung Med J* 2009;**32**:409–16; FFT). Dual administration for 2/52 then stopping first drug over one week (fast switch) or four weeks (slow switch) was equally effective for clinical response and metabolic profile over eight weeks (n=79, RCT, open, 8/52, Hwang *et al*, *J Clin Psychopharmacol* 2015;**35**:635–44). Strictly time-limited benzodiazepines (when required, for 3–4 weeks) have been used as 'glue' to help manage the initial agitation and anxiety during a switch to aripiprazole.

4a. Any to aripiprazole LAI:*

For fluphenazine to aripiprazole LAI, start aripiprazole oral when the next fluphenazine is due and start the LAI after about two weeks.

Review: * Italian consensus statement on switching to aripiprazole (Fagiolini *et al*, *Expert Opin Pharmacother* 2015;**16**:727–37).

5. Switching to/from clozapine

5a. Switching to clozapine: Care is needed with the increased risk of dyscrasias with phenothiazines, and delayed clearance of LAIs (especially risperidone, aripiprazole and olanzapine). Ideally, a previous antipsychotic should be completely withdrawn before clozapine is started, including LAIs (e.g. switch 1), but this is rarely practical. Clozapine is markedly sedative and hypotensive, and care is needed with additive effects so start with the usual gradual dose titration but monitor carefully. Warn women about the possible normalisation of prolactin and the need for adequate oral contraception if necessary.

5b. Switching from clozapine (see also 18b)

Converting clozapine to other antipsychotics is particularly problematic (n=30, RCT, Shiovitz *et al*, *Schizophr Bull* 1996;**22**:591–5; FFT). Relapse after clozapine discontinuation seems to be of a higher incidence, may be more rapid, and withdrawal symptoms may be more severe than with other drugs (see 18b). For gradual discontinuation of clozapine, it is best to introduce and escalate the doses of another antipsychotic simultaneously (switch 3).

6. Switching to/from oral olanzapine

There is a low risk of major problems with stopping olanzapine suddenly (see 18d), so any switch should be viable. When switching to olanzapine, additive EPSE, hypotension and drug interactions are unlikely to occur and so switch 3 is usually suitable. Unexpected pregnancies have occurred a couple of months after a switch from FGAs to olanzapine, despite no contraceptive use for 4–5 years (n=2, Neumann and Frasch, *Nervenarzt* 2001;**72**:876–8).

6a. Oral antipsychotics to oral olanzapine: In a comparison of four different FGA/risperidone to olanzapine switches in partially remitted, stable out-patients with schizophrenia, the most successful method was starting 10mg **olanzapine** then gradually discontinuing the original drug. The next most successful was switch 3, probably best for elderly/frail people. Most drop-outs (usually sleep-related) were with abrupt discontinuation (switch 2) and gradual olanzapine introduction (n=209[c=171], open, Kinon *et al*, *J Clin Psychiatry* 2000;**61**:833–40). Both direct switch 2 and tapered switch 3 (over 2/52) have had equivalent outcomes, both therapeutic (67–74% successful) and for adverse effects (n=108, RCT, open, 6/52, Lee *et al*, *J Clin Psychiatry* 2002;**63**:569–76).

6b. Depot/LAIs to oral olanzapine: When clinically stable, schizophrenics on depots either continued the depot or transferred to olanzapine over 4/52 the latter were clinically improved and all preferred olanzapine, so a four-week switch is clinically viable (n=26, RCT, open, 3/12, Godleski *et al*, *J Clin Psychiatry* 2003;**64**:119–22).

6c. Clozapine to oral olanzapine: In people responsive to clozapine but suffering adverse effects, a slow cross-titration over at least two weeks to olanzapine may be successful in about 90% of people (n=20, open, 24/52, Littrell *et al*, *J Clin Psychiatry* 2000;**61**:912–5).

6d. Olanzapine to risperidone: See 7a.

7. Switching to/from oral risperidone*

7a. Olanzapine to risperidone: Three **olanzapine** to risperidone switches have been studied:

1. Gradual 1; week 1 olanzapine reduced by 50% for a week and risperidone started; week 2 olanzapine stopped.
2. Gradual 2; week 1 olanzapine full dose, risperidone started; week 2 olanzapine 50%; week 3 olanzapine stopped.
3. Olanzapine stopped abruptly, risperidone started immediately and titrated as usual.

Gradual switch 2 had the least drop-outs and the best outcomes (n=123[c=97], RCT, open, 6/52, Ganguli *et al*, *BMC Med* 2008;**6**:17; FFT).

7b. Others to risperidone: An early review of switching to risperidone recommended reducing the first antipsychotic dose, then overlapping risperidone with the existing therapy, rather than making an abrupt switch (Borison *et al*, *Clin Ther* 1996;**18**:592–607). There are few obvious problems with stopping or switching risperidone (e.g. interactions), except the predictable potential for NMS, changes in prolactin, additive postural hypotension (use gradual titration) and additive EPS. Switches 2 or 3 should be possible. A sudden switch (along with gradual withdrawal of anticholinergics) may be possible in an emergency (n=36, Kirov *et al*, *Acta Psychiatr Scand* 1997;**95**:439–43). When switching to **paliperidone**, 6mg may not produce as high plasma levels as 3mg **risperidone** so a 2:1 dose equivalent may not be fully accurate (n=25, open, 6/52, Yang *et al*, *J Psychopharmacol* 2014;**28**:341–8).

8. Switching to/from Risperdal Consta® LAI*

8a. Switching to risperidone LAI:* It is vital to understand the release kinetics of RLAI before deciding a switch strategy. Therapeutic levels are not reached until week 4 (i.e. just before the third injection), but only reach optimum in weeks 5–6 (i.e. after the third injection). Assessment of the response to oral risperidone is strongly recommended before giving the first injection, then giving oral supplements for 3–4 weeks, or

Table 2.2.3: Summary of antipsychotic long-acting injections

Drug	Peak (days)	Usual frequency	Main duration	Depot/LAI half-life	Time to steady state from first dose
Aripiprazole	8–10	Monthly	6-8/52	7/52	9–10/52 if inc oral
Flupentixol	7–10	2/52	2–4/52	7/7	10–12/52
Fluphenazine	1–2	2–4/52	3–4/52	14/7	6–12/52
Fluspirilene	1–2	1/52	1/52	?	5–6/52
Haloperidol	3–9	4/52	4/52	21–28/7	10–12/52
Olanzapine	2–4	2/52 or 4/52	6/52	30 (13–42)/7	12/52
Paliperidone	13	Monthly	3 months or longer	29–45/7	2–4 weeks
Pipothiazine	9–10	4/52	4/52	21–28/7	8–12/52
Risperidone	35	2/52	2–3/52	-	12/52
Zuclopenthixol	4–9	2/52	2–4/52	7/7	10–12/52

longer. RLAI may have the best chance of success if the person has been shown to respond to oral risperidone first.

8b. Oral antipsychotics to risperidone LAI: See Table 2.2.5.

8c. FGA depot to risperidone LAI: Janssen recommend starting risperidone LAI one week before the last fortnightly injection, with oral supplementation if the risk of relapse is high, or switch on the depot due date, and supplementing with oral risperidone for 3–4 weeks. People with schizophrenia switched from **fluphenazine decanoate** (n=22) or **haloperidol decanoate** (n=40) to risperidone LAI were more likely to discontinue (30%) than those who stayed on fluphenazine or haloperidol (10%) and suffered significant weight gain and raised prolactin (n=22, RCT, 12/12, Covell *et al*, *J Clin Psychiatry* 2012;**73**:669–75; FFT).

8d. Risperidone LAI to others: The last dose of RLAI will finally stop releasing risperidone about six weeks later, so beware of using a full dose of the second drug until about day 42.

9. Switching to/from quetiapine

Quetiapine has a short receptor half-life so warn women about a possible normalisation of prolactin and the need for adequate oral contraception if necessary. A switching study from mostly FGAs and risperidone to quetiapine XL used:

- Day 1: 300mg plus 75% of first antipsychotic
- Day 2: 600mg plus 50% of first antipsychotic
- Day 3: 400–800mg/d plus 25% of first antipsychotic, then stop first antipsychotic
- Day 4: 400–800mg over four days.

Clinical benefit was achieved in 63% who switched, and tolerated the switch well (n=477[c=370], open, 12/52, Ganesan *et al*, *Curr Med Res Opin* 2008;**24**:21–3).

9a. Phenothiazine to quetiapine: Switch 3 may be reasonable. Additional initial postural hypotension may occur so start with a slightly slower dose titration or additional monitoring.

9b. D2-blocker to quetiapine: Switch 2 or 3 should be tolerable, as quetiapine's receptor blockade is quite different to standard D2-blockers.

9c. FGA depot to quetiapine: Switch 2 should be tolerable, starting quetiapine when the next depot dose would have been due.

9d. Aripiprazole to quetiapine: Quetiapine will not displace aripiprazole from receptors so quetiapine will start to act as aripiprazole dissociates from dopamine and serotonin receptors. A gradual aripiprazole discontinuation after quetiapine has reached a therapeutic level would seem reasonable.

9e. Clozapine to quetiapine: Switches 2, 3 or 4 should be tolerable, depending on the reason for the switch.

9f. Olanzapine to quetiapine: Any careful switch should be acceptable.

9g. Risperidone to quetiapine: Switches 2 or 3 should be tolerable. An abrupt switch from risperidone (mean 1.4mg/d) to quetiapine (mean 87mg/d) in elderly people with BPSD was well tolerated (n=67[c=64], open, Madhusoodanan and Bogunovic, *Am J Alzheimer's Dis Other Demen* 2006;**21**:169–74).

9h. Switching from quetiapine: There are a few problems stopping (see 18e) or switching from quetiapine, e.g. NMS, but switches 2 or 3 should be viable (for review see Weiden, *J Psychopharmacol* 2006;**20**:104–18).

10. Switching D2-blockers to phenothiazines

Switches 2 or 3 should be considered first.

11. Switching D2-blocker to D2-blocker

Consider switches 1–3 first, bearing in mind the potential for NMS and additional EPSE. For a general overview on switching to or from amisulpride, see Peuskens (*Curr Med Res Opin* 2002;**18**[Suppl 3]:S23–S28).

12. Switching to/from asenapine

12a. Asenapine to others: **Asenapine** should be gradually discontinued and overlap with other antipsychotics minimised, although there is no systematic data.

12b. Others to asenapine: Pooled data shows that a variety of switching strategies from other antipsychotics (stopping abruptly; over three days; over seven days) to asenapine are generally safe and well tolerated (s=2, n=949, RCT, d/b, 6/12, Cazorla *et al*, *Neuropsychiatr Dis Treat* 2012;**8**:247–57; FFT).

13. Switching to/from olanzapine pamoate (OLAI, see also 2.2.4)

13a. Others to OLAI: There is no systematic data available. Switching to olanzapine pamoate should present few problems as it takes 12 weeks to reach steady state, so some crossover, e.g. switches 2–4 would be viable.

13b. OLAI to others: Switching from olanzapine pamoate requires a gradual switch, as olanzapine levels can persist for up to 6–8 months after discontinuation and close supervision is required for at least two months post-switch.

14. Switching to/from ziprasidone*

14a. Others to ziprasidone:
Allowing four weeks from any of ten antipsychotics while up-titrating ziprasidone as a cross-taper can aid tolerability and success (n=67[c=42], open, 12/52, Ko *et al, Psychiatry Investig* 2014;**11**:459–66; FFT). Three one week taper/switching strategies had similar outcomes:

To ziprasidone from:	n=	c=	% completers
Haloperidol	99	67	68
Olanzapine	82	71	86
Risperidone	104	62	60

(n=285 [c=200, 68%], open, 12/52, Alptekin *et al, Int Clin Psychopharmacol* 2009;**24**:229–38).

14b. FGA to ziprasidone:

- Switch 1: Abrupt discontinuation of FGA on day 1 (n=18)
- Switch 2: FGA 50% from days 1–7, then stopped (n=18)
- Switch 3: FGA 100% days 1 and 2, 50% from days 3–7, then stopped (n=18).

One switch used ziprasidone 40mg BD for 2/7, then titrated up to 80mg BD. Switch 3 may have improved BPRS quicker, but all switches were statistically the same at the end-point (n=54, open, RCT, 6/52, Stip *et al, Prog Neuropsychopharmacol Biol Psychiatry* 2010;**34**:997–1000).

14c. Aripiprazole to ziprasidone: Cross-tapering has been used, with aripiprazole reduced stepwise over 4/52, while ziprasidone is increased to up to 160mg/d maximum over same time. Switching in non-responsive or intolerant patients improved depression, negative symptoms and metabolic symptoms, but this was balanced by sedation and raised prolactin (n=19, open, 12/52, Kim *et al, Clin Neuropharmacol* 2010;**33**:121–5).

15. Switching to/from paliperidone palmitate (PPLAI, Xeplion®, see also 2.2.4)

15a. Risperidone LAI (RLAI) to PPLAI: Start PPLAI when the next RLAI dose is due and go straight to monthly (see *Table 2.2.4* for dose equivalent). A claims database review concluded that those switching from RLAI to PPLAI had fewer events and a longer time to relapse than those switching to oral antipsychotics (n=319, Voss *et al, Int Clin Psychopharmacol* 2015;**30**:151–7).

15b. Another depot/LAI to PPLAI: Start PPLAI when the next depot dose is due and go straight to monthly.

15c. PPLAI to oral antipsychotic: Start oral antipsychotic when the next PPLAI dose is due, but titrate slowly as paliperidone levels can persist for up to six months.

15d. PPLAI to RLAI: Start risperidone LAI when the next PPLAI dose is due.

15e. PPLAI to another depot/LAI injection: There are no official recommendations, but start the new depot/LAI slowly to avoid additive ADRs and NMS as paliperidone levels can persist for up to six months.

15f. Others to PPLAI: See 2.2.5.

16. Switching to lurasidone*

16a. Aripiprazole/paliperidone to lurasidone: Stop first antipsychotic then uptitrate lurasidone over 1–2 weeks.

16b. Quetiapine/olanzapine to lurasidone: Cross-titrate over 1–2 weeks.

16c. Clozapine to lurasidone: Stop clozapine over three weeks (if possible) then increase lurasidone over 1–2 weeks.

16d. Others to lurasidone: A switching study suggested a full cross-over is possible, e.g. to 37mg/d for 2/52, 74mg/d for 2/52 or 37mg/d for 1/52 then 74mg/d for 1/52, albeit with a minor risk of NMS. Relapse rates were 12% when switching from a sedating antipsychotic (olanzapine or quetiapine) and 6% for a non-sedating antipsychotic (n=240, RCT, 6/52, McEvoy *et al, J Clin Psychiatry* 2013;**74**:170–9).

2

Reference for 16a–16d: * Stahl SM (2014) *Prescribers' Guide: Stahl's Essential Psychopharmacology*, 5th edn. Cambridge University Press.

17. Prolactin warning

Warn women about the possibility of currently raised prolactin (particularly with D2-blockers) causing amenorrhoea, and normalisation of prolactin with the new drug and, if necessary, the need for adequate oral contraception.

18. Discontinuing antipsychotics

Stopping an antipsychotic has three main risks; discontinuation symptoms, withdrawal/rebound psychosis, and relapse. Discontinuing gradually is the ideal and has the lowest incidence of these adverse outcomes.

A. Withdrawal symptoms (general)

- Cholinergic rebound (Lieberman, *Psychosomatics* 1981;**22**:253–4) from abrupt withdrawal of low-potency antipsychotics can include headache, restlessness, nausea, emesis, anorexia, diarrhoea, rhinorrhea, diaphoresis, myalgia, paraesthesia, anxiety (Dilsaver and Alessi, *Acta Psychiatr Scand* 1988;**77**:241–6) and rebound insomnia (n=3, van Sweden, *Pharmacopsychiatry* 1987;**20**:116–9)
- Insomnia, anxiety and akathisia occurs in 85% when switching to high-potency FGAs, probably due to cholinergic rebound (n=26, Chouinard *et al*, *J Clin Psychiatry* 1984;**45**:500–2)
- Cachexia (withdrawal-emergent) can be dramatic, e.g. loss of weight, appetite, muscle atrophy and wasting (n=10, Mikkelsen *et al*, *N Engl J Med* 1988;**318**:929).

B. Withdrawal psychosis

Rapid-onset psychosis (so-called 'super-sensitivity psychosis') can occur in 12–20%, peaking at 24–48 hours. It is less common with gradual compared to abrupt withdrawal (n=2, Ekblom *et al*, *Psychopharmacology [Berl]* 1984;**83**:293–4), and can occur even in bipolar patients (n=1, Witschy *et al*, *Am J Psychiatry* 1984;**141**:105–6). It usually disappears rapidly on reinstitution and may be more common with clozapine, possibly because of its short half-life (Baldessarini *et al*, *Arch Gen Psychiatry* 1995;**52**:1071–2).

C. Relapse

If an antipsychotic has been effective, discontinuation obviously risks relapse. After gradual withdrawal relapse may be heralded by anxiety, agitation, restlessness and insomnia (Dilsaver and Alessi, *Acta Psychiatr Scand* 1988;**77**:241–6). A number of studies and analyses (e.g. Moncrieff, *Acta Psychiatr Scand* 2006;**114**:3–13) conclude that:

- About 25–50% people relapse within 10–12 weeks (s=66, n=4,365), and 50% have relapsed after 6/12 (s=13, n=1,210)
- Relapse rate with slow discontinuation (32%) is half that of rapid discontinuation (65%)
- People who remain stable after 6/12 tend to remain relapse-free without medication (n=1,210, retrospective, Viguera *et al*, *Arch Gen Psychiatry* 1997;**54**:49–55).

18a. Discontinuing aripiprazole

Stopping adjunctive aripiprazole 2–5mg/d abruptly has led to nausea, lightheadedness and muscle twitching, but this began to dissipate after two weeks (n=1, Sansone and Sawyer, *Innov Clin Neurosci* 2013;**10**:10–2). Supersensitivity psychosis has been reported (n=1, Chang *et al*, *Prog Neuropsychopharmacol Biol Psychiatry* 2009;**33**:388–9).

18b. Discontinuing clozapine *

Sudden discontinuation of clozapine due to a blood dyscrasia can lead to more difficult-to-treat psychosis, e.g. in a retrospective comparison, doses on re-treatment needed to be 43% higher than the last taken dose (n=43), compared to 12.5% lower if the person (n=12) had stayed on clozapine (n=55, Miodowniok *et al*, *J Clin Psychiatry* 2006;**67**:1204–8). After sudden withdrawal of 200mg/d clozapine taken for 4/52 (in schizophrenia in remission, n=28):

- 39% had no withdrawal symptoms
- 43% had mild symptoms (agitation, headache, nausea)
- 14% had moderate symptoms (nausea, vomiting, diarrhoea)
- 4% had rebound psychosis requiring hospitalisation for manic episodes.

Most symptoms occurred within 24–36 hours and resolved over 3–7 days (n=30[c=28], 7/7, open, Shiovitz *et al*, *Schizophr Bull* 1996;**22**:591–5; FFT).

A major component of clozapine withdrawal symptoms is cholinergic rebound (see 18).

It occurs within 24–48 hours of stopping and can include limb and neck dystonias, choreoform movements, dyskinesias lasting up to 14 days (n=4, Ahmed *et al*, *J Clin Psychiatry* 1998;**59**:472–7), delirium (n=3, Stanillla *et al*, *J Clin Psychiatry* 1997;**58**:252–5), oculogyric crisis (n=1, Mendhekar and Duggal, *J Neuropsychiatry Clin Neurosci* 2006;**18**:424–5), *de novo* OCD (n=2, Poyurovsky *et al*, *Clin Neuropharmacol* 1998;**21**:97–100), Tourette-like tics (n=1, Poyurovsky *et al*, *Clin Neuropharmacol* 1998;**21**:97–100), catatonia (n=1, Yeh *et al*, *Clin Neuropharmacol* 2004;**27**:216–8), rebound insomnia (n=1, Staedt *et al*, *Eur Arch Psychiatry Clin Neurosci* 1996;**246**:79–82), serotonin syndrome (n=1, Stevenson *et al*, *JAMA Neurol* 2013;**70**:1054–5), severe akathisia (n=1, Poyurovsky *et al*, *Int Clin Psychopharmacol* 1996;**11**:283–6) and NMS (n=1, Margetic and Aukst-Margetic, *Prog Neuropsychopharmacol Biol Psychiatry*2005;**29**:14507). They may occur in 25% (<300mg/d), and most quickly resolve on restarting or use of anticholinergics (De Leon *et al*, *J Clin Psychiatry* 1994;**55**:119–20) and are reduced significantly if switched to olanzapine (n=106, RCT, d/b, p/c, Tollefson *et al*, *J Clin Psychopharmacol* 1999;**19**:435–43).

18c. Discontinuing haloperidol

Rebound psychosis (n=1, Kahne, *Can J Psychiatry* 1989;**34**:227–9) and dyskinesia (e.g. n=5, Riker *et al*, *Chest* 1997;**111**:1778–81) have been reported.

18d. Discontinuing olanzapine

There have been reports of supersensitivity psychosis 48 hours after sudden discontinuation (n=3, Llorca *et al*, *Can J Psychiatry* 2001;**46**:87–8) and myoclonus as part of a possible serotonin syndrome caused by serotonin rebound (n=1, 6/12, Nayudu and Scheftner, *J Clin Psychopharmacol* 2000;**20**:489–90).

18e. Discontinuing quetiapine

Acute withdrawal symptoms such as nausea, insomnia, diarrhoea, dizziness, irritability, headache (Jiménez-Caballero *et al*, *Rev Neurol* 2004;**38**:1094) and chorea have been reported with acute cessation of high doses. It can occur within 24 hours (where a very slow taper or ondansetron did not help, but prochlorperazine did; n=1, Kim and Staab, *Am J Psychiatry* 2005;**162**:1020). The SmPC recommends withdrawing over at least 1–2 weeks.

18f. Discontinuing risperidone

Risperidone discontinuation symptoms have included tics (Rowan and Malone, *J Am Acad Child Adolesc Psychiatry* 1997;**36**:162–3), dyskinesia (n=1, Anand and Dewan, *Ann Clin Psychiatry* 1996;**8**:179–82), respiratory dyskinesia, e.g. involuntary movements of respiratory muscles, and grunting (n=1, Ehrt *et al*, *J Clin Psychopharmacol* 2005;**25**:609) and akathisia (n=2, Bertolín Guillén *et al*, *Actas Esp Psiquiatr* 2002;**30**:195–7).

Reviews: neuroleptic discontinuation syndromes (Tranter and Healy, *J Psychopharmacol* 1998;**12**:401–6; Moncrieff, *Acta Psychiatr Scand* 2006;**114**:3–13).

2.2.1.3 ANTIPSYCHOTIC DOSE EQUIVALENTS

The antipsychotic dose(s) of each drug are approximately equivalent to others under the same heading (e.g. perphenazine 24mg/d is equivalent to chlorpromazine 300mg/d and to flupentixol 60mg 2/52), based on the references indicated. There is, however, a genuine lack of agreement about antipsychotic equivalents. This is mainly because the main methods of assessing antipsychotic equivalence (clinical studies, non-clinical/receptor binding studies, effective doses, DDD and manufacturers' information) can produce up to a five-fold difference in the equivalents calculated, especially for high-potency antipsychotics. Ranges quoted here are thus unweighted for individual variation and are valid, but imprecise. The main methods are:

1. Clinical studies — trials using active comparators or controls might give some guidance.
2. Receptor binding — antipsychotic affinity for dopamine receptors (particularly D2) to some extent correlates with their antipsychotic potency and so roughly equivalent antipsychotic doses can be calculated. However, some antipsychotic dose relationships, e.g. haloperidol, are unlikely to be linear, and sedation (to help manage disturbed behaviour; Peralta *et al*, *Acta Psychiatr Scand* 1994;**90**:354–7) may be unrelated to dopamine blockade. High-potency drugs, e.g. haloperidol and fluphenazine, have the highest quoted variance (over 1000% in some cases), which may lead to prescribing in higher doses than necessary (Dewan and Koss, *Acta Psychiatr Scand* 1995;**91**:229–32).

3. Defined daily doses (DDD) — these are an alternative to CPZ equivalents, but assume optimum doses are being used, which is not always the case (Rikcken *et al*, *J Clin Psychopharmacol* 2003;**23**:657–9).
4. Percentage of maximum dose — this is an imprecise alternative, as maximum doses may not be equivalent, e.g. is flupentixol decanoate 400mg a week is really equivalent to 50mg a week of fluphenazine decanoate?
5. Mean dose method* — this classical method (Davis, *J Psychiatr Res* 1974;**11**:65–9) has been re-evaluated (s=75, n=16555, Leucht *et al*, *Schizophr Res*;**41**:1397–402) and concludes that the equivalents are:

Drug	Olanzapine 10mg equivalents
Amisulpride	383mg
Aripiprazole	14mg
Asenapine	9mg
Chlorpromazine	389mg
Clozapine	306mg
Haloperidol	7mg
Olanzapine	10mg
Quetiapine	323mg
Risperidone	4mg
Ziprasidone	79mg

6. Minimum effective doses (MED)* — a newer method is to use MEDs as the minimum dose to be effective (drug has been significantly more effective than placebo in at least one double-blind, fixed dose, RCT as the measure). It is not applicable to specific populations, e.g. first-episode, elderly, renal or hepatic impairment, or TRS, but is a valid method as it can be applied to any antipsychotics with appropriate dose data (s=73, Leucht *et al*, *Schizophr Bull* 2014;**40**:314–26):

Antipsychotic	Minimum effective dose	Olanzapine equivalents
Aripiprazole	10mg	1.33
Asenapine	10mg	1.33
Clozapine	300mg	40
Haloperidol	4mg	0.53
Iloperidone	8mg	1.07
Lurasidone	37mg	5.33
Olanzapine	**7.5mg**	1
Paliperidone	3mg	0.4
Quetiapine	150mg	20
Risperidone	2mg	0.27
Ziprasidone	40mg	5.33

Median effective doses (ED50) and near maximal effective doses (ED85 to ED95) can also be used (systematic review and meta-analysis, Davis and Chen, *J Clin Psychopharmacol* 2004;**24**:192–208; review by Woods, *EBMH* 2004;**7**:106; FFT).

Cautions and disclaimer:

Antipsychotic equivalence is specifically quoted and the doses are as accurate as data allows, but to avoid confusion you must consider:

1. Antipsychotic equivalence must not be confused with sedation, e.g. there may be no extra antipsychotic effect from haloperidol above 8–12mg/d (see *1.10.4*) and the lack of sedation from an equivalent dose of a D2 receptor selective drug (e.g. flupentixol, sulpiride, etc) must not be interpreted as non-antipsychotic equivalence.
2. There may not be a linear relationship between dose and the antipsychotic effect.
3. Dose frequency with depots/LAIs may be important as the first pass effect may reduce the effective doses of oral preparations.
4. Differing half-lives may complicate the calculations and final dose recommendation.
5. These equivalent doses are not necessarily equivalent in terms of maximum doses.
6. For the newer antipsychotics, therapeutic doses are better defined and so no equivalent doses are appropriate.
7. Always check your answer against product information to ensure inappropriately high doses are not inadvertently used.

Review: * general (Danivas and Venkatasubramanian, *Indian J Psychiatry* 2013;**55**:207–8).

2.2.1.4 POST-SWITCHING ANTIPSYCHOTIC ISSUES

Assessing response:

1. For all drugs, aim for a minimum of three months at full therapeutic dosage.
2. Be cautious of any significant gains (e.g. reduced side-effects) within 6/52 of the last antipsychotic stopping, as drug concentrations at receptor level may outlast plasma levels (e.g. see haloperidol, *1.25*).
3. Even if gains occur, ensure a full therapeutic trial, as discontinuation of

Table 2.2.4: Antipsychotic dose estimated equivalents *

Oral	mg/d (+ range)
Chlorpromazine *	150 mg (100–194 mg; also 25–50 mg IM or 250 mg rectally)
Fluphenazine	2 mg (1.25–5 mg)
Levomepromazine	Not known
Pericyazine	24 mg
Perphenazine	8 mg (7–15 mg)
Promazine	100 mg (50–200 mg)
Trifluoperazine	2–5 mg (2–8 mg)
Benperidol	2 mg
Haloperidol §*	2.5 mg (1–5 mg), or 1.5 mg IM/IV for doses up to 20 mg
Flupentixol	2 mg
Zuclopenthixol	25 mg (25–60 mg), up to a maximum of 150 mg/d
Pimozide	2 mg (up to a maximum of 20 mg/d)
Amisulpride *	150 mg (40–190 mg)
Sulpiride	200 mg (200–333 mg)
Aripiprazole *	7 mg (6.7–7.5 mg)
Asenapine *	5 mg (4.5–6.7 mg)
Clozapine *	150 mg (30–200 mg)
Lurasidone *	18.5 mg (= 20 mg USA)
Olanzapine *	5 mg
Quetiapine *	100 mg (75–160 mg)
Paliperidone *	3mg (2.5–3 mg; based on equivalents to risperidone oral)
Risperidone *	1.5 mg (0.5–3 mg)
Ziprasidone *	40 mg (25–40 mg)
Depots and LAIs *	**mg/week**
Aripiprazole LAI *	[300–400 mg/month is the standard dose]
Flupentixol decanoate	10–20 mg (8–20 mg)
Fluphenazine decanoate	5–10 mg (1–12.5 mg)
Fluspirilene	2 mg (no evidence available)
Haloperidol decanoate	10–15 mg (5–25 mg)
Olanzapine pamoate LAI *	Via olanzapine oral: Initial 2/12 = 210 mg 4/52; maintenance 150 mg 4/52
Paliperidone palmitate LAI *	12.5 mg (around 50 mg a month, as per UK SmPC)
Pipothiazine palmitate	10 mg (5–12.5 mg)
Risperidone LAI *	12.5 mg (25 mg/fortnight, as per UK SmPC)
Zuclopenthixol decanoate	100 mg (40–100 mg)

§ The bioavailability of oral haloperidol is about 50–60% of IM, with IV approximately equivalent to IM.
90 mg (75–100) = Recommended average dose + ranges quoted in the literature. The wider the range, the greater the uncertainty about the exact equivalent.

the previous drug will lead to a gradual loss of its side-effects (including cognitive impairment), which may be interpreted as improvement.

4. If therapeutic gains occur, it has been suggested to delay discontinuing any anticholinergic and/or antiakathisia drugs until during the second month.
5. Raised prolactin levels may take over 3/12 to resolve, so women need to be warned about this, and to ensure that they have adequate contraceptive cover if needed.

6. If positive changes occur, caution the person not to risk relapse by 'over-doing it'.

Managing a sub-optimum response to a switch:

1. No improvement by 6/52 — exclude non-compliance with the switch, substance misuse and inadequate dosage. Try to work towards 12/52 at full dose.
2. Some response by 6/52 — do not get too optimistic, continue to 12/52.
3. Partial response between 6/52 and 12/52 — consider an increase in dose, and try to go for a 6/12 trial.
4. Initial response followed by worsening of positive symptoms — check deterioration is not actually improvement (e.g. previous positive symptoms hidden by the person now surfacing). Try to restabilise and aim for 12/52 at full dose.

Long-term issues:

1. With improvements in insight, increased psychosocial support and monitoring will be needed to reduce the risk of post-psychotic depression and self-harm.

2.2.1.5 DEPOT AND LAI INJECTIONS (see Table 2.2.5 on pp. 217–225)

Challenges with depot/LAIs e.g. switching and missed doses can be difficult to resolve due to the lack of reliable data, especially on multiple dosing. Table 2.2.5 is no exception, but aims to help inform discussions. The following must be considered:

- Use your own common sense and patient preference, characteristics, and symptoms when choosing a switch strategy
- Any dose suggestions must be within licensed limits, including replacement higher doses that might be calculated when a dose has been missed
- These suggestions are computer modelled and based on single dose kinetics. Half-lives tend to lengthen with chronic use
- Advice on oral to depot/LAI and vice versa is based on an assumption of exact equivalent oral/injection doses of the same drug are being used
- Plasma levels are not absolute and do not include confidence intervals or necessarily reflect CNS levels or receptor blockade
- The 'y' axis units are not established for any of the multiple dose graphs and there will, of course, be interindividual variation
- Linear kinetics (e.g. a double dose gives double the plasma levels) are assumed
- Data assume that a small test dose is given if needed, but that this is too low to have a therapeutic effect
- While double doses of depots may, thankfully, be rare events, they have been included because they happen.

2.2.2 SWITCHING BENZODIAZEPINES

Switching benzodiazepines may be advantageous for various reasons, e.g. pre-discontinuation to a drug with a longer half-life. While there is broad agreement in the literature about equivalent doses, clonazepam has a wide reported equivalence range and particular care is needed. Inter-patient variability and differing half-lives mean that the figures can never be exact and should be interpreted using your own knowledge. See *Table 2.2.6 (p. 226)*.

2.2.3 SWITCHING ANTICHOLINERGICS *

See 6.7 about the overall indications for the use of anticholinergics. Equivalent doses may be:

Orphenadrine	50 mg
Procyclidine	5 mg
Trihexyphenidyl (benzhexol)	2 mg

2.2.4 SWITCHING DRUGS OF ABUSE OR DEPENDENCE

Switching drugs of abuse/dependence, usually to methadone, is a common strategy. *Table 2.2.7* may be of some use, although caution is necessary regarding, e.g. the potency of individual samples of street drugs.

Advice:

1. Most of these equivalent doses are based on **analgesic** equivalents, which may differ by a factor of 10 from the dose needed to suppress opiate withdrawal symptoms.
2. The dose:effect relationship may be non-linear, especially at higher doses and above BNF limits.

Table 2.2.5: Depot and long-acting injections (all doses must be within licensed limits)

2.2.5.1 Weekly injection

	Flupentixol decanoate	Zuclopenthixol decanoate	Haloperidol decanoate	Pipotiazine palmitate	Fluphenazine decanoate	Risperidone LAI (Consta®, RLAI) [weekly is an unlicensed frequency]
Weekly to fortnightly	Add 25% to the final weekly dose. Miss a week, then give double the previous weekly dose fortnightly					Add up to 50% to the last weekly dose. Miss a week, then give double the previous weekly dose fortnightly
Oral to depot weekly	Stop oral on the day the depot starts		Start depot, drop oral to 66% for first week, then 33% for 2 weeks	N/A	N/A	Continue oral for 3 weeks after the first LAI dose, then stop or titrate down in week 3
Depot weekly to oral	Week one: Stop depot. Start half the oral equivalent dose on the day when the next weekly injection is due. After a week of half-dose, move to full dose equivalent daily		Start 25% oral on date next depot due for one week, then 33% for a week, then 66% for a week, then 100%. Weird but true	N/A	N/A	Plasma levels start to drop below steady state about 4–5 weeks after the last dose given. This must be considered when adding an oral or LAI antipsychotic to avoid the risk of additive ADRs and NMS
Missed dose	A dose can be given a day or two early or late without significant effects on plasma levels. If missing a week, give the next dose due on the scheduled date but add up to about 50–75% (within licensed limits), then revert to normal dose a week after that					Add up to 50% to next weekly dose, then go back to usual dose. There will be a small dip in plasma levels 3–5 weeks after the missed dose and oral supplementation may be needed
Missed two doses	Give 50% extra when restarting, then go back to original dose weekly. Blood levels return to previous within a week		Start again with the next due dose (3/52 after last dose given) at double dose, then revert to normal dose			Carry on with standard dose when next due. Be aware that levels may be lower in 3–5 weeks time. Dose adjustments do not seem to help
Missed three or more doses	Give 50% extra when restarting, then go back to the original dose weekly. Blood levels return to previous within a week or two		Start again with the next due dose (3/52 after last dose given) at double dose. The subsequent dose can have up to 25% added if felt clinically necessary, then revert to the normal dose			Start again as per normal. Will need oral cover until re-established

2.2.5.1 Weekly injections *continued*						
	Flupentixol decanoate	**Zuclopenthixol decanoate**	**Haloperidol decanoate**	**Pipotiazine palmitate**	**Fluphenazine decanoate**	**Risperidone LAI (Consta®)**
Double dose given	Omit the next due dose, then restart with the previous dose a week after the omitted dose. Beware of high plasma levels in the week after the double dose. It is possible to add up to 25% to the next dose if it is really needed for breakthrough symptoms					Carry on with usual dose next time. Plasma levels may be high 3–5 weeks later. Anticholinergics may be needed to cover additional side-effects. Dose adjustments do not seem to help
2.2.5.2 Every two weeks (fortnightly)						
Fortnightly to 3/52	Add up to 20–25% to the last fortnightly injection then move to 3/52 injection at 1.5 times the previous dose					Not recommended as plasma level variation is much higher. If essential, add 50% to the fortnightly dose from the first 3-weekly dose. Adding extra to the last fortnightly dose can lead to high levels later and is unnecessary
Fortnightly to weekly	Give the last fortnightly dose as usual, miss a week then start weekly at 50% of the previous fortnightly dose. Plasma levels may take 4–6 weeks to stabilise. No other dose adjustment seems necessary					Give the last fortnightly dose as usual, then move to weekly with the 50% fortnightly dose. There is no apparent need for any dose alterations
Oral to LAI/depot	Stop oral on the day the depot starts		Start depot, 50% oral for one week, 25% for up to two weeks	N/A	N/A	Continue oral risperidone for 3 weeks after the first fortnightly dose, and then stop or titrate down in week 3
LAI/depot to oral	Switch to oral equivalent dose on the day when the next fortnightly injection is due	Start half the oral equivalent dose on the day when the next 2/52 injection is due. After 1/52, move to full dose equivalent daily	On the date the next depot is due start 25% of the target dose for a week, then give 50% for 2 weeks, then the full dose	N/A	N/A	Plasma levels start to drop below the steady state about 5 weeks after the last dose is given and fall to near baseline by 7–8 weeks. This must be considered when adding an oral or LAI antipsychotic to avoid the risk of additive ADRs and NMS

2.2.5.2 Every two weeks (fortnightly) *continued*

	Flupentixol decanoate	Zuclopenthixol decanoate	Haloperidol decanoate	Pipotiazine palmitate	Fluphenazine decanoate	Risperidone LAI (Consta®)
Missed dose	Give the missed dose a week late, then go to fortnightly from that date if possible (which will be a different week from the previous fortnightly routine). Alternately: give 75% of the previous dose a week after the due dose was missed, then 75% again a week later, then go back to the original dose every 2 weeks. Or: add (up to) 50% to the next due fortnightly dose (i.e. 28 days after the last dose was given)		Start again with the next due dose plus (up to) about 50%, then revert to normal dose. Or: give 50% a week after the missed dose then resume the previous dose on the previous fortnightly routine. Or: give the full dose up to 6 days late			Because of the delayed release, a dose can be given as soon as possible and carried on fortnightly from that point. Do not give a double or higher dose because that could lead to toxic levels 3–5 weeks later. Oral supplementation may be needed. Or, carry on with the fortnightly dose given a week late, and carry on fortnightly from then. If you need to go back to the original fortnightly scheduled days, give 50% of the fortnightly dose on the next scheduled day (i.e. a week after the dose given a week late), then the usual dose from that point on and manage the low plasma levels 3–5 weeks later with oral supplementation
Missed 2 doses	Add 50% to the first dose given (4 weeks after the last dose), and top-up with some oral for the next two weeks if needed		Give the next dose as scheduled plus up to 75% extra (within BNF limits). Plasma levels should not rise above the previous highest			Due to the delayed release, give the dose as soon as possible and carry on from that point fortnightly. Oral supplementation may be needed. Do not give a double or higher dose as that could lead to toxic levels 3–5 weeks later

2.2.5.2 Every two weeks (fortnightly) *continued*						
	Flupentixol decanoate	**Zuclopenthixol decanoate**	**Haloperidol decanoate**	**Pipotiazine palmitate**	**Fluphenazine decanoate**	**Risperidone LAI (Consta®)**
Missed 3 or more doses	Start again but there should be no need for a test dose		Give the next dose when due, plus an extra 75% (within BNF limits). Or, if needing to get back to therapeutic plasma levels as soon as possible, restart fortnightly with the original dose, then give an extra 50% a week after the first dose. Plasma levels will be back to previous steady state in the week after the third dose			Because of the delayed release, can give a dose as soon as it can be done and carry on from that point fortnightly. Do not give a double or higher dose because that could lead to toxic levels 3–5 weeks later. Oral supplementation may be needed
Double dose given	The next fortnightly dose should be 50% of usual. Cover with (extra) anticholinergics for 2 weeks		Give the next dose as planned but only give 20–25% of the usual dose, then revert to normal dose on the routine day. High levels expected in the week after the double dose so manage with (extra) anticholinergics if needed			Choice is limited. Giving 50% of the usual dose at the next fortnightly injection will *not* help the peak level at 3–5 weeks and leads to much lower levels 6–8 weeks afterwards. Seems best to manage peaks and carry on as normal
2.2.5.3 Three-weekly						
3/52 to 4/52	Leave 4 weeks from the last dose then start with the usual dose plus 33% every 4 weeks					Not appropriate for 3–4 weekly injections
3/52 to 2/52	2 weeks after the last dose was given, start 2/52ly injection at around 66% of the previous dose					N/A
Oral to LAI/depot	Start depot, stop oral		When starting depot, reduce oral to half for a week then stop	N/A	N/A	N/A
LAI/depot to oral	Start an equivalent oral dose 3 weeks after the last depot/LAI (i.e. on the day the next depot/LAI was due)		Start half target oral dose when next depot due for a week, then move to full target oral dose	N/A	N/A	N/A

2.2.5.3 Three-weekly *continued*

	Flupentixol decanoate	Zuclopenthixol decanoate	Haloperidol decanoate	Pipotiazine palmitate	Fluphenazine decanoate	Risperidone LAI (Consta®)
Week late	Give the missed dose a week late, then carry on as before. Anticholinergic cover may be needed for a week or so after the subsequent injection		One week late — can give usual dose and resume previous routine			N/A
2 weeks late	Can give 2/52 late, then revert to the usual 3/52 days but the subsequent dose (a week after the dose given 2/52 late) should be 50% of the usual		Two weeks late — can give 75% usual dose and then resume as before (i.e. previous dose a week after the 75% dose has been given)			N/A
Missed dose	Restart at the next dose (i.e. 6/52 after the last dose given) at the usual dose plus 33–50%, then revert to the usual dose		Restart at usual dose plus 50%, then revert to previous dosage schedule			N/A
Missed 2 or more doses	Plasma levels will have dropped to low levels so start again with the usual dose					N/A
Double dose given	Give the next dose as planned, but only give 50% of the usual dose, then revert to normal dose on the routine day. Expect high levels in the week or two after the double dose so manage with (extra) anticholinergics if needed					N/A
2.2.5.4 Four-weekly or monthly						
4/52 to 3/52	3 weeks after the last dose was given, start 3/52ly injection at 75% of the previous dose					N/A
4/52 to 2/52	2 weeks after the last dose was given, start 2/52ly injection at 50% of the previous dose					N/A
Oral to LAI/depot	Stop oral on the day the depot starts		When starting the depot reduce the oral to half for a week, then stop	N/A	N/A	N/A
LAI/depot to oral	Start the full equivalent oral dose 4 weeks after the last depot (i.e. on day next depot was due)		Start half target oral dose when next depot due for a week, then move to full target oral dose	N/A	N/A	N/A

2.2.5.4 Four-weekly or monthly *continued*

	Flupentixol decanoate	Zuclopenthixol decanoate	Haloperidol decanoate	Pipotiazine palmitate	Fluphenazine decanoate	Risperidone LAI (Consta®)
Week late	Give the missed dose a week late, then carry on as before. May need (extra) anticholinergic cover for a week or so after the subsequent injection		Give the full dose and revert to routine			N/A
2 weeks late	Can give 2/52 late, then revert to the usual 4/52 days, but the subsequent dose (two weeks after the dose given 2/52 late) should be 50% of the usual		Give the full dose and revert to routine			N/A
3 weeks late	Plasma levels will have dropped to low levels so start again with the usual dose		Give 60–75% then the full dose the week after (on the routine day). Plasma levels should not rise above the previous peaks			N/A
Missed dose	Plasma levels will have dropped to low levels so start again with the usual dose		Restart at the usual dose plus up to 50%, then revert to the previous dosage schedule			N/A
Missed 2 doses	Plasma levels will have dropped to low levels, so start again with the usual dose					N/A
Missed 3 or more doses	Plasma levels will have dropped to low levels, so start again with the usual dose					N/A
Double dose given	Give the next dose as usual at the same dose. High plasma levels should be expected in the two weeks after the double dose, so manage with (extra) anticholinergics if needed		Give the next dose as planned, but only give 50–60% of the usual dose, then revert to normal dose on the routine day. High levels should be expected in the week or two after the double dose, so manage with (extra) anticholinergics if needed			N/A

2.2.5.5 Paliperidone palmitate (Xeplion®)

Four-weekly or monthly	Second dose	Maintenance
Oral to LAI/ depot	Oral antipsychotics can be stopped over 1/52 except olanzapine, quetiapine and clozapine (stop over 4/52 to minimise insomnia and cholinergic rebound)	Not applicable
Missed dose	**The second dose due on day 8 can be given four days either side, e.g. on days 4–12.** **If 13–28 days have elapsed from the initial dose:** 1. Give 100 mg in the deltoid as soon as possible as the second injection, then... 2. Give 75 mg in either the deltoid or gluteal 5 weeks after the first injection (regardless of the timing of the second injection), then... 3. Give the required maintenance dose (25–150 mg) one month after the 75 mg dose (either deltoid or gluteal) **If 28–49 days have elapsed from initial dose:** 1. Give 100 mg in the deltoid as soon as possible, then... 2. Give 100 mg in either deltoid or gluteal one week later (± 4 days), then... 3. Give the required maintenance dose (25–150 mg) one month after the second 100 mg dose (either deltoid or gluteal) **If greater than 49 days (>7 weeks) from the initial dose:** • Start again as if initiating on day one	**PPLAI can routinely be given up to seven days before, or seven days after, the monthly due date. For a missed dose:** **Up to and including 6 weeks (42 days) after the last dose:** 1. Give the usual stabilised dose as soon as possible, but 2. Move the next due date on to a month after the most recent injection **More than 6 weeks and up to 6 months since the last monthly maintenance dose:** This will depend on the maintenance dose: **For patients stabilised on 25–100 mg:** 1. Give a deltoid injection as soon as possible at the same dose the patient was previously stabilised on, then... 2. Give another deltoid injection (same dose) one week later (day 8), then... 3. Resume the normal monthly cycle of injections, in either the deltoid or gluteal muscle, as per the original maintenance dose **For patients stabilised on 150 mg:** 1. Give a deltoid injection as soon as possible at the 100 mg dose, then... 2. Give another deltoid injection 7 days later (day 8) at the 100 mg dose then... 3. Resume the normal monthly cycle of injections in either the deltoid or gluteal muscle of 25–150 mg based on individual patient tolerability and/or efficacy **Missed monthly maintenance doses (>6 months):** • Start again as if initiating on day one

2.2.5.6 Olanzapine pamoate LAI (Zypadhera®) Olanzapine pamoate is much more difficult to model and so these are little more than suggestions

Two-weekly	
2/52 to 4/52 LAI	The last dose of 2/52 given should be the predicted 4/52 dose, then leave 4/52 until the next (4/52) dose. There is not a licensed 4/52 dose equivalent to doses higher than 210mg every 2/52
LAI to oral	Olanzapine plasma levels appear not to fall to zero until around 6–8 months after the last injection, with a half-life of around 30 days for the LAI (cf 30 hours for oral olanzapine). Oral olanzapine may be reintroduced at a very low dose when the next dose is due, and gradually titrated up to an equivalent dose over the next 3–6 months, depending on response and adverse effects
Oral to 2/52 LAI	Establish oral first. Therapeutic plasma levels occur within the first week after an injection and oral olanzapine is not needed once the LAI is started. If considered essential, the combined total dose of olanzapine from both formulations (LAI dose converted to daily dosing plus oral supplementation) should not exceed the equivalent to 20mg/d (MI)
Late doses	One trial allowed dosing at 12–16 days after the previous dose. The LAI can be given a week late, but watch for slightly higher levels a week later
Missed dose	Can give up to 25% extra with the next two doses without major changes in plasma levels
Missed 2 or more doses	Modelling suggests that up to 25% extra can be given with the next two doses (assuming both are within SmPC limits), then revert to the previous dose. This may re-establish plasma levels within a month or so, although oral supplementation or restarting may be alternatives. If doses are above the SmPC limits, just carry on as before and use oral supplementation if possible and needed
Four-weekly	
4/52 to 2/52 LAI	The last dose of 4/52 given should be the predicted 2/52 dose, then continue every 2/52
LAI to oral	As for 'LAI to oral' above
Oral to 4/52 LAI	As for 'Oral to 2/52 LAI' above
Late doses	One trial allowed dosing at 24–32 days after the previous dose. Can give up to 2/52 late then continue on the usual day, or continue with 4/52 injections from the new date, where plasma levels will not rise above previous peaks
Missed dose	Can give up to 25% extra with next dose, although plasma levels may be low before that dose and oral supplementation for a few days may be useful
Missed 2 doses	Can give up to 25% extra with the next two doses, although plasma levels may be low before that first dose and oral supplementation for a few weeks may be useful
Missed 3 or more doses	Start again as if recommencing treatment

2.2.5.7 Aripiprazole LAI monthly injection *

Two-weekly	
Oral aripiprazole to aripiprazole LAI (ALAI)	Stabilise on oral aripiprazole first, then start ALAI at 400 mg. Continue oral at 10–20 mg/d for 2/52. Do not give the second injection sooner than 25 days after the first
Other oral antipsychotic to ALAI	Maintain the first antipsychotic at the previous dose. Start oral aripiprazole at 5 mg/d, increasing to 10 mg over the next week or so depending on response. Continue both for a minimum of two weeks. Adjust the aripiprazole to dose according to response and tolerability. Discontinue the first antipsychotic, and start aripiprazole LAI when stopped
Aripiprazole LAI to oral aripiprazole	Restart aripiprazole at 5–10 mg/d when the next injection would have been due. After 1–2 weeks increase the dose as needed
Missed dose	**Second or third doses missed:** If 4–5 weeks have elapsed: Restart the injection and resume on the previous planned monthly date (i.e. 3–4 weeks after the late dose) If more than five weeks have elapsed: Restart injection and resume on the previous planned monthly date (i.e. 2–3 weeks after the late dose), but oral supplementation may be needed for about two weeks **Fourth or subsequent doses missed:** Can be given up to two weeks late. If given up to two weeks late, restart monthly injection on the previous planned monthly date (i.e. 2–4 weeks after the late dose). Leaving four weeks before the next dose can lead to some sub-therapeutic levels for several months. If 6–8 weeks since the last injection, start oral aripiprazole for about four weeks while resuming the monthly injection on the previous dates
Missed 2 doses	If over eight weeks, restart as if initiating as plasma levels will have reached very low levels
Double dose	Give 20–25% of the usual dose when the next injection was due and then carry on as before. Plasma levels should not remain high for more than a few extra days and should not drop significantly below previous levels. Steady state should be regained within a few weeks

3. Analgesic equivalents are mostly derived from single-dose studies, not long-term studies where a steady state has been achieved.
4. Total daily doses should be calculated.
5. These are definitely **not** starting doses, but may give a pointer to a possible maximum or target. The person should be dose titrated and assessed, based on withdrawal symptoms and clinical response.
6. Analgesic equivalents for tramadol produce a much higher methadone equivalent. The tramadol dose here is based on a study showing tramadol 450 mg/d is equivalent to 15 mg/d methadone for suppressing opiate withdrawal symptoms (n=70, RCT, d/b, Salehi *et al*, *J Res Med Sci* 2006;**11**:185–9). NB. SR, dispersible and liquid tramadol may have different bioavailabilities.
7. Codeine is metabolised by 2D6 to active morphine, so any 2D6 slow or ultra-rapid metabolism will affect the equivalent dose.
8. Some texts recommend that if changing from less to more potent opioids, reduce the dose by up to 30–50%, as there is often incomplete cross tolerance due to different binding profiles and differential sedation.
9. Dihydrocodeine SR (DHC) is 95–100% absorbed so the total daily dose is the same as plain tablets.

TABLE 2.2.6: BENZODIAZEPINE EQUIVALENT DOSES *

See note in introduction regarding half lives

Diazepam	5 mg (oral, im, or iv)
Alprazolam	0.5 mg (0.25–0.5 mg)
Chlordiazepoxide	15 mg (10–25 mg)
Clobazam	10 mg
Clonazepam	0.5 mg (0.25–4mg)
Flunitrazepam	0.5 mg
Flurazepam	7.5–15 mg
Loprazolam	0.5–1 mg
Lorazepam	0.5 mg
Lormetazepam	0.5–1 mg
Nitrazepam	5 mg (2.5–20 mg)
Oxazepam	15 mg (10–20 mg)
Temazepam	10 mg

2.2.5 SWITCHING ADHD TREATMENTS

Methylphenidate to atomoxetine:

A slower switch is generally recommended to minimise adverse effects, although they can be given together. About 50% of methylphenidate non-responders will respond to atomoxetine and 75% methylphenidate responders will also respond to atomoxetine (Prasad and Steer, *Paediatr Drugs* 2008;**10**:39–47).

Week 1 = full-dose methylphenidate, plus atomoxetine 0.5 mg/kg/d
Weeks 2–3 = half-dose methylphenidate, plus atomoxetine 1.2 mg/kg/d
Week 4 = stop methylphenidate, atomoxetine 1.2 mg/kg/d

Reference: (n=69 [c=58], open, Quintana *et al*, *Clin Ther* 2007;**29**:1168–77).

Switching methylphenidate preparations: *

IR-MPH, Equasym XL, Medikinet XL	Concerta XL equivalent dose
10 mg/d	
15 mg	18 mg
20 mg	
30 mg	36 mg
40 mg	
45 mg	54 mg
50 mg	72 mg (unlicensed)

2.2.6 SWITCHING CHOLINESTERASE INHIBITORS (ChEIs)

Switching cholinesterase inhibitors (ChEIs):

Switching ChEIs may be needed due to poor tolerability, or lack of short- or long-term efficacy. There are subtle differences in receptor modulation between the ChEIs and so lack of response to one does not necessarily exclude response to another. There is no published data on switching to donepezil.

Donepezil to galantamine: *

In donepezil inadequate responders, a one-week gap then switching to galantamine quickly (8 mg/week increase) was as well tolerated and effective as a slow (8 mg/month increase) titration (n=89 [c=86], RCT, open, 12/52,

TABLE 2.2.7: METHADONE EQUIVALENT DOSES

Narcotics				
Drug	Total daily dose	Equivalent daily dose of methadone in mg	Range quoted	
			Lower	Upper
Buprenorphine injection	0.3 mg	8	8	8
Buprenorphine S/L	0.2 mg	5	5	8
Codeine linctus 15 mg/5 mL[7]	1 mL	0.2	0.2	0.2
Codeine phosphate[7]	15 mg	1	1	1
Dextropropoxyphene	32.5 mg	2.145	2.145	2.145
Diamorphine BP injection	5 mg	10	10	10
Diamorphine BP oral	10 mg	10	10	20
Diconal tablets	1 tab	5	4	5
Dihydrocodeine[9]	30 mg	2.5	2	3
Fentanyl patches **(mcg/hr)**	25 mcg/hr	2	1.65	2.5
Gee's Linctus	100 mL	10	10	10
Hydromorphone oral	1 mg	2.5	2.5	6.5
J Collis Brown's **(mLs)**	100 mLs	10	10	10
Morphine BP injection	10 mg	10	10	10
Morphine BP oral	15 mg	10	10	10
MST tablets	10 mg	3.25	3.25	3.25
Oxycodone	1 mg	0.8	0.4	1.32
Palfium	5 mg	5	5	10
Papaveretum	10 mg	4.4		
Pentazocine	25 mg	2	2	2
Pethidine injection/tablets	50 mg	4.25	4	5
Tramadol[6]	50 mg	1.6	1.6	8.25

Engedal *et al, Acta Neurol Scand* 2011;**126**:37–44), probably with standard response rates regardless of non-response to donepezil (Emre, *Int J Clin Pract Suppl* 2002;**127**:64–72). An abrupt switch is also possible and can help in donepezil-resistant BPSD (n=46(c=44), 3/12, Sasaki and Horie, *Dement Geriatr Cogn Dis Extra* 2014;**4**:131–9; FFT).

Donepezil to rivastigmine oral: *
In donepezil non-response, around 50% will then respond to rivastigmine (n=382, Auriacombe *et al, Curr Med Res Opin* 2002;**18**:129–38; n=188, Bartorelli *et al, Curr Med Res Opin* 2005;**21**:1809–18). Abrupt switch from donepezil to oral rivastigmine (without washout) may be effective and well tolerated (review of three switching studies; s=3, Sadowsky *et al, Int J Clin Pract* 2010;**64**:188–93).

Donepezil to rivastigmine patches: *
Immediate or seven-day delayed withdrawal switching from donepezil oral to rivastigmine patches appears equally well tolerated (n=234 [c=176], RCT, open, 25/52, Sadowsky *et al, Prim Care Companion J Clin Psychiatry* 2011;**12**:09m00852; FFT), but a slower switch might be appropriate with any pre-existing bradycardia or if concurrent beta-blockers are being taken, the incidence of nausea and vomiting being 4% and 1% respectively (open, Sadowsky *et al, Am J Alzheimer's Dis Other Demen* 2009;**24**:267–75). If switching from oral donepezil to rivastigmine patches adherence seems to improve (n=772, Tian *et al, Alzheimer Dis Assoc Disord* 2013;**27**:182–6), although this paper could be entitled 'Transdermal rivastigmine adherence to patients...' rather than 'Patient adherence to transdermal rivastigmine...'.

Galantamine plain to galantamine XL:
A manufacturer's computer simulation suggests that an abrupt switch should be acceptable (Hing *et al, Curr Med Res Opin* 2005;**21**:483–8).

Galantamine to rivastigmine patches:
Galantamine can be switched abruptly to the patch, with nausea or vomiting occurring in only 2–3% (Sadowsky *et al, CNS Neurosci Ther* 2010;**16**:51–60). Response can occur despite non-response to galantamine (n=33, Bartorelli *et al, Curr Med Res Opin* 2005;**21**:1809–18).

Rivastigmine to galantamine:
The response rate to galantamine may be the same regardless of non-response to other ChEIs (Emre, *Int J Clin Pract Suppl* 2002;**127**:64–72).

Rivastigmine oral to rivastigmine patches:
High dose oral rivastigmine can be switched abruptly to the 9.5mg/24-hour patch, but low dose should be switched to 4.6mg/24-hour for four weeks before increasing. The incidence of nausea and vomiting is 3% and 2% respectively (Sadowsky *et al, CNS Neurosci Ther* 2010;**16**:51–60). The first patch should be applied the day after the last oral dose. In people intolerant of oral rivastigmine, 70% completed an immediate switch to patches and 12% discontinued due to dermatological ADRs (n=164[c=116], open 24/52, Han *et al, J Clin Neurol* 2011;**7**:137–42; FFT).

Rivastigmine oral dose per day	Patch strength
3–6mg	4.6mg/24 hours
9mg (not stable/poorly tolerated)	4.6mg/24 hours
9mg (stable and well tolerated)	9.5mg/24 hours
12mg	9.5mg/24 hours

2.2.7 SWITCHING OR DISCONTINUING ANTIDEPRESSANTS

Switching from one antidepressant to another, either for reasons of side-effects, safety or lack of efficacy, can be problematical and present unexpected problems. Clinicians must be aware of these to eliminate avoidable adverse events. Switching may be effective if a full therapeutic trial of a previous drug has failed, although not always (s=3, d/b, Bschor and Baethge, *Acta Psychiatr Scand* 2010;**121**:174–9).

Equivalent doses (see table below):
Data from all double-blind, RCTs comparing fluoxetine or paroxetine with any other antidepressant as monotherapy in acute depression has been used to create an equivalent dose table. All results were corroborated via sensitivity analyses except for doxepin and assumes a dose-response relationship, and normal renal and hepatic function and no enzyme polymorphisms (s=83, n=11131, RCTs, d/b, Hayasaka *et al, J Affect Disord* 2015;**180**:179-84;FFT).

ANTIDEPRESSANT EQUIVALENT DOSES

Antidepressant	*Equivalent dose*
Agomelatine	25mg
Amitriptyline	60mg
Bupropion	175mg
Clomipramine	60mg
Dosulepin	75mg
Doxepin	70mg
Escitalopram	9mg
Fluoxetine	20mg
Fluvoxamine	70mg
Imipramine	70mg
Lofepramine	125mg
Maprotiline	60mg
Mianserin	50mg
Mirtazapine	25mg
Moclobemide	285mg
Nortriptyline	50mg
Paroxetine	17mg
Reboxetine	6mg
Sertraline	50mg
Trazodone	200mg
Venlafaxine	75mg

1. Agomelatine to/from others *

Agomelatine has no known problems so can be switched to and from with negligible risk, except fluvoxamine, which inhibits 1A2 and raises agomelatine levels significantly (McAllister-Williams *et al, Hum Psychopharmacol* 2010;**25**:95–102). Three switching regimens (2, 3 slow taper, 3 long taper) from paroxetine or venlafaxine to agomelatine showed similar outcomes, but SSRI/SNRI discontinuation effects were frequently interpreted as agomelatine ADRs (d/b, 8/52, Lejoyeux *et al, CNS Spectr* 2015;**20**:29–38).

2. SSRI to/from a tricyclic

Fluoxetine, paroxetine and fluvoxamine (but probably not citalopram, escitalopram or sertraline at standard doses) can double or triple tricyclic levels (particularly amitriptyline, clomipramine, imipramine and nortriptyline) by CYP2D6 inhibition and so great care is needed. Concurrent prescribing over a change-over period is not advised unless the drugs and doses are chosen carefully and specific care is taken. Ideally, 'drop-and-stop' before starting the next antidepressant is recommended (switch 1 or 2a).

Specific factors for an SSRI-tricyclic switch:

- **Speed** at which the switch is needed, e.g. faster switches can obviously be made, but additional monitoring, e.g. tricyclic levels and cardiac status is recommended.
- **Dose** — CYP2D6 inhibition is dose-related for most SSRIs, e.g. paroxetine, fluoxetine.
- **P450** status of the person, i.e. slow or rapid metaboliser (see *4.3*).
- **Tricyclic** — more potent serotonin reuptake inhibitors are more likely to produce serotonin syndrome (e.g. clomipramine). Tertiary tricyclics (e.g. imipramine, amitriptyline, clomipramine) are also metabolised by CYP3A3/4 and CYP1A2, which are inhibited by fluvoxamine.
- **Individual** susceptibility to side-effects.

Main potential problems (see introduction for more details):

- Cholinergic rebound from tricyclics (see *14*)
- TCA/SSRI discontinuation effects (see *14*)
- Serotonin syndrome (see *6.9*)
- Increased tricyclic levels via CYP2D6 inhibition by SSRIs (see *4.3.1*).

Suggested switch regimens:

Tricyclic to fluoxetine, paroxetine or fluvoxamine: Taper tricyclic dose to around 25–50 mg/d, start SSRI at usual starting dose and discontinue the tricyclic over the next 5–7 days. Be wary of serotonin syndrome, raised tricyclic levels by P450 inhibition, cholinergic rebound and tricyclic withdrawal.

Tricyclic to (es)citalopram or sertraline: As above, but this has a much lower potential for interactions so problems are less likely, although serotonin syndromes have been reported.

(Es)citalopram or sertraline to tricyclic: If necessary, reduce to minimum doses of citalopram (20 mg/d), escitalopram (10 mg) or sertraline (50 mg/d), stop the SSRI and introduce the tricyclic, titrating dose upwards as tolerated. With standard doses of these SSRIs, few problems should be seen. Be wary of SSRI withdrawal (see *14*), serotonin syndrome (e.g. clomipramine) and higher tricyclic levels via CYP2D6 inhibition (low risk).

Fluoxetine to tricyclic: Drop fluoxetine to 20 mg/d, stop, wait several days for peak levels to fall, then add the tricyclic **cautiously at low dose** and build up slowly. Care is needed for up to four weeks as the interaction potential via 2D6 inhibition may be prolonged (see *4.3.2*), e.g. an abrupt switch from fluoxetine 20 mg/d to amitriptyline 50–100 mg/d resulted in 14% dropping out due to adverse reactions, the rest tolerating the switch. Be wary of serotonin syndrome (e.g. clomipramine) and higher tricyclic levels via CYP2D6 inhibition.

Factors to consider before choosing an antidepressant switching regimen

- The speed at which the switch is needed, e.g. with less urgency a more cautious regimen can be used. Faster switches can obviously be made, but additional monitoring is recommended.
- Individual drugs and their effects, neurotransmitter effects and kinetics.
- Current dose of the first drug.
- An individuals' susceptibility to (additive) ADRs.

Potential problems

- Cholinergic rebound, e.g. headache, restlessness, diarrhoea, nausea and vomiting (see *18a*) from withdrawal of cholinergic blockers such as tricyclics.
- Antidepressant withdrawal or discontinuation symptoms (see *13*).
- Serotonin syndrome, for antidepressants affecting serotonin (see *6.9*).
- Drug–drug interactions, e.g. variable drug levels from altered metabolism (see *4.3*).
- Discontinuation effects from the first drug interpreted as side-effects of the second.

Switching drugs 'with care' means

- Drop and stop first drug.
- Leave a gap of a few days if possible before starting second drug.
- Warn the person about potential complications and what to do about them, e.g. serotonin syndrome, cholinergic rebound, toxicity and discontinuation.

Paroxetine to tricyclic: Leave a gap if possible or taper paroxetine to about 10mg/d, and introduce the tricyclic at low dose. After several days, discontinue paroxetine and increase the tricyclic dose to therapeutic levels. Be wary of SSRI withdrawal (see *14*), serotonin syndrome (especially with drugs such as clomipramine) and higher tricyclic levels via CYP2D6 inhibition.
Fluvoxamine to tricyclic: As paroxetine but also be aware of higher tricyclic levels via CYP1A2 and 3A3/4 inhibition (especially tertiary tricyclics).

3. Trazodone to/from others

Trazodone to SSRIs: Trazodone and fluoxetine have been used together, but the risks include enhanced sedation (e.g. n=8, Nirenberg *et al*, *J Clin Psychiatry* 1992;**53**:83), serotonin syndrome (n=1, George and Godleski, *Biol Psychiatry* 1996;**39**:384–5) and slightly raised trazodone levels (see *4.3.3.7*). A serotonin syndrome with low dose trazodone added to paroxetine (n=1, Reeves and Bullen, *Psychosomatics* 1995;**36**:159–60) would indicate the need for similar care. For citalopram, there is a report of lack of pharmacokinetic interaction, with plasma levels unchanged (n=81, Prapotnik *et al*, *Int J Clin Pharmacol Ther* 2004;**42**:120–4). There is no information on switching from trazodone to sertraline but a gradual switch, with close observation would seem sensible (see *5*).
Trazodone to tricyclics: Hypomania has been reported after an abrupt change to imipramine (n=2, Haggerty and Jackson, *J Clin Psychiatry* 1985;**5**:342–3), so care is needed.

4. Tricyclic to/from tricyclic

No significant problems have been reported, but a gradual switch is recommended as per normal practice (switches 1, 2 or 3).

5. SSRI to/from another SSRI*

Any combination of SSRIs could precipitate a serotonin syndrome (see *6.9*), so careful observation and a gentle changeover is recommended. A washout period would further minimise the possibility of problems.
Fluoxetine to sertraline: Be aware of fluoxetine's long half-life, e.g. in out-patients abruptly switched from fluoxetine to sertraline, 63% were successful but 37% failed, including 18% with intolerable adverse effects (nervousness, jitters, diarrhoea, nausea and headache), suggestive of a serotonin-like syndrome (n=54, Stock and Kofoed, *Am J Hosp Pharm* 1994;**51**:2279–81).
Fluoxetine to paroxetine: Abrupt switching can increase side-effects such as insomnia, nausea, dry mouth, nervousness and tremor occurred (likely to have been a serotonin syndrome) compared to a two-week washout, which was well tolerated (n=240, d/b, Kreider *et al*, *J Clin Psychiatry* 1995;**56**:142–5; n=9, Dominguez *et al*, *J Clin Psychopharmacol* 1996;**16**:320–3).
Fluvoxamine to paroxetine: There is a case of rapidly increased fluvoxamine levels when paroxetine was started during a switch, probably via 2D6 inhibition (n=1, Hori *et al*, *World J Biol Psychiatry* 2009;**10**:620–2).

> **How to use *Table 2.2.8*:**
>
> i. Look down the vertical column headed 'from' and find the drug, or drug group, the patient is currently taking.
> ii. Follow that line along until you come to the column of the drug, or drug group to which you wish to change.
> iii. The details there give the current known information. For further details look up the reference number quoted.
>
> Example: Changing from tranylcypromine to a tricyclic requires a 14-day drug-free gap (reference 9), but changing from a tricyclic to tranylcypromine only requires a seven-day drug-free gap (reference 9).

6. Duloxetine to/from SSRIs/SNRIs

SSRIs/venlafaxine to duloxetine: Abruptly stopping an SSRI and starting duloxetine was as well tolerated and safe as tapered SSRI discontinuation and immediately starting duloxetine (n=368, RCT, 10/52, Perahia *et al*, *J Clin Psychiatry* 2008;**69**:95–105).
Duloxetine to SSRIs/venlafaxine: People switching have reported less nausea when starting the SSRI than those starting *de novo*; immediate switching may be well tolerated, although fluoxetine was surprisingly excluded

Table 2.2.8: Switching antidepressants *

NSPR = no significant problems reported, careful cross-taper; OP = occasional problems; SSP = serotonin syndrome possible

To / From	MAOIs			SSRIs													
	Hydrazines	Tranyl-cypromine	Tricyclics	Citalopram/ escitalopram	Fluvoxamine	Fluoxetine	Sertraline	Paroxetine	Trazodone	Bupropion	Moclobemide	Venlafaxine	Duloxetine[6]	Mirtazapine	Agomelatine[13]	Reboxetine	Vortioxetine
MAOIs: Hydra-zines	14/7[7]	14/7[7]	7–14/7[7]	14/7[7]	14/7[7]	14/7[7]	14/7[7]	14/7[7]	14/7[7] or care	7/7[9]	See text[7]	14/7[13]	14/7[6]	2/52[7]	NSPR[1]	2/52[7]	14/7[10]
MAOIs: Tranyl-cypro-mine	14/7[7]		14/7[7]	14/7[7]	14/7[7]	14/7[7]	14/7[7]	14/7[7]	14/7[7]	7/7[9]	See text[7]	14/7[13]	14/7[6]	2/52[7]	NSPR[1]	2/52[7]	14/7[10]
Tricyclics	7/7[7]	7/7[7]	NSPR[4]	Care[2]	Great care[2]	Great care[2]	Care[2]	Great care[2]	NSPR[10]	NSPR[9]	See text[7,8]	Care[13]	SSP[5]	NSPR[11]	NSPR[1]	NSPR[12]	SSP[10]
Citalopram/ escitalopram	7/7[7]	7/7[7]	Care[2]	SSP	SSP[5]	SSP[5]	SSP[5]	SSP[5]	Care	NSPR[9]	7/7[8]	Care[13]	SSP[5]	NSPR[11]	NSPR[1]	NSPR[12]	SSP[10]
Fluvoxamine	4-5/7[7]	7–14/7[7]	Great care[2]	SSP[5]		SSP[5]	SSP[5]	SSP[5]	Care	NSPR[9]	3/7[8]	Care[13]	Care SSP[5]	NSPR[11]	Care[1]	NSPR[12]	SSP[10]
Fluoxetine	5/52[7]	5/52[7]	Great care for 28/7[2]	SSP[5]	SSP[5]		SSP[5]	SSP[5]	Care	NSPR[10]	3/52[8]	Care[13]	SSP[6]	NSPR[11]	NSPR[1]	NSPR[12]	SSP[10]
Sertraline	7-14/7[7]	7–14/7[7]	Great care[2]	SSP[5]	SSP[5]	SSP[5]		SSP[5]	Care	NSPR[9]	7–13/7[8]	Care[13]	SSP[6]	NSPR[11]	NSPR[1]	NSPR[12]	SSP[10]
Paroxetine	14/7[7]	14/7[7]	Great care[2]	SSP[5]	SSP[5]	SSP[5]	SSP[5]		Care[6]	NSPR[9]	5/7[8]	Care[13]	SSP[6]	NSPR[11]	NSPR[1]	NSPR[12]	SSP[10]
Trazodone	14/7[7]	14/7[7]	OP[3]	Care[3]	Care[3]	Care[3]	Care[3]	Care[3]		NSPR[9]	NSPR	Care[13]	SSP[6]	NSPR[11]	NSPR[1]	NSPR[12]	SSP[10]
Bupropion[10]	7/7[9]	7/7[9]	Care	NSPR[9]	NSPR[9]	NSPR[9]	NSPR[9]	NSPR[9]	NSPR[9]		NSPR[9]	NSPR[9]	NSPR[9]	NSPR[9/11]	NSPR[1]	NSPR[9]	See text[10]
Moclobemide	NSPR[7]	NSPR[7]	OP[8]	NSPR[8]	NSPR[8]	2/52[8]	NSPR[8]	NSPR[8]	NSPR[13]	NSPR		NSPR[13]	SSP[8]	NSPR[11]	NSPR[1]	NSPR[12]	SSP[10]
Venlafaxine	7/7[13]	7/7[13]	NSPR[13]	Care[13]	Care[13]	Care[13]	Care[13]	Care[13]	Care[13]	NSPR[13]	NSPR[13]		SSP[6]	NSPR[11]	NSPR[1]	NSPR[12]	SSP[10]
Duloxetine	5/7[6]	5/7[6]	SSP[5]	SSP[5] care	SSP[5]	SSP[5]	SSP[5]	SSP[5]	SSP[5]	SSP[5]	SSP[5]	SSP[5,13]		NSPR[11]	NSPR[1]	NSPR[11]	SSP[10]
Mirtazapine	7/7[7]	7/7[7]	NSPR[11]	NSPR[11]	NSPR[11]	NSPR[11]	NSPR[11]	NSPR[11]	NSPR[11]	NSPR[11]	NSPR[11]	NSPR[11]	NSPR		NSPR[1]	NSPR[12]	NSPR[10]
Agomelatine[1]	NSPR[1]	NSPR[1]	NSPR[1]	NSPR[1]	Care[1]	NSPR[1]	NSPR[1]	NSPR[1]	NSPR[1]	NSPR[1]	NSPR[1]	NSPR[1]	NSPR[1]	NSPR[1]		NSPR[1]	NSPR[10]
Reboxetine	1/52[12]	1/52[12]	NSPR[12]	NSPR[12]	NSPR[12]	NSPR[12]	NSPR[12]	NSPR[12]	NSPR[12]	NSPR[12]	NSPR[12]	NSPR[12]	NSPR[12]	NSPR[11]	NSPR[1]		NSPR[10]
Vortioxetine*	14/7[10]	14/7[10]	SSP[10]	SSP[10]	SSP[10]	SSP[10]	SSP[10]	SSP[10]	SSP[10]	Care[10]	Read text[10]	SSP[10]	SSP[10]	NSPR[10]	NSPR[10]	NSPR[10]	
Just plain stopping[17]	Over 4/52[14]	Over 4/52[14]	Over 4/52[14]	Over 4/52[14]	Over 4/52[14]	Drop and stop[14]	Over 4/52[14]	Over 4/52[14] or longer	Over 4/52[14]	Over 4/52[14]	Over 4/52[14]	Over 4/52[14] or longer	Over 4/52[14] or longer	Over 4/52[14]	NSPR[14]	Over 4/52[14]	NSPR[10]

2

from this Lilly study (n=155, Wohlreich *et al*, *Ann Clin Psychiatry* 2005;**17**:259–68, MS), as it could pose particular problems, e.g. serotonin syndrome (n=1, Liu *et al*, *J Am Geriatr Soc* 2009;**57**:2384).

7. MAOIs to/from others

MAOI to MAOI: A two-week gap is recommended, especially if switching to tranylcypromine (UK SmPC), starting tranylcypromine at half the usual dosage for one week. Careful observation is essential although tranylcypromine withdrawal or a mild serotonin syndrome can confuse the picture. A shorter gap may be feasible with full dietary control, good compliance and close monitoring (n=8, Szuba *et al*, *J Clin Psychiatry* 1997;**58**:307–10), although deaths have been reported (e.g. n=1, Bazire, *Drug Intell Clin Pharm* 1986;**20**:954–56).

SSRIs to MAOIs: The gap needed depends upon the SSRI (see below). For tranylcypromine (SmPC), leave at least a 14-day gap after stopping other antidepressants, then start tranylcypromine at half the usual dosage for one week. This would be essential for fluoxetine.

Fluvoxamine to MAOI: Fluvoxamine has a short half-life and so isocarboxazid/phenelzine may be started 4–5 days after stopping fluvoxamine (4–5 x half-life), or seven days for tranylcypromine.

Paroxetine to MAOI: A two-week gap is very cautiously recommended (SmPC).

Fluoxetine to MAOI: A serotonin syndrome has been reported with tranylcypromine six weeks after fluoxetine was stopped, due to the persistence of norfluoxetine (but not fluoxetine) in the blood (n=1, Coplan and Gorman, *Am J Psychiatry* 1993;**150**:837), so it might be best to allow six weeks after stopping fluoxetine before starting an MAOI (Anon, *Drug Ther Bull* 1990;**28**:334). The isocarboxazid SmPC recommends a 5-week gap with fluoxetine.

Sertraline to MAOI: A one-week gap should elapse before starting an MAOI. A serotonin syndrome has been reported with sertraline and tranylcypromine (see SSRI interactions 4.3.2). The SmPC states that at least a two-week gap is needed before starting sertraline after an MAOI.

Trazodone to MAOI: The literature recommends a one-week gap as combined treatment can increase in side-effects, e.g. sedation and postural hypotension (n=13, Nierenberg and Keck, *J Clin Psychopharmacol* 1989;**9**:42).

Moclobemide to MAOI: Moclobemide's half-life is 14 hours and so stopping it one day and starting an MAOI the next day seems adequate.

Mirtazapine to MAOI: A one-week washout period is recommended (SmPC), although there are no reports of problems.

Trazodone to MAOI: Trazodone's SmPC recommends a one-week gap after stopping before starting an MAOI and 2 weeks *vice versa*.

Tricyclic to MAOI: A one-week gap is recommended, particularly if imipramine, clomipramine or tranylcypromine are involved. Initial low doses of the MAOI are essential.

MAOI to SSRIs: A two-week gap has been recommended (e.g. fluoxetine SmPC), but longer may be safer as a severe serotonin syndrome has been reported with a two-week gap between stopping tranylcypromine and starting fluoxetine (n=1, Ruiz, *Ann Emerg Med* 1994;**24**:983–5), despite tranylcypromine's relatively short action and reversible MAO inhibition.

MAOI to moclobemide: A gap is not needed provided MAOI dietary restrictions are maintained for 10–14 days.

MAOI to mirtazapine: A two-week washout period is recommended.

MAOI to trazodone: The SmPC recommends a two-week gap after stopping an MAOI before trazodone is started.

MAOIs to tricyclic: A 10–14-day gap is often recommended (isocarboxazid '1–2 weeks'), particularly if imipramine, clomipramine or tranylcypromine are involved. Using initial low doses of the tricyclic is essential.

MAOIs to reboxetine: The reboxetine SmPC recommends MAOIs and reboxetine are not used together so a 7-day gap may be appropriate.

8. Moclobemide to/from others

Moclobemide to duloxetine: Immediate switching from moclobemide 400mg/d to duloxetine 60mg/d has led to a serotonin syndrome within an hour (n=1, Jimenez-Genchi, *J Clin Psychiatry* 2006;**67**:1821–2).

Moclobemide to fluoxetine: The fluoxetine SmPC states that fluoxetine can be started the day after moclobemide is stopped.

Moclobemide to tricyclic: Abrupt switching from moclobemide to tricyclics appears well tolerated, but switching to clomipramine (a serotonergic tricyclic) could cause problems.
SSRIs to moclobemide: The SmPC recommends a gap of 4–5 SSRI half-lives, as serotonin syndromes have been reported (see 4.3.3.5).
Citalopram/escitalopram to moclobemide: A seven-day gap is recommended.
Fluoxetine to moclobemide: With fluoxetine's long half-life, the gap should be as much as six weeks if five times the half-life of norfluoxetine is calculated. A three-week gap together with careful monitoring would seem a reasonably practical figure although combining moclobemide and fluoxetine seems safe (n=18, RCT, p/c, Dingemanse *et al*, *Clin Pharmacol Ther* 1998;**63**:403–13), so a more gradual switch may be tolerable.
Fluvoxamine to moclobemide: A three-day gap is recommended.
Paroxetine to moclobemide: A five-day gap is recommended, although paroxetine's half-life can be longer in the elderly. A severe serotonin syndrome has been reported when moclobemide replaced paroxetine with no washout (n=1, Wu and Deng, *J Chin Med Assoc* 2009;**72**:446–9).
Sertraline to moclobemide: With the long half-life of desmethylsertraline, the gap should be up to 13 days, but only seven days is recommended in sertraline's SmPC.
Tricyclic to moclobemide: A gap of 4–5 half-lives is recommended if the tricyclic concerned is a 5-HT reuptake inhibitor, although abruptly stopping clomipramine or amitriptyline and switching to moclobemide (150 mg first day, 300 mg/d thereafter) or placebo has shown no significant interaction (n=24, d/b, p/c, Dingemanse *et al*, *J Clin Psychopharmacol* 1995;**15**:41–8).

9. Bupropion to/from others

Bupropion is contraindicated with **MAOIs**, as animal studies show that acute bupropion toxicity is enhanced by phenelzine. Co-administration of bupropion with drugs that are metabolised by CYP2D6 (e.g. **tricyclics, paroxetine** and **fluoxetine**) should be with caution and slowly titrated if switching. If bupropion is added to the treatment regimen of a person already receiving a drug metabolised by CYP2D6, the need to decrease the dose of the original medication should be considered, particularly for those with a narrow therapeutic index.
Fluoxetine to bupropion: In fluoxetine non-responders, a switch to bupropion yielded 25% partial and 35% full responders (n=29, 12+8/52, open, Fava *et al*, *Ann Clin Psychiatry* 2003;**15**:17–22).

10. Vortioxetine *

Vortioxetine to/from MAOI: A 14-day washout period is recommended due to the risk of a serotonin syndrome (SmPC).
Vortioxetine to/from moclobemide: The combination is contraindicated but the SmPC implies that to minimise the risk of serotonin syndrome a switch using low doses and close monitoring can be used.
Vortioxetine to selegiline: As moclobemide but it is not contraindicated in the UK SmPC.
Vortioxetine to/from others: Vortioxetine has serotonergic effects and so a gap or cautious cross-titration would be needed to avoid serotonin syndrome (SmPC). Vortioxetine levels can rise with **bupropion** so extra care would be needed.

11. Mirtazapine to/from others

Mirtazapine has multiple routes of metabolism (CYP2D6, 3A4 and 1A2) so switching problems will be unlikely in terms of P450 inhibition. The only recommendation is for MAOIs (see 7). Fluoxetine 20–40 mg/d has been switched abruptly to mirtazapine 15 mg/d, without problems (n=40, Preskorn *et al*, *Biol Psychiatry* 1997;**41**:96S), although a single case of serotonin syndrome has been reported during a cross-over switch to venlafaxine (n=1, Dimellis, *World J Biol Psychiatry* 2002;**3**:167).

12. Reboxetine to/from others

Apart from MAOIs (see 7) little is published.
Fluoxetine to reboxetine: In fluoxetine non-responders, abrupt switch to reboxetine was well tolerated (n=128, open, Fava *et al*, *J Clin Psychopharmacol* 2003;**23**:365–9).

2

13. Venlafaxine to/from others

MAOI to venlafaxine: A 14-day gap is recommended between stopping an MAOI and starting venlafaxine due to reports of, e.g. extreme agitation, diaphoresis, rapid respiration and raised CPK with venlafaxine seven days after phenelzine 45 mg/d was stopped (but did not occur a further 7/7 later; n = 1, Phillips and Ringo, *Am J Psychiatry* 1995;**15**:1400–1), and serotonin syndrome (e.g. n=4, Diamond *et al*, *Neurology* 1998;**51**:274–6).

Venlafaxine to MAOI: The SmPC recommends at least a seven-day gap (see above).

Tricyclic to venlafaxine: The venlafaxine SmPC states that there is little problem between venlafaxine and tricyclics. There are no reports.

Venlafaxine to other drugs: No information is available, although agomelatine and mirtazapine have no reported or theoretical problems.

Other drugs to venlafaxine: No information.

14. Withdrawal or discontinuation

Adverse discontinuation events have been reported for many antidepressants. Such symptoms are not, however, indicative of dependence, which usually requires three of the following:

- tolerance
- withdrawal symptoms
- use greater than needed
- inability to reduce doses
- excessive time taken procuring drug
- primacy of drug-taking over other activities
- continued use despite understanding of adverse consequences.

Discontinuation symptoms usually start within 1–2 days of stopping, resolve within 2–24 hours of restarting the drug, and are more common with longer courses and higher doses. They can occur with missed doses and about 30% of people on SSRIs have dosing lapses of two or more days, long enough to produce discontinuation symptoms with some short-acting SSRIs (n=82, 3/12, Meijer *et al*, *Br J Psychiatry* 2001;**179**:519–22; FFT), but not with fluoxetine. Stopping antidepressants suddenly (over 1–7 days) increases the risk of relapse and this will occur quicker (half the time it would take otherwise) than if stopping more slowly (14 days or longer) (n=398, mean three-year follow-up, Baldessarini *et al*, *Am J Psychiatry* 2010;**167**:934–41) The *UK Drug and Therapeutics Bulletin* (1999;**37**:49–52) recommended:

- after less than eight weeks of treatment, withdraw over 1–2 weeks
- after 6–8 months of treatment, taper over 6–8-weeks
- after long-term maintenance treatment, reduce the dose by 25% every 4–6 weeks.

Options for the management of antidepressant withdrawal symptoms include:

1. Reduce the dose stepwise every 1–4 weeks or so, stabilising between reductions, e.g. paroxetine 20 mg/d, 10 mg/d, then 5mg a day or 10 mg alternate days (but not less frequently). Use of the syrup, gradually diluted, may also be effective.
2. Transfer to a long half-life antidepressant, e.g. fluoxetine (care with switching), then reduce.
3. Treat the emerging syndrome symptomatically, e.g. nausea, headache and diarrhoea have been managed with ondansetron (n = 1, Raby, *J Clin Psychiatry* 1998;**59**:621–2) and ginger root (Schechter, *J Clin Psychiatry* 1998;**59**:431–2).

Reviews: * recognition, prevention and management of antidepressant withdrawal syndromes (Haddad, *Drug Safety* 2001;**24**:183–97), general (Renoir, *Front Pharmacol* 2013;**4**:45), discontinuation symptoms (Fava *et al*, *Psychother Psychosom* 2015;**84**:72–81;FFT).

Main withdrawal symptoms

SSRIs: Symptoms can include dizziness, vertigo, lightheadedness, nausea, fatigue, headache, sensory disturbance, 'electric shocks' in the head ('brain shivers'), insomnia, abdominal cramps, chills, flu-like symptoms, increased or more vivid dreaming, anxiety/agitation and volatility, but not caused by anything else, e.g. physical illness or other drugs. Dizziness without vertigo may be caused by a sudden decrease in serotonin in the VNC (vestibular nuclear complex, also damaged in BSE/CJD), which disrupts the neurones bilaterally (Smith and Darlington, *Acta Otolaryngol* 2010;**130**:981–3). The incidence varies between SSRIs, partly due to half-life length and autoinhibition. Interruption of maintenance therapy for 5–8 days produces few discontinuation symptoms with fluoxetine (long half-life), some with sertraline and most with paroxetine (e.g. n=107, RCT, Michelson *et al*, *Br J Psychiatry* 2000;**176**:363–8; FFT).

(Es)citalopram: Even rapid citalopram discontinuation appears to produce only mild and transient effects (n=225, RCT, d/b, 10/52, Markowitz *et al*, *Int Clin Psychopharmacol* 2000;**15**:329–33). Electric shock-like sensations have been reported with escitalopram (n=1, Prakash and Dhar, *J Clin Psychopharmacol* 2008;**28**:359–60).

Fluoxetine: Discontinuation problems are rare due to its long half-life. Abrupt discontinuation can lead to slight dizziness and somnolence at weeks 2–4, but no difference at week 6, compared to continuous treatment (n=395, RCT, 12/52, Zajecka *et al*, *J Clin Psychopharmacol* 1998;**18**:193–7), although there are reports of extreme dizziness 3–14 days later (n=1, Einbinder, *Am J Psychiatry* 1995;**152**:1235), severe, dull, aching pain in the left arm, which remitted after reintroduction (n=1, Lauterbach, *Neurology* 1994;**44**:983–4), and reversible delirium (Kasantikul, *J Med Assoc Thailand* 1995;**78**:53–4).

Fluvoxamine: Slow withdrawal may be preferred (Szabadi, *Br J Psychiatry* 1992;**160**:283–4).

Paroxetine:* About 10% of people may get a significant discontinuation syndrome, more than with other SSRIs. It is more common with rapid withdrawal in people who got adverse reactions early in treatment (n=385, Himei and Okamura, *CNS Drugs* 2006;**20**:665–72). Case reports include fever, severe fatigue, headache, nausea, vomiting, agitation, electrical, shock-like sensations (Frost and Lal, *Am J Psychiatry* 1995;**152**:810), hallucinations (n=2, Yasui-Furukori and Kaneko, *Psychiatry Clin Neurosci* 2011;**65**:384–5), nocturnal enuresis (n=1, Polimeni *et al*, *J Clin Psychopharmacol* 2008;**28**:589–91), apparent stroke (n=2, Haddad *et al*, *J Psychopharmacol* 2001;**15**:139–41) and confusion with dosulepin ADRs during a switch (n=1, Haddad and Qureshi, *Acta Psychiatr Scand* 2000;**102**:466–8) probably due to its short half-life and inhibition of its own CYP2D6 metabolism leading to a rapid drop in plasma levels, although this inhibition can be as long as up to 4–6 weeks with a treatment longer than 18 weeks (s=2, n=60, Jurica and Žourková, *J Clin Pharm Ther* 2013;**38**:294–300). This inhibition dissipates much quicker than fluoxetine and sertraline (n=45, RCT, open, Liston *et al*, *J Clin Psychopharmacol* 2002;**22**:169–73). Discontinuation symptoms tend to resolve in a few days or rapidly on reintroduction of paroxetine. The CSM recommends tapering if withdrawal symptoms occur, i.e. stop and then restart and taper over 12 weeks, with either half-tablet doses or alternate day (but not less frequently) therapy. However, even a four-week gradual dose reduction is not always successful (n=5, Pacheco *et al*, *Br J Psychiatry* 1996;**169**:384).

Sertraline: Discontinuation reactions are relatively uncommon but there are reports of fatigue, cramps, insomnia (resolving on restarting and where tapering over 14 weeks was successful; Louie *et al*, *Am J Psychiatry* 1994;**151**:450–1), electrical shock-like sensations and postural hypotension (n=1, Amsden and Georgian, *Pharmacotherapy* 1996;**16**:684–6).

2

Other antidepressants

Tricyclics: Cholinergic rebound, e.g. headache, restlessness, diarrhoea, nausea and vomiting (Lieberman, *Psychosomatics* 1981;**22**:253–4), flu-like symptoms, lethargy, abdominal cramps, sleep disturbance, delirium (n=1, Alexander and Berce, *Aust N Z J Psychiatry* 2010;**44**:863) and movement disorders can occur.

MAOIs: * There have been many reports, e.g. with **phenelzine** of possible myoclonic seizures (n=1, Naylor *et al*, *J Nerv Ment Dis* 1987;**175**:111–4), psychosis (e.g. n=2, Liskin *et al*, *J Clin Psychopharmacol* 1985;**5**:46–7), nightmares (Joyce and Walshe, *J Clin Psychopharmacol* 1983;**3**:121), headache, irritability, feeling cold (n=2, Pitt, *Br Med J* 1974;**2**:332–3; FFT), disorientation, catatonia, irritability, hypomania, nausea, sweating and palpitations. **Tranylcypromine** abrupt withdrawal can lead to delirium in 50% and rapid relapse in 20% (e.g. n=25, Gahr *et al*, *Pharmacopsychiatry* 2013;**46**:123–9), especially with a longer duration of therapy (n=51, Tyrer, *J Affect Disord* 1984;**6**:1–7).

Agomelatine: No discontinuation symptoms have been seen, due to the very short half-life and so no tapering is required.

Duloxetine: * The MHRA (*MHRA Drug Safety Update* 2007;1–9) and SmPC state that duloxetine should be tapered over one to two weeks, reduced by a half on alternate days. Symptoms of abrupt withdrawal may occur in 44% people stopping duloxetine (cf 23% for placebo), with dizziness (12%), nausea, headache, paraesthesia, vomiting, irritability, shock-like sensations and nightmares being the most common (n = 1, Hou, *J Neuropsychiatry Clin Neurosci* 2014;**26**:E4). Resolution occurs within in a week in 65% (s = 6, Perahia *et al*, *J Affect Disord* 2005;**89**:207–12).

Mirtazapine: A withdrawal hypomania has been reported (n = 1, MacCall and Callender, *Br J Psychiatry* 1999;**175**:390; n = 1, Berigan, *Prim Care Companion J Clin Psychiatry* 2001;**3**:143; FFT), but that's about all.

Moclobemide: A discontinuation syndrome may present with influenza-like symptoms. Sertraline may not modify the symptoms, suggesting a non-serotonergic mechanism (n = 1, Curtin *et al*, *J Psychopharmacol* 2002;**16**:271–2).

Reboxetine: No withdrawal or discontinuation syndrome has been observed, with few additional effects on abrupt withdrawal.

St John's wort: A withdrawal syndrome has been reported (Dean *et al*, *Ann Pharmacother* 2003;**37**:150).

Venlafaxine: * If used for more than six weeks, withdrawal over at least a week is recommended (SmPC), as withdrawal reactions from abrupt cessation, dose reduction or tapering of venlafaxine can include fatigue, nausea, vomiting, dizziness, dry mouth, diarrhoea, insomnia, nervousness, confusion, paraesthesia, sweating, vertigo, headache (e.g. n = 1, Mayr and Bonelli, *Ann Pharmacother* 2003;**37**:1145–6), electric shock-like symptoms (e.g. n = 2, Reeves *et al*, *Pharmacother* 2003;**23**:678–81), pseudostroke (n = 1, Sabliji *et al*, *Psychiatr Danub* 2011; **23**;117–9; FFT), suicidal ideation (n = 2, Stone *et al*, *J Clin Psychopharmacol* 2007;**27**:94–5), delusions and psychosis (n = 1, Koga *et al*, *Acta Psychiatr Scand* 2009;**120**:329–31; FFT), mania (n = 2, Tak and Stevens, *Tijdschr Psychiatr* 2013;**55**:795–800), abdominal distension, congested sinuses (n = 1, resolving within 12 hours of restarting, Farah and Lauer, *Am J Psychiatry* 1996;**153**:576), status cataplepticus (on abrupt withdrawal; n = 1, Wang *et al*, *J Clin Sleep Med* 2013;**9**:715–6), 'brain shivers' (which have responded to atomoxetine; n = 1, Cortes and Radhakrishnan, *Prim Care Companion CNS Disord* 2013;**15**:12l01427), gastrointestinal upset (which responded to reintroduction and then slow reduction over 1–4 weeks, n = 3, Louie *et al*, *Am J Psychiatry* 1996;**153**:1652) and classic SSRI-type discontinuation symptoms (e.g. confusion, headache, agitation, abdominal distension and sweating) occurring 16 and 20 hours after stopping (n = 2, Agelink *et al*, *Am J Psychiatry* 1997;**154**:1473–4; review of similarity to SSRI symptoms, n = 13, Boyd, *Med J Aus* 1998;**169**:91–2). Discontinuation effects can adversely affect driving abilities (Campagne, *Med Gen Med* 2005;**7**:22; FFT). Interdose antidepressant discontinuation with venlafaxine XL has been resolved by using plain tablets BD, probably due to ultra-rapid metabolism (n = 1, Petit and Sansone, *Prim Care Companion CNS Disorders* 2011;**13**:11l01140; FFT).

Vortioxetine: The UK SmPC states vortioxetine can be stopped abruptly as discontinuation symptoms are no different to placebo after abrupt discontinuation after 6–12 or 24–64 weeks of treatment.

3 PSYCHOTROPICS IN PROBLEM AREAS

Contents

3.1	**Bariatric surgery**	**238**
3.1.1	Antipsychotics	238
3.1.2	Antidepressants	238
3.1.3	Mood and bipolar	239
3.1.4	Anxiolytics and hypnotics	239
3.1.5	Anticonvulsants	239
3.1.6	Others	239
3.2	**Cardiovascular disease**	**240**
3.2.1	Antipsychotics	241
3.2.2	Antidepressants	245
3.2.3	Mood and bipolar	247
3.2.4	Anxiolytics and hypnotics	248
3.2.5	Anticonvulsants	248
3.2.6	Others	248
3.3	**Diabetes**	**251**
3.3.1	Antipsychotics	252
3.3.2	Antidepressants	253
3.3.3	Mood and bipolar	254
3.3.4	Anxiolytics and hypnotics	254
3.3.5	Anticonvulsants	254
3.3.6	Others	255
3.4	**Epilepsy**	**256**
3.4.1	Antipsychotics	257
3.4.2	Antidepressants	257
3.4.3	Mood and bipolar	258
3.4.4	Anxiolytics and hypnotics	259
3.4.5	Anticonvulsants	259
3.4.6	Others	259
3.5	**Glaucoma**	**260**
3.5.1	Antipsychotics	261
3.5.2	Antidepressants	261
3.5.3	Mood and bipolar	262
3.5.4	Hypnotics	262
3.5.5	Anticonvulsants	262
3.5.6	Others	262
3.6	**Hepatic impairment**	**263**
3.6.1	Antipsychotics	264
3.6.2	Antidepressants	265
3.6.3	Mood and bipolar	266
3.6.4	Anxiolytics and hypnotics	266
3.6.5	Anticonvulsants	266
3.6.6	Others	267
3.7	**Old age**	**268**
3.7.1	Antipsychotics	269
3.7.2	Antidepressants	271
3.7.3	Mood and bipolar	273
3.7.4	Anxiolytics and hypnotics	274
3.7.5	Anticonvulsants	275
3.7.6	Others	275
3.8	**Parkinson's disease**	**276**
3.8.1	Antipsychotics	277
3.8.2	Antidepressants	277
3.8.3	Mood and bipolar	277
3.8.4	Anxiolytics and hypnotics	277
3.8.5	Anticonvulsants	278
3.8.6	Others	278
3.9	**Perinatal**	**280**
3.9.1	Antipsychotics	284
3.9.2	Antidepressants	289
3.9.3	Mood and bipolar	299
3.9.4	Anxiolytics and hypnotics	303
3.9.5	Anticonvulsants	307
3.9.6	Others	310
3.10	**Renal impairment**	**316**
3.10.1	Antipsychotics	317
3.10.2	Antidepressants	318
3.10.3	Mood and bipolar	319
3.10.4	Anxiolytics and hypnotics	320
3.10.5	Anticonvulsants	320
3.10.6	Others	321
3.11	**Sleep apnea**	**322**
3.11.1	Antipsychotics	323
3.11.2	Antidepressants	323
3.11.3	Mood and bipolar	324
3.11.4	Anxiolytics and hypnotics	324
3.11.5	Anticonvulsants	324
3.11.6	Others	324

3.1 BARIATRIC SURGERY *

There is little firm information available at the moment for the effects of bariatric surgery on the kinetics of mental health drugs.

There are two major types of bariatric surgery:

1. Restrictive — a small pouch is created at the top of the stomach, with a small hole to restrict gastric emptying and to prolong the feeling of fullness. Vitamin deficiency is less likely.
2. Restrictive-malabsorption — e.g. biliopancreatic diversion or Roux-en-Y gastric bypass (RYGB), where there is a restricted stomach volume and reduced bowel length, reducing food absorption. There is a greater risk of vitamin deficiency.

Drug considerations:

- A smaller stomach size can lead to incomplete disintegration of dosage forms
- pH tends to be higher in a gastric pouch, which may reduce absorption of acid-soluble drugs. Many alkaline-soluble drugs are absorbed in the small intestine, which may be by-passed or have a smaller surface area
- Surface area is significantly reduced and drugs mainly absorbed from the duodenum and jejunum may need to be given by a different route or doses adjusted
- Gastric side-effects may be more common
- Weight loss can occur so any drugs dosed by weight may need to be adjusted.
- Formulations — avoid MR and e/c preparations as these may reduce absorption
- Liquid dose forms are more rapidly absorbed than solid doses
- Avoid effervescent formulations or at least make sure any bubbling has fully settled
- Avoid large tablets as some openings may only be 1–1.5 cm across. Use smaller dose units, or crush or cut doses
- Non-oral routes may be needed
- Obese people may often demonstrate an acquired prolonged QTc interval due to alteration in cardiac physiology, electrolyte disturbances, and/or medication use. Bariatric surgery may further contribute additional cardiac stressors to obese people with long QT syndrome (LQTS).

Reviews: * mental health disorders among in bariatric patients (Kalarchian *et al, Am J Psych* 2007; **164**:328–34), schizophrenia and bariatric surgery (Lawlor and Rand, *Am J Psych* 1986; **143**:1321; n=5, Hamoui *et al, Obes Surg* 2004; **14**:349–52), pharmacokinetic considerations in RYGB (Smith *et al, Am J Health Syst Pharm* 2011; **68**:2241–7; Miller and Smith, *Am J Health Syst Pharm* 2006; **36**:1852–7).

3.1.1 ANTIPSYCHOTICS *

Aripiprazole: a 28-year-old male with morbid obesity suffered a ventricular non-supported polymorphic tachycardia (torsades de pointes) post-surgery, probably related to QTc prolongation from concurrent use of aripiprazole and fluoxetine (n=1, Méndez-Sánchez *et al, Actas Esp Psiquiatr* 2012; **40**:346–8).

Clozapine is mainly absorbed in the small intestine, so bariatric surgery is unlikely to significantly affect absorption, but the SmPC warns about the possible exacerbation of constipation. Pre- and post-surgery plasma levels would be prudent.

Olanzapine is absorbed from the stomach so monitor for loss of efficacy (e.g. n=1, Bechelany, *Rev Bras Psiquiatr* 2008; **30**:405–6).

Quetiapine is probably absorbed from the stomach and duodenum, so monitor for loss of efficacy.

Risperidone long-acting injection (RLAI) has been effective in a bipolar patient post-RYGB surgery who was intolerant to conventional mood stabilisers, including oral risperidone (n=1, Brietzke and Lafer, *Psychiatry Clin Neurosci* 2011; **65**:205).

3.1.2 ANTIDEPRESSANTS *

SSRIs: Fluoxetine has been used to reduce weight and the need for surgery (n=84, Dolfing *et al, Obes Surg* 2005; **15**:1185–91). **Sertraline**'s mean AUC and Cmax are significantly smaller after RYGB surgery (124±55ng-hr/mL, range 62–198) cf. a non-surgical control group (315±130ng-hr/mL, range 195–509) (n=10, Roerig *et al, Surg Obes Relat Dis* 2012; **8**:62–6). **Escitalopram** levels drop by 33% in 2 weeks post-RYGB and further decrease at 6 weeks (n=4, Marzinke *et al, Ther Drug Monit* 2015; **37**:408–12).

Duloxetine's AUC and Tmax are reduced to only 58% compared to controls, although Cmax and half-life are unchanged (n=10, Roerig *et al, J Clin Psychopharmacol* 2013; **33**:479–84).

Mirtazapine has been used for intractable nausea and vomiting post-RYGB surgery (n=1, Huerta and Siddiqui, *Obes Surg* 2006; **16**:1399; n = 2, Teixeira *et al*, *Obes Surg* 2005;**15**: 707–9).

Tricyclics have been linked to a case of cardiac arrest during laparoscopic RYGB, probably due to a tricyclic-related prolonged QTc (n = 1, Woodard *et al*, *Obes Surg* 2011;**21**:134–7).

3.1.3 MOOD AND BIPOLAR *

Lamotrigine is probably mostly absorbed from the stomach and proximal small intestine, so monitor for loss of efficacy.

Lithium should be gradually withdrawn and stopped 24 hours before major surgery and only restarted after electrolyte balance has been restored, as toxicity can occur. For example, post-gastric banding hypernatraemia has been attributed to lithium-induced renal damage from lithium stopped four years previously (n = 1, Leo *et al*, *Psychosomatics* 2013;**54**:200–4), a patient stable on 1050 mg/d developing lithium toxicity presenting as confusion 10 days post-RYGB surgery (managed by reduction of the dose to 600 mg/d; n = 1, Tripp, *J Clin Psychopharmacol* 2011; **31**:261–2) and diabetes insipidus possibly caused by delayed renal damage from previous lithium use (n = 2, Irefin *et al*, *J Clin Anesth* 2014;**26**:231–4).

Review: bariatric surgery in bipolar disorder (Davis, *Bariatr Surg Pract Patient Care* 2014;**9**:84–5).

Valproate absorption may be significantly reduced by malabsorption procedures, so monitor for loss of efficacy. Plasma levels may be useful. Gastric banding is, in theory, less likely to affect the absorption of valproate compared to RYGB. Enteric-coated valproate is released in the small intestine, so should not be affected by restrictive surgery, although there is some concern that RYGB surgery, removing some of the small intestine, reduces absorption as the transit time of the gut will be affected. IV valproate has been used successfully for maintenance in bipolar II disorder after gastric bypass surgery when complications led to non-tolerance of oral valproate (n = 1, Semion *et al*, *J Neuropsychiatry Clin Neurosci* 2005;**17**:427–9), and for acute mania after gastric bypass surgery related to clozapine therapy, being converted to oral after four days (n = 1, Kaltsounis and De Leon, *Psychosomatics* 2000;**41**:454–6).

3.2.4 ANXIOLYTICS AND HYPNOTICS *

Benzodiazepine — the time to peak levels is longer post-RYGB for oral midazolam (0.5 hours to 0.7 hours), but Cmax, AUC, half-life and oral bioavailability, were not different (n = 36, Tandra *et al*, *Ann Surg* 2013;**258**:262–9).

3.2.5 ANTICONVULSANTS *

Phenytoin levels have reduced to undetectable post-RYGB, resulting in seizures, despite the use of high doses (n = 1, Pournaras *et al*, *Obes Surg* 2011;**21**: 684–5).

Topiramate 12.5–50 mg/d can be useful for controlling binge-eating (BED) and enhance excess weight loss post-surgery (n = 16, Zilberstein *et al*, *Obes Surg* 2004;**14**:802–5). In a case series, all three patients showed complete remission of BED symptoms and lost weight with topiramate (mean dose 541 mg/d) post-bariatric surgery (n = 3, open, mean 10/12, Guerdjikova *et al*, *Obes Surg* 2005;**15**: 273–7).

3.2.6 OTHERS

Atomoxetine has no listed precautions or contraindications if there has been previous gastric surgery. There might be some gastrointestinal side-effects initially, but these should fade in a couple of weeks and may be minimised by taking atomoxetine with a little food.

Methadone — there is a case where persistent nausea and abdominal pain post-op and post-reversal turned out to be unrecognised narcotic withdrawal syndrome, reversed with regular methadone (Higa *et al*, *Obes Surg* 2001;**11**:631–4).

3

3.2 CARDIOVASCULAR DISEASE

	Lower risk	Moderate risk	Higher risk
Antipsychotics	Quetiapine[5] Sulpiride[7]	Amisulpride[7] Aripiprazole[1] Flupentixol[10] Lurasidone[3] Olanzapine[4] Paliperidone[6] Phenothiazines[9] Risperidone[6] Zuclopenthixol[10]	Clozapine[2] Haloperidol[8] Pimozide[11] Ziprasidone[11]
Antidepressants	Agomelatine[14] Duloxetine[16] Mianserin[21] Mirtazapine[17] St John's wort[21] SSRIs[12] Trazodone[20] Tryptophan[21] Vortioxetine[16]	Bupropion[15] Moclobemide[18] Reboxetine[19] Venlafaxine[22]	MAOIs[23] Tricyclics (especially dosulepin)[13]
Anxiolytics and hypnotics	Benzodiazepines[29] Buspirone[31] Melatonin [33] Z-hypnotics[35]	Beta-blockers[30] Chloral hydrate[32] Clomethiazole[32] Pregabalin[34]	
Mood and bipolar	Lamotrigine[26] Quetiapine[5] Valproate[28]	Asenapine[24] Carbamazepine[25] Lithium[27] Olanzapine[4]	
Anticonvulsants	Benzodiazepines[29] Gabapentin[37] Lamotrigine[26] Levetiracetam[38] Topiramate[41] Valproate[28]	Barbiturates[36] Carbamazepine[25] Oxcarbazepine[39] Phenytoin[40] Pregabalin[34]	
Others	Acamprosate[46a] Memantine[44] Nalmefene[46c]	Anticholinergics[45] Anticholinesterases[43] Atomoxetine[42a] Buprenorphine[47] Bupropion[15] Dexamfetamine[42b] Lisdexamfetamine[42c] Methadone[47] Methylphenidate[42d] Modafinil[48] Naltrexone[46d] Sodium oxybate[48]	Disulfiram[46b] Guanfacine[42e]

GENERAL PRINCIPLES IN CARDIAC DISEASE

1. Polypharmacy should be avoided where possible, particularly with drugs likely to effect cardiac rate and electrolyte balance.
2. Extra care and monitoring is essential with drugs likely to increase the QT interval.
3. Avoid drugs specifically contraindicated.
4. Start low and go slow is, as ever, good advice. Rapid dose escalation should be avoided.

Psychotropics in specific cardiac conditions

Angina

Avoid drugs causing orthostatic hypotension, which may exacerbate angina. Avoid drugs causing tachycardia, e.g. phenothiazines, clozapine and risperidone. Avoid tricyclics, although most other antidepressants are thought to be of a relatively low risk.

Arrhythmias

SSRIs are first choice antidepressants due to their lack of antiarrhythmic/proarrhythmic potential. Avoid phenothiazines, butyrophenones and pimozide. Sulpiride and olanzapine seem to be of low risk.

Congestive heart failure (CHF)

For chronic stable CHF, avoid beta-blockers and take care with drugs causing orthostatic hypotension, e.g. phenothiazines, clozapine, risperidone and tricyclics.

Hypertension

Drugs causing orthostatic hypotension should be monitored closely. Avoid MAOIs. Hypertension can occur with venlafaxine (high dose), clozapine, tricyclics and antipsychotics.

Myocardial infarction (MI)

If essential, use SSRIs (except perhaps fluvoxamine), agomelatine, bupropion or mirtazapine. Avoid high-dose antipsychotics and phenothiazines. Butyrophenones, thioxanthenes and benzamides appear to be lower risk.

Reviews: cardiac effects of psychotropics (Kovacs and Arora, *Am J Ther* 2008;**15**:474–83; Mackin, *Hum Psychopharmacol* 2008;**23**[Suppl 1]:3–14).

3.2.1 ANTIPSYCHOTICS *

QTc prolongation

Many antipsychotics are known to affect cardiac conduction, with a class IA antiarrhythmic-like effect presenting as lengthening of the QT interval. This may then lead onto torsade de pointes, which may be asymptomatic or, in rare cases, lead on to ventricular fibrillation and sudden death. The QT interval shortens with increased heart rate, and so a rate-corrected value QTc is usually used. A QTc prolonged to about 450 ms is considered of some concern, and above 500 ms to be of an unquantifiable risk of leading to torsade de pointes and should prompt review and action. QTc varies markedly throughout the day, and serial readings are necessary for accurate assessments.

Risk factors for antipsychotic-induced QTc prolongation: *

- The first 30 days after initiation (n = 1546, but no relationship with the class of antipsychotic; Brauer *et al*, *Eur Heart J* 2015;**36**:984–92)
- Co-prescription of other QT prolonging drugs, e.g. some antiarrhythmics, vasodilators, tricyclics, macrolides, fluoroquinolones (e.g. azithromycin), antimalarials, ketoconazole, ondansetron, methadone and antihistamines
- Underlying cardiac disease, e.g. heart-failure, angina and cardiac myopathy
- Bradycardia, or second or third-degree heart block
- Personal or family history of QTc prolongation, ventricular arrhythmias or torsade de pointes
- Severe renal or hepatic impairment
- Elderly or malnourished
- History of heavy alcohol consumption or substance misuse
- Electrolyte imbalance, especially hypokalaemia and hypomagnesaemia
- Undergoing restraint and/or severe stress
- Slow drug metabolisers
- Female gender (longer QTc more common)
- Haloperidol and phenothiazines also have a higher risk in hypokalaemia, Hep C, HIV and abnormal T-waves (n = 6790, Girardin *et al*, *Am J Psychiatry* 2013;**170**:1468–76).

Management:

1. Monitor electrolytes and ECG regularly
2. Interpret remembering results are dependent upon the timing (time since last dose, diurnal variation, postprandial state).

Risk of cardiac disease with antipsychotics: The ten-year incidence of CHD in CATIE showed:

- olanzapine *increased* the incidence by 0.5%
- quetiapine *increased* the incidence by 0.3%
- perphenazine *reduced* the incidence by 0.5%
- risperidone *reduced* the incidence by 0.6%
- ziprasidone *reduced* the incidence by 0.6%

(n=1125, 18/12–10 years, Daumit *et al*, *Schizophr Res* 2008;**105**:175–87).

- There is no difference in CV risk (based on weight and metabolic indices) between people with an untreated first episode and healthy controls, but the risk increases after first exposure to any antipsychotic drug, with no significant class differences (s=25, 4–52/52, Foley and Morley, *Arch Gen Psychiatry* 2011;**68**:609–1).
- A year after first starting olanzapine, quetiapine and risperidone, the crude rate of major cardiovascular events was one per 200 person-years and not significantly different between the drugs (n=48625, Pasternak *et al*, *CNS Drugs* 2014;**28**:963–73).

Reviews:* Extensive review of QTc prolongation and TdP (s=218, Hasnain and Vieweg, *CNS Drugs* 2014;**28**:887–920), QT alterations with psychotropics (Alvarez and Pahissa, *Curr Drug Saf* 2010;**5**:97–104).

1. **Aripiprazole** is the only SGA shown to statistically significantly lower risk of QTc prolongation (meta-analysis, s=16, n=5636, RCT, Chung and Chua, *J Psychopharmacol* 2011;**25**:646–66). The UK SmPC lists QT prolongation, ventricular arrhythmias, sudden unexplained death, cardiac arrest, TdP and bradycardia as possible unwanted effects.

2. * **Clozapine** has well-established CV side-effects, e.g. tachycardia and postural hypotension,

A review of QTc prolongation (Wenzel-Seifert *et al*, *Dtsch Arztebl Int* 2011;**108**:687–93) *

3 Severe effect (>17ms)	2 Moderate effect (>9 and <16ms)	1 Mild effect (>5 and <9ms) or only in cases of overdose or intoxication	0 No effect at therapeutic concentrations	Not Known
Melperone Pimozide Quetiapine Sertindole Thioridazine	Chlorpromazine Clozapine Levomepromazine Risperidone Sulpiride Ziprasidone	Amisulpride Flupentixol Fluphenazine Haloperidol Olanzapine Perphenazine Promethazine	Aripiprazole Benperidol Chlorprothixene Lurasidone Paliperidone Zuclopenthixol	Fluspirilene
Amitriptyline Desipramine Doxepin Imipramine Maprotiline Nortriptyline	Clomipramine Fluoxetine	Citalopram Escitalopram Mianserin Trazodone Venlafaxine	Duloxetine Fluvoxamine Mirtazapine Paroxetine Reboxetine Sertraline Trimipramine	
Lithium Methadone		Bupropion Chloral Tiapride	Atomoxetine Biperiden Carbamazepine Diazepam Hypericum Lamotrigine Methylphenidate Moclobemide Tranylcypromine Valproate	Buspirone

particularly early in treatment. There is also a risk of death from cardiovascular disease secondary to clozapine-induced obesity, diabetes, hypertension and hyperlipidaemia (n=96, 10 years, Henderson *et al*, *J Clin Psychiatry* 2005;**66**:1116–21).

Clozapine-induced myocarditis and cardiomyopathy:

- The median onset of myocarditis is 16 days, with nearly all within 6/12
- 90% occur within the dose range of 100–450mg/d (52% recovered, 38% were recovering or lost to follow-up, 10% died)
- Symptoms are diverse and non-specific so maintain a high degree of suspicion (n=116, Haas *et al*, *Drug Saf* 2007;**30**:47–57)
- The risk of myocarditis is higher with a rapid dose titration (risk increased by 26% for each additional 250mg administered in the first nine days), and doubled if used with valproate (n=401, Ronaldson *et al*, *Schizophr Res* 2012;**141**:173–8)
- Cardiomyopathy has a mean age of diagnosis of 33.5 years, a mean dose on presentation of 360mg, at an average of 14/12 after starting (n=26, Alawami *et al*, *Int J Cardiol* 2014:**176**:315–20)
- Clozapine should be discontinued if cardiomyopathy or myocarditis is suspected
- Clozapine should only be started if severe heart disease has been excluded through a full history, examination and possibly an ECG
- Persistent tachycardia at rest, especially during the first two months, should be followed up and the patient observed for other signs of cardiomyopathy or myocarditis
- It can occur even in young healthy adults
- ECG changes should be referred to a cardiologist for evaluation
- People who develop clozapine-induced cardiomyopathy should not be re-exposed to clozapine (data mining study, Coulter *et al*, *Br Med J* 2001;**322**:1207–9;FFT).

References: Myocarditis and cardiomyopathy (from Australian database of 8000, Kilian *et al*, *Lancet* 1999;**354**:1841–5; n=41 [10 fatal], La Grenade *et al*, *NEJM* 2001;**345**:224–5;FFT; Layland *et al*, *Med J Aust* 2009;**190**:190–2; De Berardis *et al*, *Curr Drug Saf* 2012;**7**:55–62).

Clozapine-induced QTc prolongation:

Prolonged QTc is also known with clozapine. Risk factors include increased age (but less so if there was a normal ECG with other antipsychotics) and dose. It often corrects itself over time, occurs mainly during the initial stages of treatment, is mostly benign, and pathological prolongation of QTc is rare (n=61, Kang *et al*, *J Clin Psychiatry* 2000;**61**:441–6). A case series has shown no significant differences in QTc before and after 18 weeks of clozapine (n=82, 18/52, Grande *et al*, *Hum Psychopharmacol* 2011;**26**:397–403), and there was no cardiomyopathy detected by cardiologists (n=125, Serrano *et al*, *Aust N Z J Psychiatry* 2014;**48**:183–92).

3. * **Lurasidone** may uncommonly cause orthostatic hypotension and syncope, perhaps due to alpha-1-adrenergic receptor antagonism, and particularly at initiation and dose changes. It has no apparent significant effect on the QTc interval.

4. **Olanzapine** can occasionally cause postural hypotension. Blood pressure monitoring is recommended periodically in people over 65. Olanzapine (mean 14mg/d) can raise fasting triglyceride levels by 37%, a significant risk factor for exacerbation of CHD (n=25, 12/52, Osser *et al*, *J Clin Psychiatry* 1999;**60**:767–70). QTc prolongation has only been seen rarely and the risk of QTc >450msec is similar to baseline (s=4, n=2700, RCTs, Czekalla *et al*, *J Clin Psychiatry* 2001;**62**:191–8). However it may be a dose-dependent effect (n=26, Suzuki *et al*, *Hum Psychopharmacol* 2011;**26**:440–3) as there can be some ECG changes in acute overdose, e.g. longer QTc (but only rarely enough for torsade de pointes) and so regular ECGs are recommended (n=23, Ciszowski and Sein Anand, *Przegl Lek* 2011;**68**:422–5). The UK SmPC cautions use of olanzapine with drugs known to increase the QTc interval.

5. * **Quetiapine**'s SmPC recommends caution with drugs known to prolong the QTc interval and in people with CV disease or conditions predisposing to hypotension. Trials have not shown sustained changes in the QTc interval, but some sources list quetiapine as a moderate-to-severe risk (review by Review of QTc prolongation and TsD (n=12, Hasnain *et al*, *Ther Adv Psychopharmacol* 2014;**4**:130–8). Orthostatic hypotension is more common in the elderly, especially initially.

6. * **Risperidone** needs caution due to orthostatic hypotension as low doses slightly drop bp and increase heart rate. It is best to introduce it slowly over several weeks. An analysis of risperidone/paliperidone studies shows the risk of cardiovascular events was significantly

3

higher than placebo, but the incidence of death was too low and similar across all groups to conclude if there was a serious problem (s=64, Gopal *et al*, *J Clin Psychopharmacol* 2013;**33**:157–61). The Medicaid cohort study (n=95,632+29,086 controls, Hennessy *et al*, *Br Med J* 2002; **325**: 1070–2;FFT) showed risperidone as the only drug that had higher rates for cardiac arrest and ventricular arrhythmia than haloperidol, especially at lower dose, although this was probably due to the frailest patients being given low doses. Serious cardiac effects at standard doses seems to be uncommon (n=107, Page *et al*, *J Clin Psychopharmacol* 2010;**30**:387–90) and any QTc prolongation with risperidone is related to paliperidone rather than risperidone plasma levels (n=61, Suzuki *et al*, *Hum Psychopharmacol* 2012;**27**:39–42). Surprisingly, risperidone had less effect on the PR interval than olanzapine in a switching study, but QTc and RR interval were unchanged (n=21, Suzuki *et al*, *Psychiatry Clin Neurosci* 2014;**68**:353–6). **Paliperidone** should be used with care in people with a familial history of CV disease or QT interval, or co-prescribed with drugs thought to prolong the QTc interval (SmPC), although it has the same effect on QTc as quetiapine (n=109, RCT, d/b, p/c, Hough *et al*, *Int Clin Psychopharmacol* 2011;**26**:25–34;MS).
Review: * cardiac effects and QTc prolongation (Vieweg *et al*, *Psychopharmacology [Berl]* 2013;**228**: 515–24).

7. **Amisulpride** overdose frequently results in QTc prolongation and torsade de pointes (n=83, Isbister *et al*, *J Clin Psychopharmacol* 2010;**30**:391–5), and it is contraindicated with drugs that could cause torsade de pointes. There are no specific problems with **sulpiride,** but prolonged QT and torsade de pointes have been reported (n=1, Chang *et al*, *Am J Emerg Med* 2009;**27**:1016).

8. **Haloperidol** is contraindicated in people with clinically significant cardiac disorders or with other QT-interval prolonging drugs (SmPC). Prolonged QT-interval has been reported (n=596, Reilly *et al*, *Lancet* 2000;**355**:1048–52) but QTc duration may change differentially, depending on pre-haloperidol QTc duration (see *table below*). Shorter QTc pre-haloperidol and surgery before use predicted a dangerously long QTc prolongation (n=97, Blom *et al*, *PloS One* 2011;**6**:e23728;FFT). Beware that people given haloperidol IV often have many risk factors for QTc prolongation (n=175, Muzyk *et al*, *Drug Saf* 2012;**35**:547–53), which may complicate the picture.

9. **Phenothiazines** can cause some ECG abnormalities, e.g. tachycardia, T-wave abnormalities, ST depression, QT prolongation and right bundle branch block. Chlorpromazine and levomepromazine significantly lengthen QTc (n=1017, Ozeki *et al*, *Prog Neuropsychopharmacol Biol Psychiatry* 2010;**34**:401–5). **Levomepromazine** causes orthostatic hypotension that can, on occasion, be prolonged and profound.

10. **Flupentixol** and **zuclopenthixol** are cautioned in susceptible individuals (hypokalaemia, hypomagnesaemia, genetic disposition), or in people with a history of CV disorders (UK SmPC).

11. **Pimozide** is contraindicated in QT prolongation, a history of cardiac arrhythmias or torsade de pointes. **Ziprasidone** causes a well-known, dose-related QTc prolongation (mean 10msec), so do not use in anyone with a known prolonged interval, recent MI or heart failure (review, Taylor, *CNS Drugs* 2003;**17**:423–30).

QTc duration during haloperidol use (n=97, Blom *et al*, *PloS One* 2011;6:e23728) *

M = male, F = female

QTc before haloperidol	QTc change with haloperidol	% of QTcs becoming abnormal with haloperidol
Normal QTc (<430ms M or <450ms F)	23ms increase	23%
Borderline QTc (430–450ms M or 450–470ms F)	15ms reduction	23%
Abnormal QTc (>450ms M or 470ms F)	46ms reduction	9%

3.2.2 ANTIDEPRESSANTS

Studies show that people with MDD:

- Are at 4–5-fold greater risk of cardiac mortality, although depression in the week preceding an MI is not a risk factor (n=588, mean 6.7 years, Dickens *et al*, *Psychosom Med* 2008;**70**:450–5; n=5936, mean 5.6 years, Nabi *et al*, *Heart* 2010;**96**:1645–50;FFT; n=489, 12/12, Parker *et al*, *Biol Psychiatry* 2008;**64**:660–6)
- May have a four-fold greater mortality over seven years if they have severe depression or fail to improve over 6/12 following ACS (acute coronary syndrome), so depression needs to be treated aggressively (n=369, seven years, Glassman *et al*, *Arch Gen Psychiatry* 2009;**66**:1022–9)
- May have a significant benefit from antidepressants without increased risk of cardiac events (meta-analysis, s=4, n=798, RCT, d/b, p/c, Dowlati *et al*, *Can J Psychiatry* 2010;**55**:91–9;FFT), as untreated depression may be a greater risk than antidepressants (n=1005, O'Connor *et al*, *Arch Intern Med* 2008;**168**:2232–7;FFT).

People with CHD and MDD are more likely to:

- Not follow recommendations to reduce their cardiac risks during recovery from an MI (n=204, Ziegelstein *et al*, *Arch Intern Med* 2000;**160**:1818–23)
- Not comply with antihypertensives (n=496, one year, Wang *et al*, *J Gen Intern Med* 2002;**17**:504–11;FFT)
- Be at greater risk of new cardiac events within the first year after a heart attack (n=528;12/12, Kaptein *et al*, *Psychosom Med* 2006;**68**:662–8)
- Be at greater risk with more severe depression, especially if they are older adults free of CHD at baseline (n=660, mean 12 years, Ahto *et al*, *Int J Ger Psychiatry* 2007;**22**:757–63), or elderly with pre-existing cardiac disease (n=652, Geerlings *et al*, *Psychol Med* 2002;**32**:609–18).

Treating depression is thus logical but curiously not yet supported by the two largest studies (CBT +/- SSRIs, n=2481, RCT, 6/12, ENRICHD, Berkman *et al*, *JAMA* 2003;**289**:3106–16; MIND-IT, n=331, RCT, 18/12, van Melle *et al*, *Br J Psychiatry* 2007; **190**:460–6; FFT; for caveats see Carney and Freedland, *Br J Psychiatry* 2007;**190**:467–8;FFT), although treatment is associated with modest improvements (s=11, Thombs *et al*, *JAMA* 2008; **300**:2161–71; FFT).

Overall, sertraline, fluoxetine, agomelatine, bupropion and mirtazapine appear safe after an MI; use of sertraline and response to mirtazapine may reduce mortality (Taylor, *Acta Psychiatr Scand* 2008;**118**:434–42).

Review: depression after acute coronary syndrome (Carney and Freedland, *Am J Psychiatry* 2009;**166**:410–7;FFT).

12. * **SSRIs** are clearly more effective than placebo for treating depression in cardiac disease, with no difference in drop-outs (meta-analysis, s=4, n=798, p/c, 9–24/52, Dowlati *et al*, *Can J Psychiatry* 2010;**55**:91–9) and show lower relapse and readmission rates than without in acute coronary syndrome (s=5, n=801, Mazza *et al*, *J Psychopharmacol* 2010;**24**:1785–92). SSRIs are consistently associated with a small but statistically significant increase in QTc interval (+6.1ms), significantly more with citalopram than the others, but 7ms less than the tricyclics (s=16, n=4292, Beach *et al*, *J Clin Psychiatry* 2014;**75**:441–9). The risk is higher with hypokalaemia, hepatitis C, HIV and abnormal T-waves (n=6790, Girardin *et al*, *Am J Psychiatry* 2013;**170**:1468–76), but not necessarily so in an elderly surgical patient cohort (n=795, van Haelst *et al*, *J Clin Psychiatry* 2014;**75**:12–21).

12a. * **Citalopram** lengthens QTc by a mean of 10–18ms at 20–40mg/d (n=38397, Castro *et al*, *BMJ* 2013;**346**:f288; n=181, RCT, d/b, p/c, Drye *et al*, *PLoS One* 2014;**9**:e98426; FFT), and is contraindicated in known prolonged QT and with other medicines known to prolong QTc, and should only be used with caution with electrolyte disturbances and bradycardia. The FDA/EMA recommend citalopram should not be used above 40mg/d due to the dose-dependent effect, or in people with CHF or bradyarrhythmias. However, a large study showed no increased risk of ventricular arrhythmia or all-cause cardiac or non-cardiac mortality with doses >40mg/d and, in fact, higher doses were associated with fewer adverse outcomes (n=984,348, Zivin *et al*, *Am J Psychiatry* 2013;**170**:642–50; see also a carefully-worded and delightfully irritated review by Vieweg *et al*, *Am J Med* 2012;**125**:859–68).

* **Escitalopram** is also contraindicated with QT prolongation, or with drugs that may cause

QT prolongation, and should only be used with caution in patients at risk of TdP, recent MI, bradyarrhythmias, hypokalaemia or hypomagnesaemia. However, several studies show **no** statistical differences between escitalopram 10 mg/d and placebo for drop-outs, any CV safety measure (including QTc), or major adverse events in people with recent ACS (n = 240, RCT, d/b, p/c, 12/12, Hanash *et al, J Cardiovasc Pharmacol* 2012;**60**:397–405; n = 3298, RCT, d/b, p/c, < 24/52, Thase *et al, Eur Neuropsychopharmacol* 2013;**23**:1391–400; review of overdoses; Hasnain *et al, J Psychiatry Neurosci* 2013;**38**:E11). It may even reduce the incidence of post-ACS from 8% to 1.5% over a year (n = 240, RCT, d/b, p/c, 12/12, Hansen *et al, J Psychosom Res* 2012;**72**:11–6).

12b. **Fluoxetine** up to 60 mg/d has been shown in several open trials to have no significant adverse cardiac effects in people with pre-existing CHF, conduction disease and/or ventricular arrhythmia (e.g. n = 27, average age 73, open, 7/52, Roose *et al, Am J Psychiatry* 1998;**155**:660–6). Fluoxetine 20 mg/d has produced a modest reduction in bp, and in people with pre-existing stable cardiovascular disease (including hypertension) showed no significant bp change (n = 796, 12/52, Amsterdam *et al, J Clin Psychopharmacol* 1999; **19**:9–14). Rare cases of, e.g. atrial fibrillation, bradycardia and syncope have been reported.

12c. **Fluvoxamine** at higher plasma levels may increase the risk of QTc prolongation.

12d. **Paroxetine** may increase cholesterol (LDL-C) concentrations by around 11%, which might increase the risk of CHD in vulnerable individuals (n = 18, Lara *et al, J Clin Psychiatry* 2003;**64**:1455). It appears to only have a minimal effect on QTc.

12e. **Sertraline** appears to be safe in people with significant CHF, although it may not be statistically significantly superior to placebo (n = 469, RCT, d/b, p/c, 12/52, SADHART-CHF, O'Connor *et al, J Am Coll Cardiol* 2010;**56**:692–9;FFT). It does not increase cardiac events in depressed people with unstable angina or recent MI, and may even cut cardiac deaths post-MI by about 10% (review by Parissis *et al, Expert Opin Pharmacother* 2007;**8**:1529–37; see also n = 5436, three years, Sauer *et al, Circulation* 2003;**108**:32–6;FFT).

13. **Tricyclics** should only be used with extreme caution in people with ischaemic heart disease, ventricular arrhythmia, angina, recent MI and hypertension. They may produce orthostatic hypotension (and hence occasional myocardial infarction), have antiarrhythmic actions (quinidine-like) and antimuscarinic (raising heart rate) actions. A large cross-sectional survey showed a modest risk of CVD with tricyclics, although the HR of 1.35 is non-significant in a non-RCT (n = 14784 [4.9% on antidepressants], Hamer *et al, Eur Heart J* 2011;**32**:437–42). Starting tricyclics increases the QTc interval by a mean of 7 msec (notably amitriptyline 8.5 ms and nortriptyline 35 msec) (n = 8222, van Noord *et al, J Clin Psychopharmacol* 2009;**29**:9–15).

Amitriptyline 150 mg/d has increased heart rate by 15 bpm and significantly worsened all other heart rate parameters (n = 48, Rechlin *et al, Psychopharmacology* 1994;**116**:110–4).

Dosulepin had a specific, significant and dose-related association for subsequently developing IHD (n = 922 with IHD, 5516 controls, Hippisley-Cox *et al, BMJ* 2001;**323**:666–9;FFT).

Doxepin has caused torsade de pointes tachycardia (n = 1, Alter *et al, Ann Intern Med* 2001;**135**:384–5).

Imipramine produced no pro-arrhythmic effect, a slightly prolonged QTc and reduced recurrent chest pain in people with normal coronary angiograms (n = 58, 9–33/12, Cannon *et al, NEJM* 1994;**330**:1411–7;FFT).

Nortriptyline has significant effects on cardiac vagal function and should only be used with care in IHD (n = 44, Yeragani *et al, Neuropsychobiology* 2002;**46**:125–35), especially in men, who may be more susceptible (n = 78, 6/52, Pomara *et al, Prog Neuropsychopharmacol Biol Psychiatry* 2001; **25**:1035–48).

14. **Agomelatine** has no effect on QTc even at supratherapeutic doses of 400mg/d (n = 60, RCT, d/b, p/c, c/o, a/c, Donazzolo *et al, J Cardiovasc Pharmacol* 2014;**64**:440–51), although there is a case of fully reversible QTc prolongation (n = 1, Kozian and Syrbe, *Psychiatr Prax* 2010;**37**:405–7).

15. * **Bupropion** may cause small rises in bp (but not always, e.g. in mild untreated hypertension, n = 300, RCT, d/b, p/c, 4/52, Thase *et al, J Clin Psychopharmacol* 2008;**28**:302–7), but without significant conduction complications, ventricular arrhythmias or orthostatic hypotension (n = 36, open, Roose *et al, Am J Psychiatry* 1991;**148**:512–6) and may even shorten QTc (n = 38397, Castro *et al, BMJ* 2013;**346**:f288). A smoking-cessation study showed bupropion well tolerated and

safe in the post-MI period, albeit ineffective for smoking cessation (n = 392, RCT, d/b, p/c, 9/52 + 2/12 follow-up, Eisenberg *et al*, *J Am Coll Cardiol* 2013;**61**:524–32).

16. * **Vortioxetine** has no effect on heart rate or blood pressure with no QTc prolongation at up to 40mg/d, double the licensed maximum (SmPC). **Duloxetine** causes no QTc prolongation (isolated case: n = 1, Stuhec, *Wien Klin Wochenschr* 2013;**125**:165–6), or major cardiac effects (n = 128, Wohlreich *et al*, *Depress Anxiety* 2007;**24**:41–52), but is contraindicated in uncontrolled hypertension (SmPC; *MHRA Drug Safety Update* 2007;1–9). High-dose duloxetine ≤400 mg/d may raise bp and pulse, which might precipitate hypertension (n = 117, RCT, d/b, p/c, c/o, 16/7, Derby *et al*, *J Cardiovasc Pharmacol* 2007;**49**:384–93; spookily similar n = 117, RCT, d/b, p/c, Zhang *et al*, *J Cardiovasc Pharmacol* 2007;**49**:146–53, MS).

17. * **Mirtazapine** is more effective than placebo for depression in cardiac disease, with no difference in drop-outs (meta-analysis, s = 4, n = 798, p/c, 9–24/52, Dowlati *et al*, *Can J Psychiatry* 2010; **55**:91–9). No ECG, bp or pulse changes have been observed in reported trials, in overdose (n = 287, Berling and Isbister, *Clin Toxicol [Phila]* 2014;**52**:20–4), or in depressed in-patients (n = 251, RCT, 6/12, Zivkov and Jongh, *Hum Psychopharmacol* 1995;**10**:173–80).

18. **Moclobemide** can cause hypertension so monitoring bp may be useful. Occasional hypertension with tyramine in people with pre-existing labile hypertension has also occurred, and so caution in cardiac disease would be sensible.

19. * **Reboxetine** increased baseline heart rate in 20% and produced tachycardia in 0.8% (cf 0.1% with placebo) of people in short-term trials. Orthostatic hypotension is dose-related and the SmPC notes close supervision would be needed if used in lower blood pressure.

20. **Trazodone** overdose can cause reversible ventricular tachycardia (n = 1, Vitullo *et al*, *Chest* 1990;**98**:247–8) and QT prolongation (e.g. n = 1, Service and Waring, *Clin Toxicol [Phila]* 2008;**46**:71–3), but it is generally considered of low risk.

21. **St John's wort** does not seem to affect heart rate variability at 75 mg/d (n = 12, RCT, d/b, c/o, 14/7 per arm, Siepmann *et al*, *Br J Clin Pharmacol* 2002;**54**:277–82; FFT). There are no known problems with **mianserin** and **tryptophan**.

22. * **Venlafaxine** has a dose-dependent effect on supine diastolic blood pressure, which can be clinically significant at high doses (200–300 mg/d), probably as a result of noradrenergic potentiation (3% incidence at less than 100 mg/d [n = 17, Emul *et al*, *J Psychopharmacol* 2009;**23**:163–7], 7% for 150–200 mg/d and 13% above 300 mg/d). However, high dose venlafaxine (mean 346 mg/d, range 225–525) did not produce any significant effects on ECG parameters, although 12.5% developed hypertension and there was a dose-related association with heart rate (n = 37, Mbaya *et al*, *Hum Psychopharmacol* 2007;**22**:129–33). A nested case-control study showed that venlafaxine (n = 19268) is not associated with an excess risk of cardiac events compared to fluoxetine, dosulepin or citalopram in depression or anxiety (n = 207 384, Martinez *et al*, *BMJ* 2010;**340**:c249; FFT). The UK SmPCs now only caution use in uncontrolled hypertension (but **not** in controlled hypertension) and in people with a recent MI or unstable CHD.

23. **Isocarboxazid, phenelzine** and **tranylcypromine** are contraindicated in severe cardiac disease.

3.2.3 MOOD AND BIPOLAR

24. **Asenapine** can cause orthostatic hypotension and syncope (UK SmPC), especially early in treatment and in the elderly. Use carefully with any other drugs with cardiac effects, e.g. QTc prolongers and in people with cardiac risk factors (n = 148, p/c, Chapel *et al*, *J Clin Pharmacol* 2009; **49**:1297–308). QTc prolongation of 2–5 msec has been shown, but with none going over 500 msec.

25. **Carbamazepine** causes a rise in cholesterol, HDL and LDL levels (n = 52 + 80 controls, Svalheim *et al*, *Acta Neurol Scand Suppl* 2010;**190**:30–3). There are rare reports of cardiac effects, e.g. cardiac conduction changes, hypertension and AV block (n = 1, Labrecque et al, *Am J Psychiatry* 1992;**149**:572–3), and pacemaker failure (n = 1, Ambrosi *et al*, *Lancet* 1993;**342**:365).

26. **Lamotrigine** ≤400 mg/d does not prolong QTc (n = 152, d/b, p/c, c/o, 11/52, Dixon *et al*, *Br J Clin Pharmacol* 2008;**66**:396–404; FFT), or raise lipid levels (n = 132, 6/12, Svalheim *et al*, *Acta Neurol Scand Suppl* 2010;**190**:30–3). Monitoring ECG is recommended in overdose (Buckley *et al*, *Lancet* 1993;**342**:1552–3).

27. * **Lithium** is contraindicated in cardiac disease and failure, and a pre-treatment ECG is essential

3

especially in the elderly. Starting lithium can increase the QTc interval by a mean of 19 msec (n=8222, van Noord *et al, J Clin Psychopharmacol* 2009;**29**:9–15), but does not seem to affect cardiac function compared to controls (n=827, Ahrens *et al, J Affect Disord* 1995;**33**:67–75). Left ventricular systolic and diastolic functions are unaffected by lithium (n=30, Zencir *et al, Int J Clin Exp Med* 2015;**8**:2915–22; FFT) but there are reports of T-wave flattening (or possibly inversion), ventricular ectopics, congestive myopathy, bradycardia (Farag *et al, Lancet* 1994;**343**:1371), ECG changes and conduction disturbances, e.g. sinus node dysfunction (Terao *et al, Acta Psychiatr Scand* 1996;**93**:407–8).

28. **Valproate** appears to have no adverse ECG effects and may even have some preventive or stabilising effects on ventricular conduction (n=55, Kurt *et al, J Psychopharmacol* 2009;**23**:328–33) and decrease the risk of MI in people with epilepsy (n=155089, 10 years, Olesen *et al, Pharmacoepidemiol Drug Saf* 2011;**20**:146–53).

3.2.4 ANXIOLYTICS AND HYPNOTICS

Phobic anxiety and depression are inter-related predictors of ventricular arrhythmias in people with coronary artery disease, and so treatment of these may be important (n=940, Watkins *et al, Psychosom Med* 2006;**68**:651–6).

29. **Benzodiazepines** are relatively safe but contraindicated in acute pulmonary insufficiency. Temazepam ≤30 mg/d may cause a fall in systolic bp and increase in heart rate (n=12, Ford, *Br J Clin Pharmacol* 1990;**29**:61–7; FFT).

30. **Beta-blocker** use would depend upon the nature of the cardiac disease. In a prospective study of people with end-stage severe HF (61% with MDD), beta-blockers had a significant effect on reducing mortality but only if used *with* SSRIs, and had a negative effect if used with SNRIs or TCAs (n=250 [c=83], 18/12, Tousoulis *et al, J Card Fail* 2008;**14**:456–64).

31. **Buspirone** may have some cardiac effects, e.g. rare cases of hypertension and tachycardia.

32. **Clomethiazole** is contraindicated in acute pulmonary insufficiency and only used with care in chronic pulmonary insufficiency. **Chloral** is contraindicated in severe cardiac disease.

33. **Melatonin** has no known problems (SmPC; s=2, n=43, RCT, Zaslavskaia *et al, Klin Med [Mosk]* 2008;**86**:64–7) and may have cardioprotective effects (Dominguez-Rodriguez, *Expert Opin Investig Drugs* 2012;**21**:1593–6) and reduce nocturnal hypertension (s=4, n=589, RCTs, 3/52, Lemoine *et al, Integr Blood Press Control* 2012;**5**:9–17; FFT).

34. * **Pregabalin** has a caution for use in severe CHF (SmPC) and there are cases of exacerbation of heart failure in people with clinically stable CHF (n=3 and review, Page *et al, J Cardiovasc Med (Hagerstown)* 2008;**9**:922–5) and cardiac decompensation (n=1, Fong and Lee, *Ann Pharmacother* 2014;**48**:1077–81).

35. **Zaleplon**, **zolpidem** and **zopiclone** have no known problems.

3.2.5 ANTICONVULSANTS

36. **Primidone** may actually shorten QTc and may be a drug of choice in QT-prolongation (Christidis *et al, Seizure* 2006;**15**:64–6; FFT).

37. **Gabapentin** has no known problems.

38. **Levetiracetam** has no known problems nor affects lipid levels (n=135, 6/12, Svalheim *et al, Acta Neurol Scand Suppl* 2010;**190**:30–3).

39. **Oxcarbazepine** needs care if used in pre-existing conduction disturbances (UK SmPC). Regular weight monitoring is needed to help detect any fluid retention if used in cardiac insufficiency and secondary heart failure.

40. **Phenytoin** injection is contraindicated in sinus bradycardia, sino-atrial block, 2nd and 3rd-degree A-V block and in Adams-Stokes syndrome.

41. **Topiramate** has no known problems.

3.2.6 OTHERS

42. * **ADHD:** The EMEA (2009) recommended screening for cardiovascular risks before prescribing, and periodically thereafter (n=125, Wilens *et al, J Clin Psychiatry* 2005;**66**:253–9), although stimulants (n=38586) and atomoxetine (n=20995) have no greater risk of cardiovascular events than matched controls (n=238183) although a small raised risk can not be excluded (Schelleman *et al, PLoS One* 2013;**8**:e52991; FFT).

42a. **Atomoxetine** should be used with caution (UK SmPC) in prolonged QT, a family history of QT prolongation, and with other drugs risking QT prolongation, electrolyte disturbances and CYP2D6 inhibition. Atomoxetine can cause modest increases in bp (mean <5 mmHg) and pulse (mean < 10 bpm), which stabilise over two years (UK SmPC) but rarely produce a dramatic rise in bp in central autonomic failure, even at very low doses (n=3, RCT, p/c, c/o, Shibao *et al, Hypertension* 2007;**50**:47–53;FFT). Atomoxetine is not associated with clinically significant changes in QTc, although there is a statistically significant prolongation with increasing plasma levels, but not dose (n=131, p/c, Loghin *et al, Br J Clin Pharmacol* 2013;**75**:538–49;FFT;MS). In children aged around 11 (range 8–14) atomoxetine had no clinically significant effects on QT/QTc, bp, pulse and left ventricular systolic functions (n=40, 5/52, Sert *et al, Cardiol Young* 2012;**22**:158–61).

42b. **Dexamfetamine** does not have any significant risk of precipitating hypertension (minimal effects from amphetamine XR preps at < 60 mg/d; n=223, <24/12, Weisler *et al, CNS Spectr* 2005;**10**[suppl 20]:35–43). Regular bp testing has been recommended (ASDA, *Sleep* 1994;**17**:348–51).

42c. **Lisdexamfetamine** (LDX) has no significant effects on cardiac measures in adult ADHD (n=15, open, 6/12, Hammerness *et al, World J Biol Psychiatry* 2013;**14**;299–306).

42d. **Methylphenidate**'s SmPC recommends caution in people with severe hypertension, and bp monitoring should be carried out in all patients. It would be prudent to check first if there is a family or personal history of cardiac problems (n=171,126, Olfson *et al, J Am Acad Child Adolesc Psychiatry* 2012;**51**:147–56; FFT). One review suggested extra care if there is an increase in resting heart rate of 5–6 bpm, as there is an increased risk of a resting pulse of > 90 bpm, or systolic bp raised by +2 mmHg (s=10, Mick, McManus *et al, Eur Neuropsychopharmacol* 2013; **23**:534–41; FFT). There is some evidence of problems, e.g. relatively high dose methylphenidate (1.5 mg/kg/d) can produce a small but significant increase in bp, especially during the first six weeks (n=114[c=57], open, 6/12, Hammerness *et al, J Pediatr* 2009;**155**:84–9) and, although there may be a 1.8-fold increase in the risk of sudden death or ventricular arrhythmia, there was no dose-response relationship so is probably not a causal effect (n=43,999+175,955, Schelleman *et al, Am J Psychiatry* 2012;**169**:178–85). Conversely, a retrospective cohort study showed no evidence that ADHD medicines are associated with an increased risk of serious cardiac events (n=1200438, n=2,579, Cooper *et al, N Engl J Med* 2011;**365**:1896–904;FFT; in children; n=241,417, Schelleman *et al, Pediatrics* 2011;**127**:1102–10; FFT), although the absolute risk was very low in both studies.

42e. * **Guanfacine** needs caution if used in someone with history of hypotension, heart block, bradycardia, cv disease, a history of syncope or with risk factors such as hypotension, postural hypotension, bradycardia or dehydration. There was no effect on QTc over 12 hours after 4mg/d or 8mg/d doses in healthy adults (n=83, d/b, c/o, p/c, a/c, Martin *et al, Int J Clin Pharmacol Ther* 2015;**53**:301–16).

43. * **Anticholinesterases** have been associated with increased rates and risk of hospitalisation for bradycardia (n=627, Park-Wyllie *et al, PloS Med* 2009;**6**:e1000157; FFT), syncope, pacemaker insertion, and hip fractures in older adults with dementia (n=81,302, Gill *et al, Arch Intern Med* 2009;**169**:867–73) and caution is advised in cardiovascular conditions, e.g. sick sinus syndrome or other supraventricular cardiac conduction disturbances. All three have similar cardiovascular risk profiles (n=76233, Fosbøl *et al, J Am Geriatrics Society* 2012;**60**:2283–9). **Donepezil** (n=71[c=52], Isik *et al, Intern Med* 2012;**51**:575–8;FFT), **galantamine** (n=64[c=51], 4/12, Isik *et al, Am J Geriatr Pharmacother* 2010;**8**:454–9) and **rivastigmine** oral (s=4, n=2149, d/b, p/c, 26/52, Morganroth *et al, J Clin Pharmacol* 2002; **42**:558–68) and patches (Riepe, *J Clin Psychiatry* 2014;**75**:288) seem to lack significant cardiac effects in elderly people. Donepezil does not affect QTc but can increase PR interval (5%; mean 10ms), so care is needed in people with AV block or if taking other PR prolongers (n=18, Igeta *et al, Hum Psychopharmacol* 2014;**29**:292–4). **Rivastigmine** can lead to a modest reduction in mean heart rate of 1.5–2 bpm, but no bradycardia or ECG abnormalities (n=661, Ballard *et al, Int J Clin Pract* 2006;**60**:639–45).

44. **Memantine** should be used with caution as it has been reported to cause bradycardia (n=36, Gallini *et al, Pharmacoepidemiol Drug Saf* 2008;**17**:877–81).

45. **Anticholinergics** should be used with caution in people with a tendency to tachycardia. Sinus bradycardia has been reported with **benzatropine** (Voinov *et al, Am J Psychiatry* 1992;**149**:711) and **trihexyphenidyl** (n=1, Blumensohn *et al, Drug*

Intell Clin Pharm 1986;**20**:786–7).

46a. **Acamprosate** has no known problems.

46b. **Disulfiram** is contraindicated in cardiac failure, coronary artery disease, previous history of CVA and hypertension. It can be cardiotoxic in overdose (n=1, Jerónimo *et al, Arq Bras Cardiol* 2009;**92**:16–18; FFT). The Antabuse-alcohol reaction can cause cardiac arrest even in healthy adults.

46c. **Nalmefene** has no clinically relevant effect on QTc and T-waves, so there are no obvious concerns (n=270, RCT, d/b, p/c, 7/7, Matz *et al, Clin Drug Investig* 2012;**31**:799–811).

46d. **Naltrexone** can cause tachycardia, palpitations and ECG changes (UK SmPC).

47a. **Buprenorphine** (n=73) and Suboxone® (n=50, 2–4/52, Baker *et al, Ann Pharmacotherapy* 2006;**40**:392–6) are not associated with QTc prolongation, unlike methadone (n=128, Fareed *et al, J Addict Dis* 2013;**32**:244–51; n=165, RCT, d/b, 17/52, Wedam *et al, Arch Intern Med* 2007;**167**:2469–75). It has been used safely in a person with methadone-induced torsade de pointes (n=1, Krantz *et al, Pharmacotherapy* 2005;**25**:611–4).

47b. * **Methadone** (n=14915) has a higher incidence of cardiac arrhythmias than buprenorphine (n=7283) and controls (n=4796017) (Kao *et al, Addiction* 2015; **110**:1468–75). Methadone also prolongs QTc. Risk factors include recent cocaine use, uncontrolled blood glucose, CHF (n=55, RCA, Fareed *et al, Am J Drug Alcohol Abuse* 2013;**39**:235–40), hypokalaemia, hepatitis C, HIV and abnormal T-waves (n=6790, Girardin *et al, Am J Psychiatry* 2013;**170**:1468–76). Methadone <100mg/d is generally not associated with a clinically significant increase in QTc (n=45, Stallvik *et al, Drug Alcohol Depend* 2013;**129**:88–93) but it can occur at lower doses, e.g. 80mg/d with no evidence of a dose-response effect (n=180, Roy *et al, Addiction* 2012;**107**:1132–9). Around 5% of **methadone**-treated patients have a QTc >500msec but the maximum mortality attributable to QTc prolongation is low at 0.06 per 100 patient-years (n=200, Anchersen *et al, Addiction* 2009;**104**:993–9). The CSAT Cardiac Expert Panel Consensus Guidelines make five recommendations:

1. Inform client of the risks of arrhythmia.
2. Enquire about any history of heart disease, arrhythmia or syncope.
3. Carry out a pre-treatment ECG to measure QTc, repeat at 30 days then annually, with additional ECGs if the dose exceeds 100mg/d or if unexplained syncope or seizures occur (see methadone QT interval screening report; Martin *et al, J Addict Dis* 2011;**30**:283–306; FFT).
4. If QTc is 451–499ms, discuss with the client and monitor more frequently. If QTc >500ms, discontinue or reduce the dose (although there is no recommendation if the QTc is *exactly* 500ms).
5. Be alert to interactions with other QT-prolonging or interacting drugs, e.g. 3A4 inhibitors and stimulants (inc. cocaine) are associated with prolonged QTc (n=155, Mayet *et al, Drug Alcohol Rev* 2011;**30**: 388–96).

Reviews: * general (Krantz *et al, Ann Intern Med* 2009;**150**:387–95:Gourevitch, *Ann Intern Med* 2009;**150**:417–8; n=109, Fonseca *et al, Drug Alcohol Depend* 2009;**99**:327–32), QTc prolongation (Mujtaba *et al, J Cardiovasc Dis Res* 2013;**4**:229–35).

48. **Modafinil** is contraindicated in severe hypertension and arrhythmia and the MHRA advises against using it in people with uncontrolled hypertension or cardiac arrhythmias. An ECG is recommended at initiation with regular pulse and bp, and discontinued if arrhythmias or moderate-to-severe hypertension develop (MHRA *Drug Safety Update* 2011;**4**:A1). **Sodium oxybate** contains a significant dose of sodium (0.75g in 4.5g dose) and so dietary restriction of sodium might be considered in hypertension and heart failure (SmPC).

3.3 DIABETES

	Lower risk	Moderate risk	Higher risk
Antipsychotics	Amisulpride[7] Aripiprazole[1] Haloperidol[8] Lurasidone[3] Paliperidone[6] Pimozide[11] Risperidone[6] Sulpiride[7] Ziprasidone[11]	Phenothiazines[9] Quetiapine[5] Thioxanthenes[10]	Clozapine[2] Olanzapine[4]
Antidepressants	Agomelatine[14] Duloxetine[16] Moclobemide[18] Reboxetine[19] SSRIs[12] Trazodone[20] Tryptophan[21] Venlafaxine[22] Vortioxetine[16]	Bupropion[15] Fluoxetine[12c] Mianserin[21] Mirtazapine[17] Tricyclics[13]	MAOIs[23]
Anxiolytics and hypnotics	Benzodiazepines[29] Buspirone[31] Chloral[32] Clomethiazole[32] Melatonin[33] Pregabalin[34] Z-hypnotics[35]	Beta-blockers[30]	
Mood and bipolar	Asenapine[24] Carbamazepine[25] Lamotrigine[26] Lithium[27]	Quetiapine[5] Valproate[28]	Olanzapine[4]
Anticonvulsants (see also mood and bipolar above)	Barbiturates[36] Benzodiazepines[29] Gabapentin[37] Oxcarbazepine[39] Pregabalin[34]	Phenytoin[40] Topiramate[41]	
Others	Acamprosate[46] Anticholinergics[45] Anticholinesterases[43] Atomoxetine[42] Buprenorphine[47] Guanfacine[42] Memantine[44] Methadone[47] Methylphenidate[42] Modafinil[48] Nalmefene[46] Naltrexone[46]	Bupropion[15] Dexamfetamine[42] Disulfiram[46] Lisdexamfetamine[42] Sodium oxybate[48]	

GENERAL PRINCIPLES IN DIABETES

1. Use drugs least likely to promote loss of diabetic control or alter glucose levels.
2. Warn that some side-effects may be interpreted as hypoglycaemia.
3. Check the family history.
4. Monitor weight and glucose parameters.

3.3.1 ANTIPSYCHOTICS *

People with schizophrenics are 2.5 times more likely to develop type II diabetes than controls (s=25, n=145718 + 4.3m controls, Stubbs *et al, Acta Psychiatr Scand* 2015;**132:**144–57) so active monitoring, screening and lifestyle interventions are essential. The risk seems greatest for olanzapine, then clozapine (n=79, Newcomer *et al, Arch Gen Psychiatry* 2002;**59**:337–45), then risperidone but not with amisulpride, quetiapine or aripiprazole (n=1,772,426, Kessing *et al, Br J Psychiatry* 2010;**197**:266–71), indicating an adverse effect by some SGAs on glucose regulation. In people with diabetes, antipsychotics can worsen metabolic control and double the need for insulin, especially in the first two years (n=2,585, Spoelstra *et al, J Clin Psychiatry* 2004;**65**:674–8). In people with diabetes over 65 years initiating any antipsychotic is associated with increased risk for hospitalisation for hyperglycaemia (n=13,817, Lipscombe *et al, Arch Int Med* 2009;**169**:1282–9).

1. * **Aripiprazole** is not thought to have any problems in diabetes (see n=345,937, Kessing *et al, Br J Psychiatry* 2010;**197**:266–71;FFT), although hyperglycaemia is listed as an ADR in the UK SmPC.

2. * **Clozapine** can elevate glucose levels (in up to 23% people with no PMH, n=121, Sernyak *et al, J Clin Psychiatry* 2003;**64**:605–8) with a dose-related effect, indicating probable insulin resistance (n=384, FDA MedWatch, Koller *et al, Am J Med* 2001;**111**:716–23; n=26, RCT, 14/7, Chiu *et al, J Clin Psychopharmacol* 2006;**26**:504–7). Clozapine can also cause metabolic syndrome, e.g. weight gain and lipid abnormalities (e.g. raised serum triglycerides), significant risk factors for developing diabetes (n=206, Zhang *et al, Hum Psychopharmacol* 2011;**26**:392–6). The risk from clozapine (but not other SGAs) may persist even after weight reduction (n=520, open, Manu *et al, Schizophr Res* 2013;**143**:358–62). Routine glucose monitoring is recommended, regardless of pre-existing diabetes (review by Mir and Taylor, *Int Clin Psychopharmacol* 2001;**16**:63–74).

3. * **Lurasidone** has a class diabetes warning and monitoring is recommended.

4. **Olanzapine** seems the most likely SGA to cause or exacerbate diabetes (see introduction), e.g. the incidence of new-onset diabetes is about 1%, but with a 20% increased risk of diabetes compared to risperidone, and 90% higher in the first three months of treatment (n=33,946, three years, Caro *et al, J Clin Psychiatry* 2002;**63**:1135–9). Routine quarterly glucose monitoring is recommended with olanzapine, regardless of pre-existing diabetes (n=590, Wirshing *et al, J Clin Psychiatry* 2002;**63**:856–65; review by Eder-Ischia *et al, Essent Psychopharmacol* 2005;**6**:112–7). Olanzapine is also linked to the metabolic syndrome via, e.g. weight gain, elevated levels of insulin, leptin and lipids (triglycerides and cholesterol), e.g. olanzapine (mean 14mg/d) can produce fasting triglyceride levels raised by a mean of 60mg/dL (37%) (n=25, 12/52, Osser *et al, J Clin Psychiatry* 1999;**60**:767–70), a risk factor for precipitating or exacerbating diabetes. Hyperglycaemia or exacerbation of pre-existing diabetes is in the 'very rare' spontaneous event (<0.01%) category in the UK SmPC.

5. **Quetiapine** may have a slightly increased risk of diabetes (n=38,632, Veterans, Sernyak *et al, Am J Psychiatry* 2002;**159**:561–6). In younger people, it has been linked to lower insulin secretion (n=54, Ngai *et al, J Clin Psychopharmacol* 2014;**34**:359–64).

6. **Risperidone** has a modest effect on blood biochemistry (n=38,632, Veterans, Sernyak *et al, Am J Psychiatry* 2002;**159**:561–6). **Paliperidone** has only a few rare reports of glucose-related adverse events (SmPC).

7. **Sulpiride** and **amisulpride** have no known problems.

8. **Haloperidol** has no apparent problems.

9. **Phenothiazines** can cause increased appetite and weight gain, which would not help diabetic control. In newly-treated diabetes there is a modest but significant increased risk of diabetes with **chlorpromazine** and **perphenazine** (n=7227+6780, Wang *et al, J Clin Psychopharmacol* 2002;**22**:236–43).

10. **Zuclopenthixol** serum levels appear not to affect plasma insulin levels (n=9, Melkersson *et al, J Clin Psychiatry* 1999;**60**:783–91). **Flupentixol** may impair diabetic control and adjustment in

antidiabetic therapy may be needed.

11. **Pimozide** has no known problems. Short-term **ziprasidone** appears to have little effect on glucose levels and may actually lower serum cholesterol and triglyceride levels (n=37, 6/52, open, Kingsbury *et al*, *J Clin Psychiatry* 2001;**62**: 347–9).

3.3.2 ANTIDEPRESSANTS *

Although diabetes is a major risk factor for depression and vice versa, depression needs to be resolved as well for diabetes to improve:

- Pain in type 2 diabetes needs treating as it inhibits antidepressant response so needs treatment (n=387, open, 16/52, Anderson *et al*, *Diabetes Care* 2010;**33**:485–9; FFT)
- Although antidepressants are linked to diabetes, causality is not proven as some are linked to worsening and some to improvement, but larger studies show only a modest effect (s=22, Barnard *et al*, *Diabetes Care* 2013;**36**:3337–45), e.g: the five-year risk for developing diabetes is:
  - ~ 1.1% for non-users/general population
  - ~ 1.7% for standard doses of antidepressants
  - ~ 2.3% for higher doses of antidepressants
  - ~ 1.1% for users of antidepressants also taking metformin (n=151,347, Kivimäki *et al Diabetes Care* 2010; **33**:2611–6; FFT)
- Depression reduces glycaemic control and adherence (n=866, 12/12, Dirmaier *et al*, *Psychother Psychosom* 2010;**79**:172–8)
- SSRIs may even decrease serum glucose levels by up to 30% and cause anorexia (reducing body weight), helping people to control hunger and eat better (n=60 [c=43], RCT, d/b, 8/52, Ghaeli *et al*, *J Clin Psychopharmacol* 2004;**24**:386–8)
- In insulin-dependent diabetics, insulin use increases by 16% in depression, remains unchanged if treated with TCAs, but is reduced by 13% with an SSRI (n=133, two years, Knol *et al*, *Pharmacoepidemiol Drug Saf* 2008;**17**: 577–86).

Fluoxetine and citalopram have been recommended to be effective antidepressants without adverse effects on glycaemic control (n=40, RCT, 12/52, Khazaie *et al*, *Neurosciences [Riyadh]* 2011;**16**:42–5).

Reviews: * treating depression in diabetes mellitus (s=14, n=1724, RCTs, van der Feltz-Cornelis *et al*, *Gen Hosp Psychiatry* 2010;**32**:380–95), psychological and pharmacological treatments for depression and diabetes (s=19, n=1592, RCTs, Baumeister *et al*, *Cochrane Database Syst Rev* 2012;**12**:CD008381).

12. * **SSRIs:**

12a. **Citalopram/escitalopram** need no dose changes e.g. citalopram had no significant effect on insulin sensitivity (n=32, RCT, open, 8/52, Kauffman *et al*, *Gynecol Endocrinol* 2005;**21**:129–37) or glycaemic control (n=15, d/b, p/c, c/o, 2x3/52, Sindrup *et al*, *Clin Pharmacol Ther* 1992;**52**:547–52).

12b. **Fluoxetine** may be one of the antidepressants of choice in diabetes, although hypoglycaemia can occur and fluoxetine's side-effects, e.g. tremor, nausea, sweating and anxiety may be mistaken for hypoglycaemia. A trend towards better glycaemic control (n=60, RCT, p/c, 8/52, Lustman *et al*, *Diabetes Care* 2000;**23**:618–23; FFT) and reversible hypoglycaemia and reduced insulin need has been reported (n=1, Biagetti and Corcoy, *World J Clin Cases* 2013;**1**:169–71). Most problems have been reported with the more common type 2 diabetes rather than the insulin-dependent type 1 disease, so warn about a possible loss of hypoglycaemic awareness and regularly check serum glucose.

12c. **Fluvoxamine** has rarely induced acute hyperglycaemia (n=1, Oswald *et al*, *Int J Neuropsychopharmacol* 2003;**6**:85–7).

12d. **Paroxetine** has no known major problems.

12e. * **Sertraline** has no significant effect on glycaemic control (n=251, RCT, s/b, 12/52+1yr, Petrak *et al*, *Diabetes Care* 2015;**38**:767–75), with a possible positive effect on the diabetes itself (n=152, RCT, d/b, p/c, Lustman *et al*, *Arch Gen Psychiatry* 2006;**63**:521–9), especially in younger people (n=152, d/b, p/c, Williams *et al*, *Diabetes Care* 2007;**30**:801–6). There are rare cases of hypoglycaemia (e.g. n=1, Pollak *et al*, *Ann Pharmacother* 2001;**35**:1371–4) and raised glucose (n=1, Sansome and Sansome, *Int J Psychiatr Med* 2003;**33**:103–5).

13. * **Tricyclics** can adversely affect diabetic control as they increase serum glucose levels by up to 150%, increase carbohydrate craving and reduce the metabolic rate, but are generally considered safe except in brittle diabetes. The

3

incidence of diabetes with **clomipramine** may be 4 x higher than controls (n=1997, Mumoli *et al, Acta Diabetol* 2014;**51**:167–8) and **nortriptyline** tends to worsen glycaemic control (n=68, RCT, d/b, p/c, 8/52, Lustman *et al, Psychosom Med* 1997;**59**:241–50).

14. **Agomelatine** may actually be beneficial, e.g. in type II DM, it was superior to sertraline on most measures, e.g. depression and anxiety, with lower HbA1C (n=40 [c=40], open, 4/12, Karaiskos *et al, Int J Clin Pract* 2013;**67**:257–60). Similarly, in type II DM response and remission with agomelatine (63%; 43%) was equivalent to paroxetine (61%, 39%) but again HbA1C was significantly lower with agomelatine (n=116[c=116], RCT, a/c, 12/52, Kang *et al, Neuropsychiatr Dis Treat* 2015;**11**:1307–11; FFT).

15. **Bupropion** has a caution for use in hypoglycaemic or insulin-treated diabetes (El-Dakhakhny *et al, Arzneimittelforschung* 1996; **46**: 667–9).

16. * **Vortioxetine** has no known problems (SmPC). **Duloxetine** has no known problems.

17. **Mirtazapine** does not seem to influence glucose homeostasis (n=14, Laimer *et al, J Clin Psychiatry* 2006;**67**:421–4) and glucose tolerance may improve, but insulin sensitivity remains unchanged (n=10, Hennings *et al, Exp Clin Endocrinol Diabetes* 2010;**118**:98–100). Mirtazapine causes increased appetite which might be counter-productive. The UK SmPC has a class labelling precaution.

18. **Moclobemide** did not modify glibenclamide's effect on plasma glucose and insulin levels in healthy individuals (Amrein *et al, Psychopharmacology* 1992;**106**:S24–S31).

19. * **Reboxetine** has no known problems.

20. **Trazodone** has no known problems.

21. **Mianserin** dose-related hyperglycaemia has been reported in a non-diabetic woman (n=1, Marley and Rohan, *Lancet* 1993;**342**:1430–1).

22. **Venlafaxine** has no known problems.

23. **MAOIs** may decrease serum glucose levels by up to 35%. Diabetes is a UK SmPC precaution for **isocarboxazid**.

3.3.3 MOOD AND BIPOLAR

24. **Asenapine** causes hyperglycaemia in less than 1%, although some care would be prudent.

25. **Carbamazepine**-induced urinary retention has been reported (n=2, Steiner and Birmanns, *Neurology* 1993;**43**:1855–6).

26. **Lamotrigine** has no known problems.

27. **Lithium** has no major problems in diabetes, but some people may develop polyuria and polydipsia, a diabetes insipidus-like syndrome via an effect on cAMP and vasopressin. This can be controlled by ensuring an adequate fluid and salt intake. Increased lithium clearance with persistent hyperglycaemia has been reported (n=1, Cyr *et al, Ann Pharmacother* 2002;**36**:427–9). Lithium may also increase insulin secretion.

28. **Valproate** may give false positives in urine tests for diabetes. Protein binding of valproate may be lower in diabetes (Doucet *et al, Eur J Clin Pharmacol* 1993;**45**:577–9).

3.3.4 ANXIOLYTICS AND HYPNOTICS

29. **Benzodiazepines**: reduced insulin requirements have been reported after discontinuing **clonazepam** (n=1, Wägner *et al, Diabetes Care* 1999;**2**:2099).

30. **Propranolol** may prolong the hypoglycaemic response to insulin and hypoglycaemic episodes.

31. **Buspirone** has no known problems.

32. **Clomethiazole** and **chloral hydrate** have no known problems.

33. **Melatonin** may improve sleep without affecting glucose or lipids, and long-term treatment significantly lowers HbA1c, suggesting *improved* glycaemic control (n=36, RCT, d/b, p/c, c/o, 7/52+5/12, Garfinkel *et al, Diabetes Metab Synd Obes* 2011;**4**:307–13; FFT).

34. **Pregabalin** has no known problems.

35. **Zaleplon**, **zolpidem** and **zopiclone** have no known problems.

3.3.5 ANTICONVULSANTS

36. **Barbiturates** have no known problems.

37. **Gabapentin** has been reported to cause blood glucose fluctuations (e.g. n=1, Penumalee *et al, Am J Kid Dis* 2003;**42**:E3–5).

38. **Levetiracetam** has no known problems.

39. **Oxcarbazepine** has no known problems.

40. **Phenytoin** may affect glucose metabolism and protein binding may be lower (Doucet *et al, Eur J Clin Pharmacol* 1993;**45**:577–9).

41. **Topiramate** has no known problems.

3.3.6 OTHERS

42. **ADHD:** * There are no apparent problems with **methylphenidate, dexamfetamine, lisdexamfetamine** or **atomoxetine,** but a transient loss of appetite may occur. There is a report of improved glucose tolerance in diabetics taking **guanfacine** for one year (n=18, Hauger-Klevene and Scornavacchi, *Eur J Clin Pharmacol* 1985;**29**:391–3).

43. **Anticholinesterases:** There are no apparent problems with **donepezil** or **galantamine**, but diabetes mellitus is a precaution for **rivastigmine**.

44. **Memantine** has no known problems.

45. **Anticholinergics** have no known problems.

46. **Disulfiram**'s UK SmPC recommends caution in diabetes mellitus. There are no known problems with **acamprosate, nalmefene** or **naltrexone**.

47. **Buprenorphine** and **methadone** have no precautions for use in diabetes (UK SmPC) although the sugar-free liquid would be the formulation of choice for the latter.

48. **Sodium oxybate** and **modafinil** have no known problems.

3

3.4 EPILEPSY

	LOWER RISK	MODERATE RISK	HIGHER RISK
Antipsychotics	Amisulpride[7] Aripiprazole[1] Flupentixol[10] Haloperidol[8] Lurasidone[3] Paliperidone[6] Pimozide[11] Risperidone[6]	Olanzapine[4] Phenothiazines (most)[9] Quetiapine[5] Sulpiride[7] Ziprasidone[11] Zuclopenthixol[10]	Chlorpromazine[9] Clozapine[2]
Antidepressants	Agomelatine[14] MAOIs[23] Moclobemide[18] Reboxetine[19] SSRIs[12] Tryptophan[21]	Duloxetine[16] Mianserin[21] Mirtazapine[17] Trazodone[20] Tricyclics (most)[13] Venlafaxine[22] Vortioxetine[16]	Bupropion[15]
Anxiolytics and hypnotics	Benzodiazepines[29] Beta-blockers[30] Chloral[32] Clomethiazole[32] Melatonin[33] Pregabalin[34] Z-hypnotics[35]	Buspirone[31]	
Mood and bipolar	Asenapine[24] Carbamazepine[25] Lamotrigine[26]	Lithium[27] Olanzapine[4] Quetiapine[5]	
Others	Acamprosate[46] Anticholinergics[45] Buprenorphine[47] Dexamfetamine[42] Guanfacine[42] Lisdexamfetamine[42] Methylphenidate[42] Modafinil[48] Methadone[47] Nalmefene[46] Naltrexone[46]	Anticholinesterases[43] Atomoxetine[42] Disulfiram[46] Memantine[44]	Bupropion[15] Sodium oxybate[48]

GENERAL PRINCIPLES FOR PRESCRIBING IN EPILEPSY

Risk factors for psychotropic-induced seizures:

- History of epilepsy (including febrile seizures) in the patient or their family
- Neurological abnormalities (e.g. brain injury, angioma cavernous, EEG alterations)
- Cerebral arteriosclerosis
- Old age and/or reduced drug clearance
- Physical illness (e.g. malignant hypertension)
- Multiple drugs.

Practical recommendations in pre-existing epilepsy:

- Use drugs with anticonvulsant properties where possible
- Avoid high-risk drugs
- Start low and go slow, monitoring plasma levels and EEG where possible
- Keep dosing simple and avoid polypharmacy.

3.4.1 ANTIPSYCHOTICS *

General principles

1. Keep the daily dose as low as possible as any proconvulsive effect may be dose-related.
2. Take extreme care where risk factors exist, including head trauma, previous seizures, concomitant drugs (especially other antipsychotics), any condition that predisposes to epilepsy and if withdrawing from central depressants, e.g. benzodiazepines and alcohol.
3. Use lowest risk drugs unless essential — antipsychotics with more antihistaminic, antiserotonergic, sedative and antiadrenergic effects may have a greater risk.
4. Use a slow rate of introduction and withdrawal.
5. Dose changes should be small and gentle.
6. Anticonvulsant cover as appropriate.

Reviews: interventions for psychosis in epilepsy (Farooq and Sherin, *Cochrane Database Syst Rev* 2008;**4**:CD006118), general (Kanner, *Semin Neurol* 2008:**28**:379–88).

1. **Aripiprazole** pre-marketing trials showed seizures occurred in only 0.1% people, but probably still needs caution in epilepsy.

2. * **Clozapine** can cause dose-related seizures, the risk rising from 1% (<300mg/d), through 2.7% (300–600mg/d) to 4.4% (>600mg/d), but is probably more plasma-level related. For advice see C6.4. EEG abnormalities have been seen in 63% of people on clozapine and slowing and epileptiform activities in 41.4% (n=87, Goyal *et al*, *Psychiatry Investig* 2011;**8**:372–6;FFT; review by Wong and Delva, *Can J Psychiatry* 2007;**52**:457–63). Rapid dose-titration increases the risk as does serum clozapine levels above 750ng/mL (n=101, Rajkumar *et al*, *Int Clin Psychopharmacol* 2013;**28**:50–6). Valproate is the routine anticonvulsant cover of choice, at clozapine doses of 600mg/d or more. See also *4.2.4* and *6.4*.

3. * **Lurasidone** had an incidence of seizures the same as placebo in schizophrenia trials (both 0.1%) and 0% in the (smaller) bipolar depression trials.

4. **Olanzapine** should be used cautiously in people with a seizure history, with a slightly higher risk in the over 65s. Unexplained seizures (i.e. people without reported risk factors) occurred in 0.9% of people during pre-marketing trials (n=2,500).

5. **Quetiapine**'s incidence of seizures appears equivalent to placebo, but a short review suggested that it may be associated with new-onset seizures in patients with seizurogenic conditions (Yalug *et al*, *J Neuropsychiatry Clin Neurosci* 2007;**19**:341–2).

6. **Risperidone** has no known problems. Pre-marketing trials showed a seizure incidence of 0.3% (n=2,607) and it has been used successfully for psychosis in epilepsy (n=1, Mahgoub, *J Neuropsychiatry Clin Neurosci* 2007;**19**:347–8). **Paliperidone** should be used with caution in people with risk factors or a history of seizures (UK SmPC).

7. **Amisulpride** has no known problems except in overdose. **Sulpiride**'s UK SmPC cautions about reduced seizure threshold so care is needed in unstable epilepsy but, with only a few cases of convulsions reported and only minimal EEG effects, it may be a drug of choice.

8. **Haloperidol** may have only mild-to-moderate effects, and may be a lower risk drug.

9. **Fluphenazine** may have a low proconvulsive effect, although status epilepticus has been reported. The incidence of seizures with **chlorpromazine** may cause in 9% at ≥1g/d and 0.5% at less than 1g/d and is best avoided.

10. **Zuclopenthixol** and **flupentixol** have few adverse reports but the UK SmPCs caution use in epilepsy, brain damage and alcohol withdrawal.

11. **Pimozide** may have a low effect (Oliver *et al*, *Arch Gen Psychiatry* 1982;**39**:206–9) and epilepsy is not mentioned in the UK SmPC. Seizures occurred in 0.4% patients during pre-marketing trials with **ziprasidone** so use with caution in epilepsy.

3.4.2 ANTIDEPRESSANTS *

Unless large scale trials are carried out (unlikely), the safest antidepressant in epilepsy will remain unknown but a review concluded that SSRIs do not significantly increase seizure threshold (s=8, n=471, Maguire *et al*, *Cochrane Database Syst Rev* 2015;**12**:CD010682). The risk of depression is doubled in seizure sufferers (13% vs 7%;

n=130,880, Fuller-Thomson and Brennenstuhl, *Epilepsia* 2009;**50**:1051–8) and the risk of suicide is high (see *C5.15*). All patients require an individual assessment of their risk factors and recognition that there is a dose-dependent relationship between antidepressants and seizures. **A slow rate of introduction** reduces the risk. In a post-hoc analysis of MDD and TLE, citalopram, reboxetine or mirtazapine were effective with no serious ADRs and no increase in seizures with (n=75, RCT, Kühn *et al*, *Epilepsy Behav* 2003;**4**:674–9).

Reviews: depression in epilepsy (Seethalakshmi and Krishnamoorthy, *Epileptic Disord* 2007; **9**:1–10;FFT;Mula *et al*, *Expert Opin Pharmacother* 2008;**9**:3159–68).

12. **SSRIs** have a low proconvulsive effect (review by Kondziella and Asztely, *Acta Neurol Scand* 2009;**119**:75–80), as serotonin function is unlikely to be of major importance in the genesis of seizures.

12a. **Citalopram** and **escitalopram** have no reports of a proconvulsive effect. Citalopram has been used for interictal (between fits) depression without an increase in seizure frequency or severity (n=43, 8/52, Hovorka *et al*, *Epilepsy Behav* 2000;**1**:444–7; n=75, RCT, Kühn *et al*, *Epilepsy Behav* 2003;**4**:674–9).

12b. **Fluoxetine** has a probable seizure incidence of 0.2%, similar to other antidepressants, and may even have a positive effect (n=17, open, add-on, Favale *et al*, *Neurology* 1995;**45**:1926–7).

12c. **Fluvoxamine** probably has a low proconvulsive effect, although this has been disputed (Vincenti, *Lancet* 1990;**336**:947).

12d. **Paroxetine** has a minimal potential for producing seizures at clinically useful doses (Milne and Goa, *Drugs* 1991;**41**:450–77).

12e. **Sertraline**-related seizures in clinical trials are at a similar frequency to placebo and only in people with a history of seizures. It has been effective for depression in younger people with epilepsy, with increased fits in only 6% (n=36, Thomé-Souza *et al*, *Epilepsy Behav* 2007;**10**:417–25).

13. **Tricyclics** seem to lower the seizure threshold, with **amitriptyline** reputed to be the most proconvulsive and **doxepin** possibly of lowest risk. TDM of tricyclics minimises the risk of toxicity.

14. **Agomelatine** is of very low risk as it reduces glutamate release, is neuroprotective, an antioxidant and stabilises circadian rhythm disturbances (Vimala *et al*, *Med Hypotheses* 2014;**82**:105–10).

15. **Bupropion**'s risk of seizures is about 0.1% up to 300mg/d (SmPC) but is contraindicated in seizures, a history of seizures or any problem lowering the seizure threshold (e.g. withdrawing from other drugs, use with any seizure threshold-lowering drug, alcohol abuse, history of head trauma, diabetes treated with hypoglycaemics or insulin, and the use of stimulants or anorectics). The effect is probably plasma level-related so doses should not exceed 450mg/d (although new-onset seizures can occur at lower doses, e.g. Pesola and Avasarala, *J Emerg Med* 2002;**22**:235–9), no single dose should be above 200mg and do not increase at more than 150mg/d.

16. * **Vortioxetine** has a class warning and care is recommended in unstable epilepsy (SmPC). **Duloxetine**'s UK SmPC cautions use in epilepsy but has no reported problems as such.

17. **Mirtazapine** high-dose has been linked to a grand mal seizure in a person with a history of seizures, but no cause-effect link could be made.

18. **Moclobemide** has no reports of problems.

19. * **Reboxetine** may be particularly useful in epilepsy with a low interaction potential and a low spontaneous incidence of seizures of <0.2% (n=1500), with no seizures in overdose.

20. **Trazodone**'s SmPC now includes a caution in epilepsy, and to avoid abrupt changes in dose.

21. **Tryptophan** has no known problems. **Mianserin** is often quoted as being relatively safe in epilepsy and in 84 overdoses of ≥1g no seizures were seen (Cassidy and Henry, *Br Med J (Clin Res Ed)* 1987;**295**:1021–4;FFT).

22. * **Venlafaxine** can be effective but trials show a seizures incidence of 0.26% and so a slow introduction and withdrawal is recommended (s=8, n=471, Maguire *et al*, *Cochrane Database Syst Rev* 2015;**12**:CD010682).

23. **MAOIs** are generally not considered epileptogenic at therapeutic doses. The UK SmPC for **isocarboxazid** notes a varying effect, with some people having decreased seizures and others increased seizures. MAOI-induced myoclonic jerks and serotonin syndrome can occasionally be interpreted as seizures.

3.4.3 MOOD AND BIPOLAR

24. **Asenapine** was linked to seizures in one

patient in trials (n=851;0.1%), compared to none with placebo (n=706), and in long-term trials in five (n=1953;0.25%), so some care would be prudent but it is not an obvious problem (UK SmPC).

25. **Carbamazepine** is an anticonvulsant.

26. **Lamotrigine** is an anticonvulsant and has proved useful for interictal depression (n=13, open, Kalogjera-Sackellares and Sackellares, *Epilepsy Behav* 2002;**3**:510–6), as well as in bipolar depression.

27. **Lithium** has a marked epileptogenic activity in overdose, but probably no effect at standard dose.

28. **Valproate** is an anticonvulsant.

3.4.4 ANXIOLYTICS AND HYPNOTICS

29. **Benzodiazepines** are obviously a treatment of choice, with established anticonvulsant activity.

30. **Beta-blockers** have no known problems.

31. **Buspirone** has no anticonvulsant activity in animal studies. The UK SmPC contraindicates use in epilepsy but there is no evidence of problems.

32. **Chloral hydrate** and **clomethiazole** have anticonvulsant properties.

33. **Melatonin** has no known problems.

34. **Pregabalin** is an anticonvulsant.

35. **Zopiclone** has a weak anticonvulsant activity, **zolpidem** has none and there is no data on **zaleplon**.

3.4.5 ANTICONVULSANTS

36–41. Considering anticonvulsants with effects on mood may be preferable.

3.4.6 OTHERS

42. * ADHD

42a. * **Atomoxetine**'s SmPC cautions use in people with a history of seizures and discontinuing considered if seizures start or increase in frequency. However, the incidence during clinical trials was 0.1–0.2%, similar to placebo and population-based data (Wernicke *et al, Dev Med Child Neurol* 2007;**49**:498–502), with no increase in the seizure risk in children aged 6–17 years with ADHD and no prior seizures (n<34,727, McAfee *et al, Curr Drug Saf* 2008;**3**:123–31) and no detrimental effect in well-controlled epilepsy (n=23, Mulas *et al, Rev Neurol* 2014;**58**[Suppl 1]:S43–9).

42b. **Dexamfetamine** has no known problems.

42c. **Lisdexamfetamine** has no known problems.

42d. * **Methylphenidate** is not associated with a significant risk of seizures at therapeutic doses so may have a good risk:benefit ratio (review by Koneski and Casella, *Arq Neuropsiquiatr* 2010;**68**:107–14; FFT). There was no increase in seizures in children aged 6–17 years with ADHD and no prior seizures (n<34,727, McAfee *et al, Curr Drug Saf* 2008;**3**:123–31), or in younger people with LD, severe refractory epilepsy and ADHD up to 1mg/kg/d (n=18, Fosi *et al, Epilepsia* 2013;**54**:2071–81; FFT) or in well-controlled epilepsy (n=23, Mulas *et al, Rev Neurol* 2014;**58**[Suppl 1]:S43–9). There are a few reports of exacerbation (e.g. Kaufmann *et al, J Child Neurol* 2009;**24**:727–33).

42e.* **Guanfacine** had a weak anticonvulsant effect in an animal test (Szot *et al, Neuroscience* 2004;**126**:795–803).

Review: ADHD treatments in epilepsy (Kattimani and Mahadevan, *Ann Indian Acad Neurol* 2011; **14**:9–11; FFT).

43. **Anticholinesterases** may have some potential for causing seizures so care is needed with all three. **Donepezil** 10mg/d had no adverse effects on seizures in one trial (n=23, RCT, s/b, p/c, c/o, 3+3/12, Hamberger *et al, Epilepsia* 2007;**48**:1283–91).

44. **Memantine** has a single case report so should be used with caution.

45. **Anticholinergics** have no known problems.

46. **Disulfiram**'s SmPC recommends caution in epilepsy. There are no known problems with **acamprosate, nalmefene** or **naltrexone**.

47. **Methadone** and **buprenorphine** appear to have no unexpected problems.

48. **Sodium oxybate** has caused seizures and use is not recommended in epilepsy (SmPC). There are no apparent problems with **modafinil,** although there are cases of *de novo* seizures and possible increased seizure frequency, albeit not dose related (n=205, 10 years, Artsy *et al, Epilepsy Behav* 2012;**23**:405–8).

3.5 GLAUCOMA (narrow-angle)

	LOWER RISK	MODERATE RISK	HIGHER RISK
Antipsychotics	Aripiprazole[3] Butyrophenones[3] Lurasidone[3] Paliperidone[3] Quetiapine[3] Risperidone[3] Sulpiride[3] Ziprasidone[3]	Clozapine[2] Phenothiazines[1] Thioxanthenes[2]	Olanzapine[2]
Antidepressants	Agomelatine[6] Bupropion[9] Vortioxetine[11]	Duloxetine[7] MAOIs[10] Mirtazapine[10] Moclobemide[10] Reboxetine[8] SSRIs[4] Trazodone[4] Venlafaxine[11]	Tricyclics[5]
Mood and bipolar	Asenapine[12] Lamotrigine[12] Lithium[12] Valproate[12]	Carbamazepine[12]	Olanzapine[2]
Others	Acamprosate[19] Anticholinesterases[18] Buprenorphine[20] Clomethiazole[13] Disulfiram[19] Gabapentin[15] Guanfacine[16] Levetiracetam[15] Lisdexamfetamine[16] Memantine[18] Melatonin[13] Methadone[20] Nalmefene[20] Naltrexone[20] Oxcarbazepine[15] Phenobarbital[15] Phenytoin[15] Tiagabine[15] Zopiclone[13]	Caffeine[15] Dexamfetamine[16] Methylphenidate[16]	Atomoxetine[16] Anticholinergics[17] Topiramate[14] Zolpidem[13]

Narrow-angle (angle closure) glaucoma occurs in eyes with a narrow anterior chamber angle, where drainage of the aqueous fluid through the anterior chamber angle is reduced or blocked. Drugs with anticholinergic effects have the potential to either induce narrow-angle glaucoma or to worsen it, although the degree of anticholinergic effect is of greater importance (review by Lam *et al*, *Curr Opin Ophthalmol* 2007;**18**:146–51).

GENERAL RECOMMENDATIONS

Patients with a shallow anterior chamber and/or narrow angles, or with previously diagnosed glaucoma may be treated with drugs with anticholinergic properties, if intraocular pressure is monitored, an ophthalmologist is involved and information is given on the symptoms of acute narrow-angle closure (blurred vision, 'coloured halos' around bright lights, intense pain, lacrimation, lid oedema, red eye, nausea, vomiting; review by Quigley, *Lancet* 2011;**377**:1367–77), including to stop the drug and seek medical attention immediately should those symptoms occur. In a person with a shallow anterior chamber and narrow angles, an ophthalmologist would normally perform an iridotomy or some type of drainage surgery to allow drug use. Treatment with miotic therapy, e.g. pilocarpine, may not necessarily protect someone with narrow angles against drug-induced angle closure, so monitoring is essential.

Risk factors include increasing age and in people unaware they have narrow iridocorneal angles. The peak effect from a drug on intraocular pressure can occur within 5–24 hours (or sooner).

Reviews: ocular ADRs of psychotropics, including glaucoma (Richa and Yazbek, *CNS Drugs* 2010;**24**:501–26), risk factors (Coleman and Kodjebacheva, *Open Ophthalmol J* 2009;**3**:38–42; FFT).

3.5.1 ANTIPSYCHOTICS

1. **Phenothiazines** have anticholinergic effects so the potential for problems exists. Screening for glaucoma has been recommended before initiating therapy, although no detectable narrow-angle glaucoma was seen with **thioridazine** (n=100), **fluphenazine** (n=98) and **chlorpromazine** (n=99) (Applebaum, *Arch Ophthalmol* 1963;**69**:578–80). See also introduction.

2. Other antipsychotics with similar anticholinergic effects would include **clozapine**, **flupentixol** and **zuclopenthixol**. **Olanzapine** is contraindicated in narrow-angle glaucoma.

3. Antipsychotics with little or no anticholinergic effects (e.g. **aripiprazole**, **haloperidol**, **lurasidone**, **paliperidone quetiapine, risperidone, sulpiride** and **ziprasidone**) must still be considered to have a potential for problems, albeit probably at a low level.

3.5.2 ANTIDEPRESSANTS

4. **SSRIs**: There have been reports of angle-closure glaucoma with **citalopram** (in younger women, n = 1, Croos *et al*, *BMC Ophthalmol* 2005;**5**:23;FFT; n = 1, Massaoutis *et al*, *Br J Ophthalmol* 2007;**91**:1086–7;FFT), **escitalopram** (n = 1, Zelefsky *et al*, *Am J Ophthalmol* 2006;**141**:1144–7), **fluvoxamine** (n = 1, Jiménez-Jiménez *et al*, *Ann Pharmacother* 2001;**35**:1565–6), **fluoxetine** (e.g. Ahmad, *DICP Ann Pharmacother* 1991;**25**:436), **paroxetine** (n=6, Sierra-Rodriguez *et al*, *Semin Ophthalmol* 2013;**28**:244–6), **sertraline** (n = 1, Ho *et al*, *Gen Hosp Psychiatry* 2013;**35**:575.e1–2; review by Costagliola *et al*, *Curr Neuropharmacol* 2008;**6**:293–310;FFT) and **trazodone** (n=1, Pae *et al*, *Psych Clin Neurosci* 2003;**57**:127–8).

5. **Tricyclics** generally have a greater anticholinergic effect than phenothiazines, although most of the data is so old it should probably be pensioned off. If people are at risk of narrow-angle glaucoma, pre-treatment examination by an ophthalmologist is recommended. People with a narrow anterior chamber angle who are receiving glaucoma treatment or who have had laser treatment should have few problems provided care (see introduction) is taken (Oshika, *Drug Saf* 1995; **12**:256–63). There is a report of people with narrow angles developing acute-angle closure glaucoma with **imipramine** (n = 4, Ritch *et al*, *Arch Ophthalmol* 1994;**112**:67–8), **clomipramine** (Schlingemann *et al*, *Lancet* 1996;**347**:465) and **amitriptyline** (review by Lieberman and Stoudemire, *Psychosomatics* 1987;**28**:145–8).

6. * **Agomelatine** can actually *reduce* intraocular pressure by about 30% in people with glaucoma (n = 10, Pescosolido *et al*, *Ophthalmic Physiol Opt* 2015;**35**:201–5).

7. **Duloxetine** may cause mydriasis so caution is necessary in people with raised intraocular pressure or at risk of acute narrow-angle glaucoma, with a case report of bilateral acute angle-closure glaucoma (n = 1, Shifera *et al*, *Ann Pharmacother* 2014;**48**:936–9).

8. **Reboxetine** has limited data but the literature recommends close supervision.

9. * **Bupropion** (for whatever indication) reduces the risk of developing OAG (Open-Angle Glaucoma) by 21% (n = 638,481, Stein *et al*, *PLoS One* 2015;**10**:e0123682; FFT) but in people

younger than 50 the risk of angle-closure glaucoma is twice as high (OR= 1.98) with bupropion (n=6110723, Symes *et al*, *JAMA Ophthalmol* 2015; **133:** 1187–9).

10. **Mirtazapine, moclobemide, trazodone** and **MAOIs** can cause dilation of the pupil.

11. **Venlafaxine** may raise intraocular pressure and rapidly developing bilateral acute narrow-angle glaucoma has been reported (n= 1, Ng *et al*, *Med J Aust* 2002; **176**:241). **Vortioxetine** has been shown to have no detectable effect on intraocular pressure or glaucoma (SmPC, EPAR).

3.5.3 MOOD AND BIPOLAR

12. There are no known problems with **asenapine, lamotrigine, lithium** and **valproate. Carbamazepine** has a precautionary warning in the SmPC.

3.5.4 HYPNOTICS

13. * No problems are expected with the **benzodiazepines, clomethiazole, melatonin, zaleplon** or **zopiclone. Zolpidem** users with an annual cumulative dose of >200mg (>15mg/month) have a significantly increased (OR= 1.3) risk of glaucoma (Ho *et al*, *J Epidemiol* 2015;**25**:15–9; FFT).

3.5.5 ANTICONVULSANTS

14. * **Topiramate** is cautioned in glaucoma (7.4-fold increased risk; n= 1956+ 15648, Ho *et al*, *Am J Ophthalmol* 2013;**155**:336–41) and the UK SmPC notes that symptoms usually start within the first month, and include decreased visual acuity and/or ocular pain. If this occurs, topiramate should be discontinued as soon as clinically feasible and appropriate measures to reduce intraocular pressure introduced (review, s=74, Abtahi *et al*, *Clin Ophthalmol* 2012; **6**:117–31; FFT). However, a case-control study concluded that there was a slight increase in the incidence of glaucoma (RR= 1.23) in regular, but higher (RR= 1.54) in new, users of topiramate, although there was no significant increase in the risk of glaucoma requiring treatment (RR= 1.09) (n=989,591, Etminan *et al*, *Am J Ophthalmol* 2012;**153**:827–30).

15. **Barbiturates, gabapentin, levetiracetam, oxcarbazepine, phenytoin** and **tiagabine** have no known problems.

3.5.6 OTHERS

16. **Atomoxetine** is contraindicated in glaucoma. **Amfetamine** causes a transient rise in intraocular pressure, which is not associated with closure of the angle although there appears no problem with **lisdexamfetamine** (SmPC) or **guanfacine. Caffeine** has been reported to cause a transient rise in intraocular pressure, or a sustained elevation at more than 180mg/d, not a lot by the author's standards (n=28, Avisar *et al*, *Ann Pharmacother* 2002;**36**:992–5). **Methylphenidate** can cause a transient rise in intraocular pressure not associated with closure of the angle. It has been used uneventfully in ADHD and primary open-angle glaucoma well-controlled by pilocarpine and betaxolol (n= 1, Bartlik *et al*, *Arch Gen Psychiatry* 1997;**54**:188–9), but 60 mg/d has precipitated severe glaucoma requiring surgery (n= 1, Lu *et al*, *J Chin Med Assoc* 2006;**69**:589–90;).

17. **Anticholinergics** are contraindicated in narrow-angle glaucoma.

18. **Donepezil** discontinuation has caused angle-closure glaucoma (n= 1, Enzenauer and Bowers, *J Geront A Biol Sci Med Sci* 2005;**60**:1083). **Memantine** has no known problems.

19. **Acamprosate, disulfiram and ginkgo biloba** (12/12, Khoury *et al*, *J Glaucoma* 2009;**18**:543–5; FFT) have no known problems.

20. **Buprenorphine, methadone nalmefene, naltrexone** have no known problems.

3.6 HEPATIC IMPAIRMENT

	Lower risk	Moderate risk	Higher risk
Antipsychotics	Amisulpride[7] Aripiprazole[1] Flupentixol[10] Haloperidol[8] Paliperidone[6] Pimozide[11] Sulpiride[7] Ziprasidone[11] Zuclopenthixol[10]	Clozapine[2] Lurasidone[3] Olanzapine[4] Phenothiazines[9] Quetiapine[5] Risperidone[6]	
Antidepressants	Mianserin[21] Paroxetine[12d] Tryptophan[21] Vortioxetine[16]	Bupropion[15] Duloxetine[16] Mirtazapine[17] Moclobemide[18] Reboxetine[19] SSRIs (most)[12] St John's wort[21] Trazodone[20] Tricyclics (most)[13] Venlafaxine[22]	Agomelatine[14] Lofepramine[13] MAOIs[23]
Anxiolytics and hypnotics	Lorazepam (low dose)[29] Melatonin[33] Oxazepam (low dose)[29] Pregabalin[34] Temazepam (low dose)[29]	Buspirone[31] Clomethiazole[32] Zaleplon[35a] Zolpidem[35b] Zopiclone[35c]	Benzodiazepines (esp. long-acting)[29] Beta-blockers[30] Chloral[32]
Mood and bipolar	Carbamazepine[25] Lithium[27]	Asenapine[24] Lamotrigine[26] Olanzapine[4] Quetiapine[5]	Valproate[28]
Anticonvulsants (see also mood & anxiety above)	Gabapentin[37] Pregabalin[34] Topiramate?[41]	Levetiracetam[38] Oxcarbazepine[39]	Barbiturates[36] Phenytoin[40] Valproate[28]
Others	Buprenorphine[47a] Dexamfetamine[42b] Donepezil[43] Lisdexamfetamine[42c] Memantine[44]	Acamprosate[46a] Anticholinergics[45] Atomoxetine[42a] Bupropion[15] Disulfiram[46b] Galantamine[43] Methadone[47b] Methylphenidate[42d] Modafinil[48] Rivastigmine[43] Sodium oxybate[48]	Guanfacine[42e] Nalmefene[46c] Naltrexone[46d]

3

GENERAL PRINCIPLES FOR PRESCRIBING IN HEPATIC IMPAIRMENT

1. The greater the degree of hepatic impairment, the greater the impairment of drug metabolism, and the greater the risk of drug toxicity. People may also be more sensitive to common or predictable side-effects.
2. Start low, go slow, and monitor LFTs regularly.
3. LFTs do not necessarily correlate well with metabolic impairment, although they can give a pointer.
4. Care is needed with drugs with a high first-pass clearance.
5. In severe liver disease, avoid drugs causing marked sedation and/or constipation.

Child-Pugh is a measure of the severity and prognosis of cirrhosis, and is calculated from the severity of ascites and encephalopathy, bilirubin, albumin and clotting times:

Child-Pugh grade	A	B	C
Child-Pugh score	5–6	7–9	10–15
Description	Cirrhosis but functioning liver	Significant functional compromise	Decom-pensation of liver

Review: general (Verbeeck, *Eur J Clin Pharmacol* 2008;**64**:1147–61).

3.6.1 ANTIPSYCHOTICS *

1. **Aripiprazole** needs no dose changes in any degree of hepatic impairment. Cmax may be lower in hepatic impairment but with no significant adverse effects (n=25, Mallikaarjun *et al, Clin Pharmacokinet* 2008;**47**:533–42).

2. **Clozapine** is contraindicated in severe hepatic disease and so lower doses, regular plasma level monitoring and LFT monitoring would be necessary if used. There are cases of reversible toxic hepatitis, with AST levels dramatically raised, and eosinophilia developing early (e.g. Thatcher *et al, Am J Psychiatry* 1995;**152**:296–7).

3. * **Lurasidone** should start at 18.5 mg/d in moderate and severe hepatic impairment. Do not go above 74 mg (moderate) or 37 mg (severe) in hepatic impairment.

4. **Olanzapine** should be started at a lower dose, e.g. 5 mg/d, as transient, asymptomatic elevations in ALT and AST have been noted and monitoring is appropriate in people with risk factors e.g. hepatic impairment, concomitant hepatotoxic drugs. A lower starting dose of 150 mg/4 weeks should be considered for **olanzapine pamoate** in people with moderate (Child-Pugh A or B) hepatic impairment (SmPC) and only increased with caution.

5. **Quetiapine**'s SmPC notes oral clearance is reduced by 25% in hepatic impairment, so start at 50 mg/d and increase at 50 mg/d according to response and tolerability. Discontinue if jaundice develops (Thyrum *et al, Prog Neuropsychopharmacol Biol Psychiatry* 2000;**24**:521–33).

6. * **Risperidone** unbound levels increase in hepatic impairment and so initial doses and dose increments should be halved, and 4 mg/d not exceeded. **Paliperidone** is not extensively metabolised by the liver, so no dose adjustments are needed in moderate hepatic impairment (n=20, Boom *et al, Int J Clin Pharmacol Ther* 2009;**47**:606–16) or cirrhosis (n=1, Chou and Chen, *J Neuropsychiatry Clin Neurosci* 2013;**25**:37), but no data is available in severe impairment so caution is recommended (SmPC).

7. **Sulpiride** and **amisulpride** are virtually un-metabolised with little or no biliary excretion. There is a low incidence of liver toxicity, with a transient rise in serum transaminase the only reported effect so dosage adjustments are not needed (SmPC).

8. **Haloperidol** has no apparent problems but the SmPC states liver disease to be a caution.

9. **Phenothiazines** (particularly **chlorpromazine,** which is contraindicated) may cause hepato-canalicular cholestasis and there may be immunological liver damage. They should be avoided where possible in hepatic dysfunction. Onset is usually during the first month of therapy. Coma may be precipitated due to increased cerebral neuronal sensitivity.

10. **Flupentixol** and **zuclopenthixol** do not need dosage changes, although both undergo hepatic metabolism.

11. **Pimozide** should be used with caution in hepatic impairment (UK SmPC). **Ziprasidone** is extensively metabolised and a longer half-life may occur in Child-Pugh A or B, but dose adjustment is not needed in mild-to-moderate impairment (n=30, open, Everson *et al, Br J Clin Pharmacol* 2000;**49**[S1]:21–6; FFT).

3.6.2 ANTIDEPRESSANTS *

12. **SSRIs:**
12a **Citalopram** and **escitalopram** are metabolised extensively, with three major metabolites. **Citalopram** should start at 10mg/d for 2/52 up to 20mg/d in mild-to-moderate hepatic impairment. **Escitalopram** should start at 5mg/d for 2/52 up to 10mg/d in mild-to-moderate hepatic impairment.
12b. **Fluoxetine** alternate day dosing is recommended in hepatic impairment. Higher plasma levels and longer half-life of fluoxetine and **norfluoxetine** occur in cirrhosis, so a 50% dose reduction is recommended, especially with low albumin levels.
12c. **Fluvoxamine** should be started at 50mg/d and monitored carefully, as raised hepatic enzymes have been reported.
12d. **Paroxetine**, at doses at the lower end of the therapeutic range, appears to be the safest option, although cases of hepatotoxicity have been reported (e.g. n=3, Azaz-Livshits *et al*, *Pharmacopsychiatry* 2002;**35**:112–5).
12e. **Sertraline** is extensively metabolised by the liver and is contraindicated in significant hepatic dysfunction. One study showed a 2.5-fold increase in half-life and a 1.6-fold increase in sertraline/desmethylsertraline peak levels in stable chronic cirrhosis (n=20, Demolis *et al*, *Br J Clin Pharmacol* 1996;**42**:394–7; FFT: n=1, Persky and Reinus, *Dig Dis Sci* 2003;**48**:939–44).
13. Most **tricyclics** have a high first-pass clearance, so lower starting doses are necessary. Increased sedation is likely due to decreased metabolism, e.g. **amitriptyline** plasma levels may be doubled or tripled in people with cirrhosis and it should be avoided. Cholestatic jaundice has occasionally been noted with tricyclics. **Lofepramine** is contraindicated in severe liver disease. Increased plasma levels may also occur with reduced plasma protein-binding if albumin levels are lower so extra monitoring would be needed. SSRIs would seem to be a better choice.
14. * **Agomelatine** is contraindicated in hepatic impairment (i.e. cirrhosis or active liver disease). Pooled data from the EMA concludes it is associated with elevated liver transaminases (>3x ULN; 2.5% at 50mg/d, 1.3% at 25mg/d and 0.5% placebo), mostly hepatocellular (Gahr *et al*, *Curr Drug Metab* 2014;**15**:694–702; see also European pharmacovigilance database; n=3300, Montastruc *et al*, *J Clin Psychopharmacol* 2014;**34**:327–30). Consider the higher risk of transaminase elevation with doses of 50mg/d (SmPC)
15. **Bupropion** is extensively metabolised and there are rare reports of abnormal LFTs, liver damage and hepatotoxicity, with some metabolite half-lives prolonged in cirrhosis. Reduced initial doses and close monitoring are required, as a prolonged half-life has been reported in hepatic failure (n=16, open, DeVane *et al*, *J Clin Psychopharmacol* 1990;**10**:328–32).
16. * **Vortioxetine** has no firm data so use with caution. A single dose study showed no effect in Child-Pugh grades A or B, but there is no data in severe hepatic impairment (SmPC). **Duloxetine** (review n=21457, Xue *et al*, *J Clin Psychopharmacol* 2011;**31**:517–22) can induce liver injury without the presence of major risk factors (Kang *et al*, *Psychiatry Investig* 2011;**8**:269–71; FFT) and is contraindicated in hepatic impairment (UK SmPC). Moderate liver disease (Child-Pugh B) increases the half-life 2.3-fold and AUC 3.7-fold.
17. **Mirtazapine** clearance is reduced by 33% in moderate hepatic impairment and so dosage reduction may be necessary. Transient asymptomatic raised liver enzymes (e.g. SGTP) have been rarely noted in early clinical trials.
18. **Moclobemide**'s clearance can be reduced and half-life increased in cirrhosis so doses should be reduced by 25–33% to avoid accumulation (Stoeckel *et al*, *Acta Psychiatr Scand* 1990;**360**:94–7).
19. **Reboxetine**'s half-life and plasma levels appear to rise in severe hepatic insufficiency and dose adjustment may be necessary. A starting dose of 2mg BD is recommended.
20. **Trazodone** should be used with care in severe hepatic impairment, as hepatotoxicity has been reported (n=1, Rettman and McClintock, *Ann Pharmacother* 2001;**35**:1559–61).
21. **Mianserin** and **tryptophan** appear to have no problems. **St John's wort** levels may rise in moderate cirrhosis, but absorption is decreased in mild cirrhosis and hepatotoxicity has been reported (n=1, Domínguez Jiménez *et al*, *Gastroenterol Hepatol* 2007;**30**:54–5).
22. **Venlafaxine** clearance is reduced by about 35% in mild-to-moderate hepatic impairment, and so doses should be reduced by about 50% (UK SmPC), although there is much interpatient variability. It is not recommended in severe hepatic impairment.

3

23. **MAOIs** are hepatotoxic and may precipitate coma. People may also be more sensitive to side-effects. If essential, start with a low dose, increase gradually and observe carefully. **Isocarboxazid** is contraindicated in any degree of impaired hepatic function.

3.6.3 MOOD AND BIPOLAR

24. **Asenapine** is not recommended in severe hepatic impairment (Child-Pugh C) as seven-fold increases in plasma levels have been shown. No dose reductions are needed in mild-to-moderate hepatic impairment (Child-Pugh A-B), (n = 30, Peeters *et al, Clin Pharmacokinet* 2011;**50**:471–81).
25. **Carbamazepine** rarely causes problems but jaundice, hepatitis and liver function disorders have been reported, and so use with caution.
26. **Lamotrigine** needs no adjustment to initial or maintenance doses in Child-Pugh grade A, but should be reduced by 50% in moderate (Child-Pugh grade B) hepatic impairment, and by 75% in severe (Child-Pugh grade C) impairment (n = 36, Marcellin *et al, Br J Clin Pharmacol* 2001;**51**:410–4;FFT).
27. **Lithium** has no known problems.
28. **Valproate** is contraindicated in active liver disease, as it can be hepatotoxic and liver failure can occur in about 0.01% (with some fatalities reported). Risk factors include early in therapy (and lessens after a couple of months; review by Eadie *et al, Med Tox* 1988;**3**:85–106), in children, and if used with other anticonvulsants. Symptoms present as worsening epilepsy, drowsiness and with biochemical and/or clinical evidence of liver failure. Valproate use may be possible in people with hepatitis C, provided ALT is closely monitored (n = 564, Felker *et al, Am J Psychiatry* 2003;**160**:174–8).

3.6.4 ANXIOLYTICS AND HYPNOTICS

29. **Long-acting benzodiazepine's** (e.g. **diazepam, chlordiazepoxide, alprazolam, clobazam** and **midazolam** [Wandel *et al, Br J Anaesthesia* 1994;**73**:658–61]) metabolism is impaired in liver disease. The half-lives of the metabolites desmethylchlordiazepoxide and demoxepam may also be longer, up to 346 hours and 150 hours respectively, which may induce coma. **Lorazepam, temazepam** and **oxazepam** metabolism is unchanged and in low dose these are probably the benzodiazepines of choice.
30. **Propranolol's** metabolism is impaired in decompensated liver disease and by portal systemic shunting. Propranolol use significantly shortens survival vs. placebo (5/12 vs. 20/12) in cirrhosis and ascites and so it should not be used (n = 151, 8/12, Sersté *et al, Hepatology* 2010;**52**:1017–22).
31. **Buspirone** Cmax and AUC are raised in hepatic failure (open, Barbhaiya *et al, Eur J Clin Pharmacol* 1994;**46**:41–7). Caution is recommended with a history of hepatic impairment and it should not be used in severe hepatic disease.
32. **Clomethiazole** clearance is reduced by 50% in moderate-to-severe hepatic impairment without greater sedation in the majority (n = 24, Centerholt *et al, Eur J Clin Pharmacol* 2003;**59**:117–22). In severe liver disease, a ten-fold increase can occur, so reduce oral doses, e.g. a third of normal, and note that sedation can mask the onset of hepatic coma. **Chloral hydrate** is contraindicated in marked hepatic impairment.
33. **Melatonin** has no known problems.
34. **Pregabalin** needs no dose adjustments.
35a. **Zopiclone** elimination can be reduced with hepatic dysfunction, increasing side effects (n = 17, open, Parker and Roberts, *Br J Clin Pharmacol* 1983;**16**:259;FFT), so use a lower dose of 3.75 mg to 7.5 mg (but no higher) with caution in hepatic disease.
35b. **Zolpidem** plasma protein binding is reduced in hepatic impairment (n = 42, open, Pacifici, *Int J Clin Pharmacol Ther Toxicol* 1988;**26**:439–43). It is contraindicated in severe hepatic insufficiency and lower doses are recommended in cirrhosis and other hepatic impairment (where half-life may rise to 10 hours).
35c. **Zaleplon** is contraindicated in severe hepatic insufficiency and the dose reduced to 5 mg in mild-to-moderate hepatic impairment.

3.6.5 ANTICONVULSANTS

Review: optimising anticonvulsants in hepatic dysfunction (Lacerda *et al, Neurology* 2006;**67**[12 Suppl 4]:S28–33).
36. **Barbiturates** can increase cerebral sensitivity and impaired metabolism may precipitate coma.
37. **Gabapentin** is virtually unmetabolised and so

no dose adjustments are necessary.

38. **Levetiracetam** needs no dose adjustment in Child-Pugh grade A-B (e.g. start at 250 mg/d and titrate to tolerance and response; n=14[c=10], open, 3/12, Bilo *et al*, *Clin Neuropharmacol* 2008;**31**:221–5), but in grade C start with half the normal dose as total clearance is reduced by about 57% (n=16, Brockmöller *et al*, *Clin Pharmacol Ther* 2005;**77**:529–41).

39. **Oxcarbazepine** is extensively metabolised, but no dose adjustments are generally needed in mild-to-moderate hepatic impairment. There is no data on severe hepatic impairment.

40. **Phenytoin** is highly protein-bound and extensively metabolised so accumulation and toxicity may occur in severe liver disease. Use reduced doses and monitor for toxicity. Active/free levels may remain unchanged so interpret plasma levels carefully.

41. * **Topiramate** is not extensively metabolised and dose adjustments are probably not needed, although care is definitely needed (Manitpisitkul *et al*, *Epilepsy Res* 2014;**108**:891–901). About 60% is excreted unchanged via the kidneys. In moderate-to-severe liver disease, clearance is reduced by about 26%.

3.6.6 OTHERS

42. ADHD:

42a. **Atomoxetine** dose modification may be needed in hepatic impairment (UK SmPC) and rare (one in 50,000) cases have been reported of severe acute hepatitis with markedly elevated hepatic enzymes and bilirubin (MHRA warning).

42b. **Dexamfetamine** has no known problems.

42c. **Lisdexamfetamine** has no known problems.

42d. **Methylphenidate** has no known problems.

42e.* At least 50% clearance of **guanfacine** is hepatic and dose reduction may be needed in hepatic impairment (UK SmPC).

43. **Anticholinesterases**: **Donepezil** 5 mg/d can be safely given in mild-to-moderate (Child-Pugh grade A-B) hepatic impairment (n=35[c=32], Reyes *et al*, *Br J Clin Pharmacol* 2004;**58**[Suppl 1]:9–17, MS:FFT; n=20, Tiseo *et al*, *Br J Clin Pharmacol* 1998;**46**[Suppl 1]:51–5; FFT). **Rivastigmine** is contraindicated in severe liver impairment. **Galantamine** is not affected in mild hepatic impairment, but clearance is reduced by 23% in moderate impairment (n=25, open, Zhao *et al*, *J Clin Pharmacol* 2002;**42**:428–36) and so start at 8 mg/d alternate days, increasing slowly up to 16 mg/d. It is contraindicated in severe impairment (Child-Pugh grade C).

44. **Memantine** lacks data in hepatic impairment, but since it is metabolised only to a minor extent to inactive metabolites, mild-to-moderate hepatic impairment is unlikely to have a significant effect.

45. **Anticholinergics** need some caution in hepatic disease (UK SmPCs).

46. **Alcohol dependence.**

46a. **Acamprosate** is contraindicated in severe hepatic failure (Child-Pugh C), but its kinetics are not altered in mild-to-moderate hepatic dysfunction and this is only an SmPC caution.

46b. **Disulfiram** needs caution in liver disease. There is some evidence of raised LFTs, but it has been used safely in people with elevated LFTs and/or evidence of hepatitis C virus, provided LFTs were monitored regularly (n=57, Saxon *et al*, *J Clin Psych* 1998;**59**:313–6).

46c. **Nalmefene** needs no dose adjustment in mild-to-moderate hepatic impairment (SmPC) although AUC may be 1.6-fold higher in mild, and 2.9-fold higher in moderate hepatic impairment.

46d. **Naltrexone** is extensively hepatically metabolised and mostly renally excreted and so care is needed in hepatic impairment, with LFTs being needed both before and during treatment.

46e. **Baclofen** is the only anti-craving drug tested in a formal RCT in cirrhosis (review: Addolorato *et al*, *CNS Drugs* 2013;**27**:287–99).

47. **Opiate dependence**

47a. **Buprenorphine** is primarily metabolised by glucuronidation (Tegeder *et al*, *Clin Pharmacokinet* 1999;**37**:17–40) and so should have a low risk in mild-to-moderate hepatic impairment. It is contraindicated in severe hepatic insufficiency.

47b. **Methadone**'s UK SmPC states to avoid or use reduced doses in hepatic impairment. QT interval prolongation and torsade de pointes have been reported (particularly at doses >100 mg/d) if used in liver disease (a risk factor for prolonged QTc).

48. **Modafinil**'s maximum dose of 400 mg/d should only be used in the absence of hepatic impairment. The starting dose of **sodium oxybate** should be halved in hepatic impairment as the elimination half-life is increased (UK SmPC).

3.7 OLD AGE

	Lower risk	Moderate risk	Higher risk
Antipsychotics	Lurasidone[3] Risperidone (but see text)[6]	Amisulpride[7] Aripiprazole[1] Olanzapine[4] Paliperidone[6] Quetiapine[5] Sulpiride[7] Thioxanthenes[10]	Clozapine[2] Haloperidol[8] Phenothiazines[9] Pimozide[11]
Antidepressants	Agomelatine[14] Duloxetine[16] Lofepramine[13] Mirtazapine[17] Moclobemide[18] SSRIs[12] Tryptophan[21] Venlafaxine[22]	MAOIs[23] Mianserin[21] Nortriptyline[13] Reboxetine[19] Trazodone[20] Vortioxetine[16]	Tricyclics (most)[13]
Anxiolytics and hypnotics	Buspirone[31] Clobazam[29] Lorazepam[29] Melatonin[33] Oxazepam[29] Oxprenolol[30] Zaleplon[35] Zopiclone[35]	Chloral[32] Clomethiazole[32] Benzodiazepines (short-acting)[29] Flunitrazepam[29] Propranolol[30] Temazepam[29] Zolpidem[35]	Benzodiazepines (long-acting)[29]
Mood and bipolar		Asenapine[24] Carbamazepine[25] Lamotrigine[26] Lithium[27] Olanzapine[4] Quetiapine[5] Valproate[28]	
Anticonvulsants	Clobazam[29]	Barbiturates[36] Benzodiazepines (short-acting)[29] Carbamazepine[25] Gabapentin[37] Lamotrigine[26] Levetiracetam[38] Oxcarbazepine[39] Pregabalin[34] Topiramate[41] Valproate[28]	Benzodiazepines (long-acting)[29] Phenytoin[40]

	Lower risk	Moderate risk	Higher risk
Others	Anticholinesterases[43] Bupropion[15] Disulfiram[46] Memantine[44] Modafinil[48] Nalmefene[46] Sodium oxybate [48]	Acamprosate?[46] Buprenorphine[47] Methadone[47] Naltrexone[46]	Anticholinergics[45] Atomoxetine[42] Dexamfetamine[42] Guanfacine[42] Lisdexamfetamine[42] Methylphenidate[42]

GENERAL PRINCIPLES FOR PRESCRIBING IN OLD AGE (adapted from *Maudsley Guidelines*)

1. Increased sensitivity to drugs occurs due to age-related changes in pharmacokinetics (ADME and protein binding) and pharmacodynamics (e.g. neuronal changes, and receptor binding). The over 70s have about twice as many ADRs as under 50s, e.g. postural hypotension, sedation and increased sensitivity to anticholinergic effects (see 8).
2. Hepatic changes (e.g. reduced metabolism) and reduced renal clearance will affect many drugs.
3. Decide a treatment aim, keep therapy simple, and discontinue gradually if no apparent benefit can be seen, as accumulation of a drug can lead to the subtle and insidious development of side-effects, especially cognitive.
4. Use the lowest effective dose (so 'start low and go slow'), avoid polypharmacy and monitor effects (both positive and negative) regularly and frequently.
5. Drugs with sedative and hypotensive effects, can create a small but consistent rise in the risk of falls (meta-analysis, s = 40, Leipzig *et al*, *J Am Geriatr Soc* 1999;**47**:30–9).
6. Avoid drugs with anticholinergic effects, which can increase the risk of cognitive decline and dementia (HR = 1.65), although discontinuing decreases the risk (n = 6,912, four years, Carrière *et al*, *Arch Intern Med* 2009;**169**:1317–24;FFT).
7. Most drugs are highly lipophilic and an increased fat to lean body mass ratio (as well as decreased metabolism and excretion) means that half-lives usually increase.
8. Consider potential poor or erratic compliance due to social or physical reasons, or use of OTC medicines.
9. Diabetes in over 66s can be exacerbated by *any* antipsychotic and can increase the risk of hospitalisation for hyperglycaemia (n = 13,817, Lipscombe *et al*, *Arch Int Med* 2009;**169**:1282–9).

3.7.1 ANTIPSYCHOTICS *

See *Table 1.13.1* (*Chapter 1*) for an extensive summary and references of the evidence for and against the use of antipsychotics in the elderly with dementia.

In summary, if antipsychotics are to be used in dementia, please note that:

- **The risk of cerebrovascular adverse events is highest in the first four weeks** (OR 9.9) and then falls to baseline after three months
- **The risk of acute MI is also 2.5 times higher** with antipsychotics up to 30/7 and at higher doses
- **The increased mortality occurs with higher doses,** e.g. haloperidol > 1 mg/d, olanzapine > 2.5 mg and risperidone > 1 mg/d, but not with quetiapine
- **Haloperidol clearly has the highest risk**
- **The risks may be due to dehydration and poor mobilisation** so ensure adequate hydration and movement in the first month
- * **Most people with BPSD can have any antipsychotic withdrawn** except perhaps where agitation or psychosis had responded well, and where relapse was quicker and more frequent.

Antipsychotics can relieve psychotic symptoms in older adults, but pre-treatment assessment, repeated every 3–6 months, is recommended to detect common side-effects such as postural hypotension, anticholinergic effects and EPSE. Single daily doses are usually appropriate once stable (as, indeed, they are in younger adults). Doses should be reviewed regularly, and a periodic reduction in dose (e.g. by 10–25% every four weeks) for some people may be indicated.

A recent systematic review and meta-analysis concluded that SGAs (aripiprazole, risperidone, olanzapine and quetiapine) were superior to placebo for psychiatric and cognitive effects with no difference in the risk of injuries, falls or death, but a higher risk of somnolence, UTI, oedema and abnormal gait (s=23, n=5819, RCTs, Tan *et al, Alzheimer's Res Treat* 2015;**7**:20).

Reviews: * general (concludes olanzapine and risperidone have the best evidence, Suzuki *et al, Drugs Aging* 2011;**28**:961–80; Trifirò and Spina, *Curr Drug Metab* 2011;**12**:611–20), use in older people with late-onset schizophrenia (s=1, n=44, Essali and Ali, *Cochrane Database Syst Rev* 2012;**2**:CD004162), antipsychotics in BPSD (Gareri *et al, J Clin Psychopharmacol* 2014;**34**:109–23).

1. **Aripiprazole** appears to be fairly well tolerated in older adults with bipolar disorder (n=20, open, 12/52, Sajatovic *et al, J Clin Psychiatry* 2008;**69**:41–6) and late-life schizophrenia (Rado and Janicak, *Clin Interv Aging* 2010;**5**:253–8;FFT). No dose adjustments are necessary in the elderly.

2. * **Clozapine** may be safe with slower dose titration, reasonably well tolerated (apart from a slightly higher risk of agranulocytosis; Bishara and Taylor, *Drugs Aging* 2014;**31**:11–20) and effective in the elderly (n=133, Barak *et al, Compr Psychiatry* 1999;**40**:320–5; n=16, Snowdon and Halliday, *Int Clin Psychopharmacol* 2011;**26**:232–5) at doses as low as 50–100mg, with 6.25–50mg/d suggested as the optimal dosage (review by Hoeh *et al, J Geriatr Psychiatry Neurol* 2003;**16**:213–8). In older people (mean 69 years) clozapine had no increase in mortality (n=43[cf. 484 controls], Pridan *et al, Int Psychogeriatr* 2015;**27**:131–4). Review plasma levels regularly as doses above 350mg/d had a 50% likelihood of plasma levels over 0.6ng/mL, potentially toxic (n=778, Bowskill *et al, Hum Psychopharmacol* 2012;**27**:277–83).

3. * **Lurasidone** has a US class dementia-related psychosis warning. Plasma levels are the similar in elderly and younger adults.

4. * **Olanzapine**'s UK CSM recommends not using in elderly demented people with behavioural problems, due to an increased risk of stroke (2% vs 1% on placebo), although the absolute risk is low, and the alternatives are not risk-free. The restriction does not apply to elderly demented people *without* behavioural problems, where a lower starting dose of 5mg/d may be appropriate, as the mean elimination half-life is 50% longer and clearance slightly reduced in otherwise healthy elderly people. Periodic blood pressure monitoring is recommended and there may be a slightly higher risk of seizures in people over 65. Transient sedation and somnolence were more marked in the elderly in pre-marketing trials. **Olanzapine pamoate** is not recommended for use in the elderly unless oral olanzapine has been used uneventfully before (SmPC), and should not be used for people over 75.

5. **Quetiapine** is not approved for the treatment of people with dementia-related psychosis due to a three-fold increased risk of cerebrovascular adverse events seen with some antipsychotics in dementia. The mean clearance in elderly people is 30–50% lower than healthy adults, so start with 25mg/d, with dose increments of 25–50mg/d (UK SmPC). Quetiapine (mean 200mg/d, range 50–800mg/d) can be effective and well tolerated but there is a wide and diagnosis-dependent (e.g. higher in functional psychosis) dosing range (n=100[c=91], Yang *et al, J Psychopharmacol* 2005;**19**:661–6). Quetiapine seems safe, effective and tolerable in the elderly with MDD (n=338, RCT, d/b, p/c, 11/52, Katila *et al, Am J Geriatr Psychiatry.* 2013;**21**:769–84) and for GAD, up to 300mg/d (n=450, RCT, d/b, p/c, 11/52, Mezhebovsky *et al, Int J Geriatr Psychiatry* 2013;**28**:615–25).

6. **Risperidone** is partially metabolised to an active metabolite and so lower doses may be needed with hepatic impairment (see *3.6.1*). Significant age-related differences have been noted, with higher plasma levels in the over 40s and with a 30% increase per decade of life (n=129, Aichhorn *et al, J Psychopharmacol* 2005;**19**:395–401). The same would apply to **paliperidone** (review by Madhusoodanan and Zaveri, *Curr Drug Saf* 2010;**5**:149–52), where renal impairment might require lower doses (see *3.10.1.1*).

7. **Amisulpride**'s plasma levels in the elderly are similar to younger adults but the elderly may respond to lower plasma levels (n=395, Müller *et al, J Psychopharmacol* 2009;**23**:278–86). Single doses of **sulpiride** are well tolerated and show a similar pharmacokinetic profile in healthy elderly and young subjects (n=20, open, Hamon-Vilcot *et al, Eur J Clin Pharmacol* 1998;**54**:405–9). However, the UK SmPCs now mentions increased mortality with sulpiride in elderly people with dementia.

8. **Haloperidol**'s UK SmPC now states that in

elderly people with dementia-related psychosis. Haloperidol has the highest risk of deaths, mostly either cardiovascular (e.g. heart failure, sudden death) or infections (e.g. pneumonia).

9. **Phenothiazine** elderly doses should be 33–50% of the adult dose due to the susceptibility to Parkinsonian side-effects (n=120, open, Caligiuri *et al*, *J Clin Psychopharmacol* 1999;**19**:322–8), and which are often then harder to manage. **Chlorpromazine** should be avoided. **Levomepromazine** is not recommended in the over 50s unless the risk of hypotension has been assessed.

10. **Zuclopenthixol** and **flupentixol** should be used with caution in renal disease, common in the elderly. The UK SmPC for zuclopenthixol now has a class warning about use in BPSD. The UK SmPC for flupentixol recommends caution in people with risk factors for stroke, and starting at 25–50% of the normal starting dose.

11. **Pimozide** should start at half the usual dose. **Ziprasidone** needs no dose changes.

3.7.2 ANTIDEPRESSANTS *

A meta-analysis of RCTs shows that antidepressants are effective for 'late-life' (ages >55 years) but less so for 'older late-life' (>65 years, although this author objects to these classifications) depression (s=74, RCT, d/b, p/c, Tedeschini *et al*, *J Clin Psychiatry* 2011;**72**:1660–8; FFT). A network meta-analysis concluded sertraline, paroxetine and duloxetine are clearly effective, with sparse reporting of outcomes for the others (s=15, RCT, Thorland *et al*, *J Am Geriatr Soc* 2015;**63**:1002–9) Poor prognosis is linked to being male, older, and with a longer duration of depression (s=34, RCT, Calati *et al*, *J Affect Disord* 2013;**147**:1–8). Lithium is difficult to use although it is the only drug with replicated evidence (Cooper *et al*, *Am J Psychiatry* 2011;**168**:681–8; FFT). SSRIs and tricyclics (but not other antidepressants) may increase the risk of non-vertebral fractures in the elderly (n=7,983, >55 years of age [mean 77 years of age], Ziere *et al*, *J Clin Psychopharmacol* 2008;**28**:411–7; comment by Diem, *EBMH* 2009;**12**:26), although the risk of falling with an antidepressant is about the same as the excess risk found in people with untreated depression (Darowski *et al*, *Drugs Aging* 2009;**26**:381–94).

Reviews: * independent (Del Casale *et al*, *Riv Psichiatr* 2012;**47**:479–88), general (Dhillon, *Drugs Aging* 2013;**30**:59–79).

12. * **SSRIs** have obvious advantages over other antidepressants in the elderly but have some increased risks, including hyponatraemia, weight loss (review: Herrmann, *Can J Clin Pharmacol* 2000;**7**:91–5), falls and osteoporotic fractures in the over 50s (n=5008, 137 on SSRIs, Richards *et al*, *Arch Int Med* 2007;**167**:188–94). The risk of GI bleed with SSRIs is higher in people over 80 and/or with a history of GI bleeds although the absolute risk remains low and can be significantly reduced by co-prescribing a PPI (e.g. lansoprazole).

12a. * **Citalopram**'s UK SmPC states it should not be used above 20 mg/d in people aged over 65 years due to the dose-dependent QT prolongation, a longer half-life and more prevalent side-effects such as bradycardia, nausea, sweating and headache, although a meta-analysis concluded that citalopram in late-life depression is equivalent to other antidepressants, with similar tolerability (s=7, n=1,288, Seitz *et al*, *Int J Geriatr Psychiatry* 2010;**25**:1296–1305). **Escitalopram**, should start at 5 mg/d for the first two weeks then increasing to 10 mg/d (UK SmPC), although age has no significant effect on plasma levels in 2D6 poor metabolisers (n=541, Waade *et al*, *Eur J Clin Pharmacol* 2014;**70**:933–40). It is well tolerated in older adults (mean 68 years), albeit not superior to placebo (n=268 [c=205], RCT, d/b, p/c, 12/52, Bose and Gandhi, *Am J Geriatr Psychiatry* 2008;**16**:14–20). Escitalopram was also modestly effective for GAD in older people, but not significantly (n=177 [c=170], RCT, p/c, d/b, 12/52, Lenze *et al*, *JAMA* 2009;**301**:295–303; FFT).

12b. **Fluoxetine**'s half-life appears not to be significantly different in the elderly and it has been claimed to be a safe and effective antidepressant in depressed and physically ill elderly people (n=20, open, Evans and Lye, *J Clin Exp Gerontol* 1992;**14**:297–307).

12c. **Fluvoxamine** has no pharmacokinetic differences in the elderly, and so no dose alterations are necessary. 200 mg/d seems as equally well tolerated and effective in old age depression as sertraline 150 mg/d (n=93, RCT, d/b, 7/52, Rossini *et al*, *J Clin Psychopharmacol* 2005;**25**:471–5).

12d. * **Paroxetine** initial lower doses of 10 mg/d are recommended, as blood levels with 20 mg/d

3

in the elderly can be similar to those of 30 mg/d in younger adults. Slower initial titration reduces anxiety and improves tolerability in over 65s (n=50, open, 8/52, Gibiino *et al*, *J Clin Psychopharmacol* 2013;**33**:565–9). Paroxetine may be associated with an increased risk of falls by impairing balance control, especially when attention is divided between two concurrent activities, presumably a particular problem in men (Hegeman *et al*, *Clin Neuropharmacol* 2011;**34**:210–5).

12e. **Sertraline**'s clearance may be slightly reduced and half-life increased in elderly volunteers, but no dose adjustments are needed. It seems safe and effective in the elderly even with significant comorbid medical problems (n=752, RCT, d/b, p/c, 8/52, Sheikh *et al*, *J Am Geriatr Soc* 2004;**52**:86–92).

13. **Tricyclics** should start at reduced doses with lower final doses, depending upon tolerance, as cognitive, anticholinergic and central effects are enhanced in the elderly. **Clomipramine** is as well tolerated in patients aged 56–70 years as in younger adults, although postural hypotension and anticholinergic side-effects are more common (n=150, Stage *et al*, *Acta Psychiatr Scand* 2002;**105**:55–9). Higher serum levels occur with standard doses of **imipramine**, with reduced clearance and doubled half-life (open, Benetello *et al*, *Int J Clin Pharmacol Res* 1990;**10**:191–5). Elderly people may respond to lower doses of **lofepramine** but in depressed elderly inpatients, low doses (70 mg/d) appear no better than placebo, indicating that full, or at least higher, doses are necessary (n=63, RCT, d/b, p/c, 4/52, Tan *et al*, *Br J Clin Pharmacol* 1994;**37**:321–4; FFT). **Nortriptyline** kinetics appear the same in the elderly as the young, although individual variation is high and the elderly may respond to lower doses (6/52, Kanba *et al*, *Prog Neuropsychopharmacol Biol Psychiatry* 1992;**16**:301–9).

14. * **Agomelatine** is not recommended in the over 75s (lack of data, SmPC), but it has shown a good clinical effect and remarkable tolerability in older people (n=23[c=23], open, 12/52, Lužný, *Actas Esp Psiquiatr* 2012;**40**:304–7; n=222, p/c, 8/52, Heun *et al*, *J Clin Psychiatry* 2013;**74**:587–94).

15. **Bupropion** can be effective and well tolerated in the elderly (n=100, RCT, d/b, a/c, Weihs *et al*, *J Clin Psychiatry* 2000;**61**:196–202:n=13, open, Bergman *et al*, *Clin Neuropharmacol* 2011;**34**:17–20), with 150–300 mg/d effective and well tolerated for MDD in over 65s (n=418[c=414], d/b, p/c, 10/52, Hewett *et al*, *J Psychopharmacol* 2010;**24**:521–9).

16. * **Vortioxetine** should be started at 5 mg/d, with caution at doses above 10 mg/d as plasma levels are 27% higher (AUC and Cmax) cf younger people (SmPC). Side-effects are more common, although it has been shown to be effective (RCT, d/b, p/c, a/c, 8/52, n=453 [c=392] Katona *et al*, *Int Clin Psychopharmacol* 2012;**27**:215–23). **Duloxetine**'s half-life is about 25% longer in the elderly, but no dose adjustment is necessary. 60 mg/d has been shown to be effective for anxiety in old age (n=291[c=220], RCT, d/b, p/c, 10/52, Alaka *et al*, *Int J Geriatr Psychiatry* 2014;**29**:978–86) and have no adverse effects on cognition and depression in elderly (65–89) people (n=311, RCT, d/b, p/c, Wise *et al*, *Int J Clin Pract* 2007;**61**:1283–93; FFT), albeit with higher drop-outs due to ADRs (RCT, d/b, 24/52, Robinson *et al*, *Am J Geriatr Psychiatry* 2014;22:34–45;MS;s=4, n=73, RCT, d/b, p/c, <10/52, Davidson *et al*, *Hum Psychopharmacol* 2008;**23**:519–26). Falls may be more common with duloxetine (25% vs 16% with placebo) so although not statistically significant some vigilance is needed in the over 65s (n=370, RCT, d/b, p/c, 24/52, Nelson *et al*, *Prim Care Companion CNS Disord* 2013;**15**:12m01419; review s=2, n=681, RCT, d/b, p/c, 8–12/52, Oakes *et al*, *Int Clin Psychopharmacol* 2013;**28**:1–11; MS).

17. **Mirtazapine** dosage can be the same in the elderly as younger adults, although the manufacturers recommend care with dosage increments. It appears to be slightly quicker acting and better tolerated than paroxetine in elderly depressed people (n=255, RCT, d/b, 8+16/52, Schatzberg *et al*, *Am J Geriatr Psychiatry* 2002;**10**:541–50), although sedation is more common in the over 80s, so use with care (Rothschild-Fuentes *et al*, *Pharmacopsychiatry* 2013;**46**:59–62).

18. **Moclobemide** appears safe, effective and having a seemingly beneficial effect on a range of cognitive functions (n=694, d/b, p/c, Roth *et al*, *Br J Psychiatry* 1996;**168**:149–57).

19. * **Reboxetine**'s side-effects are no greater in the elderly than in younger people, although the half-life may be doubled and peak plasma levels over twice that in younger people (n=12, Bergmann *et al*, *Eur J Drug Metab Pharmacokinet* 2000;**25**:195–8). Start at 2 mg BD. A delayed lowering of potassium

levels and some treatment-emergent tachycardia have been reported. Frail elderly may need dose reductions. The UK SmPC does not recommend use in the elderly, due to lack of safety data rather than the presence of negative data.

20. * **Trazodone** 50 mg at night caused no significant daytime sleepiness, naps, or effects on cognition or functionality in people with sleep problems in probable Alzheimer's (n=30, RCT, d/b, p/c, 3/52, Camargos *et al*, *Am J Geriatr Psychiatry* 2014;**22**:1565–74), but 150 mg/d may be the optimum dose in the elderly, as higher plasma levels (n=97, open, Prapotnik *et al*, *Int J Clin Pharmacol Ther* 2004;**42**:120–4) and a longer half-life can occur.

21. **Mianserin** elimination is highly variable and often prolonged in the elderly. There are no apparent problems with **tryptophan**.

22. * **Venlafaxine** clearance is reduced by about 15% in the over 65s, and levels can be eight times higher (cf under 40s) in 2D6 poor metabolisers (n=541, Waade *et al*, *Eur J Clin Pharmacol* 2014;**70**:933–40) so consider 2D6 genotype when prescribing. Venlafaxine (up to 150 mg/d) may be less well tolerated and possibly less safe than sertraline (up to 100 mg/d) in elderly frail populations (n=32, RCT, d/b, Oslin *et al*, *J Clin Psychiatry* 2003;**64**:875–82; comment by Schneider, *EBMH* 2004;**7**:47; FFT), although there were no differences in cardiac events compared to sertraline (n=41238) and actually a lower risk of heart failure (n=90114, Ho *et al*, *J Clin Psychiatry* 2014;**75**:552–8). Postural hypotension may be more common.

23. **MAOIs** are often considered to be more toxic in the elderly, mainly due to postural hypotension and dizziness, but they can be highly effective in resistant depression (review by Volz and Gleiter, *Drugs Aging* 1998;**13**:341–55).

3.7.3 MOOD AND BIPOLAR

24. **Asenapine** needs care in the elderly, as limited data is available in the over 64s (UK SmPC), and is likely to cause postural hypotension as plasma levels may be 30–40% higher than in younger adults, although it still seems tolerable and effective in older age (n=11[c=9], Baruch *et al*, *J Affect Disord* 2013;**145**:130–2). Start at 5 mg BD for 4/7 then 10 mg BD, although this slower titration is not apparently needed in people >65 with psychosis but without dementia (n=122[c=76], RCT, 6/52, Dubovsky *et al*, *Int Geriatr Psychiatry* 2012;**27**:472–82).

25. **Carbamazepine** has not been shown to produce significant changes in the elderly, including ECGs (n=108[c=75], RCT, d/b, 40/52, Saetre *et al*, *Epilepsia* 2009;**50**:1841–9), and with no effect on age, race, hepatic, renal or BMI on CBZ levels (n=121, Punyawudho *et al*, *Ther Drug Monit* 2012;**34**:176–81; FFT). The dose requirements are thus likely to be the same, or perhaps slightly lower, than adults (n=171, Bondareva *et al*, *J Clin Pharm Ther* 2006;**31**:211–21).

26. * **Lamotrigine** is hepatically metabolised and this is influenced by genetic factors more than age. Clearance (n=809) rises to a peak from mid-teens to the mid-30s, then declines gradually by about 20% in old age (Wegner *et al*, *Epilepsy Behav* 2013;**29**;217–21). Lamotrigine thus tends to be not as well tolerated in the elderly (due to increased half-life), with reduced sleep duration, dreaming and weight loss common (n=57[c=38], open, 12/52, Sajatovic *et al*, *Bipolar Disord* 2011;**13**:294–302; FFT).

27. * **Lithium** clearance is reduced in the elderly due to reduced renal function and an increased volume of distribution. There is no indication that lithium causes more neurotoxicity in the elderly than younger adults (Bogers *et al*, *Tijdschr Psychiatr* 2012;**54**:359–69; FFT) and even in octogenarians provided serum levels and renal and thyroid function are monitored frequently and regularly (n=12, Fahy and Lawlor, *Int J Geriatr Psychiatry* 2001;**16**:1000–3; n=61, RCT, d/b, p/c, 4 years, Aprahamian *et al*, *J Clin Psychiatry* 2014;**75**:e672–8). Levels of up to 0.8mmol/L may be safe in elderly people without pre-existing chronic renal failure (n=42, four years, Rej *et al*, *Drugs Aging* 2013;**30**:409–15), but there may be an increased risk of renal damage in the older age groups (HR=2.5, NNH=44[21–150]) although the absolute risk remains small (Close *et al*, *PLoS One* 2014;**9**:e90169). Hypothyroidism can also occur.
Review: lithium in late-life (D'Souza *et al*, *Curr Psychiatry Rep* 2011;**13**:488–92).

28. **Valproate**'s half-life may be doubled in the elderly and doses may need to be lower by around 25% in women, but higher if taken with concurrent carbamazepine or phenytoin and if the syrup is used (n=146, Birnbaum *et al*, *Ther Drug Monit* 2007;**29**:571–5). CNS side-effects

and nausea are likely to be increased in older people (n=6, s/b, Felix *et al*, *J Clin Psychopharmacol* 2003;**23**:471–8). There may be a change in protein binding so great care is needed in interpreting blood levels (n=102, Lampon and Tutor, *Ups J Med Sci* 2012;**117**:41–6; FFT).

3.7.4 ANXIOLYTICS AND HYPNOTICS

Review: * BDZ-reduction strategies in old age (s=18, Gould *et al*, *Br J Psychiatry* 2014;**204**:98–107).

Improvements in sleep with the use of sedatives are significant in the elderly, albeit of small magnitude, but ADRs and the risk of falls are clinically relevant (meta-analysis, s=24, n=2,417, RCT, Glass *et al*, *BMJ* 2005;**331**:1169; FFT). Z-hypnotics and benzodiazepines significantly impair body balance and standing steadiness after a single dose, aggravated by alcohol, but tolerance partially develops with time (s=57, Mets *et al*, *Sleep Med Rev* 2010;**14**:259–67). Long-term use of temazepam, zopiclone or zolpidem every night in older adults can lead to prolonged impairment of attention and cognitive functioning measurable for over at least six months after stopping (n=92[c=89], RCT, d/b, p/c, 6/12, Puustinen *et al*, *Eur J Clin Pharmacol* 2014;**70**:319–29).

29. * **Benzodiazepines** (see also above) should all be used with great care in the elderly, as side-effects are likely to be enhanced, e.g. sedation, disturbances in gait, daytime drowsiness, cognitive impairment, hypotension, memory impairment and reduced psychomotor performance. The risk of falls and hip fracture with BDZs is higher on initiation with higher doses, and when other BDZs or hypnotics are also used (n=103,188, Zint *et al*, *Pharmacoepidemiol Drug Saf* 2010;**19**:1248–55; FFT; 20/12, Uhart *et al*, *Annales Pharmaceutiques Francaises* 2012;**70**:46–52). Half-lives are generally lengthened, e.g. **bromazepam, chlordiazepoxide, clobazam, clonazepam, clorazepate, diazepam, flunitrazepam, flurazepam, midazolam** and **nitrazepam**. Normal adult doses of **oxazepam** can be used, as there are apparently no clinically significant pharmacokinetic changes in the elderly. **Lorazepam** doses as a hypnotic should probably be slightly reduced. With the exception of dual task performance, older people (n=12, mean age 64) taking lorazepam did not differ from younger people, although the abstract does not state if there was any difference in men, who are well known to only be able to do one thing at a time (n=27, RCT, d/b, p/c, c/o, Loring *et al*, *Epilepsy Behav* 2012;**25**:329–33). **Loprazolam** appears well tolerated in the elderly, with a half-life similar to young adults (n=12, Dorling and Hindmarsh, *Drugs Exp Clin Res* 2001;**27**:151–9).

30. **Propranolol** may have more side-effects in the elderly and so reduced initial doses are generally recommended. No dose reduction is necessary for **oxprenolol**.

31. **Buspirone** appears to have no significant pharmacokinetic changes in the elderly and so dose adjustments are not considered necessary (n=48, open, Gammans *et al*, *J Clin Pharmacol* 1989;**29**:72–8).

32. **Clomethiazole** doses should be lower, as its half-life can be at least doubled and plasma levels up to five times normal in the elderly (Dehlin, *Acta Psychiatr Scand* 1986;**329**:112–5). **Chloral** dosage is the same as for adults, except for frail elderly or in significant hepatic impairment, where reduced doses may be appropriate.

33. **Melatonin** has no known problems and is an ideal hypnotic in the elderly.

34. **Pregabalin** may need reduced doses due to decreased renal function, but it seems safe and effective for anxiety in older people (mean 72 years) within two weeks (n=273, RCT, d/b, p/c, 8/52, Montgomery *et al*, *Br J Psychiatry* 2008;**193**:389–94; FFT).

35. * **Z-hypnotics** (see also introduction) exposure in the previous 4/12 may increase the risk of hip fractures in elderly nursing home residents, especially in newer users and people with mild impairment (n=15528, c/o, Berry *et al*, *JAMA Intern Med* 2013;**179**:754–61). **Zopiclone** should be used at slightly lower doses e.g. 3.73–7.5 mg. **Zolpidem** is an effective hypnotic in the elderly if used at modest doses, e.g. 2.5–5 mg and could be a preferred hypnotic for this patient group (n=48, RCT, d/b, p/c, c/o, Allain *et al*, *Eur J Clin Pharmacol* 2003;**59**:179–88). However, it must be used carefully, as in the over 65s it significantly increases body sway (n=24, RCT, d/b, p/c, c/o, Otmani *et al*, *Hum Psychopharmacol* 2012;**27**:270–6) and there is a 21-fold higher incidence of hip fractures if taken for eight days or longer (Lin *et al*, *Sleep* 2014;**37**:673–9; FFT), at a similar incidence as diazepam but more than alprazolam and

lorazepam, although higher zolpidem doses may explain this (n=391609, Finkle *et al*, *J Am Geriatr Soc* 2011;**59**:1883–90). There appear to be no problems with **zaleplon** in the elderly.

3.7.5 ANTICONVULSANTS

For anticonvulsants, it is best to avoid renally excreted drugs (e.g. **gabapentin**), as renal excretion may be significantly reduced in the elderly compared with younger adults. Hepatically metabolised drugs, e.g. **carbamazepine** and **lamotrigine** may only need small dosage reductions.

Reviews: management of epilepsy in old age (Brodie et al, *Lancet Neurol* 2009;**8**:1019–30; Marasco and Ramsay, *Consult Pharm* 2009;**24** [Suppl A]:17–22).

36. **Phenobarbital** and **primidone** half-lives are longer in the elderly due to reduced metabolism and so reduced doses should be used.

37. **Gabapentin** clearance is reduced in old age, probably via reduced renal clearance, and it may cause ataxia (review by Sommer *et al*, *Expert Opin Drug Saf* 2007;**6**:133–45). It has been successful and well tolerated as add-on therapy for antipsychotics or valproate in mania in old age (n=7, open, Sethi *et al*, *J Geriatr Psychiatry Neurol* 2003;**16**:117–20).

38. **Levetiracetam** in older adults (66–80 years) may need a 30% lower dose, while those aged >81 need 50% lower doses to get the same plasma levels as adults aged 30 65 (n=272, Contin *et al*, *Epilepsy Res* 2012;**98**:130–4). However, it can be well tolerated at the right dose as an add-on in epilepsy (n=491[c=364], open, one year, Werhahn *et al*, *Seizure* 2011;**20**:305–11; FFT) with only headache and tremor occurring more frequently (n=3,352, Cramer *et al*, *Epilepsy Res* 2003;**56**:135–45).

39. **Oxcarbazepine**'s AUC may be 30–60% higher in the elderly, but tolerability is comparable to adults (n=52 cf. 1574 adults, Kutluay *et al*, *Epilepsy Behav* 2003;**4**:175–80) and no dose recommendations exist, other than gradual dose titration (n=48, van Heiningen *et al*, *Clin Pharmacol Ther* 1991;**50**:410–9) and a lower dose in compromised renal function. Monitoring is needed as it may cause hyponatraemia (review by Sommer *et al*, *Expert Opin Drug Saf* 2007;**6**:133–45).

40. **Phenytoin** needs reduced doses in the elderly, e.g. by about 20% and careful monitoring is necessary, especially with hypoalbuminaemia or renal disease as this may increase the risk of side-effects and toxicity, including cardiac arrhythmias.

41. **Topiramate** seems effective in epilepsy in elderly people, but up to 50% discontinue because of cognitive ADRs (Sommer and Fenn, *Clin Interv Aging* 2010;**5**:89–99; FFT).

3.7.6 OTHERS

42. **ADHD:** * There is no information on **atomoxetine**, **dexamfetamine**, **guanfacine**, **lisdexamfetamine** or **methylphenidate** (UK SmPCs). Methylphenidate has been used for depression in the elderly.

43. * **Anticholinesterases** have no specific problems, e.g. **donepezil, galantamine** and **rivastigmine**, provided the dose titration guidelines are followed.

44. **Memantine** has a usual maximum dose of 20mg/d.

45. **Anticholinergics** can cause confusion in the elderly by further compromising brain cholinergic activity. All should be used with extreme care and an initial very low dose is recommended.

46. **Acamprosate** should not be used in the elderly (UK SmPC), due more to a lack of data rather than specific reported problems. There are no dosage problems for **disulfiram** in the elderly. No dose adjustments seem needed for **nalmefene** (n=52, Frye *et al*, *Br J Clin Pharmacol* 1996;**42**:301–6; FFT), although transiently higher plasma levels may occur. **Naltrexone** is not recommended due to lack of data, and the risk of raised LFTs in elderly and obese people.

47.* **Methadone** needs care with repeated doses (review by Doukas, *Curr Drug Abuse Rev* 2015;**7**:65–73) but there are no recommendations for **buprenorphine**.

48. **Modafinil** starting doses of 100mg/d are recommended. **Sodium oxybate** can cause cognitive impairment so care would be needed (SmPC).

3

3.8 PARKINSON'S DISEASE (PD)

	Lower risk	Moderate risk	Higher risk
Antipsychotics	Clozapine[2]	Aripiprazole[1] Lurasidone[3] Quetiapine[5] Ziprasidone[11]	Amisulpride[7] Haloperidol[8] Olanzapine[4] Paliperidone[6] Phenothiazines[9] Pimozide[11] Risperidone[6] Sulpiride[7] Thioxanthenes[10]
Antidepressants	Agomelatine[14] Duloxetine[16] Mirtazapine[17] Reboxetine[19] SSRIs[12] Trazodone[20] Tryptophan[21] Venlafaxine[22] Vortioxetine[16]	MAOIs[23] Mianserin[21] Moclobemide[18]	Tricyclics[13]
Anxiolytics and hypnotics	Buspirone[31] Clomethiazole[32] Melatonin[33] Pregabalin[34] Z-hypnotics[35]	Benzodiazepines (short-acting)[29] Beta-blockers[30] Quetiapine[5]	Benzodiazepines (long-acting)[29]
Mood and bipolar	Carbamazepine[25] Valproate[28]	Asenapine[24] Lamotrigine[26] Quetiapine[5]	Lithium[27] Olanzapine[4]
Anticonvulsants	Barbiturates[36] Gabapentin[37] Phenytoin[40] Pregabalin[34] Topiramate[41]	Benzodiazepines (short-acting)[29] Levetiracetam[38]	Benzodiazepines (long-acting)[29]
Others	Acamprosate[46] ADHD treatments[42] Anticholinesterases[43] Buprenorphine[47] Bupropion[15] Disulfiram[46] Memantine[44] Methadone[47] Modafinil[48] Nalmefene[46] Naltrexone[46] Sodium oxybate[48]	Anticholinergics[45]	

3.8.1 ANTIPSYCHOTICS *

Introduction: All current antipsychotics block dopamine so can cause EPSE, worsen PD, antagonise levodopa and increase the risk of NMS. See *C1.21.5* for treating psychosis in PD.
1. **Aripiprazole**'s SmPC does not mention PD.
2. **Clozapine** is licensed for psychosis in PD where other treatments have failed (SmPC).
3. **Lurasidone** has class warnings for use in PD.
4. **Olanzapine** is no more effective than placebo in PD and worsens symptoms (UK SmPC).
5. **Quetiapine**'s SmPC does not mention PD.
6. **Risperidone** and **paliperidone** (see introduction).
7. **Amisulpride** and **sulpiride** (see introduction).
8. **Haloperidol** (see introduction).
9. **Phenothiazines** (see introduction).
10. **Flupentixol** and **zuclopenthixol** (see introduction).
11. **Pimozide** (see introduction).

3.8.2 ANTIDEPRESSANTS *

See *C1.14.3* for depression in Parkinson's disease.
12. * **SSRIs**: None of the SSRI SmPCs mention PD, and there are no known unexpected problems. **Fluoxetine** can be effective without impairing motor performance (n=18, open, 80/7, Kostic *et al*, *Vojnosanit Pregl* 2012;**69**:1067–75).
13. * **Tricyclics** may potentiate the effects of some anticholinergics, leading to additive confusion and hallucinations (SmPC).
14. **Agomelatine** has no known additional risks.
15. **Bupropion** can rarely cause EPSE.
16. * **Vortioxetine** and **duloxetine** have no known additional risks.
17. **Mirtazapine** appears to have no additional risks, although sedation might be a problem.
18. **Moclobemide** seems well tolerated, but slightly worsens motor symptoms in some people (e.g. n=20, open, Sternic *et al*, *Clin Neuropharmacol* 1998;**21**:93–6).
19. **Reboxetine** has no known additional risks.
20. **Trazodone** appears well tolerated (SmPC).
21. **Tryptophan** has caused a dramatic response of the 'on-off' levodopa response (n=2, Sandyk and Fisher, *Int J Neurosci* 1989;**45**:215–9).
22. **Venlafaxine** has no known additional risks.
23. **MAOIs** may potentiate some anticholinergic antiparkinsonian drugs (SmPC).

3.8.3 MOOD AND BIPOLAR

24. **Asenapine**'s SmPC notes a caution due to the risk of NMS and ADRs.
25. **Carbamazepine** has no known problems.
26. **Lamotrigine** has no antiparkinsonian effects but appears to have a high drop-out rate in PD (s=2, n=26, d/b, p/c, Shinotoh *et al*, *Neurology* 1997;**48**:1282–5).
27. **Lithium** may cause tremor, and toxicity can mimic PD so would be difficult to use, although it may have a neuroprotective effect.
28. **Valproate** may help impulse control disorder (n=3, Hicks *et al*, *Parkinsonism Relat Disord* 2012;**17**:379–81), but has very little effect on motor symptoms (n=8, Nutt *et al*, *Can J Neurol Sci* 1979;**6**:337–43).

3

3.8.4 ANXIOLYTICS AND HYPNOTICS *

Anxiety disorders are not uncommon in PD, especially panic, GAD (up to 25%) and social phobia, and may have a significant impact on quality of life (Hanna and Cronin-Golomb, *Parkinson's Dis* 2012;**2012**:640707; FFT). Anxiety that is exacerbated during 'off' periods should be managed by adjusting anti-Parkinsonian medicines (Mendis *et al*, *Can J Neurol Sci* 1999;**26**:89–103). A review of poor sleep and PD (Korczyn, *J Neurol Sci* 2006;**248**:163–6) concludes that the reasons can be because:

- Natural sleep problems in older people are exacerbated by PD making exercise more difficult and challenging
- Daytime naps occur as the person feels tired
- Social isolation leads to depression/anxiety
- Immobility makes it less easy to move in bed
- Hallucinations
- Restless legs syndrome (much more common, range 0–21%)
- REM sleep behaviour disorder can occur in 30% men (6% women) with PD (but can respond to BDZs).

Low-dose **tricyclics** (e.g. doxepin) may be useful for sleep. Although ineffective for psychosis, **quetiapine** seemed to be safe and effective for insomnia in PD (n=14[c=12], open, 12/52, Juri *et al*, *Clin Neuropharmacol* 2005;**28**:185–7).

Reviews: general (Friedman and Millman, *CNS Spectr* 2008;**13**(3 suppl 4):12–7; Jahan *et al*, *Neuropsychiatr Dis Treat* 2009;**5**:535–40; FFT).

29. **Benzodiazepines** are more likely to cause falls in people with PD especially with long-half life BDZs, so avoid or only use for short periods to avoid accumulation. One study showed no significant increase in PD drug doses in BDZ starters (n=214, van de Vijver *et al, Acta Neurol Scand* 2002;**105**:8–12).

30. **Beta-blockers** can be used for PD tremor. Cochrane concludes from the four small studies that there is a minor anti-tremor effect, but with bradycardia a limiting factor (s=4, n=72, RCT, d/b, p/c, c/o, Crosby *et al, Cochrane Database Syst Rev* 2003;**1**:CD003361).

31. **Buspirone** up to 40mg/d may be well tolerated and even reduce levodopa-induced dyskinesias (n=10, d/b, c/o, 3/52, Bonifati *et al, Clin Neuropharmacol* 1994;**17**:73–82), but worsens them at higher doses, e.g. up to 100mg/d (n=16, Ludwig *et al, Clin Neuropharmacol* 1986;**9**:373–8).

32. * **Clomethiazole** seems safe and effective for insomnia in PD (n=9, d/b, p/c, c/o, Tulloch *et al, Age Ageing* 1991;**20**:424–9). There is no information on **chloral** in PD.

33. **Melatonin** can help correct a blunted circadian rhythm in PD (n=35, 24 hours, Videnovic *et al, JAMA Neurol* 2014;**71**:463–9) and modestly improve sleep quality, with no effect on motor symptoms (n=18, RCT, d/b, p/c, 4/52, Medeiros *et al, J Neurol* 2007;**254**:459–64; c=40, d/b, p/c, c/o, 10/52, Dowling *et al, Sleep* 2005;**6**:459–66). It may even have some neuroprotective effects (Srinivasan *et al, Ther Adv Neurol Disord* 2011;**4**:297–317; FFT).

34. **Pregabalin** is ineffective for essential tremor (n=20, RCT, d/b, p/c, 6/52, Ferrara *et al, J Neurol Sci* 2009;**285**:195–7).

35. **Zolpidem** may be effective and also have some positive effect on PD symptoms (Abe, *Recent Pat CNS Drug Discov* 2008;**3**:55–60; Chen *et al, J Clin Neurosci* 2008;**15**:955–6).

3.8.5 ANTICONVULSANTS *

36. **Barbiturates** have no known problems.

37. **Gabapentin** seems to improve motor symptoms, e.g. rigidity, tremor and bradykinesia in its own right (n=19, d/b, p/c, c/o, Olson *et al, Am J Med* 1997;**102**:60–6), including enhancing the effects of levodopa (n=20[c=15], RCT, d/b, p/c, c/o, Van Blercom *et al, Clin Neuropharmacol* 2004;**27**:124–8).

38. **Levetiracetam** is poorly tolerated in PD, but if you can cope with the ADRs can occasionally help dyskinesias (n=9[c=4], open, 60/7, Zeisiewicz *et al, Mov Disord* 2005;**20**:1205–9). Up to 1–2g/d slowly titrated can help improve levodopa-induced dyskinesias (n=38, RCT, d/b, p/c, c/o, Stathis *et al, Mov Disord* 2011;**26**:264–70; n=32, RCT, d/b, p/c, 11/52, Wolz *et al, J Neural Transm* 2010;**117**:1279–86), although one study showed no antidyskinetic activity at up to 2g/d (n=16, RCT, d/b, p/c, Wong *et al, Mov Disord* 2011;**26**:1552–5).

39. **Oxcarbazepine** has no known problems.

40. **Phenytoin** has no known problems.

41. **Topiramate** has no known problems (SmPC).

3.8.6 OTHERS *

42. * ADHD:

42a. **Atomoxetine** seems tolerable in PD and can improve global cognitive performance and daytime sleepiness (n=55, RCT, d/b, p/c, 8/52, Weintraub *et al, Neurology* 2010;**75**:448–55; FFT; n=12, open, 8/12, Marsh *et al, Mov Disord* 2009;**24**:277–82; FFT).

42b. **Dexamfetamine** has no known problems.

42c. **Lisdexamfetamine** has no known problems.

42d. **Methylphenidate** seems to be generally positive, e.g. 20mg improves attention (n=21, Auriel *et al, Clin Neuropharmacol* 2006;**29**:15–7), lowers fatigue scores (n=36, RCT, d/b, p/c, 6/52, Mendonça *et al, Mov Disorder* 2007;**22**:2070–6), decreases tremor (n=13[c=12], RCT, d/b, p/c, c/o, 3/52, Nutt *et al, Arch Neurol* 2007;**64**:319–23), enhances levodopa (n=5, RCT, d/b, c/o, 3/7, Camiciolo *et al, Clin Neuropharmacol* 2001;**24**:208–13) and can improve gait hypokinesia and freezing (n=69[c=65], RCT, d/b, p/c, 90/7, Moreau *et al, Lancet Neurol* 2012;**11**:589–96). However, a longer study showed that methylphenidate did not improve gait and worsened motor function (n=23[c=17], RCT, d/b, p/c, 6/12, Espay *et al, Neurology* 2011;**76**:1256–62; FFT; review by Devos *et al, CNS Drugs* 2013;**27**:1–14).

Review: methylphenidate in PD (Auriel *et al, Clin Neuropharmacol* 2009;**32**:75–81).

42e. * **Guanfacine** has not been formally tested although alpha-2 adrenergic receptors are being investigated as a treatment for PD.

43. **Anticholinesterases** (especially **rivastigmine**)

are effective for dementia in PD, albeit with variable results (s=20, van Laar *et al, CNS Neurosci Ther* 2011;**17**:428–41), e.g. galantamine may be detrimental (n=69 [c=54], RCT, d/b, p/c, 16/52, Grace *et al, J Neurol Neurosurg Psychiatry* 2009;**80**:18–23).

44. **Memantine** may help motor fluctuations but not drug-induced dyskinesias (n=12, RCT, d/b, p/c, c/o, Merello *et al, Clin Neuropharmacol* 1999;**22**:273–6; n=3, Lökk, *Lakartidningen* 2004; **101**:2003–6).

45. **Anticholinergics** can be used but have predictable and significant adverse effects on memory (n=78, Miller *et al, Acta Neurol Scand* 1987;**76**:278–82).

46. **Acamprosate, disulfiram or nalmefene** have no known problems. High-dose **naltrexone** may help pathological gambling in PD (n=3, Bosco *et al, Clin Neuropharmacol* 2012;**35**:118–20).

47. **Buprenorphine** and **methadone** have no known problems.

48. **Modafinil** 200 mg/d is well tolerated and modestly improves excessive daytime sleepiness in PD (e.g. n=21, RCT, d/b, p/c, c/o, 9/52, Adler *et al, Mov Disord* 2003;**18**:287–93; n=10, 3/52, open, Lökk, *Neuropsychiatr Dis Treat* 2010;**7**:93–7; FFT) and may help physical fatigability (n=19, RCT, d/b, p/c, 8/52, Lou *et al, Clin Neuropharmacol* 2009;**32**:305–10) at up to 400 mg/d (n=13, open, 9/52, p/c, Tyne *et al, J Neurol* 2010;**257**:452–6). However, an RCT was unable to show a significant effect on sleep, although it was well tolerated and had no adverse motor effects (n=40 [c=37], RCT, d/b, p/c, 4/52, Ondo *et al, J Neurol Neurosurg Psychiatry* 2005;**76**:1639–9; FFT). **Sodium oxybate** (mean 7.8 g) at night improves excessive daytime sleepiness and fatigue in PD, improving nighttime sleep (n=30 [c=27], open, 12/52, Ondo *et al, Arch Neurol* 2008;**65**:1337–40).

3.9 PERINATAL

NK = NOT KNOWN; L = LOWER RISK; M = MEDIUM RISK/KNOWN BUT MANAGABLE; H = HIGHER RISK;
? = SOME DATA, E.G. ANIMAL STUDIES, CASES, LACK OF NEGATIVE REPORTS SUGGESTS THIS IS THE GRADE

	FERT-ILITY	FDA	ADEC	T1	T2-3	BIRTH	BREAST	PND
ANTIPSYCHOTICS								
Aripiprazole[1]	L	C	C	L?	M	M	M	L?
Benzamides[7]	M	NA	C	L/M	L/M	L	M	NK
Haloperidol[8]	M	C	C	L/M	M?	NK	M	M?
Clozapine[2]	L	B	C	L?	M	NK	H	L
Lurasidone[3]	L?	B	B1	L?	L?	L?	M?	NK
Olanzapine[4]	L	C	C	M	M	M	L	L?
Phenothiazines (if known)[9]	M	C	C	M	M	M	M	L?
Quetiapine[5]	L?	C	C	L?	L?	NK	L	L?
Risperidone/paliperidone[6]	M	C	C	L?	M?	NK	M?	L/M
Thioxanthenes[10]	M	NA	C	L/M	M	NK	L	L?
Pimozide[11]	M	C	C	L/M	L/M	NK	M	NK
Ziprasidone[11]	L?	C	C	M	M	NK	M?	NK
ANTIDEPRESSANTS								
SSRIs[12]								
(Es)citalopram[12a]	L?	C	C	M	M	M	L	L?
Fluoxetine[12b]	L?	C	C	M	M	M	M	L
Fluvoxamine[12c]	L?	C	C	M	M	M	L	L
Paroxetine[12d]	M	D	D	H	M	M/H	M	L?
Sertraline[12e]	L?	C	C	M	L/M	M	L	L?
Tricyclics: (all)[13]	L?	C	C	L/M	M	M	M	L
Agomelatine[14]	L?	NA	B1	L/M	NK	NK	L	NK
Bupropion[15]	L	C	B2	M?	L/M	L	L	NK
Duloxetine[16]	L	C	B3	L/M	L	M	L/M	L?
Mirtazapine[17]	L?	C	B3	L/M	L	L/M	L/M	L?
Mianserin[21]	L?	NA	B2	M	NK	NK	L	NK
Moclobemide[18]	L?	NA	B3	M	NK	NK	L	L?
Reboxetine[19]	L?	NA	B1	M	NK	NK	L	L?
Trazodone[20]	L?	C	NA	M	NK	NK	L	NK
Tryptophan[21]	L	NA	NA	L	L	L	L	L
St. John's wort[21]	L?	NA	NA	L/M?	NK	NK	L?	L?
Venlafaxine[22]	L?	C	B2	M	L/M	M/H	M/H	L?
Vortioxetine[16]	L?	C	NA	NK	NK	NK	NK	NK
MAOIs[23]	NK	C	B2/3	M	M	M/H	L/M?	NK
ANXIOLYTICS HYPNOTICS								
Benzodiazepines[29]	L?	C/D/X	C	L/M	L/M	M	M	L/M
Beta-blockers[30]	L?	C	C	M	M	M	L/M	M
Buspirone[31]	L?	B	B1	L/M	NK	NK	M/H	NK

	FERT-ILITY	FDA	ADEC	T1	T2-3	BIRTH	BREAST	PND
Chloral[32]	L?	C	A	L	NK	NK	M	NK
Clomethiazole[32]	L?	NA	A	L/M	L/M	NK	L	NK
Hydroxyzine[32]	L?	D	A	M/H	M	M	M/H	NK
Melatonin[33]	L?	NA	B3	L?	L?	L?	L/M?	L?
Pregabalin[34]	L	C	B3	L/M	NK	NK	L/M?	NK
Promethazine	L?	C	C	L/M	L/M	M	L/M	L?
Zaleplon[35a]	L?	C	C	L?	L?	NK	L/M?	NK
Zolpidem[35b]	L?	C	B3	L/M	L/M	L/M	L	NK
Zopiclone[35c]	L?	C	C	L/M	NK	L/M	H	NK
MOOD and BIPOLAR								
Asenapine[24]	L?	C	C	M	NK	NK	M	NK
Carbamazepine[25]	M?	D	D	M/H	M/H	M	M	M
Lamotrigine[26]	L	C	D	L/M	M	M	M	L
Lithium[27]	L/M	D	D	L/M	M	M	M	L?
Valproate[28]	M	D/X	D	H	M	M	L/M	H
ANTICONVULSANTS								
Barbiturates[36]	NK	D	D	M	M	M	M	M/H
Gabapentin[37]	L?	C	B1	L	NK	M	M	NK
Levetiracetam[38]	L?	C	B3	L	M	NK	M/H	L
Oxcarbazepine[39]	L?	C	D	L/M	M	NK	M	L?
Phenytoin[40]	M?	D	D	M/H	M	M	L/M	M/H
Topiramate[41]	L?	D	D	M/H	M/H	M	NK	M/H
OTHERS								
Anticholinesterases[43]	L?	B/C	B1/2/3	L/M	NK	NK	M	NK
Memantine[44]	L?	B	B2	L/M	NK	NK	M	NK
Anticholinergics[45]	L?	C	A/B1/2	NK	NK	NK	NK	NK
Acamprosate[46a]	L?	C	B2	L/M	NK	NK	L/M	NK
Disulfiram[46b]	L?	C	B2	M	M	L?	M	L?
Nalmefene[46c]	L?	B	NA	NK	NK	M	NK	NK
Naltrexone[46d]	L?	C	B3	NK	NK	M	L/M	L/M?
Buprenorphine[47a]	L/M	C	C	L/M	L/M	M	M/H	NK
Methadone[47b]	M	C	C	L/M	L/M	M/H	L/M	L/M
Modafinil[48]	L?	C	B3	L/M	L/M	NK	M/H?	NK
Sodium Oxybate[48]	L?	B	NK	L/M	L/M	NK	L/M	NK
Prazosin[48c]	L?	C	B2	M	L/M	NK	M	NK
Atomoxetine[42a]	L?	C	B3	L/M	M	L?	L/M	NK
(Lis)dexamfetamine[42bc]	L?	C	B3	L/M	M	NK	M/H	NK
Guanfacine[42e]	L?	B	NA	L/M	NK	NK	M?	NK
Methylphenidate[42d]	L?	C	B2	L/M	L/M	M	L/M	NK

3

Introduction

While drugs pose a risk in pregnancy, it is important to consider the risks of untreated mental health problems in pregnancy, e.g.:

1. Pregnancy complications, e.g. low birth weight and prematurity, possibly due to maternal stress.
2. Maternal symptoms can lead to irritation, agitation, lethargy, poverty of facial expressions.
3. Maternal symptoms can lead to lower attachment and later learning and behavioural problems.
4. Relapse can lead to the need for higher doses of drugs to facilitate stabilisation.

General advice

Reproductive toxicity falls into five domains (Wisner *et al, Am J Psychiatry* 2000;**157**:1933–40):

1. Physical malformations (T1).
2. Intrauterine fetal death/miscarriage (T2–3).
3. Growth impairment (T2–3) .
4. Neonatal toxicity, e.g. withdrawal or direct adverse effects (birth).
5. Behavioural and postnatal development.

For the record, spontaneous major congenital malformations (MCMs, usually defined as incompatible with life or requiring surgical correction) occur in 2–3% of pregnancies and spontaneous abortions in about 10–20% of clinically recognised pregnancies.

Pregnancy stages: First trimester (T1)

FDA: The US FDA has established five categories to indicate a drug's potential for teratogenicity and, where known, these are noted in the text:

- A Controlled studies in women fail to show a risk in T1 and the risk of fetal harm seems remote.
- B Either animal tests do not show a risk but there are no human studies, or animal studies show a risk but human studies have failed to show a risk.
- C Either animal studies show teratogenic or embryocidal effects but there are no controlled studies in humans, or there are no studies in either animals or humans.
- D Definite evidence of a risk to the fetus exists, but the benefits in certain circumstances (e.g. life-threatening situations) may make use acceptable.
- X Fetal abnormalities have been shown in animals or humans, or both, and the risk outweighs any possible benefits.

ADEC: The Australian Drug Evaluation Committee pregnancy category definitions (in brief) are:

- A Drug has been taken by a large number of pregnant women with no proven increase in malformations or other direct, or indirect, harmful effects on the fetus.
- B1 Drug has been taken by a limited number of pregnant women with no proven increase in malformations or other direct, or indirect, harmful effects on the fetus. Animal studies have not shown evidence of fetal damage.
- B2 As B1, but animal studies are inadequate or lacking, but other evidence shows no evidence of fetal damage.
- B3 As B1, but animal studies have shown evidence of an increased occurrence of fetal damage of uncertain significance.
- C Drug has caused, or is suspected of causing, an increase in fetal malformations or irreversible damage.
- D As 'C', but also may be expected to cause an increase in fetal malformations or irreversible damage, and have adverse pharmacological effects.
- X High risk of causing permanent damage so should not be used in pregnancy, or where there is a possibility of pregnancy.

Where known, the FDA and ADEC categories are quoted, but these may not always be a reliable source of information (Addis *et al, Drug Saf* 2000;**23**:245–53) and further information should be sought on individual drugs to balance the risk-benefit ratio in a particular individual patient.

General principles for prescribing in pregnancy

Planning for possible pregnancy allows the opportunity for informed decisions.

Pre-conception

1. For planned conception, discuss the risks and benefits of continuing or discontinuing medication, e.g. relapse, teratogenicity, etc, the unpredictability of the pre-conceptual duration, and that no decision is risk-free. Avoiding all drugs during T1 is ideal but may risk relapse. Other options include continuing at the lowest possible dose (or switching to a drug with the shortest possible half-life) until a positive pregnancy test, or continuing throughout pregnancy at the lowest viable dose.
2. Consider the risk of pregnancy even if not currently planned, e.g. carry out a pregnancy test before starting a drug in a woman of child-bearing

potential. Up to 50% of pregnancies are unplanned:

- Document any birth control method
- Document the potential risks for exposure to drug(s) during pregnancy
- Encourage proper nutrition, exercise and vitamin supplementation
- Note any other substances taken (e.g. excess caffeine, alcohol and natural products)
- Educate the patient about the risks
- Inquire about any pregnancy plans and emphasise the need for a pre-pregnancy consultation.

3. For drugs of known significant risk, or where there is little data, consider switching to a lower-risk drug before conception.

4. Avoid polypharmacy, as synergistic teratogenicity can occur.

Pregnancy

1. Avoid all drugs during T1 if possible. The maximum teratogenic potential is from days 17–60 (2–9 weeks) after conception, and decisions must balance the relative versus absolute risk.

2. Behavioural teratogenesis, subtle functional disturbances (e.g. learning difficulties, neurological deficits and developmental delay), and an effect on labour and delivery may occur with drug exposure in the second and third trimesters (T2, T3).

3. Use the lowest possible maintenance dose and monitor effects (adverse and desired) carefully with a low threshold for reintroduction or dose increase.

4. In many cases, the risk of relapse (and subsequent higher dose drug use) will be higher than the risk of fetal damage.

5. The pharmacokinetics of some drugs change during pregnancy and so doses may need to be adjusted (e.g. lithium, lamotrigine, levetiracetam)

6. Discontinuation effects have been reported in the newborn (e.g. benzodiazepines, antidepressants) so if possible gradually reduce doses or withdrawn in the weeks before delivery is due.

Unexpected pregnancy

If a woman discovers or reports that she is pregnant while taking a drug:

1. Don't panic.

2. Confirm the pregnancy.

3. If before day 17, consider immediate stopping or temporary discontinuation.

4. If after day 60, the major risk has passed and so decisions are less urgent.

5. Institute immediate nutritional supplements (e.g. an adequate dose of folic acid).

6. Reduce the dose if possible, at least during the high risk period.

7. Discontinue any non-essential drugs, particularly any that might be at sub-therapeutic doses.

8. Seek specific specialist advice, and discuss the risk of the possible consequences of relapse versus the published risk to the fetus.

Reviews: neurodevelopmental effects of prenatal exposure to psychotropics (Gentile, *Depress Anxiety* 2010;**27**:675–86), psychotropics in pregnancy in bipolar disorder (Nguyen *et al*, *Adv Ther* 2009;**26**:281–94).

Second and third trimesters (T2–3)

In pregnancy there are some important changes that may affect drug handling:

- Slower gastric emptying, slower small bowel and colonic transit time
- CYP1A2 activity is reduced by 65–70% at the end of pregnancy
- CYP3A4 activity may rise
- CYP2C19 activity is reduced by almost 50%
- CYP2D6 activity is generally induced during pregnancy so, e.g. an increased SSRI dose may often be needed
- Increased renal blood flow can increase clearance.

Birth

Poor Neonatal Adaptation (PNA) or neonatal Adaptation Syndrome (NAS) is usually mild and self-limiting, but if it occurs observe for 48–72 hours until symptoms fully subside. There is an increased risk with drug toxicity, use of several drugs and illicit drugs. PNA has 3 main causes (Kieviet *et al*, *Neuropsychiatr Dis Treat* 2013; **9**:1257–66; FFT):

1. Withdrawal of a drug, e.g. feeding problems, irritability, crying, poor sleep, tremors and vomiting, which usually occurs eight hours or so after birth.

2. Drug toxicity, e.g. jitteriness, hyperreflexia, diarrhoea, rigidity; this usually occurs straight after birth.

3. A combination of 1 and 2 or possible stress.

Breast-feeding

General principles

1. All psychotropics pass into milk, so no decision is risk-free. There have been few formal studies to guide decision-making.

2. Breast milk is more acidic than plasma, so basic compounds may be retained and accumulate in milk. Protein binding may also be a factor (in general, drug binding to milk proteins is less than

to plasma proteins). The higher lipid content of hind milk (second half of feed) makes it likely to have a higher drug concentration than the first half (fore milk).

3. Drugs should be avoided if the infant is premature, or has renal, hepatic, cardiac or neurological impairment because of an immature excretory function and the consequent risk of drug accumulation.

4. Avoid higher risk and sedating drugs and those with long half-lives. Drugs licensed for use in infants do not generally pose a hazard. Avoid new drugs if a therapeutically equivalent alternative is available that has been more widely used.

5. It is best to avoid long-acting preparations, especially those of drugs likely to cause serious side-effects as it is difficult to time feeds to minimise peak levels in the breast milk.

6. Choose a regimen and route of administration that presents the minimum amount of drug to the infant. Since nearly all psychotropics can be given as a once daily dose, this should be implemented as a single daily dose just before the infant's longest sleep period feed (e.g. for peak milk concentrations after oral administration).

7. If a mother was taking a drug during pregnancy, it will not usually be necessary to switch drugs during breast-feeding, as the amount to which the infant is exposed will be less than that *in utero*.

8. Adverse effects will often be dose-related, so use the minimum effective maternal dose.

9. Polypharmacy may lead to enhanced adverse effects in the infant. Avoiding interacting drugs that raise plasma levels (even if asymptomatically) is essential. Multiple drug regimens may pose an increased risk, especially when adverse effects such as drowsiness are additive.

10. Drug effects on the infant's brain development are not clear and so monitor biochemical and behavioural parameters, especially if the infant shows signs of possible side-effects (e.g. sedation, tremulousness, colic) and take appropriate action, e.g. dose reduction, drug change, etc.

11. Limit the use of over-the-counter (OTC) products.

A robust assessment of the balance of benefit to risk for a mother–child pair requires data both on the drug's passage into breast milk and its effects in infants: there is rarely enough information available about new drugs to allow such an assessment to be made.

Reviews: * general and extensive (Kieviet *et al*, *Neuropsychiatr Dis Treat* 2013;**9**:1257–66; FFT; Tripathi and Majumder, *Mens Sana Monogr* 2010;**8**:83–95), mood stabilisers in breast-feeding (Gentile, *Bipolar Disord* 2006;**8**:207–20), bipolar disorder treatments in puerperium (Dodd and Berk, *Curr Drug Saf* 2006;**1**:25–33), practical recommendations for treating mood disorders during lactation (Eberhard-Gran *et al*, *CNS Drugs* 2006;**20**:187–98).

Postnatal development (PND)

There is a paucity of data on neurodevelopmental effects, limited by a lack of long-term follow-up and the confounding factors of, e.g. exposure to untreated mood disorders and genetic factors. Information for individual drugs is noted where available, although this is mostly just case studies. **Reviews:** * mood disorders and effects on the child (Monk *et al*, *Pediatr Res* 2011;**69**:3R–10R; FFT; Kieviet *et al*, *Neuropsychiatr Dis Treat* 2013;**9**:1257–66; FFT), extensive review of illicit drugs (Thompson *et al*, *Nat Rev Neurosci* 2009;**10**:303–12).

3.9.1 ANTIPSYCHOTICS *

Fertility

Prolactin: Adverse effects related to hyperprolactinaemia e.g. galactorrhoea, amenorrhoea, libido decreased, erectile dysfunction and ejaculation failure, have been reported. These may have a negative impact on female and/or male sexual function and fertility.

Pre-conception: Low folate intake and low serum folate levels have been shown in women taking SGAs, increasing the risk of neural tube defects (Koren *et al*, *Am J Psychiatry* 2002;**159**:136–7) and so pre-conception dietary advice and folate supplements are essential.

T1

An extensive Swedish study (1995–2005) showed no increase in the MCM rate in women taking antipsychotics in T1, a consistent finding with other large studies, although the MCM rate was higher in women also taking anticonvulsants (infants n = 973,767, Reis and Kallen, *J Clin Psychopharmacol* 2008;**28**:279–88).

T2–3

There may be an increase in infant birth weight and a risk of larger gestational age with T2–3 use of SGAs cf FGAs (n = 108, Newham *et al*,

Br J Psychiatry 2008;**192**:333–7). The placental passage ratio (based on umbilical cord cf. maternal plasma) for the major antipsychotics (n=54[c=50], Newport *et al, Am J Psychiatry* 2007;**164**:1214–20) is:

- Olanzapine 72% (highest)
- Haloperidol 66%
- Risperidone 49%
- Quetiapine 24% (lowest).

Birth:

The FDA has added a class warning that all antipsychotics can cause EPSE in the infant if taken in T3, but advises not to stop abruptly as this can cause significant complications. The same is true of withdrawal symptoms (e.g. agitation, hypo- or hypertonia, somnolence, feeding problems, respiratory distress) after maternal use of antipsychotics in T3 (*Drug Safety Update* 2011;5), which can vary in severity and duration following delivery. Consequently, newborns should be monitored carefully.

Poor neonatal adaptation (PNA) usually develops within 48 hours and can last 2–6 days (Kieviet *et al, Neuropsychiatr Dis Treat* 2013;**9**:1257–66; FFT).

Breast-feeding

A major review (s=4 plus 41 others, Klinger *et al, Pediatr Endocrinol Rev* 2013;**10**:308–17) groups antipsychotics as follow:

- Acceptable: olanzapine and quetiapine
- Possible with close medical supervision: chlorpromazine, haloperidol, risperidone, zuclopenthixol
- Not currently recommended: aripiprazole, asenapine, clozapine, fluphenazine, flupentixol, lurasidone, paliperidone, perphenazine, pimozide, trifluoperazine, ziprasidone.

Review: general (which concludes that there is little difference between the available antipsychotics and that safety is not proven, so choose the most appropriate but avoid clozapine and olanzapine; Gentile, *J Clin Psychiatry* 2008;**69**:666–73).

Postnatal development

A prospective study showed reduced psychomotor performance (INFANIB scores) in infants aged 6/12 born to mothers taking antipsychotics during pregnancy (n=22) cf. antidepressants (n=202) or nothing (n=85) (n=309, Johnson *et al, Arch Gen Psychiatry* 2012;**69**:787–94), although numbers were very low (see individual drugs).

Reviews: general (Einarson and Boskovic, *J Psychiatr Pract* 2009;**15**:183–92; McCauley-Elsom *et al, J Psychiatr Ment Health Nurs* 2010;**17**:97–104), systematic review (Gentile, *Schizophr Bull* 2010;**36**:518–44).

1. Aripiprazole (FDA=C, ADEC=C) *

Fertility: Less effect on prolactin. No other data.

*T1–3:** Plasma levels decline and dosage may need to be increased across T1–3 (Gentile, *Expert Opin Drug Saf* 2014;**13**:1733–42). Placenta transfer is similar to other antipsychotics (n=15, Windhager *et al, J Clin Psychopharmacol* 2014;**34**:637–41).

T1: * There appears no increase in miscarriage, gestational diabetes or significant association with MCMs, but there may be increased rates of prematurity and growth retardation so more data is needed (n=86[+172 controls], Bellet *et al, Pharmacoepidemiol Drug Saf* 2015;**24**:368–80; for healthy outcomes see, e.g. n=1, Mendhekar *et al, Bipolar Disord* 2006;**8**:299–300; n=1, Widschwendter and Hofer, *Pharmacopsychiatry* 2012;**45**:299–300).

T2–3: Placental transfer occurs. The maternal concentration ratio for aripiprazole and dehydro-aripiprazole are 0.64 and 0.47 respectively, with no adverse outcomes post birth. This ratio is comparable with, e.g. risperidone (0.49), olanzapine (0.72), haloperidol (0.66) and quetiapine (0.24) (Nguyen *et al, Aust N Z J Psychiatry* 2011;**45**:500–1). There is one case report of an uneventful outcome (baby healthy, birth caesarean as mother too unwell) where the risk of aripiprazole taken in T2–3 was considered less than that of the untreated illness (n=1, Gentile *et al, J Clin Psychopharmacol* 2011;**31**:531–2).

Birth: A baby born by Caesarean at 38/52 needed short-term (1 minute) respiratory support (n=1, Watanabe *et al, J Clin Psychopharmacol* 2011;**31**:377–9).

Breast-feeding: Aripiprazole is excreted in human breast milk and so the advice should be not to breast feed (UK SmPC). Aripiprazole and dehydroaripiprazole levels peak at around three hours post-dose (80 ng/ml; 40–60 ng/ml at 10 mg/d). 320 ml/d milk may give the infant 20 mcg/d aripiprazole with no adverse events noted (n=1, multiple samples, Nordeng *et al, J Clin Psychopharmacol* 2014;**34**:272–5).

- In one human case milk levels were about 20% of maternal levels (15 mg/d producing 14 ng/mL in milk), a relatively low potential risk to the infant (n=1, Schlotterbeck *et al,*

3

Int J Neuropsychopharmacol 2007;**10**:433). Other cases had undetectable milk levels (n = 1, 3 samples, Lutz *et al*, *J Clin Psychopharmacol* 2010;**30**:204–5)

- Lactation failure has occurred due to regulation of prolactin (n = 1, Mendhekar *et al*, *Bipolar Disord* 2006;**8**:299–300).

PND: There is one case of normal development at 6/12 after aripiprazole in T1–3, except for weeks 9–19 (n = 1, Mendhekar *et al*, *Bipolar Disord* 2006;**8**: 299–300).

2. Clozapine (FDA = B, ADEC = C)

Fertility: Women are more likely to conceive on clozapine than most other antipsychotics due to a relative absence of raised prolactin.

T1: An old review quotes a 6% incidence of spontaneously reported MCMs (likely to overestimate the true incidence) and higher plasma clozapine levels in the fetus cf. the mother (Nguyen and Lalonde, *Encephale* 2003;**29**:119–24). Accumulation of clozapine has been shown in the fetus, possibly due to higher albumin concentrations (n = 1, Barnas, *Am J Psychiatry* 1994;**151**:945). No clear conclusion can be drawn, although combined with animal studies it would appear clozapine is not a major teratogen.

T2–3: A major study showed prenatal clozapine exposure (n = 338) was associated with an increased risk of gestational diabetes (OR = 1.94) compared to any other antipsychotic (n = 357696) except olanzapine (n = 169, OR = 1.77), but there were confounding factors, e.g. smoking (Bodén *et al*, *Arch Gen Psychiatry* 2012;**69**:715–21). Two women (three births, four children) took clozapine in T2–3 with entirely uneventful pregnancies and births (n = 2, Duran *et al*, *J Psychopharmacol* 2008;**22**:111–3), but there have been cases of delayed peristalsis (e.g. n = 1, Moreno-Bruna *et al*, *Arch Pediatr* 2012;**19**:913–6) and abnormal ECG after overdose in T3 (n = 1, Novikova *et al*, *Aust N Z J Obstet Gynaecol* 2009;**49**:442–4).

Birth: See introduction.

Breast-feeding: Clozapine is contraindicated, as animal studies suggest it is excreted into milk and so risks sedation and agranulocytosis in the infant and, as some accumulation can occur in breast milk (possibly due to higher lipid concentrations), doses must be kept low (Barnas *et al*, *Am J Psychiatry* 1994;**151**:945) and the infant's plasma monitored if breast-feeding is essential.

PND: * Exposure during pregnancy showed delayed development in the babies at two and six months but not by 12 months cf other SGAs, with no difference on cognitive, language, motor, social and emotions at any age (n = 63[c = 58], 12/12, Shao *et al*, *PLoS One* 2015;**10**:e0123373; FFT).

3. Lurasidone (FDA = B, ADEC = B1)

Fertility: There may be less hyperprolactinaemia but some fertility effects have been seen in animals.

T1: Lurasidone has shown no teratogenicity in animal studies and the currently unremarkable human data is limited to less than 300 pregnancies.

T2–3 and birth: See introduction.

Breast-feeding: No human data is available, but lurasidone is excreted in rats' milk.

PND: No data.

4. Olanzapine (FDA = C, ADEC = C)

Fertility: See introduction.

T1–3: A prospectively study of olanzapine (Lilly database; mean dose 10 mg/d [range 5–35], with 44% having olanzapine in all three trimesters) showed 66% normal births, 10% premature, 9% spontaneous abortions, 8% perinatal conditions, 4% congenital abnormalities and 3% other problems. These were within normal expected ranges (n = 610, Brunner *et al*, *BMC Pharmacol Toxicol* 2013;**14**:38; FFT), supporting an earlier prospective study (n = 60, McKenna *et al*, *J Clin Psychiatry* 2005;**66**:444–9).

Birth: Prenatal exposure to olanzapine (n = 169) was associated with increased risk of gestational diabetes (OR = 1.94) compared to any other antipsychotic (n = 338) except clozapine (OR = 1.77) and no antipsychotic (n = 357696), but there were many confounding factors, e.g. smoking (Bodén *et al*, *Arch Gen Psychiatry* 2012;**69**:715–21). There is a tendency for lower birth weights and SCBU admissions with olanzapine cf. other SGAs (n = 54, Newport *et al*, *Am J Psychiatry* 2007;**164**:1214–20).

Breast-feeding: Olanzapine is excreted in breast milk, with infants exposed to about 1.5% (range 0–2.5%; mbp = 5, Croke *et al*, *Int J Neuropsychopharmacol* 2002;**5**:243–7) of a weight-adjusted maternal dose of olanzapine, below the 10% nominal level of concern and with few adverse effects (eg. mbp = 7, Gardiner *et al*, *Am J Psychiatry* 2003;**160**:1428–31). In a prospective study of olanzapine (mean 7.5 mg/d, range 2.5–20) in breast-feeding, 82% of the infants had no major adverse effects, with 4% somnolence, 2% irritability, 2% tremor and 2% insomnia (n = 102, Brunner *et* *al, BMC Pharmacol Toxicol* 2013;**14**:38; FFT). Levels may decline to undetectable over the first four months, probably due to maturing of the hepatic enzymes (n = 1, Whitworth *et al, J Psychopharmacol* 2008;**22**:923–4; mbp = 1, Whitworth *et al, J Psychopharmacol* 2010;**24**:121–3).

PND: A comparative study failed to show any long-term consequences from breast-feeding with olanzapine (n = 88 [c = 37], Gilad *et al, Breastfeed Med* 2011;**6**:55–8; mbp = 1, 6/12, Aichhorn *et al, J Psychopharmacol* 2008;**22**:923–4).

5. Quetiapine (FDA = C, ADEC = C)

The SmPC recommends using only if the benefits justify the risk, but the available data shows no major cause for concern.

Fertility: See introduction.

T1–3: A prospective cohort study showed no increase in MCMs (n = 36, McKenna *et al, J Clin Psychiatry* 2005;**66**:444–9). Possible effects on the fetal eye have not been looked at. There are cases of up to 400 mg/d (e.g. n = 1, Taylor *et al, Am J Psychiatry* 2003;**160**:588–9) and 1200 mg/d (starting from week 21, n = 1, Cabuk *et al, Arch Women's Ment Health* 2007;**10**:235–6) taken throughout pregnancy without complications. The XL version may have lower peak levels (n = 1, Tényi *et al, Neuropsychopharmacol Hung* 2013;**15**:49–50).

Birth: No data.

Breast-feeding: Available reports suggest a low risk, e.g. a case series showed undetectable levels in milk, with low or undetectable levels in the infant's serum (mbp = 6, Misri *et al, J Clin Psychopharmacol* 2006;**26**:508–11). 200 mg/d produced a maximum milk level of 0.43% of the weight-adjusted maternal dose and fell to pre-dose levels within two hours, appearing to be too small for significant pharmacological effects (n = 1, Lee *et al, Am J Psychiatry* 2004;**161**:1715–6; see also infant's plasma level 6% of the mother's serum level, receiving less than 0.1% of the maternal dose; n = 1, Rampono *et al, Ann Pharmacother* 2007;**41**:711–4).

PND: Quetiapine 1200 mg/d (starting from week 21, n = 1, Cabuk *et al, Arch Women's Ment Health* 2007;**10**:235–6) has been taken throughout pregnancy without complications and with normal development at six months.

6. Risperidone/paliperidone (risperidone FDA = C; ADEC = C; paliperidone FDA = C; ADEC = C)

Fertility: See introduction.

T1–3: Risperidone has shown no evidence that *in utero* exposure increases spontaneous abortions, MCMs or teratogenicity, although self-limiting EPSEs were seen if used in T3 (n = 713, Coppola *et al, Drug Saf* 2007;**30**:247–64; see also n = 49, McKenna *et al, J Clin Psychiatry* 2005;**66**:444–9; n = 2, Mendhekar and Lohia, *J Neuropsychiatry Clin Neurosci* 2014;**20**:485–6).

Birth: See introduction.

Breast-feeding: The UK SmPCs for risperidone and paliperidone state that women should not breast-feed. The milk:plasma ratio for risperidone has been < 0.5 with a relative infant dose lower than the notional 10% level of concern (n = 2, Ilett *et al, Ann Pharmacother* 2004;**38**:273–6). In a further case, milk levels were 10 times higher than in the maternal serum but no adverse effects were seen in the infant and development was normal (n = 1, Aichhorn *et al, J Psychopharmacol* 2005;**19**:211–3).

PND: There are reports of normal pregnancies and postnatal development at 8/12 with risperidone orally (e.g. n = 1, Kim *et al, Prog Neuropsychopharmacol Biol Psychiatry* 2007;**30**:543–5; two successive pregnancies; n = 1, Mendhekar and Lohia, *J Neuropsychiatry Clin Neurosci* 2008;**20**:485–6; n = 1, Rodríguez-Salgado, *Actas Esp Psiquiatr* 2008;**36**:366–8) or RLAI at 2.5 years (n = 1, Dabbert and Heinze, *Pharmacopsychiatry* 2006; **39**:235) taken throughout pregnancy. Some reversible developmental effects have been seen with paliperidone, so it is not recommended, but should not be stopped abruptly during pregnancy (UK SmPC).

7. Benzamides (sulpiride; amisulpride ADEC = C)

Fertility: See introduction.

T1: Sulpiride has been used as an antinauseant in pregnancy. Limited human data has shown some possible adverse effects, but these are probably not drug-related and animal studies have not shown any direct or indirect adverse effects (UK SmPC recommends appropriate neonatal monitoring).

T2–3 and birth: See introduction.

Breast-feeding:

- Amisulpride may produce an infant dose intake of 10.7% of the maternal weight-adjusted dose, slightly above the usual 10% limit (mbp = 1, Teoh *et al, Breastfeed Med* 2011;**6**:85–8), but another case led to 6.1% milk levels (infant plasma level 3.9% of mothers) (mbp = 1 Ilett *et al, Ther Drug Monit* 2010;**32**:704–4)
- Sulpiride 100 mg/d is likely to give the child

3

less than 1 mg/d and no adverse effects have been reported at higher doses (n=28, p/c, d/b, 4/52, Ylikorkala *et al*, *BMJ* 1982;**285**:249–51), but it is not recommended (UK SmPC).

PND: See introduction.

8. **Butyrophenones** (**haloperidol** FDA = C, ADEC = C; **penfluridol** FDA = C)

Fertility: See introduction.

T1: Haloperidol was shown in a prospective study to have no significant increase in MCMs (cf control group) even if taken in T1, but there may be a higher incidence of therapeutic termination, preterm birth and low birth weight (n=188, Diav-Citrin *et al*, *J Clin Psychiatry* 2005;**66**:317–22). Penfluridol seems to have an incidence of MCMs similar to haloperidol in T1 (n=27, Diav-Citrin *et al*, *J Clin Psychiatry* 2005;**66**:317–22).

T2–3 and birth: See introduction.

Breast-feeding: Haloperidol is excreted in breast milk but levels are probably low, although infant levels may be the same as adults. There are isolated cases of EPSE in breast-fed children (UK SmPC).

PND: Some element of delayed development has been suggested with breast-feeding while on higher doses of haloperidol (n=5, Yoshida *et al*, *Psychol Med* 1998;**28**:81–91), and so the infant must be monitored carefully.

9. **Phenothiazines** (chlorpromazine FDA = C; ADEC = C; prochlorperazine FDA = C; levomepromazine FDA = C; fluphenazine, pericyazine, perphenazine, promazine and trifluoperazine all ADEC = C, no FDA categories available).

The phenothiazines are considered by many to be of low risk, although the potential for hypotension, sedation and anticholinergic effects means that any use must be with extreme care.

Fertility: See introduction.

T1–3: Teratogenicity data for phenothiazines is based on heritage studies and low doses and thus not necessarily applicable to higher dose use.

- Chlorpromazine and promazine (aliphatic group): in 315 pregnancies with T1 exposure there was a statistically significant difference in the malformation rate of 3.5% in the aliphatic phenothiazine-treated group (11 MCMs), compared with 1.6% in the control group, although there was no apparent trend in the type of abnormality and the risk is still considered low (n=12764, Rumeau-Rouquette *et al*, *Teratology* 1977;**15**:57–64)
- Prochlorperazine had no increased incidence of MCMs (mbp=1309, prospective, Slone *et al*, *Am J Obstet Gynecol* 1977;**128**:486–8)
- Trifluoperazine had no detectable teratogenic effects (n=700, Moriarity, *Can Med Assoc J* 1963;**88**:97; FFT)
- Phenothiazines (except prochlorperazine) at low-dose for nausea had no increased risk (n=543, Miklovich and van den Berg, *Am J Obstet Gynecol* 1976;**125**:244–8).

Birth: In the neonate, lethargy and extra-pyramidal symptoms have been reported, as has respiratory depression when given in high dose (above 500 mg chlorpromazine equivalents) close to term. Chlorpromazine crosses the placenta and may prolong labour (UK SmPC).

Breast-feeding: Phenothiazines can produce drowsiness in the infant. Chlorpromazine has an inconsistent milk/plasma ratio, and drowsiness and lethargy are possible, but not inevitable, so with careful monitoring should be safe (n=3, Yoshida *et al*, *Psychol Med* 1998;**28**:81–91). Perphenazine may become 'trapped' in milk due to its physiochemical properties and is best avoided (Olesen *et al*, *Am J Psychiatry* 1990;**10**:1378–9).

PND: A lack of impaired mental or physical development has been shown at 2–7 years follow-up (n=16, Ayd, *Int Drug Ther Newsletter* 1976;**11**:5), although some element of delayed development has been suggested (n=3, Yoshida *et al*, *Psychol Med* 1998;**28**:81–91).

10. **Thioxanthenes** (**flupentixol** ADEC = C; **zuclopenthixol** ADEC = C)

Fertility: See introduction.

T1–3: Flupentixol crosses the placenta and fetal levels are about a quarter of the mother's levels (n=5, open, Kirk and Jorgensen, *Psychopharmacology* 1980;**72**:107–8). There is no evidence of teratogenicity (three animal studies were clear), although the UK SmPC does not recommend its use. Zuclopenthixol (UK SmPC) has not shown any increase in fetal effects in animal studies, but lethargy, tremor, hyperexcitability and low Apgar scores have been reported (UK SmPC).

Birth: See introduction.

Breast-feeding:

- Zuclopenthixol (UK SmPC) appears in milk at less than 1% of the weight-related maternal dose (in mg/kg) or at less than 30% of serum levels, with the infant daily dose expected to be 0.5–5 mcg/d (equivalent to 0.01–0.1 mg to an adult), of the lowest risk (mbp = 6, Aaes-Jørgensen *et al*, *Psychopharmacology (Berl)* 1986;**90**:417–8). Monitor for adverse effects especially during the first month

- Flupentixol appears a low risk as only 0.6 mcg/kg or 1–2% of the maternal flupentixol dose might reach the infant, e.g. <2 mg/d (n = 6, Matheson and Skjaeraasen, *Eur J Clin Pharmacol* 1988;**35**:217–20).

PND: Zuclopenthixol decanoate has a report of use throughout two pregnancies with both children born healthy and developing normally (6/12 and 3.5 years) (n = 1, 2 pregnancies, Janjic *et al*, *Vojnosanit Pregl* 2013;**70**:526–9).

11a. **Pimozide** (FDA = C; ADEC = C)

Fertility: See introduction.

T1: Animal studies have shown no teratogenicity but use is not advisable (SmPC), although there is a case of 1 mg/d taken throughout T1–3 with the baby well after four days (n = 1, Bjarnason *et al*, *J Reprod Med* 2006;**51**:443–4).

T2–3 and birth: See introduction.

Breast-feeding: Pimozide may be excreted into breast milk and use is not recommended (SmPC).

PND: See introduction.

11b. **Ziprasidone** (FDA = C, ADEC = C)

Fertility: See introduction.

T1–3: No adequate human data is available.

Birth: See introduction.

Breast-feeding: There is little data apart from one report (n = 1, Schlotterbeck *et al*, *Int J Neuro-psychopharmacol* 2009;**12**:437–8).

PND: See introduction.

3.9.2 ANTIDEPRESSANTS *

The risks of untreated depression:

- A higher incidence of SIDS, poor engagement and self-care, slower rates of fetal body and head growth (n = 7,696, El Marroun *et al*, *Arch Gen Psychiatry* 2012;**69**:706–14)
- A slight but non-statistical effect on lowering birth weight (meta-analysis, s = 27, Grote *et al*, *Arch Gen Psychiatry* 2010;**67**:1012–24)
- Increased ICU admissions, pre-eclampsia and a statistical (albeit modest) increase in premature delivery (OR = 2.4) and decreased breast-feeding initiation (s = 30, Grigoriadis *et al*, *J Clin Psychiatry* 2013;**74**:321–41)
- An increased risk of vaginal bleeding in early pregnancy (OR = 1.22) and midpregnancy (OR = 1.28), but not postpartum (1.02% of 57,279 pregnancies, Lupattelli *et al*, *J Clin Psychopharmacol* 2014;**34**:143–8).

Fertility:

- Delayed orgasm or anorgasmia (especially with serotonergic agents) and erectile dysfunction may reduce fertility in men
- Some may cause hyperprolactinaemia
- SSRIs may reduce sperm motility, cause abnormal sperm DNA fragmentation and have a negative effect on semen parameters (review; Koyuncu *et al*, *Int J* 2012;**24**: 171–3)
- There is no known effect on *in vitro* fertilisation outcomes (n = 950, Friedman *et al*, *Fertil Steril* 2009;**92**:1312–4).

T1–3:

The management of depression during pregnancy

The 2009 US report (Yonkers *et al*, *Gen Hosp Psychiatry* 2009;**31**:403–13; Yonkers *et al*, *Obstet Gynecol* 2009;**114**:703–13) recommends:

1. Women thinking of getting pregnant:

- If mild or asymptomatic for 6/12 or longer, consider tapering and discontinuing before becoming pregnant. This may not be appropriate if the depression is severe or recurrent (including psychotic, bipolar and history of suicide).

2. Pregnant women currently taking antidepressants:

- Who are psychiatrically stable and want to stay on medication may be able to after discussion with a psychiatrist/obstetrician
- Who want to discontinue may attempt tapering, and stopping if no symptoms recur
- With recurrent depression, or who have symptoms despite antidepressants, may be helped by psychological therapies as a replacement or augmentation
- With severe depression (e.g. suicidal attempts, weight loss) should remain on antidepressants
- With suicidal or acute psychotic depression should be referred to secondary care for 'aggressive' treatment.

3. Pregnant women who are depressed and not currently on antidepressants:

- Psychotherapy may be helpful if the woman prefers to avoid antidepressants
- If preferring antidepressants, choose carefully based on, e.g. trimester, history of depression, comorbidity.

4. All pregnant women should:

- Seek psychiatric help urgently if suicidal or psychotic symptoms develop.

Reviews: general (Bérard *et al*, *CMAJ* 2010; **182**:1079;FFT; Byatt *et al*, *Acta Psychiatr Scand* 2013;**127**:94–114).

General risks of antidepressant-treated antenatal depression: *

The main data is:

- *There is no association with MCMs (n=27809, Reefhuis *et al*, *BMJ* 2015;**351**:h3190; FFT), although T1 exposure to fluoxetine and paroxetine might show a slight increase in some birth defects, e.g. an increase in cardiac malformations (RR 1.36) and septal heart defects (RR 1.4) for paroxetine (although the effects were marginal and may have been the result of uncontrolled confounders; meta-analysis, s=19, Grigoriadis *et al*, *J Clin Psychiatry* 2013;**74**:293–308)
- For 349,127 children born in UK between 1990–2009 (n=349127 over 20 years, Ban *et al*, *BJOG* 2014;**121**:1471–81; FFT), the absolute risks of MCMs were:
  - No diagnosed depression 2.7%
  - Unmedicated depression 2.8%
  - SSRIs or TCAs treatment 2.7%
- A Norwegian study showed that women taking SSRI/SNRI (n=527) or TCAs/others (n=59) in T1–3 were no more likely to have any obstetric complication, e.g. vaginal bleeding and postpartum haemorrhage than non-depressed, non-exposed women (n=55411) (1.02% of 57279 pregnancies, Lupattelli *et al*, *J Clin Psychopharmacol* 2014;**34**:143–8)
- The base-rate for spontaneous abortion is 11% and a large study showed no statistically significant increase with antidepressants (n=1005319, Kjaersgaard *et al*, *PLoS One* 2013;**8**:e72095;FFT)
- Of 949,504 pregnant women in US, 6.8% used antidepressants in T1 and the cardiac defect rate was 0.7% unexposed cf 0.9% exposed, but removing confounders showed no significant increase in cardiac malformations with T1 exposure to antidepressants (Huybrechts *et al*, *NEJM* 2014;**370**:2397–2407)
- Dose increases may be needed for T3 use of citalopram, clomipramine, imipramine, fluoxetine, fluvoxamine, nortriptyline, paroxetine and sertraline (Deligiannidis *et al*, *J Clin Psychopharmacol* 2014;**34**:244–55).

Birth: *

- PNAS/PNA: Postnatal adaptation syndrome (PNAS) is more likely with antidepressants (OR=5), as is respiratory distress (OR=2.2) and tremors (OR=7.9) (s=12, Grigoriadis *et al*, *J Clin Psychiatry* 2013;**74**:309–20)
- * PPHN (persistent pulmonary hypertension in newborn): SSRIs use (particularly in T3), may increase the risk of PPHN. The baseline untreated risk is small at 0.2% (1 in 500) and seems to be 1.28 higher for SSRIs and 1.14 for other antidepressants (n=3789330, n=128950 had a ppn, Huybrechts *et al*, *JAMA* 2015;**313**:2142–5; used SSRI during pregnancy=30K, n=11014 dispensed after week 20, Kieler *et al*, *BMJ* 2012;**344**:d8012)
- Withdrawal symptoms: these have been reported for many antidepressants, lasting from a few hours to weeks. See individual antidepressants for details.

Breast-feeding: The amount of antidepressant in milk varies according to the drug and what part of the milk is assayed; maternal use at normal doses does not usually lead to substantial levels in the neonate, although they should be monitored for feeding difficulties, weight gain, and sleep or state changes. A review wryly entitled a 'pooled analysis of antidepressant levels in breast milk' concluded that fluoxetine produces the highest proportion (22%) of infant levels above 10% of the average maternal level, citalopram next at 17%, and that nortriptyline, paroxetine and sertraline may be the preferred choices, with citalopram relatively safe if doses are minimised (s=67, Weissman *et al*, *Am J Psychiatry* 2004;**161**:1066–78).

Review: extensive (s=31, Lanza di Scalea and Wisner, *Clin Obstet Gynecol* 2009;**52**:483–97).

PND: A systematic review showed no difference in child outcome (cognition, motor and behaviour) with prenatal exposure to antidepressants, although two studies showed a difference in motor function (s=12, Gentile and Galbally, *J Affect Disord* 2011;**128**:1–9), e.g. use in T2–3 (n=415) resulted in the baby sitting up 15 days later and walking 29 days later cf. non-exposed (n=81042) and untreated depression (n=489), but this is all still within the normal range (19/12, Pedersen *et al*,

Pediatrics 2010;**125**:e600–8).

12. **SSRIs** (citalopram FDA = C, ADEC = C; escitalopram FDA = C, ADEC = C; fluoxetine FDA = C, ADEC = C; fluvoxamine FDA = C, ADEC = C; paroxetine FDA = D, ADEC = D; sertraline FDA = C, ADEC = C)

A systematic review and meta-analysis of SSRIs and MCMs (s = 29, Myles *et al, Aust NZ J Psychiatry* 2013;**47**:1002–12) concludes that:

- Fluoxetine (OR = 1.14) and paroxetine (OR = 1.29) are associated with an increased risk of MCMs
- Paroxetine (OR = 1.44) is associated with an increased risk of cardiac malformations
- Sertraline and citalopram are not associated with any MCMs.

Untreated MDD (n = 31) or MDD plus SSRIs (n = 46) had no effect on infant growth, length, weight or head circumference cf. controls (n = 97) through to 12 months of age (Wisner *et al, Am J Psychiatry* 2013;**170**:485–93) and that stopping SSRIs near the time of conception had a high relapse rate (n = 174, 2 years, Wisner *et al, Am J Psychiatry* 2013;**170**:485–93).

T1–3:

Miscarriage:

- A systematic review and meta-analysis showed no significant association between antidepressant exposure and spontaneous abortion (s = 23, Ross *et al, JAMA Psychiatry* 2013;**70**:436–43)
- Two newer studies shown no association with SSRIs and risk of stillbirth, and neonatal or postnatal mortality (n = 29,228 from 1633877, Stephansson *et al, JAMA* 2013; **309**:48–54), with the risk of stillbirth being 0.45% and neonatal mortality 0.34%, with no association with SSRI exposure in any combination of trimesters (n = 12425 SSRI exposures from n = 920620, Jimenez-Solem *et al, Am J Psychiatry* 2013;**170**:299–304).

Maternal hypertension: An increased incidence of gestational hypertension may occur in women taking SSRIs (19% vs 9%), especially if used in T3, although a causal link is not established (n = 5,731, Toh *et al, Am J Psychiatry* 2009;**166**:320–8; FFT; see also n = 1216, De Vera and Bérard, *Br J Clin Pharmacol* 2012;**74**:362–9; FFT).

Birth weight: Assessed from 20/52 gestation through to 12/12 postpartum neither depression nor antenatal SSRI exposure was associated with birth weight changes (n = 174, two years, Wisner *et al, Am J Psychiatry* 2013;**170**:485–93), although prenatal SSRIs were associated with reduced fetal head growth and a doubled risk of preterm birth, but not associated with reduced body growth, and not dissimilar to that with untreated maternal depression (n = 7,696, El Marroun *et al, Arch Gen Psychiatry* 2012;**69**:706–14).

Others:

- *Clubfoot:* there may be a slight increase (OR = 1.8) in the incidence of clubfoot with SSRI use for > 30/7 in pregnancy, with a higher incidence with paroxetine (OR = 9) and escitalopram (OR = 2.9) cf. sertraline (OR = 1.8) (n = 622+2002, Yazdy *et al, Epidemiology* 2014;**25**:859–65)
- *Seizures:* There may be a slightly increased risk (OR = 1.4) of infant convulsions with SSRIs taken in T3 (n = 23,280, Hayes *et al, Am J Obstet Gynecol* 2012;**207**:49.e1–9; FFT).

Birth — with SSRIs:

- About 30% (range 20–77%) babies get poor neonatal adaptation (PNA)
- PNA usually develops within 48 hours and can last 2–6 days
- PPHN is a very low risk, low enough for the FDA to advise treating depression in pregnancy with SSRIs
- May be more likely with greater duration of therapy rather than actual dose.

PPHN: See introduction.

Apgar scores: SSRIs have an association with lower Apgar scores but not other antidepressants, and independent of depression itself (n = all pregnant women in Denmark from 1996 to 2006, Jensen *et al, Br J Psychiatry* 2013;**202**:347–51).

Doses: The risk of adverse neonatal outcomes (e.g. gestation duration and low birth rate, but not length of hospital stay, convulsions or feeding difficulties) may be more related to the duration of SSRI exposure during pregnancy than the timing of the exposure, a slightly confusing finding (n = 3500, one year, Oberlander *et al, Br J Psychiatry* 2008;**192**:338–43; FFT).

Prematurity: Prenatal SSRI exposure has been associated with an increased risk of pre-term delivery (0.9 week), decreased birth weight (175 g), 0.29 decrease in mean Apgar scores at five minutes and SCBU admission (n = 329+4902 controls, Lund *et al, Arch Pediatr Adolesc Med* 2009;**163**:949–54; n = 185, controls n = 185, Simon *et al, Am J Psychiatry* 2002;**159**:2055–61).

Withdrawal symptoms: Neonatal withdrawal symptoms (irritability, constant crying, shivering, increased tonus, eating and sleeping difficulties and convulsions) have been reported after *in utero* exposure to paroxetine (n=3), citalopram (n=1) and fluoxetine (n=1), four requiring calming with chlorpromazine (Nordeng *et al, Acta Paediatrica* 2001;**90**:288–91).

Serotonergic effects: Serotonergic drugs may increase the risk of CNS serotonergic adverse effects (tremor, restlessness, rigidity), but these subside quickly without treatment and may be due to serotonergic hyperstimulation rather than withdrawal (prospective, n=40, p/c, Laine *et al, Arch Gen Psychiatry* 2003;**60**:720–6).

Birth weight: A systematic review and meta-analysis showed a significant association between antidepressant use and lower birth weight (s=23, Ross *et al, JAMA Psychiatry* 2013;**70**:436–43), although a later study contradicted this (n=174, two years, Wisner *et al, Am J Psychiatry* 2013;**170**:485–93).

Review: SSRIs, T1 exposure and birth defects (Gentile, *Acta Psychiatr Scand* 2011;**123**:266–75).

Breast-feeding: Treatment with the SSRIs seems to be compatible with breast-feeding, although fluoxetine should probably best be avoided unless also used during pregnancy. SSRIs can delay secretory activation by around 15 hours postpartum, so might delay the onset of breast-feeding (n=431, Marshall *et al, J Clin Endocrinol Metabol* 2010;**95**:837–46).

PND:

- *Autism:* * 75% studies show an association between antenatal SSRI exposure and an increased risk of ASD in children so although some signal exists it needs confirming or otherwise (s=8, Gentile, *J Affect Disord* 2015;**182**:132–7)
- *Motor skills:* Infants exposed to SSRIs *in utero* (mbp=31) had significantly lower gross motor and adaptive scales compared to controls (n=52), not explained by underlying maternal depression (Hanley *et al, Early Hum Dev* 2013;**89**:519–24)
- *Growth:* Neither depression nor SSRI use throughout pregnancy affected infant growth from birth to 12/12 (n=174, 68/52, Wisner *et al, Am J Psychiatry* 2013;**170**:485–93)
- *IQ:* There were no significant differences in IQ or development at 2–6 years if the baby had suffered PNA from SSRIs, but there was a slightly higher risk for social-behavioral abnormalities (n=30 + controls =52, Klinger *et al, J Perinatol* 2011;**31**:615–20).

12a. **Citalopram and escitalopram**

Citalopram and escitalopram seem of lower risk based on available data.

Fertility: No data, see introduction. Animal data suggests citalopram may affect sperm quality (see paroxetine). An impact on human fertility has not been observed so far.

T1–3:

- Citalopram in T1 (n=125, including 71 who also took it throughout pregnancy) led to 86% normal live births, 11% spontaneous abortions, 1.5% elective terminations and 1.5% stillbirths, plus one MCM and an overall increased rate of admission to a SCBU (n=125, Sivojelezova *et al, Am J Obstet Gynecol* 2005;**193**:2004–9)
- Citalopram may occasionally need slightly increased doses (n=11, Heikkinen *et al, Clin Pharmacol Ther* 2002;**72**:184–91)
- Escitalopram has weak evidence of increased MCMs and possibly some perinatal complications (Bellantuono *et al, Hum Psychopharmacol* 2012;**27**:534–9). However, fully normal outcomes have been reported (n=7, Bellantuono *et al, Neuropsychiatr Dis Treat* 2013;**9**:1333–7) and escitalopram (n=212) had no increase in MCMs compared to other antidepressants (n=212) or no drugs (n=212), albeit with a higher spontaneous abortion rate (15% escitalopram, 16% others, 8.5% controls), and a risk of lower birth weights (n=636, Klieger-Grossmann *et al, J Clin Pharmacol* 2012;**52**:766–70).

Birth: See introduction for withdrawal and PPHN.

Breast-feeding:

- Citalopram, escitalopram and demethyl-citalopram are excreted into milk but below the levels of concern provided doses are optimised. The mean combined dose (4.4–5.1% as citalopram equivalents) intake by infants is below the 10% notional level of concern, and infant levels appear low or undetectable (n=11, Heikkinen *et al, Clin Pharmacol Ther* 2002:**72**:184–91; n=43, Lee *et al, Am J Obstet Gynecol* 2004;**190**:218–21)

- Escitalopram appears to have no short-term adverse effects in breast-feeding (review by Bellantuono *et al*, *Neuropsychiatr Dis Treat* 2013;**9**:1333–7; see also mbp=5, Rampono *et al*, *Br J Clin Pharmacol* 2006;**62**:316–22).

PND: See introduction.

12b. **Fluoxetine**

Fertility: See introduction.

T1:

- A systematic review (s=21, Riggin *et al*, *J Obstet Gynaecol Can* 2013;**35**:362–9) calculated the odds ratios for maternal use of fluoxetine for major MCMs (OR=1.12) and cardiac malformations (s=16, OR=1.16), although two case-control studies showed the latter figure could be 0.63. The conclusion was that fluoxetine does not appear to raise the risk of MCMs
- The UK MHRA issued a warning of an increase in cardiac defects with fluoxetine taken in T1 (from 1% to 1.5%), roughly the same as paroxetine, although they noted there was no increase in non-cardiac defects, no consistent pattern and to consider the risks of untreated depression in pregnancy (see *p. 290*) (Reefhuis *et al*, *N Engl J Med* 2006;**354**:2188–90; FFT; s=7, MHRA, *Drug Safety Update* 2010;**3**:8).

T2–3:

- There is little or no increase in the rates of low birth weight and preterm births, although high-dose fluoxetine (40–80mg/d) may be associated with a risk of lower birth weight (n=138, Hendrick *et al*, *Am J Obstet Gynecol* 2003;**188**:812–15; FFT)
- Miscarriage rates with fluoxetine may be double that of a control group (n=228, Chambers *et al*, *NEJM* 1996;**335**:1010–5; FFT)
- Relatively low plasma fluoxetine levels have been reported in later pregnancy, which might lead to therapeutic failure at standard doses (n=11 + 10 controls, Heikkinen *et al*, *Clin Pharmacol Ther* 2003;**73**:330–7).

Birth:

- See introduction for PPHN
- Fluoxetine withdrawal symptoms are unusual but can include irritability, increased tonus, jitteriness and poor feeding, usually only lasting a few days (n=1, Anbu and Theodore, *Indian Pediatr* 2006;**43**:66–9), or rarely up to six weeks (n=1, Alehan *et al*, *J Matern Fetal Neonatal Med* 2008;**21**:921–3).

Breast-feeding:

- Fluoxetine levels peak in breast milk at about eight hours post-dose, with 20mg/d or less producing low infant serum levels (n=19, Hendrick *et al*, *Biol Psychiatry* 2001;**15**:775–82), probably less than 10%, below the notional level of concern (e.g. mbp=10, Suri *et al*, *Biol Psychiatry* 2002;**52**:446–51)
- Infant plasma levels (s=11, n=190, Burt *et al*, *Am J Psychiatry* 2001;**158**:1001–9) have no clear association with maternal dose, age or plasma levels, so there is clearly significant interpatient variability
- With the potential for accumulation, careful monitoring of infants is mandatory, especially if exposed *in utero* (mbp=14, Kristensen *et al*, *Br J Clin Pharmacol* 1999;**48**:521–7).

PND:

- Fluoxetine (n=55) or no drug (n=84) throughout pregnancy showed no effect on global IQ, language development or behavioural development (n=139, 18–86/12, Nulman *et al*, *NEJM* 1997;**336**:258–62; FFT), cognition or temperament, whereas untreated depression was associated with poorer cognitive and language achievement (TCA n=46, fluoxetine n=40, control n=36; open, Nulman *et al*, *Am J Psychiatry* 2002;**159**:1889–95).

12c. **Fluvoxamine**

Fertility: See introduction. The UK SmPC says it may reversibly affect sperm motility in animals.

T1–3 and birth: See introduction.

Breast-feeding: The estimated fluvoxamine daily intake by an infant is probably about 0.5% of the maternal dose (e.g. 100–200mg/d), so is thought to be of little risk (e.g. n=2, Kristensen *et al*, *J Hum Lact* 2002;**18**:139–43; n=1; Hägg *et al*, *Br J Clin Pharmacol* 2000;**49**:286–8; see also mbp=2, Piontek *et al*, *J Clin Psychiatry* 2001;**62**:111–3).

PND: See introduction. No concerns have been raised about PND (e.g. n=2, Kristensen *et al*, *J Hum Lact* 2002;**18**:139–43; n=1; Hägg *et al*, *Br J Clin Pharmacol* 2000;**49**:286–8).

12d. **Paroxetine**

Fertility: A human study showed that DNA fragmentation occurred in 30% men (cf. 14% baseline), but without effects on other semen parameters (n=35, 5/52, Tanrikut *et al*, *Fertil Steril*

3

2010;**94**: 1021–6), probably reversible. See also introduction.

T1:

- The UK SmPC states that paroxetine in T1 is associated with increased risk of cardiovascular defects (from about 1% to less than 2%), but the MHRA does not recommend stopping it abruptly if a woman is pregnant as this could precipitate discontinuation symptoms
- Two major reviews, however, conclude that the data is inconsistent and inconclusive (s=25, Gentile and Bellantuono, *J Clin Psychiatry* 2009;**70**:414–22), with no increased risk of cardiac malformations (s=9, n=97,656, O'Brien *et al, J Obstet Gynaecol Can* 2008;**30**:696–70), although a mild-to-moderate association could not be excluded (n=182 exposed infants, Davis *et al, Pharmacoepidemiol Drug Saf* 2007;**16**: 1086–94)
- Other studies showed no association with increased cardiac defects (paroxetine 0.7%, unexposed group 0.7%) (n=1174, Einarson *et al, Am J Psychiatry* 2008;**165**:749–52), but a possible association with atrial septum defects (n=1293, Bakker *et al, Birth Defects Res A Clin Mol Teratol* 2010;**88**:94–100).

T2–3:

- Paroxetine plasma levels can increase steadily throughout pregnancy (leading to accumulation) except in extensive or ultra-rapid 2D6 metabolisers where they can steadily decrease (n=74, Ververs *et al, Clin Pharmacokinet* 2009;**48**:677–83).

Birth:

- Paroxetine withdrawal symptoms may include poor neonatal adaptation, irritability and tremors from soon after birth and lasting five days (n=1, Pogliani *et al, BMJ Case Rep* 2010;**2010**:bcr1220092528)
- A prospective study showed 22% neonates had complications (9=respiratory distress, 2=hypoglycaemia) requiring intensive treatment and hospitalisation, although all symptoms had disappeared within 1–2 weeks (n=55 + controls; Costei *et al, Arch Pediatr Adolesc Med* 2002;**156**:1129–32; more severe case, n=1, Morag *et al, J Toxicol Clin Toxicol* 2004;**42**:97–100).

Breast-feeding: Paroxetine maternal doses of 10–50mg/d can lead to detectable milk levels, albeit highly variable (sample n=108, range 2–101 ng/mL), e.g. detectable in all but one milk sample but undetectable (i.e. <0.1 ng/mL) in the infants' serum, with no adverse events reported (mbp=24, Misri *et al, J Clin Psychiatry* 2000;**61**:828–32; n=6, open, Ohman *et al, J Clin Psychiatry* 1999;**60**:519–23). Hindmilk concentrations may be 78% higher than foremilk (n=16, Stowe *et al, Am J Psychiatry* 2000;**257**:185–9).

PND: Breast-feeding while on paroxetine has no effect on infant weight or milestones at one year (n=73, Merlob *et al, Eur J Pediatr* 2004;**163**:135–9).

Review: general (n=22, Wurst *et al, Birth Defects Res A Clin Mol Teratol* 2010;**88**:159–70).

12e. **Sertraline** is not contraindicated in pregnancy in the UK SmPC.

Fertility: The UK SmPC states that animal data does not show any effect on fertility parameters (see also introduction).

T1: Sertraline at recommended doses does not appear to be associated with increased teratogenicity (RR=1.06, 95% CI, 0.43–2.62) or higher rates of miscarriage, stillbirth or prematurity (n=534, Kulin *et al, JAMA* 1998;**279**:609–10), although there may be a slight increased risk of septal defects (n=2,062+213,712 controls, Kornum *et al, Clin Epidemiol* 2010;**2**:29–36; FFT;).

T2–3: Sertraline levels and AUC remain fairly constant throughout pregnancy and postpartum, although they fall slightly in T3 (n=11, Freeman *et al, J Clin Psychopharmacol* 2008;**28**:646–53).

Birth: See introduction (discontinuation, PPHN)

Breast-feeding:

- Sertraline and metabolite generally appear only at low levels in the infant (probably <2% of the maternal dose; mbp=10, Dodd *et al, Hum Psychopharmacol* 2000;**15**:161–84), unlikely to cause significant adverse effects
- Peak milk levels occur 5–9 hours post-last dose, are lowest one hour pre-next dose and discarding the peak reduces the infant's intake by 18% (mbp=26, 186 samples, Stowe *et al, J Clin Psychiatry* 2003;**64**:73–80)
- * 87% samples tested showed sertraline below detectable levels (plus 70% for weakly active desmethylsertraline) and concluded routine care is adequate, with nothing extra needed (n=167, Pinheiro *et al, Arch Women's Ment Health* 2015;**18**:139–46)
- Higher levels have been rarely reported

(mbp = 9, Wisner *et al, Am J Psychiatry* 1998;**155**:690–2; n = 1, Müller *et al, Breastfeed Med* 2013;**8**:317–9), as have rare withdrawal reactions in breast-fed children after the mother abruptly stopped sertraline suggesting enough reaches breast milk to suppress withdrawal (e.g. n = 12, Stowe *et al, Am J Psychiatry* 1997;**154**:1255–60).

PND: See introduction.

13. **Tricyclics** (amitriptyline FDA = C, ADEC = C; clomipramine FDA = C, ADEC = C; desipramine FDA = C, ADEC = C; doxepin FDA = C, ADEC = C; dosulepin/dosulepin ADEC = C; imipramine FDA = C, ADEC = C; nortriptyline FDA = not classified, ADEC = C; protriptyline ADEC = C; trimipramine FDA = C, ADEC = C)

Fertility: No data is available. Some tricyclics have serotonergic anorgasmic effects.

T1–3:

A number of studies point to a low risk:

- Prenatal tricyclic exposure was not associated with MCMs (n = 209, controls n = 209, Simon *et al, Am J Psychiatry* 2002;**159**:2055–61), and was no more likely to lead to any obstetric complications, e.g. vaginal bleeding and postpartum haemorrhage than non-depressed, non-exposed women (n = 55411) (1.02% of 57279 pregnancies, n = Lupattelli *et al, J Clin Psychopharmacol* 2014;**34**:143–8)
- Imipramine (10–40 mg/d) had no adverse consequences and was successful in 75% pregnant women with panic disorder (n = 16, Uguz *et al, J Clin Psychopharmacol* 2014;**34**:513–5)
- Doses may need to be increased in T2–3, especially later in T3, but then decreased again after birth (n=8, Wisner *et al, Am J Psychiatry* 1993;**150**:1541–2).

Birth:

- About 20–50% of infants suffer from PNA, which usually develops within 48 hours and can last 2–6 days (Kieviet *et al, Neuropsychiatr Dis Treat* 2013;**9**:1257–66; FFT)
- Discontinuation effects have been reported, some needing active treatment, e.g. clomipramine's half-life in neonates is around 42 hours (cf. 20 hours in adults) and withdrawal symptoms (e.g. short sleep, poor feeding, jittery/twitchy, abnormal movements, fetal seizures and tremors), tachycardia and cyanosis have been reported (n = 11, ter Horst *et al, Br J Clin Pharmacol* 2012;**73**:295–302; FFT)
- Urinary retention, dyspnoea, lethargy, colic, irritability, hypotension or hypertension, tremor or spasms, have been reported during the first few hours/days (UK SmPC).

Breast-feeding: This does not need to be avoided (except perhaps doxepin), as only about 1% of the maternal dose reaches the infant, with only minute amounts in the infant serum and no acute toxic effects (mbp = 10, Yoshida *et al, J Affect Disord* 1997;**43**:225–37).

- **Amitriptyline/nortriptyline** levels in the infant are probably very low (Breyer-Pfaff, *Am J Psychiatry* 1995;**152**:812–3). Two studies showed no detectable nortriptyline in infant serum, and although two infants had detectable levels of metabolites neither showed any adverse effects. The risk appears low (mbp = 12, Wisner and Perel, *Am J Psychiatry* 1996;**153**:295; see mbp = 6, Wisner *et al, Psychopharmacol Bull* 1997; **33**:249–51).
- **Clomipramine** may only reach the infant at up to 3.7% of the mother's dose (mbp = 1, Pons *et al, Clin Pharmacokinetics* 1994;**27**:270–89), with no adverse effects reported (mbp = 4, Wisner *et al, J Clin Psychiatry* 1995;**56**:17–20).
- **Doxepin**'s longer-acting metabolite N-desmethyldoxepin may accumulate in infants and has caused severe drowsiness and near fatal respiratory depression (n = 1, Frey *et al, Ann Pharmacother* 1999;**33**:690–3). Other reports have failed to replicate this (e.g. mbp = 1, Kemp *et al, Br J Clin Pharmacol* 1995;**20**:497–9; Wisner *et al, Am J Psychiatry* 1996;**153**:1132–7), so metabolic differences could explain this.
- **Imipramine** milk/plasma ratios of 0.05–0.08 (based on high dose samples), would lead to only 0.1% of the maternal daily dose appearing in milk.
- **Lofepramine** is excreted in breast milk (UK SmPC).
- **Nortriptyline** (see amitriptyline) may be the lowest risk of the tricyclics.

The general recommendation is to observe the child carefully for sedation and respiratory depression. Choosing a tricyclic with a short half-

3

life (and any active metabolites) would appear the best option. Amitriptyline and imipramine are often quoted as the preferred tricyclics.

PND: Numerous studies show a lack of effect:

- Children who were exposed to a tricyclic (n=84) in pregnancy (T1–3) showed no adverse effect on global IQ, language development or behavioural development (e.g. n=164, Nulman *et al, N Engl J Med* 1997;**336**:258–62;FFT; similar conclusions: n=209, controls n=209, Simon *et al, Am J Psychiatry* 2002;**159**:2055–61), whereas untreated depression is associated with poorer cognitive and language achievement (tricyclic n=46, fluoxetine n=40, control n=36, open, Nulman *et al, Am J Psychiatry* 2002;**159**:1889–95)
- **Dosulepin** via milk produces no detectable adverse effects on cognitive development (cf. controls, s=2, mbp=66 controls, five years, Buist and Janson, *Br J Psychiatry* 1995;**167**:370–3), and is unlikely to be a significant hazard (mbp=5, Ilett *et al, Br J Clin Pharmacol* 1992;**33**:635–9).

14. **Agomelatine** (ADEC=B1)

Fertility: No data.

T1: Little human data exists so it should be avoided in pregnancy. The UK SmPC notes limited data only (less than n=300 to 2013). Animal studies show no direct or indirect harmful effects.

T2–3 and birth: No data.

Breast-feeding: Plasma levels peak at 1–2 hours post-dose and are undetectable at 4 hours (n=1, Schmidt *et al, Int J Neuropsychopharmacol* 2013;**16**:497–9), but is not recommended (UK SmPC).

PND: No data.

15. **Bupropion** (FDA=C; ADEC=B2)

Fertility: Animal studies show no impaired fertility but there is no human data (UK SmPC).

T1: Data on teratogenicity is inconsistent.

- The risk of all CV abnormalities may be increased with T1 bupropion (0.8%) vs use outside T1 (0.5%) and the incidence of LVOTO (left ventricular outflow tract obstruction) was 0.35% vs 0.08% for T1 and post-T1 exposure (n=7005, cardiovascular MCMs=52; Thyagarajan *et al, Pharmacoepidemiol Drug Saf* 2012;**21**:1240–2; LVOTO risk; n=12,722, Alwan *et al, Am J Obstet Gynecol* 2010;**203**:e1–6)
- * Although the risk of VSD (ventricular septal defects) is raised (OR=1.6) in combination with other antidepressants and as monotherapy (OR=2.5) MCMs appear not to be raised for the 7 other cardiac sub-groups (n=16524, Louik *et al, Pharmacoepidemiol Drug Saf* 2014;**23**: 1066–75).

T2–3:

- T2–3 bupropion exposure (n=1,049) is not associated with an increased risk of cardiovascular or other malformations, compared to other antidepressants (n=4,743, Cole *et al, Pharmacepidemiol Drug Saf* 2007;**16**:474–84)
- Transient hyperinsulinism has been reported (n=1, Gisslen *et al, J Pediatr Endocrinol Metab* 2011;**24**:819–22).

Birth: There are no reports of PNA (Kieviet *et al, Neuropsychiatr Dis Treat* 2013;**9**:1257–66; FFT).

Breast-feeding:

- Bupropion 300 mg/d leads to only small amounts in milk (n=10, Haas *et al, Tob Control* 2004;**13**:52–6):
  - Average infant dose in milk 6.75mg/kg/d
  - Average infant exposure 0.14% of the standard adult dose
  - Average infant exposure to bupropion and metabolites is 2% of maternal dose
- A later study showed bupropion SR ≤300 mg/d to give milk concentrations of 9 ng/ml (trough) to 64 ng/ml (peak), but with large inter-individual variations and only detectable in one of four infant urine samples. The average infant dose was 5.7% of the mother's dose, showing limited and minimal risk of exposure (mbp=4, Davis *et al, J Clin Psychiatry* 2009;**70**:297–8)
- Bupropion peaks in milk at two hours, lasts six hours or longer and can accumulate but is not detectable in infants (e.g. mbp=1, Briggs *et al, Ann Pharmacother* 1993;**27**:431–3; mbp=2, Baab *et al, J Clin Psychiatry* 2002;**63**:910–1)
- Bupropion-related infant seizures have been reported (n=1, Chaudron and Schoenecker, *J Clin Psychiatry* 2004;**65**:881–2; n=1, *Prescrire Int* 2005;**14**:144).

PND: No data.

16. * **Vortioxetine** FDA=C

Fertility: Animal data suggests no adverse effect but

there is no human data.
T1–3: No human data is available, but animal studies show some reproductive toxicity (SmPC), so use only if vortioxetine is essential.
Breast-feeding: Animal data suggests excretion into milk but there is no human data yet.
* **Duloxetine** (FDA = C; ADEC = B3)
Fertility: Duloxetine had no effects on male fertility, and effects in females were only evident at doses that caused maternal toxicity (UK SmPC).
T1: Normal outcomes have been reported in 61% and abnormal in 39% (17% spontaneous abortions; 11% post/perinatal conditions; and 8% premature births), generally consistent with the baseline rates (n = 233, Hoog *et al, Int J Med Sci* 2013;**10**:413–9).
T2–3: Case reports show uneventful use from the middle of T2 (e.g. n = 1, Briggs *et al, Ann Pharmacother* 2009;**43**:1898–902). The cord/maternal serum concentration ratio for duloxetine was 0.12 in one well-documented case, with no adverse events (n = 1, Boyce *et al, Arch Women's Ment Health* 2011;**14**:169–72).
Birth: PPHN is possible and a withdrawal syndrome similar to SSRIs (e.g. jitteriness, poor muscle tone, weak cry, respiratory distress, hypoglycaemia, low Apgar score and seizure) has been reported, lasting several weeks (n = 1, Adby and Gerhart, *Clin Pediatr (Phila)* 2013;**52**:976–7).
Breast-feeding: Duloxetine is weakly excreted into human breast milk. Duloxetine 80 mg/d produced milk levels 25% of plasma levels with an estimated infant dose 2 mcg/kd/d (range 0.6–3 mcg/kg/d), 0.14% of maternal dose (0.8% in one case; n = 1, Boyce *et al, Arch Women's Ment Health* 2011;**14**:169–72), well below the 10% notional level (n = 6, open, Lobo *et al, Clin Pharmacokinet* 2008;**47**:103–9), but is not recommended (SmPC).
PND: Normal development has been reported (n = 1, 9/12, Bellantuono *et al, Clin Drug Investig* 2013;**33**:685–8; n = 1, two years, Eyal and Yaeger, *Am J Psychiatry* 2008;**165**:651).
17. **Mirtazapine** (FDA = C; ADEC = B3)
Fertility: No data.
T1: A comprehensive prospective study showed no increase in the baseline rate of MCMs but a slight increase in spontaneous abortions (19% vs 17% vs 11%) and preterm births (10% vs 7% vs 2%) (n = 208 vs. other antidepressants vs. controls, Djulus *et al, J Clin Psychiatry* 2006;**67**:1280–4). Animal tests do not show any teratogenicity (UK SmPC).
T2–3: Mirtazapine has been used successfully and safely as an antinauseant in severe hyperemesis gravidarum (eg. n = 3, Guclu *et al, Arch Gynecol Obstet* 2005;**272**:298–300; n = 2, Uguz, *Gen Hosp Psychiatry* 2014;**36**:e5–6).
Birth: Recurrent hypothermia lasting 10 days has been reported in a mother taking mirtazapine throughout pregnancy (n = 2, Sokolover *et al, Can J Clin Pharmacol* 2008;**15**:188–90; FFT; see also n = 1, Udechuku *et al, Aust N Z J Psychiatry* 2010;**44**:978–96).
Breast-feeding: A maximum of 1.5% of the adult mirtazapine dose (median 38 mg/d) reached the infants and only one had detectable plasma levels, well below the notional level of concern (mbp = 8, Kristensen *et al, Br J Clin Pharmacol* 2007;**63**:322–7), although much higher levels have been reported — one where infant plasma levels approached the adult range, so close monitoring is needed (mbp = 1, Tonn *et al, J Clin Psychopharmacol* 2009;**29**:191–2). Hindmilk levels are slightly higher than foremilk (mbp = 1, Klier *et al, Am J Psychiatry* 2007;**164**:348–9).
PND: Mirtazapine has been taken for resistant nausea with no problems at 6/12 (n = 1, Rohde *et al, Arch Gynaecol Obstet* 2003;**268**:219–21).
18. **Moclobemide** (ADEC = B3)
Fertility: No data.
T1: No firm data is available save for a single report of 300 mg/d taken in T1–3 with no problems (n = 1, Rybakowski, *Pharmacopsychiatry* 2001;**34**:82–3).
T2–3 and birth: No data.
Breast-feeding: The UK SmPC notes only a small amount of moclobemide passes into breast milk (approximately 3% of the maternal dose; mbp = 6, Pons *et al, Br J Clin Pharmacol* 1990;**29**:27–31).
PND: There is a case of 300 mg/d taken throughout pregnancy with normal development at 14/12 (n = 1, Rybakowski, *Pharmacopsychiatry* 2001;**34**:82–3).
19. **Reboxetine** (ADEC = B1)
Fertility: No data.
T1: No teratogenic effects have been noted and it is not contraindicated in pregnancy.
T2–3 and birth: No data.
Breast-feeding: Reboxetine hindmilk and foremilk have the same concentration, with the relative infant dose being 2% (mbp = 4, Hackett *et al, Eur J Clin Pharmacol* 2006;**62**:633–8).
PND: Some impairment of growth and development has been seen in animal studies (UK SmPC),

3

but normal development and milestones in a human case series (mbp=4, Hackett *et al*, *Eur J Clin Pharmacol* 2006;**62**;633–8).

20. **Trazodone** (FDA=C)

Fertility: No data.

T1: At very high doses (15 times maximum human dose), there may be some fetal resorption and MCMs in animals but no increase in MCMs in humans cf. controls (n=441, Einarson *et al*, *Can J Psychiatry* 2003;**48**:106–10). The UK SmPC quotes <200 known pregnancies with no adverse effects but does not approve of its use.

T2–3: Trazodone seems effective for insomnia in T3 and may reduce the risk of postpartum depression (n=54, RCT, p/c, 18/52, Khazaie *et al*, *Psychiatry Res* 2013;**210**:901–5). Plasma levels remain stable throughout pregnancy (Klier *et al*, *J Clin Psychopharmacol* 2007;**27**:720–2).

Birth: Serotonergic withdrawal symptoms can occur (UK SmPC).

Breast-feeding: A single-dose study showed 1% passes into milk (n=6, Verbeeck *et al*, *Br J Clin Pharmacol* 1986;**22**:367–70) and it would appear to be of a low risk. Drowsiness and poor feeding has been reported (mbp=1, Yapp *et al*, *Ann Pharmacother* 2000;**34**:1269–72).

PND: No data.

21a. **Mianserin** (ADEC=B2)

Fertility: No data.

T1: There is no evidence of teratogenicity in animals except at toxic doses, but little human data.

T2–3 and birth: No data.

Breast-feeding: Mianserin 40–60 mg/d may produce only low milk and infant plasma levels with no untoward effects (mbp=2, Buist *et al*, *Br J Clin Pharmacol* 1993;**36**:133–4).

PND: No data.

21b. **St. John's wort**

Fertility: No data.

T1: In St John's wort-exposed pregnancies (n=54), the MCM rate was 5%, comparable to other antidepressants (4%, n=54) and controls (0%, n=54), not considered statistically different from each other (n=162, Moretti *et al*, *Reprod Toxicol* 2009;**28**:96–9; see also n=33 cf. 132 controls, Lee *et al*, *J Clin Psychiatry* 2003;**64**:966–8).

T2–3 and birth: No data.

Breast-feeding: There were no significant problems in infants whose mothers took St John's wort while breast-feeding, e.g. no decrease in milk production or infant weight over the first year (n=33+134 controls, Lee *et al*, *J Clin Psychiatry* 2003;**64**:966–8) and hyperforin was only detected at low levels in milk, with infant exposure 0.9–2.5% of the maternal dose (n=5, Klier *et al*, *J Clin Psychiatry* 2006;**67**:305–9). However, if possible, it should probably be avoided in breast-feeding (Dugoua *et al*, *Can J Clin Pharmacol* 2006;**13**:268–76).

PND: There was no statistically significant difference in weight over first year (n=33 cf. 132 controls, Lee *et al*, *J Clin Psychiatry* 2003;**64**:966–8).

21c. **Tryptophan**

Fertility, T1–3, birth, breast-feeding and PND: No human data is available nor problems reported but tryptophan is a naturally occurring food substance.

22. **Venlafaxine** (FDA=C; ADEC=B2)

Fertility: See introduction.

T1:

- Prospective data on pregnancies showed 83% live births, 12% spontaneous abortions, 5% therapeutic abortions (two with MCMs), suggesting the base-rate of MCMs is similar to the background rate but, as with the SSRIs, the spontaneous abortion rate may be slightly higher (venlafaxine n=150; SSRIs n=150; controls n=150; Einarson *et al*, *Am J Psychiatry* 2001;**158**:1728–30)
- No consistent pattern showed in another, albeit smaller, study (n=91 from 27,045, Polen *et al*, *Birth Defects Res A Clin Mol Teratol* 2013;**97**:28–35).

T2–3: Plasma levels may drop by 13% during T3, rising again postpartum (n=7, Ter Horst *et al*, *J Clin Pharm Ther* 2014;**39**:541–4).

Birth:

- Possible withdrawal symptoms include irritability, tremor, hypotonia, persistent crying, and difficulty in sucking or in sleeping and may start as soon as infant plasma levels decline; respiratory symptoms tend to start early and may lead to PPHN (n=5, Boucher *et al*, *Ther Drug Monit* 2009;**31**:404–9; n=1, de Moor *et al*, *Ned Tijdschr Geneeskd* 2003;**147**:1370–2). These can be managed with very low doses of venlafaxine (e.g. 1 mg) or breast-feeding, and may last a week or so (e.g. de Moor *et al*, *Ned Tijdschr Geneeskd* 2003;**147**:1370–2)
- There are no reports yet of PPHN (see introduction), but it cannot be excluded.

Breast-feeding:

- Venlafaxine milk levels peak at eight hours,

with infant venlafaxine/desvenlafaxine plasma levels up to 37% of the maternal plasma levels, and highly variable but in excess of the notional 10% safety level (mbp = 13, Newport *et al*, *J Clin Psychiatry* 2009;**70**:1304–10). A previous study suggested lower milk levels and low levels in infant plasma (mbp = 6, Ilett *et al*, *Br J Clin Pharmacol* 2002;**53**:17–22; FFT)

- There may be enough venlafaxine in milk to attenuate withdrawal symptoms (mbp = 1, Koren *et al*, *J Obstet Gynaecol Can* 2006;**28**:299–302)
- Less than 5% desvenlafaxine reached milk, lower than the 10% limit and appeared of low risk (mbp = 10, Rampono *et al*, *Arch Women's Ment Health* 2011;**14**:49–53)
- Infants who cry, are irritable and have abnormal sleep patterns after stopping breast-feeding may have discontinuation effects (UK SmPC).

PND:

- Babies of mothers who took venlafaxine (n = 62) or SSRIs (n = 62), or who were depressed but untreated (n = 54) all showed significantly lower IQs at three and seven years than non-depressed untreated women (n = 62), suggesting that factors other than antidepressants predict intellect and behaviour, so treating well and early is best (n = 240, Nulman *et al*, *Am J Psychiatry* 2012;**169**:1165–74; no PND problems; n = 2, Hendrick *et al*, *Am J Psychiatry* 2001;**158**:2089–90).

Review: * general (s = 29, Bellantuono *et al*, *Hum Psychopharmacol* 2015;**30**:143–51).

23. **MAOIs**: (FDA: all = C; **phenelzine** ADEC = B3, **tranylcypromine** ADEC = B2)

Fertility: No data.

T1: There are no reports of MCMs with MAOIs although the risk may possibly be doubled with tranylcypromine taken in T1 (AAPCD, *Pediatrics* 1982;**69**:241–4; uneventful use; n = 1, Gracious and Wisner, *Depress Anxiety* 1997;**6**:124–8).

T2–3: Growth retardation and fetal toxicity have been reported. MAOIs should be avoided due to maternal toxicity and lack of published safety data.

Birth: MAOIs may interact with drugs used in labour (see also *4.3.4*).

Breast-feeding: Minimal data is available. Tranylcypromine is excreted in breast milk but levels are not thought to be significant. Some sources state that MAOI levels in milk are too small to affect the child, but this has not been supported by any studies other than with tranylcypromine.

PND: No data.

3.9.3 MOOD AND BIPOLAR

In bipolar disorder pregnancy and the postpartum can be considered as separate risk periods, and different treatment plans may be needed.

Reviews: Bipolar disorder and pregnancy (s = 70, Sharma and Pope, *J Clin Psychiatry* 2012;**73**:1447–55), pharmacotherapy in mood disorders in pregnancy (Deligiannidis *et al*, *J Clin Psychopharmacol* 2014;**34**:244–55).

24. **Asenapine** (FDA = C; ADEC = C)

Fertility: No data, see introduction.

T1: Asenapine is not teratogenic in animal studies, but human data is not yet available (UK SmPC).

T2–3 and birth: See introduction.

Breast-feeding: Asenapine is excreted in milk in animal studies, but as no human data is available it should only be used only with caution (SmPC).

PND: See introduction.

25. **Carbamazepine** (FDA = D; ADEC = D)

Carbamazepine is considered to have a higher risk than other AEDs, although most data is on use in epilepsy, which may not necessarily apply to use in mood disorders.

Fertility: Folic acid supplementation is recommended before and during pregnancy (UK SmPC) to reduce the risk of spina bifida. Epileptic men taking carbamazepine have lower testosterone levels, altered semen quality, erectile dysfunction and a reduction in coital frequency (n = 118, Reis *et al*, *J Sex Med* 2013;**10**:493–9). Switching to oxcarbazepine can help (n = 4, Sachdeo and Sathyan, *Curr Med Res Opin* 2005;**21**:1065–8).

T1:

- MCMs: The incidence of MCMs with T1 carbamazepine monotherapy is 3.3% (specifically spina bifida) but still rare, and smaller than with valproate (s = 8, n = 2,680, Jentink *et al*, *BMJ* 2010;**341**:6581; FFT). Counselling and level 2 ultrasound and fetal echocardiography are recommended for neural tube defects, which can be detected in 90–95% of such cases if carried out with AFP levels at 16–18 weeks
- The risk of cleft lip and/or palate was

actually lower than controls (good overview by Matlow and Koren, *Can Fam Physician* 2012;**58**:163–4)

- Syndromes: the incidence of carbamazepine syndrome (facial dysmorphic features and mild retardation) is 13% and does not appear to be dose-related or seizure dependent (n=47, Ornoy and Cohen, *Arch Dis Child* 1996;**75**:517–20).

Others:

- Eyes — there is no evidence of eye malformations (s=13, Kroes *et al, Epilepsia* 2002;**43**:929–31)
- Thalidomide-like phocomelia has been reported (n=1, Dursun *et al, J Obstet Gynaecol* 2012;**32**:488–9).

T2–3:

- Unbound carbamazepine levels may slightly decrease in T3, but levels remain substantially unchanged (n=15, Johnson *et al, Epilepsy Behav* 2014;**33**:49–55; n=86, Tomson *et al, Epilepsia* 1994;**35**:131–5)
- There may be a reduced gestational age at delivery
- In late T3, routine vitamin K to mothers and the neonates is usually recommended.

Birth:

- Hepatitis in the newborn may occur (n=1, Frey *et al, Ann Pharmacother* 2002;**36**:644–7)
- Birth weight reduction of 250g has occurred after T1 exposure (n=210, Diav-Citrin *et al, Neurology* 2001;**57**:321–4).

Breast-feeding:

- Carbamazepine is classed by the AAP as compatible with breast-feeding but this is only based on case reports in epilepsy, with few reports when used as a mood stabiliser
- The half-life is longer in infants, with levels in milk ranging from 7–95% of the mother's serum (e.g. mbp=13, Froescher *et al, Ther Drug Monit* 1984;**6**:266–71), but probably usually around 10%, on the cusp of the notional level of concern. There are cases of excessive somnolence, allergic skin reaction, and several of poor feeding (e.g. n=1, Merlob *et al, Ann Pharmacother* 1992;**26**:1563–5)
- The mother should be informed of the potential signs of hepatic dysfunction and CNS effects (review, Chaudron and Jefferson, *J Clin Psychiatry* 2000;**161**:79–90).

PND: Cochrane (s=28, Bromley *et al, Cochrane Database Syst Rev* 2014;**10**:CD010236; see also s=7, n=645, Banach *et al, Drug Saf* 2010;**33**:73–9) concludes that in epilepsy the developmental quotient (DQ) was:

- Lower in children exposed to carbamazepine (n=50) than in children born to women without epilepsy (n=79)
- Lower in children exposed to CBZ (n=163) compared to children of women with untreated epilepsy (n=58)
- Further analysis concluded that there was no significant association with CBZ itself
- The IQ of older children exposed to CBZ (n=313) was not lower than that of children born to women without epilepsy (n=552), or compared to the children of women with untreated epilepsy (n=87)
- There was no convincing evidence of a dose effect.

Review: general (Matlow and Koren, *Can Fam Physician* 2012;**58**:163–4; FFT).

26. **Lamotrigine** (FDA=C; ADEC=D):

Lamotrigine has consistently been shown to be among the safest AEDs in pregnancy, including for MCMs and cognitive development (Moore and Aggarwal, *Expert Opin Pharmacother* 2012;**13**:1213–6).

Fertility: Animal experiments did not show any impairment of fertility (UK SmPC).

T1:

- The 18-year International Lamotrigine Pregnancy Registry has concluded that from T1 exposures (sufficient numbers to detect MCMs), the MCM rate was 2.2%, with no pattern of malformation type, frequency or a dose-related effect (n=1,558, Cunnington *et al, Neurology* 2011;**76**:1817–23), placing it as a low risk (supported by n=1,010, Mølgaard-Nielsen and Hviid, *JAMA* 2011;**305**:1996–2002)
- Another study showed MCMs were 2.3%, and, although there was an increased risk of isolated cleft palate or cleft lip deformity (n=684, Holmes *et al, Neurology* 2008;**70**:2152–8), there was no evidence of a specific increased risk of isolated orofacial clefts (n=72, Dolk *et al, Neurology* 2008;**71**:714–22).

T2–3: Lamotrigine levels can fluctuate significantly throughout pregnancy.

Lamotrigine dosing advice in pregnancy:
Determine a baseline plasma level as soon as possible, set the reference concentration (RC) and measure every four weeks.

- *T1*: Lamotrigine and lamotrigine-n2-glucuronide clearance may double, reducing levels by about 20–38%. As levels falls below the RC, increase the dose by 20–25% (n = 19, Reimers *et al, Epilepsy Res* 2011;**94**:198–205)
- *T2*: Clearance is increased by 236%
- *T3*: Clearance is increased by 248%. The average dose increase needed to maintain therapeutic plasma levels is 250% (n=9, Fotopoulou *et al, Epilepsy Res* 2009;**85**:60–4)
- *Delivery*: Clearance is increased by 264% (perhaps up to 640%) but levels rapidly revert to normal after delivery. Measure levels in the first 1–2 weeks postpartum and if higher than the RC decrease dose by 20–25% immediately.

Birth: See above for the need to adjust doses.
Breast-feeding: See above

- Lamotrigine passes into breast milk and, as it is metabolised by glucuronidation, may lead to accumulation in infants who have reduced capacity for glucuronidation, lower plasma protein binding and maternal levels can rise rapidly after birth unless doses are reduced (Madadi and Ito, *Can Fam Phys* 2010;**56**:1132–4). Exposure via breast milk is less than placental transfer so less of an issue if taken throughout T1–3
- Premature infants should not be exposed to lamotrigine via milk because of the theoretical risk of a serious rash
- Infant plasma levels have huge interindividual variations and may be 2–43% of the mothers (peak four hours post-dose; n = 30, Newport *et al, Pediatrics* 2008;**122**:223–31; milk to maternal serum ratio a consistent 0.6; review, Chaudron and Jefferson, *J Clin Psychiatry* 2000;**161**:79–90; see also mbp = 4, Liporace *et al, Epilepsy Behav* 2004;**5**:102–5; mbp = 8, Clark *et al, Am J Psychiatry* 2013;**170**:1240–7 FFT). Some variation may be of genetic origin
- There are isolated reports of sleep apnea (Nordmo *et al, Ann Pharmacother* 2009;**43**:1893–7) and benign and symptom-less elevated platelet counts (n=8, Newport *et al, Pediatrics* 2008;**122**:223–31; FFT).

PND: *In utero* exposure to lamotrigine shows no effect on neurodevelopment in the child (ages 9–60 months) cf. controls (n=35, Cummings *et al, Arch Dis Child* 2011;**96**:643–7).

Reviews: * Sabers, *Acta Neurol Scand* 2012; **126**:1–4; n = 19, Reimers *et al, Epilepsy Res* 2011;**94**:198–205; n = 1, Nordmo *et al, Ann Pharmacother* 2009;**43**:1893–7; n = 1956, EURAP Study Group, *Neurology* 2006;**66**:354–60.

27. **Lithium** (FDA = D; ADEC = D)

Fertility: Some reduced sperm motility has been reported (e.g. Shen *et al, J Pharm Pharmacol* 1992;**44**:534–6), but it is not clear if this is relevant. Pre-conception folate may reduce the risk of Ebstein's anomaly. NICE (Antenatal and Postnatal Mental Health Guideline, 2007) recommends:

- advise woman to stop lithium if planning a pregnancy, is well and not at high risk of relapse
- if woman becomes pregnant, is well and not at high risk of relapse, lithium should be stopped gradually over four weeks, but also informed that this may not remove the risk of cardiac defects (although the logic of this escapes many, bearing in mind the fetal heart would already be formed at that point)
- if the woman is unwell or at high risk of relapse, switch to an antipsychotic, stop lithium and restart in T2, or continuing lithium if at very high risk of relapse (where rapid withdrawal would be a risk factor).

Review: Clinical decision tool (n = 1, Restrepo *et al, Rev Bras Psiquiatr* 2010;**32**:95–8).

T1: Lithium completely equilibrates across the placenta. There is much dispute about the risk of MCMs, e.g. T1 exposure to lithium (n = 165) compared to bipolar controls (n = 72) and non-exposed controls (n=748) showed no increase in MCMs but an increased rate of miscarriages (OR = 1.94) and cardiovascular anomalies (4.1% vs 0.6%) but not once spontaneously resolving anomalies were excluded, with a single case of Ebstein's anomaly (Diav-Citrin *et al, Am J Psychiatry* 2014;**171**:785–94; see also n = 225, Yacobi and Ornoy, *Isr J Psychiatry Relat Sci* 2008;**45**:95–106; FFT). Lithium thus appears not to be an important human teratogen if used with adequate screening (including level II ultrasound and fetal echocardiography) to detect Ebstein's anomaly:

- *Ebstein's anomaly* is a rare congenital

3

downward displacement of the tricuspid valve into the right ventricle, with symptoms dependent on age, severity, and other cardiac abnormalities. It can be asymptomatic until later in life, but marked symptoms in the first few days of life carry a poor prognosis. Valve repair (rather than replacement) generally has a better long-term prognosis (Osiro *et al*, *Cardiol Rev* 2013;**21**:257–63; n = 42, Oxenius *et al*, *Cardiol Young* 2013;**23**:27–34)

- An extensive review concludes that the incidence of Ebstein's anomaly with lithium is 45–76/10,000 live births (cf. baseline rate of 0.7/10,000), and so lithium appears relatively safe cf. some antipsychotics, valproate and carbamazepine, but pre-conceptual folate supplementation is highly advisable (Gentile, *Expert Opin Drug Safety* 2012;**11**:425–37).

An important study (n = 101, retrospective, Viguera *et al*, *Am J Psychiatry* 2000;**157**:179–84) noted that:

- The heart is formed by four weeks and starts beating by five weeks so stopping lithium when pregnancy is confirmed is too late
- Stopping lithium raises the risk of relapse 2–3-fold but pregnancy itself is relatively 'risk neutral'. This > 50% relapse rate in the first 40 weeks is high, and the risk from consequentially needed drugs is high
- Relapse rates are much higher with rapid rather than gradual lithium discontinuation
- Women remaining stable during the first 40 weeks post-lithium discontinuation are three times more likely to relapse than non-pregnant women during weeks 41–62 (70% vs 24%)
- An unstudied option might be to stop lithium gradually as soon as pregnancy is known, then reintroduce it in T3. This risk must be weighed against the > 50% chance of relapsing if lithium is stopped abruptly.

T2–3: As renal clearance is increased higher doses may be needed, but as clearance reduces markedly near the end of T3, doses may need to be reduced by up to 30–50% in the last few weeks, or a few doses omitted close to delivery (n = 10 + 32, Newport *et al*, *Am J Psychiatry* 2005;**162**:2162–70). NICE recommends monitoring levels every four weeks until week 36, then weekly, then within the first 24 hours after childbirth, with doses adjusted according to those serum levels, and adequate fluid intake maintained.

Birth:

- A floppy baby syndrome can occur straight after birth but seems of very low incidence
- Higher lithium levels (> 0.64 mEq/l) increase the risk of floppy baby syndrome so reduce levels gradually in T3 (see above)
- Lithium levels rapidly return to normal after birth so reduced doses and careful monitoring are essential (Kieviet *et al*, *Neuropsychiatr Dis Treat* 2013;**9**:1257–66; FFT)
- Other symptoms develop within 24 hours and can last 2–10 days.

Breast-feeding: Lithium is often contraindicated in breast-feeding, but this is based on old and limited information. It can be quite safe with extra support and education (e.g. n = 4, Bogen *et al*, *Arch Women's Ment Health* 2012;**15**:69–72). Informed choice, careful monitoring (e.g. TDM of milk or infant plasma), U&Es and use of low doses are essential (Moretti *et al*, *Ther Drug Monit* 2003;**25**:364–6).

- Lithium breast milk levels can be around 40% but with wide interindividual variability (range 24–72%), with infant serum levels 5–200% of the mother's serum levels.
- A systematic study showed relatively low milk and infant lithium plasma levels with no serious or persistent adverse events noted (mbp = 10, Viguera *et al*, *Am J Psychiatry* 2007;**164**:342–5).

Review: Chaudron and Jefferson, *J Clin Psychiatry* 2000;**161**:79–90.

PND: Two studies of children exposed to lithium *in utero* showed normal physical, mental and cognitive development (except one child with minor dysfunction) over 5–10 years (n = 60, T1, Schou, *Acta Psychiatr Scand* 1976;**54**:193–7; n = 15, van der Lugt *et al*, *Early Hum Dev* 2012;**88**:375–8; FFT).

28. **Valproate** (FDA = D for epilepsy and mania but X for migraine; ADEC = D)

Valproate crosses the placenta easily and is now well-established as both teratogenic and causing developmental problems and should not be used in women of child-bearing potential (UK MHRA enhanced warning issued January 2016). There is undoubtedly a pharmacogenetic component to these effects (Duncan, *Curr Opin Neurol* 2007;**20**:175–80).

The general advice is (n = 1,109, Mawhinney *et al*, *Seizure* 2012;**21**:215–8;FFT; CEA-ILAE and EAN recommendations; Tomson *et al*, *Epilepsia* 2015;**56**:1006–19):

- Seek specialist consultation for women who could become pregnant on valproate
- Use the lowest effective monotherapy dose (below 1000 mg/d) as higher doses increase the risk of MCMs by 1.7
- There seems no differences between rates with MR vs plain versions, or once vs four times a day, so it seems total daily dose rather than peaks may be the main effect
- Start 5 mg folic acid as soon as, or before, contraception is discontinued (Ornoy, *Reprod Toxicol* 2009;**28**:1–10).

Review: general (Duncan, *Curr Opin Neurol* 2007; **20**:175–80).

Fertility: In women, valproate can lead to menstrual cycle abnormalities, polycystic ovary syndrome (PCOS) and hyperandrogenism. PCOS may have some effect on reproductive capacity (n = 32, O'Donovan *et al*, *J Clin Psychiatry* 2002;**63**:322–30; review by Genton *et al*, *Epilepsia* 2001;**42**:295–304), but this may be because valproate causes weight gain, a risk factor for PCOS. Valproate can increase serum androgen concentrations in men with epilepsy (Rättyä *et al*, *Neurology* 2001; **57**:440–4).

T1:

- Reduced birth-weight-adjusted mean head circumference has been shown, although the significance of this is unknown, but this has not been shown for phenytoin, clonazepam, lamotrigine and gabapentin (n = 900,000, Almgren *et al*, *Seizure* 2009;**18**:672–5;FFT)
- See PND for the effects of T1 valproate exposure on lowering IQ and on mental retardation.

T2–3: Towards the end of T3 decreased serum valproate levels have been reported (Philbert *et al*, *Acta Neurol Scand* 1985;**72**:460–3) perhaps by up to 50% although unbound levels may not change (Yerby *et al* *Neurology* 1992;**42** [4 Suppl 5]:12–16).

Birth: The UK SmPC notes that there have been rare reports of haemorrhagic syndrome (possibly related to decreased vitamin K factors), as well as hypoglycaemia and hypothyroidism.

Breast-feeding:

- Valproate is classified by the AAP as compatible with breast-feeding. Infant serum levels are usually 5–12% (range detectable to 40%) of the mother's serum level (n = 16, van Unruh *et al*, *Ther Drug Monit* 1984;**6**:272–6)
- In infant exposure exclusively via breast-feeding, mothers had valproate levels in the usual range for bipolar (39–79 mcg/mL), but the infants had low levels (0.7–1.5 mcg/mL), thus presenting a relatively low risk compared to the risk of relapse in the mother (mbp = 6, Piontek *et al*, *J Clin Psychiatry* 2000;**61**:170–2)
- Valproate appears relatively safe, but with a small but finite risk of haematological effects (review, Chaudron and Jefferson, *J Clin Psychiatry* 2000;**161**:79–90).

PND: Cochrane (s = 28, Bromley *et al*, *Cochrane Database Syst Rev* 2014; **10**:CD010236) concluded (see anticonvulsants 3.9.5 for full details) that with prenatal valproate exposure for epilepsy the developmental quotient (DQ) is lower than untreated, similar to carbamazepine, and that IQ is lower than unexposed, and lower than carbamazepine and lamotrigine.

In addition:

- Mean valproate IQs were higher with preconceptual folate supplement than unexposed (n = 311[c = 224], six years, Meador *et al*, *Lancet Neurology* 2013;**12**:244–52)
- There may be a seven times higher incidence of ASD cf the control group (6.3% vs 0.9%) with valproate monotherapy (n = 620 mothers, n = 632 live births, Bromley *et al*, *Neurology* 2008;**71**:1923–24) or polytherapy but lamotrigine or carbamazepine had no effect (n = 415, six years, Bromley *et al*, *J Neurol Neurosurg Psychiatry* 2013;**84**:637–43)
- There may be a higher than expected incidence of education needs statements (n = 400 school-age children: 150 exposed to monotherapy, 74 to polytherapy and 176 to none, Adab *et al*, *J Neurol Neurosurg Psychiatry* 2001;**70**:15–21; FFT).

3.9.4 ANXIOLYTICS AND HYPNOTICS

29. **Benzodiazepines** (alprazolam FDA = D, ADEC = C; bromazepam ADEC = C; chlordiazepoxide

FDA = C, ADEC = C; clobazam ADEC = C; clonazepam FDA = D, ADEC = C; diazepam FDA = D, ADEC = C; flunitrazepam FDA = D, ADEC = C; flurazepam ADEC = C; lorazepam FDA = D, ADEC = C; midazolam FDA = D, ADEC = C; nitrazepam FDA= C, ADEC = C; oxazepam FDA = D, ADEC = C; temazepam FDA = X, ADEC = C; triazolam FDA = X, ADEC = C)

Review: Anxiety disorders in pregnancy (Vythilingum, *Curr Psychiatry Rep* 2008;**10**:331–5).

Fertility: No human data.

T1:

- Data in the last 10 years does not show any absolute contraindication for BDZs in T1 (s = 12, Bellantuono *et al, Gen Hosp Psychiatry* 2013;**35**:3–8)
- For individual BDZs, a population-based case-control study indicated that alprazolam, clonazepam, medazepam and nitrazepam taken during pregnancy did not present a detectable teratogenic risk (n = 38151 + n=351785 controls, Eros *et al, Eur J Obstet Gynecol Reprod Biol* 2002;**101**:147–54).

Alprazolam: See above.

Chlordiazepoxide may have a slight increase in MCMs with use in months two and three, but no specific type or pattern was seen so the risk is unlikely to be substantial (n = 469, Czeizel *et al, Neurotoxicol Teratol* 2004;**26**:593–8) if used at low dose and avoided in T1 (Iqbal *et al, Conn Med* 2003;**67**:259–62).

Clobazam is known to cross the placenta but no teratogenicity has been reported.

Clonazepam: See above.

Diazepam crosses the placenta in T1 and there is a varying risk of oral clefts, with the worst case scenario bringing the risk to seven in 1000 (e.g. Rosenberg *et al, N Engl J Med* 1983;**309**:1282–5), but recent data suggests minimal teratogenicity (n = 97 cf. 6876 controls, Czeizel *et al, Clin Drug Investig* 2003;**23**:451–62) with, e.g. T1 use having a MCM rate of 2.7% (n = 1159) cf. controls 2.7% (n = 360978, Ban *et al, PLoS One* 2014;**9**:e100996).

Medazepam and **nitrazepam**: See above.

Temazepam: T1 use had a MCM rate of 2.9% (n = 379) cf. controls 2.7% (n = 19193 + 351785) (Ban *et al, PLoS One* 2014;**9**:e100996).

T2–3 overdoses:

There have been a series of reports of attempted suicide by benzodiazepine overdose during pregnancy, providing unique toxicity data:

Alprazolam (mean 30 mg, range 7.5–100 mg) had no significantly higher MCM rates, albeit with only 10 live births so an association could not be excluded (n = 10, Gidai *et al, Toxicol Ind Health* 2008;**24**:53–60).

Chlordiazepoxide had no evidence of a higher MCM rate but there was a dose-dependent intrauterine growth retardation with lower birth weight newborns (n = 88, live births = 35, Gidal *et al, Toxicol Ind Health* 2008;**24**:41–51).

Diazepam (range 25–800 mg) had a higher MCM rate (13.4% cf. 7.1% matched controls), but overdoses taken during T1 did not show excess abnormalities, suggesting the MCMs were unrelated to diazepam (n = 229; 112 live births, Gidai *et al, Toxicol Ind Health* 2008;**24**:29–39).

Nitrazepam (mean 204 mg) had a higher rate of MCMs (30% cf 10% controls), although most were reported to be mild (n = 43, Gidai *et al, Pharmacoepidemiol Drug Saf* 2010;**19**:175–82).

T2–3:

- Shorter-acting benzodiazepines on a 'when required' basis may be of a low risk in T2–3
- Placental transfer of diazepam is doubled if the mother has diabetes (n = 14) or hypertension (n = 30) cf. controls (n = 31) (n = 75, Lalic-Popovic *et al, BMC Pregnancy Childbirth* 2013;**13**:188).

Birth:

- Neonatal benzodiazepine withdrawal symptoms have been reported. The 'floppy baby' syndrome includes facial features and CNS dysfunction, particularly with higher doses (eg. > 30 mg diazepam equivalent per day) of longer-acting benzodiazepines (n = 8, Laegreid *et al, J Pediatrics* 1989;**114**:126–31)
- Oral BDZ use during T3 may delay feeding in full-term infants, but premature infants may have lower Apgar scores and respiratory depression (n = 53, open, Whitelaw *et al, BMJ* 1981;**282**:1106–8; FFT)
- **Diazepam** > 30 mg IM or IV during the last 15 hours of labour can induce neonatal respiratory depression, irregular heartbeat and feeding problems, although 10 mg given IV within 10 minutes of birth appears not to affect Apgar scores (n = 23, open, McAllister, *Br J Anaesth* 1980;**52**:423–7)
- **Lorazepam** can lead to the floppy baby syndrome and respiratory depression, especially if IV doses are used close to birth.

A single dose of lorazepam 2 mg 2–9 hours before delivery showed that pregnancy increased Vd and oral clearance, and reduced half-life (n = 10, Papini *et al, J Pharm Biomed Anal* 2006;**40**:397–403).

Breast-feeding:

- Benzodiazepines are excreted in breast milk and the general recommendation is to observe the infant for sedation and poor suckling. Repeated doses of long-acting BDZs can produce lethargy and weight loss, but low and single doses are probably of low risk, provided the infant is monitored for drowsiness, e.g. BDZs were not associated with increased CNS depression (not dose, feeding or drug-related) so can be used with careful postpartum monitoring or care (mbp = 124, Kelly *et al, J Pediatr* 2012;**161**:448–51)
- **Diazepam** (Stebler and Guentert, *Pharm Res* 1992;**9** :1299–305), **flunitrazepam** Jensen *et al, Tidsskr Nor Laegeforen* 1981;**101**:504–5), **lorazepam** (Lemmer *et al, J Anal Toxicol* 2007;**31**:224–6; FFT), **nitrazepam** (n = 22, RCT, Matheson *et al, Br J Clin Pharmacol* 1990;**30**:787–93; FFT) have all been shown in breast milk
- **Alprazolam** milk levels fluctuate with plasma levels, but only 3% reaches the baby, well below the notional level of concern (n = 8, Oo *et al, Br J Clin Pharmacol* 1995;**40**:231–6)
- **Lormetazepam** may show almost no accumulation, with infant intake 0.35% of maternal dose, of low risk (n = 5, Hümpel *et al, Eur J Clin Pharmacol* 1982;**21**:421–5)
- **Midazolam** barely appears to reach breast milk (Senel and Mergan, *Braz J Anesthiol* 2014;**64**:16–21; FFT)
- **Oxazepam** has a single case suggesting 0.1% of the maternal dose is excreted in breast milk (n = 1, Wretlind, *Eur J Clin Pharmacol* 1987;**33**:209–10)
- **Temazepam** infant levels are below detection levels at maternal doses of 10–20 mg/d, with no adverse effects seen (mbp = 10, Lebedevs *et al, Br J Clin Pharmacol* 1992;**33**:204–6).

PND:

- A small number of children exposed *in utero* to benzodiazepines have shown slow development in the early years, but by four years of age have developed normally
- Diazepam during T2 + 3 leads to a lower birth weight than controls but this normalises by 8/12 (n = 484, 12/24, Czeizel *et al, Neurotoxicol Teratol* 1999;**21**:157–67).

30. **Beta-blockers:** (FDA: **propranolol** = C; ADEC = C)

Fertility: No data.

T1: Beta-blockers are not generally considered teratogens but propranolol in T1 has been postulated to be linked with tracheosophageal fistulas and intrauterine growth retardation.

T2–3: Use in T2–3 may aggravate or produce neonatal hypoglycaemia or bradycardia complicated by placental insufficiency (e.g. severe maternal hypertension).

Birth: Due to direct cardiac effects, hypoglycaemia and apnea, it may be prudent to discontinue beta-blockers 1–2 weeks before delivery. Propranolol has been used as augmentation in labour without apparent untoward effects (n = 107, RCT, d/b, Palomäki *et al, Eur J Obstet Gynecol Reprod Biol* 2006;**125**:44–9).

Breast-feeding: The amounts in breast milk are probably too small to affect a baby (<0.1% of maternal doses), but could produce bradycardia and hypoglycaemia at high doses. Propranolol milk levels peak at around 2–3 hours with a breast milk half-life of around 6.5 hours (longer than in plasma), and the child would likely receive less than 0.1% of the maternal dose of propranolol (n = 3, Smith *et al, Ther Drug Monit* 1983;**5**:87–93; n = 28, Livingstone *et al, Clin Exp Hypertens B* 1983;**2**:341–50). The UK SmPCs do not recommend use.

PND: There is an increased risk of cardiac and pulmonary complications in the neonate in the postnatal period.

31. **Buspirone** (FDA = B; ADEC = B1)

Fertility: No data.

T1: There is no evidence of teratogenicity, but effects on survival and weights have been noted in some, but not all, animal tests.

T2–3 and birth: No data.

Breast-feeding: Buspirone should be avoided, based on excretion studies in rats, although there is no specific human data to show adverse effects.

PND: No data.

32a. **Chloral** (FDA = C, ADEC = A)

Fertility: No data.

T1: Chloral appears of low risk, as no increase in MCMs was seen in women who took chloral in T1

3

or at any time in pregnancy (n=429, Heinonen *et al, Birth Defects and Drugs in Pregnancy*, Publishing Sciences Group 1977:336–7).
T2–3 and birth: No data.
Breast-feeding: Chloral is excreted in breast milk and the sedation caused in the infant makes this a precaution, although only minimal sedation after large feeds has been reported (*Adv Drug React Bull* 1976; Dec:212). The AAP recommends chloral as compatible with breast-feeding, as do the authorities in many European countries.
PND: No data.

32b. **Clomethiazole** (ADEC=A)
Fertility: No data.
T1–3: The UK SmPC states clomethiazole should not be used, particularly in T1 and T3, although it has been used widely for pre-eclampsia.
Birth: No data.
Breast-feeding: Clomethiazole is excreted in insignificant amounts (based on old IV and oral studies in pre-eclampsia) and although an infant might be sedated by active amounts from breast milk this is unlikely to be harmful (n=4, Tunstall *et al, Br J Obstet Gynaecol* 1979;**86**:793–8).
PND: No data.

32c. **Hydroxyzine** (FDA=D; ADEC=A)
Fertility: No data.
T1: Hydroxyzine is contraindicated in early pregnancy as very high-dose animal tests induce fetal abnormalities (UK SmPC).
T2–3: Sedating antihistamines in late T3 may cause adverse effects in neonates such as irritability, paradoxical excitability, and tremor.
Birth: There is a single case of hypotonia, movement disorders including EPSEs, clonic movements, tachypnea and poor feeding with a mother taking 600 mg/d during pregnancy (UK SmPC).
Breast-feeding: The UK SmPC contraindicates hydroxyzine in breast-feeding.
PND: No data.

32d. **Promethazine** (FDA=C; ADEC=C)
Fertility: No data.
T1–3: Promethazine during T1–3 (n=127) had no effect on birth weight cf. (n=358) controls (12/24, Czeizel *et al, Neurotoxicol Teratol* 1999;**21**: 157–67). In pregnant women attempting suicide by taking up to 1780 mg there was no evidence of teratogenicity, although the total MCM rate was high in the whole cohort (n=32 from 1044 overdoses, Petik *et al, Toxicol Ind Health* 2008; **24**:87–96).
Birth: Promethazine is not recommended in the two weeks before delivery because of the risk of neonatal irritability and excitement (UK SmPC).
Breast-feeding: Promethazine is excreted into milk but probably at insignificant levels (UK SmPC).
PND: There was no evidence of lower IQ or development issues after overdoses of up to 1780 mg promethazine (n=32 from 1044 overdoses, Petik *et al, Toxicol Ind Health* 2008;**24**:87–96).

33. **Melatonin** (FDA=not classified, ADEC=B3)
Fertility: No data.
T1–3: Although data is lacking, melatonin is a naturally occurring compound, albeit used at higher oral doses. It has no apparent teratogenic effects but use is not recommended (SmPC).
Breast-feeding: Melatonin is probably secreted into human breast milk and so use by lactating mothers is not recommended (SmPC).
PND: No data.

34. **Pregabalin** (FDA=C, ADEC=B3)
Fertility: The UK SmPC states that a 3/12 trial in healthy males taking pregabalin 600 mg/day showed no effects on sperm motility. Some animal studies have shown adverse reproductive effects.
T1: Animal studies have shown some animal reproductive toxicity at high dose, but the human risk is not known (SmPC).
T2–3 and birth: No data.
Breast-feeding: Pregabalin is excreted into milk in animal studies, but as no adequate human data exists it is not recommended (SmPC).
PND: No data.

35. **Z hypnotics:** None of the three Z-hypnotics are contraindicated in pregnancy and short-term 'when required' use of zolpidem would appear to present only minimal risk.

35a. **Zaleplon** (FDA=C, ADEC=C)
Fertility: No data.
T1–3: Little information is currently available, but animal studies show no teratogenicity or embryotoxic effects (UK SmPC).
Birth: No data.
Breast-feeding: Zaleplon is excreted in breast milk and should not be taken by breast-feeding mothers, although the actual amount likely to be transferred may be very low, e.g. 0.017% of the maternal dose (n=5, Darwish *et al, J Clin Pharmacol* 1999;**39**:670–4).
PND: No data.

35b. **Zolpidem** (FDA=C; ADEC=B3)

Fertility: No data.
T1: Zolpidem crosses the placenta and clears rapidly from the fetal circulation. Keep doses as low as possible in T1 as some neural tube defects have been associated with high doses (n = 1, Sharma *et al, Curr Drug Saf* 2011;**6**:128–9).
T2–3: Late T3 use risks hypothermia, hypotonia and moderate respiratory depression in the infant and severe neonatal respiratory depression if used with other CNS depressants (UK SmPC).
Birth: There is a slight risk of low birth weight (1.4x), preterm deliveries (1.5x), small size (1.3x) and caesarean delivery (1.7x) if taking zolpidem regularly (n = 2497) compared to not (n = 12485, Wang *et al, Clin Pharmacol Ther* 2010;**88**:369–74; n = 45, Juric *et al, Arch Women's Ment Health* 2009;**12**:441–6). In a unique case maternal high-dose zolpidem (at least 1000 mg over at least one month), cord levels were less than the mean maternal plasma levels likely from a single 5 mg dose, and the neonate was alert and with no apparent withdrawal symptoms over the first 48 hours (n = 1, Askew, *Pharmacotherapy* 2007;**27**:306–8). Dependence in the mother could lead to a risk of withdrawal in the infant (UK SmPC).
Breast-feeding: The AAP considers zolpidem compatible with breast-feeding, as it is found only in minute amounts in milk due to its low lipophilic properties, has a rapid onset and nearly all is excreted within three hours of a dose (n = 5, Pons *et al, Eur J Clin Pharmacol* 1989;**37**:245–8). A low dose of 5–10 mg should be relatively low risk at bedtime if avoiding breast-feeding for the next 2–3 hours.
PND: No data.
35c. **Zopiclone** (FDA = C; ADEC = C) *
Fertility: No data.
T1: Zopiclone has shown no abnormalities in animal tests with no evidence of an increase in MCMs in hypnotic use in T1 (zopiclone 2.5%), compared to unexposed but depressed/anxious 2.7% (n = 19193) and controls 2.7% (n = 351785, Ban *et al, PLoS One* 2014;**9**:e100996).
T2–3: No data.
Birth: Dependence in the mother could lead to a risk of withdrawal in the infant.
Breast-feeding: Zopiclone is not recommended in breast-feeding, as it may be excreted in appreciable amounts (up to 50% of maternal levels: n = 12, Matheson *et al, Br J Clin Pharmacol* 1990;30:267–71) although the maximum infant intake would be 1.4% weight-adjusted maternal dose and the UK SmPC states that breast milk levels are low.
PND: No data.

3.9.5 ANTICONVULSANTS *

Pregnant women with epilepsy are at increased risk of complications, seizures and MCMs (6% polytherapy; 3.7% monotherapy; n = 3,607, Morrow *et al, J Neurol Neurosurg Psychiatry* 2006;**77**:193–8; FFT).

Summary of risk minimisation strategies

1. Pre-conception:

- Diagnosis should be verified and the need for anticonvulsants confirmed.
- Use adequate oral contraceptive dosage (see *C4.5*) until conception is planned
- Start regular multivitamins with folate (4–5 mg/d from before oral contraceptives are stopped, until at least 12 weeks of gestation) to reduce the risk of spina bifida, cardiovascular birth defects and oral clefts (n = 6932, Hernández-Díaz *et al, N Engl J Med* 2000;**343**:1608–14; FFT)
- Minimise exposure to AEDs with known risks. Use lowest dose monotherapy (Vajda *et al, Epilepsia* 2010;**51**:805–10) and avoid any AEDs in a second pregnancy if that AED caused a birth defect in the first pregnancy, especially valproate (n = 1,243, Vajda *et al, Epilepsia* 2013;**54**:181–6).

2. After conception:

- Risk minimisation, e.g. vitamin supplements.

3. Seizure control without toxicity:

- Do not switch drugs if stabilised
- Continue multivitamins with folate
- Continue monotherapy if possible and monitor free anticonvulsant concentrations frequently and adjust doses if necessary
- Vitamin K should be given during the last week of pregnancy if possible
- Ultrasound and AFPs should be carried out.

Reviews: AEDs in pregnancy (De Santis *et al, Curr Pharm Biotechnol* 2011;**12**:781–8), EURAP registry (Tomson *et al, Lancet Neurol* 2011;**10**:609–17), extensive (Hill *et al, Expert Rev Neurother* 2010;**10**:943–59;FFT), teratogenicity (Tomson and Battino, *Neurol Clin* 2009;**27**:993–1002), postnatal development (Meador *et al, N Engl J Med* 2009;**360**:1597–605; FFT), 2nd generation AEDs

3

in pregnancy (Reimers and Brodtkorb, *Expert Rev Neurother* 2012;**12**:707–17).

Fertility: Reproductive endocrine problems, e.g. PCOS, amenorrhea, premature menopause and hyperprolactinemia are reported to be more common in women with epilepsy than in the general female population.

T1–3: A major review (n=2600 cf. 711412 controls, Veiby *et al*, *J Neurol* 2014;**261**:579–88) concluded MCM rates were:

- Low with carbamazepine, lamotrigine, levetiracetam, oxcarbazepine, gabapentin, pregabalin
- Elevated with topiramate (substantially higher risk of fetal growth restriction) and valproate monotherapy, especially in repeated pregnancies.

Review: AEDs in pregnancy, including pharmacokinetics (Tomson *et al*, *Epilepsia* 2013;**54**:405–14).

Breast-feeding: Extensive reviews conclude that:

- Compatible with breast-feeding: carbamazepine, valproate and phenytoin
- Potentially unsafe: ethosuximide, levetiracetam, phenobarbital and primidone, so close clinical monitoring is recommended
- Data on the newer drugs is too sparse for reliable recommendations
- Occasional or short-term treatment with benzodiazepines could be considered compatible with breast-feeding (see benzodiazepines).

Reviews: general (Sabers and Tomson, *Curr Opin Neurol* 2009;**22**:157–61; Harden *et al*, *Epilepsia* 2009;**50**:1247–55; Davanzo *et al*, *Ital J Pediatr* 2013;**39**:50; FFT).

PND: An important longitudinal study of mothers taking AEDs during pregnancy and then when breast-feeding (mean 7/12) reported IQ and cognitive outcomes at six years:

- There was no adverse effects from AED exposure (CBZ, lamotrigine, phenytoin, valproate)
- IQ with valproate was 7–13 points lower
- Breast-fed infants had higher IQs at six years and enhanced verbal communication cf. non-breastfed infants.

(n=181, six years, Meador *et al*, *JAMA Pediatr* 2014; **168**:729–36; FFT).

Cochrane (s=28, Bromley *et al*, *Cochrane Database Syst Rev* 2014;**10**:CD010236) concluded that in epilepsy:

- Developmental quotient (DQ) is lower in children exposed to valproate (n=199) than children of women with untreated epilepsy (n=58) and children born to women without epilepsy (n=552)
- There is no significant difference in the DQ of children exposed to CBZ (n=210) versus VPA (n=160)
- IQ in children exposed to valproate (n=89) was lower than children born to women with untreated epilepsy (n=87)
- IQ of children exposed to VPA (n=112) was significantly lower than for those exposed to CBZ (n=191); lower with valproate (n=74) than lamotrigine (n=84); and lower with valproate (n=61) than phenytoin (n=45)
- A dose effect for valproate was reported in six studies, with higher doses (>800 mg/d or above) associated with a poorer cognitive outcome in the child.

36. **Barbiturates** (**phenobarbital** FDA=D, ADEC=D, **primidone** ADEC=D)

Fertility: No data.

T1: The incidence of MCMs with phenobarbital is very low (n=149 from 11,843 cases, Czeizel *et al*, *ISRN Obstet Gynecol* 2011;**2011**:719675; FFT), even in large overdoses (e.g. n=88, Timmermann *et al*, *Pharmacoepidemiol Drug Saf* 2009;**18**:815–25). The UK SmPC lists a range of MCMs. Folic acid can reduce the risks.

T2–3: See introduction.

Birth: Withdrawal symptoms, e.g. seizures and irritability, have been reported, some delayed by up to two weeks after birth, as have neonatal bleeding and respiratory depression.

Breast-feeding: Larger doses of phenobarbital and primidone may accumulate in breast milk and cause unacceptable drowsiness.

PND: There is evidence of poorer neurodevelopmental outcomes at two years than with levetiracetam (Maitre *et al*, *J Perinatol* 2013;**33**:841–6), and lower verbal intelligence, especially if used in T3 (s=2, n=267, Reinisch *et al*, *JAMA* 1995;**274**:1518–25).

37. **Gabapentin** (FDA=C, ADEC=B1)

Fertility: No human data is available, but adverse effects on sperm motility may occur in rats.

T1: Exposure to gabapentin in T1 has not been associated with an increased risk of MCMs cf no exposure (n=59, Mølgaard-Nielsen and Hviid, *JAMA* 2011;**305**:1996–2002; n=446, Fujii *et al, Neurology* 2013;**80**:1565–70; Southampton PMSS, n=3100, Wilton and Shakir, *Epilepsia* 2002;**43**:983–92). Gabapentin levels in the fetus were estimated to be 0.2–1.3 mg/kg/d (1.3–3.8% of mother's dose), with no adverse effects detected (n=6, Ohman *et al, Epilepsia* 2005;**46**:1621–4).

T2–3: No data.

Birth: There may be an increased risk of preterm births, lower birth weight and the need for special monitoring after birth (38% vs 3% unexposed; n=446, Fujii *et al, Neurology* 2013;**80**:1565–70).

Breast-feeding: Gabapentin crosses into breast milk but appears of lower risk, e.g. levels were estimated to be 6–12% of the mother's plasma level, but with no adverse effects detected (mbp=6, Ohman *et al, Epilepsia* 2005;**46**:1621–4; mbp=1, Kristensen *et al, J Hum Lact* 2006;**22**:426–8).

PND: No data.

38. **Levetiracetam** (FDA=C, ADEC=B3)

Fertility: No problems have been reported in animal (UK SmPC) or human studies (e.g. n=56, Svalheim *et al, Epilepsy Behav* 2009;**16**:281–7).

T1: Exposure in T1 does not appear to be associated with increased risk of MCMs cf no exposure (n=58, Mølgaard-Nielsen and Hviid, *JAMA* 2011;**305**:1996–2002). The UK SmPC notes over 1000 exposures in T1 and that the data does not suggest a substantial increase in MCMs.

T2–3: Levetiracetam crosses the placenta (the infant dose is equivalent to 7.9% of weight-normalised maternal dose), with plasma concentrations in the infant around 13% of mother's plasma levels (n=15, Abou-Khalil, *Epilepsy Curr* 2008;**8**:62–3; FFT). A significant fall in levetiracetam levels may occur during pregnancy (Tomson and Battino, *Clin Pharmacokinet* 2007;**46**:209–19) and BD dosing may be needed to maintain plasma levels (n=1, Garrity *et al, Pharmacotherapy* 2014;**34**:e128–32).

Birth: No data.

Breast-feeding: Levetiracetam is excreted in milk and unusually high levels can occur (Pennell, *Neurology* 2003;**61**[6 Suppl 2]:S35–S42), so breast-feeding is not recommended.

PND: Levetiracetam during pregnancy appears to have no effect on the development of the child, at least up to the age of two (n=192, Shallcross *et al, Neurology* 2011;**76**:383–9; FFT), and is a better option than valproate (n=228, Shallcross *et al, Neurology* 2014;**82**:213–21).

39. **Oxcarbazepine** (FDA=C, ADEC=D)

Oxcarbazepine is closely related to carbamazepine.

Fertility: No data.

T1: There is significant placental transfer in humans but no association with increased risk of MCMs cf no exposure (n=393, Mølgaard-Nielsen and Hviid, *JAMA* 2011;**305**:1996–2002). See also below for plasma level advice.

T2–3: Plasma levels may decrease markedly during pregnancy so careful monitoring throughout pregnancy and immediately afterwards is essential (n=5, Mazzucchelli *et al, Epilepsia* 2006;**47**:504–9).

- 1st trimester: levels 70–75% of baseline
- 2nd trimester: levels 60–75% of baseline
- 3rd trimester: levels 60–65% of baseline
- Postnatal: levels 108% of baseline.

Birth: No data.

Breast-feeding: Oxcarbazepine is excreted into breast milk; the breast milk/plasma ratio for drug and metabolite being about 0.5, similar to carbamazepine (n=1, Bülau *et al, Eur J Clin Pharmacol* 1988;**34**:311–3). It is not recommended.

PND: Normal development has been reported at 6/12 when taken thought pregnancy (n=2, Eisenschenk, *Neurologist* 2006;**12**:249–54).

Reviews: (n=10 [13 pregnancies], Petrenaite *et al, Epilepsy Res* 2009;**84**:245–9; n=1,956, EURAP Study Group, *Neurology* 2006;**66**:354–60; n=13, Petrenaite *et al, Epilepsy Res* 2009;**84**:245–9).

40. **Phenytoin** (FDA=D, ADEC=D)

Phenytoin is higher risk but withdrawal may be a greater risk than continued use, so the following precautions are recommended:

1. Use minimal effective doses, at least monthly blood level monitoring (including free levels) during T1–3 and for six months afterwards.
2. Use folic acid 5 mg/d from before conception (e.g. n=1,935, Morrow *et al, J Neurol Neuro surg Psychiatry* 2009;**80**:506–11).

Fertility: Epileptic fathers taking phenytoin may have increased rates of malformed children (Friis, *Acta Neurol Scand* 1983;**94**[Suppl]:39–43).

T1: Phenytoin teratogenicity is well-established, particularly the 'fetal hydantoin syndrome', e.g. growth retardation, microcephaly, mental retardation, facial defects, and others. The full syndrome occurs in about 8–10% of children (n=88, Rodríguez-Palomares *et al, Arch Med Res* 1995;**26**:371–7), and a part syndrome in a further 30% of children (n=34, Nulman *et al, Am J Med Genet* 1997;**68**:18–24) and appears not to be

3

dose-related (n=88, Rodriguez-Palomares *et al*, *Arch Med Res* 1995;**26**:371–7).

T2–3: Phenytoin elimination increases and plasma levels fall steadily as pregnancy progresses, but free (i.e. active) levels may be unchanged, so care is needed with plasma level interpretation (Eadie *et al*, *Eur J Clin Pharmacol* 1992;**43**:389–92).

Birth: Phenytoin inhibits vitamin K-dependent clotting factors synthesis so neonatal haemorrhage may occur. Early vitamin K supplementation to the neonate is recommended after birth.

Breast-feeding: Small amounts of phenytoin are excreted in breast milk (SmPC), peaking at three hours, and have been considered clinically safe.

PND: Phenytoin is associated with a subtle but significant reduction in locomotor development at five years (n=133, 15 years, Wide *et al*, *Acta Paediatr* 2002;**91**:409–14), and significantly lower mean IQ and language ability (n=34, Scolnik *et al*, *JAMA* 1994;**271**:767–70).

41. **Topiramate** * (FDA=D; ADEC=D)

Despite conflicting data the general consensus is that topiramate is associated with significant risks in T1.

Fertility: No data.

Plasma levels: TDM and dose adjustment is advised to avoid the risk of increased seizures (n=12, Westin *et al*, *Epilepsia* 2009;**50**:480–5), as there is significant interindividual variation (n=10, Ohman *et al*, *Epilepsy Res* 2009;**87**:124–9). In general:

- T1 maternal levels may rise by around 32%
- T2 maternal levels may rise by 81%
- T3 maternal levels may rise by 75%.

T1: Topiramate crosses the placenta and most data suggests a problem, especially with polytherapy and if used for epilepsy rather than for migraines (n=1163, Castilla-Puentes *et al*, *Epilepsy Res* 2014;**108**:717–24):

- Monotherapy has a three-fold increased risk of MCMs, e.g. cleft lip/palate, hypospadias (SmPC). The FDA states the risk of oral clefts with topiramate is 1.4% vs. 0.38–0.55% with other AEDs, and 0.07% with no AED
- *Oral clefts:* There is a clear risk of cleft lip (OR=5.4) with or without cleft palate (n=3068) cf. controls (n=15480) (n=18548, Margulis *et al*, *Am J Obstet Gynaecol* 2012;**207**:405.e1–7). The UK Epilepsy and Pregnancy Register showed 17% abnormalities with oral clefts at 2.2%, about 11 times the background rate (n=203, Hunt *et al*, *Neurology* 2008;**71**:272–6). The most recent study showed a five-fold increase (never exposed=0.07%; stopped topiramate or other AEDs before pregnancy=0.14%; topiramate 0.36%; n=29071, Mines *et al*, *Pharmacoepidemiol Drug Saf* 2014;**23**:1017–25).

But not all data supports this:

- Topiramate monotherapy MCM rates were 2.4%, not statistically different to background rates (e.g. n=108, Mølgaard-Nielsen and Hviid, *JAMA* 2011;**305**:1996–2002), but the polytherapy rate was higher (14%), which may be dose-related in T1 (n=1625, Vajda *et al*, *Acta Neurol Scand* 2014;**130**:234–8)
- There was no significantly increased risk of cleft lip (0.23% vs 0.17% other AEDs vs 0.26 for diabetics) or other MCMs (n=146,770, Green *et al*, *Headache* 2012;**52**:1070–84).

T2–3:

- Up to 79% have a low birth weight (<2500 grams) cf. controls (UK SmPC; n=52, Ornoy *et al*, *Reprod Toxicol* 2008;**25**:388–9) and mean 1 cm lesser neonatal length (n=347, Hernández-Díaz *et al*, *Obstet Gynaecol* 2014;**123**:21–8), although a causal relationship has not been established
- Plasma levels may rise (see above).

Birth: No data. Plasma levels may fall (see above).

Breast-feeding: Topiramate is not recommended as no systematic human information is currently available, although there is one report of a healthy outcome with breast-feeding (n=1, Gentile, *Clin Drug Investig* 2009;**29**:139–41).

PND: Topiramate exposure in T1–3 may lead to worse cognitive functioning at 3–7 years, as well as motor function and behaviour, suggesting subtle effects (n=21, Rihtman *et al*, *Reprod Toxicol* 2012;**34**:308–11).

3.9.6 OTHERS *

42. **ADHD:**

ADHD treatments (n=480) may double the risk of miscarriage (n=1054494, Haervig *et al*, *Pharmacoepidemiol Drug Saf* 2014;**23**:526–33).

Review: ADHD treatments and pregnancy (Besag, *Drug Saf* 2014;**37**:397–408).

42a. **Atomoxetine** (FDA=C, ADEC=B3)

Fertility: No data.

T1: Animal studies show no harmful effects. Human

data is lacking (UK SmPC) apart from some unpublished reports (mentioned in Humphreys *et al, Can Fam Physician* 2007;**53**:1153–5).
T2–3: See introduction.
Birth: Animal data suggests no problems (US PI).
Breast-feeding: Animal studies show excretion into breast milk but human data is not available (UK SmPC).
PND: No data.

42b. **Dexamfetamine** (FDA=C, ADEC=B3)
Fertility: no data
T1: There was no increased risk of MCMs shown in women taking dexamfetamine for weight loss (n=1694) and not abusing other drugs, compared to controls (n=8989) (Milkovich and van der Berg, *Am J Obstet Gynecol* 1977;**129**:637–42).
T2–3: Amfetamines are associated with adverse outcomes (s=10, n=92,585, Ladhani *et al, Am J Obstet Gynecol* 2011;**205**:219.e1–7), including significantly lower birth weight, e.g. 4% lower if dexamfetamine is taken after week 28 but with no change in birth length or head circumference (Golub *et al, Birth Defects Res B Dev Reprod Toxicol* 2005;**74**:471–584).
Birth: No data
Breast-feeding: Dexamfetamine readily transfers to breast milk, but the relative infant dose is <10%, below the nominal level of concern (n=4 pairs, Ilett *et al, Br J Clin Pharmacol* 2007;**63**:371–5).
PND: No data

42c. **Lisdexamfetamine** (FDA=C, ADEC=B3)
Fertility: A rat study showed no harmful effects (UK SmPC).
T1–3: See dexamfetamine.
Birth: No data.
Breast-feeding: Lisdexamfetamine is excreted in milk and use is not recommended (UK SmPC).
PND: No data.

42d. **Methylphenidate** (FDA=C; ADEC=B2)
Fertility: No data is available but no relevant effects were observed in non-clinical studies (UK SmPC).
T1: A recent systematic review concluded that concomitant drugs and poor data mean that no conclusions can be drawn about MTH in pregnancy and lactation, and of the 41 reported cases there were five MCMs but it was unclear if there was selective reporting (s=3, n=41, Bolea-Alamañac *et al, Br J Clin Pharmacol* 2014;**77**:96–101). The Swedish (n=180, Dideriksen *et al, Basic Clin Pharmacol Toxicol* 2013;**112**:73–6) and Danish Birth Registry studies showed no statistically significant increase in MCMs or cardiac malformations with T1 exposure (n=222 vs n=2220 controls, Pottegård *et al, J Clin Psychiatry* 2014;**75**:e88–93).
T2–3: See introduction.
Birth: Neonatal cardiorespiratory toxicity (specifically tachycardia and respiratory distress) have been reported (UK SmPC).
Breast-feeding: Data is limited, but of the reported cases there were no problems (n=4, Bolea-Alamañac *et al, Br J Clin Pharmacol* 2014;**77**:96–101), with no methylphenidate detectable in breast milk 20–21 hours after the last dose of a plain tablet (probably because of its short half-life of 2–3 hours), so breast-feeding before a morning dose should have a low risk (n=1, Spigset *et al, Am J Psychiatry* 2007;**164**:348). The UK SmPC quotes an infant who experienced an unspecified decrease in weight during the period of exposure, but recovered and gained weight after the mother discontinued treatment (UK SmPC).
PND: No human data.

42e.* **Guanfacine** (FDA=B)
Fertility: No female human data is available but animal studies suggest no effect at toxic doses. In males some reduced male fertility occurred in rats at 10 times the human dose.
T1: Not recommended. There is some animal data for reproductive toxicity but only at toxic doses. US FDA shows no proven risk in humans.
T2–3: No data.
Birth: No data.
Breast-feeding: Not known, animal studies suggest it is excreted in milk.
PND: No data.

43–44. **Anticholinesterases and memantine**
Donepezil (FDA=C; ADEC=B3), **rivastigmine** (FDA=B; ADEC=B2), **galantamine** (FDA=B; ADEC=B1), **memantine** (FDA=B, ADEC=B2)
Fertility: No data.
T1–3: Very high doses of donepezil may have some minor effects in pregnancy, but no noted teratogenicity. The safety of rivastigmine or galantamine in pregnancy have not been established, although animal studies show a slight delay in fetal and neonatal development. Human data is lacking with memantine, but animal data suggest potentially reduced interuterine growth.
Breast-feeding: There is no information available on donepezil, galantamine, rivastigmine and memantine (which may appear in milk), so they

should not be used in breast-feeding mothers.
PND: No data.
45. **Anticholinergics** (**benzatropine** ADEC=B2; **biperiden** FDA=C, ADEC=B2; **orphenadrine** FDA=C; **procyclidine** FDA=C, ADEC=A; **trihexyphenidyl/benzhexol** FDA=C, ADEC=B1)
Fertility: No data
T1–3: There is little data available apart from an uncomplicated outcome from higher dose trihexyphenidyl in pregnancy (n=2, Robottom and Reich, *Neurologist* 2011;**17**:340–1). The UK SmPC notes that there are no studies with orphenadrine, so it should only be used if there is no safer alternative.
Birth: No data
Breast-feeding: There is no data for anticholinergics, but the UK SmPC for orphenadrine notes that mothers should not breast-feed.
PND: No data.
46. **Alcohol dependence:**
46a. **Acamprosate** (FDA=C, ADEC=B2)
Fertility: Animal data shows no problems but no human data is available (UK SmPC).
T1: Acamprosate is contraindicated in pregnancy (SmPC), but animal studies show no problems.
T2–3 and birth: No data.
Breast-feeding: Acamprosate is excreted in milk in some animal studies but human data is lacking (UK SmPC).
PND: No data.
46b. **Disulfiram** (FDA= C, ADEC=B2)
Fertility: No data.
T1–3: For disulfiram there have been isolated reports of MCMs (e.g. Reitnauer *et al*, *Teratology* 1997;**56**:358–62), although other drugs were often taken and the symptoms were similar to the fetal alcohol syndrome. Disulfiram is embryotoxic in some animals.
Birth: See PND.
Breast-feeding: No information is available to date on disulfiram in breast milk, so use with great caution. There is the possibility of interaction with alcohol in paediatric medicines (see *4.7.1*).
PND: There are cases of normal birth and PND after T1 disulfiram exposure (n=2, Helmbrecht and Hoskins, *Am J Perinatol* 1993;**10**:5–7).
46c. **Nalmefene** (FDA=B)
Fertility: Animal data shows no reduction in fertility (US PI, UK SmPC).
T1–3: There are fewer than 300 pregnancy outcomes known and no data is available.
Birth: There is a risk of acute withdrawal syndrome (UK SmPC) and antagonism of opiate analgesics.
Breast-feeding: Nalmefene is excreted in rat milk, but no human data is available.
PND: No human data is available but any risk would need to be balanced against the risk of alcohol.
46d. **Naltrexone** (FDA=C, ADEC=B3)
Fertility and T1: no data
T2–3: Naltrexone has no formal data but reproductive toxicity has been shown in animals. Use in late pregnancy would risk a withdrawal syndrome and antagonising opiate analgesics.
Birth: See above.
Breast-feeding: There is limited clinical data so is not recommended. One infant received about 1% of the mother's naltrexone dose over 24 hours (n=1, Chan *et al*, *J Hum Lact* 2004;**20**:322–6).
PND: A case series showed no problems and normal development with T1–3 naltrexone (n=7, Hulse *et al*, *Aust N Z J Obstet Gynaecol* 2001;**41**:424–8).
47. **Opiate dependence**
The risks of **methadone** and **buprenorphine** need to be compared to untreated substance misuse, with its low birth weight pre-term births (31% vs 8%) and growth restriction (n=247 vs 741, four years, Pinto *et al*, *Eur J Obstet Gynecol Reprod Biol* 2010;**150**:137–41). Methadone maintenance throughout pregnancy is associated with reduced risk of poor quality street drug use, earlier and better antenatal care and improved treatment retention (n=2,993, Burns *et al*, *Addiction* 2007;**102**:264–70), cf. tapered withdrawal (n=175, Jones *et al*, *Am J Addict* 2008;**17**:372–86).
47a. **Buprenorphine** * (FDA=C; ADEC=C) may have some advantages over methadone in pregnancy (review by Soyka, *CNS Drugs* 2013;**27**: 653–62). See also 47c.
An extensive review concludes that in opioid-dependent pregnant women buprenorphine:
- Is comparable in efficacy with methadone
- Causes less suppression of the fetal heart rate than methadone
- Produces less severe NAS than methadone
- Is compatible with breast-feeding
- Has no deleterious effects *in utero* (s=3 RCTs, s=44 non-RCTs, Jones *et al*, *Addiction* 2012;**107**(Suppl 1):5–27).

Fertility: Buprenorphine (13%) may cause less sexual dysfunction than methadone (52%) (s=16, n=1570, Yee *et al*, *J Sex Med* 2014;**11**:22–32).

Substances of misuse in pregnancy *

The general principles (Keen, *PharMag* 2012;**11**:3–4) are that two people (mother and baby) are involved:

1. Illicit and prescribed drugs can be harmful to the developing fetus, and so their effects must be minimised — relapse to heroin should be avoided at almost all costs.
2. Dose adjustments may be necessary due to changes in maternal metabolism.
3. NAS is a risk after delivery with all opiates (illicit or otherwise).
4. Overall poor health and nutrition may also adversely affect outcomes and engagement.
5. Pregnancy may present a window of opportunity to achieve dose reduction or abstinence.
6. Breast-feeding should be encouraged (except if HIV-positive), as it can ameliorate NAS.
7. Dose increases may be necessary in some people during the third trimester due to increased blood volume, haemodilution and altered liver metabolism. BD dosage may be useful.
8. Dose reductions may be necessary after pregnancy due to reduced blood volumes.
9. Buprenorphine can present problems with analgesia during delivery.

T1: Surprisingly, little data is available on T1 exposure, although there are uneventful cases of buprenorphine taken before and throughout pregnancy (n=2, Schindler *et al*, *Addiction* 2003;**98**:103–10). Buprenorphine with naloxone seems to have no differential effects to pure buprenorphine in pregnancy (n=10 vs + s=7, Lund *et al*, *Subst Abuse* 2013;**7**:61–74; n=62, Weigand *et al*, *Obstet Gynaecol* 2015;**125**:363–8).
T2–3: Increased buprenorphine renal elimination in T3 may require higher doses, but with significant intrasubject differences (n=9, Kacinko *et al*, *Clin Chem* 2009;**55**:1177–87; FFT).
Birth:

- High-dose buprenorphine (n=159) throughout T1–3 showed that, like methadone, there was no relationship between dose and duration or severity of NAS (n=251, Simmat-Durand *et al*, *Eur J Obstet Gynecol Reprod Biol* 2008:**142**:119–23)
- There are low buprenorphine levels in the mothers' serum at standard doses and low transfer to the infant at birth (mbp=10, Bartu *et al*, *Aust N Z J Obstet Gynaecol* 2012;**52**:342–7).

Breast-feeding:

- Buprenorphine is contraindicated in breast-feeding (UK SmPC) as buprenorphine and norbuprenorphine are detectable in infant's urine. The infant-exposed dose has been calculated at under 1%, supporting use during breast-feeding (mbp=7, Lindemalm *et al*, *J Hum Lact* 2009;**25**:199–205)
- Breast-fed infants have less severe NAS and are less likely to need pharmacological treatment (mbp=85, O'Connor *et al*, *J Midwifery Women's Health* 2013;**58**:383–8) and no adverse effect were seen at four weeks in one cohort (mbp=7, Gower *et al*, *J Hum Lact* 2014;**30**:217–23)
- * NAS may be prolonged if buprenorphine is taken with concurrent antidepressants (n=148, O'Connor *et al*, *J Matern Fetal Neonatal Med* 2016;**29**:112–4)
- A mean dose of 7 mg/d (range 2.4–24) buprenorphine and norbuprenorphine via milk is unlikely to cause any acute ADRs in breast-fed infants (mbp=7, Ilett *et al*, *Breastfeed Med* 2012;**7**:269–74).

PND: No data. See also 47c.

47b. **Methadone** (FDA=C, ADEC=C)

Fertility: No data, see also buprenorphine.

T1:

- With potentially illicit drug-using mothers, the teratogenicity of methadone will be difficult to ascertain, but there does not appear to be a clear association with MCMs. Stopping opiates abruptly is dangerous, as withdrawal reactions can damage the fetus more than methadone
- Multiple drug exposure may potentiate the effects of methadone on the fetus (n=49, Jansson *et al*, *Drug Alcohol Depend* 2012;**122**:213–9; FFT)
- Therapeutic opiates in T1 have been linked with some birth defects especially heart anomalies, but the absolute risk is still low (n=24,150, Broussard *et al*, *Am J Obstet Gynecol* 2011:**204**:e1–11)
- Methadone clearance can be increased,

with trough plasma levels dropping to 58% of baseline, which may require higher doses (n = 9, Wolff *et al*, *Eur J Clin Pharmacol* 2005;**61**:763–8).

T2–3:

- Methadone exposure may be associated with a 2.5x greater risk of very pre-term birth (<32/52), small for gestational age (3x), and MCMs (2x) (n = 618 cf. 61030, Cleary *et al*, *Am J Obstet Gynecol* 2011;**204**:139e1–9)
- Sub-therapeutic dosing in T2–3 may lead to withdrawal symptoms and use of additional illicit opiates (n = 904, Delano *et al*, *PLoS One* 2013;**8**:e82647), so adequate dosing is needed to avoid risky behaviour
- Methadone clearance may be increased (see T1 above).

Review: general (s = 10, Shiu and Ensom, *Can J Hosp Pharm* 2012;**65**:380–6).

Birth: The symptoms of NAS (neonatal absence syndrome; Bio *et al*, *J Perinatol* 2011;**31**:692–701) include tremor, irritability, hyperactivity, jitteriness, shrill cry, vomiting, diarrhoea and convulsions. About 45% of infants develop NAS with maternal methadone requiring treatment (median stay 10/7), but the incidence can be reduced by breast-feeding (n = 450, Dryden *et al*, *BJOG* 2009;**116**:665–71) and using a set protocol (McCarthy *et al*, *J Addict Med* 2015;**9**:105–10).

- *NAS duration:* each 1 mg/d of methadone taken before delivery adds an extra 0.18 days to the duration of NAS or, to put it another way, each 5.5 mg/d adds a day to NAS (n = 68, retrospective, Lim *et al*, *Am J Obstet Gynecol* 2009;**200**:70.e1–5).
- *Dose relationship:* NAS has been reported to be higher with 40 mg/d methadone than 20 mg/d, and >40 mg/d than 40 mg/d, but a meta-analysis showed no significant association so methadone dose is only one factor in development of NAS (meta-analysis, s = 29, Cleary *et al*, *Addiction* 2010;**105**:2071–84), along with overall maternal drug use (n = 81, McCarthy *et al*, *Am J Obstet Gynecol* 2005;**193**:606–10) and illicit drug use (n = 330, offspring n = 300, Seligman *et al*, *J Pediatr* 2010;**157**:428–33), such as opiates, benzodiazepines or cocaine (n = 117, Cleary *et al*, *Addiction* 2012;**107**:1482–92).
- *Infant adverse effects:* At lower doses, there may be a linear relationship between dose and infant ADRs (n = 32 + 42 controls, Wouldes and Woodward, *Neurotoxicol Teratol* 2010;**32**:406–13). Maternal methadone-exposed infants usually show excessive early weight loss, peaking at day five and more marked in formula-fed infants (n = 354, Dryden *et al*, *Arch Dis Child Fetal Neonatal Ed* 2012;**97**:F214–6). Head circumference and birth weight may be slightly lower compared to controls (n = 32, Brown *et al*, *Am J Obstet Gynecol* 1998;**179**:459–63).
- *Infant mortality:* There may be a six times higher risk of mortality in infants (especially SIDS) of mothers on methadone maintenance than all other mothers (Burns *et al*, *Drug Alcohol Rev* 2010;**29**:551–6).

Breast-feeding: Methadone is now generally considered compatible with breast-feeding:

- Methadone concentrations in milk seem unrelated to maternal dose, may peak about three hours post-dose, but are small (at 21–314 ng/mL; n = 12, Jansson *et al*, *J Hum Lact* 2007;**23**:184–90), increase gradually over 30 days (e.g. n = 16, 30/7, Jansson *et al*, *Pediatrics* 2008;**121**:106–14) and are insufficient to prevent the development of NAS (mbp = 8, Begg *et al*, *Br J Clin Pharmacol* 2001;**52**:681–5), although they might help
- Breast-feeding by drug-dependent mothers reduces NAS, delays the onset of NAS and decreases the need for pharmacological interventions, regardless of gestation and type of drug
- Stopping methadone is also dangerous as withdrawal reactions can damage the fetus.

PND:

- *Long-term development:* Outcomes at six months seem unaffected by methadone (n = 268, 6/12, Kaltenbach and Finnegan, *Neurotoxicol Teratol* 1987;**9**:311–3; effect in the first year see mbp = 190, Abdel-Latif *et al*, *Pediatrics* 2006;**117**:1163–9)
- *Mortality:* Children under one year are at no greater risk of dying after T1–3 methadone than matched controls (Kelly *et al*, *J Popul Ther Clin Pharmacol* 2012;**19**:e160–5)
- *Eyesight:* There may be an eyesight risk for children of mothers taking methadone in pregnancy, e.g. acuity (95%), nystagmus (70%), delayed visual maturation (50%),

strabismus (30%), refractive errors (30%), and cerebral visual impairment (25%), although the underlying causes are unclear (n=20, Hamilton *et al, Br J Ophthamol* 2010;**94**:696–700).

47c. **Buprenorphine vs methadone**

T1–3:

- Both appear viable in pregnancy, but buprenorphine may be the drug of choice due to a lesser effect on neonatal growth parameters (n=139, Welle-Strand *et al, Drug Alcohol Depend* 2013;**127**:200–6)
- Cochrane (s=4, n=271, Minozzi *et al, Cochrane Database Syst Rev* 2013;**12**:CD006318) could find no significant differences between methadone, buprenorphine and morphine MR in pregnancy. Methadone had slightly higher treatment-retention and buprenorphine had less severe and later-onset NAS, and may cause less suppression of spontaneous motor activity in fetuses compared to methadone (n=13, Jansson *et al, Neurotoxicol Teratol* 2011;**33**:240–3; FFT).

Birth:

- Cochrane concludes there is no proven significant difference between the available opiate agonists regarding NAS and birth weight, but the data sample was still small (s=4, n=271, Minozzi *et al, Cochrane Database Syst Rev* 2013;**12**:CD006318).

Neonatal Abstinence Syndrome (NAS):

- Infants exposed to buprenorphine need significantly less morphine for NAS (mean 1.1 mg vs 10.4 mg), hospital stays are shorter by 43% (21 vs 14 days; n=152, Pritham *et al, J Obstet Gynecol Neonatal Nurs* 2012;**41**:180–90), and NAS duration is shorter by 41% than those exposed to methadone, although the incidence of NAS was the same, just less severe with buprenorphine (n=175 [c=131], RCT, d/b, Jones *et al, N Engl J Med* 2010;**363**:2320–31; FFT)
- *The incidence of NAS with buprenorphine-naloxone is 25–26% cf. 52–80% with methadone (n=62, Wiegand *et al, Obstet Gynecol* 2015;**125**:363–8; Nanda *et al, W V Med J* 2015;**111**:16–21).

PND: Over the first month, buprenorphine-exposed babies showed better neurobehavioural scores and less severe withdrawal than methadone (n=39, RCT, d/b, 1/12, Coyle *et al, Addiction* 2012;**107** Suppl 1:63–73).

Reviews: extensive review of methadone, naltrexone and buprenorphine (Farid *et al, Curr Neuropharmacol* 2008;**6**:125–50; FFT), naltrexone in pregnancy (Jones *et al, Addiction* 2013;**108**:233–47), methadone vs buprenorphine (Konijnenberg and Melinder, *Child Neuropsychol* 2011;**17**:495–519; Jones *et al, Drugs* 2012;**72**:747–57), management of NAS (Grim *et al, Clin Perinatol* 2013;**40**:509–24).

48a. **Modafinil** (FDA=C, ADEC=B3)

Fertility: No data is available but modafinil may reduce the effect of OCs (UK SmPC).

T1–3: Modafinil is contraindicated in pregnancy (*Drug Safety Update* 2011;**4**:A1). Animal studies have shown some reproductive toxicity (UK SmPC).

Birth: No data.

Breast-feeding: Modafinil is not recommended.

PND: No data.

48b. **Sodium oxybate** (FDA=B)

Fertility: Rat studies show no adverse effects (UK SmPC).

T1: No data.

T2–3 and birth: There is limited data on oxybate, with no evidence of malformations or toxicity with T2–3 exposure, but it is not recommended. The UK SmPC notes a possible increased risk of spontaneous abortions.

Breast-feeding: Oxybate is not recommended but there is no human data available (SmPC).

PND: No data.

48c. **Prazosin** (FDA=C, ADEC=B2)

Fertility: No data.

T1–3: Prazosin has been linked with increased risk of intrauterine deaths (RCT, Hall *et al, BJOG* 2000;**107**:759–65), but there is no evidence of teratogenicity as monotherapy or in combination in T2–3.

Birth: No data.

Breast-feeding: Prazosin is excreted in small amounts in human milk so some caution would be needed (UK SmPC).

PND: No data.

3.10 RENAL IMPAIRMENT (SEE ALSO BNF)

	Lower risk	Moderate risk	Higher risk
Antipsychotics		Aripiprazole[1] Butyrophenones[8] Clozapine[2] Lurasidone[3] Olanzapine[4] Phenothiazines[9] Pimozide[11] Quetiapine[5] Thioxanthenes[10] Ziprasidone[11]	Amisulpride[7] Paliperidone[6] Risperidone[6] Sulpiride[7]
Antidepressants *	Agomelatine[14] Mianserin[21] Moclobemide[18] Tricyclics[13] Trazodone[20] Tryptophan[21] Vortioxetine[16]	Bupropion[15] Duloxetine[16] MAOIs[23] Mirtazapine[17] Reboxetine[19] SSRIs (most)[12]	Fluoxetine[12c] Sertraline[12e] Venlafaxine[22]
Anxiolytics and hypnotics	Zaleplon[35] Zopiclone[35]	Benzodiazepines[29] Beta-blockers[30] Clomethiazole[32] Hydroxyzine[32] Melatonin[33] Zolpidem[35]	Buspirone[31] Chloral[32] Pregabalin[34]
Mood and bipolar	Asenapine[24]	Carbamazepine[25] Lamotrigine[26] Olanzapine[4] Quetiapine[5]	Lithium[27] Valproate[28]
Anticonvulsants	Phenytoin[40]	Barbiturates[36] Benzodiazepines[29] Carbamazepine[25] Lamotrigine[26] Topiramate[41]	Gabapentin[37] Levetiracetam[38] Midazolam[29] Oxcarbazepine[39] Pregabalin[34] Valproate[28]
Others	Anticholinesterases[43] Sodium oxybate[48]	Anticholinergics[45] Atomoxetine[42] Buprenorphine[47] Bupropion[15] Disulfiram[46] Memantine[44] Modafinil[48] Nalmefene[46] Naltrexone[46]	Acamprosate[46] Dexamfetamine[42] Guanfacine[42] Lisdexamfetamine[42] Lithium[27] Methylphenidate[42]

Grade	GFR ml/min	Serum creatinine micromo/L
Mild	20–50	150–300
Moderate	10–20	300–700
Severe	<10	>700

GENERAL PRINCIPLES FOR PRESCRIBING IN RENAL IMPAIRMENT (adapted from *Maudsley Guidelines*)

1. The greater the renal impairment, the greater the potential for drug accumulation. ADRs such as confusion, postural hypotension and sedation may be more common.
2. Serum creatinine levels may be normal in the elderly, despite renal impairment.
3. Care is needed with drugs or active metabolites predominantly cleared by the kidney, e.g. antidepressants and antipsychotics (except aripiprazole).
4. Start low and go slow, adjusting doses to tolerance.
5. Care is needed with markedly anticholinergic drugs, which may cause urinary retention and interfere with U&E measurements.

3.10.1 ANTIPSYCHOTICS *

Lower doses of all antipsychotics should be used, due to increased cerebral sensitivity and EPSE. In adults over 64 SGAs (quetiapine, risperidone and olanzapine) are associated with a higher risk of acute kidney injury (RR=1.7), hypotension (RR=1.9), acute urinary retention (RR=1.98), and all-cause mortality (RR=2.39) (n=97,777+97,777 controls, 10 years, Hwang *et al, Ann Intern Med* 2014;**161**:242–8).

1. **Aripiprazole** needs no dose adjustment even in severe renal impairment. Although the Cmax for a stat dose of aripiprazole was 40% higher in severe renal impairment, there were no significant adverse effects (n=13, Mallikaarjun *et al, Clin Pharmacokinet* 2008;**47**:533–42).

2. * **Clozapine** is contraindicated in severe renal disease. In mild-to-moderate renal failure start at 12.5 mg/d and increase more slowly. Acute renal failure has been reported with clozapine and so people must be monitored for early symptoms of hypersensitivity, e.g. fever and eosinophilia (n=8, Kanofsky *et al, Prim Care Companion CNS Disorders* 2011;**13**:10br01091; FFT).

3. * **Lurasidone** should start at 18.5 mg and not go above 74 mg in moderate and severe renal impairment (CrCl <50mL/min).

4. * **Olanzapine** is excreted primarily (57%) via the renal pathway and 30% in faeces so a lower starting dose of 5 mg/d may be appropriate in renal impairment. If creatinine clearance is <10 mL/min, there is only a slight (11%) increase in half-life and 17% reduction in clearance. There are reports of prolonged hypothermia with olanzapine in renal failure (n=2, Kansagra *et al, Ther Adv Psychopharmacol* 2013;**3**:335–9). **Olanzapine pamoate** needs a lower starting dose of 150 mg/4 weeks in renal impairment (SmPC).

5. **Quetiapine**'s oral clearance is reduced by 25% in renal impairment, so start at 50 mg/d (25 mg/d if severe) and increase at 50 mg/d according to response and tolerability (e.g. n=8, Thyrum *et al, Prog Neuropsychopharmacol Biol Psychiatry* 2000;**24**:521–33).

6. **Risperidone** elimination is reduced in renal impairment so initial doses and dose increments should be halved, up to a maximum of about 4 mg/d. Haemodialysis can result in reduced risperidone levels and relapse (n=1, Railton *et al, Ther Drug Monit* 2005;**27**:558–61). In mild renal impairment (Ccr 50–79 mL/min), start **paliperidone** at 3 mg/d and increase carefully. If 30–49 mL/min stay at 3 mg/d; if 10–29 mL/min use 3 mg on alternate days; and it is not recommended for <10 mL/min. **Paliperidone palmitate** needs no dose adjustment in mild-to-moderate renal impairment, but there is no data in severe impairment (Gopal *et al, Curr Med Res Opin* 2010;**26**:377–87).

7. **Sulpiride** is mainly cleared by the kidneys with a half-life ranging from 6–25 hours, depending upon renal function. Reduce the dose by 35–70% or extend the dosage interval by a factor of 1.5–3 if necessary (n=24, open, Bressolle *et al, Clin Pharmacokinet* 1989;**17**:367–73). **Amisulpride** is principally cleared unchanged through the kidneys, so care is needed in moderate-to-severe renal insufficiency (GFR 10–30 mL/min), but is not appreciably removed by haemodialysis.

8. **Haloperidol** has no apparent problems, although some accumulation might occur.

9. **Phenothiazines** have little data but excretion may be slower and accumulation may occur, causing sedation or postural hypotension. **Levomepromazine** should be used with care in renal disease, and chlorpromazine avoided.

10. **Zuclopenthixol** should be used at half-dose in renal impairment. **Flupentixol** has not been studied in renal impairment, but use with caution as increased cerebral sensitivity has been reported with other antipsychotics.

11. **Pimozide**'s UK SmPC recommends caution in renal impairment. **Ziprasidone** needs no dose adjustments in renal impairment.

3.10.2 ANTIDEPRESSANTS *

Depression in renal impairment can lead to a three-fold greater risk of death in people with stage 5 diabetic chronic kidney disease cf. non-depressed people (n = 110, five years, Young *et al*, *Gen Hosp Psychiatry* 2010;**32**:119–24; FFT). **Omega-3 fatty acids** may reduce depression in people undergoing haemodialysis (n=54, RCT, p/c, 4/12, Gharekhani *et al*, *Eur J Clin Pharmacol* 2014;**70**:655–65).

Review: Recommendations by European Renal Best Practice for antidepressants in stage 3–5 chronic renal disease (Nagler *et al*, *Nephrol Dial Transplant* 2012;**27**:3736–45;FFT).

12. **SSRIs:**

12a. **Citalopram**'s renal clearance is about 20% of its total elimination and, although half-life increases slightly, no reduction of dosage is needed in moderately impaired renal function, but a slight reduction in severe renal failure may be prudent. Haemodialysis has an insignificant effect on citalopram plasma levels (n = 12, open, Spigset *et al*, *Eur J Clin Pharmacol* 2000;**56**:699–703). **Escitalopram** dose adjustment is not needed in mild-moderate impairment. Caution is advised in severe renal impairment (CrCl < 30 mL/min).

12b. **Fluoxetine**'s SmPC notes caution in severe renal failure (GFR < 10 mL/min) requiring dialysis. There was no difference in plasma levels of fluoxetine or norfluoxetine compared to controls with normal renal function.

12c. **Fluvoxamine** needs care, starting at 50 mg/d and increasing only slowly. Plasma levels are reduced by about 22% by haemodialysis, so higher doses might be needed (n=7, Kamo *et al*, *Psychiatr Clin Neurosci* 2004;**58**:133–7).

12d. **Paroxetine** should start at 10 mg/d in moderate renal impairment and increase only if necessary.

12e. **Sertraline** can be used in peritoneal dialysis (n = 25, 12/52, Atalay *et al*, *Int Urol Nephrol* 2010;**42**:527–36), but in maintenance haemodialysis for end-stage renal disease serotonin syndrome even 25 mg/d led to 92% discontinuing within three weeks, and there was one near-fatal outcome (n = 12, Chandler *et al*, *J Indian Med Assoc* 2011;**109**:36–7).

13. **Tricyclics** should be started at low dose and increased slowly, with divided doses. Avoid **lofepramine** in severe renal impairment, as 50% is renally excreted.

14. **Agomelatine** needs no dose adjustments.

15. **Bupropion** and metabolites are almost exclusively (85%) excreted via the kidneys and so, in renal failure, the initial dose should be reduced and close monitoring for toxicity carried out.

16. * **Vortioxetine** has limited data. Caution is recommended but dose adjustment is unlikely to be needed in severe impairment. A single dose study showed only a modest (30%) increase in exposure. Only a small amount is lost during dialysis in ESRD (SmPC). **Duloxetine** needs no dose adjustment in mild-to-moderate renal disease (CrCl 30–80 mL/min), but is contraindicated in severe (CrCl < 30 mL/min) renal disease where plasma levels are doubled.

17. **Mirtazapine** clearance is reduced by 33% in moderate and by 50% in severe renal failure, but not in mild renal impairment (n=40, Bengtsson *et al*, *Hum Psychopharmacol* 1998;**13**:357–65). Mirtazapine is largely unaffected by haemodialysis as, since 85% is protein-bound, only 15% is likely to be dialysed (n = 1, Schlotterbeck *et al*, *Pharmacopsychiatry* 2008;**41**:259–60).

18. **Moclobemide** needs no dosage adjustments in renal disease (n = 12, open, Stoeckel *et al*, *Acta Psychiatr Scand* 1990;**360**:94–97).

19. **Reboxetine**'s half-life and plasma levels appear to rise (up to two-fold) in severe renal impairment, where dose adjustment may be necessary. A starting dose of 2 mg BD in people with moderate-to-severe renal impairment has been suggested (n = 18, open, Coulomb *et al*, *J Clin Pharmacol* 2000;**40**:482–7).

20. **Trazodone** needs no dosage adjustments.

21. **Mianserin** and **tryptophan** need no dosage adjustments.

22. **Venlafaxine** partly cleared unchanged by the kidney (1–10%) and 30% renally excreted as the major metabolite. Total clearance is reduced by about 35% in mild-to-moderate renal impairment (GFR 10–30 mL/min) and so doses should be reduced by about 25–50%, although there is much inter-patient variability (Anon, *J Clin Psychiatry* 1993;**54**:119–26). Clearance is reduced by about 55% in moderate-to-severe renal disease, and a

50% reduction in dose is recommended, given once a day where GFR is less than 30 mL/min (n = 38, open, Troy *et al*, *Clin Pharmacol Therapeut* 1994;**56**:14–21). Daily doses should also be reduced by 50% in dialysis and doses withheld until after dialysis is complete. Venlafaxine is not recommended in severe renal failure.

23. **MAOIs** usually need no dosage adjustments, although **isocarboxazid** may accumulate with lower renal function.

3.10.3 MOOD AND BIPOLAR

24. **Asenapine** is 50% renally excreted but no dose reductions are needed in any degree of renal failure (n = 33, Peeters *et al*, *Clin Pharmacokinet* 2011;**50**:471–81).

25. **Carbamazepine** doses may need to be reduced by 25% in severe renal failure (renal impairment is a precaution in the SmPC).

26. **Lamotrigine** may need a reduced maintenance dose in severe renal impairment, but the dose probably needs little adjustment in mild-to-moderate impairment (n = 21, Wootton *et al*, *Br J Clin Pharmacol* 1997;**43**:23–7), and even in end-stage renal failure although the major glucuronide metabolite levels may increase eight-fold due to reduced renal clearance.

27.* **Lithium** can be used in renal impairment with great care and close monitoring. The prevalence of chronic renal disease (plasma creatinine > 150 micromol/l) with lithium is about 1.2% (n = 3,369, mean 10 years, Bendz *et al*, *Kidney Int* 2010;**77**:219–24), although there are apparently no reported cases of renal failure indisputably caused by properly monitored lithium, with no toxicity. A Swedish study showed people taking lithium (n = 3836) had no evidence of renal damage if starting lithium after 1980, suggesting more recent monitoring and plasma levels may have eliminated the risk of ESRD (n = 2,823,626, Aiff *et al*, *J Psychopharmacol* 2014;**28**:151–4).

Minimising lithium's renal effects:*

- avoid acute episodes of lithium toxicity
- ensure regular (3-monthly) and frequent plasma monitoring to get the optimum dose
- use a single daily dose at night
- avoid any possible drug interactions.

Risk factors for further reduced glomerular function:

- duration of treatment (Bocchetta *et al*, *BMC Med* 2013;**11**:33; Rej *et al*, *Am J Geriatr Psychiatry* 2014;22:1075–82)
- older users (>65 years old) (40% in lithium, 30% in matched controls; n = 282, Rej *et al*, *Aging Ment Health* 2014;**18**:847–53)
- male gender (n = 80, Rybakowski *et al*, *Med Sci Monit* 2012;**18**:CR656–60; FFT)
- toxicity (a *single* lithium level > 1.0 mmol/L causes an acute decline in eGFR over the next year; n=699, 10yrs, Kirkham *et al*, *BMJ Open* 2014;**4**:e006020; FFT).

Lithium in chronic renal disease:
A review (Kripalani *et al*, *Br Med J* 2009;**339**:b2452) notes that the renal markers that should prompt nephrology advice and (consideration of) stopping lithium include:

- GFR falling (rapidly) to < 45mL/min/1.732 body surface, or heavy proteinuria
- a steady or persistent fall in GFR (rather than a single measurement)
- stages 4 and 5 of chronic kidney disease.

A decision analysis tool concludes that **lithium** is still a treatment of choice even in the presence of long-term renal effects, *unless* the likelihood of progressing to end-stage renal disease exceeds 41.3%, and that any nephrologist consulted should help with *management* of the associated risks of continuing lithium, rather than the decision of whether to stop lithium (Werneke *et al*, *Acta Psychiatr Scand* 2012;**126**:186–97; FFT).

Lithium in end-stage renal disease (ESRD):
ESDR occurs in < 1% people taking lithium for more than 15 years, and classifies as being extremely rare (n = 114, mean 16 years, Tredget *et al*, *J Affect Disord* 2010;**126**:436–40). If lithium is essential, use alternate-day dosing (e.g. 125 mg on alternate days, n = 1, Gash *et al*, *J Affect Disord* 1995;**34**:51–3), very low doses (25–75% normal), and frequently estimate levels; use in chronic renal failure (n = 1, Belgamwar *et al*, *Gen Hosp Psychiatry* 2010;**32**:341.e3–5) especially with haemodialysis in ESRD (n = 1, Knebel *et al*, *Am J Psychiatry* 2010;**167**:1409–10).

Reviews: * lithium nephrotoxicity (Ibbeken *et al*, *Dtsch Med Wochenschr* 2012;**137**:143–8: Gahr *et al*, *Psychiatr Prax* 2014;**41**:15–22), general (McKnight *et al*, *Lancet* 2012;**379**:721–8; FFT; but may underestimate renal side-effects; Müller-Uerlinghausen *et al*, *BMC Med* 2012;**10**:132), use in renal impairment (Severus and Bauer, *BMC Med* 2013;**11**:34), renal side-effects (Albert *et al*,

3

Riv Psychiatry 2014;**49**:12–21).

28. **Valproate** is mainly eliminated renally and it may be necessary to decrease dosage in renal insufficiency. It has been used successfully in haemodialysis (n=2, Gupta and Annadatha, *Clin Pract Epidemol Ment Health* 2008;**4**:21; FFT).

3.10.4 ANXIOLYTICS AND HYPNOTICS

29. **Benzodiazepines** in low doses may be acceptable, as higher doses in renal impairment produce an increase in CNS sedative side-effects. **Chlordiazepoxide** can be given in normal doses and is not affected by haemodialysis (review, Bennett *et al*, *Am J Kidney Dis* 1983;**3**:155). **Oxazepam** doses should be reduced to 75% in severe renal failure. In end-stage renal failure and haemodialysis, **clobazam** and metabolite concentrations appear no different to those with normal renal function (n=1, Roberts and Zoanetti, *Ann Pharmacother* 1994;**28**:966–7) or in haemodialysis. **Clonazepam** 5–10mg (sic) has been used successfully for insomnia (n=23, RCT, c/o, 5/52, Dashti-Khavidaki *et al*, *Iran J Kidney Dis* 2011;**5**:404–9; FFT). **Midazolam** metabolites accumulate and may lead to prolonged sedation in severe renal failure, not reversible by flumazenil (n=5, Bauer *et al*, *Lancet* 1995;**346**:145–7).

30. **Beta-blocker** plasma levels may be higher in severe renal disease, and so starting doses should be lower. Beta-blockers may also reduce renal blood flow and adversely affect renal function.

31. **Buspirone** plasma levels appear higher in renal failure, with a good correlation between steady-state levels and serum albumin (n=54, open, Barbhaiya *et al*, *Eur J Clin Pharmacol* 1994;**46**:41–7). It is contraindicated in moderate or severe renal impairment. **Hydroxyzine** doses should be reduced by a half in renal impairment (UK SmPC).

32. **Clomethiazole** should be used in caution in chronic renal disease. **Chloral** is contraindicated in moderate to marked renal impairment.

33. **Melatonin** has not been studied in renal impairment (SmPC), but 3mg/d improves sleep-wake rhythm in people undergoing haemodialysis (c=20, RCT, d/b, p/c, c/o, 3x6/52, Koch *et al*, *Br J Clin Pharmacol* 2009;**67**:68–75; FFT; Aperis *et al*, *J Ren Care* 2012;**38**:86–92).

34. **Pregabalin** is mainly excreted unchanged by the kidney, clearance being directly proportional to creatinine clearance (n=50, Randinitis *et al*, *J Clin Pharmacol* 2003;**43**:277–83), so doses in renal impairment must be individually calculated (see SmPC), as a few cases of reversible renal failure have been reported. Supplementary doses are necessary after every four-hour haemodialysis.

35. **Zolpidem** plasma protein-binding is reduced in renal failure (n=54, open, Pacifici, *Int J Clin Pharmacol Ther Toxicol* 1988;**26**:439–43) and the half-life may be doubled, but no dosage adjustments are recommended in mild renal dysfunction. Zolpidem 1mg is well tolerated and effective in people undergoing maintenance haemodialysis (n=23, RCT, c/o, Dashti-Khavidaki *et al*, *Iran J Kidney Dis* 2011;**5**:404–9; FFT). **Zaleplon** and **zopiclone** do not need dose alterations.

3.10.5 ANTICONVULSANTS

Review: AEDs in renal dysfunction (Lacerda *et al*, *Neurology* 2006;**67**(12 Suppl 4):S28–33).

36. **Phenobarbital** causes increased sedation and the dosage interval should be no more frequently than 12–16 hours in severe renal failure. Large doses of **primidone** should be avoided.

37. **Gabapentin** is mainly excreted unchanged in the urine and the UK SmPC now recommends dose reductions as follows:

Creatine clearance	Gabapentin dosage and frequency
≥80mL/min	300–1200mg TDS
50–79 mL/min	200–600mg TDS
30–49mL/min	100–300mg BD
15–29mL/min	300mg on alternative days, up to 200mg/d TDS
<15mL/min	300mg on alternative days, up to 100mg/d TDS

Patients undergoing haemodialysis should receive a loading dose of 300–400mg, plus 200–300mg for every four hours of dialysis, with no treatment on dialysis-free days (see SmPC for full details). Gabapentin toxicity in renal impairment is often unrecognised, leading to unnecessary morbidity (n=729, Zand *et al*, *Am J Med* 2010;**123**:367–73).

38. **Levetiracetam** is 66% excreted unchanged in the urine. Dose reductions are necessary in impaired renal function as follows (UK SmPC):

Renal function	Creatinine clearance	Levetiracetam max. dose
Normal	≥80 mL/min	500–1500 mg BD
Mild	50–79 mL/min	500–1000 mg BD
Moderate	30–49 mL/min	250–750 mg BD
Severe	<30 mL/min	250–500 mg BD
ESRD and undergoing dialysis	–	500–1000 mg OD

Following dialysis, a 250–500 mg supplemental dose is recommended.

39. **Oxcarbazepine** should start at half the usual dose (300 mg/day) in renal impairment (Ccr <30 mL/min), increasing at no more often than weekly intervals. Monitor serum sodium in people with pre-existing renal conditions associated with low sodium or in people treated concomitantly with sodium-lowering drugs (e.g. diuretics, desmopressin) as well as NSAIDs.

40.* **Phenytoin** needs no specific dose adjustments but protein-binding is altered in uraemia, which can hinder accurately assessing serum levels, and care is needed in hemodialysis (Bezzaoucha *et al, Eur J Clin Pharmacol* 2014;**70**:499–500).

41. **Topiramate** is about 60–70% excreted unchanged via the kidneys. Time to steady state may be 10–15 days in severe renal impairment instead of 4–8 days with normal renal function. Start topiramate at half the usual dose in moderate or severe renal impairment, plus use a lower maintenance dose. Supplemental doses of 50% of the daily dose should be given on haemodialysis days (Manitpisitkul *et al, Epilepsy Res* 2014;**108**:891–901). There is an increased risk of renal stone formation so ensure adequate fluid throughput, especially in higher risk people.

3.10.6 OTHERS

42.* **Atomoxetine** is 80% renally excreted and dose reduction may be needed (UK SmPC). There is no information for **methylphenidate** or **lisdexamfetamine** in renal failure. **Guanfacine's** clearance is 30% renal and unchanged. Dose reduction may be needed in severe renal impairment (GFR 29–15 ml/min; Carchman *et al, Nephron* 1989;**53**:18–23) and ESRD requiring dialysis.

43. **Anticholinesterases**: No dose changes are needed with **donepezil** in mild-to-moderate renal impairment and even moderate-to-severe renal impairment did not significantly alter its kinetics (open, n=22, Tiseo *et al, Br J Clin Pharmacol* 1998;**46**[Suppl 1]:56–60;FFT). There are no reported problems with **rivastigmine**. **Galantamine** needs no dosage reduction with a CrCl >9 mL/min but is contraindicated in severe impairment (<9 mL/min).

44. **Memantine** is eliminated unchanged by the kidneys but with significant interindividual variation (Noetzli *et al, Clin Pharmacokinet* 2013;**52**:211–23). In severe renal failure 5 mg BD is recommended (n=32[c=31], Periclou *et al, Clin Pharmacol Ther* 2006;**79**:134–43; FFT), but care is needed as AUC can be 1.6, 2 and 2.3 times higher in mild, moderate and severe renal impairment respectively (n=25, Moritoyo *et al, J Pharmacol Sci* 2012;**119**:324–9;FFT), a study remarkable for having nearly twice as many authors (n=46) as patients.

45. **Anticholinergics** need some caution in renal disease. **Orphenadrine** is mainly renally excreted.

46a. **Acamprosate** is contraindicated in renal insufficiency (serum creatinine >120 micromol/L).

46b. **Disulfiram**'s SmPC recommends caution in renal disease.

46c. **Nalmefene** AUC increases 1.6-fold and Cmax reduces in severe or ESRD and the half-life increases from 10 to 26 hours in renal impairment and so extended dose intervals may be needed to avoid the risk of accumulation (Matzke *et al, J Clin Pharmacol* 1996;**36**:144–51). Haemodialysis seems not to have a significant effect.

46d. **Naltrexone** is primarily renally excreted, 60% within 48 hours. It is contraindicated in severe renal impairment and care is needed in other grades.

47. * **Methadone** elimination is reduced in renal impairment but haemodialysis does not require dose adjustment (n=4, Opdal *et al, Clin Ther* 2015;**37**:1594–9). **Buprenorphine**'s renal excretion is only about 30% of the total. Caution is recommended in severe renal impairment.

48. The maximum **modafinil** dose of 400 mg/d should only be used in the absence of renal impairment. **Sodium oxybate** contains a significant dose of sodium (0.75 g in 4.5 g dose) and so dietary restriction of sodium might be considered, but since the kidney is not involved in excretion no dose reduction is thought to be necessary (SmPC).

3.11 SLEEP APNEA (APNOEA)

	LOWER RISK (BUT SEE TEXT)	MODERATE RISK (BUT SEE TEXT)	HIGH RISK
Antipsychotics	All others[3,6–11]	Aripiprazole[1] Clozapine[2] Olanzapine[4] Quetiapine[5]	
Antidepressants	Agomelatine[14]	Most antidepressants[12–23] Mirtazapine[17]	
Mood and bipolar	Most[24–28]	Lithium[27]	
Anxiolytics and hypnotics	All[29–35], including benzodiazepines[29]	Midazolam[29]	
Anticonvulsants	All others[7–8]		
Others	Anticholinesterases[43] All others[42–48]	Lithium[27]	

Sleep apnea (SA) can have several forms, of which obstructive sleep apnea (OSA) is predominant (75% cases). It is defined as periods of stopping breathing while asleep, clinically significant if lasting for more than 10 seconds and for more than 5–10 times an hour. Symptoms include loud snoring, daytime sleepiness, irritability, changes in mood or behaviour (n=79, Peng *et al, Chin Med Sci J* 2004;**19**:262–5), unexplained fatigue and tiredness (n=64, Jackson *et al, Sleep Breath* 2011;**15**:439–45), anxiety and depression (n=1408, Peppard *et al, Arch Intern Med* 2006;**166**:1709–15; 0.8% of the population have both, with a 20% comorbidity, Schröder and O'Hara, *Ann Gen Psychiatry* 2005;**4**:13; FFT). It occurs naturally in about 4% of men and 2% of women, and is associated with being overweight, smoking, older age and having type 2 diabetes (n=90, Lecube *et al, PLoS One* 2009;**4**:e4692; FFT). OSA is more common (10%) in psychiatric outpatients than the general population (3%) (n=330, Nasr *et al, Ann Clin Psychiatry* 2010;**22**:29–32), especially in people with depression (22%), anxiety (17%), PTSD (12%), psychosis (5%) and bipolar (3.3%) (n=4,060,504, Sharafkhaneh *et al, Sleep* 2005;**28**:1405–11).

First-line treatment of OSA is continuous positive airway pressure (CPAP). Severity is measured using the Respiratory Disturbance Index (RDI) or the apnea-hypopnea index (AHI; higher score is worse).

Treating OSA with CPAP has resulted in remission of psychosis (n=1, Karanti and Landén, *Psychopharmacol Bull* 2007;**40**:113–7), TRS (n=1, Boufidis *et al, Int J Psychiatry Med* 2003;**33**:305–10), depression (n=50, Schwartz *et al, Chest* 2005;**128**:1304–9) and suicidal ideation (n=1, Krahn *et al, J Clin Sleep Med* 2008;**4**:64–5;FFT). However, CPAP is not risk-free, as psychotic mania (e.g. n=1, Bergé *et al, Psychosomatics* 2008;**49**:447–9: n=1, Trakada *et al, Psychopharmacol Bull* 2008;**41**:89–92), and psychosis (n=1, Chiner *et al, Eur Respir J* 2001;**17**:313–5;FFT) have been reported. CPAP itself has, however, no effect on mood (n=71 [c=56], RCT, d/b, p/c, 3/52, Lee *et al, Sleep Med* 2012;**13**:161–6; FFT).

If OSA is being properly managed with CPAP (or BiPAP as an alternative), then prescribing any drug should have no more problems than in a person without OSA. However, as not everyone can tolerate CPAP, the potential effects on respiration or sleep architecture need to be considered.

Reviews: * general (Lin *et al, Expert Opin Pharmacother* 2012;**13**:841–57; Paiva and Attarian, *Handb Clin Neurosci* 2014;**119**:251–71; Young and Collop, *Curr Treat Options Neurol* 2014;**16**:305), adjunctive use of rhubarbic acid (Hannant, *J Irreprod Med* 2014;**3**:27–31).

3.11.1 ANTIPSYCHOTICS *

Obesity, male gender and chronic antipsychotics appear to be risk factors for OSA and so overweight people should be evaluated for OSA (n=364, Winkelman, *J Clin Psychiatry* 2001;**62**:8–11). Logically, antipsychotics causing sedation and weight gain can exacerbate or precipitate OSA (Wirshing *et al, J Clin Psychiatry* 2002;**63**:369–70). SGAs have been associated with a greater risk of severe OSA (n=68, Rishi *et al, Clin Neuropharmacol* 2010;**33**:109–13). ECT is a viable alternative for mania (n=1, Bastiampillai *et al, J ECT* 2011;**27**:15–6).

Review: * OSA and schizophrenia (Kalucy *et al, Sleep Med Rev* 2013;**17**:357–65).

1. **Aripiprazole** has been linked with CSA in a man with psychotic depression (n=1, Kohen and Sarcevic, *Am J Ther* 2009;**16**:197–8).
2. **Clozapine** weight gain would be detrimental.
3. **Lurasidone** has no known problems.
4. **Olanzapine** weight gain would be detrimental.
5. **Quetiapine** may exacerbate OSA in obese people, e.g. in combination with previously tolerated lorazepam, and so use should only be with full monitoring (n=2, Freudenmann *et al, Pharmacopsychiatry* 2008;**41**:119–21).
6. **Risperidone/paliperidone** — no information.
7. **Benzamines** — no information.
8. **Haloperidol** has had no adverse effect on OSA (n=1, Sobel *et al, Am J Psychiatry* 1985; **142**:775–6).
9. **Phenothiazines** — no information.
10. **Thioxanthenes** — no information.
11. **Pimozide and ziprasidone** — no information.

3.11.2 ANTIDEPRESSANTS *

Depression can be a symptom of OSA and up to 32–53% of people with sleep apnea and snoring have depression (n=233, Douglas *et al, Intern Med J* 2013;**43**:630–4). Many people with residual depressive symptoms may have OSA and treatment with CPAP may improve these, probably by improving daytime sleepiness (n=17, Habukawa *et al, Sleep Med* 2010;**11**:552–7). People with OSA and daytime sleepiness are more likely to have depression (n=53, Ishman *et al, Laryngoscope* 2010;**120**:2331–5).

12. * **SSRIs** disrupt sleep architecture so are best avoided if possible, or use a short-acting SSRI as a morning dose. Intuitively, avoiding **fluoxetine** with its long half-life would be appropriate. There are, however, some suggestions that boosting serotonin with SSRIs can have modest benefits on OSA during non-REM sleep, and one trial showed fluoxetine plus ondansetron to be well tolerated and improved AHI compared to placebo (n=35, RCT, p/c, 4/52, Prasad *et al, Sleep* 2010;**33**:982–9; FFT). **Paroxetine** 20 mg/d seems to reduce apnea or improve breathing in non-REM sleep but not during REM sleep (n=20 [c=17], RCT, d/b, p/c, 16/52, Kraiczi *et al, Sleep* 1999;**22**:61–7). OSA has been associated with a relatively poor response to **sertraline** (n=30, RCT, d/b, p/c, 10/52, Roest *et al, J Clin Psychiatry* 2012;**73**:31–6; FFT).
13. **Tricyclics:** abrupt **amitriptyline** withdrawal has precipitated OSA, probably due to cholinergic rebound, which may be detrimental to OSA (n=1, Musa, *J Clin Pharmacol* 1988; **28**:1038–9). A case series suggested that **imipramine** 25–50 mg/d may improve OSA (n=31, Rubin *et al, Eur Neurol* 1986;**25**:81–5).
14. **Agomelatine** does not cause drowsiness and improves sleep architecture, so would seem a good option.
15. **Bupropion** — no information.
16. **Duloxetine** — no information.
17. **Mirtazapine** 4.5–15 mg/d may reduce AHI scores by a half in adults with OSA, but is not recommended as a treatment (n=12, RCT, d/b, p/c, c/o, 3/52, Carley *et al, Sleep* 2007;**30**:35–41) Two studies with different designs failed to show an improvement in OSA with mirtazapine 7.5–45 mg/d, but caused excessive sedation, and weight gain which may worsen OSA (s=2, n=64 [c=46], RCT, d/b, p/c, Marshall *et al, Sleep* 2008;**31**:824–31; FFT). In non-depressed stroke patients who refused CPAP, mirtazapine can have a mixed effect, improving RDI in six but deteriorating it in four, so monitor carefully (n=10, 9/52, Brunner, *Sleep Breath* 2008;**12**:281–5).
18. **Moclobemide** — no information.
19. **Reboxetine** — no information.
20. **Trazodone** has increased arousal thresholds in OSA, allowing higher CO_2 levels to be tolerated (n=9, RCT, p/c, d/b, c/o, 2/7, Heinzer *et al, Eur Respir J* 2008;**31**:1308–12; FFT; n=7, c/o, Eckert *et al, Sleep* 2014;**37**:811–9).

21. **Tryptophan, mianserin** and **St. John's wort** — no information.
22. **Venlafaxine** — no information.
23. **MAOIs** — no information.

3.11.3 MOOD AND BIPOLAR

24. **Asenapine** has no known problems.
25. **Carbamazepine** has no known problems.
26. **Lamotrigine** has no known problems.
27. **Lithium** has been linked to OSA in treatment-resistant mania (n=4, Strakowski *et al*, *J Clin Psychiatry* 1991;**52**:156–8).
28. **Valproate** has no known problems.

3.11.4 ANXIOLYTICS AND HYPNOTICS

Insomnia and OSA frequently co-occur. 39–58% of people with OSA also have insomnia, and 29–67% of people with insomnia also have OSA (s=12, Luyster *et al*, *J Clin Sleep Med* 2010;**6**:196–204; FFT). Thus, it is essential to ensure when treating insomnia that OSA has been excluded as a cause (e.g. n=90, Sivertsen *et al*, *J Clin Sleep Med* 2009;**5**:349–54;FFT).

Review: comorbid insomnia and OSA including differential diagnosis (Luyster *et al*, *J Clin Sleep Med* 2010;**6**:196–204).

29. **Benzodiazepines** are contraindicated in OSA. **Flumazenil** has no effect, either positive or negative (n=10, RCT, s/b, p/c, c/o, Schönhofer and Köhler, *Eur Respir J* 1996;**9**:1816–20;FFT). **Temazepam** 15–30mg/d may cause no change in RDI in mild apnea (n=15, RCT, p/c, Camacho and Morin, *Sleep* 1995;**18**:644–5). **Nitrazepam** 5–10mg/d had no significant effect in mild-to-moderate OSA (n=14[c=11], RCT, d/b, p/c, 3/52, Höijer *et al*, *Eur Respir J* 1994;**7**:2011–5;FFT). **Midazolam** 15mg orally has caused rapid and life-threatening sedation and apnea in OSA (n=1, Bezel *et al*, *Schweiz Med Wochenschr* 1987;**117**:579–83). There is a case of OSA induced by **clonazepam** (n=1, Schuld *et al*, *J Sleep Res* 1999;**8**:321–2;FFT). In treated arterial hypertension and obesity (BMI >25), BDZ use was not associated with an increase in apnea indices (n=30, Nunes *et al*, *Int J Cardiol* 2007;**114**:416–8).
30. **Beta-blockers** have no consistent associations with changes in sleep architecture in untreated OSA (n=1,779, Smith *et al*, *J Clin Sleep Med* 2006;**2**:156–62).
31. **Buspirone** has no known problems.
32. **Clomethiazole and chloral** have no known problems.
33. **Melatonin** has no relevant adverse effects, or acts by causing sedation and so might be a good choice.
34. **Pregabalin** has no known problems.
35. **Zolpidem** is a very short-acting hypnotic and would probably be preferred as OSA is a whole night problem, e.g. zolpidem 10mg at night had no effect on the Apnea-Hypopnea Index, nor did it impair the efficacy of CPAP in severe OSA (n=16, RCT, d/b, p/c, c/o, 3/52, Berry and Patel, *Sleep* 2006;**29**:1052–6), but improved sleep continuity (n=20, open, 9/52, Quadri *et al*, *J Clin Sleep Med* 2009;**5**:122–9;FFT) possibly because of its short duration of effect. **Zaleplon** may be an alternative (Coyle *et al*, *J Clin Sleep Med* 2005;**1**:97). In one study, 41% of chronic **zopiclone** users had OSA as the probable underlying cause (n=90, Sivertsen *et al*, *J Clin Sleep Med* 2009;**5**:349–54; FFT).

3.11.5 ANTICONVULSANTS *

There is little published on AEDs in OSA, but comorbidity may occur in 10% adult epileptics, 20% children with epilepsy and in 30% with drug-resistant epilepsy (Manni and Terzaghi, *Epilepsy Res* 2010;**90**:171–7). There is a case of carbamazepine and tiapride being successfully used for AWS in someone with OSA (n=1, Gartenmaier *et al*, *Pharmacopsychiatry* 2005;**38**:96–8).

36. **Phenobarbital** withdrawal has improved alertness but unmasked OSA (n=1, Takhar and Bishop, *J Psychiatry Neurosci* 2000;**25**:321–4; FFT).
37. **Gabapentin** has no known problems.
38. **Levetiracetam** has no known problems.
39. **Oxcarbazepine** has no known problems.
40. **Phenytoin** has no known problems.
41. **Topiramate** initiation in bipolar disorder has led to marked improvement in OSA (n=1, Weber, *Am J Psychiatry* 2002;**159**:872–3).

3.11.6 OTHERS *

42. ADHD * There is no information on **atomoxetine, dexamfetamine, lisdexamfetamine** or **methylphenidate**. **Guanfacine** can suppress REM sleep.

43. **Anticholinesterases**: There is a strong link between severe OSA and severe dementia (n=235, Ancoli-Israel *et al, J Am Geriatr Soc* 1991; **39**:258–63), which may be as high as 43% (n=61, Reynolds *et al, J Clin Psychiatry* 1985;**46**:257–61). **Donepezil** appears to actually improve OSA parameters and a similar effect would be expected from other cholinergic enhancers (n=21, RCT, d/b, p/c, 4/52, Sukys-Claudion *et al, Sleep Med* 2012;**13**:290–6).

44. **Memantine** has no known problems.

45. * **Anticholinergics:** Excess acetylcholine increases REM sleep so, in theory, anticholinergics might not be detrimental.

46. There is no information on **acamprosate, disulfiram, nalmefene** or **naltrexone**.

47. * **Methadone** maintenance can lead to 30% having central sleep apnea (CSA) (n=70, Wang et al, Chest 2005;128:1348–56), which would not help OSA (n=19, Teichtahl *et al, Addiction* 2001; **96**:395–403). The same would be expected for **buprenorphine,** but there is nothing published as such although there is a case of reversal of methadone-induced CSA with a switch to buprenorphine-naloxone (n=1, Wang *et al, Eur Respir* 2015;**46:** 1202–5).

48. **Modafinil** seems safe in OSA as it can maintain the effects of CPAP (n=21, RCT, d/b, c/o, Williams *et al, Am J Respir Crit Care Med* 2010;**181**:825–31). When used for excessive sleepiness, it can lead to improvements in daytime functioning in OSA (s=2, n=480, RCT, p/c, Weaver *et al, J Clin Sleep Med* 2009;**5**:499–505; FFT; n=114[c=114], RCT, d/b, p/c, 4/52, Inoue *et al, J Clin Sleep Med* 2013;**15**:751–7; n=32, RCT, p/c, c/o, 4/52, Chapman *et al, Thorax* 2014;**69**:274–9). **Sodium oxybate** 4.5 g at night has significantly improved AHI (n=48, p/c, 3/52, George *et al, Sleep Breath* 2011;**15**:13–20; FFT) and 9 g at night had no detrimental effect in mild-to-moderate OSA, but should still be used with caution (n=60[c=42], RCT, d/b, c/o, p/c, George *et al, Sleep Med* 2010;**11**:38–42).

3

4 DRUG INTERACTIONS

Contents

4.1	**Anxiolytics and hypnotics**	**327**
4.1.1	Benzodiazepines	327
4.1.2	Buspirone	330
4.1.3	Chloral hydrate	331
4.1.4	Melatonin	332
4.1.5	Pregabalin	332
4.1.6	Zaleplon	333
4.1.7	Zolpidem	333
4.1.8	Zopiclone	334
4.2	**Antipsychotics**	**335**
4.2.1	General	335
4.2.2	Aripiprazole	338
4.2.3	Asenapine	339
4.2.4	Clozapine	339
4.2.5	Lurasidone	342
4.2.6	Olanzapine	343
4.2.7	Quetiapine	345
4.2.8	Risperidone	346
4.2.9	Ziprasidone	348
4.3	**Antidepressants**	**348**
4.3.1	Tricyclic antidepressants	348
4.3.2	SSRIs	352
4.3.2.1	*Citalopram and escitalopram*	*352*
4.3.2.2	*Fluoxetine*	*354*
4.3.2.3	*Fluvoxamine*	*357*
4.3.2.4	*Paroxetine*	*360*
4.3.2.5	*Sertraline*	*362*
4.3.3	Other antidepressants	364
4.3.3.1	*Agomelatine*	*364*
4.3.3.2	*Duloxetine*	*365*
4.3.3.3	*Mianserin*	*366*
4.3.3.4	*Mirtazapine*	*366*
4.3.3.5	*Moclobemide*	*368*
4.3.3.6	*Reboxetine*	*369*
4.3.3.7	*Trazodone*	*370*
4.3.3.8	*Venlafaxine*	*371*
4.3.3.9	*Vortioxetine* *	*373*
4.3.3.10	*St John's wort*	*373*
4.3.4	MAOIs	376
4.4	**Mood stabilisers**	**381**
4.4.1	Carbamazepine	381
4.4.2	Lamotrigine	387
4.4.3	Lithium	389
4.4.4	Valproate	393
4.5	**Anticonvulsants**	**395**
4.5.1	Gabapentin	395
4.5.2	Levetiracetam	396
4.5.3	Oxcarbazepine	396
4.5.4	Phenobarbital/primidone	397
4.5.5	Phenytoin	400
4.5.6	Topiramate	405
4.6	**Other drugs**	**406**
4.6.1	Acamprosate	406
4.6.2	Anticholinergics	406
4.6.3	Anticholinesterases	407
4.6.3.1	*Donepezil*	*407*
4.6.3.2	*Galantamine*	*408*
4.6.3.3	*Rivastigmine*	*408*
4.6.4	Atomoxetine	408
4.6.5	Buprenorphine	409
4.6.6	Bupropion	410
4.6.7	Clomethiazole	412
4.6.8	Disulfiram	412
4.6.9	Guanfacine	413
4.6.10	Lisdexamfetamine	413
4.6.11	Memantine	413
4.6.12	Methadone	414
4.6.13	Methylphenidate	417
4.6.14	Modafinil	417
4.6.15	Nalmefene	418
4.6.16	Naltrexone	419
4.6.17	Pirenzepine	419
4.6.18	Sodium oxybate	419
4.7	**Non-prescribed drugs and 'vices'**	**420**
4.7.1	Alcohol	420
4.7.2	Cannabis	423
4.7.3	Cocaine	423
4.7.4	Smoking	424
4.8	**Cytochrome P450 drug metabolism**	**426**
	CYP1A2	427
	CYP2B6	428
	CYP2C9	429
	CYP2C19	430
	CYP2D6	431
	CYP3A3/4	433

Absolute classification of interactions is impossible. Many individual factors, e.g. age, concurrent illness and P450 status are important. Single case reports merely suggest a possible interaction. To give some guidance, interactions with the drugs in CAPITAL LETTERS are those that could be:

- potentially hazardous
- where dosage adjustment may be needed
- well-established and documented
- rare but important.

How to use this section:

1. Look up the psychotropic drug or group.
2. Look up the group of the interacting drug e.g. macrolides, triazoles, antiretrovirals, carbapenems, calcium-channel blockers etc.
3. If no entry there, look up the actual drug.
4. If still no entry, little has been reported.

4.1 ANXIOLYTICS AND HYPNOTICS

Reviews: clinically important drug interactions with zopiclone, zaleplon and zolpidem (Hesse *et al*, *CNS Drugs* 2003;**17**:513–32), pharmacokinetics and pharmacodynamics (Drover, *Clin Pharmacokinet* 2004;**43**:227–38).

4.1.1 BENZODIAZEPINES *

Benzodiazepines are mainly metabolised by CYP2C19 and CYP3A3/4. Clobazam metabolised by 3A4 to desmethylclobazam which is inactivated by 2C19 to inactive metabolites, and 2C19 is significantly affected by polymorphisms (n =50, Hashi *et al*, *Eur J Clin Pharmacol* 2015;**71**:51–8).

Review: herbal medication interactions with midazolam (Tweddell and Boyle, *Dent Update* 2009;**36**:175–8).

Acamprosate + benzodiazepines

See acamprosate (*4.6.1*).

Agomelatine + benzodiazepines

See agomelatine (*4.3.3.1*).

ALCOHOL + BENZODIAZEPINES

See alcohol (*4.7.1*).

Alosetron + alprazolam

Alosetron has no effect on alprazolam (n=12, RCT, open, D'Souza *et al*, *J Clin Pharmacol* 2001;**41**:452–4).

Amfetamines + benzodiazepines

Amfetamine significantly reverses the sedative and memory-impairing effects of triazolam (n=20, p/c, d/b, c/o, Mintzer and Griffiths, *J Psychopharmacol* 2003;**17**:17–29).

Amiodarone + clonazepam

Amiodarone has caused clonazepam toxicity at low dose (n=1, Witt *et al*, *Ann Pharmacother* 1993;**27**:1463–4).

Antacids + benzodiazepines

Benzodiazepine absorption is slightly delayed by antacids, but total absorption remains the same.

Anticholinergics + benzodiazepines

Benzodiazepine absorption may be delayed by anticholinergics, but the AUC remains unchanged.

Anticoagulants + benzodiazepines

No interaction has been reported with warfarin but is theoretically possible (mentioned in Sayal *et al*, *Acta Psychiatr Scand* 2000;**102**:250–5).

Antihistamines + benzodiazepines

Enhanced sedation is possible.

Antihypertensives + benzodiazepines

Enhanced hypotension is possible.

Antipsychotics + benzodiazepines

See individual drugs and antipsychotics (*4.2.1*).

ANTIRETROVIRALS + BENZODIAZEPINES

Maraviroc has no effect on midazolam (UK SmPC). The UK SmPC contraindicates **ritonavir** with diazepam, flurazepam, oral midazolam (parenteral is just a warning) and triazolam due to the risk of extreme sedation and respiratory depression. Increased **clobazam** levels causing neurotoxicity have been reported (n=1, Naccarato *et al*, *Antivir Ther* 2012;**17**:589–92).

Atomoxetine + benzodiazepines

See atomoxetine (*4.6.4*).

Baclofen + benzodiazepines

Enhanced sedation can occur.

Barbiturates + benzodiazepines

Enhanced sedation and increased benzodiazepine clearance may occur via CYP3A4 induction. Dose adjustment may be necessary.

Beta-blockers + benzodiazepines

Propranolol and **metoprolol** produce a small but significant increase in diazepam levels. Propranolol and **labetolol** have no effect on oxazepam (n=6, Sonne *et al*, *Br J Clin Pharmacol* 1990;**29**:33–7; FFT) and metoprolol has no effect on lorazepam (n=12, open, Scott *et al*, *Eur J Clin Pharmacol* 1991;**40**:405–9).

Brivanib + midazolam

Brivanib has no effect on midazolam (n=24[c=21], Syed *et al*, *J Clin Pharmacol* 2012;**52**:914–21).

4

Buprenorphine + benzodiazepines
Buprenorphine does not inhibit the metabolism of flunitrazepam but deaths have been reported with buprenorphine and benzodiazepines (n=6, Reynaud *et al*, *Addiction* 1998;**93**:1385–92).

Buspirone + benzodiazepines
See buspirone (*4.1.2*).

CALCIUM-CHANNEL BLOCKERS + BENZODIAZEPINES
Diltiazem significantly increases diazepam levels (n=13, RCT, d/b, c/o, Kosuge *et al*, *Drug Metab Dispos* 2001;**29**:1284–9; FFT, UK SmPC) and both diltiazem and **verapamil** significantly raise midazolam levels and half-life, probably via 3A4 inhibition and a 50% midazolam dose reduction has been recommended (n=9, RCT, d/b, c/o, 2/7, Backman *et al*, *Br J Clin Pharmacol* 1994;**37**:221–5; FFT).

Cannabis + benzodiazepines
See cannabis (*4.7.2*).

Carbamazepine + benzodiazepines
See carbamazepine (*4.4.1*).

Charcoal, activated + benzodiazepines
25 g of activated charcoal given 30 minutes after diazepam 5 mg reduces diazepam AUC by 27%, but not the peak levels. Concurrent gastric lavage does not provide any additional reductions (n=9, RCT, Lapatto-Reiniluoto *et al*, *Br J Clin Pharmacol* 1999;**48**:148–53; FFT).

Citalopram + benzodiazepines
See citalopram/escitalopram (*4.3.2.1*).

Clarithromycin + benzodiazepines
Clarithromycin (2.5 g/d) may increase midazolam's availability, probably via CYP3A4 inhibition (n=16, open, 8/7, Gorski *et al*, *Clin Pharmacol Ther* 1998;**64**:133–43).

CLOZAPINE + BENZODIAZEPINES
See clozapine (*4.2.4*).

Cyclophosphamide + benzodiazepines
Cyclophosphamide toxicity has been suggested in animals but not reported in humans.

Dehydroepiandrosterone + benzodiazepines
Alprazolam rapidly and significantly increases dehydroepiandrosterone levels (n=38, Kroboth *et al*, *J Clin Psychopharmacol* 1999;**19**:114–24).

Dextropropoxyphene + alprazolam
Increased sedation can occur with alprazolam.

Digoxin + benzodiazepines
Lack of interaction has been shown.

Disulfiram + benzodiazepines
See disulfiram (*4.6.8*).

Duloxetine + benzodiazepines *
See benzodiazepines + duloxetine (*4.3.3.2*).

Escitalopram + benzodiazepines
See citalopram/escitalopram (*4.3.2.1*).

Ethambutol + diazepam
Lack of interaction has been shown.

Fluoxetine + benzodiazepines
See fluoxetine (*4.3.2.2*).

Fluvoxamine + benzodiazepines
See fluvoxamine (*4.3.2.3*).

Food + benzodiazepines
Food delays the absorption of benzodiazepines; only significant if rapid onset of action is needed.

Gabapentin + benzodiazepines
See gabapentin (*4.5.1*).

Ginkgo biloba + benzodiazepines
GB may inhibit CYP3A4 and increase midazolam's AUC by 25–30%, possibly significantly (n=14, 2/52, Robertson *et al*, *Curr Med Res Opin* 2008;**24**:591–9), but has no effect on diazepam (n=12, Zuo *et al*, *Eur J Clin Pharmacol* 2010;**66**:503–9).

Grapefruit juice + benzodiazepines
200 mL normal-strength grapefruit juice increases plasma triazolam levels, and chronic use produces a greater increase (n=12, RCT, Lilja *et al*, *Eur J Clin Pharmacol* 2000;**56**:411–5).

Guanfacine + benzodiazepines
See benzodiazepines + guanfacine (*4.6.9*).

H2-blockers + benzodiazepines
Cimetidine slightly inhibits the metabolism of long-acting benzodiazepines, but not lorazepam, oxazepam or temazepam. Ranitidine may slightly reduce the absorption of diazepam (n=30, RCT, open, 3/7, O'Connor-Semmes *et al*, *Clin Pharmacol Ther* 2001;**70**:126–31).

Heparin + benzodiazepines
A transient rise in benzodiazepine levels could occur (n=14, open, Desmond *et al*, *Br J Clin Pharmacol* 1980;**9**:171–5; FFT).

Indometacin + diazepam
Increased dizziness may occur (d/b, Nuotto and Saariolho, *Pharmacol Toxicol* 1988;**62**:293–7).

Isoniazid + benzodiazepines
Isoniazid reduces the clearance of diazepam but not oxazepam (n=9, Ochs *et al*, *Clin Pharmacol Ther* 1981;**29**:671–8).

Lamotrigine + benzodiazepines
See lamotrigine (*4.4.2*).

LEVODOPA + BENZODIAZEPINES
Levodopa can be antagonised by diazepam,

nitrazepam and chlordiazepoxide (Yousselson *et al*, *Ann Intern Med* 1982;**96**:259–60).

Lithium + benzodiazepines
See lithium (*4.4.3*).

MAOIs + benzodiazepines
See MAOIs (*4.3.4*).

Melatonin + benzodiazepines
See melatonin (*4.1.4*).

Methadone + benzodiazepines
See methadone (*4.6.12*).

Methamphetamine + benzodiazepines
Alprazolam can produce 'small, but orderly, reductions in some subjective effects' of intranasal methamphetamine (n=8, Lile *et al*, *Drug Alcohol Depend* 2011;**119**:187–93).

Metronidazole + benzodiazepines
Lack of interaction has been reported.

Mianserin + benzodiazepines
See mianserin (*4.3.3.3*).

Mirtazapine + benzodiazepines
See mirtazapine (*4.3.3.4*).

Moclobemide + benzodiazepines
See moclobemide (*4.3.3.5*).

Modafinil + benzodiazepines
See modafinil (*4.6.14*).

Muscle relaxants + benzodiazepines
Diazepam may hasten the onset and prolong the duration of action of vecuronium (n=20, RCT, Yuan *et al*, *Chunghua Yi Xue Za Zhi (Taipei)* 1994;**54**:259–64), but midazolam appears not to do this (n=10, Husby *et al*, *Acta Anaesthesiol Scand* 1989;**33**:280–2).

Nimodipine + benzodiazepines
Lack of a clinically significant interaction has been reported (n=24, RCT, c/o, 3x5/7, Heine *et al*, *Br J Clin Pharmacol* 1994;**38**:39–43; FFT).

Olanzapine + benzodiazepines
See olanzapine (*4.2.6*).

Ondansetron + benzodiazepines
Lack of interaction has been shown with temazepam (n=24, RCT, d/b, c/o, 2/7, Preston *et al*, *Anesthesia* 1996;**51**:827–30).

Opioids + benzodiazepines
Synergism (e.g. n=95, RCT, d/b, Kissin *et al*, *Anesth Analg* 1990;**71**:65–9) and changes in haemodynamic status have been reported, as has a fatal interaction with clonazepam and oxycodone (n=1, Burrows *et al*, *J Forensic Sci* 2003;**48**:683–6).

Oral contraceptives + benzodiazepines
OCs may increase the effects of longer-acting benzodiazepines, probably of minimal significance.

Orlistat + benzodiazepines
Loss of BDZ efficacy has occurred (SmPC).

Paraldehyde + benzodiazepines
Enhanced sedation would be expected.

Paroxetine + benzodiazepines
See paroxetine (*4.3.2.4*).

Passiflora incarnata + benzodiazepines
See valerian + benzodiazepines.

Phenytoin + benzodiazepines
See phenytoin (*4.5.5*).

Physostigmine + benzodiazepines
Physostigmine may reverse diazepam (Speeg *et al*, *J Neurochem* 1980;**34**:856–5) and midazolam-induced somnolence (Ho *et al*, *Ma Zui Xue Za Zhi* 1991;**29**:643–7).

Pomegranate juice + benzodiazepines
A 'small Japanese adult' study showed that 200 mL pomegranate juice twice a day for two weeks had no significant effect on the kinetics of a single dose of midazolam (n=16, RCT, open, c/o, Misaka *et al*, *Clin Ther* 2011;**33**:246–52).

Pregabalin + benzodiazepines
See pregabalin (*4.1.5*).

Probenecid + lorazepam
Probenecid speeds the onset and prolongs the effect of lorazepam so doses should be reduced by 50% (SmPC).

Progabide + clonazepam
Lack of interaction has been reported.

Propofol + benzodiazepines
Propofol increases midazolam's half-life by 61%, probably by inhibiting CYP3A4 (n=24, RCT, Hamaoka *et al*, *Clin Pharmacol Ther* 1999;**66**:110–7).

Proton-pump inhibitors + benzodiazepines
Omeprazole and esomeprazole (review: Steinijans *et al*, *Int J Clin Pharmacol Ther* 1996;**34**:S31–S50), can reduce diazepam clearance by up to 50% (n=12, 1/52, Andersson *et al*, *Eur J Clin Pharmacol* 1990;**39**:51–4), AUC (28%), Cmax (31%) and half-life (41%) probably by 3A4 inhibition. Pantoprazole does not and is a safer alternative (n=24, RCT, d/b, c/o, Drewelow *et al*, *Arzneimittelforschung* 2010;**60**:483–91).

Quetiapine + benzodiazepines
See quetiapine (*4.2.7*).

Reboxetine + benzodiazepines
See reboxetine (*4.3.3.6*).

4

Rifampicin + benzodiazepines
CYP3A4 induction by rifampicin can lead to reduced levels of diazepam (n=21, 7/7, Ohnhaus, *Clin Pharmacol Ther* 1987;**42**:148) and midazolam (n=9, 9/7, Backman *et al*, *Eur J Clin Pharmacol* 1998;**54**:53–8).

Rivastigmine + benzodiazepines
See rivastigmine (*4.6.3.3*).

Rufinamide + benzodiazepines
Rufinamide induces CYP3A4 and reduces levels of, e.g. triazolam (UK SmPC) but rufinamide is unaffected.

Selegiline + benzodiazepines
Selegiline transdermal system (STS) had no effects on alprazolam (open, RCT, c/o, Azzaro *et al*, *J Clin Pharmacol* 2007;**47**:146–58).

Sertraline + benzodiazepines
See sertraline (*4.3.2.5*).

Smoking + benzodiazepines
See smoking (*4.7.4*).

Sodium oxybate + benzodiazepines
See sodium oxybate (*4.6.18*).

St John's wort + benzodiazepines
See St John's wort (*4.3.3.10*).

Statins + benzodiazepines *
Fatal rhabdomyolysis has been reported with midazolam and high dose atorvastatin (n=1, Gigante *et al*, *World J Gastrointest Pharmacol Ther* 2014; **5**:196–9; FFT).

Tiagabine + benzodiazepines
No interaction with triazolam has been detected (n=12, RCT, Richens *et al*, *Drug Metabol Drug Interact* 1998;**14**:159–77).

Ticagrelor + midazolam *
Ticagrelor reduces midazolam's AUC by 30% via other mechanisms so is a complicated interaction (s=2, n=56, RCT, d/b, p/c, c/o, 6/7, Teng and Butler, *Clin Ther* 2013;**35**:1025–37).

Triazole antifungals + benzodiazepines
Increased chlordiazepoxide oral bioavailability and midazolam AUC can be up to eight-fold higher with **ketoconazole**, (e.g. n=10, RCT, 12/7, Lam *et al*, *J Clin Pharmacol* 2003;**43**:1274–82). Midazolam levels were significantly higher with **itraconazole** 200mg/d, the effect being detectable up to four days after cessation of treatment (n=9, open, Backman *et al*, *Eur J Clin Pharmacol* 1998;**54**:53–8). **Posaconazole** is a less potent 3A4 inhibitor but can cause an up to 2.4-fold increase in midazolam levels (n=12, open, Krishna *et al*, *Clin Ther* 2009;**31**:286–98).

Tricyclics + benzodiazepines
Enhanced sedation would be expected. Clomipramine dose reduction may be necessary (Anon, *Pharmaceutisch Weekblad* 1992;**14**[4] Suppl D:D3).

Valerian + benzodiazepines
Tremor, dizziness and fatigue have been reported in someone on lorazepam after taking valerian *officinalis* and *Passiflora* incarnate (n=1, Carrasco *et al*, *Phytother Res* 2009;**23**:1795–6).

Valproate + benzodiazepines *
Valproate displaces diazepam from plasma protein-binding sites and so lower diazepam doses may be needed. Valproate increases lorazepam levels by up to 20–40% (SmPC) via reduced clearance (n=1, Lee *et al*, *Seizure* 2002;**11**:124–5) and stupor has been reported (n=2, Uz *et al*, *Turk Psikiyatri Derg* 2012;**23**:281–3). Valproate increases clonazepam clearance by 14% and clonazepam reduces valproate clearance by 18% (n=317, Yukawa *et al*, *J Clin Pharm Ther* 2003;**28**:497–504), probably of minimal significance (n=4, Wang and Wang, *Ther Drug Monit* 2002;**24**:532–6).

Venlafaxine + benzodiazepines
See venlafaxine (*4.3.3.8*).

Vortioxetine + benzodiazepines *
See vortioxetine (*4.3.3.9*).

Xanthines + benzodiazepines
Xanthines, e.g. **theophylline**, **aminophylline** and **caffeine** antagonise the sedative (and possibly anxiolytic) effects of benzodiazepines (e.g. midazolam is moderately antagonised by 250mg caffeine, n=114, Mattila *et al*, *Int J Clin Pharmacol Ther* 2000;**38**:581–7). This can be useful in the treatment of benzodiazepine overdose, but take care if a patient on a benzodiazepine has theophylline stopped, as respiratory depression could occur.

Ziprasidone + benzodiazepines
See ziprasidone (*4.2.9*).

4.1.2 BUSPIRONE

Buspirone is metabolised by CYP3A4 and has an active metabolite 6-hydroxybuspirone (n=13, Dockens *et al*, *J Clin Pharmacol* 2006;**46**:1308–12).

Alcohol + buspirone
See alcohol (*4.7.1*).

Antiretrovirals + buspirone
The combination has been used safely (n=2,

Batki, *J Clin Psychopharmacol* 1990;**10**[Suppl 3]:111S–5S) but severe EPSE have occurred after **ritonavir** was added to buspirone (n=1, Clay and Adams, *Ann Pharmacother* 2003;**37**:202–5).

Benzodiazepines + buspirone

Three studies with diazepam and alprazolam have shown a minimal enhanced sedation (n=24, 7/7, Buch *et al*, *J Clin Pharmacol* 1993;**33**:1104–9).

Beta-blockers + buspirone

Buspirone appears not to displace propranolol from plasma-binding sites (review: Gammans *et al*, *Am J Med* 1986;**80**[Suppl 3B]:41–51).

Calcium-channel blockers + buspirone

Verapamil and **diltiazem** increase buspirone plasma concentrations 3-fold and 5-fold respectively, probably by CYP3A4 inhibition, potentially enhancing buspirone's side-effects (n=9, RCT, p/c, c/o, Lamberg *et al*, *Clin Pharmacol Ther* 1998;**63**:640–5).

Cimetidine + buspirone

No interaction occurs (n=10, open, Gammans *et al*, *Pharmacotherapy* 1987;**7**:72–9).

Citalopram + buspirone

See citalopram/escitalopram (*4.3.2.1*).

Clozapine + buspirone

Near fatal gastrointestinal bleeding and hyperglycaemia occurred one month after buspirone was added to a stable clozapine regimen (n=1, Good, *Am J Psychiatry* 1997;**154**:1472–3).

ERYTHROMYCIN + BUSPIRONE

Erythromycin may increase plasma buspirone levels dramatically, probably via CYP3A4 inhibition, with increased side-effects noted (n=8, Kivisto *et al*, *Clin Pharmacol Ther* 1997;**62**:348–54).

Escitalopram + buspirone

See citalopram/escitalopram (*4.3.2.1*).

Fluoxetine + buspirone

Reduced anxiolytic effect, dystonia and akathisia (e.g. n=1, Metz, *Can J Psychiatry* 1990;**35**:722–3) have been reported.

Fluvoxamine + buspirone

Fluvoxamine raises buspirone levels, probably via CYP3A4 inhibition, of limited significance (n=10, RCT, Lamberg *et al*, *Eur J Clin Pharmacol* 1998;**54**:761–6).

Grapefruit juice + buspirone

200mL double-strength grapefruit juice may raise peak buspirone plasma levels four-fold, so avoid buspirone and, at least, large amounts of grapefruit juice, or adjust doses (n=10, RCT, Lilja *et al*, *Clin Pharmacol Ther* 1998;**64**:655–60).

MAOIs + BUSPIRONE

See MAOIs (*4.3.4*).

NSAIDs + buspirone

GI side-effects and headache may be slightly more common with the combination.

Phenytoin + buspirone

Buspirone does not appear to displace phenytoin from plasma-binding sites (review: Gammans *et al*, *Am J Med* 1986;**80**[Suppl 3B]:41–51).

Rifampicin + buspirone

Rifampicin decreases buspirone plasma levels, probably via CYP3A4 induction (UK SmPC). Significant changes in psychomotor tests have been noted so adjust doses when necessary (n=10, Lamberg *et al*, *Br J Clin Pharmacol* 1998;**45**:381–5; FFT).

St John's wort + buspirone

There is a possible case of serotonin syndrome (n=1, Dannawi, *J Psychopharmacol* 2002;**16**:401).

Terfenadine + buspirone

No interaction occurs (n=10, RCT, p/c, c/o, 3/7, Lamberg *et al*, *Pharmacol Toxicol* 1999;**84**:165–9).

Trazodone + buspirone

There are isolated reports of raised SGPT/ALT levels and serotonin syndrome (n=1, Goldberg and Huk, *Psychosomatics* 1992;**3**:235–6).

Triazole antifungals + buspirone

Itraconazole may increase plasma buspirone levels dramatically, probably via CYP3A4 inhibition, with increased side-effects noted (n=8, Kivistö *et al*, *Clin Pharmacol Ther* 1997;**62**:348–54).

Warfarin + buspirone

Buspirone does not appear to displace warfarin from plasma-binding sites (review: Gammans *et al*, *Am J Med* 1986;**80**[3B]:41–51).

4.1.3 CHLORAL HYDRATE

Chloral is probably metabolised by CYP2E1.

Acenocoumarol + chloral hydrate

An enhanced anticoagulant effect can occur. See also warfarin + chloral hydrate.

ALCOHOL + CHLORAL HYDRATE

See alcohol (*4.7.1*)

Fluvoxamine + chloral hydrate

See fluvoxamine (*4.3.2.3*).

Furosemide + chloral hydrate

Rapidly reversible diaphoresis, facial flushing and agitation have occurred with chloral hydrate and IV furosemide (n=1, Dean *et al*, *Clin Pharm* 1991;**10**:385–7).

MAOIs + chloral hydrate
See MAOIs (*4.3.4*).

Methadone + chloral hydrate
See methadone (*4.6.12*).

Methotrexate + chloral *
The AUC of methotrexate was nearly twice as high with chloral (n = 1, Dao *et al*, *Pediatr Blood Cancer* 2013;**60**:518–20).

Phenytoin + chloral hydrate
See phenytoin (*4.5.5*).

Warfarin + chloral hydrate
The anticoagulant effect of warfarin is slightly increased by chloral, probably by plasma protein displacement (BCDSP, *N Engl J Med* 1972;**286**:53–5). This can be important if chloral hydrate is given as a "when required" hypnotic.

4.1.4 MELATONIN

Melatonin is metabolised by 1A2 and possibly 2C9/19 (Facciola *et al*, *Eur J Clin Pharmacol* 2001;**56**:881–8). It induces 3A4, and possibly 2C19, but has no effect on 1A2.

Review: * general (Papagiannidou *et al*, *Physiol Behav* 2014;**131**:17–24).

Alcohol + melatonin
Alcohol reduces the effect of melatonin (SmPC).

Antipsychotics + melatonin
Muzzy-headedness has been reported with thioridazine and melatonin (SmPC).

Benzodiazepines + melatonin
Melatonin enhances the sedative effects of benzodiazepines (SmPC).

Carbamazepine + melatonin
Carbamazepine may decrease melatonin levels (SmPC) via 1A2 induction.

Cimetidine + melatonin
Cimetidine may raise melatonin levels (SmPC).

Citalopram/escitalopram + melatonin
See citalopram/escitalopram (*4.3.2.1*).

Estrogens + melatonin
Estrogens (e.g. oral contraceptives or HRT) may increase melatonin levels (SmPC).

FLUVOXAMINE + MELATONIN
Fluvoxamine may raise melatonin levels, with AUC 17-fold higher and Cmax 12-fold higher (UK SmPC) (e.g. n=5, open, Hartter *et al*, *Clin Pharmacol Ther* 2000;**67**:1–6).

Methoxypsoralen + melatonin
Melatonin levels can be raised (SmPC).

Quinolones + melatonin
Quinolones may increase melatonin levels via 1A2 inhibition (SmPC).

Rifampicin + melatonin
Rifampicin may decrease melatonin levels (SmPC) via 1A2 induction.

Smoking + melatonin
Smoking may decrease melatonin levels (SmPC) via 1A2 induction.

Tricyclics + melatonin
Increased feelings of tranquility may occur with imipramine and melatonin (SmPC).

Zaleplon + melatonin
Melatonin can enhance the sedative effects of zaleplon (SmPC).

Zolpidem + melatonin
Melatonin can enhance the sedative effects of zolpidem (SmPC).

Zopiclone + melatonin
Melatonin can enhance the sedative effects of zopiclone (SmPC).

4.1.5 PREGABALIN

Pregabalin is excreted by the kidneys, undergoes little metabolism, has no effect on P450 enzymes, and is not plasma protein so significant interactions are unlikely. Lack of interaction has also been shown with antidiabetics, diuretics and insulin.

Review: interactions with other AEDs (Bockbrader *et al*, *Epilepsia* 2011;**52**:405–9).

Alcohol + pregabalin
Pregabalin may potentiate the sedative effects of alcohol (SmPC).

Benzodiazepines + pregabalin
Pregabalin may potentiate the sedative effects of lorazepam (SmPC).

Carbamazepine+ pregabalin
Lack of interaction has been shown (UK SmPC).

Clozapine + pregabalin
See pregabalin + clozapine (*4.2.4*).

Gabapentin + pregabalin
Lack of interaction has been shown (UK SmPC), but pregabalin displaces gabapentin from receptors.

Lacosamide + pregabalin
Enhanced PR prolongation can occur (SmPC).

Lamotrigine + pregabalin
Lack of interaction has been shown (UK SmPC).

Oral contraceptives + pregabalin
Lack of interaction has been shown (UK SmPC).

Oxycodone + pregabalin *

Pregabalin may enhance the cognitive and motor effects of oxycodone (SmPC) and serotonin syndrome has been reported (n=1, Song, *Pain Physician* 2013;**16**:E632–3).

Phenobarbital + pregabalin
Lack of interaction has been shown (UK SmPC).

Phenytoin + pregabalin
Lack of interaction has been shown (UK SmPC).

Tiagabine + pregabalin
Lack of interaction has been shown (UK SmPC) although increased tiagabine clearance is possible (Bockbrader *et al*, *Epilepsia* 2011;**52**:405–9).

Topiramate + pregabalin
Lack of interaction has been shown (UK SmPC).

Simvastatin + pregabalin *
Rhabdomyolysis has been reported (n=1, Kaufman and Choy, *PT* 2012;**37**:579–95).

Valproate + pregabalin
Lack of interaction has been shown (UK SmPC).

4.1.6 ZALEPLON

Zaleplon is primarily metabolised by aldehyde oxidase, and a small amount by CYP3A4, to inactive metabolites.

Alcohol + zaleplon
See alcohol (*4.7.1*).

Antipsychotics + zaleplon
Additive psychomotor effects may occur with thioridazine (n=12, RCT, Hetta *et al*, *Eur J Clin Pharmacol* 2000;**56**:211–7).

Carbamazepine + zaleplon
Co-administration may reduce zaleplon's efficacy through CYP3A4 induction.

Cimetidine + zaleplon
Raised zaleplon levels can occur with cimetidine, via aldehyde oxidase and CYP3A4 inhibition.

Digoxin + zaleplon
Lack of interaction has been shown (n=20, Sanchez-Garcia *et al*, *Am J Health Syst Pharm* 2000;**57**:2267–70).

Erythromycin + zaleplon
Raised zaleplon levels can occur, via 3A4 inhibition.

Ibuprofen + zaleplon
Lack of significant interaction has been shown (n=17, open, Sanchez Garcia *et al*, *Am J Health Syst Pharm* 2000;**57**:1137–41).

Ketoconazole + zaleplon
Raised zaleplon levels can occur, via 3A4 inhibition.

Melatonin + zaleplon
See melatonin (*4.1.4*).

Opioids + zaleplon
Enhanced euphoria is possible.

Phenobarbital + zaleplon
Reduced zaleplon levels can occur, via CYP3A4 induction.

Rifampicin + zaleplon
A four-fold reduction in zaleplon levels can occur, via CYP3A4 induction.

Warfarin + zaleplon
Lack of interaction has been shown.

4.1.7 ZOLPIDEM

Zolpidem is mainly metabolised by CYP3A4 and has no effect on 1A2, 2B6, 2C9, 2D6 and 3A4. Enhanced sedation would be expected with concurrent use with any CNS depressant.

Alcohol + zolpidem
See alcohol (*4.7.1*).

Antipsychotics + zolpidem
Excessive sedation has been reported with chlorpromazine (n=6, d/b, single-dose, Desager *et al*, *Psychopharmacol* 1988;**96**:63–6).

Bupropion + zolpidem
See bupropion (*4.6.6*).

Caffeine + zolpidem
While antagonism would be expected, 300 mg caffeine did not antagonise the sedative effects of zolpidem given during the day (n=45+, d/b, p/c, Mattila *et al*, *Eur J Clin Pharmacol* 1998;**54**:421–5), and there are even cases of paradoxically enhanced sedation (discussion of putative mechanisms; Myslobodsky, *Curr Drug Targets* 2009;**10**:1009–20).

Carbamazepine + zolpidem
Carbamazepine can produce a 57% reduction in zolpidem plasma levels and shorten the half-life (Vlase *et al*, *J Clin Pharmacol* 2011;**51**:1233–6).

Ciprofloxacin + zolpidem
Ciprofloxacin 500 mg can increase zolpidem's half-life by an hour, lengthen time to Tmax and increase AUC by 46%, potentially significant (Vlase *et al*, *Eur J Drug Metab Pharmacokinet* 2011;**35**:83–7).

Clarithromycin + zolpidem
Clarithromycin has no effect on the kinetics or dynamics of zolpidem (n=10, c/o, Farkas *et al*, *Clin Pharmacol Ther* 2009;**85**:644–50).

4

Food + zolpidem
The rate of absorption of zolpidem is slowed significantly by food.

Gabapentin + zolpidem *
Lack of interaction has been shown (n=40, Galitz *et al, Drugs R D* 2015; **15**:71–7; FFT).

H2-blockers + zolpidem
Lack of interaction has been shown with cimetidine and ranitidine (n=6, c/o, 18/7, Hulhoven *et al, Int J Clin Pharmacol Res* 1988;**8**:471–6).

Melatonin + zolpidem
See melatonin (*4.1.4*).

Oral Contraceptives + zolpidem
Zolpidem clearance is slightly higher and half-life slightly shorter in women using OCs (n=16, Olubodun *et al, J Clin Pharmacol* 2002;**42**:1142–6).

Rifampicin + zolpidem
Rifampicin significantly reduces zolpidem's plasma levels and therapeutic effect, via CYP3A4 induction (n=8, RCT, Villikka *et al, Clin Pharmacol Ther* 1997;**43**:629–34).

Smoking + zolpidem
Zolpidem's half-life may be 30% shorter in smokers than non-smokers, of low clinical significance (due to CYP1A2 induction; n=16, Olubodun *et al, J Clin Pharmacol* 2002;**42**:1142–6).

Sodium oxybate + zolpidem
See sodium oxybate (*4.6.18*).

SSRIs + zolpidem *
SSRIs may enhance zolpidem-associated hallucinations (n=5, Elko *et al, J Toxicol Clin Toxicol* 1998;**36**:195–203; n=1 Coleman and Ota, *J Forensic Sci* 2004;**49**:392–3). There is a minimal interaction between **fluoxetine** and regular zolpidem, although zolpidem's half-life increases slightly (n=29, 5/52, Allard *et al, Drug Metab Dispos* 1998;**26**:617–22; FFT). **Fluvoxamine** increases zolpidem plasma levels and AUC by about 150% (Vlase *et al, Clin Exp Pharmacol Physiol* 2012;**39**:9–12) and visual hallucinations and amnesia have been reported (n=1, Kito and Koga, *Int Psychogeriatr* 2006;**18**:749–51) e.g. with paroxetine (n=1, Skourides and Samartzis, *Prim Care Companion CNS Disord* 2012;**14**:12i01361). **Sertraline** may lead to a shorter onset of action and an increased effect from zolpidem (n=28, RCT, Allard *et al, J Clin Pharmacol* 1999;**39**:184–91).

St John's wort + zolpidem
In most people SJW reduces zolpidem AUC and Cmax by 30% but can slightly increase it in a few (n=3) people (n=14, 14/7, Hojo *et al, J Clin Pharm Ther* 2011;**36**:711–5).

Triazole antifungals + zolpidem
Itraconazole or **fluconazole** slightly lengthen zolpidem's half-life (n=12, RCT, Greenblatt *et al, Clin Pharmacol Ther* 1998;**64**:661–71), although not inevitably (n=10, RCT, c/o, 4/7, Luurila *et al, Eur J Clin Pharmacol* 1998;**54**:163–6).

Valproate + zolpidem
Somnambulism has been reported with the combination (n=1, Sattar *et al, Ann Pharmacother* 2003;**37**:1429–33).

4.1.8 ZOPICLONE

Zopiclone is mainly metabolised by CYP3A4 to active metabolites, with 2C8 a minor metaboliser. It is excreted via the urine (80%) and faeces (16%).

Alcohol + zopiclone
See alcohol (*4.7.1*).

Aspirin + zopiclone
Lack of interaction has been shown.

Caffeine + zopiclone
Caffeine moderately antagonises the psychomotor impairment caused by zopiclone (d/b, Mattila *et al, Pharmacol Toxicol* 1992;**70**:286–9).

Erythromycin + zopiclone
Erythromycin accelerates zopiclone absorption, leading to a more rapid onset, which could be clinically significant in the elderly (n=10, Aranko *et al, Br J Clin Pharmacol* 1994;**38**:363–7; FFT).

Itraconazole + zopiclone
Itraconazole may significantly increase zopiclone plasma levels by 28% and half-life by 40%, but not clinically significantly (n=10, d/b, p/c, c/o, Jalava *et al, Eur J Clin Pharmacol* 1996;**51**:331–4).

Melatonin + zopiclone
See melatonin (*4.1.4*).

Ranitidine + zopiclone
Lack of interaction has been shown.

Rifampicin + zopiclone
Rifampicin significantly reduces zopiclone plasma levels and effect (n=8, RCT, Villikka *et al, Br J Clin Pharmacol* 1997;**43**:471–4; FFT).

Tricyclics + zopiclone
One study showed minimally decreased levels of trimipramine and zopiclone (n=10, RCT, Caille *et al, Biopharm Drug Dispos* 1984;**5**:117–25).

4.2 ANTIPSYCHOTICS

Aripiprazole (4.2.2), asenapine (4.2.3) clozapine (4.2.4), lurasidone (4.2.5) olanzapine (4.2.6), quetiapine (4.2.7), risperidone/ paliperidone (4.2.8) and ziprasidone (4.2.9) also have their own sections.

4.2.1 ANTIPSYCHOTICS — GENERAL

There are few specific interactions reported for some antipsychotics, other than additive sedation. **Phenothiazines** have multiple metabolites and multiple metabolism, with 1A2 the prominent enzyme (Wójcikowski *et al, Biochem Pharmacol* 2010;**80**:1252–9). **Sulpiride** has no significant effect on 1A2, 2C9, 2C19, 2D6 2E1 or 3A4 enzymes (Niwa *et al, Biol Pharm Bull* 2005;**28**:188–91; FFT). **Haloperidol** is metabolised by 3A4, 2D6 and by glucuronidation. Use of **haloperidol** with other drugs known to prolong the QTc interval is not recommended (UK SmPC, 2009), e.g:

- Class 1A (quinidine, disopyramide, procainamide)
- Class III (e.g. amiodarone, sotalol, dofetilide)
- Some antimicrobials (moxifloxacin, IV erythromycin)
- Tricyclics, other antipsychotics (e.g. pimozide, phenothiazines), bretylium, quinine, mefloquine.

Review: * Clinically relevant interactions between newer antidepressants and SGAs (Spina and de Leon, *Expert Opin Drug Metab Toxicol* 2014;**10**:721–46).

ACE inhibitors + antipsychotics

Enhanced hypotension has been reported, e.g. captopril plus chlorpromazine (n = 1, White, *Arch Int Med* 1986;**146**:1833–4).

Activated charcoal + phenothiazines

Decreased antipsychotic absorption is likely.

ALCOHOL + ANTIPSYCHOTICS

See alcohol (*4.7.1*).

Amfetamines + antipsychotics

Antipsychotic effects can be antagonised by amfetamines.

Amiodarone + antipsychotics

There is an increased risk of ventricular arrhythmias and a small but potentially significant QTc prolongation (but not ventricular arrhythmia) has been seen with haloperidol (n=49, Bush *et al, Am J Health Syst Pharm* 2008;**65**:2232–6).

Antacids + antipsychotics

Antacids may reduce chlorpromazine and possibly haloperidol serum levels. Sulpiride absorption may be reduced by sucralfate or aluminium-containing antacids. Separating doses by a couple of hours minimises the effect.

Anticholinergics + antipsychotics

Anticholinergics may reduce the efficacy of antipsychotics, probably by lowering their serum levels (n = 25, Bamrah *et al, Br J Psychiatry* 1986;**149**:726–33). Additive anticholinergic effects, e.g. acute intestinal pseudo-obstruction have been reported with benzatropine and haloperidol (n = 1, Sheikh *et al, Am J Gastroenterol* 2001;**96**:934–5). The UK SmPC recommends anticholinergics are not used with **olanzapine.**

ANTICONVULSANTS + ANTIPSYCHOTICS

Antipsychotics lower the seizure threshold and may thus antagonise anticonvulsant actions. See also individual anticonvulsants (*4.5*).

ANTIHISTAMINES + ANTIPSYCHOTICS

Loratadine and **fexofenadine** are currently considered suitable, although there are three unproven reports of arrhythmia with loratadine.

Antimalarials + chlorpromazine

One study showed markedly increased chlorpromazine levels with e.g. chloroquine and 'Fansidar' (open, Makanjuola *et al, Trop Geogr Med* 1988;**40**:31–3).

Aripiprazole + antipsychotics (other)

See aripiprazole (*4.2.2*).

BARBITURATES + ANTIPSYCHOTICS

Additive sedative effects can occur acutely and death has been reported (n = 1, Hino *et al, Leg Med [Tokyo]* 1999;**1**:48–51). Barbiturates may induce the metabolism of many antipsychotics, e.g. haloperidol levels are reduced by 40–75%.

Benzodiazepines + antipsychotics

Enhanced sedation and impaired psychomotor function can occur (see *1.1*) and a death has been reported with an overdose of triazolam and promazine (n = 1, Rossi *et al, Med Sci Law* 2009;**49**:65–8).

Beta-blockers + antipsychotics

Raised antipsychotic plasma levels may occur, possibly clinically significant, e.g. chlorpromazine levels may rise by up to 500% with **propranolol** (Peet *et al, Lancet* 1980;**2**:978), although **pindolol** has no significant effect on haloperidol levels (n = 26, open, Greendyke and Gulya, *J Clin Psychiatry* 1988;**49**:105–7).

4

Betel nut + antipsychotics
Betel nut (*Areca catechu*) contains the cholinergic alkaloid arecoline, and has caused EPSE and bradykinesia with flupentixol and fluphenazine (n=1, Deahl, *Mov Disord* 1998;**4**:330–3).

Bromocriptine + antipsychotics
Predictable antagonism of antipsychotic and hypoprolactinaemic and antiparkinsonian effects may occur.

Calcium-channel blockers + antipsychotics
Increased antipsychotic levels or enhanced hypotension might occur (review by Markowitz *et al*, *Ann Pharmacother* 1995;**29**:603–9).

Cannabis + antipsychotics
See cannabis (*4.7.2*).

CARBAMAZEPINE + ANTIPSYCHOTICS
See carbamazepine (*4.4.1*).

Citalopram + antipsychotics
See antipsychotics + (es)citalopram (*4.3.2.1*).

Clonidine + antipsychotics
Phenothiazines and haloperidol (but not pimozide) may antagonise the hypotensive effect of clonidine and severe hypotension and delirium have been reported (review by Markowitz *et al*, *Ann Pharmacother* 1995;**29**:603–9).

CLOZAPINE + ANTIPSYCHOTICS (other)
See clozapine (*4.2.4*).

Cocaine + antipsychotics
See cocaine (*4.7.3*).

Desferrioxamine + prochlorperazine
Prolonged unconsciousness may occur.

Diazoxide + chlorpromazine
Enhanced hypoglycaemia has been reported (n=1, Aynsley-Green and Illig, *Lancet* 1975;**2**:658).

Disopyramide + antipsychotics
Increased anticholinergic effects may occur.

Disulfiram + antipsychotics
See disulfiram (*4.6.8*).

Domperidone + antipsychotics
There is an enhanced risk of EPSE.

Donepezil + antipsychotics
See donepezil (*4.6.3.1*).

Escitalopram + antipsychotics
See citalopram/escitalopram (*4.3.2.1*).

FLUOXETINE + ANTIPSYCHOTICS
Severe EPSE have been reported with fluoxetine and **haloperidol** (n=1, Tate, *Am J Psychiatry* 1989;**146**:399–400), dystonia with **fluphenazine**, and stupor, confusion, and severe bradycardia and drowsiness (n=1, Friedman, *Can J Psychiatry* 1994;**39**:634) with **pimozide**. **Zuclopenthixol** levels are increased by around 93% by fluoxetine, in a dose-dependent manner (n=923 samples, Davies *et al*, *Acta Psychiatr Scand* 2010;**122**:444–53). This has led to laryngeal dystonia (n=1, Hood *et al*, *Australas Psychiatry* 2010;**18**:174–6), so the combination should be avoided if possible (n=1, Ahmed *et al*, *Can J Psychiatry* 1993;**38**:62–3). Citalopram, escitalopram and sertraline would be suitable alternatives.

Fluvoxamine + antipsychotics
See fluvoxamine (*4.3.2.3*).

Ginseng + haloperidol
Ginseng may potentiate the effects of haloperidol (Mitra *et al*, *Indian J Exp Biol* 1996;**34**:41–7).

Guanfacine + antipsychotics
See antipsychotics + guanfacine (*4.6.9*).

H2-blockers + antipsychotics
Chlorpromazine levels may be reduced by 30% by **cimetidine** (Howes *et al*, *Eur J Clin Pharmacol* 1983;**24**:99–102), but not **ranitidine**.

Haloperidol + chlorpromazine
Chlorpromazine may significantly raise haloperidol levels, probably via CYP2D6 inhibition (n=43, Suzuki *et al*, *Ther Drug Monit* 2001;**23**:363–8).

Hydroxyzine + phenothiazines
The effect of phenothiazines may be decreased (Ross and Priest, *Dis Nerv Syst* 1970;**31**:412).

Hypoglycaemics + chlorpromazine
Chlorpromazine can induce hyperglycaemia and disrupt the control of diabetes (Schwarz and Munoz, *Am J Psychiatry* 1968;**125**:253).

Indometacin + haloperidol
Profound drowsiness and confusion can occur (Bird *et al*, *Lancet* 1983;**1**:830–1).

Letrozole + zuclopenthixol *
Apparent zuclopenthixol toxicity has been reported developing over 6/12 and dramatic reversal over 2/7 when letrozole was stopped (n=1, Lertxundi *et al*, *Nord J Psychiatry* 2015;**69**:79–80).

LEVODOPA + ANTIPSYCHOTICS
The therapeutic effect of levodopa is antagonised by antipsychotics and vice versa. Levodopa may worsen antipsychotic-induced EPSE.

Levomepromazine + zuclopenthixol
Zuclopenthixol levels are increased by around 46% by levomepromazine, in a dose-dependent manner (n=923 samples, Davies *et al*, *Acta Psychiatr Scand* 2010;**122**:444–53).

Lithium + antipsychotics

See antipsychotics + lithium (*4.4.3*).

MACROLIDE ANTIBIOTICS + ANTIPSYCHOTICS

There are reports of an increased risk of arrhythmias with **clarithromycin** and phenothiazines and the combination should be avoided as death has been reported with clarithromycin and pimozide (n=1, Flockhart *et al*, *J Clin Psychopharmacol* 2000;**20**:317–24).

MAOIs + antipsychotics

See antipsychotics + MAOIs (*4.3.4*).

Melatonin + antipsychotics

See melatonin (*4.1.4*).

Memantine + antipsychotics

See memantine (*4.6.11*).

Methadone + sulpiride

The sulpiride SmPC now states that it should be used with caution with drugs that can prolong QTc, e.g. methadone and halofantrine.

Metirosine + antipsychotics

An enhanced risk of EPSE exists.

Metoclopramide + antipsychotics

An enhanced risk of EPSE exists.

Minocycline + phenothiazines

Pigmented galactorrhoea has been reported with the combination (n=1, Basler and Lynch, *Arch Dermatol* 1985;**121**:417–8).

Naltrexone + phenothiazines

See naltrexone (*4.6.16*).

Olanzapine + antipsychotics (other)

See olanzapine (*4.2.6*).

Oral contraceptives + chlorpromazine

There is a report of a combined OC raising chlorpromazine levels six-fold (n=1, Chetty and Miller, *Ther Drug Monit* 2001;**23**:556–8).

Orlistat + haloperidol *

A small trial suggested a lack of interaction (n=8, open, 8/52, Hilger *et al*, *J Clin Psychopharmacol* 2002;**22**:68–70) but loss of antipsychotic efficacy has occurred (SmPC).

Oxcarbazepine + antipsychotics

See oxcarbazepine (*4.5.3*).

Paroxetine + antipsychotics

See antipsychotics + paroxetine (*4.3.2.4*).

Pethidine + phenothiazines

Increased CNS toxicity and hypotension can occur (n=10, open, c/o, Stambaugh and Wainer, *J Clin Pharmacol* 1981;**21**:140–6).

PHENYTOIN + ANTIPSYCHOTICS

Phenytoin may reduce **haloperidol** levels by 40–75%, probably via enzyme induction (n=30, open, Linnoila *et al*, *Am J Psychiatry* 1980;**137**:819). **Chlorpromazine** may increase phenytoin levels by up to 50% (n=27, open, Sands *et al*, *Drug Intell Clin Pharm* 1987;**21**:267–72). Other studies show a nil or opposite effect. Antipsychotics may antagonise the anticonvulsant effect of phenytoin.

Polymyxins + phenothiazines

The neuromuscular blocking effects of polymyxin antibiotics may be increased by phenothiazines with prolonged respiratory depression possible (n=1, Pohlmann, *JAMA* 1966;**196**:181).

Procarbazine + antipsychotics

Enhanced sedation is possible.

Quetiapine + antipsychotics (other)

See quetiapine (*4.2.7*).

Reboxetine + antipsychotics

See reboxetine (*4.3.3.6*).

RIFAMPICIN + HALOPERIDOL

Rifampicin may reduce haloperidol serum levels by a third (n=17, Kim *et al*, *J Clin Psychopharmacol* 1996;**16**:247–52), a clinically significant effect. Care would be needed if rifampicin were stopped.

Sertraline + antipsychotics

See sertraline (*4.3.2.5*).

Smoking + antipsychotics

See smoking (*4.7.4*).

Suxamethonium + promazine

Prolonged apnoea has been reported (n=1, Regan and Aldrete, *Anesth Analg* 1967;**46**:315–8).

Sucralfate + antipsychotics

See antacids + antipsychotics (*4.2.1*).

Tea or coffee + antipsychotics

Phenothiazines may precipitate out of solution to form a tannin complex with tea and coffee, almost certainly of minimal clinical significance (Bowen *et al*, *Lancet* 1981;**i**:1217–8).

Terbinafine + perphenazine *

Perphenazine toxicity lasting 5–6 weeks has been reported after a week's course of terbinafine (n=1, Park, *Psychiatry Investig* 2012;**9**:422–4).

Tetrabenazine + antipsychotics

Enhanced EPSE in a Huntington's patient has been reported (n=1, Moss and Stewart, *Can J Psychiatry* 1986;**31**:865–6).

Trazodone + antipsychotics

See trazodone (*4.3.3.7*).

Triazole antifungals + haloperidol

Itraconazole 200mg/d for seven days significantly increases haloperidol levels, leading to increased side-effects, presumably via CYP3A4 inhibition (n=13, Yasui *et al*, *J Clin Psychopharmacol* 1999; **19**:149–54).

Tricyclics + antipsychotics
See tricyclics (*4.3.1*).
Valproate + antipsychotics *
Valproate may lower **aripiprazole** levels by 23%, probably clinically insignificant (n=69, Eryılmaz *et al, Int J Psychiatry Clin Pract* 2014;**18**:288–92). **Chlorpromazine** may inhibit valproate's metabolism so monitor valproate levels (open, Ishizaki *et al, J Clin Psychopharmacol* 1984;**4**:254–61). Valproate has no significant effect on **haloperidol** plasma levels (n=27, 4/52, Hesslinger *et al, J Clin Psychopharmacol* 1999;**19**:310–5) or **risperidone** and **paliperidone** (e.g. n=12, Yoshimura *et al, Pharmacopsychiatry* 2007;**40**:9–13), but there are cases of dose-related generalised oedema with risperidone and valproate (n=2, Sanders and Lehrer, *J Clin Psychiatry* 1998;**59**:689–90). However, risperidone plus valproate may cause less weight gain and metabolic abnormalities than risperidone monotherapy, the opposite to valproate's effect on olanzapine (n=160, RCT, open, 12/12, Meltzer *et al, J Clin Psychiatry* 2011;**72**:1602–10). Risperidone might be a risk factor for valproate-induced encephalopathy (n=1, Rodrigues-Silva *et al, Gen Hosp Psychiatry* 2013;**35**:452.e5–6). Valproate is often used as anticonvulsant cover for higher doses of **clozapine**, but a careful study showed valproate to produce a 15% drop in clozapine levels and a 65% drop in norclozapine levels (eg. n=151, Diaz *et al, Pharmacopsychiatry* 2014;**47**:89–96), although raised clozapine levels have been reported (n=1, Costello and Suppes, *J Clin Psychopharmacol* 1995;**15**:139–41). Since norclozapine is more toxic than clozapine, this may be a useful effect with careful manipulation of the dose. Clozapine may, of course, lower the seizure threshold and antagonise the anticonvulsant effect of valproate. Valproate increases paliperidone Cmax and AUC by 50%, but paliperidone has no effect on valproate (18/7, Remmerie *et al, J Clin Pharmacol* 2015; in press).
Venlafaxine + antipsychotics
See venlafaxine (*4.3.3.8*).
Warfarin + antipsychotics
An interaction is theoretically possible (see Sayal *et al, Acta Psychiatr Scand* 2000;**102**:250–5).
Zaleplon + antipsychotics
See zaleplon (*4.1.6*).
Zolpidem + antipsychotics
See zolpidem (*4.1.7*).

4.2.2 ANTIPSYCHOTICS — ARIPIPRAZOLE

Aripiprazole is metabolised mainly by CYP2D6 (n=80, Kim *et al, Br J Clin Pharmacol* 2008;**66**:802–10;FFT) and 3A4, but not CYP1A1, 1A2 or 2C9/19. It has no effect on CYP2C9, 2C19, 2D6 and 3A4. Inducers of 3A4 may lower aripiprazole levels by about 60%, while 3A4 inhibitors increase levels by about 45% (samples=361, Waade *et al, Ther Drug Monit* 2009;**31**:233–8). The UK SmPC now states that caution is necessary with drugs that cause QTc prolongation or electrolyte imbalance.
Alcohol + aripiprazole
See alcohol (*4.7.1*).
Antipsychotics (other) + aripiprazole *
There is a theoretical interaction between aripiprazole and potent D2 antagonists, as aripiprazole has a very high affinity for D2 receptors and displaces almost any other antipsychotic from D2 receptors. There is a case of asymptomatic QTc prolongation with aripiprazole and **haloperidol** (n=1, Leo *et al, J Clin Psychiatry* 2008;**69**:327–8). Exacerbation of tics has been reported with pimozide (n=1, Mazium *et al, J Clin Psychopharmacol* 2015;**35**:350–1). See also combinations in *C1.23*.
CARBAMAZEPINE + ARIPIPRAZOLE
See antipsychotics + carbamazepine (*4.4.1*).
Citalopram + aripiprazole
See antipsychotics + citalopram (*4.3.2.1*).
Dextromethorphan + aripiprazole
Lack of interaction has been shown.
Duloxetine + aripiprazole
See aripiprazole + duloxetine (*4.3.3.2*).
Escitalopram + aripiprazole
See antipsychotics + escitalopram (*4.3.2.1*).
Fluoxetine + aripiprazole *
Pooled data shows no substantial effect from aripiprazole on fluoxetine and norfluoxetine kinetics (s=2, n=55, d/b, p/c, Boulton *et al, J Psychopharmacol* 2010;**24**:537–46; MS), although there are reports of leucopenia (n=1, Huang and Chiang, *J Clin Psychopharmacol* 2011;**31**:376–7) and dyskinesia (n=1, Patra, *Curr Drug Saf* 2015; in press).
Fluvoxamine + aripiprazole
See antipsychotics + fluvoxamine (*4.3.2.3*).
H2-blockers + aripiprazole
Lack of significant interaction has been shown with famotidine.

Lamotrigine + aripiprazole
See aripiprazole + lamotrigine (see *4.4.2*).
Lithium + aripiprazole
See antipsychotics + lithium (*4.4.3*).
Omeprazole + aripiprazole
Lack of interaction has been shown.
Paroxetine + aripiprazole
See antipsychotics + paroxetine (*4.3.2.4*).
Quinidine + aripiprazole
Quinidine decreases aripiprazole metabolism and so aripiprazole doses should be halved.
Smoking + aripiprazole
See smoking (*4.7.4*)
Sertraline + aripiprazole
See antipsychotics + sertraline (*4.3.2.5*).
Tamoxifen + aripiprazole
Tardive dyskinesia has been reported (n=1, Evcimen *et al, Am J Psychiatry* 2007;**164**:1436–7).
Triazole antifungals + aripiprazole
Although **itraconazole** is a potent CYP3A4 inhibitor, it made no clinically significant difference to aripiprazole levels in one study (n=24, Kubo *et al, Drug Metab Pharmacokinet* 2005;**20**:55–64; FFT). **Ketoconazole** decreases aripiprazole metabolism and so aripiprazole doses should be decreased by a half during co-administration.
Valproate + aripiprazole
See valproate + antipsychotics (*4.2.1*).
Venlafaxine + aripiprazole
See antipsychotics + venlafaxine (*4.3.3.8*).
Warfarin + aripiprazole
Lack of interaction has been shown.

4.2.3 ANTIPSYCHOTICS — ASENAPINE

Asenapine is extensively and rapidly metabolised by UGT1A4 and CYP1A2 (van de Wetering-Krebbers *et al, Drug Metab Dispos* 2011;**39**:580–90; FFT).
Cimetidine + asenapine
Lack of interaction has been shown (UK SmPC).
Carbamazepine + asenapine
See antipsychotics + carbamazepine (*4.4.1*).
Fluvoxamine + asenapine
See antipsychotics + fluvoxamine (*4.3.2.3*).
Imipramine + asenapine
Lack of interaction has been shown (UK SmPC).
Paroxetine + asenapine
Lack of interaction has been shown, although asenapine may enhance the inhibitory effects of paroxetine on its own metabolism (UK SmPC).
Smoking + asenapine
Lack of interaction has been shown (UK SmPC).
Valproate + asenapine
Valproate almost completely inhibits the glucuronidation of asenapine, but this seems to have no effect on the actual pharmacokinetics of asenapine (n=24, RCT, open, c/o, Gerrits *et al, J Clin Pharmacol* 2012;**52**:757–65; see also UK SmPC).

4.2.4 ANTIPSYCHOTICS — CLOZAPINE

See *4.2.1* for other, more general interactions

CYP1A2 is clozapine's major metabolising enzyme, with 2D6, 3A4, 2C9/19 and FMO enzymes also involved (Urichuk *et al, Curr Drug Metab* 2008;**9**:410–8). The major metabolic route is to norclozapine, which is more stable but more toxic to stem cells (Gerson *et al, Br J Haematology* 1994;**86**:555–61).
ACE inhibitors + clozapine
Clozapine plus **diltiazem**, **enalapril** (Aronowitz *et al, J Clin Psychopharmacol* 1994;**14**:429–30) and **lisinopril** (n=1, Abraham *et al, Am J Psychiatry* 2001;**158**:969) may produce additional hypotension, and clinically important rises in clozapine and norclozapine levels.
Alcohol + clozapine
See antipsychotics + alcohol (*4.7.1*).
Amiodarone + clozapine
Raised clozapine levels have been reported (n=1, Stevens *et al, Psychosomatics* 2008;**49**:255–7).
ANTIBIOTICS/FUNGALS/VIRALS + CLOZAPINE *
1. Antibiotics: Some have been reported to cause leucopenia/neutropenia and may enhance the likelihood of clozapine-induced neutropenia and so should, if possible, be avoided. Note, however, that respiratory infections can themselves inhibit CYP1A2, raising clozapine levels, so antibiotics may not always be the cause of apparent interactions (de Leon, *J Clin Psychiatry* 2004;**65**:1144–5).
Where possible, choose antibiotics from the first list and be aware of the potential for problems if drugs from the second list must be used.
1a. Antibiotics LESS likely to cause neutropenia (safer to use): penicillins (all except benzylpenicillin G), tetracyclines, aminoglycosides, macrolides, clarithromycin, some anti-TBs (ethambutol, pyrazinamide, streptomycin), clofazimide, hexamine, sodium fusidate, spectinomycin, colistin, polymixin B and cycloserine.
1b. Antibiotics MORE likely/CAN cause

leucopenia and/or neutropenia (less safe to use): cephalosporins and cephamycins, clindamycin, lincomycin, sulphonamides (precaution in SmPC), trimethoprim, some anti-TBs (capreomycin, isoniazid [n=1, Angelini *et al, J Clin Psychopharmacol* 2009;**29**:190–1], rifampicin [e.g. 600% reduction in clozapine levels; n=1, Joos *et al, J Clin Psychopharmacol* 1998;**18**:83–5]), co-trimoxazole, dapsone, metronidazole, tinidazole, nitrofurantoin, **chloramphenicol**, erythromycin (e.g. raised levels and seizures; n=1, Funderburg *et al, Am J Psychiatry* 1994;**151**:1840–1); somnolence and leukocytosis; n=1, Cohen *et al, Arch Intern Med* 1996;**156**:675–7), vancomycin, teicoplanin and the 4-quinolones (ciprofloxacin [50% reduction in clozapine levels e.g. n=1, Markowitz *et al, Am J Psychiatry* 1997;**154**:881; n=2, Brouwers *et al, Clin Drug Invest* 2009;**29**:59–63], nalidixic acid, etc). However, a case-note review of 93 antibiotic regimens supported the use of ciprofloxacin or moxifloxacin as having the lowest risk of dyscrasias e.g. cf. penicillins, cephalosporins and others (n=42, Shuman *et al, Innov Clin Neurosci* 2012;**9**:18–30) although see below for potential interactions.

2. Antifungals: **itraconazole** 200mg/d (RCT, n=7, 7/7, Raaska and Neuvonen, *Eur J Clin Pharmacol* 1998;**54**:167–70), and **ketoconazole** have no effect on clozapine (Lane *et al, Drug Metabol Drug Interact* 2001;**18**:263–78).

3. Antivirals: Although absolute neutrophil counts can be significantly different with oseltamivir this is not considered significant and stopping clozapine is not warranted (n=32, Demler and Trigoboff, *Psychiatry (Edgmont)* 2009;**11**:29–33; FFT), e.g. **oseltamivir** had no impact on mental health symptoms when given with clozapine (n=31, Allen *et al, Innov Clin Neurosci* 2011;**8**:12–3; FFT).

Anticholinergics + clozapine

See antipsychotics (*4.2.1*).

Antihypertensives + clozapine

Potentiation of the antihypertensive effects may occur. This can be particularly important during the upward dose titration period.

ANTIPSYCHOTICS (other) + CLOZAPINE *

A 15% reduction in clozapine levels has been reported with **aripiprazole** (n=94, Englisch and Zink, *Prog Neuropsychopharmacol Biol Psychiatry* 2008;**32**:1386–92). **Amisulpride** has no apparent effect on clozapine levels (Bergemann *et al, J Clin Psychopharmacol* 2005;**25**:494–7). There is an enhanced risk of agranulocytosis with some antipsychotics, e.g. **phenothiazines**, (which would additionally be complicated by the long-term nature of any given as a depot) e.g. thrombocytopenia with **fluphenazine** (n=1, Mihaljevic-Peles *et al, Nord J Psychiatry* 2001;**55**:449–50) and significantly lower clozapine plasma levels with **levomepromazine** (n=2, Bugamelli *et al, Prog Neuropsychopharmacol Biol Psychiatry* 2007;**31**:567–70) but raised clozapine levels with perazine, a phenothiazine (n=1, Fischer *et al, Psychopharmacology [Berl]* 2013;**226**:623–5). Elevated **haloperidol** levels have been reported in combination with clozapine (n=1, Allen, *J Clin Pharmacol* 2000;**40**:1296–7), as have myoclonic and GTC seizures (n=1, Haberfellner, *Eur Psychiatry* 2002;**17**:55–6). **Risperidone** has no kinetic interactions with clozapine (n=20, Chetty *et al, Br J Clin Pharmacol* 2009;**68**:574–9; FFT), although there are case reports, e.g. (n=18, Raaska *et al, Eur J Clin Pharmacol* 2002;**58**:587–91; n=1, Kontaxakis *et al, Prog Neuropsychopharmacol Biol Psychiatry* 2002;**26**:407–9). The mechanism cannot be explained by inhibition of CYP1A2, 2D6 or 2C19 (n=8, Eap *et al, Ther Drug Monit* 2001;**23**:228–31). See also antipsychotics + quetiapine (4.2.7) and combinations (*1.23*).

Azathioprine + clozapine

There is a report of successful and uneventful use with no dyscrasias (n=1, De Berardis *et al, Gen Hosp Psychiatry* 2012;**35**:213.e9–11).

BENZODIAZEPINES + CLOZAPINE

There are rare cases of severe hypotension and respiratory depression (e.g. n=1, Friedman *et al, N Engl J Med* 1991;**325**:518–9; FFT), sedation (n=2, Cobb *et al, Am J Psychiatry* 1991;**148**:1606–7), delirium (n=3, Jackson *et al, Ann Clin Psychiatry* 1995;**7**:139–41) and sudden death (after IV **lorazepam**; n=1, Klimke and Klieser, *Am J Psychiatry* 1994;**151**:780). Monitor for enhanced sedation and take particular care when a clozapine dose is being increased.

Bupropion + clozapine *

Seizures and visual hallucinations have been reported when bupropion was added to clozapine (n=1, Castelnovo *et al, J Clin Psychopharmacol* 2015;**35**:97–9)

Buspirone + clozapine

See buspirone (*4.1.2*).

Caffeine + clozapine

Caffeine and clozapine are both metabolised by CYP1A2 and so some competitive inhibition of metabolism may occur. Caffeine 400–1000mg inhibits the metabolism of clozapine, which might be significant in some people (n=12, RCT, open, Hagg *et al*, *Br J Clin Pharmacol* 2000;**49**:59–63; FFT), e.g. mean serum trough levels of clozapine increased by about 26% have been reported (n=12[c=6], RCT, d/b, Raaska *et al*, *Basic Clin Pharmacol Toxicol* 2004;**94**:13–8), causing drowsiness and siallorrhoea, with clozapine levels halving when caffeine was stopped (n=1, Odom-White and de Leon, *J Clin Psychiatry* 1996;**57**:175–6).

Cannabis + clozapine

See antipsychotics + cannabis (*4.7.2*).

CARBAMAZEPINE + CLOZAPINE

See antipsychotics + carbamazepine (*4.4.1*).

Citalopram + clozapine

See antipsychotics + citalopram/escitalopram (*4.3.2.1*).

Clonidine + clozapine

See clonidine + antipsychotics (*4.2.1*).

Cocaine + clozapine

See antipsychotics + cocaine (*4.7.3*).

Cola + clozapine

Clozapine levels might be affected by excessive cola consumption, probably via 1A2 inhibition (Al Hadithy *et al*, *J Clin Psychopharmacol* 2012;**32**:717–9).

Cytotoxic agents + clozapine

Although there is an increased risk of neutropenia, there may be no need to discontinue clozapine if people needing chemotherapy are assessed on an individual basis and special monitoring carried out, e.g. monitor for symptoms of infection, increase the frequency of testing and establish thresholds for stopping treatments, in collaboration with medical and haematological specialists.

Digoxin + clozapine

The SmPC for clozapine advises caution with highly bound drugs, which would include digoxin. Monitor and adjust doses as necessary.

Escitalopram + clozapine

See antipsychotics + (es)citalopram (*4.3.2.1*).

FLUOXETINE + CLOZAPINE

Fluoxetine produces significant increases in plasma clozapine and norclozapine levels, with some inter-individual variation (n=80, open, Centorrino *et al*, *Am J Psychiatry* 1996;**153**:820–2). There are many case reports (e.g. n=6, Centorrino *et al*, *Am J Psychiatry* 1994;**151**:123–5), including death (n=1, Ferslew *et al*, *J Forensic Sci* 1998;**43**:1082–5) and uncontrollable myoclonic jerks (n=1, Kingsbury and Puckett, *Am J Psychiatry* 1995;**152**:473–2). The mechanism is possibly CYP2D6 inhibition so clozapine toxicity must be considered and levels measured.

FLUVOXAMINE + CLOZAPINE *

This is an important and significant interaction. Although it has been suggested that reducing norclozapine levels will help efficacy and tolerability, it is a high-risk strategy (review by Légaré *et al*, *Med Hypotheses* 2013;**80**:689–91). Fluvoxamine inhibition of CYP1A2 leads to clozapine levels increased by up to 900% and AUC by 40% (e.g. n=1, Armstrong and Stephans, *J Clin Psychiatry* 1997;**58**:499), although peak levels may remain unchanged (n=9, Wang *et al*, *J Clin Pharmacol* 2004;**44**:785–92). Fluvoxamine has been used to counteract 1A2 induction by smoking, which can lead to clozapine non-response (n=3, Bender and Eap, *Arch Gen Psychiatry* 1998;**55**:1048–50) in 1A2 ultra-rapid metabolisers. Close pharmacokinetic monitoring is thus necessary, as the effect can be dramatic over a few days in some patients even with very low doses, e.g. 10–20mg/d fluvoxamine.

Review: * general (Wigard *et al*, *Tijdschr Psychiatr* 2013;**55**:113–21).

Grapefruit juice + clozapine

Grapefruit juice has no effect on clozapine levels (n=15, open, 12/52, Lane *et al*, *Drug Metabol Drug Interact* 2001;**18**:263–78).

H2-blockers + clozapine *

Clozapine levels may rise 2–3-fold with cimetidine (n=1, Watras and Taylor, *Ther Adv Psychopharmacol* 2013;**3**:294–7). Ranitidine is a safer alternative.

Influenza vaccine + clozapine

Influenza vaccine has no effect on clozapine levels (n=14, Raaska *et al*, *Eur J Clin Pharmacol* 2001;**57**:705–8).

Lamotrigine + clozapine

Lamotrigine has no effect on stable clozapine levels (n=11, 8/52, Spina *et al*, *Ther Drug Monit* 2006;**28**:599–602), although a three-fold increase has occurred two weeks after lamotrigine was added to a stable clozapine regimen (n=1, Kossen *et al*, *Am J Psychiatry* 2001;**158**:1930) as has late-onset agranulocytosis (n=1, Tourian and

4

Margolese, *J Clin Psychopharmacol* 2011;**31**:665–7) have been reported.

Lithium + clozapine

See antipsychotics + lithium (*4.4.3*).

MAOIs + clozapine

See antipsychotics + MAOIs (*4.3.4*).

Mirtazapine + clozapine

See mirtazapine (*4.3.3.4*).

Oral contraceptives + clozapine *

Elevated plasma clozapine levels have been reported with **norethindrone**, resolving on OC discontinuation (n=1, Gabbay *et al*, *J Clin Psychopharmacol* 2002;**22**:621–2; Bookholt and Bogers, *J Clin Psychopharmacol* 2014;**34**:389–90).

Orlistat + clozapine

A small trial suggested lack of interaction (8/52, Hilger *et al*, *J Clin Psychopharmacol* 2002;**22**:68–70).

Oxcarbazepine + clozapine

See antipsychotics + oxcarbazepine (*4.5.3*).

PAROXETINE + CLOZAPINE

Paroxetine significantly increases plasma clozapine and norclozapine levels (n=60, open, Centorrino *et al*, *Am J Psychiatry* 1996;**153**:820–2), and so risks clozapine toxicity. NMS with no leukocytosis and normal CPK has also been reported (n=1, Gambassi *et al*, *Aging Clin Exp Res* 2006;**18**:266–70).

Penicillamine + clozapine

There is an enhanced risk of agranulocytosis (mandatory precaution in SmPC).

Phenobarbital + clozapine

Elevated plasma clozapine levels (requiring dose reduction) have occurred after stopping phenobarbital, presumably from removal of CYP1A2 induction (n=1, Lane *et al*, *J Clin Psychiatry* 1998;**59**:131–3).

Phenylbutazone + clozapine

There is an enhanced risk of agranulocytosis (mandatory precaution in SmPC).

PHENYTOIN + CLOZAPINE

Plasma clozapine levels may be markedly reduced by phenytoin (n=2, Miller *et al*, *J Clin Psychiatry* 1991;**52**:23–5) via CYP1A2 induction, so monitor for reduced effect.

Pregabalin + clozapine

There are cases of raised clozapine serum levels (n=1, Gahr *et al*, *Pharmacopsychiatry* 2012;**45**:297–9; n=1, Englisch *et al*, *J Clin Psychopharmacol* 2012;**32**:127).

Proton-pump inhibitors + clozapine

A switch from **omeprazole** to **pantoprazole** does not alter mean clozapine plasma levels, although some individual increases may be seen (n=13, Mookhoek and Loonen, *Pharm World Sci* 2004;**26**:180–2).

Pyrazolone analgesics + clozapine

There is an enhanced risk of agranulocytosis (mandatory precaution in SmPC).

Quetiapine + clozapine

See quetiapine (*4.2.7*).

Reboxetine + clozapine

See reboxetine (*4.3.3.6*).

SERTRALINE + CLOZAPINE

Sertraline may significantly increase plasma clozapine and norclozapine levels, with some inter-individual variation (n=80, Centorrino *et al*, *Am J Psychiatry* 1996;**153**:820–2) and sudden death has been reported, probably as a result of cardiac arrhythmia (n=1, Hoehns *et al*, *Ann Pharmacother* 2001;**35**:862–6). The risk of clozapine toxicity must be considered.

Smoking + clozapine

See antipsychotics + smoking (*4.7.4*).

St. John's wort + clozapine

Reduced clozapine levels have occurred after SJW was started as self-medication (n=1, Van Strater and Bogers, *Int Clin Psychopharmacol* 2012;**27**:121–4).

Topiramate + clozapine

See antipsychotics + topiramate (*4.5.6*).

Tricyclics + clozapine

See antipsychotics + tricyclics (*4.3.1*).

Valproate + clozapine

See valproate + antipsychotics (*4.2.1*).

Venlafaxine + clozapine

See venlafaxine (*4.3.3.8*).

Warfarin + clozapine

The SmPC for clozapine advises caution with highly bound drugs, including warfarin (mentioned in Sayal *et al*, *Acta Psychiatr Scand* 2000;**102**:250–5), so monitor and adjust doses.

4.2.5 ANTIPSYCHOTICS — LURASIDONE *

Lurasidone is metabolised by 3A4 and is highly bound to plasma proteins but has no significant effect on other P450 enzymes. Lurasidone is contraindicated with moderate 3A4 inducers such as avasimibe, St. John's wort, phenytoin, rifampicin and carbamazepine. Lurasidone is contraindicated with strong 3A4 inhibitors such as boceprevir, clarithromycin, cobicistat, indinavir, itraconazole, ketoconazole, nefazodone, nelfinavir, posaconazole, ritonavir, saquinavir, telaprevir, telithromycin, voriconazole. Keep the dose to a maximum of 40 mg/d with concurrent 3A4 inhibitors e.g. diltiazem. See the SmPC for a full list and exact details of possible interactions.

Carbamazepine + lurasidone *

Carbamazepine is contraindicated with lurasidone.

Calcium-channel blockers + lurasidone

Start at 20 mg/d (maximum 80 mg/d) if using with moderate 3A4 inhibitors such as diltiazem and verapamil.

Digoxin + lurasidone *

Lurasidone increases digoxin's Cmax and AUC by 9% and 13% respectively but dose adjustments would not be needed (Chui *et al, Drug Metabol Drug Interact* 2014;**29**:191–202).

Ethinylestradiol/norelgestromin + lurasidone*

Lack of interaction has been shown (Chui *et al, Drug Metabol Drug Interact* 2014;**29**:191–202).

Fluoxetine + lurasidone *

Glossopharyngeal dystonia has been reported (n=1, Paul *et al, Case Rep Psychiatry* 2013;**2013**: 136194).

Food + lurasidone

Food increases lurasidone absorption, e.g. Cmax is 1.5–2-fold higher and AUC 2–3-fold higher cf no food. A minimum 350 calories is needed, regardless of fat content.

Grapefruit juice + lurasidone *

The SmPC says avoid the combination.

Lithium + lurasidone *

No interaction or dose adjustments are needed (SmPC, Chui *et al, Drug Metabol Drug Interact* 2014;**29**:191–202).

Midazolam + lurasidone *

Lurasidone increases midazolam's Cmax and AUC by 21% and 44% respectively (Chui *et al, Drug Metabol Drug Interact* 2014;**29**:191–202).

Rifampicin + lurasidone *

Rifampicin decreases lurasidone's Cmax and AUC by 14% and 20% respectively and dose adjustment may be needed (Chui *et al, Drug Metabol Drug Interact* 2014;**29**:191–202).

Smoking + lurasidone *

No interaction is known.

Triazole antifungals + lurasidone *

Lurasidone is contraindicated with strong 3A4 inhibitors such as ketoconazole and voriconazole. Repeated doses of ketoconazole can lead to a 6.8-fold increase in lurasidone's Cmax and a 9.3-fold increase in AUC (Chui *et al, Drug Metabol Drug Interact* 2014;**29**:191–202).

Valproate + lurasidone *

Lack of interaction has been shown (SmPC, Chui *et al, Drug Metabol Drug Interact* 2014;**29**: 191–202).

4.2.6 ANTIPSYCHOTICS — OLANZAPINE

See *4.2.1* for other, more general, interactions

Olanzapine is metabolised by CYP1A2 and 2D6, 2D6 and 3A4 (Urichuk *et al, Curr Drug Metab* 2008;**9**:410–8), with little or no effect on 1A2, 2D6, 2C19, 2C9 and 3A4 at normal doses. It is highly bound to albumin (90%) and alpha 1-acid glycoprotein (77%). Olanzapine also undergoes N-glucuronidation by UGT1A4 (Haslemo *et al, Clin Pharmacol Ther* 2012;**92**:221–7). Olanzapine is approximately 60% excreted in urine and 30% in faeces. Fixed doses appear to give higher levels in women. The UK SmPC cautions about use with known QTc-interval prolonging drugs.

Reviews: * extensive, of pharmacokinetics and pharmacodynamics (Schwenger *et al, Clin Pharmacokinet* 2011;**50**:415–28), pharmacogenetics of metabolism (Söderberg and Dahl, *Pharmacogenomics* 2013;**14**:1319–36).

Alcohol + olanzapine

See antipsychotics + alcohol (*4.7.1*).

Antacids + olanzapine

Antacids have no effect on olanzapine.

Anticholinergics + olanzapine

The UK SmPC now recommends that anticholinergics are not used with olanzapine.

Antipsychotics (other) + olanzapine

An interaction has been suggested with **haloperidol** (Gomberg, *J Clin Psychopharmacol* 1999;**19**:272–3) and NMS has been reported (n=1, Mujica and Weiden, *Am J Psychiatry* 2001;**158**:650–1). Seizures have been reported with **quetiapine** and olanzapine (n=1, Hedges and Jeppson, *Ann Pharmacother* 2002;**36**:437–9). Unchanged olanzapine levels with **flupentixol** were mentioned in one study (Bergemann *et al, Pharmacopsychiatry* 2004;**37**:63–8).

Benzodiazepines + olanzapine

Olanzapine has no effect on **diazepam** and although mild increases in pulse, sedation and

4

dry mouth have been noted, no dose adjustment is usually necessary. Unchanged olanzapine levels with **lorazepam** were mentioned in one study (Bergemann *et al*, *Pharmacopsychiatry* 2004;**37**:63–8). Concomitant IM olanzapine and IM BDZs are contraindicated (UK SmPC) and must be separated by at least one hour. Hypotension (down to 66/30 within four hours) lasting 12 hours was seen in a patient given olanzapine IM with lorazepam 2 mg IM 30 minutes later (n=1, Zacher and Roche–Desilets, *J Clin Psychiatry* 2005;**66**:1614–5).

Carbamazepine + olanzapine
See antipsychotics + carbamazepine (*4.4.1*).

Charcoal (activated) + olanzapine
Activated charcoal reduces olanzapine bio-availability by 50–60%.

Cimetidine + olanzapine
Cimetidine has no effect on olanzapine.

Ciprofloxacin + olanzapine
Raised olanzapine levels have been reported, (n=1, Markowitz and DeVane, *J Clin Psychophamacol* 1999;**19**:289–91).

Duloxetine + olanzapine
Urinary retention has been reported, resolving when duloxetine was switched to venlafaxine (n=1, Englisch *et al*, *Clin Neuropharmacol* 2008;**31**:307–9).

Fosamprenavir/ritonavir + olanzapine *
A 50% olanzapine dosage increase has been recommended when used with fosamprenavir/ritonavir (n=24, RCT, c/o, open, Jacobs *et al*, *Int J Antimicrob Agents* 2014;**44**:173–7).

Lamotrigine + olanzapine
Lamotrigine for 2 months has produced a statistically significant but probably clinically insignificant rise in stable olanzapine levels (n=11, Spina *et al*, *Ther Drug Monit* 2006;**28**:599–602).

Lisinopril + olanzapine
A woman taking olanzapine for bipolar developed acute pancreatitis 3/12 after starting lisinopril (n=1, Bracamonte *et al*, *Am J Health-Syst Pharm* 2010;**67**:214–6).

Lithium + olanzapine
See antipsychotics + lithium (4.4.3).

MAOIs + olanzapine
See antipsychotics + MAOIs (4.3.4).

Mirtazapine + olanzapine
See olanzapine + mirtazapine (4.3.3.4).

Opioids + olanzapine
Opioid-induced delirium has been reported with the combination (n=2, Estfan *et al*, *J Pain Symptom Manage* 2005;**29**:330–2).

Oxcarbazepine + olanzapine
See antipsychotics + oxcarbazepine (4.5.3).

Pramipexole + olanzapine *
There is a case of acute mania (n=1, Bet *et al*, *Bipolar Disord* 2013;**15**:446–8).

Probenecid + olanzapine
Probenecid appears to decrease olanzapine glucuronidation (n=12, RCT, d/b, c/o, Markowitz *et al*, *Clin Pharmacol Ther* 2002;**71**:30–8).

Reboxetine + olanzapine
See antipsychotics + reboxetine (*4.3.3.6*).

Rufinamide + olanzapine
Rufinamide has no effect on olanzapine (SmPC).

Selegiline + olanzapine
Selegiline transdermal system (STS) had no effects on olanzapine (open, RCT, c/o, Azzaro *et al*, *J Clin Pharmacol* 2007;**47**:146–58).

Smoking + olanzapine
See antipsychotics + smoking (*4.7.4*).

SSRIs + olanzapine
Fluvoxamine (but not **sertraline**) inhibits the metabolism of olanzapine (n=165, Weigmann *et al*, *Ther Drug Monit* 2001;**23**:410–13; Bergemann *et al*, *Pharmacopsychiatry* 2004;**37**:63–8), with 100 mg/d raising olanzapine Cmax by 49%, AUC by 70%, half-life by 40% and steady-state levels by 12–112% and so care is needed (e.g. n=12, Wang *et al*, *J Clin Pharmacol* 2004;**44**:785–92). Fluvoxamine 25 mg/d has allowed a 26% reduction in olanzapine dose for the same plasma level, or could allow increasing OLZ levels by 25% without increasing the dose (n=10, 6/52, open, Albers *et al*, *J Clin Psychopharmacol* 2005;**25**:170–4). **Fluoxetine** at higher dose may slightly increase olanzapine levels, probably via CYP2D6 inhibition (n=15, Gossen *et al*, *AAPS Pharm-Sci* 2002;**4**:E11; FFT) and melancholic depression has been reported (n=1, Nelson and Swartz, *Ann Clin Psychiatry* 2000;**12**:167–70). There is a case of hyperprolactinaemia and breast enlargement with olanzapine and **sertraline** (n=1, Praharaj, *Indian J Pharmacol* 2011;**43**:739–40; FFT).

Topiramate + olanzapine
See antipsychotics + topiramate (4.5.6).

Tricyclics + olanzapine
See antipsychotics + tricyclics (*4.3.1*).

Valproate + olanzapine *
Valproate reduces olanzapine levels by up to 32%, equivalent to smoking's effect (e.g. n=429,

Haslemo *et al, Ther Drug Monit* 2012;**34**:512–7), although hypersalivation (n=1, Kieling *et al, CNS Spectr* 2011;**16**:83) and NMS (n=1, Verma *et al, BMJ Case Rep* 2014;**2014**:bcr2013202578) have been reported. Greater weight gain and metabolic abnormalities may occur with the combination than olanzapine monotherapy, the opposite to valproate's effect on risperidone (n=160, RCT, open, 12/12, Meltzer *et al, J Clin Psychiatry* 2011;**72**:1602–10).

Warfarin + olanzapine

Single dose studies show no effect of olanzapine on the metabolism of warfarin, although it could be possible (mentioned in Sayal *et al, Acta Psychiatr Scand* 2000;**102**:250–5).

Xanthines + olanzapine

Lack of interaction has been shown with aminophylline and theophylline (n=19, RCT, Macias *et al, Pharmacotherapy* 1998;**18**:1237–48).

4.2.7 ANTIPSYCHOTICS — QUETIAPINE

See *4.2.1* for other, more general, interactions

Quetiapine is metabolised primarily by CYP3A4. N-desalkylquetiapine is metabolised predominantly by 2D6 to active metabolites and by 3A4 to inactive metabolites (Bakken *et al, Drug Metab Dispos* 2012;**40**:1778–84; FFT). The UK SmPC contraindicates quetiapine with 3A4 inhibitors and advises caution with drugs known to increase the QTc interval or cause electrolyte imbalances.

Review: kinetics review (Bakken *et al, Ther Drug Monit* 2011;**33**:222–6).

Alcohol + quetiapine

See alcohol (*4.7.1*).

Armodafinil + quetiapine

Armodafinil may decrease quetiapine's AUC by 42%, probably by 3A4 induction (n=37[c=25], open, 6/52, Darwish *et al, J Clin Pharmacol* 2012;**52**:1399–409).

Antipsychotics (other) + quetiapine

Haloperidol and **risperidone** have no effect on quetiapine (n=36, RCT, 9/7, Potkin *et al, J Clin Psychopharmacol* 2002;**22**:121–30). Lower quetiapine doses have been recommended when used with **clozapine** in a TDM service analysis (n=1,179, Castberg *et al, J Clin Psychiatry* 2007;**68**:1540–5). See also *4.2.4*.

Antiretrovirals + quetiapine *

The UK SmPC states that caution is necessary with antiretrovirals, as quetiapine levels can rise via CYP3A4 induction by, e.g. **fosamprenavir**, **indinavir**, **nelfinavir** and **ritonavir**. There are many case reports, e.g. rapid but reversible weight gain and sedation with **atazanavir/ritonavir** (n=2, Pollack *et al, Pharmacother* 2009;**29**:1386–91), and deep coma and sustained hypotension with **lamuvidine, ritonavir, atazanavir** (see UK SmPC) and **tenofovir** (n=1, Hantson *et al, Drug Metab Lett* 2010;**4**:7–8). The UK SmPC contraindicates quetiapine with **fosamprenavir** and **darunvir**.

Baclofen + quetiapine

There is a case of cranial diabetes insipidus after an overdose of baclofen and quetiapine (n=1, Silverstone and Scott, *Anaesth Intensive Care* 2009;**37**:319–20).

Barbiturates + quetiapine

Lower levels of quetiapine would be expected, due to CYP3A4 induction by barbiturates.

Benzodiazepines + quetiapine

Single doses of lorazepam and diazepam are unaffected by quetiapine.

Binding resins + quetiapine *

Polystyrene sulfonate (for hyperkalaemia) and sevelamer (for hyperphosphataemia) taken with quetiapine have led to low serum levels and treatment failure, and separating ingestion times partly resolved the problem (n=1, Hoge *et al, J Clin Pharm Ther* 2015;**40**:355–7).

Carbamazepine + quetiapine

See antipsychotics + carbamazepine (*4.4.1*).

Cimetidine + quetiapine

No interaction occurs (n=13, open, Strakowski *et al, J Clin Psychopharmacol* 2002;**22**:201–5).

KETOCONAZOLE + QUETIAPINE

Ketoconazole increases quetiapine plasma levels 3.5-fold, by CYP3A4 inhibition, potentially clinically significant (n=12, Grimm *et al, Br J Clin Pharmacol* 2006;**61**:58–69; FFT).

Lamotrigine + quetiapine

Lamotrigine can reduce quetiapine levels by 58%, potentially clinically significant (n=44, Andersson *et al, Br J Clin Pharmacol* 2011;**72**:153–6; FFT).

Lithium + quetiapine

See antipsychotics + lithium (*4.4.3*).

Lovastatin + quetiapine

A prolonged QTc interval has been reported with the combination (n=1, Furst *et al, Biol Psychiatry* 2002;**51**:264–5).

Macrolide antibiotics + quetiapine

A major increase in quetiapine plasma levels has

4

occurred with **clarithromycin** (n=1, Schulz-Du Bois *et al, Pharmacopsychiatry* 2008;**41**:258–9). Raised quetiapine levels are likely with **erythromycin** via CYP3A4 inhibition.

MAOIs + quetiapine

See antipsychotics + MAOIs (*4.3.4*).

Methadone + quetiapine

See quetiapine + methadone (*4.6.12*).

Phenytoin + quetiapine

Lower levels of quetiapine would be expected, due to CYP3A4 induction by phenytoin.

Reboxetine + quetiapine

See antipsychotics + reboxetine (*4.3.3.6*).

Rifampicin + quetiapine

Lower levels of quetiapine would be expected, due to CYP3A4 induction by rifampicin.

Smoking + quetiapine

See quetiapine + smoking (*4.7.4*).

SSRIs + quetiapine

Fluoxetine 60 mg/d has no significant effect on quetiapine kinetics (n=26, RCT, Potkin *et al, J Clin Psychopharmacol* 2002;**22**:174–82) although rhabdomyolysis (n=1, Himmerrich *et al, J Clin Psychopharmacol* 2006;**26**:676–7) has been reported, as has restless legs with **paroxetine** (n=1, Chou *et al, Prog Neuropsychopharmacol Biol Psychiatry* 2010;**34**:1139–40). Lower doses have been recommended with **fluvoxamine** (n=1,179, Castberg *et al, J Clin Psychiatry* 2007;**68**:1540–5).

Topiramate + quetiapine

See antipsychotics + topiramate (*4.5.6*).

Tricyclics + quetiapine

Imipramine 150 mg/d has no significant effect on quetiapine (n=26, RCT, Potkin *et al, J Clin Psychopharmacol* 2002;**22**:174–82) but quetiapine has caused a falsely elevated estimation of nortriptyline levels (n=1, Schussler *et al, Am J Psychiatry* 2003;**160**:589).

Valproate + quetiapine *

There are reports of cervical dystonia (n=1, Habermeyer *et al, J Clin Psychopharmacol* 2007;**27**:396–7), delirium (n=2, Huang and Wei, *Gen Hosp Psychiatry* 2010;**32**:446), neutropenia (incidence of neutropenia with combination in acquired brain injury was 32% cf. 13% with either as monotherapy; n=101, Park and Kim, *Arch Phys Med Rehabil* 2016;**97**:183–8), reversible EPSE and cognitive decline (n=1, De Dios *et al, J Clin Pharm Ther* 2011;**36**:430–2), rapid and severe hypertriglyceridemia and hypercholesterolemia (n=1, Liang *et al, J Clin Psychopharmacol* 2011;**31**:242–3) and hyperammonemia (n=2, Halaby *et al, Curr Drug Saf* 2013;**8**:284–6).

Venlafaxine + quetiapine *

See quetiapine + venlafaxine (*4.3.3.8*).

Warfarin + quetiapine *

No interaction is likely to occur routinely (mentioned in Sayal *et al, Acta Psychiatr Scand* 2000;**102**:250–5), but enhanced bleeding has been reported (e.g. n=1, Chen *et al, J Neuropsychiatry Clin Neurosci* 2013;**25**:E25).

4.2.8 ANTIPSYCHOTICS — RISPERIDONE AND PALIPERIDONE

See *4.2.1* for other, more general, interactions

Risperidone is metabolised by 3A4 (n=130, Du *et al, J Psychopharmacol* 2010;**24**:1115–20) and by 2D6 to 9-hydroxyrisperidone (n=218, Mannheimer *et al, Ther Drug Monit* 2008;**30**:565–9) where CYP2D6 genotype affects response (Novalbos *et al, J Clin Psychopharmacol* 2010;**30**:504–11).

Armodafinil + risperidone *

Armodafinil reduces the Cmax and AUC of risperidone and paliperidone by about 48% (n=36[c=34], open, Darwish et al, *Clin Drug Investig* 2015;**35**:725–33).

Antiretrovirals + risperidone/paliperidone

Addition of **ritonavir/indinavir** to risperidone has led to severe EPSE, dystonia (n=1, Kelly *et al, Ann Pharmacother* 2002;**36**:827–30) and reversible coma (n=1, Jover *et al, Clin Neuropharmacol* 2002;**25**:251–3), probably via risperidone toxicity.

Aripiprazole + risperidone/paliperidone

See antipsychotics (other) + aripiprazole (*4.2.2*).

Bupropion + risperidone *

See bupropion + antipsychotics (*4.6.6*).*

Caffeine + risperidone/paliperidone

Caffeine appears to have no effect on plasma risperidone levels (n=136, Kakihara *et al, Int Clin Psychopharmacol* 2005;**20**:71–8).

CARBAMAZEPINE + RISPERIDONE/ PALIPERIDONE

See antipsychotics + carbamazepine (*4.4.1*).

Citalopram/escitalopram + risperidone/ paliperidone

See citalopram/escitalopram (*4.3.2.1*).

Clindamycin + risperidone/paliperidone

Abnormal movements have been seen when clindamycin was added to risperidone (n=1,

Malone and Harvery, *J Child Adolesc Psychopharmacol* 2008;**18**:221–2).

CLOZAPINE + RISPERIDONE/PALIPERIDONE

See antipsychotics + clozapine (*4.2.4*).

Co-trimoxazole + risperidone *

Sudden cardiac death has been reported with co-trimoxazole and low dose risperidone (n=1, Rajabi *et al, Asian J Psychiatr* 2011;**4**:218–20).

Dexamfetamine + risperidone

Acute dystonia has occurred when dexamfetamine was stopped from this combination (e.g. n=1, Keshen and Carandang, *J Child Adolesc Psychopharmacol* 2007;**17**:867–70).

Donepezil + risperidone/paliperidone

See antipsychotics + donepezil (*4.6.3.1*).

Duloxetine + risperidone

See risperidone + duloxetine (*4.3.3.2*).

5-fluorouracil + paliperidone *

5-fluorouracil can reduce paliperidone levels (n=1, Yasui-Furukori *et al, Neuropsychiatr Dis Treat* 2013;**9**:317–20).

FLUOXETINE + RISPERIDONE/PALIPERIDONE

Fluoxetine has caused a 75% increase in risperidone levels over four weeks, resulting in side-effects in 30% (n=10, Spina *et al, J Clin Psychopharmacol* 2002;**22**:419–23) and there are reports of severe EPSEs, urinary retention (n=1, Bozikas *et al, J Psychopharmacol* 2001;**15**:142–3) and nasal bleeding (n=1, Mowla *et al, Pharmacopsychiatry* 2009;**42**:204–5).

Fluvoxamine + risperidone/paliperidone

See antipsychotics + fluvoxamine (*4.3.2.3*).

Galantamine + risperidone/paliperidone

See antipsychotics + galantamine (*4.6.3.2*).

Ginkgo biloba + risperidone/paliperidone

Priapism has been reported (n=1, Lin *et al, Mayo Clin Proc* 2007;**82**:1289–90).

Lamotrigine + risperidone/paliperidone

Lamotrigine 200mg/d for 8/52 had no effect on stable risperidone levels (n=10, Spina *et al, Ther Drug Monit* 2006;**28**:599–602) but there is a case of increasing lamotrigine from 175mg/d to 225mg/d led to a 5-fold rise in risperidone levels in someone also on clozapine, although the mechanism was unknown (n=1, Bienentreu and Kronmüller, *Am J Psychiatry* 2005;**162**:811–2). This has been disputed (n=226, Castberg and Spigset, *J Clin Psychiatry* 2006;**67**:1159).

Lithium + risperidone/paliperidone

See antipsychotics + lithium (*4.4.3*).

Methadone + risperidone/paliperidone

See methadone (*4.6.12*).

MAOIs + risperidone/paliperidone

See antipsychotics + MAOIs (*4.3.4*).

Mirtazapine + risperidone/paliperidone

See mirtazapine (*4.3.3.4*).

Oxcarbazepine + risperidone/paliperidone

See antipsychotics + oxcarbazepine (*4.5.3*).

Paroxetine + risperidone/paliperidone

Paroxetine causes a dose-dependent rise in risperidone and metabolite levels (up to double with paroxetine 40mg/d), so a risperidone dose reduction might be needed (e.g. n=12, open, 12/52, Saito *et al, J Clin Psychopharmacol* 2005;**25**:527–32). There seems to be no clinically relevant interaction with single paliperidone doses (RCT, c/o, Berwaerts *et al, Pharmacopsychiatry* 2009;**42**:158–63).

Phenothiazines + risperidone/paliperidone

Levomepromazine has no effect on risperidone plasma levels (n=20, 2/52, Yoshimura *et al, Pharmacopsychiatry* 2005;**38**:98–100).

Phenytoin + risperidone/paliperidone

Severe EPSE have been reported (n=1, Sanderson, *J Clin Psychiatry* 1996;**57**:177).

Probenecid + risperidone/paliperidone

Probenecid has no effect on risperidone kinetics (n=12, RCT, d/b, c/o, Markowitz *et al, Clin Pharmacol Ther* 2002;**71**:30–8).

Quetiapine + risperidone/paliperidone

See antipsychotics + quetiapine (*4.2.7*).

Reboxetine + risperidone/paliperidone

See antipsychotics + reboxetine (*4.3.3.6*)

RIFAMPICIN + RISPERIDONE/PALIPERIDONE

Rifampicin reduces risperidone AUC by 72% and Cmax by 50%, probably by 3A4/2D6 induction (n=10, RCT, open, c/o, 2x5/7, Mahatthanatrakul *et al, J Clin Pharm Ther* 2007;**32**:161–7).

Selegiline + risperidone/paliperidone

Selegiline transdermal system (STS) had no effects on risperidone (open, RCT, c/o, Azzaro *et al, J Clin Pharmacol* 2007;**47**:146–58).

Sertraline + risperidone/paliperidone

Sertraline 150mg/d can elevate risperidone levels by about 40%, presumably via 2D6 inhibition (n=11, open, Spina *et al, Ther Drug Monit* 2004;**26**:386–90), and priapism has been reported (n=1, Salawu *et al, Ann African Med* 2010;**9**:195; FFT). Risperidone has no effect on sertraline (n=10, 4/52, Yoshimura *et al, Hum Psychopharmacol* 2008;**23**:707–13).

4

Smoking + risperidone/paliperidone
See antipsychotics + risperidone (*4.7.4*).
Topiramate + risperidone/paliperidone
See antipsychotics + topiramate (*4.5.6*).
Triazole antifungals + risperidone/paliperidone
Itraconazole raises risperidone and metabolite levels by around 70–75%, presumably via 3A4 inhibition, returning to normal over the next week (n=19, 2/52, Jung *et al*, *Clin Pharmacol Ther* 2005;**78**:520–8).
Tricyclics + risperidone/paliperidone
See antipsychotics + tricyclics (*4.3.1*).
Valproate + risperidone/paliperidone
See antipsychotics (*4.2.1*).
Venlafaxine + risperidone/paliperidone
See antipsychotics + venlafaxine (*4.3.3.8*).

4.2.9 ANTIPSYCHOTICS — ZIPRASIDONE

Ziprasidone is partly metabolised by CYP3A4 (and a minor amount from 1A2), plus around 65% via aldehyde reductase. It has no effect on CYP1A2, 2C9/19, 2D6 or 3A4. It is 99% plasma bound. Due to its QTc-prolonging effect, ziprasidone should not be used with drugs also known to prolong QTc, e.g. sotalol, quinidine, other class Ia and III anti-arrhythmics, phenothiazines, tricyclics, pimozide, mefloquine and dolasetron.

Antacids + ziprasidone
Lack of interaction has been shown (n=11, RCT, Wilner *et al*, *Br J Clin Pharmacol* 2000;**49**[S3]:57–60; FFT).
Armodafinil + ziprasidone *
No interaction occurs (n=35[c=5], open, Darwish *et al*, *Clin Drug Investig* 2014;**34**:691–9).
Anticholinergics + ziprasidone
Lack of interaction has been shown.
Benzodiazepines + ziprasidone
Lack of interaction has been shown.
Beta-blockers + ziprasidone
Lack of interaction has been shown.
Carbamazepine + ziprasidone
See antipsychotics + carbamazepine (*4.4.1*).
Cimetidine + ziprasidone
Lack of interaction has been shown (n=11, RCT, Wilner *et al*, *Br J Clin Pharmacol* 2000;**49**[S3]:57–60; FFT).
Dextromethorphan + ziprasidone
Lack of interaction has been shown (Wilner *et al*, *Br J Clin Pharmacol* 2000;**49**(S3):43–8; FFT).
Triazole antifungals + ziprasidone
Ketoconazole decreases ziprasidone AUC by about 35%, requiring slightly raised doses.
Levodopa + ziprasidone
Ziprasidone may antagonise the effects of levodopa and other dopaminergic agents.
Lithium + ziprasidone
See antipsychotics + lithium (*4.4.3*).
Oral contraceptive + ziprasidone
Lack of interaction has been shown with combined OCs (n=19, d/b, p/c, c/o, Muirhead *et al*, *Br J Clin Pharmacol* 2000;**49**[S1]:49–56; FFT).
Sertraline + ziprasidone *
Serotonin Syndrome has been reported (n=1, Palekar and Eisman, *J Neuropsychiatry Clin Neurosci* 2013;**25**:E1).
Smoking + ziprasidone
See antipsychotics + smoking (*4.7.4*).
Warfarin + ziprasidone
Lack of interaction has been shown.

4.3 ANTIDEPRESSANTS *

Reviews: general (Spina *et al*, *CNS Drugs* 2012;**26**:39–67), interactions between newer antidepressants and SGAs (Spina and de Leon, *Expert Opin Drug Metab Toxicol* 2014;**10**:721–46), and antineoplastics (Miguel and Albuquerque, *Pharmacology* 2011;**88**:333–9; FFT).

4.3.1 TRICYCLIC ANTIDEPRESSANTS

Tricyclics are metabolised by a range of P450 enzymes, e.g. CYP1A2, 2D6 and 3A3/4. Some tricyclics have several metabolic routes, which may vary with concentration and where another might take over should one be inhibited.

Acamprosate + tricyclics
See acamprosate (*4.6.1*).
Acetazolamide + tricyclics
An interaction is unlikely to occur.
Adrenaline + tricyclics
Tricyclics may potentiate the effects of adrenaline injection increasing the risk of hypertension and cardiac arrhythmias (SmPC).
ALCOHOL + TRICYCLICS
See alcohol (*4.7.1*).
Amiodarone + tricyclics
The literature notes an increased risk of ventricular arrhythmias with tricyclics.
Anaesthetics + tricyclics

Halothane and pancuronium should be used with care with tricyclics with strong anticholinergic actions. Enflurane may be a safer alternative.

Anticholinergics + tricyclics

Enhanced anticholinergic effects may occur, especially in the elderly.

Antihistamines + tricyclics

Enhanced sedative and anticholinergic effects are possible.

Antipsychotics + tricyclics *

Desipramine, nortriptyline and imipramine levels may be up to twice as high with **haloperidol**. Tricyclic levels may also rise with phenothiazines, e.g. **perphenazine** increased nortriptyline levels by about 25%, probably by CYP2D6 inhibition (n=25, Mulsant *et al*, *J Clin Psychopharmacol* 1997;**17**:318–21). No significant interaction has been reported with the **thioxanthenes**, although **flupentixol** has raised imipramine levels (n=1, Cook *et al*, *Can J Psychiatry* 1986;**31**:235–7). **Olanzapine** has no effect on imipramine (n=9, open, Callaghan *et al*, *J Clin Pharmacol* 1997;**37**:971–8), although seizures have been reported with olanzapine and clomipramine (Deshauer *et al*, *J Clin Psychopharmacol* 2000;**20**:283–4). Lower olanzapine levels with trimipramine, but unchanged levels with amitriptyline, were mentioned in one study (Bergemann *et al*, *Pharmacopsychiatry* 2004;**37**:63–8). Up to 100mg/d amitriptyline may have no effect on **risperidone** (n=12, open, Sommers *et al*, *Int Clin Psychopharmacol* 1997;**12**:141–5) but risperidone may raise **maprotiline** levels, not a thing you would want to do accidentally (Normann *et al*, *J Clin Psychopharmacol* 2002;**22**:92–4). Severe ADRs have occurred with **melperone** and nortriptyline (n=1, Hefner *et al*, *J Clin Psychopharmacol* 2014;**34**:394–6).

Asenapine + imipramine

See imipramine + asenapine (*4.2.3*).

Aspirin + imipramine

Imipramine plasma levels may rise and ADRs increase when aspirin is added (n=20, Juarez-Olguin *et al*, *Clin Neuropharmacol* 2002;**25**:32–6).

Atomoxetine + tricyclics

See atomoxetine (*4.6.4*).

Baclofen + tricyclics

A person with MS lost muscle tone when nortriptyline and imipramine were added to baclofen (n=1, Silverglat, *JAMA* 1981;**246**:1659).

BARBITURATES + TRICYCLICS

Barbiturates can reduce the serum levels of amitriptyline, protriptyline and nortriptyline by 14–60%, via CYP3A4 induction.

Benzodiazepines + tricyclics

See benzodiazepines (*4.1.1*).

Beta-blockers + tricyclics

Labetolol increases imipramine plasma levels by 28% (n=12, RCT, p/c, c/o, Hermann *et al*, *J Clin Pharmacol* 1992;**32**:176–83) and **propranolol** might raise imipramine levels (n=2, Gillette and Tannery, *J Am Acad Child Adolesc Psychiatry* 1994;**33**:223–4), possibly via 2D6 inhibition. This would appear to be a rare but possible interaction.

Buprenorphine + amitriptyline

No enhanced CNS or respiratory depression has been seen (n=12, d/b, p/c, c/o, Saarialho-Kere *et al*, *Eur J Clin Pharmacol* 1987;**33**:139–46).

Bupropion + tricyclics

See bupropion (*4.6.6*).

Calcium-channel blockers + tricyclics

Amitriptyline plasma levels can be increased by **diltiazem** (n=1, Krahenbuhl *et al*, *Eur J Clin Pharmacol* 1996;**49**:417–9) and **verapamil**, with ADRs increased (n=32, Hermann *et al*, *J Clin Pharmacol* 1992;**32**:176–83). Enhanced cardiac side-effects are also possible.

Cannabis + tricyclics

See antidepressants + cannabis (*4.7.2*).

CARBAMAZEPINE + TRICYCLICS

See carbamazepine (*4.4.1*).

Charcoal, activated + tricyclics

5–10g may reduce the absorption of tricyclics by up to 75% if given within 30 minutes and may be an effective treatment for overdose, even up to two hours after the overdose is taken (open, Dawling *et al*, *Eur J Clin Pharmacol* 1978;**14**:445–7).

Cholestyramine + doxepin

Plasma levels of doxepin have been reduced to a third by cholestyramine (n=1, Geeze *et al*, *Psychosomatics* 1988;**29**:233–6).

CLONIDINE + TRICYCLICS

Tricyclics can be expected to antagonise the hypotensive effects of clonidine (e.g. Hui, *J Am Geriatr Soc* 1983;**31**:164–5).

Cocaine + tricyclics

See antidepressants + cocaine (*4.7.3*).

Codfish + clomipramine

In the never-ending quest for completeness, it may be worth noting that a generalised urticaria

(Naranjo 'probable') occurred after someone ate codfish while taking clomipramine (n=1, Gallelli *et al*, *Pharmacopsychiatry* 2006;**39**:154–6).

Co-trimoxazole + tricyclics

Relapse has been reported (n=5, Brion *et al*, *Encephale* 1987;**13**:123–6).

Dextropropoxyphene + doxepin

There have been reports of doxepin plasma levels raised by up to 150% with dextropropoxyphene, via 2D6 inhibition.

Disopyramide + tricyclics

Increased anticholinergic effects may occur (Hartel *et al*, *Clin Pharmacol Ther* 1974;**15**:551–5) and the BNF notes an increased risk of ventricular arrhythmias.

Disulfiram + tricyclics

Amitriptyline may enhance the effects of disulfiram (MacCallum, *Lancet* 1969;**i**:313) and tricyclic levels may be increased by about 30% via CYP1A2 inhibition (n=2, Ciraulo *et al*, *Am J Psychiatry* 1985;**142**:1373–4).

Duloxetine + tricyclics

See duloxetine (*4.3.3.2*).

Fibre + tricyclics

There are several cases of a high fibre diet reducing doxepin levels by up to a third (and hence to inactive levels). This might explain non-response in some patients.

Glyceryl trinitrate + tricyclics

See nitrates + tricyclics (below).

H2-blockers + tricyclics

CYP1A2 inhibition by **cimetidine** may decrease the metabolism and increase the half-life and plasma levels of tricyclics, e.g. amitriptyline (by 37–80%, Curry *et al*, *Eur J Clin Pharmacol* 1985;**29**:429–33), doxepin (by 30%, n=10, RCT, Abernethy and Todd, *J Clin Psychopharmacol* 1986;**6**:8–12) and imipramine (by over 100%, n=12, RCT, d/b, p/c, c/o, Wells *et al*, *Eur J Clin Pharmacol* 1986;**31**:285–90). Other H2-blockers, e.g. **ranitidine**, do not appear to interact this way (n=6, open, Sutherland *et al*, *Eur J Clin Pharmacol* 1987;**32**:159–64).

Hypoglycaemics + tricyclics

Enhanced hypoglycaemia has been reported with doxepin and nortriptyline (n=2, True *et al*, *Am J Psychiatry* 1987;**144**:1220–1), so monitor blood glucose regularly.

Levodopa + tricyclics

A small reduction in the effect of levodopa may be seen (open, Morgan *et al*, *Neurology* 1975;**25**:1029–34), of minimal significance.

Levothyroxine + tricyclics

This is usually a synergistic combination (see *1.14*) but a few isolated cases of tachycardia and hypothyroidism have been reported.

Lithium + tricyclics

Some ADRs have been reported, e.g. myoclonus (Devanand *et al*, *J Clin Psychopharmacol* 1988;**8**:446–7), neurotoxicity with motor symptoms and seizures (e.g. Austin *et al*, *J Clin Psychiatry* 1990;**51**:344–5) and NMS (n=1, Gupta and Racaniello, *Ann Clin Psychiatry* 2000;**12**:107–9).

MAOIs + TRICYCLICS

See MAOIs (*4.3.4*).

Melatonin + tricyclics

See melatonin (*4.1.4*).

Methadone + tricyclics

See methadone (*4.6.12*).

Methylene blue + clomipramine

See methylene blue + paroxetine (*4.3.2.4*).

Methylphenidate + tricyclics

See methylphenidate (*4.6.13*).

Mirtazapine + tricyclics

See mirtazapine (*4.3.3.4*).

Moclobemide + tricyclics

See moclobemide (*4.3.3.5*).

Modafinil + tricyclics

See modafinil (*4.6.14*).

Morphine + tricyclics

Tricyclics may increase the bioavailability of morphine and potentiate the analgesic effect, usually beneficial (Ventafridda *et al*, *Lancet* 1987;**i**:1204).

Nitrates (sublingual) + tricyclics

Tricyclic-induced dry mouth may reduce the dissolution of sublingual nitrates.

Olanzapine + tricyclics

See olanzapine (*4.2.6*).

Oral contraceptives/estrogens + tricyclics

Akathisia (n=3, Krishnan *et al*, *Am J Psychiatry* 1984;**141**:696–7), reduced tricyclic effectiveness and enhanced tricyclic toxicity have been reported. Best to monitor the tricyclic closely.

Orlistat + tricyclics

A small trial suggested lack of interaction with clomipramine (n=8, 8/52, Hilger *et al*, *J Clin Psychopharmacol* 2002;**22**:68–70).

Phenindione + tricyclics

An enhanced risk of bleeding may occur.

Phenylbutazone + tricyclics

Tricyclic absorption may be delayed or reduced (Consolo *et al*, *Eur J Pharmacol* 1970;**10**:239–42).

PHENYTOIN + TRICYCLICS
See phenytoin (*4.5.5*).

Quetiapine + tricyclics
See quetiapine (*4.2.7*).

Quinine/quinidine + tricyclics
Raised nortriptyline levels may occur (n=10, Steiner *et al*, *Clin Pharmacol Ther* 1988;**43**:577–81), via 2D6 inhibition. Best to monitor tricyclic levels.

Reboxetine + tricyclics
See reboxetine (*4.3.3.6*).

Smoking + tricyclics
See smoking (*4.7.4*).

Sodium oxybate + tricyclics
See sodium oxybate (*4.6.18*).

SSRIs + TRICYCLICS
Tricyclics are predominantly metabolised by CYP2D6. Fluoxetine, paroxetine and fluvoxamine all cause significant inhibition of 2D6 at therapeutic doses, risking serotonin syndrome (see *5.13*) and other events. (Es)citalopram and sertraline cause little clinically significant 2D6 inhibition at standard doses.

Citalopram and escitalopram have no effect on most tricyclic levels (n=5, Baettig *et al*, *Eur J Clin Pharmacol* 1993;**44**:403–5), although desipramine (but not imipramine) levels may rise slightly (e.g. n=1, Ashton, *J Clin Psychiatry* 2000;**61**:144).

Fluoxetine may double or triple tricyclic levels, e.g. with amitriptyline (e.g. fatal, n=1, Preskorn and Baker, *JAMA* 1997;**277**:1682; n=29, open, Vandel *et al*, *Pharmacol Res* 1995; **31**:347–53), clomipramine (n=4, Vandel *et al*, *Neuropsychobiology* 1992;**25**:202–7), and imipramine (Leroj and Walentynowicz, *Can J Psychiatry* 1996;**41**:318–9), even if the tricyclic is used after an extended interval (Extein, *Am J Psychiatry* 1991;**148**:1601–2). Tricyclic doses should be reduced by up to 75% with fluoxetine (n=3, Westermeyer, *J Clin Pharmacol* 1991;**31**:388–92).

Fluvoxamine increases amitriptyline (n=22, Vezmar *et al*, *J Pharmacol Sci* 2009;**110**:98–104; FFT), clomipramine (n=1, Bertschy *et al*, *Eur J Clin Pharmacol* 1991;**40**:119–20) and imipramine levels (Maskall and Lam, *Am J Psychiatry* 1993;**50**:1566).

Paroxetine significantly inhibits the metabolism of amitriptyline and imipramine (e.g. Skjelbo and Brosen, *Br J Clin Pharmacol* 1992;**34**:256–61; FFT), resulting in enhanced tricyclic toxicity.

Sertraline 50mg/d may produce a 31–60% increase in desipramine levels (n=18, RCT, 7/52, Preskorn *et al*, *J Clin Psychopharmacol* 1994;**14**:90–8) but a 200–300% increase has been seen (e.g. n=12, RCT, open, Kurtz *et al*, *Clin Pharmacol Ther* 1997;**62**:145–56).

St John's wort + tricyclics
See St John's wort (*4.3.3.10*).

Sucralfate + amitriptyline
A small study showed a marked reduction in amitriptyline absorption (*Fed Proc* 1986;**45**:205).

Tea or coffee + tricyclics
Some tricyclics (e.g. amitriptyline and imipramine) precipitate out of solution to form a tannin complex with tea and coffee (Lasswell *et al*, *J Pharm Sci* 1984;**73**:1056–8) but the clinical significance is thought to be minimal (Bowen *et al*, *Lancet* 1981;**i**:1217–8).

TERBINAFINE + TRICYCLICS
Terbinafine, a potent 2D6 inhibitor, may triple desipramine plasma levels (n=1, O'Reardon *et al*, *Am J Psychiatry* 2002;**159**:492) and lead to imipramine (e.g. n=1, Teitelbaum and Pearson, *Am J Psychiatry* 2001;**158**:2086) and nortriptyline toxicity (n=1, Van Der Kuy *et al*, *Ann Pharmacother* 2002;**36**:1712–4). A significant rise may occur in amitriptyline levels, an effect that may, extraordinarily, last for up to three to six months after stopping terbinafine (n=1, Castberg *et al*, *Ther Drug Monit* 2005;**27**:680–2).

Triazole antifungals + tricyclics
Inhibition of CYP3A4 by fluconazole has resulted in cases of elevated, toxic nortriptyline levels (n=1, Gannon, *Ann Pharmacother* 1992;**26**:1456–7), syncope (Robinson *et al*, *Ann Pharmacother* 2000;**34**:1406–9) and delirium with amitriptyline (Duggal, *Gen Hosp Psychiatry* 2003;**25**:297–8).

Valproate + tricyclics
See antidepressants + valproate (*4.4.4*).

VASOCONSTRICTOR SYMPATHOMIMETICS + TRICYCLICS
A greatly enhanced response, e.g. hypertension and arrhythmias, to norepinephrine and phenylephrine has been shown in people taking tricyclics. Doxepin may have a lesser effect. Local anaesthetics with epinephrine appear safe. Moderate doses of cold cures containing sympathomimetics should present little risk in healthy people.

4

Venlafaxine + tricyclics
Venlafaxine increases imipramine levels, with a consistent but probably clinically modest effect (n=8, Albers *et al*, *Psychiatr Res* 2000;**96**:235–43). There are reports of serotonin syndrome with venlafaxine and amitriptyline (n=1, Perry *et al*, *Postgrad Med J* 2000;**76**:254–6; FFT) and a GTC fit with venlafaxine and trimipramine (n=1, Schlienger *et al*, *Ann Pharmacother* 2000;**34**:1402–5).

Warfarin + tricyclics
Normally there is no problem, but occasional control problems have been reported with lofepramine (see Sayal *et al*, *Acta Psychiatr Scand* 2000;**102**:250–5).

Yohimbine + tricyclics
Tricyclics can potentiate the blood pressure changes caused by yohimbine, especially if blood pressure is already raised (mentioned in Fugh Berman, *Lancet* 2000;**355**:134–8).

Zopiclone + tricyclics
See zopiclone (*4.1.8*).

4.3.2 SSRIs (SELECTIVE SEROTONIN REUPTAKE INHIBITORS)

All SSRIs inhibit P450 enzymes but there are significant differences in the isoenzymes inhibited and the degree of inhibition. The most potent 2D6 inhibitor is paroxetine, followed by norfluoxetine, fluoxetine, sertraline, fluvoxamine and escitalopram/citalopram (least potent).

Reviews: general (Hemeryck and Belpaire, *Curr Drug Metab* 2002;**3**:13–37; Mandrioli *et al*, *Curr Med Chem* 2012;**19**:1846–63).

4.3.2.1 CITALOPRAM AND ESCITALOPRAM *

Citalopram is a weak inhibitor of CYP2D6 and is metabolised mainly by 3A4 (also 2D6 and 2C19). Citalopram is unlikely to be a source or a cause of clinically important drug–drug interactions (Brosen and Naranjo, *Eur Neuropsychopharmacol* 2001;**11**:275–83). Escitalopram is metabolised by CYP1A2 to two metabolites (n=158, Kuo *et al*, *Pharmacogenomics* 2013;**14**:1191–201).

Acenocoumarol/nicoumalone + citalopram/escitalopram
There is some evidence that there is no interaction (Teichert *et al*, *Br J Clin Pharmacol* 2011:**72**:798–805; FFT), but there is one reported case (n=1, Borras-Blasco *et al*, *Ann Pharmacother* 2002;**36**:345).

Alcohol + citalopram/escitalopram
See alcohol (*4.7.1*).

Alimemazine (trimeprazine) + citalopram/escitalopram
See antipsychotics + citalopram/escitalopram.

Antipsychotics + citalopram/escitalopram *
Aripiprazole has no substantial effect on escitalopram (s=2, n=163, d/b, p/c, Boulton *et al*, *J Psychopharmacol* 2010;**24**:537–46), although urinary obstruction has been reported (n=1, Padala *et al*, *J Clin Psychopharmacol* 2006;**26**:667–8). Escitalopram has no effect on aripiprazole or dehydroaripiprazole levels (n=13, 6/52, Nemoto *et al*, *Pharmacopsychiatry* 2014;**47**:101–4).
Levomepromazine may increase plasma levels of citalopram by about a third (Milne and Goa, *Drugs* 1991;**41**:450–77), possibly via enzyme inhibition albeit of minimal clinical significance.
Levosulpiride has caused QT prolongation (650ms) with citalopram (n=1, Agosti *et al*, *Am J Emerg Med* 2013;**31**:1624).
Risperidone and citalopram have caused torsades de pointes (n=1, Blaschke *et al*, *Pharmacopsychiatry* 2007;**40**:294–5).
Citalopram has no detectable effects on the plasma levels of other antipsychotics (n=90, d/b, Syvalahti *et al*, *J Intern Med Res* 1997;**25**:24–32). The FDA issued a warning about citalopram raising **clozapine** levels by clinically significant levels.

Antiretrovirals + citalopram/escitalopram
No pharmacokinetic interaction occurs with **ritonavir** (n=21[c=18], RCT, open, c/o, Gutierrez *et al*, *Clin Ther* 2003;**25**:1200–10).

Atomoxetine + citalopram/escitalopram
See SSRIs + atomoxetine (*4.6.4*).

Benzodiazepines + citalopram/escitalopram
Lack of interaction has been shown between citalopram and the CYP3A4 substrate **triazolam** (n=18, open, Nolting and Abramowitz, *Pharmacother* 2000;**20**:750–5) and citalopram does not prolong the half-life of **alprazolam** (Hall *et al*, *J Clin Psychopharmacol* 2003;**23**:349–57).

Beta-blockers + citalopram/escitalopram
A review concludes that (es)citalopram produces a 2–3 fold increase in **metoprolol**'s effective plasma levels, not expected to cause clinically relevant changes (Molden and Spigset, *Tidsskr Nor Laegeforen* 2011;**131**:1777–9; FFT).

Buspirone + citalopram/escitalopram

Hyponatraemia and serotonin syndrome has been reported (Spigset and Adielsson, *Int Clin Psychopharmacol* 1997;**12**:61–3).

Carbamazepine + citalopram/escitalopram
Carbamazepine may reduce the proportion and concentration of the escitalopram isomer (n=6, Steinacher *et al*, *Eur Neuropsychopharmacol* 2002;**12**:255–60). Citalopram has no effect on carbamazepine kinetics (n=12, open, Møller *et al*, *J Clin Psychophamacol* 2001;**21**:493–9).

Charcoal + citalopram/escitalopram
25g activated charcoal given 30 minutes after citalopram overdose reduced AUC by 51%, and peak levels by over 50%. Concurrent gastric lavage did not provide any additional reductions (n=9, RCT, Lapatto-Reiniluoto *et al*, *Br J Clin Pharmacol* 1999;**48**:148–53; FFT).

Ciclosporin + citalopram/escitalopram
Citalopram has no effect on ciclosporin kinetics (Liston *et al*, *Psychosomatics* 2001;**42**:370–2).

Cimetidine + citalopram/escitalopram
Cimetidine can moderately raise (es)citalopram levels, but this is unlikely to be clinically significant (n=16, RCT, p/c, Malling *et al*, *Br J Clin Pharmacol* 2005;**60**:287–90; FFT; UK SmPC).

Cocaine + citalopram/escitalopram *
See cocaine + modafinil (*4.7.3*).

Cyproheptadine + citalopram
A death occurred after intoxication with these two serotonergic agents (n=1, Hargrove and Molina, *J Anal Toxicol* 2009;**33**:564–7; FFT).

Digoxin + citalopram/escitalopram
Steady state citalopram 40mg/d had no effect on the kinetics of single doses of digoxin 1mg (n=11, open, c/o, 50/7, Larsen *et al*, *J Clin Pharmacol* 2001;**41**:340–6).

Donepezil + citalopram/escitalopram
See SSRIs + donepezil (*4.6.3.1*).

Duloxetine + citalopram/escitalopram
See SSRIs + duloxetine (*4.3.3.2*).

Fluvoxamine + citalopram/escitalopram
Fluvoxamine may increase the escitalopram to R-citalopram ratio (n=7, open, Bondolfi *et al*, *Psychopharmacol [Berl]* 1996;**128**:421–5).

Itopride + escitalopram
Tardive dyskinesia has been reported with escitalopram and the antinauseant itopride (n=1, Park *et al*, *Prog Neuropsychopharmacol Biol Psychiatry* 2009;**33**:380–1).

Ketoconazole + citalopram/escitalopram
Single doses of ketoconazole have no effect on citalopram (n=18, RCT, d/b, c/o, Gutierrez and Abramowitz, *Pharmacotherapy* 2001;**21**:163–8).

Lamotrigine + citalopram/escitalopram
Myoclonus has been reported (n=1, Rosenhagen *et al*, *J Clin Psychopharmacol* 2006;**26**:346–7).

Linezolid + citalopram/escitalopram
In people taking SSRIs, serotonin syndrome may occur around nine days after starting linezolid (longer the older you are). If stopped symptoms may resolve in three days or longer (eg. n=12, Morales–Molina *et al*, *J Antimicrob Chemother* 2005;**56**:1176–8; FFT n=1, McClean *et al*, *Ir J Med Sci* 2011;**180**:285–6).

Lithium + citalopram/escitalopram
No pharmacokinetic interaction was noted in one study (n=24, open, Gram *et al*, *Ther Drug Monit* 1993;**15**:18–24).

MAOIs + citalopram/escitalopram
See MAOIs (*4.3.4*).

Melatonin + citalopram/escitalopram
Citalopram may slow the metabolism of exogenous melatonin (n=15, RCT, d/b, p/c, 21/7, Huuhka *et al*, *Methods Find Exp Clin Pharmacol* 2006;**28**:447–50).

Methylene blue + citalopram/escitalopram
See methylene blue + paroxetine (*4.3.2.4*).

Metoclopramide + citalopram/escitalopram
See metoclopramide + fluvoxamine (*4.3.2.3*).

Miconazole + escitalopram
A serotonin syndrome has been reported with oral miconazole (n=1, Baptista *et al*, *Int Psychogeriatr* 2012;**24**:845–7).

Mirtazapine + escitalopram *
There is a case of serotonin toxicity (n=1, Ansermot *et al*, *J Clin Psychopharmacol* 2014;**34**:540–1).

Moclobemide + citalopram/escitalopram
See SSRIs + moclobemide (*4.3.3.5*).

NSAIDs + citalopram/escitalopram
See NSAIDs + fluoxetine (*4.3.2.2*).

Omeprazole + citalopram/escitalopram
Omeprazole increases escitalopram levels, unlikely to be clinically significant (n=16, RCT, p/c, Malling *et al*, *Br J Clin Pharmacol* 2005;**60**:287–90; FFT).

Oxcarbazepine + citalopram/escitalopram
See oxcarbazepine (*4.5.3*).

Perhexiline + citalopram/escitalopram
Perhexiline toxicity with citalopram has been reported (n=1, Nyfort–Hansen, *Med J Aust* 2002;**176**:560–1).

4

Propafenone + citalopram/escitalopram
There is a case of citalopram enhancing propafenone's side-effects such as dizziness, and mimicking coronary artery disease (n=1, Garcia, *Am J Geriatr Pharmacother* 2008;**6**:96–9).

Proton-pump inhibitors + (es)citalopram *
Citalopram (n=459) and escitalopram (n=660) levels are higher with **omeprazole** (+35%; +94% respectively), **esomeprazole** (+33%; +82%) and **lansoprazole** (+15%; +20%) and **pantoprazole** (0%, +22%) and so dose reductions may be needed (Gjestad *et al*, *Ther Drug Monit* 2015;**37**; 90–7; FFT).

Rasagiline + escitalopram
Lack of significant interaction has been shown, although rasagiline's AUC was increased by 42% (n=12, 17/7, Hilli *et al*, *Prog Neuropsychopharmacol Biol Psychiatry* 2009;**33**:1526–32). Confusion and hallucinations have also been reported (n=1, Bandrés Liso *et al*, *Farm Hosp* 2009;**33**:173–5).

Rifampicin + citalopram *
Recurrence of panic attacks has occurred when rifampicin was started (n=1, Khalili *et al*, *J Clin Psychopharmacol* 2012;**32**:842–4).

Selegiline + citalopram/escitalopram
One study showed the lack of a clinically significant interaction (n=18, RCT, Laine *et al*, *Clin Neuropharmacol* 1997;**20**:419–33).

Sibutramine + citalopram/escitalopram
Hypomania has been reported (n=1, Benazzi, *J Clin Psychiatry* 2002;**63**:165). A serotonin syndrome is also possible.

St John's wort + citalopram/escitalopram
See SSRIs + St John's wort (*4.3.3.10*).

Statins + (es)citalopram *
See statins + fluvoxamine (*4.3.2.3*).

Sympathomimetics + citalopram/escitalopram
Augmentation of amfetamines is theoretically possible (see sympathomimetics + fluoxetine).

Tamoxifen + citalopram/escitalopram
A nested case-control study showed that long-term citalopram does not reduce tamoxifen's breast cancer protective effect (n=732, Lash *et al*, *Acta Oncol* 2010;**49**:305–12; FFT).

Topiramate + citalopram/escitalopram
See citalopram + topiramate (*4.5.6*).

Tramadol + citalopram/escitalopram *
There is a risk of serotonin syndrome (n=1, Mahlberg *et al*, *Am J Psychiatry* 2004;**161**:1129), so monitor, counsel and take extra care with older age, higher doses and concomitant 2D6 inhibitors (review of n=10, Park *et al*, *J Pharm Pract* 2014;**27**:71–8).

Trazodone + citalopram/escitalopram
No pharmacokinetic interaction occurs (n=41, Prapotnik *et al*, *Int J Clin Pharmacol Ther* 2004; **42**:120–4).

Triazole antifungals + citalopram/escitalopram
Serotonin syndrome has been reported with **fluconazole**, probably via 2C19 inhibition (n=2, Levin *et al*, *Gen Hosp Psychiatry* 2008;**30**:372–7).

Tricyclics + citalopram/escitalopram
See SSRIs + tricyclics (*4.3.1*).

Triptans + citalopram/escitalopram
There may be an increased risk of CNS toxicity with triptans. See triptans + fluoxetine (*4.3.2.2*).

Vortioxetine + citalopram/escitalopram *
See SSRIs + vortioxetine (*4.3.3.9*).

Warfarin + citalopram/escitalopram
Citalopram 40mg/d may produce a small increase in prothrombin time (n=12, Priskorn *et al*, *Br J Clin Pharmacol* 1997;**44**:199–202; FFT), probably clinically insignificant (Sayal *et al*, *Acta Psychiatr Scand* 2000;**102**:250–5).

Zolpidem + citalopram/escitalopram
See SSRIs + zolpidem (*4.1.7*).

4.3.2.2 FLUOXETINE

Fluoxetine is 95% protein bound and substantially inhibits CYP2D6 and probably 2C9/10, moderately inhibits 2C19 and weakly inhibits 3A3/4 and so has a higher incidence of interactions with drugs metabolised by these enzymes. Norfluoxetine is a potent CYP3A4 inhibitor and a moderate inhibitor of 2D6.

Acenocoumarol/nicoumalone + fluoxetine
There is some evidence that there is no interaction (n=1, Teichert *et al*, *Br J Clin Pharmacol* 2011:**72**:798–805; FFT).

Alcohol + fluoxetine
See alcohol (*4.7.1*).

Alosetron + fluoxetine
There is no significant effect from the 5-HT3 antagonist alosetron on fluoxetine kinetics (n=12, D'Souza *et al*, *J Clin Pharmacol* 2001; **41**:455–8).

Amfetamines + fluoxetine
See sympathomimetics + fluoxetine.

ANTIPSYCHOTICS + FLUOXETINE
See antipsychotics (*4.2.1*), aripiprazole (*4.2.2*),

asenapine (4.2.3), clozapine (4.2.4), lurasidone (4.2.5), olanzapine (4.2.6), quetiapine (4.2.7), risperidone and paliperidone (4.2.8).

Atomoxetine + fluoxetine

See SSRIs + atomoxetine (4.6.4).

Benzodiazepines + fluoxetine

Fluoxetine may slightly increase the plasma levels of some benzodiazepines (e.g. **diazepam**: n=10, Lemberger *et al*, *Clin Pharmacol Ther* 1988;**43**:412–9), although probably not **midazolam** (n=10, RCT, 12/7, Lam *et al*, *J Clin Pharmacol* 2003;**43**:1274–82). Desmethyldiazepam levels may be lower, which may explain the lack of additive psychomotor impairment (Ciraulo and Shader, *J Clin Psychopharmacol* 1990;**10**:213–7). Fluoxetine increases **alprazolam's** half-life by 16% (Hall *et al*, *J Clin Psychopharmacol* 2003;**23**:349–57) due to decreased clearance.

Beta-blockers + fluoxetine

Fluoxetine produces a 4–6-fold increase in **metoprolol**'s effective plasma levels (Molden and Spigset, *Tidsskr Nor Laegeforen* 2011;**131**:1777–9; FFT). Dose reduction may be prudent as bradycardia may occur. **Atenolol**, **sotalol** (n=2, Proudlove, *Lancet* 1993;**341**:967–8) and **nebivolol** (Lindamood *et al*, *J Clin Pharmacol* 2011;**51**:575–85) may be suitable alternatives. Fluoxetine may inhibit the metabolism of R-**carvedilol** (rather than S-carvedilol), but this appears to have little clinical significance (n=10, RCT, d/b, c/o, 28/7, Graff *et al*, *J Clin Pharmacol* 2001;**41**:97–106).

Bupropion + fluoxetine

See bupropion (4.6.6).

Buspirone + fluoxetine

See buspirone (4.1.2).

Calcium-channel blockers + fluoxetine

Oedema, weight gain and headache have occurred with **verapamil** and fluoxetine (n=2, Sternbach, *J Clin Psychopharmacol* 1991;**11**:390–1). Lowering doses is recommended if an interaction is suspected.

Cannabis + fluoxetine

See antidepressants + cannabis (4.7.2).

Carbamazepine + fluoxetine

Fluoxetine and norfluoxetine inhibit carbamazepine metabolism, increasing levels by up to 25% (e.g. n=14, Gidal *et al*, *Ther Drug Monit* 1993;**15**:405–9), but a smaller study showed fluoxetine 20mg/d to have no effect on carbamazepine levels (n=8, open, Spina *et al*, *Ther Drug Monit* 1993;**15**:247–50). A toxic serotonin syndrome has been reported (n=1, Dursun *et al*, *Lancet* 1993;**342**:442–3).

Ciclosporin + fluoxetine

Ciclosporin plasma concentrations were nearly doubled by fluoxetine 20mg/d in one report, probably by CYP3A4 inhibition (n=1, Holton and Bonser, *Br Med J* 1995;**311**:422; FFT).

Clopidogrel + fluoxetine *

Clopidogrel's AUC and Cmax can be reduced by 21% and 25% respectively by fluoxetine (n=8, open, c/o, 5/7, Delavenne *et al*, *Fundam Clin Pharmacol* 2013;**27**:683–9).

Cocaine + fluoxetine

See antidepressants + cocaine (4.7.3).

Cyproheptadine + fluoxetine

People taking cyproheptadine for fluoxetine-induced anorgasmia may relapse (n=3, Feder, *J Clin Psychiatry* 1991;**52**:163–4), and interaction has been reported in bulimia (n=2, Goldbloom and Kennedy, *J Clin Psychiatry* 1991;**52**:261–2).

Dextromethorphan + fluoxetine

Visual hallucinations lasting 6–8 hours occurred in a person taking fluoxetine 20mg/d who also took a cough mixture containing dextromethorphan (n=1, Achamallah, *Am J Psychiatry* 1992;**149**:1406). Serotonin syndrome has been reported (n=1, Navarro *et al*, *Gen Hosp Psychiatry* 2006;**28**:78–80).

Digoxin + fluoxetine

There is no apparent increased risk of digoxin toxicity after initiation of SSRIs compared to tricyclics and benzodiazepines (n=3,144, Juurlink *et al*, *Br J Clin Pharmacol* 2005;**59**:102–7, FFT) provided compliance is appropriate (n=1, Yasui-Fukukori and Kaneko, *Lancet* 2006;**367**:788; Bateman *et al*, *Lancet* 2006;**368**:1962–3).

Donepezil + fluoxetine

See SSRIs + donepezil (4.6.3.1).

Duloxetine + fluoxetine

See SSRIs + duloxetine (4.3.3.2).

Lamotrigine + fluoxetine

Delirium has occurred within two weeks of a lamotrigine dose being increased from 200mg/d to 400mg/d in a lady taking fluoxetine 40mg/d (n=1, Chistyakova and Amos, *Am J Psychiatry* 2008;**165**:918–9).

Lansoprazole + fluoxetine

Fluoxetine significantly increases lansoprazole levels by 68% and AUC by 259%, potentially significant (n=18, c/o, 10/7, Vlase *et al*, *Clin Drug Investig* 2011;**31**:727–33).

4

Lithium + fluoxetine
See lithium (*4.4.3*).

LSD + fluoxetine
GTC convulsions occurred in someone who took a double dose of LSD while on fluoxetine 20mg/d, having previously taken single doses of LSD uneventfully (n=1, Picker *et al, Am J Psychiatry* 1992;**149**:843–4).

Macrolide antibiotics + fluoxetine
Acute delirium has been reported with **clarithromycin** and fluoxetine (e.g. n=1, Pollak *et al, Ann Pharmacother* 1995;**29**:486–8), probably via CYP3A4 inhibition.

MAOIs + FLUOXETINE
See MAOIs (*4.3.4*)

Methadone + fluoxetine
See methadone (*4.6.12*).

Methylene blue + fluoxetine
See methylene blue + paroxetine (*4.3.2.4*).

Methylphenidate + fluoxetine
See fluoxetine + methylphenidate (*4.6.13*).

Metoclopramide + fluoxetine
Fluoxetine increases metoclopramide plasma levels, increasing Cmax by 42% and half-life by 53% (n=24, c/o, Viase *et al, Biopharm Drug Dispos* 2006;**27**:285–9). See also fluvoxamine.

Mirtazapine + fluoxetine
See mirtazapine (*4.3.3.4*).

Moclobemide + fluoxetine
See SSRIs + moclobemide (*4.3.3.5*).

Morphine + fluoxetine
Fluoxetine may mildly enhance the analgesic effects of morphine and reduce its side-effects (n=15, d/b, Erjavec *et al, J Clin Pharmacol* 2000;**40**:1286–95).

NSAIDs + SSRIs
A recent extensive review concludes that SSRI use roughly doubles the risk of upper GI bleeds and this is increased to 3-fold by concurrent NSAIDs, but reduced by concurrent PPIs (Andrade *et al, J Clin Psychiatry* 2010;**71**:1565–75), although the absolute risk remains low, e.g. NNH=411 for SSRIs alone, NNH=106 for an SSRI plus NSAID (s=4, n=153,000, Loke *et al, Aliment Pharmacol Ther* 2008;**27**:31–40; FFT). It is best to use NSAIDs and SSRIs together with caution in the over 80s, especially in those with a history of GI bleeding.

Olanzapine + fluoxetine
See SSRIs + olanzapine (*4.2.6*).

Oral contraceptives + fluoxetine
Lack of interaction has been shown (n=1,698, Koke *et al, Am J Obstet Gynecol* 2002;**187**:551–5).

Pentazocine + fluoxetine
Rapid toxicity has been reported, although an interaction was not proven (n=1, Hansen *et al, Am J Psychiatry* 1990;**147**:949–50).

PHENYTOIN + FLUOXETINE
See phenytoin (*4.5.5*).

Quetiapine + fluoxetine
See SSRIs + quetiapine (*4.2.7*).

Reboxetine + fluoxetine
See reboxetine (*4.3.3.6*).

RISPERIDONE + FLUOXETINE
See risperidone (*4.2.8*).

Rivastigmine + fluoxetine
See rivastigmine (*4.6.3.3*).

Selegiline + fluoxetine
There are isolated cases of toxic reactions, e.g. ataxia (n=1, Jermain *et al, Ann Pharmacother* 1992;**26**:1300) and hypertension (Montastruc *et al, Lancet* 1993;**341**:555).

Sertraline + fluoxetine
See sertraline (*4.3.2.5*).

Sibutramine + fluoxetine
Serotonin syndrome is possible.

St John's wort + fluoxetine
See SSRIs + St John's wort (*4.3.3.10*).

Statins + fluoxetine *
See statins + fluvoxamine (*4.3.2.3*).

Sympathomimetics + fluoxetine
There are reports of extreme restlessness, agitation and psychotic symptoms apparently caused by fluoxetine augmentation of amfetamines (n=2, Barrett *et al, Br J Psychiatry* 1996;**168**:253).

Tamoxifen + fluoxetine
See tamoxifen + paroxetine (*4.3.2.4*).

Tolterodine + fluoxetine
Fluoxetine inhibits the 2D6 metabolism of tolterodine (n=13, open, Brynne *et al, Br J Clin Pharmacology* 1999;**48**:553–63; FFT).

Tramadol + fluoxetine *
Serotonin syndrome and mania have been reported (n=1, Kesavan and Sobala, *J Roy Soc Med* 1999;**92**:474–5; FFT; n=1, Gonzalez-Pinto *et al, Am J Psychiatry* 2001;**158**:964–5). SSRIs may inhibit 2D6 metabolism of tramadol but the variability of the interaction may be due to 2D6 poor metabolisers. If concomitant use is needed, monitor, counsel and take extra care with older age, higher doses and other 2D6

inhibitors (review of n=10, Park *et al*, *J Pharm Pract* 2014;**27**:71–8).

Trazodone + fluoxetine

No pharmacokinetic interaction occurs (n=16, Prapotnik *et al*, *Int J Clin Pharmacol Ther* 2004;**42**:120–4), although trazodone toxicity (e.g. Neirenberg *et al*, *J Clin Psychiatry* 1992;**53**:83–5) and myoclonus have been reported (n=1, Darko *et al*, *Vet Hum Toxicol* 2001;**43**:214–5).

TRICYCLICS + FLUOXETINE

See SSRIs + tricyclics (*4.3.1*).

Triptans + fluoxetine

The literature notes an increased risk of CNS toxicity with all SSRIs and triptans and recommends avoiding the combination. However, the American Headache Society position statement reviews 25 published cases and concludes that none satisfied the Hunter Serotonin Toxicity Criteria, so the evidence for limiting SSRIs with triptans is lacking, although some caution is still prudent (Evans *et al*, *Headache* 2010;**50**:1089–99). Activation of 5HT2A may be the predominant cause, so there is neither clinical nor theoretical reason to suggest serious SS is likely from triptans and SSRIs (Gillman, *Headache* 2010;**50**:264–72) and denies a highly effective drug for a disabling (for a day or so) and painful condition (and the author is speaking here from personal experience). Triptans with low lipid solubility and a short half-life (e.g. **sumatriptan**, **rizatriptan** or **zolmitriptan**) may in theory be a safer choice than others (e.g. **frovatriptan**, which has a long half-life).

Tryptophan + fluoxetine

Central toxicity has been reported (n=5, Steiner and Fontaine, *Biol Psychiatry* 1986;**21**:1067–71).

Valproate + fluoxetine

Valproate levels may rise by up to 50% if fluoxetine is added, although the mechanism is unclear (e.g. Lucena *et al*, *Am J Psychiatry* 1998;**155**:575), although reduced valproate levels have also been reported (Droulers *et al*, *J Clin Psychopharmacol* 1997;**17**:139–40).

Venlafaxine + fluoxetine

Serotonin syndrome has been reported when venlafaxine was started immediately after fluoxetine was discontinued (n=1, Bhatara *et al*, *Ann Pharmacother* 1998;**32**:432–6), as have severe anticholinergic side-effects (n=4, Benazzi, *J Clin Psychopharmacol* 1999;**19**:96–8).

Vortioxetine + fluoxetine *

See SSRIs + vortioxetine (*4.3.3.9*).

WARFARIN + FLUOXETINE

An *in vitro* study indicated fluoxetine has a potentially significant effect on warfarin (Schmider *et al*, *Br J Clin Pharmacol* 1997;**44**:495–8; FFT). Raised INR has been reported within ten days of starting fluoxetine (n=2, Woolfrey *et al*, *Br Med J* 1993;**307**:241; FFT), and fluoxetine has led to dramatic increases in INR (n=2, Hanger and Thomas, *N Z Med J* 1995;**108**:157), and one death from cerebral haemorrhage (n=1, Dent and Orrock, *Pharmacotherapy* 1997;**17**:170–2).

Zolpidem + fluoxetine

See SSRIs + zolpidem (*4.1.7*).

4.3.2.3 FLUVOXAMINE

Fluvoxamine is 80% protein bound and strongly inhibits CYP1A2, 2D6, 3A4 and 2C19 (and possibly 2C8 weakly) and may have a high incidence of interactions with drugs metabolised by these enzymes (n=20, Kashuba *et al*, *Clin Pharmacol Ther* 1998;**64**:257–68). It is probably only metabolised by CYP2D6 to fluvoxamino alcohol, then by alcohol dehydrogenase (Miura and Ohkubo, *Xenobiotica* 2007;**37**:169–79).

Acenocoumarol/nicoumalone + fluvoxamine

There is an increased risk (HR 2.63) of over-anticoagulation with concomitant fluvoxamine (n=14926, Teichert *et al*, *Br J Clin Pharmacol* 2011:**72**:798–805; FFT).

AGOMELATINE + FLUVOXAMINE

See agomelatine (*4.3.3.1*).

Alcohol + fluvoxamine

See alcohol (*4.7.1*).

AMINOPHYLLINE + FLUVOXAMINE

See theophylline + fluvoxamine (*4.3.2.3*).

Antipsychotics + fluvoxamine

Asenapine plasma levels may rise by up to 29% (UK SmPC).

Aripiprazole clearance is decreased by about 40%, the same in both extensive and intermediate CYP2D6 metabolisers (n=28, Azuma *et al*, *Eur J Clin Pharmacol* 2012;**68**:29–37; FFT).

Clozapine — see *4.2.4*.

Haloperidol levels are increased by fluvoxamine, and dose-dependent with 150mg/d raising levels by 60%, without additional side-effects at 6mg/d (n=12, Yasui-Furukori *et al*, *Psychopharmacology [Berl]* 2003;**171**:223–7).

4

Levomepromazine and fluvoxamine have caused seizures (n=1, Grinshpoon *et al*, *Int Clin Psychopharmacol* 1993;**8**:61–2), although levomepromazine has no effect on fluvoxamine levels (n=15, Yoshimura *et al*, *Int Clin Psychopharmacol* 2000;**15**:233–5).

Risperidone is not affected by fluvoxamine. 100mg/d but 200mg/d increased risperidone levels by 26% (n=11, open, 8/52, D'Arrigo *et al*, *Pharmacol Res* 2005;**52**:497–501), and rapid neurotoxicity (e.g. confusion, diaphoresis and myoclonus) has been reported (n=1, Reeves *et al*, *Ann Pharmacother* 2002;**36**:440–3).

Benzodiazepines + fluvoxamine

Lorazepam is unaffected (van Harten *et al*, mentioned in *Clin Pharmacokinet* 1993;**24**:203–20). Fluvoxamine 100mg/d increases **alprazolam** levels by 100%, and so reduce doses of alprazolam (n=60, Fleishaker and Hulst, *Eur J Clin Pharmacol* 1994;**46**:35–9). The effect may be 30% greater in non-smokers compared to smokers (n=49, Sugahara *et al*, *Eur J Clin Pharmacol* 2009:**65**:699–704). A slight increase (66%) in **midazolam** (n=10, RCT, 12/7, Lam *et al*, *J Clin Pharmacol* 2003;**43**:1274–82) and **quazepam** levels (n=12, RCT, d/b, c/o, p/c, 14/7, Kanda *et al*, *J Clin Pharmacol* 2003;**43**:1392–7) has been reported.

Beta-blockers + fluvoxamine

Lack of significant interaction has been shown with **atenolol**. **Propranolol** plasma levels can be raised by fluvoxamine by up to 500%, but apparently without major clinical effect (reviewed by Benfield and Ward, *Drugs* 1988;**32**:313–34).

Buspirone + fluvoxamine

See buspirone (*4.1.2*).

Caffeine + fluvoxamine

Even low-dose fluvoxamine (10–20mg/d) inhibits the metabolism of caffeine, via 1A2 inhibition (n=10, Christensen *et al*, *Clin Pharmacol Ther* 2002;**71**:141–52), and its half-life may rise from five hours to 22 hours (Slaughter and Edwards, *Ann Pharmacother* 1995;**29**:619–24), although unlikely to be significant (n=10, Spigset, *Eur J Clin Pharmacol* 1998;**54**:665–6). Caffeine decreases plasma levels of fluvoxamine but not its effects (n=12, RCT, 11/7, d/b, p/c, c/o, Fukasawa *et al*, *Ther Drug Monit* 2006;**28**:308–11).

Carbamazepine + fluvoxamine

Fluvoxamine 100mg/d has no effect on carbamazepine levels (n=15, RCT, Spina *et al*, *Ther Drug Monit* 1993;**15**:247–50), although increased carbamazepine levels and toxicity have been reported (e.g. n=1, Martinelli *et al*, *Br J Clin Pharmacol* 1993;**36**:615–6; FFT).

Celecoxib + fluvoxamine *

Agitation and delirium has been reported (n=1, Hori *et al*, *Psychiatry Clin Neurosci* 2013;**67**:363).

Ciclosporin + fluvoxamine

Ciclosporin levels have been elevated by fluvoxamine in a ciclosporin-treated allograft recipient, probably via CYP3A4 inhibition. Intensive monitoring of the serum creatinine and ciclosporin level was recommended, along with appropriate dose reductions (n=2, Vella and Sayegh, *Am J Kidney Dis* 1998;**31**:320–3).

Citalopram/escitalopram + fluvoxamine

See citalopram/escitalopram (*4.3.2.1*).

CLOZAPINE + FLUVOXAMINE

See clozapine (*4.2.4*).

Digoxin + fluvoxamine

See digoxin + fluoxetine (*4.3.2.2*).

Donepezil + fluvoxamine

See SSRIs + donepezil (*4.6.3.1*).

DULOXETINE + FLUVOXAMINE

See SSRIs + duloxetine (*4.3.3.2*).

Enoxacin + fluvoxamine

Enoxacin appears to increase the sleepiness caused by fluvoxamine (n=10, RCT, d/b, c/o, 11/7, Kunii *et al*, *Ther Drug Monit* 2005;**27**:349–53).

Fexofenadine + fluvoxamine

Fluvoxamine and paroxetine significantly increases fexofenadine's AUC and Tmax (n=12, RCT, c/o, Saruwatari *et al*, *J Clin Psychopharmacol* 2012;**32**:195–9), but sertraline doesn't.

Glimepiride + fluvoxamine

Fluvoxamine may modestly increase glimepiride plasma levels (n=12, RCT, d/b, c/o, 4/7, Niemi *et al*, *Clin Pharmacol Ther* 2001;**69**:194–200).

Lansoprazole + fluvoxamine

Fluvoxamine increases lansoprazole levels 2–3-fold in extensive (but not poor) metabolisers, probably by 2C19 inhibition (n=18, RCT, p/c, Yasui-Furukori *et al*, *J Clin Pharmacol* 2004;**44**:1223–9; n=18, Miura *et al*, *Br J Clin Pharmacol* 2005;**60**:61–8; FFT).

Lidocaine + fluvoxamine

Lidocaine metabolism is reduced by fluvoxamine, leading to potential toxicity (n=8, RCT, d/b, p/c, c/o, Isohanni *et al*, *Basic Clin Pharmacol Toxicol* 2006;**99**:168–72), although the effect of the interaction lessens as liver function worsens (n=30, RCT, d/b, c/o, Orlando *et al*, *Clin Pharmacol Ther* 2004;**75**:80–8).

Lithium + fluvoxamine

Case reports exist of serotonin syndrome (n=1, Ohman and Spigset, *Pharmacopsychiatry* 1993;**26**:263–4), irresistible somnolence (n=1, Evans and Marwick, *Br J Psychiatry* 1990;**156**:286) and diurnal somnolence (n=1, Marchesi *et al*, *Pharmacopsychiatry* 2005;**38**:145–6).

MAOIs + FLUVOXAMINE

See MAOIs (*4.3.4*).

MELATONIN + FLUVOXAMINE

See melatonin (*4.1.4*).

Methadone + fluvoxamine

See methadone (*4.6.12*).

Metoclopramide + fluvoxamine

The combination metoclopramide with **fluoxetine, sertraline** (n=1, Fisher and Davies, *Ann Pharmacother* 2002;**36**:67–71) or **fluvoxamine** may increase the incidence of serotonin syndrome (SmPC). Acute dystonia has occurred with the combination (n=1, Palop *et al*, *Ann Pharmacother* 1999;**33**:382).

MIRTAZAPINE + FLUVOXAMINE

See mirtazapine (*4.3.3.4*).

Moclobemide + fluvoxamine

See SSRIs + moclobemide (*4.3.3.5*).

NSAIDs + FLUVOXAMINE

See NSAIDs + fluoxetine (*4.3.2.2*).

Olanzapine + fluvoxamine

See olanzapine (*4.2.6*).

Oxycodone + fluvoxamine

Serotonin syndrome has been reported (n=1, Karunatilake and Buckley, *Ann Pharmacother* 2006;**40**:155–7).

PHENYTOIN + FLUVOXAMINE

See phenytoin (*4.5.5*).

Pipamperone + fluvoxamine

ECG changes have occurred as a result of acute overdose with this combination (Gallerani *et al*, *Clin Drug Invest* 1998;**15**:64–8).

Quetiapine + fluvoxamine

See quetiapine (*4.2.7*).

Quinidine + fluvoxamine

Fluvoxamine significantly inhibits the 3A4 clearance of quinidine (n=6, open, Damkier *et al*, *Eur J Clin Pharmacol* 1999;**55**:451–6).

Ramosetron + fluvoxamine

Fluvoxamine increases ramosetron Cmax and AUC 1.42-fold and 2.78-fold respectively (open, 11/7, Kadokura et *al*, *Eur J Clin Pharmacol* 2008;**64**:691–5).

Reboxetine + fluvoxamine

See reboxetine (*4.3.3.6*).

Risperidone + fluvoxamine

See antipsychotics + risperidone (*4.2.8*).

Rosiglitazone + fluvoxamine

There appears no significant interaction, although rosiglitazone levels may rise in some people (n=23, open, c/o, Pedersen *et al*, *Br J Clin Pharmacol* 2006;**62**:682–9; FFT).

Sibutramine + fluvoxamine

Serotonin syndrome is possible.

Sildenafil + fluvoxamine

Fluvoxamine increases sildenafil AUC by 40% and half-life by 19%, probably via CYP3A4 inhibition (n=12, Hesse *et al*, *J Clin Psychopharmacol* 2005;**25**:589–92).

Smoking + fluvoxamine

See smoking (*4.7.4*).

St John's wort + fluvoxamine

See SSRIs + St John's wort (*4.3.3.10*).

Statins + fluvoxamine *

SSRIs might inhibit statin metabolism and increase ADRs, especially myopathy. Escitalopram, citalopram and paroxetine are almost certainly safe with all statins. Rosuvastatin and pravastatin are almost certainly safe with all SSRIs so any risk (if at all) lies with fluvoxamine with atorvastatin, simvastatin or lovastatin and even that can be minimised by using the lowest statin dose (Andrade, *J Clin Psychiatry* 2014;**75**:e95–9).

Sympathomimetics + fluvoxamine

Augmentation of amfetamines is theoretically possible (see also fluoxetine, *4.3.2.2*).

THEOPHYLLINE + FLUVOXAMINE

Several cases of theophylline toxicity have been reported (e.g. Devane *et al*, *Am J Psychiatry* 1997;**154**:1317–18), probably via CYP1A2 inhibition. The literature recommends avoiding the combination (*Curr Prob* 1994;**20**:12).

TIZANIDINE + FLUVOXAMINE

Fluvoxamine increases tizanidine's AUC 33-fold and peak levels 12-fold, a dramatic and important interaction (n=10, RCT, d/b, c/o, 4/7, Granfors *et al*, *Clin Pharmacol Ther* 2004;**75**:331–41).

Tolbutamide + fluvoxamine

Fluvoxamine 150mg/d may increase tolbutamide levels by about 20% (n=14, RCT, Madsen *et al*, *Clin Pharmacol Ther* 2001;**69**:41–7).

4

Topiramate + fluvoxamine
There is a case of rapidly reversible tremor and myoclonus with the combination (n=1, Oulis *et al*, *Clin Neuropharmacol* 2008;**31**:366–7).

Tramadol + fluvoxamine *
Although there is a risk of serotonin syndrome, this does not need to be a reason not to use tramadol. Monitor and counsel and take extra care with older age, higher doses and with concomitant 2D6 inhibitors (review of n=10, Park *et al*, *J Pharm Pract* 2014;**27**:71–8).

TRICYCLICS + FLUVOXAMINE
See SSRIs + tricyclics (*4.3.1*).

Triptans + fluvoxamine
See triptans + fluoxetine (*4.3.2.2*).

Tryptophan + fluvoxamine
Central toxicity has been suggested with fluvoxamine (n=5, Steiner and Fontaine, *Biol Psychiatry* 1986;**21**:1067–71).

Valproate + fluvoxamine
Augmentation of fluvoxamine has been claimed for valproate (Corrigan, *Biol Psychiatry* 1992;**31**: 1178–9).

Vortioxetine + fluvoxamine *
See SSRIs + vortioxetine (*4.3.3.9*).

WARFARIN + FLUVOXAMINE
Fluvoxamine has the most potent effect of the SSRIs on warfarin (n=6, Schmider *et al*, *Br J Clin Pharmacol* 1997;**44**:495–8; FFT), e.g. it can increase warfarin levels by up to 65%, increasing prothrombin time (Benfield and Ward, *Drugs* 1986;**32**:313–34; n=1, Limke *et al*, *Ann Pharmacother* 2002;**36**:1890–2). Elevated INR has occurred two weeks after fluvoxamine was stopped, a prolonged effect (n=1, Yap and Low, *Singapore Med J* 1999;**40**:480–2).

Zolpidem + fluvoxamine
See SSRIs + zolpidem (*4.1.7*).

4.3.2.4 PAROXETINE *

Paroxetine is 95% protein-bound and probably the most potent SSRI inhibitor of CYP2D6, albeit rapidly reversible. It does not appear to inhibit any other P450 enzyme. The main metabolite has approximately one third the CYP2D6 inhibition potency of paroxetine. After short-term paroxetine (<6/52) enzyme inhibition wanes in 4/52 but takes 6/52 if paroxetine was taken for more than 10/52 (n=30, Jurica and Žourková, *J Clin Pharm Ther* 2013;**38**:294–300).

Acenocoumarol/nicoumalone + paroxetine
There seems to be sufficient evidence that there is no interaction (Teichert *et al*, *Br J Clin Pharmacol* 2011:**72**:798–805; FFT).

Agomelatine + paroxetine
See agomelatine (*4.3.3.1*).

Alcohol + paroxetine
See alcohol (*4.7.1*).

Anticholinergics + paroxetine
See SSRIs + anticholinergics (*4.6.2*).

Antipsychotics + paroxetine *
Asenapine does not interact (SmPC).
Aripiprazole has no significant effect on paroxetine (s=2,n=38, d/b, p/c, Boulton *et al*, *J Psychopharmacol* 2010;**24**:537–46; MS), but paroxetine increases aripiprazole levels 1.5–1.7-fold, but less so in intermediate metabolisers (n=28, Azuma *et al*, *Eur J Clin Pharmacol* 2012;**68**:29–37; FFT; n=14, 2/52, Nemoto *et al*, *Ther Drug Monit* 2012;**34**:188–92; n=13, 6/52, Nemoto *et al*, *Pharmacopsychiatry* 2014;**47**:101–4).
Haloperidol appears not to interact with paroxetine (Cooper *et al*, *Acta Psychiatr Scand* 1989;**350**:53–5).
Zuclopenthixol levels are increased by around 78% by paroxetine, in a dose-dependent manner (n=923 samples, Davies *et al*, *Acta Psychiatr Scand* 2010;**122**:444–53).
See also **clozapine** (*4.2.4*) and **quetiapine** (*4.2.7*).

Atomoxetine + paroxetine
See SSRIs + atomoxetine (*4.6.4*).

Benzodiazepines + paroxetine
Lack of interaction has been shown, e.g. with **oxazepam** (Cooper *et al*, *Acta Psychiatr Scand* 1989;**350**:53–5) and **alprazolam** (n=25, d/b, p/c, c/o, 4x15/7, Calvo *et al*, *J Clin Psychopharmacol* 2004;**24**:268–76), but NMS has been reported with alprazolam (n=1, Naranjo=6, Tanii *et al*, *Prog Neuropsychopharmacol Biol Psychiatry* 2006;**30**:1176–8) and serotonin syndrome with **clonazepam** (Rella and Hoffman, *J Toxicol Clin Toxicol* 1998;**36**:257–8).

Beta-blockers + paroxetine *
Metoprolol's effective plasma levels can be increased 4–6-fold by paroxetine (probably via 2D6 inhibition) which might lead to greater beta-blockade, complete AV block (n=1, Onalan *et al*, *Mayo Clin Proc* 2008;**83**:595–9). and lost cardioselectivity (n=10, Stout *et al*, *J Clin Pharmacol* 2011;**51**:389–96; FFT), and so dose

reduction may be prudent (Molden and Spigset, *Tidsskr Nor Laegeforen* 2011;**131**:1777–9; FFT).
Pindolol can increase paroxetine levels, probably via 2D6 inhibition (n = 1, Olver and Burrows, *Int J Psychiatry Clin Pract* 1998;**2**:225–7).
Carvedilol kinetics are unaffected by paroxetine (n = 12, RCT, c/o, Stout *et al*, *J Cardiovasc Pharmacol Ther* 2010;**15**:373–9; FFT).
Nebivolol (a highly selective beta-blocker) exposure can be increased 6-fold but apparently with no significant effect on its pharmacodynamics (n = 23, open, Briciu *et al*, *J Clin Pharm Ther* 2014;**39**:535–40).

Bupropion + paroxetine
See bupropion (*4.6.6*).

Carbamazepine + paroxetine
Lack of significant interaction has been shown (n = 20, s/b, p/c, c/o, 23/7, Andersen *et al*, *Epilepsy Res* 1991;**10**:201–4), although hyponatraemia has been reported (n = 1, Sempere i Verdú *et al*, *Aten Primaria* 2004;**33**:473–4).

CLOZAPINE + PAROXETINE
See clozapine (*4.2.4*).

Dextromethorphan + paroxetine
Paroxetine would be expected to increase dextromethorphan levels via CYP2D6 inhibition (see reported case with fluoxetine, *4.3.2.2*).

Digoxin + paroxetine
See digoxin + fluoxetine (*4.3.2.2*).

Donepezil + paroxetine
See SSRIs + donepezil (*4.6.3.1*).

Duloxetine + paroxetine
See SSRIs + duloxetine (*4.3.3.2*).

Ecstasy (MDMA) + paroxetine
Paroxetine significantly attenuates the physiological and psychological effects of ecstasy, which could lead users to take higher (and hence toxic) doses to achieve the same effects (n = 12, RCT, d/b, p/c, c/o, 2x3/7, Farré *et al*, *J Pharmacol Exp Ther* 2007;**323**:954–62; FFT).

Fexofenadine + paroxetine
See fexofenadine + fluvoxamine (*4.3.2.3*).

Flecainide + paroxetine
Paroxetine inhibits flecainide's metabolism, which may be related to 2D6 genotype (n = 21, open, Lim *et al*, *Clin Ther* 2010;**32**:659–66) and led to flecainide toxicity as delirium (n = 1, Tsao and Gugger, *Ann Pharmacother* 2009;**43**:1366–9).

Galantamine + paroxetine
See galantamine (*4.6.3.2*).

H2-blockers + paroxetine
Cimetidine increases paroxetine's bioavailability by up to 50% (Bannister *et al*, *Acta Psychiatr Scand* 1989;**350**:102–6), so use ranitidine instead.

Hydrocodone + paroxetine*
Lack of interaction has been shown (n = 24, RCT, d/b, c/o, 12/7, Kapil *et al*, *Clin Ther* 2015;**37**:2286–96; FFT).

Interferon alfa + paroxetine
A previous good response to paroxetine and trazodone was reversed by interferon alfa, which has anti-serotonergic actions (n = 1, McAllister-Williams *et al*, *Br J Psychiatry* 2000;**176**:93).

Lithium + paroxetine
There are some cases of a possible serotonin syndrome (n = 17, Fagiolini *et al*, *J Clin Psychopharmacol* 2001;**21**:474–8).

Methadone + paroxetine
Steady-state plasma methadone levels may rise with paroxetine, but only in poor 2D6 metabolisers (n = 10, 12/7, Begre *et al*, *J Clin Psychopharmacol* 2002;**22**:211–5).

Methylene blue + paroxetine
Postoperative serotonin syndrome has been reported after methylene blue use in someone taking paroxetine (systematic review of SSRIs, n = 25, Ng and Cameron, *Psychosomatics* 2010;**51**:194–200). The FDA has warned methylene blue should not generally be used with SSRIs, but if urgent or life-threatening then the risk:benefit must be clearly assessed.

Methylphenidate + paroxetine
See paroxetine + methylphenidate (*4.6.13*).

Metoclopramide + paroxetine
See metoclopramide + fluvoxamine (*4.3.2.3*).

Mirtazapine + paroxetine
See mirtazapine (*4.3.3.4*).

Moclobemide + paroxetine
See SSRIs + moclobemide (*4.3.3.5*).

MAOIs + PAROXETINE
See MAOIs (*4.3.4*).

NSAIDs + paroxetine
See NSAIDs + fluoxetine (*4.3.2.2*).

Oral contraceptives + paroxetine
Lack of interaction has been shown (Boyer and Blumhardt, *J Clin Psychiatry* 1992;**53**[Suppl 2]:61–6).

Oxycodone + paroxetine
Paroxetine has no clinical effect on oxycodone (n = 12, p/c, Kummer *et al*, *Eur J Clin Pharmacol* 2011;**67**:63–71; n = 12, RCT, p/c, c/o, Grönlund *et al*, *Clin Drug Invest* 2011;**31**:143–53).

4

Phenytoin + paroxetine
Paroxetine bioavailability may be decreased slightly (n=20, s/b, p/c, c/o, 23/7, Andersen *et al, Epilepsy Res* 1991:**10**:201–4).

Phenobarbital + paroxetine
Paroxetine bioavailability may be decreased slightly, with a 25% decrease in plasma concentrations (Bannister *et al, Acta Psychiatr Scand* 1989;**350**:102–6).

Risperidone + paroxetine
See risperidone (*4.2.8*).

Sertraline + paroxetine *
See paroxetine + sertraline (*4.3.2.5*).

Sibutramine + paroxetine
Serotonin syndrome is possible.

St John's wort + paroxetine
See SSRIs + St John's wort (*4.3.3.10*).

Statins + paroxetine *
A US FDA Adverse Event Reporting System (AERS) analysis showed a unique increase in glucose levels with **pravastatin** and paroxetine (mean 1 mmol/l), higher in diabetics at 2.7 mmol/l (n=239, Tatonetti *et al, Clin Pharmacol Ther* 2011;**90**:133–42; FFT), although a larger study showed no effect (n=2149, Orrico *et al, Ann Pharmacother* 2014;**48**:1172–6). See also statins + fluvoxamine (*4.3.2.3*).

Sympathomimetics + paroxetine
Augmentation of amfetamines is theoretically possible (see sympathomimetics + fluoxetine *4.3.2.2*).

TAMOXIFEN + PAROXETINE *
Paroxetine may increase the risk of recurrence of breast cancer when given with tamoxifen, but no increase is seen with other SSRIs (including fluoxetine), venlafaxine and mirtazapine (n=2,430, <14 years, Kelly *et al, BMJ* 2010;**340**:c693; FFT; s=7, Desmarais and Looper, *J Clin Psychiatry* 2009;**70**:1688–97), although bupropion might (*Drug Safety Update* 2010;**4**:A1).

Tamsulosin + paroxetine
Paroxetine can raise tamsulosin levels by around a third via 2D6 inhibition (n=24, RCT, c/o, Troost *et al, Br J Clin Pharmacol* 2011;**72**:247–56; FFT).

Terbinafine + paroxetine
Terbinafine 150 mg/d increases paroxetine's Cmax 2-fold and half-life by 48% from 15–23 hours (n=12, 2×6/7, Yasui-Furukori *et al, Eur J Clin Pharmacol* 2007;**63**:51–6).

Tramadol + paroxetine *
Although there is a risk of serotonin syndrome, this is not a reason not to use tramadol. Monitor and counsel and take extra care with older age, higher doses and with concomitant 2D6 inhibitors (review of n=10, Park *et al, J Pharm Pract* 2014;**27**:71–8).

TRICYCLICS + PAROXETINE
See SSRIs + tricyclics (*4.3.1*).

Triptans + paroxetine
The literature notes an increased risk of CNS toxicity and recommends avoiding **sumatriptan** with paroxetine, although almost complete lack of interaction has been shown with **rizatriptan** and paroxetine (n=12, RCT, 14/7, Goldberg *et al, J Clin Pharmacol* 1999;**39**:192–9). See also fluoxetine (*4.3.2.2*).

Valproate + paroxetine
No significant interaction occurs (n=20, s/b, p/c, c/o, 23/7, Andersen *et al, Epilepsy Res* 1991;**10**:201–4).

Warfarin + paroxetine
An *in vitro* study indicated that all SSRIs have an effect on warfarin (n=6, Schmider *et al, Br J Clin Pharmacol* 1997;**44**:495–8; FFT), e.g. up to a three-point rise in INR has been reported in several patients (mentioned by Askinazi, *Am J Psychiatry* 1996;**153**:135–6).

Venlafaxine + paroxetine *
There are cases of rapid weight gain and oedema within 2–3 weeks of starting the combination (n=2, Uguz, *Clin Neuropharmacol* 2014;**37**:34–5).

Vortioxetine + paroxetine *
See SSRIs + vortioxetine (*4.3.3.9*).

Zolpidem + paroxetine
See SSRIs + zolpidem (*4.1.7*).

4.3.2.5 SERTRALINE

Sertraline is 98% protein-bound and has a minor (at 50–100 mg/d) but dose-related inhibition of CYP2D6 but little, if any, effect on CYP1A2, 2C9/10, 2C19 or 3A3/4. It is metabolised mainly by 3A4 but also other P450 enzymes, plus monoamine oxidase and UGT2B7 (Obach *et al, Drug Metab Disp* 2005;**33**:262–70; FFT).

Acenocoumarol/nicoumalone + sertraline
There is some evidence that there is no interaction (Teichert *et al, Br J Clin Pharmacol* 2011:**72**:798–805; FFT).

Alcohol + sertraline
See alcohol (*4.7.1*).

Anticholinergics + sertraline
See SSRIs + anticholinergics (*4.6.2*).

Antipsychotics + sertraline
There were no changes in a range of antipsychotic levels when sertraline 50–100mg/d was added (n=48, RCT, d/b, p/c, 6/52, Pierson *et al, Can J Psychiatry* 2006;**51**:715–8). Sertraline (up to 200mg/d) may cause **pimozide** levels to rise by 35%, but with no prolonged QTc (n=15, Alderman, *Clin Ther* 2005;**27**:1050–63). **Aripiprazole** has no substantial effect on sertraline (s=2, n=90, d/b, p/c, Boulton *et al, J Psychopharmacol* 2010;**24**:537–46; MS), although life-threatening myxedema coma (responding to dexamethasone and IV levothyroxine) has been reported (n=1, Church and Callen, *Ann Pharmacother* 2009;**43**:2113–6). See also individual antipsychotics e.g. ziprasidone + SSRIs.

Atomoxetine + sertraline
See SSRIs + atomoxetine (*4.6.4*).

Ayurvedic medicines + sertraline
There is a case of a person twice suffering relapses after starting Ayurvedic herbal mixtures, probably due to either Terminalia chebula or Commiphora wighteii (n=1, Prasad *et al, J Psychopharmacol* 2009;**23**:216–9).

Benzodiazepines + sertraline
Sertraline has no significant effect on **diazepam** and other benzodiazepines (n=20, RCT, d/b, p/c, c/o, Gardner *et al, Clin Pharmacokinetics* 1997;**31**[Suppl 1]:43–9).

Beta-blockers + sertraline
No pharmacodynamic interaction has been found with **atenolol** (e.g. n=10, RCT, Ziegler and Wilner, *J Clin Psychiatry* 1996;**57**[Suppl 1]:12–15). Sertraline produces little or no change in **metoprolol**'s effective plasma levels (Molden and Spigset, Tidsskr *Nor Laegeforen* 2011;**131**:1777–9; FFT), although its AUC can increase by 48–67% (17/7, Preskorn et al, *J Clin Psychopharmacol* 2007;**27**:28–34).

Bupropion + sertraline
See bupropion (*4.6.6*).

Carbamazepine + sertraline
Lack of significant interaction has been reported, but there are cases where sertraline 100mg/d increased carbamazepine plasma levels, probably via 3A4 inhibition (d/b, p/c, Joblin, *N Z Med J* 1994;**107**:43; Lane, *N Z Med J* 1994;**107**:209). Non-response to sertraline has been due to low plasma levels associated with carbamazepine CYP3A4 induction (n=2, Khan *et al, J Clin Psychiatry* 2000;**61**:526–7).

Clozapine + sertraline
See clozapine (*4.2.4*).

Digoxin + sertraline
See digoxin + fluoxetine (*4.3.2.2*).

Dolasetron + sertraline
Serotonin syndrome has been reported (n=1, Sorscher, *J Psychopharmacol* 2002;**16**:191).

Donepezil + sertraline
See SSRIs + donepezil (*4.6.3.1*).

Duloxetine + sertraline
See SSRIs + duloxetine (*4.3.3.2*).

Erythromycin + sertraline
Serotonin syndrome has been reported with the combination, maybe via CYP3A4 inhibition (n=1, Lee and Lee, *Pharmacother* 1999;**19**:894–6).

Fexofenadine + sertraline
See fexofenadine + fluvoxamine (*4.3.2.3*).

Fluoxetine + sertraline
A possible serotonin syndrome has been reported (see switching antidepressants, *2.2.5*).

Indometacin + sertraline
Serotonin syndrome has been reported (n=1, Coster *et al, J Clin Psychopharmacol* 2010;**30**:468–70).

Lamotrigine + sertraline
See lamotrigine (*4.4.2*).

Linezolid + sertraline
Serotonin syndrome has been reported (n=1, Clark *et al, Pharmacotherapy* 2006;**26**:269–76).

Lithium + sertraline
See SSRIs + lithium (*4.4.3*).

MAOIs + SERTRALINE
See MAOIs (*4.3.4*).

Methylene blue + sertraline
See methylene blue + paroxetine (*4.3.2.4*).

Methylphenidate + sertraline
See sertraline + methylphenidate (*4.6.13*).

Metoclopramide + sertraline
See metoclopramide + fluvoxamine (*4.3.2.3*).

Mirtazapine + sertraline
See SSRIs + mirtazapine (*4.3.3.4*).

Moclobemide + sertraline
See SSRIs + moclobemide (*4.3.3.5*).

Naltrexone + sertraline
See naltrexone (*4.6.16*).

NSAIDs + sertraline
See NSAIDs + fluoxetine (*4.3.2.2*).

Olanzapine + sertraline
See SSRIs + olanzapine (*4.2.6*).

Oxycodone + sertraline
Visual hallucinations and tremor have been

reported with the combination (n=1, Rosebraugh *et al*, *J Clin Pharmacol* 2001;**41**:224).

Paroxetine + sertraline *

There is a case of NMS with the combination (n=1, Uguz and Sonmez, *Gen Hosp Psychiatry* 2013;**35**:327).

Phenytoin + sertraline

Lack of significant interaction has been shown (n=30, RCT, Rapeport *et al*, *J Clin Psychiatry* 1996;**57**[Suppl 1]:24–8), but dramatically raised phenytoin levels have been reported after the addition of sertraline (n=2, Haselberger *et al*, *J Clin Psychopharmacol* 1997;**17**:107–9), as has a significant reduction in sertraline levels by phenytoin (Pihlsgard and Eliasson, *Eur J Clin Pharmacol* 2002;**57**:915–6). Monitoring levels would seem sensible.

Proton-pump inhibitors + sertraline *

Sertraline levels are 39% higher with esomeprazole but not with other PPIs (Gjestad *et al*, *Ther Drug Monit* 2015;**37**:90–7).

Risperidone + sertraline

See risperidone (*4.2.8*).

Sibutramine + sertraline

Serotonin syndrome is possible.

Statins + sertraline *

See statins + fluvoxamine (*4.3.2.3*).

St John's wort + sertraline

See SSRIs + St John's wort (*4.3.3.10*).

Sympathomimetics + sertraline

Augmentation of amfetamines is theoretically possible (see sympathomimetics + fluoxetine, *4.3.2.2*).

Tamoxifen + sertraline

See tamoxifen + paroxetine (*4.3.2.4*).

Tolbutamide + sertraline

Sertraline 200mg/d decrease tolbutamide clearance by 16%, possibly via inhibition of CYP2C9 (e.g. n=25, RCT, Tremaine *et al*, *Clin Pharmacokinet* 1997;**31**[Suppl 1]:31–6).

Tramadol + sertraline *

Although there is a risk of serotonin syndrome (n=1, Mason and Blackburn, *Ann Pharmacother* 1997;**31**:175–7), this does not necessarily rule out the use tramadol. Monitor, counsel and take extra care with older age, higher doses and with concomitant 2D6 inhibitors (review of n=10, Park *et al*, *J Pharm Pract* 2014;**27**:71–8).

Tricyclics + sertraline

See SSRIs + tricyclics (*4.3.1*).

Triptans + sertraline

The literature notes an increased risk of CNS toxicity with sumatriptan and recommends avoiding the combination. See also fluoxetine (*4.3.2.2*).

Venlafaxine + sertraline

Acute liver damage possibly related to sertraline and venlafaxine ingestion has been reported (n=1, Kim *et al*, *Ann Pharmacother* 1999;**3**:381–2).

Vortioxetine + sertraline *

See SSRIs + vortioxetine (*4.3.3.9*).

Warfarin + sertraline

An *in vitro* study indicated that, of the SSRIs, sertraline had the least potent effect on warfarin (Schmider *et al*, *Br J Clin Pharmacol* 1997;**44**:495–8; FFT), with only a modest and clinically insignificant increase in prothrombin time (n=12, RCT, 22/7, Apseloff *et al*, *Clin Pharmacokinet* 1997;**32**[Suppl 1]:37–42). However, an up to three-point rise in INR has been reported in several patients (mentioned by Askinazi, *Am J Psychiatry* 1996;**153**:135–6).

Zolpidem + sertraline

See SSRIs + zolpidem (*4.1.7*).

4.3.3 OTHER ANTIDEPRESSANTS

4.3.3.1 AGOMELATINE

Agomelatine is metabolised by CYP1A2 (90%) and CYP9/19 (10%). 2D6 and 3A4 are not involved.

Alcohol + agomelatine

Concurrent use is not advisable (SmPC) but there is no kinetic interaction, and a very minor effect in only one of 23 psychometric tests (MI).

Benzodiazepine + agomelatine

Lack of kinetic interaction has been shown (SmPC) and there was no interaction between agomelatine 50mg/d and lorazepam 2.5mg for seven days (MI).

CIPROFLOXACIN + AGOMELATINE

This combination is an SmPC contraindication.

Duloxetine + agomelatine

See agomelatine + duloxetine (*4.3.3.2*).

Enoxacin + agomelatine

This combination is a UK SmPC caution.

Estrogens + agomelatine

Estrogens can be moderate 1A2 inhibitors and may raise agomelatine levels several-fold (SmPC).

Fluconazole + agomelatine

Fluconazole does not affect the pharmacokinetics of agomelatine (SmPC).

FLUVOXAMINE + AGOMELATINE
Fluvoxamine (a 1A2 and 2C9 inhibitor) may increase agomelatine Cmax and AUC 47-fold and 61-fold respectively, although agomelatine may still be well tolerated (SmPC).

Lithium + agomelatine
Lack of significant interaction has been shown (SmPC), although agomelatine exposure was insignificantly increased.

Paroxetine + agomelatine
Paroxetine does not affect the pharmacokinetics of agomelatine (SmPC).

Propranolol + agomelatine
This combination is a UK SmPC caution.

Smoking + agomelatine
Smoking induces 1A2 and reduces agomelatine bioavailability by 33%, seen as insignificant (MI).

Tamoxifen + agomelatine *
These have been used together successfully and safely (n=1, De Berardis *et al, Clin Neuropharmacol* 2014;**37**:31–3).

Theophylline + agomelatine
Lack of interaction has been shown (SmPC).

4.3.3.2 DULOXETINE

Duloxetine is 95% protein-bound and metabolised by 1A2, a moderate inhibitor and substrate for 2D6 (s=2, Skinner *et al, Clin Pharmacol Ther* 2003;**73**:170–7), but appears to have no effect on 1A2 or 3A4. Caution is recommended with sedative drugs, e.g. alcohol, benzodiazepines, antipsychotics and sedative antihistamines. Elimination is primarily renal (review of kinetics, Wernicke *et al, Expert Opin Drug Saf* 2005;**4**:987–93).

Review: kinetics and interactions (Knadler *et al, Clin Pharmacokinet* 2011;**50**:281–94; MS)

Agomelatine + duloxetine *
There are cases of akathisia, which ceased once agomelatine was stopped (n=1, Imboden and Hatzinger, *Pharmacopsychiatry* 2012;**45**:162–3) and excessive sweating (n=1, Stuhec, *Wien Klin Wochenschr* 2015;**127**:703–6).

Antacids + duloxetine
Lack of interaction has been shown with a single 40 mg dose of duloxetine (UK SmPC).

Aripiprazole + duloxetine
Duloxetine does not seem to affect the plasma levels of aripiprazole (n=7, Hendset *et al, Ther Drug Monit* 2010;**32**:787–90).

Benzodiazepines + duloxetine *
There is a case of visual hallucinations in prodromal Lewy Body dementia (n=1, Rolma *et al, Gen Hosp Psychiatry* 2013;**35**:678.e7–9).

Beta-blockers + duloxetine
A review concludes that duloxetine produces a 2–3-fold increase in **metoprolol**'s effective plasma levels (via 2D6 inhibition), not expected to be clinically relevant (Molden and Spigset, *Tidsskr Nor Laegeforen* 2011;**131**:1777–9; FFT).

CIPROFLOXACIN + DULOXETINE
This combination is a UK SmPC contraindication due to the potential for raised duloxetine levels from 1A2 inhibition by ciprofloxacin.

Ecstasy (MDMA) + duloxetine
Duloxetine can reduce the subjective effects of MDMA despite raised MDMA levels (n=16, RCT, d/b, p/c, c/o, Hysek *et al, PLoS One* 2012;**7**:e36476; FFT).

ENOXACINE + DULOXETINE
This combination is a UK SmPC contraindication due to the potential for raised duloxetine levels from 1A2 inhibition by enoxacine.

H2-blockers + duloxetine
Lack of interaction has been shown with a single 40 mg dose of duloxetine (UK SmPC).

MAOIs + DULOXETINE
This combination is a UK SmPC contraindication, due to the risk of serotonin syndrome. Do not use duloxetine within 14 days of stopping an MAOI, or use an MAOI for five days after stopping duloxetine.

Moclobemide + duloxetine
The UK SmPC recommends caution, due to the risk of serotonin syndrome.

NSAIDs + duloxetine *
An analysis of placebo-controlled trials and spontaneously reported post-marketing adverse events shows no increase in bleeding with NSAIDs and duloxetine cf NSAID alone (Perahia *et al, Drug Health Patient Saf* 2013;**5**:211–9).

Olanzapine + duloxetine
See olanzapine (*4.2.6*).

Oral contraceptives + duloxetine
There is no reason to suspect an interaction would occur, but there are no formal studies.

Pethidine + duloxetine
Due to the risk of serotonin syndrome, the combination should only be used with great care.

Quetiapine + duloxetine *
Severe urinary retention has been reported (n=1, Wang *et al, Psychiatry Clin Neurosci* 2013;**67**:191).

4

Risperidone + duloxetine
Duloxetine does not seem to affect the plasma levels of risperidone (n=8, Hendset *et al*, *Ther Drug Monit* 2010;**32**:787–90).

SMOKING + DULOXETINE
Smokers may have duloxetine plasma levels 50% lower than non-smokers (UK SmPC).

SSRIs + DULOXETINE
Due to the risk of serotonin syndrome, duloxetine should only be used with care with SSRIs. **Fluvoxamine** is contraindicated with duloxetine as duloxetine levels can increase up to 3-fold (range 50–506%), probably by 1A2 inhibition (n=13, Paulzen *et al*, *Pharmacopsychiatry* 2011;**44**:317–23).

St John's wort + duloxetine
The UK SmPC recommends caution when duloxetine is used with St John's wort.

Theophylline + duloxetine
Duloxetine had no effect on theophylline in a study in male patients (UK SmPC).

Tilidine/naloxone + duloxetine *
Severe postoperative hyperthermia has been reported (n=1, Vinetti *et al*, *Clin Toxicol (Phila)* 2013;**51**:516–7).

Tolterodine + duloxetine
There is no significant interaction (n=16, RCT, d/b, c/o, 2x5/7, Hua *et al*, *Br J Clin Pharmacol* 2004;**57**:652–6; FFT).

Tramadol + duloxetine *
Although there is a risk of serotonin syndrome, they can be used with care if monitored, counselled and extra care taken with older age, higher doses and concomitant 2D6 inhibitors (review of n=10, Park *et al*, *J Pharm Pract* 2014; **27**:71–8).

Tricyclics + duloxetine
Due to the risk of serotonin syndrome, duloxetine should only be used with care with tricyclics.

Triptans + duloxetine
Due to the risk of serotonin syndrome, duloxetine should only be used with care with triptans.

Tryptophan + duloxetine
Due to the risk of serotonin syndrome, duloxetine should only be used with care with tryptophan.

Venlafaxine + duloxetine
Due to the risk of serotonin syndrome, duloxetine should only be used with care with venlafaxine.

Warfarin + duloxetine
Duloxetine has no significant effect on the kinetics of steady-state warfarin (n=30, 14/7, Chappell *et al*, *J Clin Pharmacol* 2009;**49**:1456–66), although there are cases of severe elevation of INR (n=3, Glueck *et al*, *JAMA* 2006;**295**:1517–8).

4.3.3.3 MIANSERIN

ALCOHOL + MIANSERIN
See alcohol (*4.7.1*).

Benzodiazepines + mianserin
Enhanced sedation may occur.

Beta-blockers + mianserin
Mianserin produces minimal change in **metoprolol**'s effective plasma levels (Molden and Spigset, *Tidsskr Nor Laegeforen* 2011;**131**:1777–9; FFT).

Carbamazepine + mianserin
Plasma levels of mianserin may be halved by carbamazepine, probably via 3A4 induction (n=12, Eap *et al*, *Ther Drug Monit* 1999;**21**:166–70).

Warfarin + mianserin
There is normally no problem but occasional control difficulties have been reported (Warwick and Mindham, *Br J Psychiatry* 1983;**143**:308).

4.3.3.4 MIRTAZAPINE

Mirtazapine does not inhibit CYP2D6, 1A2 nor 3A. Mirtazapine is mainly metabolised by CYP2D6 and 1A2 (Montgomery, *Int Clin Psychopharmacol* 1995;**10**[Suppl 4]:37–45) and if one enzyme is inhibited, the other takes over, so mirtazapine is less susceptible to P450 interactions. It is 85% protein bound, has linear kinetics from 15–75mg/d, and is 100% excreted via the urine and faeces.

Review: clinical pharmacokinetics (Timmer *et al*, *Clin Pharmacokinet* 2000;**38**:461–74).

Alcohol + mirtazapine
See alcohol (*4.7.1*).

Atomoxetine + mirtazapine
See atomoxetine (*4.6.4*).

Benzodiazepines + mirtazapine
Diazepam and mirtazapine, not surprisingly,, produce additive sedation (n=12, RCT, d/b, c/o, Mattila *et al*, *Pharmacol Toxicol* 1989;**65**:81–8).

Beta-blockers + mirtazapine
Mirtazapine produces little or no change in **metoprolol**'s plasma levels (Molden and Spigset, *Tidsskr Nor Laegeforen* 2011;**131**:1777–9; FFT).

Carbamazepine + mirtazapine
Mirtazapine has no significant effect on carbamazepine levels, but carbamazepine decreases mirtazapine levels by 60%, probably by CYP3A4 induction, and mirtazapine doses may need to be increased (RCT, 4/52, Sitsen *et al*, *Eur J Drug Metab Pharmacokinet* 2001;**26**:109–21).

Cimetidine + mirtazapine
Mirtazapine has no effect on cimetidine but mirtazapine levels may be higher (probably by CYP3A4 inhibition), but not enough to require dose reduction (n=12, d/b, p/c, c/o, Sitsen *et al*, *Eur J Clin Pharmacol* 2000;**56**:389–94).

Citalopram/escitalopram + mirtazapine *
See mirtazapine + citalopram (*4.3.2.1*).

Clozapine + mirtazapine
Lack of significant interaction has been shown (n=9, 6/52, Zoccali *et al*, *Pharmacol Res* 2003;**48**:411–4).

Fluoxetine + mirtazapine
Fluoxetine caused a clinically insignificant 32% increase in mirtazapine plasma levels after an abrupt switch (n=40, Preskorn *et al*, *Biol Psychiatry* 1997;**41**:96S). Mania has been reported (n=1, Ng, *Depress Anxiety* 2002;**15**:46–7), suggesting a combined effect (n=1, Liu *et al*, *J Psychopharmacol* 2009;**23**:220–2).

FLUVOXAMINE + MIRTAZAPINE
Fluvoxamine 50–100mg/d may increase mirtazapine serum levels 3–4-fold, a significant effect (n=2, Anttila *et al*, *Ann Pharmacother* 2001;**35**:1221–3). Serotonin syndrome has been reported (n=1, Demers and Malone, *Ann Pharmacother* 2001;**35**:1217–20).

Levodopa + mirtazapine
Psychosis has been reported (n=1, Normann *et al*, *Pharmacopsychiatry* 1997;**30**:263–5).

Lithium + mirtazapine
Lack of pharmacokinetic interaction has been shown (n=12, 10/7, Sitsen *et al*, *J Clin Psychopharmacol* 2000;**14**:172–6).

MAOIs + mirtazapine
The UK SmPC cautiously recommends a two-week gap between stopping an MAOI and starting mirtazapine.

Olanzapine + mirtazapine
Lack of significant interaction has been shown (n=7, 6/52, Zoccali *et al*, *Pharmacol Res* 2003;**48**:411–4), although status epilepticus has been reported (n=1, Spyridi *et al*, *Int J Clin Pharmacol Ther* 2009;**47**:120–3).

Ondansetron + mirtazapine *
Mirtazapine seems to block the antinauseant effect of ondansetron (n=1, Koch and Nanev, *Afr J Psychiatry [Johannesbg]* 2012;**15**:160; FFT; Lozano, *Afr J Psychiatry [Johannesbg]* 2013;**16**:56).

Paroxetine + mirtazapine
Mirtazapine had no effect on the kinetics of paroxetine and the combination was better tolerated than either alone, suggesting a lack of clinically relevant interaction (n=24, RCT, c/o, 6/7 per arm, Ruwe *et al*, *Hum Psychopharmacol* 2001;**16**:449–59).

Phenytoin + mirtazapine
Mirtazapine has no effect on the steady-state of phenytoin, but phenytoin may reduce mirtazapine levels by a mean of 46%, possibly clinically significant (n=17, RCT, open, Spaans *et al*, *Eur J Clin Pharmacol* 2002;**58**:423–9).

Propafenone + mirtazapine *
There is a case of seizures, bradycardia and prolonged QT and QRS, possibly due to 2D6 inhibition (n=1, Rajpurohit *et al*, *S D Med* 2014; **67**:137–9).

Risperidone + mirtazapine
Mirtazapine 30mg/d has no effect on risperidone 2–6mg/d (e.g. n=8, 6/52, Zoccali *et al*, *Pharmacol Res* 2003;**48**:411–4).

Sertraline + mirtazapine *
Hypomania has been reported with adjunctive mirtazapine 15mg/d (n=1, Soutullo *et al*, *J Clin Psychiatry* 1998;**59**:320) and ventricular tachycardia and cardiac arrest has been reported with the combination (n=1, Atmaca and Mermi, *Iran J Psychiatry* 2014;**9**:45–6; FFT).

Smoking + mirtazapine
See mirtazapine + smoking (*4.7.4*).

Tacrolimus + mirtazapine
Rapid onset of hypotension with raised tacrolimus levels has been reported (n=1, Fraile *et al*, *Nephrol Dial Transplant* 2009;**24**:1999–2001; FFT).

Tamoxifen + mirtazapine
See tamoxifen + paroxetine (*4.3.2.4*).

Tramadol + mirtazapine *
Although there is a risk of serotonin syndrome, they can be used with care if monitored, counselled and extra care taken with older age, higher doses and concomitant 2D6 inhibitors (review of n=10, Park *et al*, *J Pharm Pract* 2014;**27**:71–8).

Tricyclics + mirtazapine
Amitriptyline causes clinically insignificant increases in mirtazapine plasma levels and vice

4

versa (n=24, Sennef *et al*, *Hum Psychopharmacol* 2003;**38**:91–101).

Venlafaxine + mirtazapine

Serotonin syndrome has been reported during a cross-over (n=1, Dimellis, *World J Biol Psychiatry* 2002;**3**:167), as has angiodema (n=1, Lin and Chen, *Gen Hosp Psychiatry* 2010;**32**:341) and when both were also combined with tramadol (n=1, Houlihan, *Ann Pharmacother* 2004;**38**:411–3). See also *1.14* for rational use of this combination.

Warfarin + mirtazapine

No interaction is known or suspected, but there is insufficient information to confirm this (Sayal *et al*, *Acta Psychiatr Scand* 2000;**102**:250–5).

4.3.3.5 MOCLOBEMIDE

Moclobemide is metabolised by CYP2C19, and inhibits 2D6, 2C19 and 1A2. Use with other serotonergic drugs is not recommended due to the risk of serotonin syndrome.

Alcohol + moclobemide

See alcohol (*4.7.1*).

Benzodiazepines + moclobemide

No significant interaction occurs (Zimmer *et al*, *Acta Psychiatr Scand* 1990;**360**:84–6).

Beta-blockers + moclobemide

Concurrent **metoprolol** and moclobemide result in further lowering of blood pressure, although postural hypotension was not reported (Zimmer *et al*, *Acta Psychiatr Scand* 1990;**360**:84–6).

Bupropion + moclobemide

See MAOIs + bupropion (*4.6.6*).

Carbamazepine + moclobemide

Carbamazepine can reduce moclobemide's levels by about 35% (n=21, open, 4/52, Rakic Ignjatovic *et al*, *Br J Clin Pharmacol* 2009;**67**:199–208; FFT).

Digoxin + moclobemide

Lack of interaction has been reported (Zimmer *et al*, *Acta Psychiatr Scand* 1990;**360**:84–6).

Duloxetine + moclobemide

See duloxetine (*4.3.3.2*).

Ecstasy (MDMA) + moclobemide *

Deaths have been reported, with the victims apparently taking moclobemide in an attempt to enhance the effects of MDMA (n=4, Vuori *et al*, *Addiction* 2003;**98**:365–8; n=4, Pilgrim *et al*, *Forensic Sci Int* 2012;**215**:184–8).

H2-BLOCKERS + MOCLOBEMIDE

Cimetidine may reduce the clearance and prolong the half-life of moclobemide, so start with lower doses and monitor closely (n=8, open, Schoerlin *et al*, *Clin Pharmacol Ther* 1991;**49**:32–8)

Ibuprofen + moclobemide

Moclobemide is alleged to potentiate the effect of ibuprofen, but lack of interaction has been reported (Zimmer *et al*, *Acta Psychiatr Scand* 1990;**360**:84–6).

Nifedipine + moclobemide

No significant interaction occurs, apart from a slight reduction in blood pressure (Zimmer *et al*, *Acta Psychiatr Scand* 1990;**360**:84–6).

Opiates + moclobemide

Moclobemide is alleged to potentiate the effect of opiates, and dose reductions of morphine and fentanyl may be considered necessary.

Oral contraceptives + moclobemide

No significant interaction has been detected (Zimmer *et al*, *Acta Psychiatr Scand* 1990; **360**: 84–6).

Pethidine + moclobemide *

This is an SmPC contraindication and there is a possible serotonin syndrome reported (n=1, Gillman, *Med J Aust* 1995;**162**:554).

SELEGILINE + MOCLOBEMIDE

Selegiline is an MAO-B inhibitor and if combined with an MAO-A inhibitor, such as moclobemide, could produce full MAO inhibition, albeit reversible. The combination is not recommended but, if the two need to be used together, full MAOI dietary precautions might be required.

SSRIs + moclobemide

Citalopram and moclobemide have been linked with a fatal possible serotonin syndrome (n=1, Dams *et al*, *J Anal Toxicol* 2001;**25**:147–51; FFT; disputed by Isbister *et al*, *J Anal Toxicol* 2001;**25**:716–7; FFT).

Fluoxetine may not interact with up to 600 mg/d moclobemide and even marked inhibition of moclobemide's metabolism did not lead to excessive accumulation or suggestion of serotonin syndrome (n=18, RCT, open, Dingemanse *et al*, *Clin Pharmacol Ther* 1998;**63**:403–13), although it would be a possibility (UK SmPC).

Fluvoxamine and moclobemide have caused headaches, fatigue (review, Dingemanse, *Int Clin Psychopharmacol* 1993;**7**:167–80), excitation, insomnia and dysphoria (n=36, open, 6/52, Ebert, *Psychopharmacology* 1995;**119**:342–4).

Paroxetine and moclobemide have been linked

with a fatal serotonin syndrome (Singer and Jones, *J Anal Toxicol* 1997;**21**:518–20; FFT).

Sympathomimetics + moclobemide

The UK SmPC recommends avoiding this combination. **Phenylephrine** may slightly raise bp in people taking high dose (600 mg/d) moclobemide (Amrein *et al*, *Psychopharmacology* 1992;**106**:S24–S31), but **ephedrine** produces a greater rise in bp (Dingemanse, *Int Clin Psychopharmacol* 1993;**7**:167–80). An earlier study noted no clinically significant interaction, although the pressor effect may be slightly enhanced (review: Zimmer *et al*, *Acta Psychiatr Scand* 1990;**360**:84–6).

Tricyclics + moclobemide

The UK SmPC contraindicates the combination if the tricyclic (or metabolite) is a serotonin reuptake inhibitor, e.g. **clomipramine** or **imipramine**. Serotonin syndrome has been reported with moclobemide and clomipramine, imipramine (Brodribb *et al*, *Lancet* 1994;**343**:475–6) and after moclobemide plus clomipramine overdoses (n=5, fatal, Neuvonen *et al*, *Lancet* 1993;**342**:1419), where aggressive therapy may be needed. Lack of interaction has been noted with **amitriptyline** 150 mg/d (e.g. n=21, Amrein *et al*, *Psychopharmacology* 1992;**106**:S24–S31).

Triptans + moclobemide

There may be an increased risk of CNS toxicity with **sumatriptan** (n=14, open, Blier and Bergeron, *J Clin Psychopharmacol* 1995;**15**:106–9), **rizatriptan** (n=12, RCT, Van Haarst *et al*, *Br J Clin Pharmacol* 1999;**48**:190 6; FFT) and **zolmitriptan** with moclobemide (e.g. Morales Asín, *Neurologia* 1998;**13**[Suppl 2]:25–30), and that lower doses should be used. **Almotriptan** may be the triptan of choice (n=12, RCT, open, c/o, Fleishaker *et al*, *Br J Clin Pharmacol* 2001;**51**:437–41; FFT).

Tyramine + moclobemide

Minor pressor effects are not seen with moclobemide until about 100 mg tyramine (Zimmer *et al*, *Acta Psychiatr Scand* 1990;**360**:84–6) and even 150 mg tyramine is suggested by some as being safe (n=8, Zimmer *et al*, *Acta Psychiatr Scand* 1990;**360**:78–80). Dietary restrictions are generally not required, but patients should avoid eating excessive amounts of tyramine-containing foods, especially if they have pre-existing hypertension. The combination has been used to treat severe postural hypotension (e.g. n=1, Karet *et al*, *Lancet* 1994;**344**:1263–5) and for clozapine-induced hypotension (n=1, Taylor *et al*, *Br J Psychiatry* 1995;**167**:409–10).

Venlafaxine + moclobemide

See venlafaxine (*4.3.3.8*).

Valproate + moclobemide

Valproate 1 g/d has no effect on moclobemide levels (n=21, open, 4/52, Rakic Ignjatovic *et al*, *Br J Clin Pharmacol* 2009;**67**:199–208; FFT).

Vortioxetine + moclobemide *

See vortioxetine (*4.3.3.9*).

Warfarin + moclobemide

No interaction has been reported, but moclobemide inhibits CYP1A2 and 2C19 and so the potential for warfarin potentiation exists (Sayal *et al*, *Acta Psychiatr Scand* 2000;**102**:250–5).

4.3.3.6 REBOXETINE

Reboxetine is predominantly metabolised *in vitro* via CYP2D6 and 3A4 (n=51, Kuhn *et al*, *Int J Clin Pharmacol Ther* 2007;**45**:36–46). It inhibits CYP2D6 and CYP3A4, but has no effect on CYP1A2, CYP2C9, CYP2C19, and CYP2E1. Care is needed with potent inhibitors of CYP3A4. It is extensively (97%) bound to plasma proteins (particularly the alpha-1 acid glycoprotein fraction) and may interact with drugs with a high affinity for this fraction, e.g. dipyridamole, propranolol, methadone, imipramine, chlorpromazine (see antipsychotics below) and local anaesthetics.

Alcohol + reboxetine

See alcohol (*4.7.1*).

Antipsychotics + reboxetine

An interaction is possible (see above). Reboxetine has no effect on **clozapine** or **risperidone** plasma levels (n=7, Spina *et al*, *Ther Drug Monit* 2001;**23**;675–8).

Benzodiazepines + reboxetine

Lack of interaction has been reported, although some mild-to-moderate drowsiness and transient increases in heart rate have been noted.

Carbamazepine + reboxetine

Low serum concentrations of reboxetine have been reported with carbamazepine (n=1, Helland and Spigset, *J Clin Psychopharmacol* 2007;**27**:308–10).

Dipyridamole + reboxetine

An interaction is possible (see introduction).

Disopyramide + reboxetine

The UK SmPC advises caution with the combination.

Diuretics + reboxetine

4

There may be an increased risk of hypokalaemia with loop diuretics or thiazides (BNF).

Ecstasy (MDMA) + reboxetine

Reboxetine reduces the subjective and physical effects of ecstasy (n=16, d/b, p/c, c/o, Hysek *et al*, *Clin Pharmacol Ther* 2011;**90**:246–55).

Erythromycin + reboxetine

The literature advises caution (UK SmPC).

Flecainide + reboxetine

The literature advises caution (UK SmPC).

Fluoxetine + reboxetine

There are no statistically significant effects of reboxetine on fluoxetine or norfluoxetine pharmacokinetics although urinary retention has been reported (n=1, Benazzi, *Can J Psychiatry* 2000;**45**:936).

Fluvoxamine + reboxetine

The literature advises caution with combination.

Ketoconazole + reboxetine

Ketoconazole decreases the clearance of reboxetine, with no adverse effects, but some caution may be advisable (n=11, open, Herman *et al*, *Clin Pharmacol Ther* 1999;**66**:374–9)

Lidocaine + reboxetine

An interaction is possible (see introduction), and with other local anaesthetics. The literature advises caution with the combination.

MAOIs + reboxetine

This has not been evaluated so best to avoid and leave a two-week gap after an MAOI and one week after reboxetine before switching to the other.

Methadone + reboxetine

An interaction is possible (see introduction).

Phenobarbital + reboxetine

Low reboxetine plasma levels have been reported with phenobarbital (n=1, Helland and Spigset, *J Clin Psychopharmacol* 2007;**27**:308–10).

Potassium-losing diuretics + reboxetine

See diuretics (introduction to *4.3.3.6*).

Propafenone + reboxetine

The literature advises caution with the combination.

Propranolol + reboxetine

An interaction is possible (see introduction).

Tricyclics + reboxetine

An interaction is possible (see introduction).

Triiodothyronine + reboxetine

Noradrenergic adverse effects have been reported (n=1, Cooper-Kazaz *et al*, *J Clin Psychopharmacol* 2010;**30**:211–2).

Warfarin + reboxetine

No interaction is known or suspected, but there is insufficient information to confirm this (Sayal *et al*, *Acta Psychiatr Scand* 2000;**102**:250–5).

4.3.3.7 TRAZODONE

Trazodone is metabolised by CYP2D6 and inhibits 3A4.

ALCOHOL + TRAZODONE

See alcohol (*4.7.1*).

Antipsychotics + trazodone

Enhanced hypotension may occur when trazodone is added to either **chlorpromazine** or **trifluoperazine** (n=2, Asayesh, *Can J Psychiatry* 1986;**31**:857–8).

Buspirone + trazodone

See buspirone (*4.1.2*).

Carbamazepine + trazodone

See carbamazepine (*4.4.1*).

Citalopram/escitalopram + trazodone

See citalopram (*4.3.2.1*).

Clarithromycin + trazodone

Clarithromycin increases the AUC and half-life of trazodone, enhancing sedative effects (n=10, c/o, Farkas *et al*, *Clin Pharmacol Ther* 2009;**85**:644–50).

Cocaine + trazodone

See antidepressants + cocaine (*4.7.3*).

Digoxin + trazodone

Cases of digoxin toxicity exist (n=2, Rauch and Jenike, *Psychosomatics* 1984;**25**:334–5).

Fluoxetine + trazodone

See fluoxetine (*4.3.2.2*).

Ginkgo biloba + trazodone

Coma has been reported with concomitant use in an Alzheimer's patient (n=1, Galluzzi *et al*, *J Neurol Neurosurg Psychiatry* 2000;**68**:679–80; FFT).

Interferon alfa + trazodone

See interferon alfa + paroxetine (*4.3.2.4*).

MAOIs + trazodone

See MAOIs (*4.3.4*).

Omeprazole + trazodone *

AV block and syncope have occurred with the combination (n=1, Akinseye *et al*, *Am J Case Rep* 2015;**16**:319–21; FFT).

Phenytoin + trazodone

See phenytoin (*4.5.5*).

Tramadol + trazodone *

Although there is a risk of serotonin syndrome, this is not a reason not to use tramadol. Monitor, counsel and take extra care with older age, higher doses and with concomitant 2D6 inhibitors (review of n=10, Park *et al, J Pharm Pract* 2014;**27**:71–8).

Venlafaxine + trazodone

See venlafaxine (*4.3.3.8*).

Warfarin + trazodone

INR and PT can fall when trazodone is added to warfarin, and rise when trazodone is stopped, and so caution is necessary (adjust doses and/or monitor), especially if trazodone is used as a PRN hypnotic (e.g. n=1, Jalili and Dehpour, *Arch Med Res* 2007;**38**:901–4).

4.3.3.8 VENLAFAXINE

Venlafaxine is metabolised by CYP2D6 to O-desmethylvenlafaxine, a major active metabolite and by CYP3A4 to N-desmethylvenlafaxine. Other, minor, metabolic pathways exist. Venlafaxine has a low potential for CYP2D6 and 3A4 inhibition (Ball *et al, Br J Clin Pharmacol* 1997;**43**:619–26; FFT) and has no significant effect on other P450 enzymes. 2D6 polymorphism has no effect on desvenlafaxine metabolism, but has significant and predictable effects on venlafaxine (n=14, open, c/o, Preskorn *et al, J Clin Psychopharmacol* 2009;**29**:39–43).

Review: * interactions (Magalhães *et al, Drug Metabol Drug Interact* 2014;**30**:3–17).

Acenocoumarol/nicoumalone + venlafaxine

There is an increased risk (HR 2.19) of over-anticoagulation with venlafaxine (Teichert *et al, Br J Clin Pharmacol* 2011:**72**:798–805; FFT).

Alcohol + venlafaxine

See alcohol (*4.7.1*).

Anticholinergics + venlafaxine

See anticholinergics (*4.6.2*).

Antipsychotics + venlafaxine

Aripiprazole has no apparent effect on venlafaxine and its metabolite's kinetics (s=2, n=152, d/b, p/c, Boulton *et al, J Psychopharmacol* 2010;**24**:537–46; MS).

Clozapine levels can be increased and adverse effects have been reported, although one study showed that even only moderate doses of venlafaxine had no significant effect on clozapine plasma levels (n=11, Repo-Tiihonen *et al, Neuropsychobiol* 2005;**51**:173–6).

Haloperidol AUC and Cmax are increased by 70% and 88% respectively by venlafaxine (SmPC) and urinary retention has been reported (Benazzi, *Pharmacopsychiatry* 1997;**30**:27).

Quetiapine and venlafaxine have caused NMS (n=1, Woods *et al, Ther Adv Psychopharmacol* 2013;**3**:53–5).

Risperidone is not affected by venlafaxine, although some enzyme inhibition led to slightly raised risperidone plasma levels (n=30, open, Amchin *et al, J Clin Pharmacol* 1999;**39**:297–309).

ANTIRETROVIRALS + VENLAFAXINE

Neither venlafaxine nor desvenlafaxine produced any changes in **indinavir** kinetics (n= 24, RCT, open, 12/7, Jann *et al, Eur J Clin Pharmacol* 2012;**68**:715–21), although an earlier study showed venlafaxine reduces indinavir's peak plasma levels by 36% and AUC by 28%, a potentially clinically significant effect (n=9, Levin *et al, Psychopharmacol Bull* 2001;**35**:62–71).

Atomoxetine + venlafaxine

See atomoxetine (*4.6.4*).

Benzodiazepines + venlafaxine

Diazepam 10mg has no significant effect on venlafaxine or metabolite kinetics, but venlafaxine slightly increased diazepam clearance (n=17, Troy *et al, J Clin Pharmacol* 1995;**35**:410–9).

Beta-blockers + venlafaxine

Venlafaxine produced little or no change in **metoprolol**'s plasma levels (Molden and Spigset, *Tidsskr Nor Laegeforen* 2011;**131**:1777–9; FFT).

Bupropion + venlafaxine

See bupropion (*4.6.6*).

Carbamazepine + venlafaxine

Carbamazepine does not appear to effect venlafaxine plasma levels (n=10, open, 8/52, Ciusani *et al, J Psychopharmacol* 2004;**18**:559–66).

Cimetidine + venlafaxine

A 45% reduction in venlafaxine clearance via reduced first-pass metabolism can result in increased venlafaxine levels. The major metabolite, O-desmethylvenlafaxine, is unaffected.

Co-amoxiclav + venlafaxine

Serotonin syndrome has been reported after single doses of co-amoxiclav with venlafaxine (n=1, Connor, *J R Soc Med* 2003;**96**:233–4; FFT).

Co-trimoxazole + venlafaxine *

There is a report of severe tremor, probably from elevated venlafaxine levels (n=1, Geber *et al, Ther Drug Monit* 2013;**35**:279–82).

Duloxetine + venlafaxine

See duloxetine (*4.3.3.2*).

ERYTHROMYCIN + VENLAFAXINE

Potent CYP3A4 inhibitors (e.g. erythromycin) should only be prescribed with venlafaxine if strictly indicated (UK SmPC).

4

Fluoxetine + venlafaxine
See fluoxetine (*4.3.2.2*).

Ketoconazole + venlafaxine
Ketoconazole increases venlafaxine's AUC and Cmax by about 30% in CYP3A4 extensive metabolisers, but the effect appears erratic in poor metabolisers, variably increasing AUC (0–206%) and Cmax (0–119%), so it's a good job they're relatively rare (n=21, open, Lindh *et al*, *Eur J Clin Pharmacol* 2003;**59**:401–6).

Linezolid + venlafaxine
There are several reports of serotonin syndrome (e.g. n=1, Bergeron *et al*, *Ann Pharmacother* 2005;**39**:956–61).

Lisdexamfetamine + venlafaxine
See lisdexamfetamine (*4.6.10*).

Lithium + venlafaxine *
Venlafaxine has no significant effect on lithium kinetics in a single dose study (open, Troy *et al*, *J Clin Pharmacol* 1996;**36**:175–81), but there are cases of raised lithium levels and of serotonin syndrome (e.g. n=1, Adan-Manes *et al*, *J Clin Pharm Ther* 2006;**31**:397–400; n=1, Shahani, *J Neuropsychiatry Clin Neurosci* 2012;**24**:E47). Lithium reduces the renal clearance of venlafaxine, but without apparent clinical significance.

MAOIs + VENLAFAXINE
The SmPCs state that venlafaxine and MAOIs should not be used together and recommend a 14-day gap after stopping an MAOI and starting venlafaxine, and a seven-day gap after stopping venlafaxine and starting an MAOI. This may not be enough in some people as hypotension has been reported four weeks after phenelzine was discontinued (n=1, Yates *et al*, *Ther Adv Psychopharmacol* 2011;**1**:125–7; FFT). There are many reported cases of severe reactions, e.g. extreme agitation, diaphoresis, rapid respiration and raised CPK levels (n=1, Phillips and Ringo, *Am J Psychiatry* 1995;**152**:1400–1), hypomania, heavy perspiration, shivering and dilated pupils (n=1, Klysner *et al*, Lancet 1995;**346**:1298–9), and serotonin syndrome (e.g. n=1, Weiner *et al*, *Pharmacotherapy* 1998;**18**:399–403).

Mirtazapine + venlafaxine
See mirtazapine (*4.3.3.4*).

Moclobemide + venlafaxine
The UK SmPC for venlafaxine states very cautiously that these should not be used together and recommends a 14-day gap after stopping moclobemide before starting venlafaxine, and a seven-day gap after venlafaxine before moclobemide is used. This seems overcautious, although a serotonin syndrome has been reported (n=1, Fisher and Davies, *Ann Pharmacother* 2002;**36**:67–71).

Paroxetine + venlafaxine *
See venlafaxine + paroxetine (*4.3.2.4*).

Propafenone + venlafaxine
An organic psychosis has been reported, with raised venlafaxine levels (n=1, Pfeffer and Grube, *Int J Psychiatr Med* 2001;**31**:427–32).

Selegiline + venlafaxine
The UK SmPC for venlafaxine states the combination should not be used and recommends a 14-day gap after stopping selegiline before starting venlafaxine, and a seven-day gap after venlafaxine before selegiline is used.

Sertraline + venlafaxine
See sertraline (*4.3.2.5*).

Sour date nut + venlafaxine
A severe serotonin syndrome with anaphylactic features has been reported with combined sour date nut (jujube) and venlafaxine 37.5 mg/d (n=1, Stewart, *Am J Psychiatry* 2004;**161**:1129–30).

Tamoxifen + venlafaxine
See tamoxifen + paroxetine (*4.3.2.4*).

Ticagrelor + venlafaxine *
Ticagrelor has no clinically relevant effect on venlafaxine or metabolite, or vice versa (n=25, Teng *et al*, *Clin Ther* 2014;**36**:1217–25).

Tramadol + venlafaxine *
Although there is a risk of serotonin syndrome, this is not a reason *not* to use tramadol. Monitor, counsel and take extra care with older age, higher doses and with concomitant 2D6 inhibitors (review of n=10, Park *et al*, *J Pharm Pract* 2014;**27**:71–8).

Trazodone + venlafaxine
Serotonin syndrome (n=1, McCue and Joseph, *Am J Psychiatry* 2001;**158**:2088–9) and fulminant hepatic failure have been reported (n=1, Detry *et al*, *Transplant Proc* 2009;**41**:3435–6).

Tricyclics + venlafaxine
See tricyclics (*4.3.1*).

Valproate + venlafaxine *
See venlafaxine + valproate (*4.4.4*).

Verapamil + venlafaxine
A fatality has been reported (n=1, Kusman *et al*, *J Forensic Sci* 2000;**45**:926–8).

Warfarin + venlafaxine
Potentiation of warfarin's anticoagulant effects

has been reported, including increased PT or INR (UK SmPC).

4.3.3.9 VORTIOXETINE *

Vortioxetine is metabolised mainly by 2D6 plus a minor effect from 3A4/5 and 2C9. Lower doses are needed if used with 2D6 inhibitors, especially in 2D6 poor metabolisers. Higher doses may be needed with P450 inducers, e.g. rifampicin, carbamazepine and phenytoin, with a 72% decrease in AUC possible. Vortioxetine has no effect on 2D6, 2C9, 2C19, 3A4, 2B6, 1A2 or 2D6. Care is needed with SGAs, phenothiazines, tricyclics, NSAIDs, anticoagulants, and in known bleeding tendencies/disorders as risk of haemorrhage. There is a risk of serotonin syndrome with tramadol, sumatriptan and other triptans, St John's wort and SSRIs. A lower seizure threshold is possible with antidepressants, antipsychotics, mefloquine, bupropion and tramadol.

Alcohol + vortioxetine *

There is no effect on cognition, but it is not advised (SmPC).

Aspirin + vortioxetine *

Lack of interaction has been shown (p/c, c/o, 20/7, Chen *et al*, *J Clin Pharmacol* 2015;**55**:671–9).

Benzodiazepines + vortioxetine *

Lack of interaction has been noted (SmPC).

Bupropion + vortioxetine *

Bupropion 300 mg/d can increase vortioxetine AUC by 2.3-fold leading to increased ADRs (SmPC).

Ketoconazole/fluconazole + vortioxetine *

Vortioxetine AUC is raised 1.3–1.5-fold, but no dose adjustment needed (SmPC).

Linezolid + vortioxetine *

These are contraindicated but can be used with minimal doses and close monitoring. (SmPC).

Lithium + vortioxetine *

Lack of interaction has been noted (SmPC).

MAOIs + vortioxetine *

The combination is contraindicated with 14 days of either (SmPC).

Moclobemide + vortioxetine *

These are contraindicated but can be used with minimal doses and close monitoring. (SmPC).

OCs + vortioxetine *

Lack of interaction has been noted (SmPC).

Omeprazole + vortioxetine *

Lack of interaction has been noted (SmPC).

Quinidine + vortioxetine *

Care is needed as raised levels of vortioxetine can occur (SmPC).

Selegiline/rasagiline + vortioxetine *

These can be used with minimal doses and close monitoring. (SmPC).

SSRIs + vortioxetine *

Care with fluoxetine and paroxetine (SmPC).

Warfarin + vortioxetine *

Lack of interaction has been shown (p/c, c/o, 20/7, Chen *et al*, *J Clin Pharmacol* 2015;**55**:671–9).

4.3.3.10 ST JOHN'S WORT

SJW is unlicensed but widely used as self-medication, so remember to ask about it as up to 7% may be taking it at any one time (n=101, Redvers *et al*, *Psychiatr Bull* 2001;**25**:254–6). Minor serotonin, norepinephrine and dopamine reuptake inhibition activity has been shown with St John's wort (SJW) and might thus potentiate any antidepressants, and so any combinations should in theory be avoided, particularly at high dose. SJW at standard doses is unlikely to inhibit CYP2D6 or 3A4 activity (n=7, open, Markowitz *et al*, *Life Sci* 2000;**66**:133–9), but is probably a CYP3A4 and 2C9 inducer (n=2, Ruschitzka *et al*, *Lancet* 2000;**355**:548–9). SJW increases the expression of P-glycoprotein, which may have implications for drug interactions (n=22, Hennessy *et al*, *Br J Clin Pharmacol* 2002;**53**:75–82; FFT).

Review: general interactions (Borrelli and Izzo, *AAPS J* 2009;**11**:710–27; FFT).

Alitretinoin + St John's wort

The SmPC for alitretinoin states that it should not be used with SJW.

Ambrisentan + St John's wort *

SJW reduces ambrisentan exposure by 17–26%, but SJW has little effect on ambrisentan except in poor metabolisers (n=20, 20/7, Markert *et al*, *Basic Clin Pharmacol Toxicol* 2015;**116**:423–8).

Androgens + St John's wort

Short-term SJW does not significantly alter circulating androgen levels in men and women, although 5-alpha-reduced-androgen levels may drop (n=12, 14/7, Donovan *et al*, *Phytother Res* 2005;**19**:901–6).

ANTIRETROVIRALS + ST JOHN'S WORT *

SJW induces the metabolism of antiretrovirals and so they should not be taken together (CSM warning). The UK SmPC for **atazanavir** contraindicates it with any products containing SJW, with a similar warning for **maraviroc** (UK SmPC). SJW may reduce the levels of **indinavir** (AUC reduced by 57%), reducing efficacy, and so these should not be taken together (n=8, Piscitelli *et al, Lancet* 2000;**355**:547–8). The same would probably be true for other protease inhibitors, e.g. **ritonavir** and **saquinavir**. Suddenly stopping SJW may require dose adjustment of any anti-HIV drug.

Benzodiazepines + St John's wort

SJW halves **alprazolam's** half-life (n=12, open, Markowitz *et al, JAMA* 2003;**290**:1500–2), but there was no significant interaction between stat doses of alprazolam 1 mg and the Esbericum brand of SJW (n=28, RCT, p/c, Arold *et al, Planta Med* 2005;**71**:331–7).

Boceprevir + St. John's wort *

No clinically significant interaction occurs (n=17, open, c/o, 8/52, Jackson *et al, J Antimicrob Chemother* 2014;**69**:1911–5).

Bosentan + St. John's wort *

There is no significant interaction in most people but 2C9 genotype may have some effect (n=13, Markert *et al, Int J Clin Pharmacol Ther* 2014;**52**:328–36).

Bupropion + St John's wort

St John's wort can decrease bupropion and hydrobupropion plasma levels, probably via 2B6 induction (n=18, Lei *et al, Xenobiotica* 2010;**40**:275–81).

Buspirone + St John's wort

See buspirone (*4.1.2*).

Caffeine + St John's wort

There was no significant interaction between stat doses of caffeine 100 mg and the Esbericum brand of SJW (n=28, RCT, p/c, Arold *et al, Planta Med* 2005;**71**:331–7).

Carbamazepine + St John's wort

Carbamazepine reduces hypericum levels by 30%, probably clinically insignificant (n=33, RCT, p/c, 7/7, Johne *et al, Eur J Clin Pharmacol* 2004;**60**:617–22). SJW may have no effect on carbamazepine clearance (n=8, 5/52, Burstein *et al, Clin Pharmacol Ther* 2000;**68**:605–12), but the CSM (2000) warned that SJW may induce the metabolism of carbamazepine, increasing the risk of seizures, and so should not be taken together. Suddenly stopping SJW may require dose adjustment of carbamazepine so check levels before and after stopping SJW.

CICLOSPORIN + ST JOHN'S WORT

SJW causes rapid (within three days) and significant (60%) reduction in ciclosporin plasma levels and may alter the metabolite ratio as well (n=11, open, 14/7, Bauer *et al, Br J Clin Pharmacol* 2003;**55**:203–11; FFT), so these should not be taken together (CSM warning, 2000; Moschella and Jaber, *Am J Kidney Dis* 2001;**38**:1105–7). Heart transplant rejection has been reported (n=2, Ruschitzka *et al, Lancet* 2000;**355**:548).

Cimetidine + St John's wort

Cimetidine increases hypericum levels by 25%, probably insignificant (n=33, RCT, p/c, 7/7, Johne *et al, Eur J Clin Pharmacol* 2004;**60**:617–22).

Clozapine + St John's wort

See clozapine (*4.2.4*).

DIGOXIN + ST JOHN'S WORT

SJW reduces digoxin's AUC by up to 25%, and so avoid the combination (n=25, 10/7, s/b, p/c, Johne *et al, Clin Pharmacol Ther* 1999;**66**:338–45), although stat doses are probably safe (n=28, RCT, p/c, Arold *et al, Planta Med* 2005;**71**:331–7). Suddenly stopping SJW may also require dose adjustment of digoxin.

Docetaxel + St John's wort *

SJW reduces docetaxel's AUC by 12%, which might be significant (n=10, Goey *et al, Clin Pharmacokinet* 2014;**53**:103–10).

Duloxetine + St John's wort

See duloxetine (*4.3.3.2*).

Fexofenadine + St John's wort

SJW may inhibit the metabolism of fexofenadine (open, c/o, Wang *et al, Clin Pharmacol Therapeutics* 2002;**71**:414–20).

Finasteride + St John's wort

SJW induces the metabolism of finasteride and reduces its AUC and half-life (n=12, 2/52, Lundahl *et al, Eur J Pharm Sci* 2009;**36**:433–43).

Fingolimod + St John's wort *

Concurrent use is not recommended (SmPC).

Ibuprofen + St John's wort

SJW appears to have no significant effect on ibuprofen (n=8, 21/7, Bell *et al, Ann Pharmacother* 2007;**41**:229–34).

Ketamine + St John's wort

SJW can significantly reduce ketamine's AUC by 58%, and peak by 66% (n=12, RCT, d/b, p/c, c/o, 14/7, Peltoniemi *et al, Fundam Clin Pharmacol* 2012;**26**:743–50).

Lacosamide + St John's wort

SJW induces lacosamide's metabolism (SmPC).

MAOIs + St John's wort
Minor MAOI activity has been detected from SJW, which might potentiate existing MAOI therapy, and should be avoided, particularly at high dose.

Methadone + St John's wort
SJW induces methadone metabolism, decreasing levels by up to 47% and may precipitate withdrawal symptoms (n=4, Eich-Höchli *et al*, *Pharmacopsychiatry* 2003;**36**:35–7).

Methylphenidate + St John's wort
See methylphenidate (*4.6.13*).

Omeprazole + St John's wort
SJW may produce 'enormously' decreased omeprazole levels (n=12, RCT, c/o, Wang *et al*, *Clin Pharmacol Ther* 2004;**75**:191–7).

Oral contraceptives + St John's wort *
The UK CSM recommends that since SJW reduces the effectiveness of oral contraceptives, the two should not be taken together (e.g. n=12, open, Hall *et al*, *Clin Pharmacol Ther* 2003;**74**:525–35). However, a small study showed no loss of efficacy of Loestrin 1/20® (Galen), with no significant change in serum androgen levels (n=15, open, Fogle *et al*, *Contraception* 2006;**74**:245–8). For **Emergency Hormonal Contraception** the RCOG advises that the use of a copper intrauterine device is most effective if taking (or within 28 days of stopping) SJW. If not, levonorgestrel 3mg stat within 120 hours is possible, albeit unlicensed and with limited efficacy data.

Oxycodone + St. John's wort
SJW reduces oral oxycodone's AUC by 50% and shortens the half-life (n=12, RCT, p/c, c/o, 15/7, Nieminen *et al*, *Eur J Pain* 2010;**14**:854–9).

PHENOBARBITAL + ST JOHN'S WORT
SJW may induce the metabolism of phenobarbital, increasing the risk of seizures, and so should not be taken together. Suddenly stopping SJW may require dose adjustment of phenobarbital so check levels before and after stopping SJW.

PHENYTOIN + ST JOHN'S WORT
SJW may induce the metabolism of phenytoin, increasing the risk of seizures, and so should not be taken together. Suddenly stopping SJW may require dose adjustment of phenytoin so check levels before and after stopping SJW.

Prednisone + St John's wort
Lack of interaction has been shown (n=8, 28/7, Bell *et al*, *Ann Pharmacother* 2007;**41**:1819–24).

RASAGILINE + ST JOHN'S WORT
Combined use (14-day gap required) is a contra-indication (UK SmPC, 2010).

SSRIs + St John's wort
Minor serotonin reuptake inhibition activity has been detected from SJW which might potentiate existing SSRI therapy and so should, in theory, be avoided, particularly at high dose.

Statins + St John's wort
SJW may decrease **rosuvastatin** (n=1, Gordon *et al*, *Am J Med* 2009;**122**:e1–2), **simvastatin** and **atorvastatin** (but not **pravastatin**) plasma levels (n=16, d/b, c/o, 14/7, Sugimoto *et al*, *Clin Pharmacol Ther* 2001;**70**:518–24).

TACROLIMUS + ST JOHN'S WORT
SJW induces tacrolimus metabolism via 3A4, which has led to organ rejection (n=10, Hebert *et al*, *J Clin Pharmacol* 2004;**44**:89–94).

Theophylline + St John's wort
SJW may induce the metabolism of theophylline, reducing efficacy, and so these should not be taken together (SmPC). Suddenly stopping SJW may require dose adjustment of theophylline (n=1, Nebel *et al*, *Ann Pharmacother* 1999;**33**:502), although not in everyone (n=12, open, RCT, c/o, 15/7, Morimoto *et al*, *J Clin Pharmacol* 2004;**44**:95–101). Check theophylline levels before and after stopping SJW.

Tolbutamide + St John's wort
There was no significant interaction between stat doses of tolbutamide 500mg and the Esbericum brand of SJW (n=28, RCT, p/c, Arold *et al*, *Planta Med* 2005;**71**:331–7)

Tricyclics + St John's wort
Minor SNRI activity has been detected from SJW, which might thus potentiate tricyclics and so should, in theory, be avoided, particularly at high dose. Amitriptyline and nortriptyline levels reduced by 22% have been reported (n=12, Johne *et al*, *J Clin Psychopharmacol* 2002;**22**:46–54).

Triptans + St John's wort
The CSM has warned that SJW may increase the serotonergic effects of **sumatriptan**, **naratriptan**, **rizatriptan** and **zolmitriptan**, with increased adverse effects so avoid the combination.

Tyramine + St John's wort
There is not thought to be an interaction (Cupp, *Am Fam Physician* 1999;**59**:1239–45; FFT).

Verapamil + St John's wort
SJW significantly reduces verapamil bioavailability

4

(AUC 50–60% decreased) via increased first-pass gut metabolism (n=8, open, Tannergren *et al*, *Clin Pharmacol Ther* 2004;**75**:298–309).

WARFARIN + ST JOHN'S WORT

SJW may induce the metabolism of warfarin, reducing efficacy, and so these should not be taken together (SmPC). Suddenly stopping SJW may require dose adjustment of warfarin so check INR before and after stopping SJW and adjust doses as necessary.

Zolpidem + St John's wort

See zolpidem (*4.1.7*).

4.3.4 MONOAMINE OXIDASE INHIBITORS (MAOIs)

Reviews: dietary restrictions (Flockhart, *J Clin Psychiatry* 2012;**73**[Suppl 1]:17–24), in primary care (Culpepper, *J Clin Psychiatry* 2012;**73**[Suppl 1]:37–41).

Adrenaline + MAOIs

See norepinephrine + MAOIs.

ALCOHOL + MAOIs

See alcohol (*4.7.1*).

Amantadine + MAOIs

Hypertension occurred in someone taking amantadine two days after starting phenelzine (n=1, Jack and Daniel, *Arch Gen Psychiatry* 1984;**41**:726), with one reported safe use of both (n=1, Greenberg and Meyers, *Am J Psychiatry* 1985;**142**:273).

AMFETAMINE + MAOIs

See dexamfetamine + MAOIs.

Anaesthetics + MAOIs *

With proper monitoring, general and local anaesthesia can be given safely with MAOIs (n=27, el-Ganzouri *et al*, *Anesth Analg* 1985;**64**:592–6), although occasional cases of reactions have been reported (e.g. Sides, *Anesthesia* 1987;**42**:633–5). Regional or spinal anaesthesia may be safe with care (n=1 with tranylcypromine, Krings-Ernst *et al*, *Int J Clin Pharmacol Ther* 2013;**51**:763–70).

Anticholinergics + MAOIs

Enhanced anticholinergic effects might occur.

Anticoagulants + MAOIs

An enhanced anticoagulant effect has been shown in animals.

Antipsychotics + MAOIs

Unexplained deaths with **levomepromazine** exist, probably not a drug-related interaction. The combination is a risk factor for NMS and may enhance anticholinergic and EPSEs. Enhanced sedation could occur. There is a case of serotonin syndrome with **phenelzine** and **quetiapine** (n=1, Kohen *et al*, *CNS Spectr* 2007;**12**:596–8).

Aspartane + MAOIs

Recurrent headaches following aspartane ingestion have been reported (n=1, Ferguson, *Am J Psychiatry* 1985;**142**:271).

ATOMOXETINE + MAOIs

See atomoxetine (*4.6.4*).

Atracurium + MAOIs

Atracurium-induced hypertension has occurred (n=1, Sides, *Anesthesia* 1987;**42**:633–5).

Barbiturates + MAOIs

Barbiturate sedation may be prolonged. Although little human data exists, be aware of the potential for toxicity as one fatality has been reported.

Benzodiazepines + MAOIs

Although there are isolated cases of MAOI toxicity, oedema and hepatotoxicity (e.g. Young and Walpole, *Med J Aust* 1986;**144**:166–7), this is normally considered a safe combination.

Beta-blockers + MAOIs

Propranolol used with MAOIs has caused severe hypertension (Risch *et al*, *J Clin Psychiatry* 1982;**43**:16–31) and slight bradycardia (n=1, Reggev and Vollhardt, *Psychosomatics* 1989;**30**:106–8), although not inevitably (review: Davidson *et al*, *J Clin Psychiatry* 1984;**45**:81–4). Best to monitor bp carefully, especially in the elderly.

Bretylium + MAOIs

Bretylium might increase heart rate with MAOIs, but it is only dangerous if other sympathomimetics are present. There are no case reports.

Bupropion + MAOIs

See bupropion (*4.6.6*).

BUSPIRONE + MAOIs

There are four unpublished reports of increased bp and possible CVA, although the combination has been used safely.

Caffeine + MAOIs *

Severe hypertension has been reported with caffeinated coffee and tranylcypromine (n=1, van der Hoeven *et al*, *Ann Intern Med* 2014;**160**:657–8), as has increased jitteriness (Berkowitz *et al*, *Eur J Pharmacol* 1971;**16**:315–21).

Carbamazepine + MAOIs

Carbamazepine is contraindicated with MAOIs. There have been reports of raised carbamazepine levels but a lack of interaction with **tranylcypromine** (Lydiard *et al*, *J Clin Psychopharmacol* 1987;**7**:360) and **phenelzine** (Yatham *et al*, *Am J Psychiatry* 1990;**147**:367).

Chloral hydrate + MAOIs

There are two poorly documented case reports of fatal hyperpyrexia and hypertension with chloral hydrate and **phenelzine**. This is not thought to be an important interaction.

Citalopram + MAOIs

There are many reported cases of serotonin syndrome with other SSRIs and MAOIs and so care is needed (review: Graber *et al*, *Ann Pharmacother* 1994;**28**:732–5).

Clozapine + MAOIs

See clozapine (4.2.4).

Cocaine + MAOIs

See cocaine (4.7.3).

Cyproheptadine + MAOIs

An isolated case exists of hallucinations with cyproheptadine and phenelzine (Hahn, *Am J Psychiatry* 1987;**144**:1242–3).

DEXAMFETAMINE + MAOIs

There is a report of a death with phenelzine and dexamfetamine (n = 1, Lloyd and Walker, *Br Med J* 1965;ii:168–9; FFT) and one with amfetamine.

Dextromethorphan + MAOIs

Case reports exist with cough mixtures containing dextromethorphan but, since all also contained sympathomimetics, these are questionable. Two were fatal, so care is advised. Dizziness and muscle spasms have been reported (Harrison *et al*, *J Clin Psychiatry* 1989;**50**:64–5), as has a serotonin syndrome (Nierenberg *et al*, *Clin Pharmacol Ther* 1993;**53**:84–8).

Dextropropoxyphene + MAOIs

Dextropropoxyphene plus **phenelzine** may produce sedation (n = 1, Garbutt, *Am J Psychiatry* 1987;**144**:251–2), severe hypotension, ataxia and impaired coordination (n = 1, Zornberg and Hegarty, *Am J Psychiatry* 1993;**150**:1270–1).

Disulfiram + MAOIs

See disulfiram (4.6.8).

DOPAMINE/DOXAPRAM + MAOIs

The SmPCs recommend that dopamine or doxapram can be used if their initial dose is reduced to one tenth the normal dose and great care taken.

DULOXETINE + MAOIs

See duloxetine (4.3.3.2).

Ecstasy (MDMA) + MAOIs

Hypertensive crisis has been reported with MDMA and phenelzine (n = 1, Smilkstein *et al*, *J Toxicol Clin Toxicol* 1987;**25**:149–59), as has muscle tension, coma, hypertension and delirium (n = 2, Kaskey, *Am J Psychiatry* 1992;**149**:411–2).

Escitalopram + MAOIs

See citalopram + MAOIs.

FLUOXETINE + MAOIs

There are several reported interactions (e.g. Sternbach, *Lancet* 1988;**2**:850–1), including four deaths. A gap must be left when switching from one to the other (see 2.2.5).

FLUVOXAMINE + MAOIs

The SmPC recommends allowing a two-week gap between therapies. There are many reports of serotonin syndrome with other SSRIs and MAOIs and so care is needed.

Ginseng + MAOIs

There are cases of headache, tremor (Shader and Greenblatt, *J Clin Psychopharmacol* 1985;**5**:65) and mania (Jones and Runikis, *J Clin Psychopharmacol* 1987;**7**:201–2) with ginseng and **phenelzine**.

Hypoglycaemics + MAOIs

An enhanced hypoglycaemic effect with insulin and sulphonylureas has been noted.

INDORAMIN + MAOIs

The combination is contraindicated (indoramin's SmPC) as indoramin antagonises alpha-receptors, thus competing with norepinephrine for post-synaptic alpha-receptors, which could cause vasoconstriction and raised blood pressure.

Isoprenaline + MAOIs

This is a postulated interaction, but with no evidence or case reports.

Patient information: warning signs of a reaction with MAOIs

If a patient experiences any of the following symptoms, especially after eating, taking drugs of any type or if unexpected or severe, a reaction should be suspected and appropriate medical attention sought immediately: headache (especially at the back of the head), lightheadedness or dizziness, flushing of the face, pounding of the heart, numbness or stiffness in the neck, photophobia, chest pain or nausea and vomiting. It usually occurs within about two hours of the ingestion of the compound.

4

LEVODOPA + MAOIs

Low dose levodopa with carbidopa or benserazide seems safe but higher doses should be avoided, as should levodopa on its own (n=4, Teychenne *et al*, *Clin Pharmacol Ther* 1975;**18**:273).

LISDEXAMFETAMINE + MAOIs

See MAOIs + lisdexamfetamine (*4.6.10*).

Lithium + MAOIs

Lack of an interaction has been reported (n=4, Fein *et al*, *Am J Psychiatry* 1988;**145**:249–50).

MAOIs + MAOIs

It is possible for different MAOIs to interact with each other, especially if abruptly changed, e.g. **isocarboxazid** to **tranylcypromine** (n=1, Bazire, *Drug Intell Clin Pharm* 1986;**20**:954–6) and **phenelzine** to **isocarboxazid** (Safferman and Masiar, *Ann Pharmacother* 1992;**26**:337–8). Tranylcypromine is metabolised to an amfetamine and an internal autoreaction (i.e. interacts with itself) has been postulated (n=1, Gunn *et al*, *BMJ* 1989;**298**:964; FFT).

Methadone + MAOIs

Lack of an interaction has been reported (Mendelson, *Med J Aust* 1979;**1**:400).

Methyldopa + MAOIs

There is a single case report of hallucinations with methyldopa and pargyline.

METHYLPHENIDATE + MAOIs

A single case of headaches and hyperventilation has been reported.

Mirtazapine + MAOIs

See mirtazapine (*4.3.3.4*).

Modafinil + MAOIs

There is a report of safe use of tranylcypromine and modafinil for refractory narcolepsy (n=1, Clemons *et al*, *Sleep Med* 2004;**5**:509–11).

Morphine + MAOIs

Cases exist of hypotension and loss of consciousness with IV morphine (n=2, Barry, *Anaesth Intensive Care* 1979;**7**:194), responsive to naloxone. Low dose morphine and other narcotics, e.g. codeine and fentanyl are probably safe. **Methadone** may be a suitable alternative. If opiates are used, it is best to start at a third or half the normal dose of opiate and titrate carefully, noting blood pressure and levels of consciousness. See also pethidine.

NEFOPAM + MAOIs

The UK SmPC for nefopam recommends avoiding this combination.

Norepinephrine + MAOIs

Although unlikely to cause problems if care is used, norepinephrine is potentially dangerous by injection if other sympathomimetics are present.

Oxcarbazepine + MAOIs

See oxcarbazepine (*4.5.3*).

Oxymetazoline/xylometazoline + MAOIs

There is little systemic effect when these drugs are used nasally, but there are no formal studies.

Paraldehyde + MAOIs

Enhanced CNS sedation and respiratory depression have been suggested.

Paroxetine + MAOIs

Nothing has been reported, but see other SSRIs in this MAOI section.

PETHIDINE + MAOIs

This is a well-documented, rapid, severe and potentially fatal interaction, although not inevitable (Evans-Prosser, *Br J Anaesth* 1968;**40**:279–82).

RASAGILINE + MAOIs

Combined use (14-day gap required) is a contra-indication (UK SmPC).

Reboxetine + MAOIs

See reboxetine (*4.3.3.6*).

Salbutamol + MAOIs

No interaction occurs.

SERTRALINE + MAOIs

Sertraline is contraindicated with MAOIs (UK SmPC) with a one-week washout period after sertraline before an MAOI is used. Serotonergic syndrome has been reported, so care is essential (e.g. cases and review, Graber *et al*, *Ann Pharmacother* 1994;**28**:732–5).

St John's wort + MAOIs

See St John's wort (*4.3.3.10*).

Sulphonamides + MAOIs

An isolated case exists of adverse effects with sulphafurazole and phenelzine (n=1, Boyer and Lake, *Am J Psychiatry* 1983;**140**:264–5).

Suxamethonium + MAOIs

There are cases of enhancement of suxamethonium by phenelzine (n=3, Bodley *et al*, *BMJ* 1969;**3**:510–2; FFT).

SYMPATHOMIMETICS + MAOIs

Hypertension has been reported with many indirectly-acting sympathomimetic amines, e.g. ephedrine, metaraminol, pseudoephedrine and phenylpropanolamine. Phenylephrine is found in many OTC cough and cold remedies and can cause a massive rise in blood pressure with MAOIs. Although no case reports, use in nasal sprays and drops is not recommended.

Tetrabenazine + MAOIs

Reports exist of a central excitation and hypertension with tetrabenazine.

Trazodone + MAOIs

There are many reported cases of serotonin syndrome with SSRIs and MAOIs (see *C5*) and so care is needed (n = 1, Graber *et al*, *Ann Pharmacother* 1994;**28**:732–5).

TRICYCLICS + MAOIs

Tranylcypromine has caused four deaths with **clomipramine** and one with **imipramine** (n = 1, Birkenhager and van den Broek, *Eur Psychiatry* 2003;**18**:264–5). There are cases of excitation, seizures, hyperpyrexia and a serotonin syndrome after a clomipramine overdose (325–750 mg) with phenelzine (Nierenberg *et al*, *Clin Pharmacol Ther* 1993;**53**:84–8). The dangers could have been exaggerated and the combination may be relatively event-free if the following precautions are taken:

- avoid imipramine, desipramine, clomipramine and tranylcypromine
- prefer amitriptyline
- start both drugs simultaneously at low dose, increase slowly and monitor closely.

See also combinations in depression (*1.14*) for a review of the potentially beneficial effects.

TRIPTANS + MAOIs

The SmPCs recommend **sumatriptan** is not used with MAOIs, or for two weeks after an MAOI has stopped. The UK SmPC contraindicates MAOIs with **rizatriptan**.

Tryptophan + MAOIs

Hypomania and behavioural and neurological toxicity have been reported, mostly with **tranylcypromine** (n = 8, Pope *et al*, *Am J Psychiatry* 1985:**142**:491–2). Potentiation of the therapeutic effect is well known so monitor carefully.

TYRAMINE + MAOIs

Ingestion of dietary tyramine by someone on an MAOI can produce a hypertensive crisis, e.g. headache, rapid and prolonged rise in blood pressure, intracranial haemorrhage, acute cardiac failure and death. The effect is probably only seen with slow acetylators, as fast acetylators seem able to handle tyramine and other monoamines better. The effect is hugely variable, but 8 mg tyramine can produce a 30 mmHg rise in bp in about 50% people, and 25 mg and above is potentially dangerous (e.g. n=16, d/b, p/c, Berlin *et al*, *Clin Pharmacol Ther* 1989;**46**:344–51). In a normal person, bp rises within 10–20 minutes (range 0–60) of tyramine ingestion, peaking at 20–110 minutes, prolonged if an MAOI is taken. For advice on dietary tyramine, see the following section.

L-tyrosine + phenelzine *

Despite many warnings an interesting review found no reported cases and complete lack of evidence for an interaction (Hinz *et al*, *Clin Pharmacol* 2014;**6**:107–10).

VENLAFAXINE + MAOIs

See venlafaxine (*4.3.3.8*).

Vortioxetine + MAOIs *

See vortioxetine (*4.3.3.9*).

Warfarin + MAOIs

No interaction is known, although tranylcypromine inhibits CYP2C19 and so some minor potential exists (Sayal *et al*, *Acta Psychiatr Scand* 2000;**102**:250–5).

Xylometazoline + MAOIs

See oxymetazoline + MAOIs.

FOOD

Reviews: User-friendly MAOI diet (Gardner *et al*, *J Clin Psychiatry* 1996;**57**:99–104), dietary restrictions (Rapaport, *J Clin Psychiatry* 2007;**68**[suppl 8]:42–6).

1. General principles

Freshness of food is vital. Do not eat if there is any sign of spoilage. Avoid foods that are matured or might be 'spoiling'. Generally, the more 'convenience' the food, the safer it is, e.g. packet soups are generally safe. Although many foods have only small amounts of tyramine, it is possible to have local concentrations, which might give a reaction.

2. Tyramine-containing foods to avoid

The following may be useful guidelines:

- Dairy products

Avoid hard cheeses and soft cheeses. Special care is needed with salty, bitter tasting, refrigerated cheese. Avoid foods containing cheese (e.g. pizzas and pies, see below) as these are a known cause of inadvertent ingestion and death. However, cottage cheese, cream cheeses (e.g. Philadelphia), Ricotta and processed cheese contain only minute amounts of tyramine and large quantities would be needed to produce a reaction.

- Fruit and vegetables

Avoid broad bean pods (but not the beans), banana skins (occasionally cooked as part of whole unripe bananas in a stew) and avocado.

4

- **Game, meat and fish**

Avoid pickled or salted dried herrings and any hung or badly stored game, poultry or other meat that might be 'spoiling'. NB. reports with pickled herrings were probably spoilage in the brine surrounding the fish, and are probably safe.

- **Meat products**

Avoid chicken liver pâté, liver pâté and any other liver that is not fresh. Avoid aged and cured meats (e.g. salami, mortadella, pastrami). Fresh chicken liver, fresh beef liver and fresh pâté should be safe.

- **Pizzas**

Commercially available pizzas from large chain outlets seem safe (analysis by Shulman and Walker, *J Clin Psychiatry* 1999;**60**:191–3; comment by Feinberg and Holzer, reply by Shulman and Walker, *J Clin Psychiatry* 2000;**61**:145–6). Gourmet pizzas from smaller outlets may have higher tyramine contents, especially if mature cheeses are used.

- **Soy and soybean**

Some samples of soy sauce and soybean preparations may have very high tyramine levels. Either avoid entirely or limit intake to a 10mL maximum (Shulman and Walker, *J Clin Psychiatry* 1999;**60**:191–3):

Soy sauce (Pearl River, etc) — some have high quantities, i.e. up to 3.4mg/15mL, and so double or triple helpings could be well above the threshold for a reaction

Soybean curd (e.g. Tofu) — some have high quantities, especially if kept refrigerated for seven days or longer, i.e. up to 5mg per 300mg helping, and so double or triple helpings could well be above the threshold for a reaction.

- **Yeast and meat extracts**

Avoid 'Oxo', 'Marmite', 'Bovril' and other meat or yeast extracts. Gravy made with 'Bisto' is safe (all contain less than 0.0022mg/g tyramine and a half-pint of gravy would contain less than 0.05mg tyramine). Gravy made from juices of the roast or fresh meat should be safe. Brewers yeast (Shulman *et al*, *J Clin Psychopharmacol* 1989;**9**:397–402) and bread are safe.

3. Foods known to contain some tyramine where excessive consumption is not advisable, albeit unlikely

Plums, matured pork, sauerkraut, spinach.

4. Foods thought to contain only minute amounts of tyramine

Banana pulp (skins unsafe), chocolate (one anecdotal report of headache), cottage cheese, cream cheese, eggplant, fruit juices, octopus, peanuts, raspberries (minor reports of raised tyramine), sausages, soy milk, tomato, vinegar, yoghurt (commercial), Worcester sauce, eg. Lee and Perrins and others (very low, Shulman and Walker, *J Clin Psychiatry* 1999;**60**:191–3).

5. Other foods with isolated reports

Chicken nuggets, chapatti, protein dietary supplement, sea kale.

6. Alcoholic drinks

Patient instructions usually state that all alcoholic and some non-alcoholic drinks must be avoided. Real ales may contain up to 110mg/L, with reports of hypertensive crisis after 0.6 pint (79 brand study, Tailor *et al*, *J Clin Psychopharmacol* 1994;**14**:5–14). Low or non-alcoholic beers may have a significant tyramine content (Murray *et al*, *Lancet* 1988;**i**,1167–8), shown by three reactions to less than two-thirds of a pint of alcohol-free and 'de-alcoholised' beer (n=3, Thakore *et al*, *Int Clin Psychopharmacol* 1992;**7**:59–60). There is a large variation in other beers, so take in moderation (i.e. 1–2 bottles a day maximum), prefer canned beers from major brewers and take care with de-alcoholised beers. The maximum reported level in Chianti wine is 12mg/L, likely to be dangerous only in overdose. The following may, however, be of use where a particular patient wishes to drink.

Avoid:

- Chianti
- Home-made beers and wines
- Real ales
- Red wines

True moderation (e.g. one unit):

- White wines
- Non-alcoholic beers and lagers

Safest:

- Gin, vodka, other clear spirits

Red wines contain phenolic flavanoids, which inhibit the enzymes that metabolise catecholamines, including tyramine.

Over-the-counter medicines

Each person should be warned about the possibility of interactions with over-the-counter medicines. The general advice for people is:

1. Only buy medicines from a pharmacy
Do not use medicines from supermarket shelves, drug stores or newsagents. Do not take medicines given to you by friends or relatives. Do not take medicines taken before the MAOI was prescribed until advice has been sought.
2. Carry an MAOI card and show it to any doctor, dentist or pharmacist who may treat you.
3. Take special care over any medicines for coughs, colds, 'flu, hay fever, asthma and catarrh.

4.4 MOOD STABILISERS

4.4.1 CARBAMAZEPINE *

Carbamazepine is principally metabolised by CYP3A4 (also CYP2C8), but is also a potent inducer of CYP3A4 and other oxidative mechanisms in the liver. This auto-induction takes up to four weeks to stabilise, although it is practically complete after a week. Carbamazepine (CBZ) is metabolised to carbamazepine epoxide (CBZ-E), which may be more toxic than carbamazepine itself and so alteration of the CBZ:CBZ-E ratio by another drug would alter toxicity. Carbamazepine is extensively plasma protein-bound, from 75–80% of total plasma concentration. Major diurnal variations in plasma levels occur, which can be as much as 90% during polytherapy compared to monotherapy (Höppener *et al*, *Epilepsia* 1980;**21**:341–50).

Reviews: * general (Tolou Ghamari *et al*, *J Res Med Sci* 2013;**18**(Suppl 1):S81–5) interactions with herbs, dietary supplements and food (s=74, Fong *et al*, *Evid Based Complement Alternat Med* 2013;**2013**:898261).

ACENOCOUMAROL + CARBAMAZEPINE

The metabolism of acenocoumarol is accelerated by carbamazepine to give a reduced effect.

Acetazolamide + carbamazepine

CYP3A4 inhibition may raise carbamazepine levels (mentioned in Spina *et al*, *Clin Pharmacokinet* 1996;**31**:198–214).

Alcohol + carbamazepine

See alcohol (*4.7.1*).

ANTIPSYCHOTICS + CARBAMAZEPINE *

Antipsychotics lower the seizure threshold, antagonising carbamazepine's anticonvulsant effects, amongst other drug-drug interactions.

Aripiprazole levels are about 70% lower, probably by CYP3A4 induction, so doses may need to be doubled with carbamazepine, and halved if carbamazepine is discontinued (n=9[c=6], 8/52, Citrome *et al*, *J Clin Psychopharmacol* 2007;**27**:279–83), although one study did not find a loss of efficacy despite the dramatic plasma level drop (n=18, Nakamura *et al*, *Ther Drug Monit* 2009;**31**:575–8).

Asenapine appears not to interact (UK SmPC).

Clozapine and carbamazepine are contra-indicated (SmPC) due to the very real enhanced risk of agranulocytosis. Clozapine levels have nearly doubled after carbamazepine was stopped (Raitasuo *et al*, *Am J Psychiatry* 1993;**150**:169).

Haloperidol levels are reduced by up to 50% (n=11, Yasui-Furukori *et al*, *J Clin Psychopharmacol* 2003;**23**:435–40). The effect is dose-dependent (e.g. n=27, 4/52, Hesslinger *et al*, *J Clin Psychopharmacol* 1999;**19**:310–5). A significantly extended QT interval has been shown, probably by increased haloperidol metabolite concentrations (n=2, Iwahashi *et al*, *Am J Psychiatry* 1996;**153**:135).

Olanzapine's clearance is increased by 44% and half-life reduced by 20% (n=47, Linnet and Olesen, *Ther Drug Monit* 2002;**24**:512–7), probably by CYP1A2 induction, but dose adjustment is not needed as olanzapine has a wide therapeutic index (n=11, Lucas *et al*, *Eur J Clin Pharmacol* 1998;**54**:639–43).

Quetiapine plasma levels can be decreased by 80% (eg. n=18, Grimm *et al*, *Br J Clin Pharmacol* 2006;**61**:58 69; FFT), or even to undetectable (n=1, Nickl-Jockschat *et al*, *Clin Neuropharmacol* 2009;**32**:55), presumably by CYP3A4 induction, potentially clinically significant. CBZ (n=2, Fitzgerald and Okos, *Pharmacother* 2002;**22**:1500–3) and CBZ-epoxide (SmPC) levels can be raised 3–4-fold.

Risperidone (n=34, Spina *et al*, *Ther Drug Monit* 2000;**22**:481–5; n=11, Ono *et al*, *Psychopharmacol [Berl]* 2002;**162**:50–4) and **paliperidone** (by 45% at 200mg/d, by 65% at >400mg/d and is only dose-dependent to 400mg/d; n=6, Yasui-Furukori *et al*, *Ther Drug Monit* 2013;**35**:649–52) levels can be halved, probably via 2D6 and 3A4 induction. EPSE have occurred after carbamazepine discontinuation (n=2, Takahashi *et al*, *Clin Neuropharmacol* 2001;**24**:358–60). Risperidone can increase steady-state carbamazepine levels by 10% over 24 hours and 20% over two weeks

4

(n=8, Mula and Monaco, *Clin Neuropharmacol* 2002;**25**:97–100), and has caused complex but reversible cardiac effects, e.g. arrhythmia (n=1, Hydzik *et al, Przegl Lek* 2011;**68**:499–502).

Ziprasidone's AUC can be reduced by about 35%, which may require slightly raised doses (n=25, RCT, 4/52, Miceli *et al, Br J Clin Pharmacol* 2000;**49**[S3]:65–70; FFT).

ANTIRETROVIRALS + CARBAMAZEPINE *

The UK SmPC notes the possibility of reduced plasma **indinavir** (n=36, open, L'homme *et al, J Acquir Immune Defic Syndr* 2006;**43**:193–6), **ritonavir, saquinavir, efavirenz** (RCT, c/o, open, 6/52, Ji *et al, J Clin Pharmacol* 2008;**48**:948–56) and **atazanavir** levels, probably by 3A4 induction. Carbamazepine toxicity (levels increased by 53%) has been reported with **lopinavir/ritonavir, nelfinavir** (n=1, Bates and Herman, *Ann Pharmacother* 2006;**40**:1190–5), **ritonavir** (n=1, Kato *et al, Pharmacother* 2000;**20**:851–4; Antonio *et al, Ann Pharmacother* 2001;**35**:125–6) and **darunavir** (carbamazepine AUC increased by 45%) and a 25–50% dose reduction of carbamazepine is recommended. Efavirenz significantly *reduces* carbamazepine (but not CBZ-E) levels (RCT, c/o, open, 6/52, Ji *et al, J Clin Pharmacol* 2008;**48**:948–56).

Benzodiazepines + carbamazepine

Carbamazepine increases clonazepam clearance by 22% and clonazepam decreases carbamazepine clearance by 22% (n=183, Yukawa *et al, J Clin Psychopharmacol* 2001;**21**:588–93), so slightly higher benzodiazepine doses may be needed (n=17, Baba *et al, Br J Clin Pharmacol* 1990;**29**:766–9; FFT). Carbamazepine toxicity has occurred with **clobazam** (n=1, Genton *et al, Epilepsia* 1998;**39**:1115–8), probably due to progressive increases in norclobazam levels.

Bupropion + carbamazepine

See bupropion (*4.6.6*).

Caffeine + carbamazepine

Carbamazepine induces the CYP1A2 metabolism of caffeine (n=5, Parker *et al, Br J Clin Pharmacol* 1998;**45**:176–8; FFT).

CALCIUM-CHANNEL BLOCKERS + CARBAMAZEPINE

Verapamil increases carbamazepine plasma levels by 50%, via CYP3A4 inhibition (n=43, open, Bahls *et al, Neurology* 1991;**41**:740–2) as does **diltiazem** (postoperative ophthalmoplegia and ataxia, n=1, Wijdicks *et al, J Neuroophthalmol* 2004;**24**:95), suggesting a substantial risk of toxicity. The antihypertensive effect of **nilvadipine** (n=1, Yasui-Furukori and Tateishi, *J Clin Pharmacol* 2002;**42**:100–3) and **isradipine** may be reduced. No interaction occurs with **nifedipine** (n=43, open, Bahls *et al, Neurology* 1991;**41**:740–2), it is the calcium-channel blocker of choice, although the BNF notes the efficacy of nifedipine may be reduced, so care is needed.

Charcoal, activated + carbamazepine

Carbamazepine absorption may be almost completely stopped if activated charcoal is given five minutes after ingestion, with a lesser effect if given after an hour (Neuvonen and Elonen, *Eur J Clin Pharmacol* 1980;**17**:51–7).

Chinese medicines + carbamazepine

Paeoniae Radix, a traditional Chinese medicine, may increase carbamazepine absorption (in rats, Chen *et al, Biol Pharm Bull* 2002;**25**:532–5; FFT).

CICLOSPORIN + CARBAMAZEPINE

Ciclosporin metabolism is accelerated by carbamazepine, reducing plasma levels.

Cilostazol + carbamazepine

A hypersensitivity syndrome with eosinophilia and systemic symptoms has been reported (n=1, Kang *et al, J Dermatol* 2012;**39**:723–4).

Ciprofloxacin + carbamazepine

Ciprofloxacin significantly increases the plasma levels of CBZ, probably by 1A2 inhibition (n=8, Shahzadi *et al, Pak J Pharm Sci* 2011;**24**:63–8).

Cisplatin + carbamazepine

The UK SmPC notes that cisplatin might decrease carbamazepine plasma levels.

Citalopram + carbamazepine

See citalopram/escitalopram (*4.3.2.1*).

Cocaine + carbamazepine

See cocaine (*4.7.3*).

CORTICOSTEROIDS + CARBAMAZEPINE

Corticosteroid CYP3A4 metabolism is accelerated by carbamazepine, giving a reduced effect (n=15, open, Bartoszek *et al, Clin Pharmacol Ther* 1987;**42**:424–32).

DANAZOL + CARBAMAZEPINE

Danazol inhibits carbamazepine metabolism (n=6, open, Zielinski *et al, Ther Drug Monit* 1987;**9**:24–7), so monitor levels.

Dantrolene + carbamazepine

Carbamazepine toxicity has been reported when dantrolene and oxybutinin were added to a stable carbamazepine dose (n=1, Vander *et al, Spinal Cord* 2005;**43**:252–5).

DEXTROPROPOXYPHENE + CARBAMAZEPINE
Dextropropoxyphene enhances carbamazepine toxicity via CYP3A4 inhibition and levels may rise by 44–77% or more (4-fold over 24 hours; n=1, Allen, *Postgrad Med J* 1994;**70**:764; FFT). Monitor closely if used together, especially in the elderly (n=84, open, Bergendal *et al*, *Eur J Clin Pharmacol* 1997;**53**:203–6).

Digoxin + carbamazepine
An isolated case exists of bradycardia with digitalis and carbamazepine but not with digoxin.

Disulfiram + carbamazepine
See disulfiram (*4.6.8*).

Diuretics + carbamazepine
Hyponatraemia has occurred with furosemide or thiazides (eg. n=1, Ranta and Wooten, *Epilepsia* 2004;**45**:879).

Doxorubicin + carbamazepine
The UK SmPC notes doxorubicin might decrease carbamazepine plasma levels, and vice versa.

DOXYCYCLINE + CARBAMAZEPINE
Doxycycline metabolism is accelerated by carbamazepine, reducing efficacy and halving its half-life (Penttilå *et al*, *Br Med J* 1974;**2**:470–2; FFT). Other tetracyclines appear not to interact.

Enteral feeds + carbamazepine
Carbamazepine suspension absorption has been shown to be slightly slowed and reduced during nasogastric feeding (n=8, RCT, c/o, Bass *et al*, *Epilepsia* 1989;**30**:364–9), so take care with dosing after enteral feeding is stopped.

Escitalopram + carbamazepine
See citalopram/escitalopram (*4.3.2.1*).

Ethosuximide + carbamazepine
Carbamazepine induces ethosuximide's metabolism, reducing plasma levels by about 17% (n=6, open, 55/7, Warren *et al*, *Clin Pharmacol Ther* 1980;**28**:646–51), probably of minor significance.

Etretinate + carbamazepine
One girl treated with the combination only responded to etretinate when her carbamazepine was withdrawn (n=1, Mohammed, *Dermatology* 1992;**185**:79).

Fexofenadine + carbamazepine
Carbamazepine may significantly decrease the AUC of fexofenadine (n=12, Akamine *et al*, *Br J Clin Pharmacol* 2012;**73**:478–81; FFT).

Fluoxetine + carbamazepine
See fluoxetine (*4.3.2.2*).

Fluvoxamine + carbamazepine
See fluvoxamine (*4.3.2.3*).

Gabapentin + carbamazepine
See gabapentin (*4.5.1*).

Gestrinone + carbamazepine
The UK SmPC states that carbamazepine may reduce the activity of gestrinone.

Grapefruit juice + carbamazepine
300 mL grapefruit juice increased carbamazepine levels by 40% and AUC by 41%, probably by CYP3A4 inhibition (n=10, RCT, Garg *et al*, *Clin Pharmacol Ther* 1998;**64**:286–8).

Griseofulvin + carbamazepine
A reduced griseofulvin level by enzyme induction may occur (see Albengres *et al*, *Drug Saf* 1998;**18**:83–97).

H2-BLOCKERS + CARBAMAZEPINE
Studies show no interaction with **ranitidine** (e.g. n=8, RCT, Dalton *et al*, *Drug Intell Clin Pharm* 1985;**19**:941–4), whereas **cimetidine** can increase CBZ levels (eg. n=8, open, 7/7, Dalton *et al*, *Epilepsia* 1986;**27**:553–8) via CYP3A4 inhibition.

Herbal tea + carbamazepine
Rats drinking herbal tea may have raised carbamazepine levels (Thabrew *et al*, *Drug Metabol Drug Interact* 2003;**19**:177–87). No human studies are yet available.

Honey + carbamazepine
It is reassuring to discover there is no interaction (n=10, RCT, c/o, 1/52, Malhotra *et al*, *Methods Find Exp Clin Pharmacol* 2003;**25**:537–40).

Influenza vaccine + carbamazepine
A transient 10% increase in carbamazepine levels has occurred (n=55, open, Jann and Fidone, *Clin Pharm* 1986;**5**:817–20), with one report of carbamazepine toxicity (n=1, Robertson, *Pediatr Neurol* 2002;**26**:61–3).

ISONIAZID + CARBAMAZEPINE
Potentially rapid and serious carbamazepine toxicity may occur via 3A4 inhibition (n=13, Valsalan and Cooper, *Br Med J* 1982;**285**:261–2; FFT). Monitor carefully for toxicity.

Isotretinoin + carbamazepine
Isotretinoin may slightly reduce CBZ plasma levels and alter the CBZ:CBZ-E ratio (n=1, Marsden *et al*, *Br J Dermatol* 1988;**119**:403).

Ivabradine + carbamazepine
Carbamazepine can lower the bioavailability of the antianginal ivabradine by 80%, clinically significant (n=18, Vlase *et al*, *J Clin Pharm Ther* 2011;**36**:225–9).

Lacosamide + carbamazepine

4

Caution is needed as enhanced PR prolongation could occur (lacosamide SmPC) and lacosamide levels may be reduced by 25% (n=37, Cawello *et al*, *J Clin Pharmacol* 2010;**50**:459–71).

Lamotrigine + carbamazepine
See lamotrigine (*4.4.2*).

Levetiracetam + carbamazepine
See levetiracetam (*4.5.2*).

Levothyroxine (thyroxine) + carbamazepine
Levothyroxine metabolism is accelerated by carbamazepine, increasing the levothyroxine requirements in hypothyroidism.

Lithium + carbamazepine
Neurotoxicity has occurred without increased plasma levels (Marcoux, *Ann Pharmacother* 1996;**30**:547), albeit mostly in people with pre-existing brain damage (n=5, Shukla *et al*, *Am J Psychiatry* 1984;**141**:1604–6). EPSE has been reported, which resolved when the CBZ was stopped (n=1, Palma *et al*, *Clin Neuropharmacol* 2010;**33**:102–3). An additive anti-thyroid effect can occur, lowering T4 and free T4 levels (n=23, open, Kramlinger and Post, *Am J Psychiatry* 1990:**147**:615–20). Lithium intoxication has led to carbamazepine-induced renal failure (n=1, Mayan *et al*, *Ann Pharmacother* 2001;**35**:560–2). Monitor carefully and regularly for signs of toxicity.

MACROLIDE ANTIBIOTICS + CARBAMAZEPINE
A rapid 100–200% rise in carbamazepine levels has been reported with oral (n=4, Wroblewski *et al*, *JAMA* 1986;**255**:1165–7; n=1, Tatum and Gonzalez, *Hosp Pharm* 1994;**29**:45) and with IV **erythromycin**, probably via CYP3A4 inhibition. The greatest risk is with high doses of both drugs, and least with **clarithromycin** (Pauwels, *Pharmacol Res* 2002;**45**:291–8), although clarithromycin has raised CBZ levels significantly, leading to toxicity (n=10, Gélisse *et al*, *Rev Neurol [Paris]* 2007;**163**:1096–9) and hyponatraemia (n=1, Kanbay *et al*, *South Med J* 2007;**100**:222). Monitor levels or use an alternative antibiotic.

MAOIs + carbamazepine
See MAOIs (*4.3.4*).

Mefloquine + carbamazepine
The SmPC states that mefloquine may antagonise the anticonvulsant effect of carbamazepine.

Melatonin + carbamazepine
See melatonin (*4.1.4*).

Methadone + carbamazepine
See methadone (*4.6.12*).

Methylphenidate + carbamazepine
See methylphenidate (*4.6.13*).

Metoclopramide + carbamazepine
Neurotoxicity has been reported after metoclopramide 30mg/d was added to CBZ, which resolved when metoclopramide was stopped (n=1, Sandyk, *BMJ* 1984;**288**:830; FFT).

Metronidazole + carbamazepine
Plasma carbamazepine levels rose by 60% in one case when metronidazole was added, resulting in toxicity (n=1, Patterson, *Ann Pharmacother* 1994;**28**:1303–4).

Mianserin + carbamazepine
See mianserin (*4.3.3.3*).

Miconazole + carbamazepine
An isolated case report of an adverse response has appeared (n=1, Loupi *et al*, *Therapie* 1982;**37**:437–41).

Mirtazapine + carbamazepine
See mirtazapine (*4.3.3.4*).

Moclobemide + carbamazepine
See moclobemide (*4.3.3.5*).

Modafinil + carbamazepine
See modafinil (*4.6.14*).

Neuromuscular blocking agents + carbamazepine
Reduced responses and recovery times to NMBAs are known, e.g. **vecuronium** doses need to be significantly higher in patients on maintenance carbamazepine (n=8, open, Whalley and Ebrahim, *Br J Anaesth* 1994;**72**:125–6) and recovery times can be 40–60% faster with **atracurium** and **pancuronium** (n=53, open, Tempelhoff *et al*, *Anesth Analg* 1990;**71**:665–9).

Nicotinamide + carbamazepine
The UK SmPC notes that high-dose nicotinamide can raise CBZ/CBZ-epoxide levels in adults.

ORAL CONTRACEPTIVES + CARBAMAZEPINE
The CYP3A4 metabolism of OCs is accelerated by carbamazepine to give a **reduced contraceptive effect.** In women taking enzyme-inducing AEDs (e.g. carbamazepine, phenobarbital or phenytoin), the choice of a Combined Oral Contraceptive requires 50–60mcg/d estrogen (ethinylestradiol, EE). In the UK there is no suitable product at the time of writing, but this dose can be achieved by a daily combination of:

- Leostrin 20® and Loestrin 30® daily (norethisterone)
- Mercilon® and Marvelon® (desogesterol)
- Femodette® and Femodene® (gestodene)

- Sunya 20/75® and Katya 30/75® (gestodene). Alternatively, two tablets daily of, e.g. Microgynon 30®, Ovranette®, Loestrin 30®, Marvelon®, Femodene® or Katya 30/75® can be used, but provide 60 mcg ethinyloestradiol. The NELM (National Electronic Library for Medicines, UKMI Q&A 43.4, Sept 2010) recommend three successive packets without a pill-free interval (PFI), followed by a shorter four-day PFI, as well as additional non-hormonal contraception. This is unlicensed and there is no formal evidence to support this. First choice remains an IUD or depot, e.g. medroxyprogesterone given every 10 rather than 12 weeks has been suggested (Crawford, *CNS Drugs* 2002;**16**:263–72).

Orlistat + carbamazepine
A small trial suggested lack of interaction (n=8, open, 8/52, Hilger *et al*, *J Clin Psychopharmacol* 2002;**22**:68–70).

Oxcarbazepine + carbamazepine
See oxcarbazepine (*4.5.3*).

Oxybutynin + carbamazepine
See dantrolene + carbamazepine.

Paracetamol + carbamazepine
Carbamazepine may reduce the bioavailability of paracetamol (UK SmPC). Hepatotoxicity (n=1, Parikh *et al*, *Intern Med J* 2004;**34**:441–2), acute liver and renal failure have been reported (n=1, Jickling *et al*, *Epilept Disord* 2009;**11**:329–32).

Paroxetine + carbamazepine
See paroxetine (*4.3.2.4*).

Phenobarbital + carbamazepine
Phenobarbital induces carbamazepine CYP3A4 metabolism, slightly reducing plasma levels (Christianssen and Dam, *Acta Neurol Scand* 1973;**49**:543–6). Carbamazepine may raise phenobarbital levels but not by a clinically significant amount (d/b, c/o, 4x21/7, Cereghino *et al*, *Clin Pharmacol Ther* 1975;**18**:733–41).

PHENYTOIN + CARBAMAZEPINE
Phenytoin induces carbamazepine CYP3A4 metabolism, reducing levels, often dramatically and with some evidence of increased CBZ-E in the CSF. Raised carbamazepine levels may result from withdrawal of phenytoin via removal of enzyme induction (n=2, Chapron *et al*, *Ann Pharmacother* 1993;**27**:708–11). Raised phenytoin concentrations may occur due to CYP2C19 inhibition (Lakehal *et al*, *Epilepsy Res* 2002;**52**:79–83) and mean serum levels increase by up to 100%, producing neurotoxicity (Browne *et al*, *Neurology* 1988;**38**:1146–50). The overall clinical effect may be limited but best to monitor levels of both drugs.

Piperine + carbamazepine
Piperine (used as a spice and adjuvant in traditional Indian medicines) can significantly raise carbamazepine levels (n=20, Pattanaik *et al*, *Phytother Res* 2009;**23**:1281–6).

Pregabalin + carbamazepine
See pregabalin (*4.1.5*).

Primidone + carbamazepine
The UK SmPC notes that primidone can increase the levels of CBZ-E.

Probenecid + carbamazepine
Probenecid has a minimal effect on CBZ kinetics, but can increase the proportion of CBZ-E via enzyme induction (n=10, RCT, open, Kim *et al*, *Eur J Clin Pharmacol* 2005;**61**:275–80).

Progabide + carbamazepine
Progabide has no effect on carbamazepine (n=24, open, Bianchetti *et al*, *Epilepsia* 1987;**28**:68–73), but may slightly increase CBZ-E levels.

Protein kinase inhibitors + carbamazepine
Carbamazepine decreases **lapatinib** AUC, Cmax and absorption by 72%, 59% and 28% respectively, probably by CYP3A4 induction, but with no change in half-life (n=24, 20/7, Smith *et al*, *Br J Clin Pharmacol* 2009;**67**:421–6; FFT). Mean trough levels of **imatinib** are reduced up to 2.9-fold by carbamazepine (n<224, p/c, Pursche *et al*, *Curr Clin Pharmacol* 2008;**3**:198–203; FFT).

PROTON-PUMP INHIBITORS + CARBAMAZEPINE
Carbamazepine induces the CYP3A4 metabolism of **omeprazole**, but has little or no effect on hydroxylation via CYP2C19 (n=5, open, Bertilsson *et al*, *Br J Clin Pharmacol* 1997;**44**:186–9; FFT). **Pantoprazole** appears to have no effect on carbamazepine (n=20, RCT, Huber *et al*, *Int J Clin Pharmacol Ther* 1998;**36**:521–4).

Reboxetine + carbamazepine
See reboxetine (*4.3.3.6*).

RIFAMPIN + CARBAMAZEPINE
Rapid CYP3A4 induction may lower carbamazepine levels (n=1, Zolezzi, *Am J Psychiatry* 2002;**159**:874).

Rivaroxaban + carbamazepine *
Pulmonary embolism has been reported, probably due to lower levels of rivaroxaban via enzyme induction (n=1, Risselada *et al*, *Ned Tijdschr Geneeskd* 2013;**157**:A6568).

4

Rufinamide + carbamazepine
The plasma levels of rufinamide are reduced by carbamazepine, but carbamazepine is unaffected by rufinamide (UK SmPC).

Sertraline + carbamazepine
See sertraline (*4.3.2.5*).

Simethicone + carbamazepine
There is a report of carbamazepine toxicity after simethicone was started (n=1, Guneysel *et al*, *J Med Case Rep* 2008;**2**:242; FFT).

Smoking + carbamazepine
See carbamazepine + smoking (*4.7.4*).

St John's wort + carbamazepine
See St John's wort (*4.3.3.10*).

Statins + carbamazepine
Transient carbamazepine toxicity has been reported with **atorvastatin** and roxithromycin (n=1, Corbin *et al*, *Therapie* 2004;**59**:267–9). Carbamazepine reduces **simvastatin**'s AUC by 75% and Cmax 68%, so increased doses would be needed (n=12, RCT, c/o, Ucar *et al*, *Eur J Clin Pharmacol* 2004;**59**:879–82).

Stiripentol + carbamazepine
Stiripentol is a potent inhibitor of CBZ–E formation (Cazali *et al*, *Br J Clin Pharmacol* 2003;**56**:526–36; FFT).

Tacrolimus + carbamazepine
Tacrolimus levels have been reduced by 50% (after 11/7) and 70% (after 3/12) by carbamazepine (n=1, Wada *et al*, *J Heart Lung Transplant* 2009;**28**:409–11).

Terfenadine + carbamazepine
There is a case of raised CBZ levels leading to toxicity after starting terfenadine (n=1, Naranjo=6, Baath *et al*, *Can J Clin Pharmacol* 2006;**13**:e228–31; FFT).

Thiazides + carbamazepine
Hyponatremia has been reported (n=1, Ranta and Wooten, *Epilepsia* 2004;**45**:879).

Tiagabine + carbamazepine
Carbamazepine reduces tiagabine levels 1.5–3-fold, probably by CYP3A4 induction. Tiagabine has no effect on carbamazepine.

Tibolone + carbamazepine
The carbamazepine SmPC states that CBZ may reduce the activity of tibolone.

Topiramate + carbamazepine
See topiramate (*4.5.6*).

Tramadol + carbamazepine
Carbamazepine may reduce the effectiveness of tramadol.

Trazodone + carbamazepine
Raised carbamazepine levels and toxicity have been reported (n=1, Romero *et al*, *Ann Pharmacother* 1999;**33**:1370), reversed if trazodone is stopped (n=1, Sánchez-Romero *et al*, *Pharmacopsychiatry* 2011;**44**:158–9).

Triazole antifungals + carbamazepine
Sub-therapeutic **itraconazole** levels may occur with carbamazepine, so monitor for lack of efficacy (n=12, open, Tucker *et al*, *Clin Infect Dis* 1992;**14**:165–74). **Fluconazole**-induced carbamazepine toxicity has been reported (eg. n=1, Finch *et al*, *South Med J* 2002;**95**:1099–100; Ulivelli *et al*, *J Neurol* 2004;**251**:622–3). There is a case of **voriconazole** failure in an ultra-rapid 2C19 metaboliser caused by carbamazepine (n=1, Malimgré *et al*, *Br J Clin Pharmacol* 2012; **74**:205–6; FFT).

TRICYCLICS + CARBAMAZEPINE
CBZ may induce the CYP3A4 metabolism of imipramine, doxepin and amitriptyline, reducing plasma levels by 42–50% (e.g. n=51, Leinonen *et al*, *J Clin Psychopharmacol* 1991;**11**:313–8), clinically significant, although the free fraction may remain unchanged, so dose increases may not be necessary (n=13, Szymura-Oleksiak *et al*, *Psychopharmacology [Berl]* 2001;**154**:38–42). NMS has been reported with amitriptyline and carbamazepine (n=1, Janati *et al*, *Case Report Neurol Med* 2012;**2012**:183252).

VALPROATE + CARBAMAZEPINE
Valproate inhibits several carbamazepine metabolic pathways, resulting in raised CBZ-E levels (which has led to CBZ-E-induced psychosis, n=1, McKee *et al*, *Lancet* 1989;**1**:167), but sometimes with unchanged or lower carbamazepine levels (n=27, Bernus *et al*, *Br J Clin Pharmacol* 1997;**44**:21; FFT). Valproate may also displace carbamazepine from binding sites on plasma proteins (n=8, open, Macphee, *Br J Clin Pharmacol* 1988;**25**:59–66; FFT). Conversely, carbamazepine induces valproate metabolism, reducing plasma levels by about 20% (n=8, RCT, d/b, c/o, Larkin *et al*, *Br J Clin Pharmacol* 1989;**27**:313–22; FFT). This is probably minor but a mean 59% increase in valproate levels can occur on carbamazepine withdrawal (n=6, open, Jann *et al*, *Epilepsia* 1988;**29**:578–81). No adjustments in carbamazepine doses are generally necessary, but be aware of the altered metabolite ratio and monitor if clinical symptoms change.

Venlafaxine + carbamazepine

See venlafaxine (*4.3.3.8*).

Vigabatrin + carbamazepine

A 10% rise in carbamazepine levels (n=66, Jedrzejczak *et al*, *Epilepsy Res* 2000;**39**:115–20) and an 18% reduction in steady-state carbamazepine levels have been reported (n=15, Sanchez-Alcaraz et al, *J Clin Pharm Ther* 2002;**27**:427–30).

Vincristine + carbamazepine

Carbamazepine significantly reduces the plasma levels of vincristine, probably by CYP3A4 induction (n=15, open, Villikka *et al*, *Clin Pharmacol Therapeut* 1999;**66**:589–93).

WARFARIN + CARBAMAZEPINE

The metabolism of warfarin is accelerated by carbamazepine, reducing efficacy. Warfarin doses may need to be doubled (n=59, Herman *et al*, *Eur J Clin Pharmacol* 2006;**62**:291–6), monitored frequently and reduced carefully if carbamazepine is discontinued (n=1, Denbow and Fraser, *South Med J* 1990;**83**:981).

Xanthines + carbamazepine

Theophylline metabolism is accelerated by carbamazepine to give a reduced effect (Mitchell *et al*, *N Z Med J* 1986;**99**:69–70).

Zaleplon + carbamazepine

See zaleplon (*4.1.6*).

Ziprasidone + carbamazepine

See ziprasidone (*4.2.9*).

Zonisamide + carbamazepine

Zonisamide does not significantly effect carbamazepine, but 3A4 induction by CBZ reduces zonisamide half-life from 65 to 36 hours (n=18, Ragueneau-Majlessi *et al*, *Epilepsy Res* 2004;**62**:1–11), and an NMS-like state has been reported (n=1, Azuma *et al*, *Epilepsia* 2007;**48**:1999–2001).

4.4.2 LAMOTRIGINE

Lamotrigine seems to have no effect on P450 enzymes.

Review: pharmacokinetics (n=65, Brzakovic *et al*, *J Clin Pharm Ther* 2012;**37**:693–7).

ANTIRETROVIRALS + LAMOTRIGINE *

Lopinavir/ritonavir (Kaletra® Abbott) reduces lamotrigine levels by 55%, with a doubling of lamotrigine dose needed to compensate (n=24, 31/7, van der Lee *et al*, *Clin Pharmacol Ther* 2006;**80**:159–68). **Atazanavir** is now listed as an interaction in the UK SmPC.

Aripiprazole + lamotrigine *

Aripiprazole has no significant effect on lamotrigine (n=18, open, 2/52, Schieber *et al*, *Hum Psychopharmacol* 2009;**24**:145–52), although intention tremor has been reported (n=1, Ali *et al*, *Prim Care Companion CNS Disorders* 2012;**14**:11l01236; FFT) as has akathisia, anxiety and suicidal thoughts (n=2, Pondé and Freire, *Case Rep Psychiatry* 2015;**2015**:419746; FFT).

Barbiturates + lamotrigine

Lamotrigine has no significant effect on primidone and phenobarbital (n=158, Manon-Espaillat *et al*, *Epilepsia* 1991;**32**:96–100), although a blood dyscrasia has been reported (n=1, Siniscalchi *et al*, *Ann Pharmacother* 2010;**44**:2031–4).

Benzodiazepines + lamotrigine

Lamotrigine has no significant effect on clonazepam (n=158, Manon-Espaillat *et al*, *Epilepsia* 1991;**32**:96–100).

Bupropion + lamotrigine

Steady-state bupropion had no effect on a single 10 mg dose of lamotrigine (n=12, RCT, Odishaw and Chen, *Pharmacotherapy* 2000;**20**:1448–53).

Carbamazepine + lamotrigine *

Carbamazepine toxicity appears more likely to occur when lamotrigine is added to carbamazepine if the initial CBZ level is greater than 8 mg/L (n=47, open, Besag *et al*, *Epilepsia* 1998;**39**:183–7). Lamotrigine does not seem to raise the levels of CBZ-E and, in fact, may reduce the levels of this active but toxic metabolite (n=14, open, Eriksson and Boreus, *Ther Drug Monit* 1997;**19**:499–501). Carbamazepine reduces the half-life of lamotrigine from 29 hours to about 15 hours via enzyme induction (n=23, open, 4/52, Jawad *et al*, *Epilepsia Res* 1987;**1**:194–201), with clinically important reductions in lamotrigine plasma concentrations reported (Koch et al, *Eur Psychiatry* 2003;**18**:42). Serious lamotrigine rash has been reported after carbamazepine was stopped, presumably as lamotrigine levels increased (n=1, Surja *et al*, *J Clin Psychiatry* 2005;**66**:400–1), as has a case of toxic epidermal necrolysis associated (n=1, Mansouri *et al*, *Arch Dermatol* 2005;**141**:788–9).

Citalopram/escitalopram + lamotrigine

See citalopram/escitalopram (*4.3.2.1*).

Clozapine + lamotrigine

See clozapine (*4.2.4*).

Eslicarbazepine + lamotrigine

Lack of interaction has been reported (n=16,

4

open, 27/7, Almeida *et al, Acta Neurol Scand* 2010;**121**:257–64).

Fosphenytoin + lamotrigine
See phenytoin + lamotrigine.

Imatinib + lamotrigine
Plasma levels of imatinib do not appear to be affected by lamotrigine (n<224, p/c, Pursche *et al, Curr Clin Pharmacol* 2008;**3**:198–203; FFT).

Lacosamide + lamotrigine
Caution is necessary with this combination as enhanced PR prolongation could occur (SmPC).

Levetiracetam + lamotrigine
See levetiracetam (*4.5.2*).

Lithium + lamotrigine
See lithium (*4.4.3*).

Olanzapine + lamotrigine
See lamotrigine + olanzapine (*4.2.6*).

ORAL CONTRACEPTIVES + LAMOTRIGINE
Lamotrigine reduces the effectiveness of hormonal contraceptives. OCs may reduce lamotrigine AUC by at least 52% and Cmax by 39% (eg. with Microgynon 30® [Schering Health]; n=7, Sabers *et al, Epilepsy Res* 2001;**47**:151–4; n=24, open, Herzog *et al, Neurology* 2009;**72**:911–4) even higher during pill-free weeks and on discontinuation; n=21, Wegner *et al, Neurology* 2009;**73**:1388–93). The advice is:

- In women starting lamotrigine while on OCs, the normal dose titration should be used
- In women starting OCs while on lamotrigine, the dose of lamotrigine may need to be increased two-fold (unless also taking any drug that induces lamotrigine glucuronidation)
- In women stopping OCs, lamotrigine levels may double, mostly during the first week, a rapid and significant effect (RCT, 2/12, d/b, p/c, c/o, Christensen *et al, Epilepsia* 2007;**48**:484–9). Lamotrigine doses may need to be halved (unless also taking any drug-inducing lamotrigine glucuronidation).

In a controlled study, only the ethinylestradiol component of OCs reduced lamotrigine serum levels, but progestogens did not alter the levels (n=45, Reimers *et al, Epilepsia* 2005;**46**:1414–7), so advice may need to be considered carefully.

Oxcarbazepine + lamotrigine
See oxcarbazepine (*4.5.3*).

Phenytoin + lamotrigine
Phenytoin increases lamotrigine's clearance by 125% and reduces half-life from 29 hours to 15 hours (n=570, chart analysis, Weintraub *et al, Arch Neurol* 2005;**62**:1432–6). Lamotrigine has no effect on phenytoin

Pregabalin + lamotrigine
See pregabalin (*4.1.5*).

Risperidone + lamotrigine
See risperidone (*4.2.8*).

Rufinamide + lamotrigine
No significant interaction occurs (UK SmPC).

Sertraline + lamotrigine
Lamotrigine levels might be about 18% higher (n=51, Christensen *et al, Pharmacopsychiatry* 2012;**45**:119–21), but there are case reports, e.g. sertraline 25 mg/d doubled lamotrigine levels and where a 25 mg/d dose reduction halved lamotrigine levels, despite a 33% lamotrigine dose increase (n=2, Kaufman and Gerner, *Seizure* 1998;**7**:163–5; FFT).

Smoking + lamotrigine
See lamotrigine + smoking (*4.7.4*).

Statins + lamotrigine
Lamotrigine has no apparent effect on atorvastatin (n=119, Bullman *et al, Epilepsia* 2011;**52**:1351–8).

Topiramate + lamotrigine
Topiramate does not cause a significant change in lamotrigine levels (n=24, Berry *et al, Epilepsia* 2002;**43**:818–23) at standard doses (n=13, open, 22/52, Doose *et al, Epilepsia* 2003;**44**:917–22).

VALPROATE + LAMOTRIGINE *
Lamotrigine can significantly affect valproate levels, but the effect is variable (n=76, Martin *et al, Curr Drug Saf* 2011;**6**:23–9), e.g:

- 34% had a >25% *increase* in valproate levels
- In 14% the increase was >50%
- 5% had a >25% *decrease* in valproate levels.

Valproate inhibits lamotrigine glucuronidation, doubling plasma levels (n=38, RCT, Lalic *et al, Eur J Drug Metab Pharmacokinet* 2009;**34**:93–9), reducing clearance (by 21%) and lengthening half-life from 29 hours to about 59 hours (e.g. n=570, chart analysis, Weintraub *et al, Arch Neurol* 2005;**62**:1432–6), probably in a dose-dependent (n=28, open, Kanner and Frey, *Neurology* 2000;**55**:588–91), rather than in a concentration-dependent way (n=62, open, Gidal *et al, Epilepsy Res* 2000;**42**:23–31). Lamotrigine should thus start at half the usual dose when used with valproate (see the SmPC for exact dosing schedules). Numerous ADRs have been reported and can even be delayed by up to two years after starting the combination (n=4, Thome-Souza *et al*, *Pediatr Neurol* 2012;**47**:47–50).

Zonisamide + lamotrigine

Lack of clinically significant interaction has been shown (n=20 [c=18], open, Levy *et al*, *Ther Drug Monit* 2005;**27**:193–8).

4.4.3 LITHIUM

ACE INHIBITORS + LITHIUM *

There are many cases of lithium toxicity with ACE inhibitors (eg. n=9, open, DasGupta *et al*, *J Clin Psychiatry* 1992;**53**:398–400), especially in the elderly (n=20, Finley *et al*, *J Clin Psychopharmacol* 1996;**16**:68–71), so either monitor very carefully (review: Lehmann and Ritz, *Am J Kidney Dis* 1995;**25**:82–7) or use an alternative, e.g. beta-blockers. ACE inhibitors are most likely to increase lithium toxicity within a month of starting (Juurlink *et al*, *J Am Geriatr Soc* 2004;**52**:794–8). **Fosinopril** has caused a 5-fold increase in lithium levels so monitor carefully for 4–6 weeks after any change (n=1, Meyer *et al*, *Int Clin Psychopharmacol* 2005;**20**:115–8).

Acetazolamide + lithium

Lithium excretion may be increased or, less likely, possibly decreased by acetazolamide (n=2, Gay *et al*, *Encephale* 1985;**11**:261–2).

Agomelatine + lithium

See agomelatine (*4.3.3.1*).

Alcohol + lithium

See alcohol (*4.7.1*).

Amfetamines + lithium

Lithium may suppress amfetamine 'highs' (n=3, Flemenbaum, *Am J Psychiatry* 1974;**131**:820–1).

AMINOPHYLLINE + LITHIUM

See xanthines + lithium.

Amiodarone + lithium

The SmPCs note an increased risk of QT prolongation and this is a contraindication.

Angiotensin II antagonists + lithium

There are cases of lithium toxicity with **candesartan** (n=1, 8/52, Zwanzger *et al*, *J Clin Psychiatry* 2001;**62**:208–9), **losartan** 50 mg/d (n=1, 5/52, Blanche *et al*, *Eur J Clin Pharmacol* 1999;**52**:501) and **telmisartan** (n=1, Ma *et al*, *Psychiatry Clin Neurosci* 2012;**66**:165–6). **Valsartan** has increased lithium levels when lithium was taken twice a day but not when taken once a day provided the dose was separated from valsartan, so the recommendation is to not take the two together and don't take lithium twice a day (n=1, Lazarczyk and Giannakopoulos, *Bipolar Disord* 2014;**16**:662–6).

Antacids + lithium

See sodium + lithium.

Antibiotics + lithium

Antibiotics may lead to raised lithium levels (cases within n=102, Wilting *et al*, *Bipolar Disord* 2005;**7**:274–80).

Antipsychotics + lithium *

Reports of mostly reversible neurotoxicity in the 1980s were probably lithium toxicity. The main risk factors seem to be high doses of both and signs of impending toxicity are ignored.

Amisulpride has no effect on lithium (n=24, RCT, d/b, p/c, Canal *et al*, *Int J Neuropsychopharmacol* 2003;**6**:103–9).

Aripiprazole has no effect on lithium (e.g. n=32 [c=23], open, 26/7, Boulton *et al*, *J Clin Pharm Ther* 2012;**37**:565–70)

Chlorpromazine levels may be lowered by up to 40% by lithium, with enhanced EPSE and rarely neurotoxicity.

Clozapine appears safe with lithium, within moderate dose limits and without co-prescription of serotonergic or 1A2-inhibiting drugs (n=44, Bender *et al*, *Int J Neuropsychopharmacol* 2004;**7**:59–63), although there are reports of NMS and reversible neurotoxicity (n=1, Blake *et al*, *J Clin Psychopharmacol* 1992;**12**:297–9), including one where lithium levels were below 0.5 mEq/L (n=1, Lee and Yang, *Zhonghua Yi Xue Za Zhi [Taipei]* 1999;**62**:184–7). Diabetic ketoacidosis has also been reported (e. g. n=1, Peterson and Byrd, *Am J Psychiatry* 1996;**153**:737–8), and so glucose monitoring might be indicated with this particular combination.

Haloperidol — case on NMS (n=1, Yang *et al*, *Shanghai Arch Psychiatry* 2014;**26**:368–70; FFT).

Olanzapine levels may be lower (Bergemann *et al*, *Pharmacopsychiatry* 2004;**37**:63–8), NMS is possible (n=1, Berry *et al*, *Pharmacother* 2003;**23**:255–9) and severe delirium and EPSE have occurred (n=1, Tuglu *et al*, *J Korean Med Sci* 2005;**20**:691–4; FFT).

Quetiapine has no significant effect on lithium kinetics (n=10, open, 4/52, Potkin *et al*, *Clin Ther* 2002;**24**:1809–23), but rapidly developing delirium has occurred (n=1, Miodownik *et al*, *Clin Neuropharmacol* 2008;**31**:176–9).

4

Risperidone has little effect on lithium (n=13, open, 9/7, Demling *et al, Pharmacopsychiatry* 2006;**39**:230–1), but there are reports of delirium (n=1, Chen and Cardasis, *Am J Psychiatry* 1996;**153**:1233–4), diabetic ketoacidosis, rabbit syndrome (n=1, Mendhekar, *Can J Psychiatry* 2005;**50**:369), encephalopathy (e.g. n=1, Boora *et al, Acta Psychiatr Scand* 2008;**117**:394–6) and myocardial infarction (n=1, Ananth *et al, J Clin Psychiatry* 2004;**65**:724).
Sulpiride may lead to an increased risk of EPSEs (SmPC).
Ziprasidone has no significant effect on lithium (n=25, RCT, Apseloff *et al, Br J Clin Pharmacol* 2000;**49**[S3]:61–4; FFT), although lithium toxicity (n=2, Miodownik *et al, Clin Neuropharmacol* 2005;**28**:295–7) and NMS (n=1, Borovicka *et al, Ann Pharmacother* 2006;**40**:139–42) have been reported.

Baclofen + lithium
Aggravation of Huntington's disease has occurred (n=2, Andén *et al, Lancet* 1973;**2**:93).

Benzodiazepines + lithium
There have been a few anecdotal reports of e.g. hypothermia and neurotoxicity (n=5, Koczerginski *et al, Int Clin Psychopharm* 1989;**4**: 195–9). Routine use of this usually beneficial combination suggests it to be safe.

Beta-blockers + lithium
Bradycardia with **propranolol** and lithium has been reported (n=1, Becker, *J Clin Psychiatry* 1989;**50**:473), although propranolol and **nadolol** (n=1, Dave and Langbart, *Ann Clin Psychiatry* 1994;**6**:51–2) have been used uneventfully for lithium-induced tremor.

Bumetanide + lithium
Bumetanide has rarely caused lithium toxicity (n=2, Kerry *et al, Br Med J* 1980;**281**:371; FFT).

Calcium-channel blockers + lithium *
Cases of enhanced effect and toxicity with unchanged plasma levels have been reported with **verapamil** (Price and Giannini, *J Clin Pharmacol* 1986;**26**:717–9), as have reduced lithium levels (Weinrauch *et al, Am Heart J* 1984;**108**:1378–80). Acute EPSE and bradycardia have been reported with **diltiazem** (n=1, Binder *et al, Arch Intern Med* 1991;**151**:373–4).

Cannabis + lithium
See cannabis (*4.7.2*).

Carbamazepine + lithium
See carbamazepine (*4.4.1*), plus 'combinations' in bipolar disorder (*1.10*).

Cisplatin + lithium
Cisplatin has reduced lithium levels by up to 64% (e.g. Vincent *et al, Cancer Chemother Pharmacol* 1995;**35**:533–4).

Clonidine + lithium
Lithium may reduce the hypotensive effect of clonidine (Goodnick and Meltzer, *Biol Psychiatry* 1984;**19**:883–9), so monitor carefully.

Coca-cola Zero® + lithium
Low serum lithium levels have occurred in someone drinking large amounts of Coke-Zero® (n=1, Kralovec *et al, J Clin Psychopharmacol* 2011;**31**:543–4).

Cocaine + lithium
See cocaine (*4.7.3*).

Corticosteroids + lithium
An isolated case exists of lithium reducing the effect of fludrocortisone on the kidneys (n=1, Stewart *et al, Clin Endocrinol* 1987;**27**:63).

Co-trimoxazole + lithium
Cases exist of enhanced toxicity with reduced levels (n=2, Edwards, *N Z Med J* 1984;**97**:729–32).

COX-2 inhibitors + lithium
See NSAIDs + lithium.

Dextromethorphan + lithium
Serotonin syndrome has been reported (n=1, Navarro *et al, Gen Hosp Psychiatry* 2006;**28**:78–80).

Digoxin + lithium
Lack of interaction has been shown (n=6, open, Cooper *et al, Br J Clin Pharmacol* 1984;**18**:21–5).

Dipyridamole + lithium
Lack of interaction has been shown (n=6, Wood *et al, Br J Clin Pharmacol* 1989;**27**:749–56; FFT).

Disulfiram + lithium
See disulfiram (*4.6.8*).

Domperidone + lithium
An enhanced risk of EPSE exists.

Fluoxetine + lithium
Lack of significant pharmacokinetic interaction has been shown (e.g. n=110, open, Bauer *et al, J Clin Psychopharmacol* 1996;**16**:130–4), although it may be poorly tolerated (n=14, open, Hawley *et al, Int Clin Psychopharmacol* 1994;**9**:31–3), with isolated reports of e.g. serotonin syndrome and acute confusion or lithium toxicity (review by Levinson *et al, DICP* 1991;**25**:657–61).

Furosemide + lithium
Furosemide is probably the safest diuretic with

lithium (e.g. n=13, RCT, Crabtree *et al*, *Am J Psychiatry* 1991;**148**:1060–3). Loop diuretics are most likely to increase lithium toxicity within a month of starting (Juurlink *et al*, *J Am Geriatr Soc* 2004;**52**:794–8).

Gabapentin + lithium

Gabapentin seems to have no effect on lithium (n=13, Frye *et al*, *J Clin Psychopharmacol* 1998; **18**:461–4).

Herbal diuretics + lithium

There is a clear case of life-threatening lithium toxicity (4.5 mmol/L) induced by a herbal diuretic preparation (n=1, Pyevich and Bogenschutz, *Am J Psychiatry* 2001;**158**:1329).

Hypoglycaemics + lithium

Lithium has been used to improve glucose metabolism and assist the effects of oral hypoglycaemics and insulin (n=38, Hu *et al*, *Biol Trace Elem Res* 1997;**60**:131–7).

Iodides + lithium

Enhanced antithyroid and goiter effects of lithium have been reported.

Isotretinoin + lithium *

Mild lithium toxicity has been reported (n=1, Lambe, *Aust N Z J Psychiatry* 2014;**48**:1066).

Ispaghula husk + lithium

A single case exists of reduced lithium levels (n=1, Perlman, *Lancet* 1990;**335**:416).

Lamotrigine + lithium

Lamotrigine has no significant effect on lithium's pharmacokinetics (n=20, RCT, 6/7, Chen *et al*, *Br J Clin Pharmacol* 2000;**50**:193–6; FFT).

Levodopa + lithium

Lithium has been used to treat levodopa-induced side-effects, e.g. psychosis and mania (n=1, Braden, *Am J Psychiatry* 1977;**134**:808). Reversible CJD-like syndrome has been reported (n=1, Broussolle *et al*, *J Neurol Neurosurg Psychiatry* 1989;**52**:686–7; FFT).

Levofloxacin + lithium

A case has been reported of severe lithium toxicity (with plasma levels more than doubled) two days after starting levofloxacin in a stable bipolar patient (n=1, Takahashi *et al*, *J Clin Psychiatry* 2000;**61**:949–50).

Lithium + lisdexamfetamine

See lisdexamfetamine (*4.6.10*).

MAOIs + lithium

See MAOIs (*4.3.4*).

METHYLDOPA + LITHIUM

Many cases of rapidly appearing lithium toxicity with normal plasma levels have been reported (e.g. n=1, Yassa, *CSAJ* 1986;**134**:141–2; FFT).

Metoclopramide + lithium

Enhanced risk of EPSE and of neurotoxicity exists.

Metronidazole + lithium

Lithium toxicity has been reported (n=1, Teicher *et al*, *JAMA* 1987;**257**:3365–6).

Mirtazapine + lithium

See mirtazapine (*4.3.3.4*).

Neuromuscular blocking agents + lithium *

The UK SmPC now notes that lithium can prolong the effects of NMBAs so the last dose or two of lithium could be omitted before the use of an NMBA.

NON-STEROIDAL ANTI-INFLAMMATORY DRUGS/COX-2 INHIBITORS + LITHIUM

This is a well-known interaction, probably due to inhibition of renal prostaglandin PGE2 and reduced blood flow. Lithium levels should be monitored frequently if the combination is used. **Review:** NSAIDs and COX-2 inhibitors (Phelan *et al*, *J Clin Psychiatry* 2003;**64**:1328–34).

Avoid:

- Indometacin: lithium levels may rise by 61% (e.g. n=10, open, Reimann *et al*, *Arch Gen Psychiatry* 1983;**40**:283–6).

Extra care:

- Ibuprofen: * studies show a variable effect, with a 25% increase in lithium levels possible (e.g. n=9, open, Ragheb, *J Clin Psychiatry* 1987;**48**:161–3), although a 3-fold rise has been reported with ibuprofen 2400 mg/d for 5/7 (n=1, Hassan *et al*, *Case Rep Nephrol* 2013;**2013**:839796). As ibuprofen is available over-the-counter, this interaction should be remembered
- Diclofenac: lithium levels may rise by up to 23% (n=5, Reimann and Frolich, *Clin Pharmacol Ther* 1981;**30**:348–52)
- Piroxicam: several cases exist of a slow-onset (e.g. several months) lithium toxicity (e.g. n=1, Walbridge and Bazire, *Br J Psychiatry* 1985;**147**:206–7).

Care (raised lithium levels are possible with):

- Azapropazone: raised lithium levels (SmPC)
- Celecoxib: (e.g. Gunja *et al*, *Intern Med J* 2002;**32**:494; life-threatening n=1, Slørdal *et al*, *Br J Clin Pharmacol* 2003;**55**:413–4)
- Etodolac: raised lithium possible (SmPC)
- Ketoprofen: (n=1, Singer *et al*, *Therapie* 1981;**36**:323–6)

4

- **Ketorolac:** lithium levels have been nearly doubled (n=5, Cold *et al*, *J Clin Psychopharmacol* 1998;**18**:33–7)
- **Mefenamic acid:** (n=2, MacDonald and Neale, *BMJ* 1988;**297**:1339; FFT)
- **Meloxicam:** (n=16, Türck *et al*, *Br J Clin Pharmacol* 2000;**50**:197–204; FFT)
- **Naproxen:** short-term naproxen has little effect on lithium levels (n=12, Levin *et al*, *J Clin Psychophamacol* 1998;**18**:237–40), but increased lithium levels have been reported (n=7, Ragheb and Powell, *J Clin Psychopharmacol* 1986;**6**:150–4)
- **Phenylbutazone:** doubled lithium levels possible (see Ragheb, *J Clin Psychopharmacol* 1990;**10**:149–50)
- **Rofecoxib:** (e.g. n=1, Lundmark *et al*, *Br J Clin Pharmacol* 2002;**53**:403–4; FFT; n=1, Bravo *et al*, *Ann Pharmacother* 2004;**38**:1189–93)
- **Tiaprofenic acid:** (n=1, Alderman and Lindsay, *Ann Pharmacother* 1996;**30**:1411–3).

Least risk:

- **Aspirin:** 4g/d had no effect on lithium levels (n=10, open, 7/7, Reimann *et al*, *Arch Gen Psychiatry* 1983;**40**:283–6), and other studies have only shown a mildly variable effect (e.g. Ragheb, *J Clin Psychiatry* 1987;**48**:425)
- **Sulindac:** case reports show either a slightly reduced level of lithium (n=2, Furnell and Davies, *Drug Intell Clin Pharm* 1986;**19**:374–6), no effect (n=4, Ragheb and Powell, *J Clin Psychiatry* 1986;**47**:33–4) or raised levels (n=2, Jones and Stoner, *J Clin Psychiatry* 2000;**61**:527–8).

Orlistat + lithium *

Loss of BDZ efficacy has occurred (SmPC).

Oxcarbazepine + lithium

See oxcarbazepine (*4.5.3*).

Phenytoin + lithium

There are several reports of lithium neurotoxicity, without increased lithium levels (e.g. Raskin, *J Clin Psychopharmacol* 1984;**4**:120).

Potassium iodide + lithium

An additive effect may cause hypothyroidism.

Psyllium + lithium

See Ispaghula husk + lithium.

Quetiapine + lithium

See quetiapine (*4.2.7*).

Smoking + lithium

See smoking (*4.7.4*).

Sodium + lithium

Excess sodium (e.g. as bicarbonate in antacids) can reduce lithium levels (e.g. McSwiggan, *Med J Aust* 1978;**1**:38–9) and sodium restriction can lead to lithium intoxication (e.g. Baer *et al*, *J Psychiatr Res* 1971;**8**:91–105).

Spironolactone + lithium

A rise in lithium levels has been reported (Baer *et al*, *J Psychiatr Res* 1971;**8**:91–105), as has synergism (see combinations, *1.10*).

SSRIs + lithium

See citalopram/escitalopram (*4.3.2.1*), fluoxetine (*4.3.2.2*), fluvoxamine (*4.3.2.3*) and paroxetine (*4.3.2.4*). No interaction has been seen yet with sertraline.

Tetracyclines + lithium

Lithium intoxication (e.g. n=1, McGennis, *Br Med J* 1978;**2**:1183; FFT) has been reported, so monitor lithium regularly.

THIAZIDE DIURETICS + LITHIUM

Thiazides reduce lithium's renal clearance and levels can rise within a few days. Thiazides should only be used where unavoidable and where strict monitoring is used, although the effect on lithium is not invariably dramatic:

- **Bendroflumethiazide:** a 24% reduction in lithium excretion has been shown (n=22, Petersen *et al*, *Br Med J* 1974;**2**:143–5; FFT), leading to lithium toxicity (n=1, Vipond *et al*, *Anesthesia* 1996;**51**:1156–8)
- **Co-amilozide:** case report (n=1, Dorevitch and Baruch, *Am J Psychiatry* 1986;**143**:257–8)
- **Hydrochlorthiazide:** a minor effect (n=13, RCT, Crabtree *et al*, *Am J Psychiatry* 1991;**148**:1060–3)
- **Hydroflumethiazide:** a 24% reduction in lithium excretion may occur (Petersen *et al*, *Br Med J* 1974;**2**:143–5; FFT)
- **Triamterene:** increased lithium clearance may occur (n=8, open, Wetzels *et al*, *Nephrol Dial Transplant* 1989;**4**:939–42).

Topiramate + lithium

Toxic lithium levels have been reported with higher (800mg/d) dose topiramate, but not with 500mg/d (Pinninti and Zelinski, *J Clin Psychopharmacol* 2002;**22**:340; Abraham and Owen, *J Clin Psychopharmacol* 2004;**24**:565–7).

Tricyclics + lithium

See tricyclics (*4.3.1*).

Trimethoprim + lithium

Lithium toxicity has been reported (n=1, de

Vries, *Ned Tijdschr Geneeskd* 2001;**145**:539–40).

Triptans + lithium

The literature notes an increased risk of CNS toxicity with sumatriptan.

Venlafaxine + lithium

See venlafaxine (*4.3.3.8*).

Vortioxetine + lithium *

See vortioxetine (*4.3.3.9*).

Warfarin + lithium

No interaction is suspected or reported (Sayal *et al, Acta Psychiatr Scand* 2000;**102**:250–5).

XANTHINES + LITHIUM

Theophylline may reduce lithium levels by 20–30% (Cook *et al, J Clin Psychiatry* 1985;**46**:278–9), as may **aminophylline**, probably by increased excretion. Extra care is needed if the xanthine is stopped as toxicity can occur.

Ziprasidone + lithium

See ziprasidone (*4.2.9*).

4.4.4 VALPROATE (SODIUM VALPROATE, VALPROIC ACID, DIVALPROEX SODIUM) *

Valproate has a complex metabolism; about 50% is by glucuronidation, 40% by mitochondrial beta-oxidation and 10% by P450 (CYP2C9 and 2C19) enzymes (Sheehan *et al, Ann Pharmacother* 2006;**40**:147–50), and some by UGT2B7 (Me *et al, Zhong Nan Da Xue Xue Bao Yi Xue Ban* 2013; **38**:766–72).

Review: DeVane, *Psychopharmacol Bull* 2003;**37** (Suppl 2):25–42.

Antacids + valproate

A slight decrease in valproate absorption has been noted (n=7, open, May *et al, Clin Pharm* 1982;**1**:244–7).

Antiretrovirals + valproate

Lopinavir/ritonavir (Kaletra®, Abbott) can reduce valproate levels by 48%, probably via glucuronidation-induction (n=1, Sheehan *et al, Ann Pharmacother* 2006;**40**:147–50). **Zidovudine** levels can be raised by valproate via a dose-dependent inhibition of glucuronidation (Trapnell *et al, Antimicrob Agents Chemother* 1998;**42**:1592–6; FFT), possibly up to three-fold (n=1, Akula *et al, Am J Med Sci* 1997;**31**:244–6). Severe anaemia has been reported (n=1, Antoniou *et al, Clin Infect Dis* 2004;**38**:38–40; FFT).

Asenapine + valproate

See valproate + asenapine (*4.2.3*).

Aspirin + valproate

Valproate's levels may rise by 12–43% (n=3, Goulden *et al, Neurology* 1987;**37**:1392–4; n=6, open, Orr *et al, Clin Pharmacol Ther* 1982;**31**:642–9).

Benzodiazepines + valproate

See benzodiazepines (*4.1.1*).

Bupropion + valproate

See bupropion (*4.6.6*).

CARBAMAZEPINE + VALPROATE

See carbamazepine (*4.4.1*).

CARBAPENEM ANTIBIOTICS + VALPROATE *

Carbapenems (e.g. doripenem, ertapenem, imipenem, meropenem) can induce a rapid and significant drop in valproate levels, often not correctable by dose increases, so do not use these together (*Drug Safety Update* 2010;**3**:4):

- **Doripenem** can reduce valproate levels by 62–69% (n=2, Hellwig *et al, Curr Drug Saf* 2011;**6**:54–8)
- **Ertapenem** * can reduce valproate to almost undetectable levels (n=2, Liao *et al, Am J Health Syst Pharm* 2010;**67**:1260–4; n=1, Park *et al, Ther Drug Monit* 2012;**34**:599–603) and where even increasing the dose may not return levels to normal, with deaths reported (n=2, Spriet *et al, Am J Health Syst Pharm* 2007;**64**:54–8). There is a case of valproate levels increased by ertapenem but not meropenem (n=1, Yoon and Kim, *Int J Clin Pharm* 2013;**35**:316–8)
- **Imipenem** can reduce valproate levels by 73% (n=1, Park *et al, Ther Drug Monit* 2012;**34**:599 603)
- **Meropenem** can rapidly reduce valproate levels by about 82% (n=26, Vélez-Díaz-Pallarés *et al, Neurologia* 2012;**27**:34–38; FFT) and remain low for a week after meropenem is stopped, gradually returning to normal over the next week (e.g. n=36, Haroutiunian *et al, J Clin Pharmacol* 2009;**49**:1363–9; n=3, Park *et al, Ther Drug Monit* 2012;**34**:599–603). The decline can be unpredictable and rapid (Naranjo=7, n=1, Gu and Huang, *Am J Geriatr Pharmacother* 2009;**7**:26–33).

Charcoal, activated + valproate

Activated charcoal reduces the absorption of valproate by 65% (n=6, Neuvonen *et al, Eur J Clin Pharmacol* 1983;**24**:243–6), but has no effect on its elimination (n=8, al-Shareef *et al, Br J Clin Pharmacol* 1997;**43**:109–11).

CHITOSAN + VALPROATE
Chitosan (a weight-loss product) has reduced valproate to almost undetectable levels, with resultant seizures (n=2, Striano *et al*, *BMJ* 2009;**339**:b3751).

Clozapine + valproate
See clozapine (*4.2.4*).

Erythromycin + valproate
Valproate levels have risen three-fold with erythromycin, resulting in CNS toxicity (n=1, Redington *et al*, *Ann Intern Med* 1992;**116**:877–8).

Ethosuximide + valproate
Valproate may transiently increase ethosuximide plasma levels by up to 50% via enzyme inhibition (n=6, Pisani *et al*, *Epilepsia* 1984;**25**:229–33). Ethosuximide may reduce valproate levels by 28% (n=4) and stopping ethosuximide has led to valproate levels rising by 36% (n=9). The mechanism is unknown (open, Sälke–Kellermann *et al*, *Epilepsy Res* 1997;**26**:345–9).

Fluoxetine + valproate
See fluoxetine (*4.3.2.2*).

Fluvoxamine + valproate
See fluvoxamine (*4.3.2.3*).

Gabapentin + valproate
See gabapentin (*4.5.1*).

Ginkgo biloba + valproate
A fatal seizure has been reported, probably due to reduced valproate levels via CYP2C19 induction (n=1, Kupiec and Raj, *J Anal Toxicol* 2005;**29**:755–8; FFT).

Guanfacine + valproate
See valproate + guanfacine (*4.6.9*).

H2-blockers + valproate
Cimetidine prolongs valproate's half-life but ranitidine does not (n=12, RCT, Webster *et al*, *Eur J Clin Pharmacol* 1984;**27**:341–3).

Imatinib + valproate
Plasma levels of imatinib do not appear to be affected by valproate (n<224, p/c, Pursche *et al*, *Curr Clin Pharmacol* 2008;**3**:198–203; FFT).

Isoniazid + valproate *
Enhanced hepatotoxicity (n=1, Dockweiler, *Lancet* 1987;**2**:152) and valproate toxicity (n=1, Stewart *et al*, *J Clin Psychopharmacol* 2012;**32**:840–1) have been reported.

Lacosamide + valproate *
There is no significant interaction (n=32, RCT, open, Cawello and Bonn, *J Clin Pharmacol* 2012;**52**:1739–48), although lacosamide levels may be reduced by 25% and valproate toxicity has been reported (n=1, Jones *et al*, *Pediatr Neurol* 2013;**48**:308–10).

LAMOTRIGINE + VALPROATE
See lamotrigine (*4.4.2*).

Levetiracetam + valproate
See levetiracetam (*4.5.2*).

Methylphenidate + valproate
See methylphenidate (*4.6.13*).

Moclobemide + valproate
See valproate + moclobemide (*4.3.3.5*).

Olanzapine + valproate
See valproate + olanzapine (*4.2.6*).

Oral contraceptives + valproate
A reduced contraceptive effect has not been reported with valproate but valproate plasma levels may be 23% lower with a combined hormonal oral contraceptives (n=24, open, Herzog *et al*, *Neurology* 2009;**72**:911–4). There is a wide inter-individual variation and monitoring valproate may be prudent if adding or discontinuing OCs or steroids (n=9, RCT, c/o, Galimberti *et al*, *Epilepsia* 2006;**47**:1569–72).

Oxcarbazepine + valproate
See oxcarbazepine (*4.5.3*).

Paroxetine + valproate
See paroxetine (*4.3.2.4*).

PHENOBARBITAL + VALPROATE
See phenobarbital (*4.5.4*).

PHENYTOIN + VALPROATE
See phenytoin (*4.5.5*).

Pregabalin + valproate
See pregabalin (*4.1.5*).

Quetiapine + valproate
See quetiapine (*4.2.7*).

Riluzole + valproate
Increased valproate levels have been reported (n=1, Veenstra-VanderWeele, *J Child Adolesc Psychopharmacol* 2010:**20**:163–5).

Risperidone + valproate
See valproate + antipsychotics (*4.2.1*).

Rufinamide + valproate
Rufinamide plasma levels may be increased by valproate (UK SmPC), especially if body weight is <30kg, so use lower doses. Rufinamide has no effect on valproate (UK SmPC).

Smoking + valproate
See smoking (*4.7.4*).

Sodium oxybate + valproate
See sodium oxybate (*4.6.18*).

Tiagabine + valproate
Tiagabine can reduce steady-state valproate

levels by 10–12%, while valproate increases free tiagabine levels by about 40% (n=12, open, Gustavson *et al*, *Am J Ther* 1998;**5**:73–9).

Topiramate + valproate

See topiramate (4.5.6).

TRICYCLICS + VALPROATE *

Valproate can double tricyclic levels e.g. **amitriptyline, nortriptyline** (n=66, retrospective, Unterecker *et al*, *J Clin Psychopharmacol* 2013;**33**:561–4) and **doxepin** (2.2-fold, dose-related, n=41, Unterecker *et al*, *Int Clin Psychopharmacol* 2014;**29**:206–11; FFT), a remarkable finding, so cautious use of the combination is essential. Status epilepticus has been reported with **clomipramine** (eg. n=1, DeToledo *et al*, *Ther Drug Monit* 1997;**19**:71–3; Fehr *et al*, *J Clin Psychopharmacol* 2000;**20**:493–4).

Venlafaxine + valproate *

Valproate has no effect on venlafaxine levels but desmethylvenlafaxine levels may be 27% higher (n=41, Unterecker *et al*, *Int Clin Psychopharmacol* 2014;**29**:206–11; FFT).

Vigabatrin + valproate

Lack of interaction has been shown (e.g. McKee *et al*, *Epilepsia* 1993;**34**:937–43).

Warfarin + valproate

Rapidly raised INR (to 3.9) has been reported after a single dose of valproate (Guthrie *et al*, *J Clin Psychopharmacol* 1995;**15**:138–9) and with IV valproate (n=1, Yoon *et al*, *Neurocrit Care* 2011;**15**:182–5).

Zolpidem + valproate

See zolpidem (4.1.7).

Zonisamide + valproate

Lack of significant interaction has been shown (n=22 [c=17], open, Ragueneau-Majlessi *et al*, *Clin Pharmacokinet* 2005;**44**:517–23).

4.5 ANTICONVULSANTS

Combining anticonvulsants can be an essential strategy but knowledge of interactions is vital, both when adding drugs (or increasing doses) or stopping drugs (or decreasing doses).

Reviews: AEDs and antimicrobials (Desai, *Epilepsia* 2008;**49**(Suppl 6):47–9), AEDs and cancer chemotherapy (Yap *et al*, *Clin Ther* 2008;**30**:1385–407), P450 interactions with AEDs (Mula, *Curr Drug Metab* 2008;**9**:730–7) and AEDs with other drugs (Díaz *et al*, *Neurologist* 2008;**14** [6 suppl 1]:S55–65).

4.5.1 GABAPENTIN

Gabapentin is not metabolised or protein-bound, so has little chance of interactions by these mechanisms. Excretion is almost completely renal.

Antacids + gabapentin

A magnesium oxide-containing antacid significantly has reduced gabapentin plasma levels (n=13, RCT, open, c/o, Yagi *et al*, *Drug Metab Pharmacokinet* 2012;**27**:248–54; FFT).

Benzodiazepines + gabapentin

No significant interaction has been noted with clonazepam (n=127, d/b, p/c, UKGSG, *Lancet* 1990;**335**:1114–7).

Carbamazepine + gabapentin

Lack of significant interaction has been noted (e.g. n=26, open, Radulovic *et al*, *Epilepsia* 1994;**35**:155–61).

Cimetidine + gabapentin

Cimetidine may reduce gabapentin clearance by about 10%.

Levetiracetam + gabapentin

See levetiracetam (4.5.2).

Lithium + gabapentin

See lithium (4.4.3).

Omeprazole + gabapentin

Omeprazole has no significant effect on gabapentin (n=13, RCT, open, c/o, Yagi *et al*, *Drug Metab Pharmacokinet* 2012;**27**:248–54; FFT).

Oral contraceptives + gabapentin

No change in the kinetics of norethisterone and ethinylestradiol were seen with gabapentin (Busch *et al*, *Epilepsia* 1993;**34**[Suppl 2]:158).

Phenobarbital + gabapentin

One study showed no significant interaction (n=12, open, 52/7, Hooper *et al*, *Br J Clin Pharmacol* 1991;**31**:171–4; FFT).

Phenytoin + gabapentin

Phenytoin levels can be raised, but rarely to toxic levels (e.g. n=1, Sánchez-Romero *et al*, *Rev Neurol* 2002;**34**:952–3; FFT).

Pregabalin + gabapentin

See pregabalin (4.1.5).

Valproate + gabapentin

Lack of significant interaction has been noted (n=127, d/b, p/c, UKGSG, *Lancet* 1990;**335**:1114–7).

Zolpidem + gabapentin *

See gabapentin + zolpidem (4.1.7).

4

4.5.2 LEVETIRACETAM

Levetiracetam is not plasma protein-bound or extensively metabolised. It does not inhibit or induce CYP1A2, 2A6, 2C8/9/10, 2C19, 2D6, 2E1 and 3A4, nor UGT enzymes. There appears no need to adjust levetiracetam doses if prescribed with any other AED (n=590, Perucca *et al*, *Epilepsy Res* 2003;**53**:47–56).

Review: May *et al*, *Ther Drug Monit* 2003;**25**:690–9).

Alcohol + levetiracetam

No data is available (UK SmPC).

Carbamazepine + levetiracetam

Lack of interaction has been shown, although disabling symptoms consistent with carbamazepine toxicity (but with unchanged levels) have been reported (n=4, Sisodiya *et al*, *Epilepsy Res* 2002;**48**:217–9).

Ciclosporin + levetiracetam

Lack of interaction has been suggested (n=1, Franzoni *et al*, *J Child Neurol* 2007;**22**:440–2).

Digoxin + levetiracetam

Lack of pharmacokinetic interaction has been demonstrated (n=11, RCT, Levy *et al*, *Epilepsy Res* 2001;**46**:93–9).

Food + levetiracetam

Levetiracetam absorption is slightly slowed by food, but total absorption remains unchanged.

Gabapentin + levetiracetam

Lack of interaction has been shown (UK SmPC).

Imatinib + levetiracetam

Plasma levels of imatinib do not appear to be affected by levetiracetam (n<224, p/c, Pursche *et al*, *Curr Clin Pharmacol* 2008;**3**:198–203; FFT).

Lamotrigine + levetiracetam

Lack of interaction has been shown (UK SmPC).

Oral contraceptives + levetiracetam

Lack of interaction has been shown (n=18, RCT, d/b, c/o, Ragueneau-Majlessi *et al*, *Epilepsia* 2002;**43**:697–702). OCs have no effect on levetiracetam kinetics (n=53, Sabers and Christensen, *Epilepsy Res* 2011;**95**:277–9).

Phenobarbital + levetiracetam

Lack of interaction has been shown (UK SmPC).

Phenytoin + levetiracetam

Levetiracetam has no effect on the kinetics of phenytoin (n=6, open, Browne *et al*, *J Clin Pharmacol* 2000;**40**:590–5).

Probenecid + levetiracetam

Probenecid may inhibit the clearance of the primary (inactive) metabolite of levetiracetam, but not of the parent drug.

Valproate + levetiracetam

Lack of interaction has been shown (UK SmPC. n=16, open, c/o, Coupez *et al*, *Epilepsia* 2003;**44**:171–8).

Warfarin + levetiracetam

Lack of pharmacokinetic interaction has been demonstrated (n=42, RCT, Ragueneau-Majlessi *et al*, *Epilepsy Res* 2001;**47**:55–63).

4.5.3 OXCARBAZEPINE

Oxcarbazepine and its metabolite MHD inhibit 2C19 and induce 3A4 and 3A5 at higher (n=4, open, Patsalos *et al*, *Eur J Clin Pharmacol* 1990;**39**:187–8), but probably not at lower doses (n=8, Larkin *et al*, *Br J Clin Pharmacol* 1991;**31**:65–71; FFT).

Alcohol + oxcarbazepine

Caution should be exercised if alcohol is taken, as additive sedation can occur.

Antipsychotics + oxcarbazepine

Carbamazepine reduces the plasma levels of many antipsychotics eg. **olanzapine** (n=13) and **risperidone** (n=12) (5/52, Rosaria Muscatello *et al*, *Epilepsia* 2005;**46**:771–4). However, as oxcarbazepine seems to have less enzyme-inducing activity when substituted for carbamazepine, it can lead to plasma levels of some antipsychotics (e.g. **haloperidol**, **chlorpromazine** and **clozapine**) increasing by 50–200% over 2–4 weeks (n=6, Raitasuo *et al*, *Psychopharmacology [Berl]* 1994;**16**:115–6). Addition of oxcarbazepine to **amisulpride** has caused NMS (n=1, Angelopoulos *et al*, *Gen Hosp Psychiatry* 2008;**30**:482–4).

Carbamazepine + oxcarbazepine

Addition of oxcarbazepine to carbamazepine has resulted in a ≤22% decrease in carbamazepine levels and a 40% reduction in MHD levels (UK SmPC), important during a switch.

Ciclosporin + oxcarbazepine

Trough levels of ciclosporin may fall slightly with oxcarbazepine (n=1, Rosche *et al*, *Clin Neuropharmacol* 2001;**24**:113–6).

Cimetidine + oxcarbazepine

Cimetidine has no effect on the kinetics of oxcarbazepine (n=8, c/o, Keränen *et al*, *Acta Neurol Scand* 1992;**85**:239–42).

Citalopram + oxcarbazepine
Citalopram plasma levels may rise if oxcarbazepine replaces carbamazepine (n=2, Leinonen *et al*, *Pharmacopsychiatry* 1996;**29**:156–8).

Corticosteroids + oxcarbazepine
Oxcarbazepine induces 3A4, reducing hydrocortisone levels. This might be relevant at higher doses or in critical care (n=12, p/c, Högler *et al*, *Arch Dis Child* 2010;**95**:1065).

Erythromycin + oxcarbazepine
Erythromycin has no effect on the kinetics of oxcarbazepine (n=8, c/o, Keränen *et al*, *Acta Neurol Scand* 1992;**86**:120–3).

Escitalopram + oxcarbazepine
See citalopram + oxcarbazepine.

Felodipine + oxcarbazepine
Oxcarbazepine can reduce felodipine AUC and plasma levels by 28% and 34% respectively, which might slightly reduce its clinical effect (n=8, open, Zaccara *et al*, *Ther Drug Monit* 1993;**15**:39–42).

Fosphenytoin + oxcarbazepine
See phenytoin + oxcarbazepine.

Furosemide + oxcarbazepine
Acute encephalopathy has occurred (n=1, Siniscalchi *et al*, *Ann Pharmacother* 2004;**38**:509–10).

Imatinib + oxcarbazepine
Mean trough levels of imatinib are reduced up to 2.9-fold by oxcarbazepine (n<224, p/c, Pursche *et al*, *Curr Clin Pharmacol* 2008;**3**:198–203; FFT).

Lamotrigine + oxcarbazepine
There appears to be no significant interaction (n=47, RCT, s/b, Theis *et al*, *Neuropsychopharmacol* 2005;**30**:2269–74; FFT), although ADRs may be more common and a retrospective review suggested that lamotrigine levels may fall by 29% and that reduced lamotrigine doses may be needed if oxcarbazepine is discontinued (n=222, May *et al*, *Therap Drug Monit* 1999;**21**:175–81).

Lithium + oxcarbazepine
The combination of lithium and oxcarbazepine might theoretically cause enhanced neurotoxicity.

MAOIs + oxcarbazepine
A theoretical risk of interaction exists.

ORAL CONTRACEPTIVES + OXCARBAZEPINE
Oxcarbazepine can produce significant reductions in some OC plasma levels, with reports of breakthrough bleeding (eg. n=16, RCT, Fattore *et al*, *Epilepsia* 1999;**40**:783–7). See oral contraceptives + carbamazepine for advice.

Phenobarbital + oxcarbazepine
Phenobarbital levels may be raised by 14% and oxcarbazepine/MHD levels reduced by 30%.

Phenytoin + oxcarbazepine
Oxcarbazepine >1200mg/d may increase phenytoin levels by up to 40% (less than 10% for doses below 1200mg/d), probably due to CYP2C19 inhibition (e.g. n=1, Soskin *et al*, *Psychosomatics* 2010;**51**:532–5; Lakehal *et al*, *Epilepsy Res* 2002;**52**:79–83). Close monitoring of phenytoin is essential, especially at higher doses.

Propoxyphene + oxcarbazepine
Propoxyphene has no significant effect on oxcarbazepine kinetics (n=8, open, Mogensen *et al*, *Acta Neurol Scand* 1992;**85**:14–7).

Smoking + oxcarbazepine
See smoking (*4.7.4*).

Temozolomide + oxcarbazepine
Temozolomide seems not to affect oxcarbazepine pharmacokinetics (n=8, Maschio *et al*, *J Neurooncol* 2008;**90**:217–21).

Valproate + oxcarbazepine
Valproate free levels (n=1, Xiong *et al*, *J Clin Psychopharmacol* 2008;**28**:472–3) may rise if oxcarbazepine replaces carbamazepine (n=4, Patsalos *et al*, *Eur J Clin Pharmacol* 1990;**39**:187–8). There is also a theoretical increase in the risk of teratogenicity, due to increased metabolite levels.

Verapamil + oxcarbazepine *
Verapamil increases the AUC of oxcarbazepine's metabolites by about 10%, a minor effect (n=12, 10/7, de Jesus Antunes *et al*, *Eur J Clin Pharmacol* 2016;**72**:195–201).

Warfarin + oxcarbazepine
Oxcarbazepine does not appear to affect the anticoagulant activity of warfarin (n=10, 1/52, Krämer *et al*, *Epilepsia* 1992;**33**:1145–8).

4.5.4 PHENOBARBITAL AND PRIMIDONE

Alcohol + barbiturates
See alcohol (*4.7.1*).

ANTICOAGULANTS + BARBITURATES
Anticoagulant effects can be significntly reduced by concurrent barbiturates so anticoagulant doses may need to be raised by up to 60%.

ANTIPSYCHOTICS + BARBITURATES
See antipsychotics (*4.2.1*) and quetiapine (*4.2.7*).

4

Antiretrovirals + barbiturates
The plasma levels of **indinavir** may be reduced by barbiturates via CYP3A4 induction.

Benzodiazepines + barbiturates
See benzodiazepines (*4.1.1*).

Beta-blockers + barbiturates
Metoprolol and **propranolol** plasma levels are reduced by barbiturates (open, Seideman *et al*, *Br J Clin Pharmacol* 1987;**23**:267–71; FFT), but **timolol** (n = 12, RCT, c/o, Mantyla *et al*, *Eur J Clin Pharmacol* 1983;**24**:227–30), **atenolol** and **nadolol** appear to be unaffected.

Bupropion + phenobarbital
See bupropion (*4.6.6*).

CALCIUM-CHANNEL BLOCKERS + BARBITURATES
Phenobarbital may reduce the efficacy of **verapamil** (open, Rutledge *et al*, *J Pharmacol Exp Therap* 1988;**246**:7–13), **diltiazem**, **isradipine**, **nicardipine** and **nifedipine**, via 3A4 inhibition so some care is needed.

Carbamazepine + phenobarbital
See carbamazepine (*4.4.1*).

Charcoal, activated + barbiturates
If given within five minutes, activated charcoal can be an effective adjunct in overdose treatment (Neuvonen and Elonen, *Eur J Clin Pharmacol* 1980;**17**:51–7).

Chloramphenicol + barbiturates
Chloramphenicol's metabolism is accelerated by barbiturates, reducing its efficacy (n = 1, Koup *et al*, *Clin Pharmacol Ther* 1978;**24**:571–5).

CICLOSPORIN + PHENOBARBITAL
Even low dose phenobarbital induces the CYP3A4 metabolism of ciclosporin (n=1, Carstensen, *et al*, *Br J Clin Pharmacol* 1986;**21**:550–1; FFT).

Cimetidine + phenobarbital
Reduced actions of both can occur, of very limited significance (n = 8, open, 6/52, Somogyi *et al*, *Eur J Clin Pharmacol* 1981;**19**:343–7).

Clozapine + phenobarbital
See clozapine (*4.2.4*).

CORTICOSTEROIDS + PHENOBARBITAL
CYP3A4 induction reduces the effect of some corticosteroids (Brooks *et al*, *NEJM* 1972;**286**:1125–8).

Digoxin + phenobarbital
Digitoxin (but not digoxin) levels can be reduced by up to 50% by phenobarbital (Káldor *et al*, *Int J Clin Pharmacol Biopharm* 1975;**12**:403–7).

Disopyramide + phenobarbital
Barbiturates induce disopyramide's CYP3A4 metabolism, reducing plasma levels (n = 14, open, Kapil *et al*, *Br J Clin Pharmacol* 1987;**24**:781–91; FFT).

Doxorubicin + phenobarbital
Doxorubicin clearance may be increased by barbiturates and so doses may need to be increased.

Doxycycline + phenobarbital
Doxycycline levels are reduced via CYP3A4 induction (n=5, Neuvonen and Penttilä, *Br Med J* 1974;**2**:535–6; FFT), unlike other tetracyclines.

Ethosuximide + phenobarbital
Reduced phenobarbital and ethosuximide effectiveness has been reported (n = 198, Battino *et al*, *Clin Pharmacokinet* 1982;**7**:176–80).

Fenoprofen + phenobarbital
Phenobarbital may slightly increase fenoprofen metabolism, reducing its efficacy (Helleberg *et al*, *Br J Clin Pharmacol* 1974;**1**:371–4; FFT).

Furosemide + phenobarbital
Barbiturates have no effect on furosemide (n = 10, open, Lambert *et al*, *Clin Pharmacol Ther* 1983;**34**:170–5).

Gabapentin + phenobarbital
See gabapentin (*4.5.1*).

Glyceryl trinitrate + phenobarbital
A reduced nitrate effect may occur via enzyme induction.

Griseofulvin + phenobarbital
Griseofulvin levels can be reduced by up to 45% by phenobarbital, either by enzyme induction or reduced absorption.

Influenza vaccine + phenobarbital
A transient 20% rise in barbiturate levels has been reported (n = 35, open, Jann and Fidone, *Clin Pharm* 1986;**5**:817–20).

Isoniazid + primidone
Primidone levels might rise by 80% (n = 1, Sutton and Kupferberg, *Neurology* 1975;**25**:1179–81).

Ketoconazole + phenobarbital
Reduced ketoconazole levels have been reported (n = 1, Brass *et al*, *Antimicrob Agents Chemother* 1982;**21**:151–8; FFT).

Lacosamide + phenobarbital
There is no significant pharmacokinetic interaction, although lacosamide levels may reduce by 25%.

Lamotrigine + phenobarbital
See lamotrigine (*4.4.2*).

Levetiracetam + phenobarbital

See levetiracetam (4.5.2).

Levonorgestrel + phenobarbital
There is a case of a levonorgestrel implant (Norplant) failing twice in a woman also taking phenobarbital (n=1, Shane-McWhorter *et al*, *Pharmacotherapy* 1998;**18**:1360–4).

Levothyroxine (thyroxine) + barbiturates
Levothyroxine metabolism is accelerated and so may require increase doses in hypothyroidism.

Lidocaine + barbiturates
Serum lidocaine levels may be lower in people taking barbiturates (LeLorier, *Toxicol Appl Pharmacol* 1978;**44**:657–9), via CYP3A4 induction.

MAOIs + phenobarbital
See MAOIs (4.3.4).

Memantine + phenobarbital
See memantine (4.6.11).

Methadone + phenobarbital
See methadone (4.6.12).

Metronidazole + phenobarbital
Metronidazole metabolism may be accelerated (n=7, Loft *et al*, *Eur J Clin Pharmacol* 1987;**32**:35–41).

Modafinil + phenobarbital
See modafinil (4.6.14).

Nicotinamide + primidone
There are reports of reduced conversion from primidone to phenobarbital (n=1, Bourgeois *et al*, *Neurology* 1982;**32**:1122–6).

ORAL CONTRACEPTIVES + PHENOBARBITAL
See oral contraceptives + carbamazepine.

Oxcarbazepine + phenobarbital
See oxcarbazepine (4.5.3).

Paracetamol + phenobarbital
An isolated case of enhanced hepatotoxicity exists (Pirotte, *Ann Int Med* 1984;**101**:403).

Paroxetine + phenobarbital
See paroxetine (4.3.2.4).

Pethidine + phenobarbital
Severe sedation has been reported (n=12, open, c/o, Stambaugh *et al*, *J Clin Pharmacol* 1978;**18**:482–90).

Phenylbutazone + phenobarbital
Reduced levels of phenylbutazone may occur (Levi *et al*, *Lancet* 1968;**1**:1275–9).

Phenytoin + phenobarbital
See barbiturates + phenytoin (4.5.5).

Pregabalin + phenobarbital
See pregabalin (4.1.5).

Pyridoxine + phenobarbital
Large doses of pyridoxine (e.g. 200mg/d) can reduce phenobarbital levels by up to 40–50% (Hansson and Sillanpaa, *Lancet* 1976;**1**:256).

Quetiapine + phenobarbital
See quetiapine (4.2.7).

Quinidine + phenobarbital
CYP3A4 induction may reduce quinidine levels by up to 50% (Rogers and Blackman, *Drug Intell Clin Pharm* 1983;**17**:819–20).

Reboxetine + phenobarbital
See reboxetine (4.3.3.6).

Rifampicin + barbiturates
Rifampicin can induce barbiturate metabolism (n=40, open, see Richter *et al*, *Eur J Clin Pharmacol* 1980;**17**:197–202).

Rufinamide + phenobarbital
The plasma levels of rufinamide are reduced but rufinamide has no effect on barbiturates (SmPC).

Smoking + phenobarbital
See smoking (4.7.4).

St John's wort + phenobarbital
See St John's wort (4.3.3.10).

Testosterone + phenobarbital
CYP3A4 induction can reduce steroid effects.

THEOPHYLLINE + BARBITURATES
Theophylline metabolism can be accelerated, reducing its effect (n=24, Kandrokas *et al*, *Ther Drug Monit* 1990;**12**:139–43).

Tiagabine + phenobarbital
Tiagabine plasma levels can be reduced by a factor of 1.5–3, probably by CYP3A4 induction. There is no effect on phenobarbital.

Topiramate + phenobarbital
See topiramate (4.5.6).

TRICYCLICS + BARBITURATES
See tricyclics (4.3.1).

Tropisetron + phenobarbital
Phenobarbital reduces the plasma levels of tropisetron (BNF).

VALPROATE + PHENOBARBITAL
Valproate increases phenobarbital plasma concentrations by up to 25% (n=20, Bernus *et al*, *Br J Clin Pharmacol* 1994;**38**:411–6; FFT), increasing side-effects, although this may only be transient. There are cases of hyper-ammonaemic encephalopathy (eg. n=3, Cano-Zuleta *et al*, *Farm Hosp* 2012;**36**:441–2), so monitor blood levels regularly.

Vigabatrin + phenobarbital
There are non-clinically significant 7–11% reductions in barbiturate levels (n=89, s/b, 12/52, Browne *et al*, *Neurology* 1987;**37**:184–9).

4

Zaleplon + phenobarbital
See zaleplon (*4.1.6*).

4.5.5 PHENYTOIN

Phenytoin has a narrow therapeutic index. It is primarily metabolised by 2C9, and partly by 2C19, with genetic polymorphism affecting levels. It is extensively bound to plasma proteins, induces CYP3A4 and has a saturable metabolism. It can be displaced, giving an increased proportion of free active phenytoin, significant where TDM just measures total phenytoin rather than the proportion of free (hence active) phenytoin. Low concentrations may appear below the normal therapeutic range, but free (active) levels are appropriate, prompting inappropriately increased doses or discontinuation (see Toler, *Ann Pharmacother* 1994;**28**:808–9).

ACENOCOUMAROL + PHENYTOIN
Acenocoumarol metabolism is induced by phenytoin, reducing its effect, although enhancement has also been reported.

Acetazolamide + phenytoin
Acetazolamide has enhanced the osteomalacia secondary to phenytoin (n=2, Mallette, *Arch Intern Med* 1977;**137**:1013–7).

ALCOHOL + PHENYTOIN
See alcohol (*4.7.1*).

Allopurinol + phenytoin
Phenytoin toxicity may occur with repeated high-dose allopurinol (Ogiso *et al*, *J Pharmacobiodyn* 1990;**13**:36–43).

AMIODARONE + PHENYTOIN
Amiodarone reduces phenytoin metabolism, toxicity developing over two weeks (n=7, open, 8/52, Nolan *et al*, *Am J Cardiol* 1990;**65**:1252–7), so reduce phenytoin doses by at least 25%.

Anaesthetics + phenytoin
Case reports exist of phenytoin toxicity following halothane (Karlin and Kutt, *J Pediatr* 1970;**76**:941–4), and so caution is needed.

Antacids + phenytoin
Antacids probably reduce phenytoin levels, shown in several studies (e.g. n=6, McElnay *et al*, *Br J Clin Pharmacol* 1982;**13**:501; FFT), so separate doses by about three hours or use ranitidine.

ANTIPSYCHOTICS + PHENYTOIN
See antipsychotics (*4.2.1*), clozapine (*4.2.4*), quetiapine (*4.2.7*) and risperidone/paliperidone (*4.2.8*).

ANTIRETROVIRALS + PHENYTOIN
Phenytoin increases **lopinavir** clearance. Phenytoin levels are reduced by **lopinavir, ritonavir** (n=24, Lim *et al*, *J Acquir Immune Defic Syndr* 2004;**36**:1034–40), **efavirenz** (Spak *et al*, *AIDS* 2008;**22**:164–5), **indinavir** (BNF) and **nevirapine** (n=36, open, L'homme *et al*, *J Acquir Immune Defic Syndr* 2006;**43**:193–6), probably by 2C9 induction.

Atomoxetine + phenytoin
See atomoxetine (*4.6.4*).

Ayurvedic herbal mixtures + phenytoin
See shankhapushpi + phenytoin.

Barbiturates + phenytoin
Phenobarbital probably induces phenytoin's metabolism, slightly reducing levels but at very high doses phenytoin serum levels are increased, a dose-dependent effect (n=1, Kuranari *et al*, *Ann Pharmacother* 1995;**29**:83–4). Phenytoin can raise phenobarbital levels by up to 100%, resulting in increased sedation (n=1, Porro *et al*, *Br J Clin Pharmacol* 1982;**14**:294–7; FFT), so regular monitoring should still be done.

Benzodiazepines + phenytoin
Some benzodiazepines have been reported to potentiate phenytoin but other studies have not shown this effect. Phenytoin induces clonazepam's metabolism, reducing levels by up to 50% (n=27, open, Sjo *et al*, *Eur J Clin Pharmacol* 1975;**8**:249–54).

Bupropion + phenytoin
See bupropion (*4.6.6*).

Buspirone + phenytoin
See buspirone (*4.1.2*).

Calcium-channel blockers + phenytoin
Phenytoin levels are increased by higher doses of **diltiazem and verapamil**, n=43, Bahls *et al*, *Neurology* 1991;**41**:740–2), **isradipine** (n=1, Cachat and Tufro, *Ann Pharmacother* 2002;**36**:1399–402) but not by **nifedipine** (e.g. n=8, open, Schellens *et al*, *Br J Clin Pharmacol* 1991;**31**:175–8; FFT). Phenytoin toxicity has been reported (n=1, Ahmad *et al*, *J Am Coll Cardiol* 1984;**3**:1582) as has almost complete lack of verapamil absorption (at up to 400mg/d; n=1, Woodcock *et al*, *N Engl J Med* 1991;**325**:1179; FFT). The effects of **isradipine** and **nicardipine** may be reduced by phenytoin.

Capecitabine + phenytoin *
Phenytoin toxicity and seizures developing over 4/52 and taking 9/52 to resolve after dose

changes has been reported (e.g. n = 1, Ciftci *et al*, *Am J Ther* 2015;**22**;e17–9; n = 1, Taguchi *et al*, *Brain Nerve* 2015;**67**:213–7).

CARBAMAZEPINE + PHENYTOIN

See carbamazepine (*4.4.1*).

Charcoal, activated + phenytoin

Phenytoin absorption is almost completely (98%) prevented if activated charcoal is taken within five minutes and reduced by about 80% if given after one hour (n=6, open, c/o, Neuvonen *et al*, *Eur J Clin Pharmacol* 1978;**13**:213–8). Multiple-doses have been used successfully over several days, and may even have some use up to a week after phenytoin ingestion (n=1, Howard *et al*, *Ann Pharmacother* 1994;**28**:201–3).

Chinese medicines + phenytoin

Phenytoin poisoning after using Chinese proprietary medicines has been reported (n = 1, Lau *et al*, *Hum Experimental Toxicol* 2000;**19**:385–6).

Chloral + phenytoin

Dichloralphenazone has decreased phenytoin levels (n=5, Riddell *et al*, *Br J Clin Pharmacol* 1980;**9**:118P), although whether the chloral part of the molecule was responsible is not known.

CHLORAMPHENICOL + PHENYTOIN

Phenytoin toxicity may occur with oral chloramphenicol via enzyme inhibition, a serious effect.

Chlorphenamine + phenytoin

Isolated cases exist of phenytoin toxicity (n=2, Pugh *et al*, *Br J Clin Pharmacol* 1975;**2**:173–5; FFT).

CICLOSPORIN + PHENYTOIN

Ciclosporin levels can be reduced by 80% by phenytoin, by enzyme induction (n=6, Freeman *et al*, *Br J Clin Pharmacol* 1984;**18**:887–93; FFT).

Ciprofloxacin + phenytoin *

Although raised phenytoin levels with oral ciprofloxacin have been reported (n=1, Hull, *Ann Pharmacother* 1993;**27**:1283). IV ciprofloxacin has halved phenytoin levels (e.g. n=1, Brouwers and de Boer, *Ann Pharmacother* 1997;**31**:498). Even ciprofloxacin eye-drops have led to subtherapeutic phenytoin levels and seizures (n=1, Malladi *et al*, *Singapore Med J* 2014;**55**:114–5).

Cisplatin/S-1 + phenytoin

Phenytoin toxicity has occurred about two months after Cisplatin was started (n = 1, Mimatsu *et al*, *Gan To Kagaku Ryoho* 2011;**38**:1003–6).

Clinafloxacin + phenytoin

Phenytoin has no effect on clinafloxacin kinetics. Phenytoin clearance is 15% lower with clinafloxacin (Randinitis *et al*, *Antimicrob Agents Chemother* 2001;**45**:2543–52; FFT).

CLOZAPINE + PHENYTOIN

See clozapine (*4.2.4*).

CORTICOSTEROIDS + PHENYTOIN

Phenytoin may induce the metabolism of steroids and so higher doses may be needed. Hydrocortisone may be less affected than other steroids. Phenytoin levels may also be changed.

Co-trimoxazole + phenytoin

Raised phenytoin levels have occurred (n=1, Gillman and Sandyk, *Arch Intern Med* 1985;**102**:559).

DEXAMETHASONE + PHENYTOIN

Phenytoin levels may be halved by dexamethasone (e.g. n=1, Griffiths and Taylor, *Can J Hosp Pharm* 1999;**52**:96–8), and very high doses of phenytoin may be necessary (e.g. 900mg/d) to maintain levels (review by Recuenco *et al*, *Ann Pharmacother* 1995;**29**:935). Regular and frequent monitoring of phenytoin levels is essential.

Dexibuprofen + phenytoin

Acute phenytoin toxicity has been reported (n=1, Llinares–Tello *et al*, *Med Clin [Barc]* 2007;**128**:239).

Dextropropoxyphene + phenytoin

See propoxyphene + phenytoin.

DIAZOXIDE + PHENYTOIN

Reduced phenytoin levels occur via increased metabolism (Turck *et al*, *Presse Med* 1986;**15**:31).

DICOUMAROL + PHENYTOIN

Phenytoin levels may rise rapidly by over 100% (Hansen *et al*, *Acta Med Scand* 1971;**189**:15 9), so avoid the combination or monitor carefully.

Digoxin + phenytoin

Phenytoin reduces digoxin half-life by 30% (n=6, RCT, open, c/o, Rameis *et al*, *Eur J Clin Pharmacol* 1985;**29**:49–53;), so monitor carefully.

DISOPYRAMIDE + PHENYTOIN

Phenytoin reduces the plasma levels of disopyramide, possibly to below therapeutic levels (Kessler *et al*, *Clin Pharm* 1982;**1**:263–4).

Disulfiram + phenytoin

Phenytoin toxicity and delirium may occur via enzyme inhibition (e.g. n=1, Brown *et al*, *Ann Emerg Med* 1983;**12**:310–3).

Dopamine + phenytoin

Hypotension may occur (n=5, Bivins *et al*, *Arch Surg* 1978;**113**:245–9), although not invariably (n=1, Torres *et al*, *Ann Pharmacother* 1995;**29**:1300–1).

4

Doxifluridine + phenytoin
Elevated phenytoin levels have occurred (n=1, Konishi *et al*, *Ann Pharmacother* 2002;**36**:831–4).

DOXYCYCLINE + PHENYTOIN
Doxycycline metabolism is induced by phenytoin with a halved half-life (n=4, Penttilá *et al*, *Br Med J* 1974;**2**:470–2; FFT). Other tetracyclines appear not to interact, so make dosage adjustments or use an alternative.

Enteral feeds + phenytoin
See nasogastric feeds + phenytoin.

Ethosuximide + phenytoin
Phenytoin may reduce ethosuximide plasma levels (n=198, retrospective, Battion *et al*, *Clin Pharmacokinet* 1982;**7**:176–80).

Fluorouracil + phenytoin
Elevated phenytoin levels have occurred 11 weeks after starting fluorouracil and leucovorin, possibly via CYP2C9 inhibition (n=1, Gilbar and Brodribb, *Ann Pharmacother* 2001;**35**:1367–70; n=1, Rosemergy and Findlay, *N Z Med J* 2002;**115**:U124).

FLUOXETINE + PHENYTOIN *
Phenytoin levels raised by 66% have been reported two weeks after fluoxetine was added, resolving within a week of stopping fluoxetine (n=1, Woods *et al*, *N Z Med J* 1994;**107**:19) a potentially serious interaction (Lance and Ternouth, *N Z Med J* 2015;**128**:78–9).

FLUVOXAMINE + PHENYTOIN
Fluvoxamine may triple phenytoin levels, probably by 2C9/19 inhibition (n=1, Mamiya *et al*, *Ther Drug Monit* 2001;**23**:75–7).

Folic acid + phenytoin
Serum folate decreases when phenytoin is started. Folic acid supplementation should be started with phenytoin as folic acid supplementation in folate-deficient people lowers phenytoin levels (n=4, open, Berg *et al*, *Ther Drug Monit* 1983;**5**:389–99). If started later, phenytoin levels should be monitored and changes in seizure activity monitored (extensive review by Lewis *et al*, *Ann Pharmacother* 1995;**29**:726–35).

Furosemide + phenytoin
The diuretic effect may be reduced by up to 50% (e.g. Bissoli *et al*, *Recenti Prog Med* 1996;**87**:227–8), so larger doses may be needed.

Gabapentin + phenytoin
See gabapentin (*4.5.1*).

Ginkgo biloba + phenytoin
A fatal seizure has occurred, probably due to reduced phenytoin levels via CYP2C19 induction by GB (n=1, Kupiec and Raj, *J Anal Toxicol* 2005;**29**:755–8; FFT).

Glucagon + phenytoin
Patients on phenytoin may get false negatives with glucagon stimulation tests.

Glucocorticoids + phenytoin
A reduced steroid effect via enzyme induction is possible.

H2-blockers + phenytoin
Cimetidine can rapidly raise phenytoin levels (e.g. n=9, Rafi *et al*, *Ann Pharmacother* 1999;**33**:769–74). Use **famotidine** (n=10, RCT, open, c/o, Sambol *et al*, *Br J Clin Pharmacol* 1989;**27**:83–7; FFT), **nizatidine** (n=18, Bachmann *et al*, *Br J Clin Pharmacol* 1993;**36**:380–2; FFT) or **ranitidine** (e.g. n=4, Watts *et al*, *Br J Clin Pharmacol* 1983;**15**:499–500), although there have been reports of elevated phenytoin levels with ranitidine (e.g. n=1, Tse *et al*, *Ann Pharmacother* 1993;**27**:1448–51; n=1, Tse and Iagmin, *Ann Intern Med* 1994;**120**:892–3).

Influenza vaccine + phenytoin
Influenza vaccine may reduce total and free phenytoin levels (Smith *et al*, *Clin Pharm* 1988;**7**:828–32), although it may only be transient in 60% (Jann and Fidone, *Clin Pharm* 1986;**5**:817–20).

Irinotecan + phenytoin
Irinotecan plasma levels can fall (Murry *et al*, *J Pediatr Hematol Oncol* 2002;**24**:130–3).

ISONIAZID + PHENYTOIN
Phenytoin toxicity may occur via enzyme inhibition (n=1, Witmer and Ritschel, *Drug Intell Clin Pharm* 1984;**18**:483–6).

Ivabradine + phenytoin
Phenytoin reduces the Cmax and AUC of ivabradine by around 70% (n=18, c/o, Vlase *et al*, *Clin Drug Investig* 2012;**32**:533–8).

Lacosamide + phenytoin
Lacosamide levels may be reduced by 25%, probably not clinically significant.

Lamotrigine + phenytoin
See lamotrigine (*4.4.2*).

Levetiracetam + phenytoin
See levetiracetam (*4.5.2*).

Levodopa + phenytoin
Levodopa can be completely antagonised by phenytoin (Mendez *et al*, *Arch Neurol* 1975;**32**:44–6).

Levothyroxine (thyroxine) + phenytoin

Levothyroxine's metabolism is accelerated by phenytoin, increasing requirements (Blackshear *et al*, *Ann Int Med* 1983;**99**:341–2).

Lidocaine + phenytoin

Phenytoin's central effects may be enhanced by lidocaine (Karlsson *et al*, *Eur J Clin Pharmacol* 1974;**7**:455–9). Sinoatrial arrest has been reported (n=1, Wood, *Br Med J* 1971;**i**:645).

Lithium + phenytoin

See lithium (*4.4.3*).

Losartan + phenytoin

Losartan has no effect on phenytoin, but losartan levels may rise via 2C9 inhibition (n=16, RCT, c/o, Fischer *et al*, *Clin Pharmacol Ther* 2002;**72**:238–46).

Memantine + phenytoin

See memantine (*4.6.11*).

Methadone + phenytoin

See methadone (*4.6.12*).

Methaqualone (Mandrax) + phenytoin

Phenytoin toxicity has been reported (n=1, Verma and Tiwari, *Epilepsy Res* 2012;**98**:281–2).

Methotrexate + phenytoin

An increased antifolate effect with phenytoin may occur.

Methylphenidate + phenytoin

See methylphenidate (*4.6.13*).

METRONIDAZOLE + PHENYTOIN

Phenytoin toxicity has been reported (Blyden *et al*, *J Clin Pharmacol Ther* 1988;**28**:240–5).

MEXILITINE + PHENYTOIN

Mexilitine levels may be reduced by up to 50% via enzyme induction (n=6, open, Begg *et al*, *Br J Clin Pharmacol* 1982;**14**:219–23).

Mirtazapine + phenytoin

See mirtazapine (*4.3.3.4*).

Modafinil + phenytoin

See modafinil (*4.6.14*).

Nasogastric feeds + phenytoin

Reduced phenytoin levels have been reported with nasogastric feeds (e.g. Osmolite®, Ensure® [Abbott]) and other enteral feeds and that the absorption patterns were significantly different, with phenytoin sodium more rapidly absorbed (n=10, RCT, Doak *et al*, *Pharmacotherapy* 1998;**18**:637–45). Phenytoin dosage should be spaced to one hour before feeding or two hours after feeding (tube may need to be clamped). Monitor plasma levels frequently (see Au Yeung and Ensom, *Ann Pharmacother* 2000;**34**:896–905).

Neuromuscular blocking agents + phenytoin

Phenytoin reduces the effects of most NMBAs, e.g. **pancuronium** (eg. n=1, Hickey *et al*, *Anesthesia* 1988;**43**:757–9; n=1, Liberman *et al*, *Int J Clin Pharmacol Ther Toxicol* 1988;**26**:371–4) and **vecuronium** (n=22, Wright *et al*, *Anesthesiology* 2004;**100**:626–33; n=1, Chowdhury *et al*, *Indian J Pharmacol* 2011;**43**:214–5; FFT). **Atracurium** appears unaffected.

Nitrofurantoin + phenytoin

There is a report of seizures, requiring increased phenytoin dosage (n=1, Heipertz and Pilz, *J Neurol* 1978;**218**:297–301).

NSAIDs + phenytoin

Ibuprofen appears to have no interaction (n=10, open, Bachmann, *Br J Clin Pharmacol* 1986;**21**:165–9; FFT), but toxicity has been reported (n=1, Sandyk, *S Afr Med J* 1982;**62**:592). **Aspirin** may increase phenytoin levels via binding displacement (n=10, open, 11/7, Leonard *et al*, *Clin Pharmacol Ther* 1981;**29**:56–60), and transient toxicity may occur, as it can with **azapropazone** (n=5, open, Geaney *et al*, *Br J Clin Pharmacol* 1983;**15**:727–34; FFT) and **phenylbutazone** (n=6, open, Neuvonen *et al*, *Eur J Clin Pharmacol* 1979;**15**:263–8).

ORAL CONTRACEPTIVES + PHENYTOIN

Contraceptive failure via enzyme induction is well established. See oral contraceptives + carbamazepine for advice (see *4.4.1*).

Oxcarbazepine + phenytoin

See oxcarbazepine (*4.5.3*).

Paroxetine + phenytoin

See paroxetine (*4.3.2.4*).

Pethidine + phenytoin

A reduction of pethidine's effect is possible, with increased pethidine metabolite levels (n=4, open, Pond and Kretschzmar, *Clin Pharmacol Ther* 1981;**30**:680–6).

Phenindione + phenytoin

No interaction is thought to occur (n=54, open, Skovsted *et al*, *Acta Med Scand* 1976;**199**:513–5).

Pregabalin + phenytoin

See pregabalin (*4.1.5*).

PROGABIDE + PHENYTOIN

Phenytoin levels may rise by up to 40% (n=6, open, Bianchetti *et al*, *Epilepsia* 1987;**28**:68–73).

Propoxyphene + phenytoin

Phenytoin levels can be raised by high doses (Kutt *et al*, *Ann N Y Acad Sci* 1971;**179**:705–

4

22), but not normal doses of propoxyphene (n=16, open, Hansen *et al*, *Acta Neurol Scand* 1980;**61**:357–67).

Protein kinase inhibitors + phenytoin

Phenytoin decreases **gefitinib**'s levels by about 26% (n=18, RCT, open, c/o, Chhun *et al*, *Br J Clin Pharmacol* 2009;**68**:226–37; FFT) and **imatinib**'s by up to 2.9-fold (n<224, p/c, Pursche *et al*, *Curr Clin Pharmacol* 2008;**3**:198–203; FFT).

Proton-pump inhibitors + phenytoin

Omeprazole (n=10, RCT, d/b, c/o, 9/7, Prichard *et al*, *Br J Clin Pharmacol* 1987;**24**:543–5; FFT) and **pantoprazole** (n=23, RCT, d/b, p/c, c/o, Middle *et al*, *Int J Clin Pharmacol Ther* 1996;**34**:S72–S75) have no significant effect on phenytoin kinetics.

Pyridoxine + phenytoin

Large doses of pyridoxine (e.g. 200mg/d) can reduce phenytoin levels by up to 40–50% (Hansson and Sillanpaa, *Lancet* 1976;**1**:256).

Quetiapine + phenytoin

See quetiapine (*4.2.7*).

QUINIDINE + PHENYTOIN

A reduced quinidine effect may occur via enzyme induction (Anon, *N Engl J Med* 1983;**308**:724–5).

RIFAMPICIN + PHENYTOIN *

Significant reductions in phenytoin levels may occur via enzyme induction (eg. n=1, Van Berkel *et al*, *Pharmacotherapy* 2013;**33**:e96–100).

Rufinamide + phenytoin

Rufinamide plasma levels are reduced by phenytoin (UK SmPC) and phenytoin clearance is reduced by rufinamide.

Sertraline + phenytoin

See sertraline (*4.3.2.5*).

Shankhapushpi + phenytoin

Avoid the Ayurvedic herbal mixture shankhapushpi, as decreased phenytoin levels may occur (see Fugh-Berman, *Lancet* 2000; **355**:134–8).

Sodium oxybate + phenytoin

See sodium oxybate (*4.6.18*).

Statins + phenytoin *

Phenytoin can reduce **atorvastatin** levels by about 54% and Cmax by 24% (n=119, Bullman *et al*, *Epilepsia* 2011;**52**:1351–8) and significantly reduce the therapeutic effect of **simvastatin** probably via CYP3A4 induction (e.g. n=1, Khandwala, *South Med J* 2006;**99**:1385–7).

St John's wort + phenytoin

See St John's wort (*4.3.3.10*).

SUCRALFATE + PHENYTOIN

A small reduction in phenytoin absorption (n=9, open, Hall *et al*, *Drug Intell Clin Pharm* 1986;**20**:607–11) can be avoided by giving phenytoin two hours or more after sucralfate.

Sulphonamides + phenytoin

Phenytoin toxicity can occur with co-trimoxazole (Gillman and Sandyk, *Ann Intern Med* 1985;**102**:559) and other sulphonamides.

Temozolomide + phenytoin

There is a reported case of delirium (n=1, Levy, *Psychosomatics* 2007;**48**:359–60).

Theophylline + phenytoin

Phenytoin increases theophylline's clearance by 45% (n=8, open, Adebayo, *Clin Exp Pharmacol Physiol* 1988;**15**:883–7). Phenytoin absorption may also be reduced, avoidable by separating the doses by 1–2 hours.

Tiagabine + phenytoin

Tiagabine levels are reduced by up to 3-fold, probably by CYP3A4 induction. There is no effect on phenytoin.

Ticlopidine + phenytoin

Ticlopidine inhibits phenytoin clearance so dose adjustment may be needed (n=6, Donahue *et al*, *Clin Pharmacol Therapeut* 1999;**66**:563–8).

Tolbutamide + phenytoin

Mild phenytoin toxicity may occur via increased free levels (n=18, Tassaneeyakul *et al*, *Br J Clin Pharmacol* 1992;**34**:494–8; FFT).

Topiramate + phenytoin

See topiramate (*4.5.6*).

Trazodone + phenytoin

Phenytoin toxicity has occurred with high-dose trazodone (n=1, Dorn, *J Clin Psychiatry* 1986;**47**:89–90).

TRIAZOLE ANTIFUNGALS + PHENYTOIN

Continuous phenytoin plasma monitoring is recommended with higher doses of **ketoconazole, miconazole** and **fluconazole** (n=20, RCT, p/c, Blum *et al*, *Clin Pharmacol Ther* 1991;**49**:420–5) as rapid and severe toxicity has been reported (e.g. n=1, Helldén *et al*, *Eur J Clin Pharmacol* 2010;**66**:791–5; review by Cadle *et al*, *Ann Pharmacother* 1994;**28**:191–5). Ketoconazole may also have a reduced effect. **Voriconazole** may decrease phenytoin levels dramatically, where even doubling phenytoin dose is insufficient (n=3, Alffenaar *et al*, *Br J Clin Pharmacol* 2009;**68**:462–3; FFT).

TRIMETHOPRIM + PHENYTOIN

Plasma phenytoin levels and the antifolate effect may be increased by trimethoprim.

TRICYCLICS + PHENYTOIN
Phenytoin levels may be raised by **imipramine** (n=2, Perucca and Richens, *Br J Clin Pharmacol* 1977;**4**:485–6), but not **nortriptyline** (Houghton and Richens, *Int J Clin Pharmacol* 1975;**12**:210–6) or **amitriptyline** (Pond *et al*, *Clin Pharmacol Ther* 1975;**18**:191–9), probably due to CYP2C19 inhibition (Shin *et al*, *Drug Metab Dispos* 2002;**30**:1102–7; FFT). Monitor phenytoin levels frequently. Tricyclics may also lower the seizure threshold.

VALPROATE + PHENYTOIN
This interaction is complex and not entirely predictable. Competition for binding sites, saturable metabolism and different ratios of free and bound phenytoin mean standard plasma levels may be misleading. Close and regular monitoring of free levels of phenytoin are essential to avoid toxicity.

VIGABATRIN + PHENYTOIN
Vigabatrin reduces phenytoin levels by 20–30% (n=8, open, Rimmer and Richens, *Br J Clin Pharmacol* 1989;**27**:27S–33S; FFT).

Vincristine + phenytoin
Phenytoin significantly lowers vincristine levels, probably by CYP3A4 induction (n=15, open, Villikka *et al*, *Clin Pharmacol Ther* 1999;**66**:589–93).

WARFARIN + PHENYTOIN
Warfarin metabolism is accelerated by phenytoin reducing its effect, although enhanced levels of both and deaths have been reported (n=1, Panegyres and Rischbieth, *Postgrad Med J* 1991;**67**:98; FFT; Meisheri, *J Ass Physicians India* 1996;**44**:661–23).

Zonisamide + phenytoin
Lack of clinically relevant interaction has been shown (SmPC), although a delayed-onset psychosis has been reported (n=1, Abdoh *et al*, *Am J Ther* 2013;**21**:e15–6).

4.5.6 TOPIRAMATE

Topiramate is 13–17% bound to plasma proteins (and unlikely to interact with highly bound drugs) and not extensively metabolised with no major effect on P450 enzymes. Excretion is mainly via the kidneys. It is not recommended to use topiramate with drugs predisposing to nephrolithiasis (renal stone formation), e.g. **acetazolamide**, **allopurinol**, megadose **ascorbic acid**, **furosemide**, **methyldopa**, **phenolphthalein** abuse, **steroids** and **Worcester sauce** overdose.

Review: Bialer *et al*, *Clin Pharmacokinet* 2004;**43**:763–80.

Antipsychotics + topiramate
Topiramate had no significant effect on the plasma levels of **clozapine** and norclozapine (n=10), **olanzapine** (n=12), **risperidone** and **paliperidone** (n=9), or **quetiapine** (n=7) and was well tolerated (n=38, 6/52, Migliardi *et al*, *Clin Neuropharmacol* 2007;**30**:107–13).

Barbiturates + topiramate
Topiramate has no effect on plasma levels of barbiturates but the effect of barbiturates on topiramate has not been studied.

Carbamazepine + topiramate
Topiramate has no major effect on the plasma levels of CBZ or CBZ-E, although it may increase CBZ levels (n=25, Mack *et al*, *Seizure* 2002;**11**:464–7). Topiramate clearance is increased two-fold by CBZ and half-life reduced (n=12 open, Britzi *et al*, *Epilepsia* 2005;**46**:378–84), and so topiramate doses may need to be lowered if CBZ is reduced or discontinued (n=12, open, Sachdeo *et al*, *Epilepsia* 1996;**37**:774–80).

Citalopram + topiramate
Acute glaucoma has been reported (n=1, Spaccapelo *et al*, *Cases J* 2009;**2**:87; FFT).

Digoxin + topiramate
Topiramate may decrease peak digoxin plasma levels by 16%, possibly by reduced bioavailability.

Eslicarbazepine + topiramate
Lack of significant interaction has been reported (n=32, open, 27/7, Nunes *et al*, *Curr Med Res Opin* 2010;**26**:1355–62).

Fluvoxamine + topiramate
See topiramate + fluvoxamine (*1.3.2.3*).

GHB + topiramate *
Coma and raised GHB levels have been reported (n=1, Weiss *et al*, *Eur J Clin Pharmacol* 2013;**69**:1193–4).

Lamotrigine + topiramate
See lamotrigine (*4.4.2*).

Lithium + topiramate
See lithium (*4.4.3*).

Metformin + topiramate *
There is a modest increase in metformin, and decrease in topiramate levels (open, 10/7, Manitpisitkul *et al*, *Epilepsy Res* 2014;**108**:1519–32).

4

ORAL CONTRACEPTIVES + TOPIRAMATE
Serum estrogen levels are reduced by topiramate in women taking combined oestrogen/progesterone oral contraceptives (see SmPC). See oral contraceptives + carbamazepine for additional advice (see *4.4.1*).

Phenytoin + topiramate
Decreased phenytoin clearance may occur probably via CYP2C19 inhibition (n=12, Sachdeo *et al*, *Epilepsia* 2002;**43**:691–6). Con-versely, topiramate plasma levels are reduced by about 40% by phenytoin, if phenytoin is withdrawn.

Pioglitazone + topiramate *
There is a notable decrease in pioglitazone levels with topiramate (open, 10/7, Manitpisitkul *et al*, *Epilepsy Res* 2014;**108**:1519–32).

Pregabalin + topiramate
See pregabalin (*4.1.5*).

Rufinamide + topiramate
No significant interaction has been seen (SmPC).

Temozolomide + topiramate
Temozolomide does not seem to affect topiramate pharmacokinetics (n=14, Maschio *et al*, *J Neurooncol* 2008;**90**:217–21).

Triamterene + topiramate
There may be an increased risk of renal stone formation in susceptible patients.

Triazole antifungals + topiramate
Posaconazole has been implicated in inducing topiramate toxicity (n=1, Marriott *et al*, *Ann Intern Med* 2009;**151**:143).

Valproate + topiramate *
Topiramate may produce a small but significant increase in valproate clearance, reducing plasma levels, although there may be enhanced valproate side-effects and there are reports of, e.g. apathy, hypothermia and raised LFTs (n=3, Longin *et al*, *Epilepsia* 2002:**43**:451–4), reversible hepatic failure (n=1, Bumb *et al*, *Epileptic Disord* 2003;**5**:157–9), hyperammonaemic encephalopathy (many cases eg. n=11, Noh *et al*, *Epilepsia* 2013;**54**:e1–4; n=1, Blackford *et al*, *J Pediatr Pharmacol Ther* 2013;**18**:128–36) and hypothermia (n=19, Knudsen *et al*, *J Clin Pharm Ther* 2008;**33**:513–9). Topiramate plasma levels are increased by about 15% by valproate, which could be important if valproate is withdrawn.

Zonisamide + topiramate
The UK SmPC recommends caution with the use of zonisamide with carbonic anhydrase inhibitors such as topiramate.

4.6 OTHER DRUGS

4.6.1 ACAMPROSATE

Acamprosate is not protein-bound, is renally excreted and is not significantly metabolised and so has a low liability for drug–drug interactions.

Alcohol + acamprosate
See alcohol (*4.7.1*).

Benzodiazepines + acamprosate
Lack of interaction with diazepam has been shown.

Disulfiram + acamprosate
Lack of interaction has been shown (n=118, RCT, p/c, two years, Besson *et al*, *Alcohol Clin Exp Res* 1998;**22**:573–9).

Food + acamprosate
Food reduces acamprosate's oral absorption.

Naltrexone + acamprosate
See naltrexone (*4.6.16*).

Tricyclics + acamprosate
There is a lack of interaction with imipramine.

4.6.2 ANTICHOLINERGIC OR ANTIMUSCARINIC AGENTS

The antimuscarinic effects of anticholinergics can be enhanced by other drugs with antimuscarinic effects, e.g. antihistamines, tricyclics, phenothiazines, dopaminergic antiparkinsonian agents (e.g. amantadine), antispasmodics and antiarrhythmics (e.g. disopyramide).

Anticholinesterases + anticholinergics
Some antagonism would be expected.

Antipsychotics + anticholinergics
See antipsychotics (*4.2.1*).

Benzodiazepines + anticholinergics
See benzodiazepines (*4.1.1*).

Beta-blockers + anticholinergics
Propantheline increases **atenolol** bioavailability by 36%, increasing its effect (open, Regårdh *et al*, *Biopharm Drug Dispos* 1981;**2**:79–87), but not that of **metoprolol** (n=15, open, Briant *et al*, *Eur J Clin Pharmacol* 1983;**25**:353).

Betel nut + anticholinergics
Heavy betel nut consumption has resulted in severe EPSE, possibly by antagonising procyclidine's effect (n=1, Deahl, *Mov Disord* 1989;**4**:330–2).

H2-blockers + anticholinergics
Cimetidine absorption is reduced (n=8, Kanto *et*

al, *Br J Clin Pharmacol* 1981;**11**:629–31; FFT), but not **ranitidine** (n=12, open, Donn *et al*, *Pharmacother* 1984;**4**:89–92) or **nizatidine** (Knadler *et al*, *Clin Pharmac Ther* 1987;**42**:514–20).

MAOIs + anticholinergics
See MAOIs (*4.3.4*).

Memantine + anticholinergics
See memantine (*4.6.11*).

Nitrofurantoin + anticholinergics
Nitrofurantoin bioavailability may be increased by anticholinergics (n=10, Mannisto, *Int J Clin Pharmacol Biopharm* 1978;**16**:223–8).

Paracetamol + anticholinergics
Propantheline delays paracetamol's absorption (n=6, Nimmo *et al*, *Br Med J* 1973;**1**:587–9; FFT).

Procarbazine + anticholinergics
Increased sedation could occur.

SSRIs + anticholinergics
There are reports of delirium, e.g. with **sertraline** and benzatropine (n=1, Byerly *et al*, *Am J Psychiatry* 1996;**153**:965–6), **paroxetine** and benzatropine (Armstrong and Schweitzer, *Am J Psychiatry* 1997;**154**:581–2) and other SSRIs (n=5, Roth *et al*, *J Clin Psychiatry* 1994;**55**:492–5). CYP2D6 inhibition seems the likely mechanism.

Thiazide diuretics + anticholinergics
Thiazide bioavailability may be enhanced (open, Beermann *et al*, *Eur J Clin Pharmacol* 1978;**13**:385–7).

Tricyclics + anticholinergics
See tricyclics (*4.3.1*).

Venlafaxine + anticholinergics
An acute adverse cutaneous reaction has been reported with venlafaxine and orphenadrine (n=1, Papadimitriou *et al*, *J Eur Acad Dermatol Venereol* 2006;**20**:1019).

Ziprasidone + anticholinergics
See ziprasidone (*4.2.9*).

4.6.3 ANTICHOLINESTERASES

Review: anticholinesterase interactions (Bentué-Ferrer *et al*, *CNS Drugs* 2003;**17**:947–63).

4.6.3.1 DONEPEZIL

Donepezil is metabolised slowly by CYP2D6 and 3A4 to multiple metabolites, only one of which appears to be pharmacologically active.

Anticholinergics + donepezil
See anticholinesterases + anticholinergics (*4.6.2*).

Antipsychotics + donepezil
Donepezil has no effect on **risperidone** pharmacokinetics and is well tolerated (n=31, open, 7/7, Reyes *et al*, *Br J Clin Pharmacol* 2004;**58**[Suppl 1]:50–7; FFT), although severe EPSE (n=1, Magnuson *et al*, *Am J Psychiatry* 1998;**155**:1458–9) have been reported.

Cimetidine + donepezil
Lack of significant pharmacokinetic interaction has been reported (n=19, open, Tiseo *et al*, *Br J Clin Pharmacol* 1998;**46**[Suppl 1]:25–9; FFT).

Clarithromycin + donepezil
Although donepezil levels may be increased by clarithromycin via 3A4 inhibition, there did not seem to be any additional cardiovascular effects (n=59, Hutson *et al*, *Drugs Aging* 2012;**29**:205–11).

Digoxin + donepezil
Lack of significant pharmacokinetic interaction has been reported (n=12, open, Tiseo *et al*, *Br J Clin Pharmacol* 1998;**46**[Suppl 1]:40–4; FFT).

Ketoconazole + donepezil
Donepezil levels may rise by around 25% over a week (n=21, open, Tiseo *et al*, *Br J Clin Pharmacol* 1998;**46**[Suppl 1]:30–4; FFT).

Memantine + donepezil
See anticholinesterases + memantine (*4.6.11*).

NMBAs + donepezil
A synergistic effect could be predicted.

NSAIDs + donepezil
The donepezil SmPC recommends additional monitoring of people at risk of developing ulcers, e.g. if taking concomitant NSAIDs.

SSRIs + donepezil
Lack of interaction has been shown with **sertraline** (n=19 [c=16], RCT, open, c/o, Nagy *et al*, *Br J Clin Pharmacol* 2004;**58**(Suppl 1):25–33; FFT), although reports exist with **paroxetine** (n=1, Carrier, *J Am Geriatr Soc* 1999;**47**:1037) and cholinergic toxidrome with **fluoxetine** (n=1, Marshall *et al*, *J Neuropsychiatry Clin Neurosci* 2012;**24**:E50).

Suxamethonium + donepezil
Donepezil is a cholinesterase inhibitor and would be likely to enhance the effect of suxamethonium-type muscle relaxants (n=1, Crowe and Collins, *Anesthiology* 2003;**98**:574–5), e.g. during ECT (Walker and Perks, *Anesthesia* 2002;**57**:1041).

Theophylline + donepezil
Lack of significant pharmacokinetic interaction has been reported (n=12, open, Tiseo *et al*, *Br J*

4

Clin Pharmacol 1998;**46**[Suppl 1]:35–9; FFT).

Warfarin + donepezil

A lack of significant pharmacokinetic interaction has been reported (n=12, open, Tiseo *et al, Br J Clin Pharmacol* 1998;**46**[Suppl 1]:45–50; FFT).

4.6.3.2 GALANTAMINE

Galantamine is 90% bioavailable, has a large Vd, low protein binding, and is metabolised by CYP2D6 and 3A4. Galantamine has a minimal effect on P450 enzymes (review by Farlow, *Clin Pharmacokinet* 2003;**42**:1383–92).

Anticholinergics + galantamine

See anticholinesterases + anticholinergics (*4.6.2*).

Antipsychotics + galantamine

Lack of interaction has been reported with risperidone (n=16, RCT, open, c/o, Huang *et al, J Clin Pharmacol* 2002;**42**:1341–51).

Beta-blockers + galantamine

As galantamine may cause bradycardia, the SmPC recommends care with drugs that significantly reduce heart rate, e.g. beta-blockers.

Digoxin + galantamine

As galantamine may cause bradycardia, the SmPC recommends care with drugs that significantly reduce heart rate, e.g. digoxin. Galantamine has no effect on digoxin.

Erythromycin + galantamine

A 12% increase in galantamine levels has been reported, probably by CYP3A4 inhibition.

Ketoconazole + galantamine

A 30% increase in galantamine levels has been reported, probably by CYP3A4 inhibition and a reduced dose might be appropriate.

Memantine + galantamine

See memantine (*4.6.11*).

Paroxetine + galantamine

A 40% increase in galantamine plasma levels has been reported, probably by CYP2D6 inhibition, and so a reduced dose might be appropriate.

Suxamethonium + galantamine

Galantamine is likely to enhance the effect of suxamethonium-type muscle relaxants.

Warfarin + galantamine

Galantamine has been shown to have no effect on the kinetics of warfarin.

4.6.3.3 RIVASTIGMINE

Rivastigmine has minimal protein binding, a short half-life, is metabolised by esterases (but with little effect on P450 enzymes) and a lack of significant interaction has been shown with 22 different therapeutic classes (Grossberg *et al, Int J Geriatr Psychiatry* 2000;**15**:242–7).

Anticholinergics + rivastigmine

See anticholinesterases + anticholinergics (*4.6.2*).

Atenolol + rivastigmine

There is a case of true syncope (n=1, Paulison and Léos, *Cardiovasc Toxicol* 2010;**10**:306–10).

Benzodiazepines + rivastigmine

Lack of interaction has been seen (UK SmPC).

Digoxin + rivastigmine

Lack of interaction has been seen (UK SmPC).

Fluoxetine + rivastigmine

Lack of interaction has been seen (UK SmPC).

Memantine + rivastigmine

See anticholinesterases + memantine (*4.6.11*).

Suxamethonium + rivastigmine

Rivastigmine may enhance the effect of suxamethonium-type muscle relaxants during anaesthesia.

Warfarin + rivastigmine

Lack of interaction has been seen (UK SmPC).

4.6.4 ATOMOXETINE *

Atomoxetine is metabolised by 2D6. In poor metabolisers there may be increased ADRs (but moderate to ultra-rapid do not; Fijal *et al, J Clin Pharmacol* 2015; **55**:1167–74), the half-life may be longer (five hours vs 21 hours) and peak levels five times higher, and accumulation can occur (Sauer *et al, Clin Pharmacokinet* 2005;**44**:571–90). 2C19 polymorphisms may affect metabolism (Choi *et al, J Clin Psychopharmacol* 2014;**34**:139–42). It has no clinically significant effect on CYP1A2, 3A4, 2D6 or 2C9. The UK SmPC recommends caution with the potential for potentiation with other noradrenergic drugs, e.g. tricyclics, venlafaxine, reboxetine, mirtazapine, pseudoephedrine or phenylephrine.

ADHD + atomoxetine *

See ADHD + alcohol (*4.7.1*).

Antacids + atomoxetine

Antacids and omeprazole have no effect on atomoxetine bioavailability (UK SmPC).

Aspirin + atomoxetine

Lack of interaction has been shown (UK SmPC).

Benzodiazepines + atomoxetine

Lack of interaction has been shown with diazepam (UK SmPC).

Linezolid + atomoxetine *

Any interaction can be avoided by stopping atomoxetine for four weeks (n=1, Aggarwal *et al, J Child Adolesc Psychopharmacol* 2012;**22**:405).

MAOIs + ATOMOXETINE

A two-week gap is recommended after stopping an MAOI before starting atomoxetine (UK SmPC).

Methylphenidate + atomoxetine

Lack of additive cardiovascular effects has been shown (UK SmPC).

Mirtazapine + atomoxetine

See introduction to *4.6.4*.

Phenytoin + atomoxetine

Lack of interaction has been shown (UK SmPC).

Proton-pump Inhibitors + atomoxetine

See antacids + atomoxetine.

Salbutamol + atomoxetine

Caution is needed with high-dose salbutamol (any route) or other beta-blockers, as the cardiovascular effects can be potentiated (UK SmPC).

SSRIs + atomoxetine

Fluoxetine and paroxetine may increase atomoxetine levels via 2D6 inhibition (UK SmPC).

Tricyclics + atomoxetine

See introduction to *4.6.4*.

Venlafaxine + atomoxetine

There is a case of tic, tremor and speech disturbance, resolving when atomoxetine was discontinued (n=1, Bond *et al, Clin Toxicol [Phila]* 2007;**45**:182–5). See also introduction to *4.6.4*.

Warfarin + atomoxetine

Lack of interaction has been shown (UK SmPC).

4.6.5 BUPRENORPHINE

Buprenorphine has an extensive first-pass metabolism, but sublingual bioavailability is sufficient to allow administration by this route. Half-life can vary widely (3–44 hours), it is highly protein bound (96%), and metabolised by CYP2D6 and 3A4. It is a major inhibitor of 2D6 and 3A4, and probably a weak inhibitor of 1A2, 2B6, 2C9, 2C19 and 2E1 (review by Elkader and Sproule, *Clin Pharmacokinet* 2005;**44**:661–80).

Antiretrovirals + buprenorphine *

Choose your drugs with care (review by Bruce *et al, Clin Infect Dis* 2006;**43**[Suppl 4]:S216–23; FFT):

Antiretrovirals not interacting with buprenorphine:

- Darunavir-ritonavir (n=11, Gruber *et al, Clin Infect Dis* 2012;**54**:414–23; FFT)
- Delavirdine (n=10, McCance-Katz *et al, Clin Infect Dis* 2006;**43**[Suppl 4]:S224–34; FFT)
- Efavirenz (UK SmPC)
- Fosamprenavir-ritonavir (n=10, Gruber *et al, Clin Infect Dis* 2012;**54**:414–23; FFT)
- Lopinavir-ritonavir (e.g. n=12, open, Bruce *et al, J Acquir Immune Defic Syndr* 2010;**54**:511–4)
- Maraviroc
- Nelfinavir (n=7, 15/7, McCance-Katz *et al, Am J Addict* 2010;**19**:30–7; FFT)
- Raltegravir * (n=12, Bruce *et al, Am J Drug Alcohol Abuse* 2013;**39**:80–5)
- Telaprevir: no dose adjustments are needed for either drug, despite a slight reduction in buprenorphine levels (n=14[c=13], open, 7/7, Luo *et al, Antimicrob Agents Chemother* 2012;**56**:3641–7; FFT)
- Tipranavir-ritonavir (n=12[c=10], Bruce *et al, Drug Alcohol Depend* 2009;**105**:234–9; FFT) but see below.

Antiretrovirals interacting with buprenorphine:

- Atazanavir-ritonavir (n=3, Bruce and Altice, *AIDS* 2006;**20**:783–4)
- Elvitegravir-cobicistat: * Buprenorphine AUC and Cmax are modestly increased (n=12, Bruce *et al, J Acquir Immune Defic Syndr* 2013;**63**:480–4)
- Ritonavir can significantly increase buprenorphine's AUC, albeit asymptomatically (n=7, 15/7, McCance-Katz *et al, Am J Addict* 2010;**19**:30–7; FFT)
- Tipranavir levels may be substantially reduced, leading to potential loss of efficacy (n=12[c=10], Bruce *et al, Drug Alcohol Depend* 2009;**105**:234–9; FFT).

Review: Gruber and McCance-Katz, *Curr HIV/AIDS Rep* 2010;**7**:152–60, FFT.

Antivirals + buprenorphine/naloxone *

Lack of interaction has been shown with faldaprevir (n=19[c=14], 8/7, Joseph *et al, Antimicrob Agents Chemother* 2015;**59**:498–504; FFT) and daclatasvir (n=11, open, 10/7, Garimella *et al, J Int AIDS Soc* 2014;**17**(4 Suppl 3):19628; FFT).

Benzodiazepines + buprenorphine

See benzodiazepines (*4.1.1*).

Cocaine + buprenorphine

Regular cocaine users have lower buprenorphine AUC and Cmax (s=90, McCance-Katz *et al, Am J Addict* 2010;**19**:38–46).

4

Codeine + buprenorphine
Buprenorphine does not inhibit codeine transformation to the active morphine-6-glucuronide, and does not reduce its analgesic effects (n=8, Gelston *et al, Br J Clin Pharmacol* 2012;**73**:786–94; FFT).

Ketoconazole + buprenorphine
Start with half doses of buprenorphine due to ketoconazole's CYP3A4 inhibition (SmPC). although there was no interaction between ketoconazole and a once weekly buprenorphine patch (n=20, RCT, d/b, p/c, c/o, 4/52, Kapil *et al, Clin Drug Investig* 2012;**32**:583–92).

Methadone + buprenorphine
See methadone (*4.6.12*).

Tramadol + buprenorphine
Buprenorphine does not seem to inhibit the 2D6-mediated metabolism of tramadol to M1, the major analgesic component, unlike methadone (n=9, Coller *et al, Br J Clin Pharmacol* 2012;**74**:835–41; FFT).

Tricyclics + buprenorphine
See tricyclics (*4.3.1*).

4.6.6 BUPROPION

Bupropion is 84% protein bound and primarily metabolised by CYP2B6, with a significant first-pass metabolism, although poor metabolisers may accumulate hydroxybupropion, leading to reduced efficacy (n=12, Pollock *et al, Ther Drug Monit* 1996;**18**:581–5).

Alcohol + bupropion
There is an increased risk of seizures, so alcohol should be avoided or minimised. There is a case of unexpected aggression (n=1, Chandler and Herxheimer, *Int J Risk Saf Med* 2011;**23**:133–7). Extreme care is needed in overdose, chronic use and alcohol withdrawal states.

Antipsychotics + bupropion *
The CSM recommends caution due to an increased risk of seizures. Delirium has been reported with bupropion and **risperidone** (n=1, Lu *et al, J Clin Psychopharmacol* 2014;**34**:161–2).

Antiretrovirals + bupropion
Single doses of bupropion have no effect on **lopinavir/ritonavir** but **lopinavir/ritonavir** reduces bupropion levels, probably via 2B6 and UGT induction (n=12, 4/52, Hogeland *et al, Clin Pharmacol Ther* 2007;**81**:69–75). **Ritonavir** HD (1200 mg/d) and LD (200 mg/d) decreases bupropion AUC and Cmax by about 65% and 22% respectively, and so increased bupropion dose (by up to 100%) may be needed, but not above the BNF maximum (Park *et al, J Clin Pharmacol* 2010;**50**:1180–7).

Baicalin + bupropion
Baicalin (a Chinese herbal medicine) significantly reduces the plasma levels of bupropion via 2B6 induction (n=17, Fan *et al, Eur J Clin Pharmacol* 2009;**65**:403–9).

Beta-blockers + bupropion
Bupropion produces a 4–6-fold increase in **metoprolol**'s effective plasma levels and so dose reduction may be prudent (Molden and Spigset, *Tidsskr Nor Laegeforen* 2011;**131**:1777–9; FFT).

Carbamazepine + bupropion
Carbamazepine induces bupropion metabolism, markedly decreasing its plasma levels (n=17, RCT, Ketter *et al, J Clin Psychopharmacol* 1995;**15**:327–33).

Ciclosporin + bupropion
A life-threatening decrease in ciclosporin levels has been reported (n=1, Lewis *et al, J Child Adolesc Psychopharmacol* 2001;**11**:193–8).

Cimetidine + bupropion
Cimetidine may inhibit the metabolism of bupropion, although no effect on bupropion SR was seen in one study (n=24, RCT, open, Kustra *et al, J Clin Pharmacol* 1999;**39**:1184–8).

Clonidine + bupropion
Lack of interaction has been reported (n=8, RCT, d/b, c/o, Cubeddu *et al, Clin Pharmacol Ther* 1984;**35**:576–84).

Clopidogrel + bupropion
A single-dose study showed clopidogrel to significantly inhibit bupropion's 2B6 metabolism, increasing AUC by 60% (n=12, Turpeinen *et al, Clin Pharmacol Ther* 2005;**77**:553–9).

Clozapine + bupropion *
See bupropion + clozapine (*4.2.4*).

Escitalopram/dosulepin + bupropion *
Hyponatraemia occurred when bupropion was added to citalopram and dosulepin, the authors concluding this was an interaction rather than a direct side effect of bupropion (n=1, Wiggins *et al, Australas Psychiatry* 2015;**23**:507–9).

Fluoxetine + bupropion
Bupropion produces no significant changes in fluoxetine levels (n=24, open, 8/52, Kennedy *et al, J Clin Psychiatry* 2002;**63**:181–6), but there are reports of panic disorder (n=1, Young, *J Clin*

Psychiatry 1996;**57**: 177–8) and delirium (n=1, Chan *et al*, *J Clin Psychopharmacol* 2006;**26**:677–9).

Fosphenytoin + bupropion
See phenytoin + bupropion.

Ginkgo biloba + bupropion
There is no significant interaction, although hydroxybupropion levels may be reduced (n=14, 2/52, Lei *et al*, *Br J Clin Pharmacol* 2009;**68**:201–6; FFT).

Guanfacine + bupropion
There is a report of a grand mal seizure (n=1, Tilton, *J Am Acad Child Adolesc Psychiatry* 1998;**37**:682–3).

MAOIs + bupropion
Acute bupropion toxicity might occur, and the combination is contraindicated.

Lamotrigine + bupropion
See lamotrigine (*4.4.2*).

Levodopa + bupropion
An increased incidence of side-effects has been reported with the combination.

Moclobemide + bupropion
See MAOIs + bupropion.

Paroxetine + bupropion
Bupropion produces no significant changes in paroxetine levels (open, 8/52, Kennedy *et al*, *J Clin Psychiatry* 2002;**63**:181–6), but the CSM recommends caution.

Phenobarbital + bupropion
Phenobarbital may induce the metabolism of bupropion, which would reduce its efficacy.

Phenytoin + bupropion
Phenytoin may induce the metabolism of bupropion, which would reduce its efficacy.

Pseudoephedrine + bupropion
There is a report of acute myocardial ischaemia (n=1, Pederson *et al*, *Can J Cardiol* 2001;**17**:599–601).

Rifampicin + bupropion
Rifampicin may shorten bupropion's half-life by 50%, probably by CYP2B6 induction (n=18, Loboz *et al*, *Clin Pharmacol Ther* 2006;**80**:75–84).

Selegiline + bupropion
See MAOIs + bupropion.

Sertraline + bupropion
Serotonin syndrome has been reported (n=1, Munhoz, *Clin Neuropharmacol* 2004;**27**:219–22).

Smoking + bupropion
In a single-dose study, cigarettes had no detectable effect on bupropion kinetics (open, Hsyu *et al*, *J Clin Pharmacol* 1997;**37**:737–43).

St John's wort + bupropion
See bupropion + St. John's wort (*4.3.3.10*).

Tamoxifen + bupropion
See tamoxifen + paroxetine (*4.3.2.4*).

Ticlopidine + bupropion
Ticlopidine significantly inhibits bupropion's meta-bolism, increasing its AUC by 85% (n=12, Turpeinen *et al*, *Clin Pharmacol Ther* 2005;**77**:553–9).

Tramadol + bupropion *
There is a risk of serotonin syndrome so monitor, counsel and take extra care with older age, higher doses and with concomitant 2D6 inhibitors (review of n=10, Park *et al*, *J Pharm Pract* 2014;**27**:71–8).

Tricyclics + bupropion
Bupropion may increase **imipramine** and **desipramine** levels, through decreased clearance (n=1, Shad and Preskorn, *J Clin Psychopharmacol* 1997;**17**:118–9). Seizures have also been reported with **trimipramine** (n=1, Enns, *J Clin Psychiatry* 2001;**62**:476–7), **clomipramine** (n=1, Shin *et al*, *Clin Neuropharmacol* 2004;**27**:192–4) and **nortriptyline** (n=1, Weintraub, *Depress Anxiety* 2001;**13**:50–2).

Valproate + bupropion
Valproate does not seem to induce bupropion metabolism, but raised metabolite levels are possible (n=17, RCT, Ketter *et al*, *J Clin Psychopharmacol* 1995;**15**:327–33).

Varenicline + bupropion *
When used together for smoking cessation there is an increased risk of depression at 2 weeks (but not 4/52) compared to varenicline monotherapy (n=505, RCT, 12/52, Hong *et al*, *J Subst Abuse Treat* 2015;**52**:78–81).

Venlafaxine + bupropion
Bupropion can significantly increase venlafaxine levels, sometimes dramatically and requiring dose reduction (n=3, Paslakis *et al*, *J Clin Psychopharmacol* 2010;**30**:473–4), but decrease O-desmethylvenlafaxine levels (open, 8/52, Kennedy *et al*, *J Clin Psychiatry* 2002;**63**:181–6). See also sertraline + bupropion.

Vortioxetine + bupropion *
See vortioxetine (*4.3.3.9*).

Warfarin + bupropion *
Stopping bupropion has led to a doubling of INR, reversible on restarting, when used with warfarin (n=1, Bavle and Phatak, *Indian J Psychol Med* 2013;**35**:311–3).

4

Zolpidem + bupropion
Short-lived visual hallucinations have been reported (e.g. n=5, Elko *et al*, *Clin Toxicol* 1998;**36**:195–203).

4.6.7 CLOMETHIAZOLE

Clomethiazole inhibits CYP2E1.

Alcohol + clomethiazole
See alcohol (*4.7.1*).

Cimetidine + clomethiazole
Cimetidine inhibits the metabolism of clomethiazole, raising plasma levels.

Methadone + clomethiazole
See methadone (*4.6.12*).

4.6.8 DISULFIRAM

Disulfiram is a potent inhibitor of CYP1A2, 2B6 and 2E1 (the enzyme that metabolises ethanol), but chronic use might also alter other enzymes too (n=7, Frye and Branch, *Br J Clin Pharmacol* 2002;**53**:155–62; FFT).

Review: interactions (Enghusen Poulsen *et al*, *Acta Psychiatr Scand* 1992;**86**[Suppl 369]:59–66).

Acamprosate + disulfiram
See acamprosate (*4.6.1*).

ACENOCOUMAROL + DISULFIRAM
An enhanced anticoagulant effect is possible.

ALCOHOL + DISULFIRAM
See disulfiram under 'Alcohol abuse and dependence' (*1.4*) and alcohol (*4.7.1*).

Antipsychotics + disulfiram
Increased first-pass metabolism of perphenazine can lead to relapse of psychosis (n=1, Hansen and Larsen, *Lancet* 1982;**2**:1472).

Antiretrovirals + disulfiram *
Efavirenz increases disulfiram's effect (possibly by 3A4 induction) whereas **atazanavir** decreases disulfiram's effect (possibly by 3A4 inhibition) but disulfiram has no effect on any antiretroviral tested (n=40, McCance-Katz *et al*, *Am J Addict* 2014;**23**:137–44).

Benzodiazepines + disulfiram
Disulfiram may inhibit the metabolism of **diazepam, chlordiazepoxide** and **temazepam** (n=1, Hardman *et al*, *Lancet* 1994;**344**:1231–2), leading to lengthened half-lives, but not with **oxazepam** (open, MacLeod, *Clin Pharmacol Ther* 1978;**24**:583–9) or **alprazolam** (n=11, 2/52, Diquet *et al*, *Eur J Clin Pharmacol* 1990;**38**:157–60).

Caffeine + disulfiram
Disulfiram may reduce caffeine clearance by 50% (n=21, open, Beach *et al*, *Clin Pharmacol Ther* 1986;**39**:265–70).

Cannabis + disulfiram
See cannabis (*4.7.2*).

Carbamazepine + disulfiram
Lack of interaction has been shown (n=7, open, Krag *et al*, *Acta Neurol* 1981;**63**:395–8).

Cocaine + disulfiram
Disulfiram does not seem to enhance to c/v effects of cocaine and might reduce the subjective high (n=22, RCT, d/b, p/c, Roache *et al*, *Drug Alcohol Depend* 2011;**119**:37–45; FFT), although there is a case of pronounced paranoia (n=1, Mutschler *et al*, *J Clin Psychopharmacol* 2009;**29**:99–101).

Colchicine + disulfiram
A potentially fatal interaction has been reported (Chen *et al*, *Prog Neuropsychopharmacol Biol Psychiatry* 2009;**33**:1281).

Griseofulvin + disulfiram *
Delirium has been reported with the combination (n=1, Cheng *et al*, *J Clin Psychopharmacol* 2015;**35**:477–8).

Isoniazid + disulfiram
CNS toxicity has been reported (Rothstein, *JAMA* 1972;**219**:1216).

Lithium + disulfiram
There is no theoretical or clinical reasons why an interaction should occur.

MAOIs + disulfiram
Delirium has been reported (e.g. n=1, Blansjaar and Egberts, *Am J Psychiatry* 1995;**152**:296).

Methadone + disulfiram
See methadone (*4.6.12*).

Methylphenidate + disulfiram
See methylphenidate (*4.6.13*).

Metronidazole + disulfiram *
Psychosis has been reported (eg. n=1, Luykx *et al*, *J Clin Psychopharmacol* 2013;**33**:136–7).

Omeprazole + disulfiram
There is a report of confusion, disorientation and catatonia with the combination (n=1, Hajela *et al*, *CMAJ* 1990;**143**:1207–8; FFT).

Paraldehyde + disulfiram
An enhanced disulfiram reaction is possible (mentioned in Hadden and Metzner, *Am J Med* 1969;**47**:642–7).

Phenytoin + disulfiram
See phenytoin (*4.5.5*).

Theophylline + disulfiram
Theophylline levels may be increased via enzyme inhibition. Monitor and reduce the theophylline dose if necessary (n=20, RCT, Loi *et al, Clin Pharmacol Ther* 1989;**45**:476–86).

Tricyclics + disulfiram
See tricyclics (*4.3.1*).

WARFARIN + DISULFIRAM
Prothrombin time can fall by about 10%, with one study showing a marked effect with reduced warfarin doses sometimes necessary (n=7, open, O'Reilly, *Clin Pharmacol Ther* 1981;**29**:332).

4.6.9 GUANFACINE

Guanfacine is a substrate of CYP3A4 but has no effect on major CYP enzymes. Use with 3A4 inhibitors or inducers may require guanfacine dose reduction or increases respectively. Additive sedation can occur with other sedative drugs.

Antihypertensives + guanfacine
Potentiation of hypotension can occur (SmPC).

Antipsychotics + guanfacine
Additive sedation can occur (SmPC).

Benzodiazepines + guanfacine
Additive sedation can occur (SmPC).

KETOCONAZOLE + GUANFACINE
Ketoconazole inhibits CYP3A4 leading to potentially toxic guanfacine levels (SmPC).

Lisdexamfetamine + guanfacine
Although guanfacine's Cmax may be increased by 17% and AUC by 7%, dose adjustment is not considered necessary (SmPC).

Methylphenidate + guanfacine
Lack of interaction has been shown (SmPC).

QT-prolonging drugs + guanfacine
Guanfacine can slow the heart rate and so use with QT-prolonging drugs is not recommended (SmPC).

Rifampicin + guanfacine
Rifampicin induces CYP3A4, leading to potentially sub-therapeutic guanfacine levels (SmPC).

Valproate + guanfacine *
Raised valproate levels can occur, possibly via an effect on glucuronidation so monitor valproate carefully (SmPC).

4.6.10 LISDEXAMFETAMINE (LDX)

Lisdexamfetamine has minor inhibiting effect on CYP1A2, 2D6 and 3A4. All antipsychotics can block the dopaminergic effects of LDX and LDX could counteract the dopamine blockade from antipsychotics.

Alcohol + lisdexamfetamine *
See ADHD + alcohol (*4.7.1*).

Ascorbic acid + lisdexamfetamine
Ascorbic acid acidifies urine and can decrease the half-life of lisdexamfetamine.

Guanfacine + lisdexamfetamine
See lisdexamfetamine + guanfacine (*4.6.9*).

Lithium + lisdexamfetamine
Lithium may inhibit the anorectic and stimulatory effects of lisdexamfetamine (UK SmPC).

MAOIs + LISDEXAMFETAMINE
LDX should not be used with MAOIs, or for 14 days after stopping them.

Venlafaxine + lisdexamfetamine
Lack of a clinically significant interaction has been shown (UK SmPC).

4.6.11 MEMANTINE

Memantine is only minimally metabolised, does not inhibit CYP1A2, 2A6, 2C9, 2D6, 2E1 or 3A, the FMO system, or epoxide hydrolase or sulphation, and so metabolic interactions are unlikely. Raised urinary pH (e.g. infections, diet change, excessive alkalising gastric buffers, etc) may significantly reduce excretion. Plasma protein binding is 45%.

Alcohol + memantine
See alcohol (*4.7.1*).

Amantadine + memantine
Both are NMDA-antagonists and the combination should be avoided as CNS ADRs may be more frequent. The same may be true with ketamine and dextromethorphan.

Anticholinergics + memantine
The anticholinergic's effects may be enhanced by memantine.

Anticholinesterases + memantine *
Lack of interaction has been shown with **donepezil** (n=19, open, Periclou *et al, Ann Pharmacother* 2004;**38**:1389–94) or **rivastigmine** (n=16, open, c/o, 7/52, Shua-Haim *et al, Clin Drug Investig* 2008;**8**:361–74), but PR prolongation has been reported (n=1, Igeta *et al, Gen Hosp Psych* 2013;**35**:680.e-680.e10). See *C1* for the positive effects of the combination. Donepezil 28mg and memantine 10mg are available as a combined product in USA (Namzaric®) (Greig,

4

CNS Drugs 2015;**29**:963–70).

Antipsychotics + memantine

The antipsychotic effects may be reduced by memantine.

Antispasmodic agents + memantine

The effects may be modified by memantine and dose adjustment may be necessary.

Baclofen + memantine

Baclofen's effects may be modified by memantine and dose adjustment may be necessary (SmPC).

Dantrolene + memantine

Dantrolene's effects may be modified by memantine and dose adjustment necessary.

Dextromethorphan + memantine

See amantadine + memantine.

Dopamine agonists + memantine

Dopamine antagonists such as bromocriptine may be enhanced by memantine.

H2-blockers + memantine

A theoretical interaction via competition for cationic transport system exists and there is the potential for increased memantine plasma levels.

Hydrochlorthiazide + memantine

There is a theoretical possibility of a reduced diuretic effect.

Ketamine + memantine

See amantadine + memantine.

Levodopa + memantine

The effects of levodopa may be enhanced by memantine.

Phenobarbital + memantine

The barbiturate's effects may be reduced by memantine.

Phenytoin + memantine

There is one case report of interaction (SmPC).

Procainamide + memantine

See H2-blockers + memantine.

Quinidine/quinine + memantine

See H2-blockers + memantine.

Smoking + memantine

See H2-blockers + memantine.

4.6.12 METHADONE *

Methadone is probably metabolised mainly by CYP3A4 (or not, as the case may be; Kharasch *et al, Clin Pharmacol Ther* 2008;**84**:506–12; FFT) and partly by 2D6 (but genotype has no apparent effect on clearance; Coller *et al, Int J Clin Pharmacol Ther* 2007;**45**:410–7), 1A2 and possibly by 2B6 and 2C19 (n=366, Tsai *et al, Pharmacogenomics* 2014;**15**:977–86). It inhibits CYP2D6, 3A4, UGT2B4 and UGT2B7. Absorption is also variable according to P-glycoprotein status. The (R)-methadone is the active moiety, (S)-methadone being inactive.

Alcohol + methadone

See alcohol (*4.7.1*).

Antipsychotics + methadone

See methadone + antipsychotics (*4.2.1*).

Antiretrovirals + methadone

Antiretrovirals and methadone are not an uncommon combination, and some (but not all) retrovirals can reduce methadone levels significantly, by 3A4 induction and *vice versa*:

Antiretrovirals not interacting with methadone:

- Elvitegravir-cobicistat (n=11, 2/52, Bruce *et al, Antimicrob Agents Chemother* 2013;**57**:6154–7)
- Fosamprenavir-ritonavir can reduce methadone AUC by 18%, considered insignificant (n=26, 18/7, Cao *et al, Pharmacotherapy* 2008;**28**:863–74)
- Indinavir (n=12, c/o, Kharasch *et al, Anesthesiology* 2012;**116**:432–47; FFT)
- Maraviroc (SmPC)
- Raltegravir (n=12, Anderson *et al, J Clin Pharmacol* 2010;**50**:1461–6)
- Saquinavir-ritonavir (n=12, Gerber *et al, J AIDS* 2001;**27**:153–60).

Antiretrovirals interacting with methadone:

- Atazanavir is a potent CYP3A4 inhibitor. One study showed no clinically relevant interaction and no dose adjustments needed (n=16, 2/52, Friedland *et al, AIDS* 2005;**19**:1635–41), but in another methadone reduced atazanavir plasma levels and AUC by around 40%, which may well be clinically significant (n=24, Haberl *et al, Eur J Clin Pharmacol* 2010;**66**:375–81)
- Didanosine levels can be reduced by about 40% by methadone (n=27, open, Rainer *et al, J AIDS* 2000;**24**:241–8)
- Efavirenz can induce (and inhibit) CYP3A4 and decrease methadone levels by 50–70% (Kharasch *et al, Clin Pharmacol Ther* 2012;**91**:673–84; FFT) which can produce withdrawal symptoms (e.g. n=9+52 controls, Esteban *et al, Drug Metab Lett* 2008;**2**:269–79)
- Nelfinavir can induce methadone metabolism, with levels reduced by 40–50%

(n = 12, Kharasch *et al*, *Drug Alcohol Depend* 2009;**101**:158–68; FFT)

- **Nevirapine** can reduce methadone levels and AUC by 47% (UK SmPC) via CYP3A4 induction, precipitating withdrawal (e.g. n = 57 controls, Esteban *et al*, *Drug Metab Lett* 2008;**2**:269–79). In patients receiving HAART, monitor levels and withdrawal carefully (n = 9, Pelet *et al*, *Am J Drug Alcohol Abuse* 2011;**37**:264–8)
- **Ritonavir** may reduce methadone levels by 40–50% (Kharasch *et al*, *Clin Pharmacol Ther* 2008;**84**:497–505; FFT; n = 1, Geletko and Erickson, *Pharmacother* 2000;**20**:93–4)
- **Zidovudine** levels can be raised by methadone, with AUC increased by 41% (n = 8, McCance-Katz *et al*, *J Acquir Immune Defic Synd Hum Retrivirol* 1998;**18**:435–43).

Review: Gruber and McCance-Katz, *Curr HIV/AIDS Rep* 2010;**7**: 152–60; FFT.

Antivirals + methadone *

Lack of clinically meaningful interaction has been shown with daclatasvir (n = 14, open, 10/7, Garimella *et al*, *J Int AIDS Soc* 2014;**17**(4 Suppl 3): 19628; FFT) and faldaprevir (n = 15[c = 15], 8/7, Joseph *et al*, *Antimicrob Agents Chemother* 2015; **59**:498–504; FFT).

Ascorbic acid + methadone

Vitamin C and other urine acidifiers (e.g. ammonium chloride) can decrease methadone plasma levels via increased renal excretion if the pH is less than 6. Methadone's half-life can be halved to around 19–20 hours.

Azithromycin + methadone *

Death from sudden cardiac arrest has been reported, probably due to QTc prolongation (n = 1, 3/7, Winton and Twilla, *Am J Med Sci* 2013; **345**:160–2).

Benzodiazepines + methadone *

Apart from additive sedation (e.g. n = 5, RCT, Preston *et al*, *Drug Alc Dep* 1986;**18**:195–202) illicit BDZ use with methadone is associated with higher hospitalisation rates, greater ICU use and worse medical outcomes than non-BDZ use (n = 744, Lee *et al*, *Drug Alcohol Depend* 2014;**138**:118–23), as well as a greater QTc prolongation than methadone alone (n = 421, Peles *et al*, *J Addict Med* 2013;**7**:428–34).

Buprenorphine + methadone

An antagonistic effect would be predicted and buprenorphine might displace methadone from Mu-opioid receptors, precipitating withdrawal. Enhanced sedation and respiratory depression may occur.

Cannabis + methadone *

There is no major interaction, although cannabis may reduce methadone withdrawal symptoms (n = 91, RCT, Pani *et al*, *Cochrane Database Syst Rev* 2013;**6**:CD008939).

Carbamazepine + methadone

Reduced methadone levels can occur through CYP3A4 induction (Ketter *et al*, *J Clin Psychopharmacol* 1991;**11**:198–203; n = 43, Bell *et al*, *Clin Pharmacol Ther* 1988;**43**:623–9), and methadone-induced respiratory depression has been reported after withdrawal of carbamazepine (n = 1, Benítez-Rosario *et al*, *J Pain Symptom Manage* 2006;**32**:99–100).

Chloral + methadone

Additive sedation can occur (SmPC).

Cimetidine + methadone

Raised methadone levels can occur (SmPC).

CIPROFLOXACIN + METHADONE

A course of ciprofloxacin has caused sudden and profound methadone toxicity (n = 1, Herrlin *et al*, *Lancet* 2000;**356**:2069–70) and QTc prolongation leading to torsades de pointes (n = 1, Nair *et al*, *Addiction* 2008;**103**:2062–4). The UK SmPC now says to avoid the combination.

Clomethiazole + methadone

Additive sedation can occur.

Cocaine + methadone *

Regular cocaine users show lower methadone Cmax and AUC (n = 39, retrospective, McCance-Katz *et al*, *Am J Addict* 2010;**19**:47–52) possibly by accelerated methadone elimination (review by Moolchan *et al*, *J Addict Dis* 2001;**20**:55–73). Although methadone causes prolonged QTc, addition of cocaine does not seem to increase the risk (n = 180, Roy *et al*, *Addiction* 2012;**107**:1132–9; n = 421, Peles *et al*, *J Addict Med* 2013;**7**:428–34).

Codeine + methadone

Methadone inhibits codeine metabolism to active morphine-6-glucuronide, possibly reducing the analgesic effects (n = 10, Gelston *et al*, *Br J Clin Pharmacol* 2012;**73**:786–94; FFT).

Cyclizine + methadone

There are rare reports of hallucinations.

Dextromethorphan + methadone

Delirium, hypersomnia and confusion has been reported (n = 1, Lotrich *et al*, *Am J Geriatr Pharmacother* 2005;**3**:17–20).

Diphenhydramine + methadone
There are rare reports of additional CNS effects.

Disulfiram + methadone
Lack of kinetic interaction has been shown (n=7, Tong *et al, J Clin Pharmacol* 1980;**20**:506–13).

Domperidone + methadone
Increased absorption has been reported.

Erythromycin + methadone
Raised methadone levels could occur through CYP3A4 inhibition and the UK SmPC now says to avoid the combination.

Fluoxetine + methadone
Lack of significant interaction has been shown (n=16, open, 9/52, Batki *et al, J Clin Psychopharmacol* 1993;**13**:243–50).

Fluvoxamine + methadone
Fluvoxamine may inhibit methadone metabolism leading to raised levels (n=1, DeMaria and Serota, *J Addict Dis* 1999;**18**:5–12) and severe hypoventilation has been reported (n=1, Alderman and Frith, *Aust N Z J Psychiatry* 1999; **33**:99–101).

Fosphenytoin + methadone
See phenytoin.

Grapefruit juice + methadone
Raised methadone levels through CYP3A4 inhibition could theoretically occur.

Hypnotics + methadone
Enhanced sedation can occur.

Letrozole + methadone
Letrozole reduces methadone clearance by 22%, suggesting that methadone may be metabolised by aromatase and this may explain the unpredictable variation in methadone levels (n=15, Lu *et al, J Clin Psychopharmacol* 2012;**32**:511–7), e.g. two reported cases of co-administration produced marked methadone toxicity in one and no change in the other (n=2, Lu *et al, J Med Case Reports* 2011;**5**:513; FFT).

Lofexidine + methadone
Lofexidine decreases sitting systolic and diastolic bp by 27 and 15 mmHg respectively, and reduced cognitive efficiency compared to placebo when given with methadone, so monitor for cardiovascular and cognitive changes if using the combination (n=14, d/b, p/c, 11/52, Schroeder *et al, Pharmacotherapy* 2007;**27**:1111–9).

MAOIs + methadone
See MAOIs (*4.3.4*).

Metyrapone + methadone
Metyrapone can cause a withdrawal-like syndrome with methadone (n=15, open, Kennedy *et al, Br J Addict* 1990;**85**:1133–40).

Naloxone + methadone
This opiate antagonist can block the effect of methadone within 5–10 minutes if given by injection (Tornabene, *Ann Intern Med* 1974;**81**:785–7).

Naltrexone + methadone
This opiate antagonist would block the effect of methadone.

Paroxetine + methadone
See paroxetine (*4.3.2.4*).

Phenobarbital + methadone
Enhanced sedation and respiratory depression may occur. Reduced methadone levels have been reported with phenobarbital (e.g. n=43, Bell *et al, Clin Pharmacol Ther* 1988;**43**:623–9).

PHENYTOIN + METHADONE
Reduced methadone levels can occur through CYP3A4 induction, with withdrawal symptoms occurring within four days (n=43, Bell *et al, Clin Pharmacol Ther* 1988;**43**:623–9). Dosage adjustment may be needed.

Quetiapine + methadone
Quetiapine increases the plasma levels of the active R-methadone enantiomer by about 20%, possibly by CYP2D6 inhibition, but this is highly variable and probably not clinically significant, (n=14, Uehlinger *et al, J Clin Psychopharmacol* 2007;**27**:273–8).

Reboxetine + methadone
See reboxetine (*4.3.3.6*).

Rifampicin + methadone
Methadone levels reduce by 30–65% within 4–5 days in 70% patients given rifampicin, via CYP3A4 induction (n=30, Kreek *et al, N Engl J Med* 1976;**294**:1104–6).

Risperidone + methadone
There is a report of possible interaction, resulting in irritability and aches (n=1, Wines and Weiss, *J Clin Psychopharmacol* 1999:**19**:65–7).

Sodium bicarbonate + methadone
Sodium bicarbonate and other urinary alkalinisers can increase plasma levels via decreased renal excretion.

St John's wort + methadone
See St John's wort (*4.3.3.10*).

Telaprevir + methadone *
Although methadone exposure is reduced (by about 30%) dose reduction is probably not required (n=16, 1/52, van Heeswijk *et al,*

Antimicrob Agents Chemother 2013;**57**:2304–9).

Ticlopidine + methadone *

Ticlopidine (related to clopidogrel) increases the AUC for R- and S-methadone by 20% and 60% respectively (Kharasch *et al*, *J Clin Pharmacol* 2013; **53**:305–13).

Tramadol + methadone

Methadone inhibits the 2D6-mediated metabolism of tramadol to M1, the major analgesic component, unlike buprenorphine (n=9, Coller *et al*, *Br J Clin Pharmacol* 2012;**74**:835–41; FFT).

TRIAZOLE ANTIFUNGALS + METHADONE

Methadone levels can rise by a mean of 27% through CYP3A4 inhibition, although one study did not detect any signs of toxicity with **fluconazole** (n=25, RCT, d/b, p/c, 14/7, Cobb *et al*, *Clin Pharmacol Ther* 1998;**63**:655–62). Torsade de pointes has been reported after two doses of **itraconazole** in someone taking methadone (n=1, NoorZurani *et al*, *Drug Alcohol Rev* 2009;**28**:688–90). The UK SmPC now says to avoid the combination of methadone and any triazole.

Tricyclics + methadone

Additive sedation might occur and methadone can double desipramine blood levels (n=5, Maany *et al*, *Am J Psychiatry* 1989;**146**:1611–3).

4.6.13 METHYLPHENIDATE

Alcohol + methylphenidate *

See ADHD + alcohol (*4.7.1*).

Atomoxetine + methylphenidate

See atomoxetine (*4.6.4*).

Carbamazepine + methylphenidate

Carbamazepine has been reported to cause an extreme reduction of methylphenidate levels (n=1, Behar *et al*, *J Am Acad Child Adolesc Psychiatry* 1998;**37**:1128–9).

Ciclosporin + methylphenidate

A rise in ciclosporin levels has been reported with methylphenidate (n=1, Lewis *et al*, *J Child Adolesc Psychopharmacol* 2001;**11**:193–8).

Cocaine + methylphenidate

No pharmacokinetic or physiological interaction seems to occur (n=7, p/c, Winhusen *et al*, *Pharmacol Biochem Behav* 2006;**85**:29–38), but psychosis has been reported (n=1, Delavenne *et al*, *Gen Hosp Psychiatry* 2013;**35**:451.e7–9).

Disulfiram + methylphenidate

There is a case of an acute-onset psychotic episode after a single dose of methylphenidate in someone taking disulfiram 400mg/d (n=1, Caci and Baylé, *Am J Psychiatry* 2007;**164**:1759).

Fluoxetine + methylphenidate

Hallucinations have been reported (n=1, Coskun and Zoroglu, *J Clin Psychopharmacol* 2008;**28**:723–5).

Glipizide + methylphenidate

A 26% reduction in plasma glucose has been reported when methylphenidate was started in a woman on glipizide (n=1, Gontkovsky *et al*, *Clin Drug Investig* 2007:**27**:719–25).

Guanfacine + methylphenidate

See methylphenidate + guanfacine (*4.6.9*).

MAOIs + methylphenidate

See MAOIs (*4.3.4*).

Modafinil + methylphenidate

See modafinil (*4.6.14*).

Paroxetine + methylphenidate

Manic switch and serotonin syndrome has been reported (n=1, Park and Jung, *Prog Neuropsychopharmacol Biol Psychiatry* 2010;**34**:719–20).

Phenytoin + methylphenidate

Phenytoin toxicity has been reported (n=3, Ghofrani, *Dev Med Child Neurol* 1988;**30**:267–8).

Sertraline + methylphenidate

Seizures (n=1, Schertz and Steinberg, *J Child Adolesc Psychopharmacol* 2008;**18**:301–3) and serotonin syndrome (n=1, Ishii *et al*, *Psychiatry Clin Neurosci* 2008;**62**:246) have been reported.

St John's wort + methylphenidate

It has been suggested that SJW may reduce the efficacy of methylphenidate in ADHD (Niederhofer, *Med Hypotheses* 2007;**68**:1189).

Tricyclics + methylphenidate

Methylphenidate may inhibit the metabolism of **imipramine** producing up to a four-fold increase in levels, with mood and cognitive impairment (e.g. n=2, Grob and Coyle, *J Dev Behav Pediatrics* 1986;**7**:265–7).

Valproate + methylphenidate

Rapid onset severe dyskinesia and bruxism have been reported (n=2, Gara and Roberts, *J Child Adolesc Psychopharmacol* 2000;**10**:39–43).

4.6.14 MODAFINIL

Modafinil is moderately bound to plasma proteins (62%), essentially to albumin. Renal excretion is the main route of elimination, but it is also metabolised by CYP3A4. It inhibits

4

2C19, 2D6 and has a small and concentration-dependent induction of 1A2, 2B6 and 3A4 (Robertson and Hellriegel, *Clin Pharmacokinet* 2003;**42**:123–37). It has two inactive metabolites.

Amfetamines + modafinil

Low dose amfetamines e.g. dexamfetamine have no significant effects on steady-state modafinil levels (n=32, RCT, open, Hellriegel *et al*, *J Clin Pharmacol* 2002;**42**:450–60).

Benzodiazepines + modafinil

Triazolam levels may be significantly reduced, probably via 3A4 induction (n=41, RCT, 4/52, Robertson, *Clin Pharmacol Ther* 2002;**71**:46–56).

Carbamazepine + modafinil

Carbamazepine might reduce plasma modafinil levels (SmPC).

Ciclosporin + modafinil

The UK SmPC reports a case of a 50% reduction in ciclosporin levels with modafinil.

Cocaine + modafinil *

IV cocaine has no apparent medical or cardiac interaction with modafinil (e.g. n=12, Malcolm *et al*, *Am J Drug Alcohol Abuse* 2006;**32**:577–87). Modafinil blunts the euphorant effects of cocaine, but escitalopram does not enhance this (n=64, RCT, d/b, p/c, 5/7, Verrico *et al*, *Drug Alcohol Depend* 2014;**141**:72–8).

Ethinylestradiol + modafinil

Ethinylestradiol levels may be reduced by modafinil, probably via 3A4 induction (n=41, RCT, 4/52, Robertson, *Clin Pharmacol Ther* 2002;**71**:46–56).

MAOI + modafinil

See MAOIs (*4.3.4*).

Methylphenidate + modafinil

Low-dose methylphenidate does not appear to interact with modafinil (n=32, RCT, open, Hellriegel *et al*, *J Clin Pharmacol* 2002;**41**:895–904), although modafinil absorption may be reduced (open, RCT, c/o, Wong *et al*, *J Clin Pharmacol* 1998;**38**:276–82).

ORAL CONTRACEPTIVES + MODAFINIL

Modafinil can reduce OC efficacy via 3A4 induction (and for up to two months after stopping). Alternative contraceptive methods or higher dose oral contraceptives containing 50mcg ethinylestradiol should be used.

Phenobarbital + modafinil

Phenobarbital might reduce plasma modafinil levels (SmPC).

Phenytoin + modafinil

Phenytoin's clearance might be reduced by modafinil (SmPC).

Sodium oxybate + modafinil

See sodium oxybate (*4.6.18*).

Tricyclics + modafinil *

A single dose study showed a clinically important interaction with clomipramine 50mg/d (n=1, Grozinger *et al*, *Clin Neuropharmacol* 1998;**21**:127–9).

Warfarin + modafinil

A single-dose study suggested no interaction (n=28, Robertson *et al*, *J Clin Pharmacol* 2002;**42**:205–14), but additional monitoring is needed as warfarin clearance may be reduced (SmPC).

4.6.15 NALMEFENE

Nalmefene is about 45% bound to plasma proteins, is metabolised primarily by glucuronidation to inactive or minimally active metabolites, and 5% is excreted unchanged in the urine. There may be some enterohepatic recycling. Lack of significant interaction has been shown with UGT2B7 inhibitors and inducers.

Alcohol + nalmefene

Lack of interaction has been shown (UK SmPC).

Benzodiazepines + nalmefene

Lack of interaction has been shown (US PI).

Fentanyl intranasal + nalmefene

Nalmefene decreases the effects of fentanyl intranasal by pharmacodynamic antagonism. This might be significant and may precipitate withdrawal in opioid-dependent patients, so avoid the combination.

Flumazenil + nalmefene

No adverse effects are anticipated but care would be prudent as animal studies show an unpredictable effect on seizures (SmPC).

Inhaled anaesthetics + nalmefene

Lack of interaction has been shown (US PI).

Muscle relaxants + nalmefene

Lack of interaction has been shown (US PI).

Opioid agonists + nalmefene

Nalmefene decreases the effects of opioid agonists by pharmacodynamic antagonism, a generally minor or non-significant interaction. Such agonists include alfentanil, buprenorphine, butorphanol, codeine, dextromoramide, diamorphine, diphenoxylate, dipipanone, fentanyl, hydrocodone, hydromorphone, levorphanol, meperidine/pethidine, methadone, morphine, nalbuphine, oxycodone, oxymorphone, pentazocine, (dextro)propoxyphene, tapentadol and tramadol.

4.6.16 NALTREXONE

Naltrexone is extensively metabolised by the liver (but not the P450 system) and is mostly renally excreted.

Review: Saber-Tehrani *et al*, *Am J Drug Alcohol Abuse* 2011;**37**:1–11.

Acamprosate + naltrexone

Naltrexone may significantly increase acamprosate plasma levels by 33% and AUC by 25% (UK SmPC; n=23, RCT, d/b, p/c, c/o, 23/7, Johnson *et al*, *J Clin Psychopharmacol* 2003;**23**:281–93).

Alcohol + naltrexone

There are no known interactions between naltrexone and alcohol. Impaired hepatic function has been reported rarely with naltrexone and alcohol, so monitor LFTs.

Cannabis + naltrexone

Naltrexone/opioid receptor blockers seem to increase the subjective effects of oral THC without affecting plasma levels (s=3, n=39, Haney *et al*, *Psychopharmacology [Berl]* 2003;**166**:77–85), although a later publication concludes naltrexone has no effects on cannabis' central effects (Ranganathan *et al*, *Int J Neuropsychopharmacol* 2012;**15**:1251–64).

Cocaine + naltrexone

No interaction between cocaine and naltrexone has been described.

Opiates + naltrexone

See naltrexone + methadone (*4.6.12*).

Phenothiazines + naltrexone

One case of lethargy and somnolence has been reported with naltrexone and thioridazine.

Sertraline + naltrexone

There is no evidence of an adverse interaction (n=113, RCT, d/b, p/c, 10/52, Farren *et al*, *Drug Alcohol* Depend 2009;**99**:317–21; FFT).

Tramadol + naltrexone

Naltrexone does not reduce tramadol's central effects, but has some complex pharmacodynamic interactions (c=10, RCT, d/b, Stoops *et al*, *Psychopharmacol [Berl]* 2012;**223**:427–38; FFT).

4.6.17 PIRENZEPINE

Pirenzepine is a selective M1 receptor antagonist, but little is documented about its interactions or metabolism — or anything else for that matter.

Cimetidine + pirenzepine

Lack of interaction has been shown (n=8, c/o, Jamali *et al*, *Clin Pharmacol Ther* 1985;**38**:325–30).

Theophylline + pirenzepine

Lack of interaction has been shown (n=5, 1/52, Sertl *et al*, *Int J Clin Pharmacol Ther Toxicol* 1987;**25**:15–7).

4.6.18 SODIUM OXYBATE (GHB)

Sodium oxybate is metabolised by GHB dehydrogenase, eventually to carbon dioxide and water, with no active metabolites. It does not significantly inhibit P450 enzymes 1A2, 2C9, 2C19, 2D6, 2E1, and 3A4 at therapeutic doses.

Alcohol + sodium oxybate *

Enhanced CNS depression can occur (SmPC). The FDA contraindicates alcohol while taking oxybate due to respiratory depression, loss of consciousness, coma and death.

Benzodiazepines + sodium oxybate

Respiratory depression might be increased and so the combination should be avoided (SmPC).

Ethosuximide + sodium oxybate *

Ethosuximide inhibits GHB dehydrogenase. The UK SmPC notes an interaction but not any need for dose changes.

Modafinil + sodium oxybate

Lack of interaction has been reported (SmPC), although there is a case of rapid onset depression (n=1, Rossetti *et al*, *Sleep Med* 2010;**11**:500–1).

NSAIDs + sodium oxybate *

There is no interaction with either diclofenac or ibuprofen (UK SmPC).

Phenytoin + sodium oxybate *

Phenytoin inhibits GHB dehydrogenase, and the UK SmPC notes an interaction but not any need for dose changes.

Proton-pump inhibitors + sodium oxybate

Lack of interaction has been reported with omeprazole (SmPC).

Tricyclics + sodium oxybate

Lack of interaction has been reported with protriptyline, but adverse effects may be increased with this combination (SmPC).

Valproate + sodium oxybate *
Valproate inhibits GHB dehydrogenase, and the UK SmPC now states a 20% decreased oxybate dose is recommended.

Zolpidem + sodium oxybate
Lack of interaction has been reported (SmPC).

4.7 NON-PRESCRIBED DRUGS AND 'VICES'

4.7.1 ALCOHOL

Alcohol-psychotropic drug interactions can occur frequently and with varied outcome, depending upon:

- alcohol usage (e.g. chronic and/or acute, leading to altered enzymes)
- consumption (amount, time span)
- type of interaction (e.g. additive sedation, antagonism or cross-tolerance)
- what the individual then tries to do (e.g. sleep, drive)
- comorbidity (e.g. breathing problems).

These variables need to be considered when assessing the effect, or potential effect, of the interaction. Alcohol distribution is wide, with the direct central depressant effect impairing all central functions (e.g. cognition and respiration) which contribute to many of the drug–drug interactions. Alcohol also promotes the action of GABA and may release other amines such as dopamine and endorphins.

Reviews: general (Jang and Harris, *Expert Opin Drug Metab Toxicol* 2007;**3**:719–31), in older adults (Moore *et al*, *Am J Geriatr Pharmacother* 2007;**5**:64–74; FFT).

Acamprosate + alcohol
Continued alcohol consumption may negate the therapeutic effect of acamprosate. There is no detectable pharmacokinetic interaction (review by Nalpas *et al*, *Encephale* 1990;**16**:175–9).

ADHD + alcohol *
A systematic review concluded that there was only a minimal increase in side effects when alcohol is consumed with ADHD treatments, with no severe sequalae, even in overdose (s=20, Barkla *et al*, *BMC Psychiatry* 2015;**15**:270; FFT).

Agomelatine + alcohol
See agomelatine (*4.3.3.1*).

ANTIPSYCHOTICS + ALCOHOL
There is no clear evidence that alcohol reduces antipsychotic efficacy. However, enhanced CNS depression is well-documented, resulting in impaired concentration, coordination, judgment, drowsiness and lethargy, as well as hypotension and respiratory depression. Alcohol-related drowsiness is significant with **phenothiazines** and **flupentixol**. EPSE may also be enhanced (Freed, *Med J Aust* 1981;**2**:44–5), as can hepatotoxicity with, e.g. **chlorpromazine** (Strubelt, *Biochem Pharmacol* 1980;**29**:1445–9). Single oral doses of **amisulpride** do not seem to enhance the effects of alcohol on the performance and memory of healthy subjects (n=18, RCT, Mattila *et al*, *Eur J Clin Pharmacol* 1996;**51**:161). No significant difference in performance or gross motor skills has been shown with **aripiprazole,** although 2.5–10mg/d increases sedation from alcohol (n=18, p/c, Kranzler *et al*, *Alcohol Clin Exp Res* 2008;**32**:573–9; FFT). Enhanced CNS sedation would be expected with **olanzapine**, and raised heart rate and increased postural hypotension have been reported. Overall, this is a potentially important interaction, especially in the community. Accidental alcohol over-dosage, especially in people with asthma, respiratory depression or chest infections, could prove fatal if combined with antipsychotics.

Baclofen + alcohol
There is a case of *de novo* seizures following taking alcohol with high dose baclofen 240mg/d (n=1, Rolland *et al*, *Alcohol Alcohol* 2012;**47**:577–80; FFT).

BARBITURATES + ALCOHOL
Enhanced or prolonged CNS and respiratory depression can occur, seriously impairing concentration and performance. Acute alcohol ingestion may increase barbiturate levels but chronic alcohol use may decrease barbiturate levels (Mezey and Robles, *Gastroenterology* 1974;**66**:248–53). The lethal dose of barbiturates is reported to be up to 50% lower when alcohol is also present (Bogan and Smith, *J Forensic Sci* 1967;**7**:37–45). This is mainly due to additive respiratory depression.

BENZODIAZEPINES + ALCOHOL
Alcohol can enhance the sedation caused by benzodiazepines by 20–30%, a well-established, documented and predictable interaction. Synergistic sedation has been reported with **lorazepam** (d/b, c/o, Lister and File, *J Clin Psychopharmacol* 1983;**3**:66–71), **clorazepate** and **diazepam**. Larger quantities of alcohol may

inhibit benzodiazepine metabolism, especially in those with impaired or borderline hepatic function (review by Guthrie and Lane, *Alcoholism* 1986;**10**:686–90). At low dose, alcohol and **temazepam** appear not to interact adversely (n=24, p/c, c/o, Martin and Siddle, *Brain Cogn* 2003;**53**:58–65).

Beta-blockers + alcohol

Alcohol may slightly reduce **propranolol** absorption and increase clearance (Sotaniemi *et al*, *Clin Pharmacol Ther* 1981;**29**:705–10).

Bupropion + alcohol

See bupropion (*4.6.6*).

Buspirone + alcohol

A minimal interaction and slightly increased sedation have been reported (n=24, RCT, Erwin *et al*, *J Clin Psychopharmacol* 1986;**6**:199–209).

BZP (benzylpiperazine) and TFMPP (trifluoromethylphenylpiperazine) + alcohol

Severe adverse reactions (agitation, anxiety, hallucinations, vomiting, insomnia, migraine) have been reported with tablets containing BZP and TFMPP, possibly slightly enhanced by alcohol, and so this appears to hold a significant risk (n=35, RCT, d/b, p/c, Thompson *et al*, *J Psychopharmacol* 2010;**24**:1299–308).

Cannabis + alcohol

See cannabis (*4.7.2*).

Carbamazepine + alcohol

There is virtually nothing published but additive sedation would be expected. In acute carbamazepine intoxication, alcohol does not seem to affect CBZ kinetics (n=158, Piekoszewski *et al*, *Pharmacol Rep* 2010;**62**:398–404; FFT).

CHLORAL HYDRATE + ALCOHOL

Additive CNS depressant effects occur when alcohol is taken with chloral hydrate. Tachycardia, impaired concentration, disulfiram-like effects and profound vasodilation may also occur (Owen and Taberner, *Br J Pharmacol* 1978;**64**:400; FFT).

Clomethiazole + alcohol

Alcohol increases the bioavailability of oral clomethiazole, probably via inhibition of first-pass metabolism.

Citalopram + alcohol

There is little published at present on this. The UK SmPC notes that citalopram should not enhance the sedation caused by alcohol.

Cocaine + alcohol

See cocaine (*4.7.3*).

DISULFIRAM + ALCOHOL

Disulfiram inhibits the aldehyde dehydrogenase enzyme, leading to accumulation of acetaldehyde from incomplete alcohol metabolism. The main symptoms of the 'Antabuse reaction' are flushing, sweating, palpitations, hyperventilation, increased pulse, hypotension, nausea and vomiting (often in that order). Arrhythmias and shock can follow. The reaction occurs within 5–15 minutes and can be fatal. Factors affecting the severity of the reaction include the dose of disulfiram, rate and dose of alcohol ingestion, sensitivity, individual aldehyde dehydrogenase activity, concurrent medication (see disulfiram, *4.6.4*) and co-existing pulmonary or cardiac disease. Patients should be warned that reactions can occur with disguised sources of alcohol, e.g. Listerine® mouthwashes (which can contain up to 21–27% alcohol), sauces, pharmaceuticals (e.g. cough mixtures) and topical preparations (e.g. shampoo, Stoll and King, *JAMA* 1980;**244**:2045). Delirium has also been reported with the combination (Park and Riggio, *Ann Pharmacother* 2001;**35**:32–5).

Escitalopram + alcohol

See citalopram + alcohol.

Fluoxetine + alcohol

Alcohol has no additional significant effect on drowsiness, sedation or task performance tests with fluoxetine 40 mg/d, compared with fluoxetine alone (e.g. Shaw *et al*, *Hum Psychopharmacol* 1989;**4**:113–20).

Fluvoxamine + alcohol

There appears no significant potentiation of the cognitive effects of 40 g IV alcohol by single and multiple doses of 50 mg fluvoxamine (n=24, van Harten *et al*, *Clin Pharmacol Ther* 1992;**52**:427–35).

Lacosamide + alcohol

There is no data on the interaction (SmPC).

Levetiracetam + alcohol

See levetiracetam (*4.5.2*).

Lithium + alcohol

Impaired driving skills have been suggested and alcohol may produce a slight (12%) increase in peak lithium levels (n=10, RCT, d/b, p/c, c/o, Anton *et al*, *Clin Pharmacol Ther* 1985;**38**:52–5).

MAOIs + ALCOHOL

As well as an interaction occurring with alcoholic and low alcoholic drinks (see MAOIs, *4.3.4*), alcohol may increase central catecholamine

4

synthesis and release, and MAOIs may inhibit alcohol dehydrogenase, potentiating alcohol (comprehensive review by Weller *et al*, *Psychosomatics* 1984;**25**:301–9).

MDMA (ecstasy) + alcohol
People aged 18–29 taking both substances become more aroused when intoxicated, but psychomotor accuracy is significantly impaired compared to placebo or either substance alone (n=16, RCT, d/b, p/c, c/o, Dumont *et al*, *J Psychopharmacol* 2010;**24**:155–64).

Melatonin + alcohol
See melatonin (*4.1.4*).

Memantine + alcohol
Memantine has no effect on alcohol-induced performance impairment, but may increase some subjective symptoms (n=18, 3x3/7, d/b, Bisaga and Evans, *Psychopharmacol [Berl]* 2003;**172**:16–24).

Methadone + alcohol
Predictably, increased sedation and respiratory depression may occur, especially in overdose, as could hepatotoxicity. Chronic high use of alcohol may induce enzymes requiring higher methadone doses and binge drinking may increase methadone excretion via an enhanced diuretic effect.

MIANSERIN + ALCOHOL
Mianserin causes drowsiness, which is enhanced considerably by alcohol (n=13, RCT, Seppälä *et al*, *Eur J Clin Pharmacol* 1984;**27**:181–9).

Mirtazapine + alcohol
Lack of pharmacokinetic interaction has been shown, but additive sedation noted (see Timmer *et al*, *Clin Pharmacokinet* 2000;**38**:461–74).

Moclobemide + alcohol
Some degree of potentiation of the effects of alcohol has been noted (Zimmer *et al*, *Acta Psychiatr Scand* 1990;**360**[Suppl]:84–6). There has also been a case of a fatality with a moclobemide overdose, plus half a bottle of whisky (n=1, Bleumink *et al*, *Neth J Med* 2003;**61**:88–90; FFT).

Nalmefene + alcohol
See nalmefene (*4.6.15*).

Naltrexone + alcohol
See naltrexone (*4.6.16*).

Oxcarbazepine + alcohol
See oxcarbazepine (4.5.3).

Paraldehyde + alcohol
An enhanced sedative effect can be expected.

Paroxetine + alcohol
Lack of interaction has been shown (review by Boyer and Blumhardt, *J Clin Psychiatry* 1992;**53**[Suppl]:61–6).

PHENYTOIN + ALCOHOL
Alcohol has a variable effect on phenytoin so monitor plasma levels regularly. The half-life of phenytoin can be up to 50% shorter in an abstaining alcoholic than in a non-drinker (see also n=1, Bellibas and Tuglular, *Therapie* 1995; **50**:487–8).

Pregabalin + alcohol
See pregabalin (*4.1.5*).

Quetiapine + alcohol
Additive sedation would be expected.

Reboxetine + alcohol
No potentiation of alcohol's cognitive effects has been reported (UK SmPC), and up to 4mg/d showed no interaction with alcohol in one trial (n=10, d/b, Kerr *et al*, *Br J Clin Pharmacol* 1996;**42**:239–41; FFT).

Rufinamide + alcohol
No information is available (UK SmPC).

Sertraline + alcohol
There is evidence for a lack of interaction (review, Warrington, *Int Clin Psychopharmacol* 1991;**6**[Suppl 2]:11–21).

Sodium oxybate + alcohol
See sodium oxybate (*4.6.18*).

Tiagabine + alcohol
Lack of interaction has been suggested (n=20, RCT, d/b, p/c, c/o, Kastberg *et al*, *Drug Metabol Drug Interact* 1998;**14**:259–73).

TRAZODONE + ALCOHOL
Additive sedation has been reported (n=26, d/b, c/o, Warrington *et al*, *Neuropsychobiology* 1986;**15**[Suppl 1]:31–7).

TRICYCLICS + ALCOHOL
Enhanced sedation with most tricyclics is known, but surprisingly little has been published. Most studies refer to the effect on driving performance. Sedation caused by **amitriptyline** and **doxepin** is enhanced by alcohol, but less, or minimally so, with **nortriptyline** and **clomipramine**. Both alcohol and tricyclics lower the seizure threshold and care is needed in patients susceptible to seizures. Concurrent alcohol may also increase the oral bioavailability of tricyclics by reducing first-pass metabolism (n=5, open, Dorian *et al*, *Eur J Clin Pharmacol* 1983;**25**:325–31).

Venlafaxine + alcohol
There appears to be no significant additive

effect between alcohol and venlafaxine (n=16, RCT, d/b, p/c, c/o, Troy *et al*, *J Clin Pharmacol* 1997;**37**:1073–81).

Vortioxetine + alcohol *

See vortioxetine (*4.3.3.9*).

Zaleplon + alcohol

While zaleplon enhances alcohol performance impairment, the effect appears short-lived and less than with zolpidem, albeit less potent on a mg for mg basis (n=10, RCT, c/o, Drover *et al*, *Clin Ther* 2000;**22**:1443–61).

Zolpidem + alcohol

There is no published information available indicating an interaction (and see above).

Zopiclone + alcohol

It appears not to be a good idea to take zopiclone, drink alcohol and then try to drive up to 6.5 hours later (n=16, RCT, d/b, p/c, Gustavsen *et al*, *Addiction* 2012;**107**:925–32; spookily similar publication as n=16, RCT, d/b, p/c, Gustavsen *et al*, *J Clin Psychopharmacol* 2011;**31**:481–8), although there may be no significant kinetic interaction (n=9, RCT, Hindmarch, *Int Clin Psychopharmacol* 1990;**5**[Suppl 2]:105–13).

4.7.2 CANNABIS (TETRAHYDRO-CANNABINOL, SEE ALSO SMOKING)

Cannabis/marijuana is a frequently (and usually secretively) used drug but, with the exception of perhaps tricyclics, has few known important adverse drug interactions.

Alcohol + cannabis

Decreased ethanol metabolism may occur, with enhanced CNS depression (n=10, RCT, p/c, d/b, c/o, Consroe *et al*, *Psychopharmacol* 1979;**66**:45–50). Cannabis may also reduce peak alcohol levels in modest doses (n=15, RCT, p/c, Lukas *et al*, *Neuropsychopharmacology* 1992;**7**:77–81).

Antidepressants + cannabis

Delirium, tachycardia (e.g. n=1, Hillard and Vieweg, *Am J Psychiatr* 1983;**140**:626–7), mania (**fluoxetine**, n=1, Stoll *et al*, *J Clin Psychiatry* 1991;**52**:280–1) and other clinically significant adverse events have been reported following use of marijuana and **tricyclics** (n=4, Wilens *et al*, *J Am Acad Child Adolesc Psychiatry* 1997;**36**:45–8).

Antipsychotics + cannabis

Chlorpromazine clearance is increased by cannabis smoking, although the clinical significance is not known (n=31, Chetty *et al*, *Eur J Clin Pharmacol* 1994;**46**:523–6). Cessation of cannabis smoking can lead to **clozapine** intoxication through removal of CYP1A2 induction (n=1, Zullino *et al*, *Int Clin Psychopharmacol* 2002;**17**:141–3). **Olanzapine** reduces feelings of high from cannabis (n=49, p/c, c/o, Kleinloog *et al*, *J Psychopharmacol* 2012;**26**:1307–16). Craving for cannabis is lower with clozapine and olanzapine compared to risperidone (n=264, Machielsen *et al*, *J Psychopharmacol* 2012;**26**:189–95). Additive drowsiness has been reported.

Antiretrovirals + cannabis

Although strong CYP3A4 inhibitors might increase cannabis levels, there appears to be no significant interaction (n=67, RCT, p/c, Abrams *et al*, *Ann Intern Med* 2003;**139**:258–66; review by Gruber and McCance-Katz, *Curr HIV/AIDS Rep* 2010;**7**:152–60; FFT).

Benzodiazepines + cannabis

Additive drowsiness has been reported (review by Benowitz and Jones, *Clin Pharmacol Ther* 1977;**22**:259–68).

Cocaine + cannabis

See cocaine (*4.7.3*).

CNS depressants + cannabis

The combination has resulted in additive drowsiness (review by Benowitz and Jones, *Clin Pharmacol Ther* 1977;**22**:259–68), e.g. anticholinergics and barbiturates.

Disulfiram + cannabis

A hypomanic episode (n=1, Lacoursiere and Swatek, *Am J Psychiatry* 1983;**140**:242–4) and an acute confusional state (n=1, Mackie and Clark, *Br J Psychiatry* 1994;**164**:421) have been reported.

Lithium + cannabis

Lithium levels have been raised into the toxic range by secretive use of cannabis (n=1, Ratey *et al*, *J Clin Psychopharmacol* 1981;**1**:32–3) and additive drowsiness has occurred (review by Benowitz and Jones, *Clin Pharmacol Ther* 1977;**22**:259–68).

Methadone + cannabis

See methadone (*4.6.12*).

Naltrexone + cannabis

See naltrexone (*4.6.16*).

4.7.3 COCAINE

Cocaine is metabolised by plasma and hepatic esterases, and 10% by CYP3A4 (Gruber and

4

McCance-Katz, *Curr HIV/AIDS Rep* 2010;**7**:152–60).

Alcohol + cocaine

Simultaneous cocaine and alcohol may produce changes in heart rate and blood pressure, increasing the risk of cardiovascular toxicity (Farré *et al, J Pharmacol Exp Ther* 1993;**166**:1364–73). Combined use has led to enhanced cocaine-induced hepatotoxicity.

Antidepressants + cocaine

Desipramine has reduced the effects of cocaine, **fluoxetine** has no significant effect (n=5, Walsh *et al, J Clin Psychopharmacol* 1994;**14**:396–407), trazodone has minor physiological effects and MAOIs probably augment the pressor effect.

Antipsychotics + cocaine

Flupentixol may reduce cocaine craving and **haloperidol** may moderate the stimulant effects. **Clozapine** increases cocaine levels but reduces the cocaine 'high', and some cardiac events (near-syncopal episode) have been reported, so caution is necessary (n=8, Farren *et al, Drug Alcohol Depend* 2000;**59**:153–63).

Antiretrovirals + cocaine

For a review see (Gruber and McCance-Katz, *Curr HIV/AIDS Rep* 2010;**7**:152–60).

Buprenorphine + cocaine

See buprenorphine (*4.6.5*).

Cannabis + cocaine

Enhanced cardiotoxicity (e.g. increased heart rate) may occur.

Carbamazepine + cocaine

Cocaine may enhance the cardiac effects of carbamazepine.

Disulfiram + cocaine

See cocaine + disulfiram (*4.6.8*).

Lithium + cocaine

Lithium probably has little effect on cocaine.

Methadone + cocaine

See methadone (*4.6.12*).

Methylphenidate + cocaine

See methylphenidate (*4.6.13*).

Modafinil + cocaine

See modafinil (*4.6.14*).

Naltrexone + cocaine

See naltrexone (*4.6.16*).

4.7.4 SMOKING

There are over 3000 different known chemicals in cigarette smoke, but which ones are significant is not fully known. A few smoking drug interactions are significant, and only brief details of the more significant psychotropic ones are included here. The major enzyme metabolising nicotine is probably CYP2A6, with 2B6 and 2D6 playing lesser, but still substantial, roles. Cigarette smoke contains polycyclic aromatic hydrocarbons, which are potent inducers of CYP1A2.

Reviews: general (Zevin and Benowitz, *Clin Pharmacokinet* 1999;**36**:425–38; Desai *et al, CNS Drugs* 2001;**15**:469–94).

Agomelatine + smoking

See agomelatine (*4.3.3.1*).

Antipsychotics + smoking

Amisulpride: lack of interaction has been shown (n=85, Bergemann *et al, Eur Neuropsychopharmacol* 2004;**14**:245–50).

Aripiprazole: no dose adjustments needed (UK SmPC).

Chlorpromazine clearance may be increased by cigarette smoking, but the clinical significance is unclear (n=31, Chetty *et al, Eur J Clin Pharmacol* 1994;**46**:523–6).

Clozapine * levels can be significantly lowered by smoking (n=148, open, Haring *et al, Am J Psychiatry* 1990;**147**:1471–5), via 1A2 induction, and this usually takes two to four weeks to manifest itself (Zullion *et al, Int Clin Psychopharmacol* 2002;**17**:141–3). Stopping smoking can be dangerous for someone taking clozapine, e.g. one study showed a mean 72% **increase** in stable clozapine levels on smoking cessation, with one case so extreme it caused a significant ADR (n=11, open, Meyer, *J Clin Psychopharmacol* 2001;**21**:569–74). A meta-analysis concludes that smokers need twice the dose of clozapine than non-smokers, and have the dose reduced by a half if stopping smoking (s=4, n=196, Tsuda *et al, BMJ Open* 2014;**4**:e004216). The change in plasma clozapine levels can, in 80% of cases, be predicted by using the formula:

> Non-smoking level = 45.3 + (1.474 x smoking level)

In a smoker, taking a constant dose of clozapine, on average plasma levels:

- Are17% higher in women than men
- Are 48% higher than in non-smokers

- Change by +/-4% for every five years over 40
- Change by +/-5% for every 10kg over 80kg.

But:

- These may be dose-dependent (i.e. number of cigarettes smoked, up to 10 cigarettes a day). After that, levels do not change, so dropping to 10 a day is the easy part
- If stopping smoking suddenly, significant plasma changes can occur within 3–5 days
- If starting smoking suddenly, significant plasma changes can also occur within 3–5 days
- Smoking cannabis has the same effect but NRT, chewing tobacco or snuff have no effect.

(Flanaghan, *Br J Clin Pharmacy* 2011;**3**:18–20)

Nomograms exist to help predict doses in people on clozapine who smoke, but you will need a colour copy of the best paper (Rostami-Hodjegan *et al*, *J Clin Psychopharmacol* 2004;**24**:70–80) to make sense of it (reviews by Lowe and Ackman, *Ann Pharmacother* 2010;**44**:727–32; and for our Norwegian readers; Molden and Spigset, *Tidsskr Nor Laegeforen* 2009;**129**:623–3; FFT).

Valproate has a variable effect on smoking and clozapine (n=255, Diaz *et al*, *Pharmacopsychiatry* 2008;**41**:81–91):

- Valproate inhibits clozapine metabolism in non-smokers (levels can rise by 16%)
- Valproate induces clozapine metabolism in smokers (levels can fall by 22%)
- Smoking induces clozapine and reduces plasma levels by 20% (if not also taking valproate)
- Smoking induces clozapine and reduces plasma levels by 46% if taking valproate.

In summary, smoking induces clozapine metabolism and this induction may be stronger when the person is taking valproate; so the effect may be even more marked when stopping smoking.

Haloperidol plasma levels are around 23% lower in smoking than in non-smoking schizophrenics (n=66, open, Shimoda *et al*, *Ther Drug Monit* 1999;**21**:293–6; confirmed by another study, n=63, Pan *et al*, *Ther Drug Monit* 1999;**21**:489–97).

Olanzapine * clearance may be higher and half-life 21% shorter in smokers compared to non-smokers, probably via CYP1A2 induction (review by Lowe and Ackman, *Ann Pharmacother* 2010;**44**:727–32). Smoking cessation can lead to olanzapine toxicity through removal of CYP1A2 induction (n=1, Zullino *et al*, *Int Clin Psychopharmacol* 2002;**17**:141–3). A meta-analysis concludes that smokers should have their olanzapine dose reduced by 30% if stopping smoking (s=7, n=1094, Tsuda *et al*, *BMJ Open* 2014;**4**: e004216).

Perphenazine clearance is increased by smoking, reducing levels (n=156, Jin *et al*, *J Clin Pharmacol* 2010;**50**:73–80; FFT).

Risperidone: no dose adjustments needed (UK SmPC).

Ziprasidone: no interaction reported.

Benzodiazepines + smoking

Early studies suggested an increased clearance of benzodiazepines in smokers (review by Schein, *Ann Pharmacother* 1995;**29**:1139–48). One review noted increased clearance by smoking of alprazolam, lorazepam, oxazepam and diazepam but not chlordiazepoxide (mentioned in Desai *et al*, *CNS Drugs* 2001;**15**:469–94).

Beta-blockers + smoking

Nicotine may negate the effects of beta-blockers on heart rate and blood pressure. Steady-state propranolol levels may be reduced in smokers, via 1A2 induction.

Bupropion + smoking

See bupropion (4.6.6).

Carbamazepine + smoking

Carbamazepine seems likely to induce 2A6 and lowers nicotine levels, which may lead to increased smoking and exposure to tobacco toxins (n=8, open, Williams *et al*, *Cancer Epidemiol Biomarkers Prev* 2010;**19**:2582–9).

DULOXETINE + SMOKING

See duloxetine (4.3.3.2).

Fluvoxamine + smoking

Fluvoxamine levels are significantly lower in smokers, probably due to induction of CYP1A2 (n=30, open, Yoshimura *et al*, *Neuropsychobiology* 2002;**45**:32–5), and/or CYP2D6 (n=32, >4/52, Katoh *et al*, *Biol Pharm Bull* 2010;**33**:285–8; FFT).

Lamotrigine + smoking

Lamotrigine levels are about 16% lower in smokers compared to non-smokers, probably via UDPGT2B7 induction (n=44, Reinsberger *et al*, *Seizure* 2008;**17**:651–3; FFT).

Lithium + smoking

Smoking induces CYP1A2 and caffeine is

4

metabolised by CYP1A2. Theoretically, ceasing smoking could raise xanthine levels, which could increase lithium excretion (as with theophylline), lowering levels.

Melatonin + smoking

See melatonin (*4.1.4*).

Memantine + smoking

See memantine (*4.6.11*).

Mirtazapine + smoking

Mirtazapine levels are significantly (25%) lower in smokers than non-smokers (n=95, Lind *et al*, *Clin Pharmacokinet* 2009;**48**:63–70).

Oxcarbazepine + smoking

Oxcarbazepine seems likely to induce 2A6 and lowers nicotine levels, which may lead to increased smoking and exposure to tobacco toxins (n=6, open, Williams *et al*, *Cancer Epidemiol Biomarkers* Prev 2010;**19**:2582–9).

Phenobarbital + smoking

Smoking has been shown not to affect the drowsiness caused by phenobarbital (n=12, d/b, Mirfazaelian *et al*, *Biopharm Drug Dispos* 2001;**22**:403–6).

Tricyclics + smoking

Although serum levels of tricyclics fall in smokers, free levels rise, minimising the clinical significance (n=24, open, Perry *et al*, *Ther Drug Monit* 1986;**8**:279–84).

Valproate + smoking

Valproate does not seem to induce CYP2A6 and does not alter nicotine levels (n=40, open, Williams *et al*, *Cancer Epidemiol Biomarkers Prev* 2010;**19**:2582–9; FFT). See antipsychotics + smoking for effect on clozapine.

Zolpidem + smoking

See zolpidem (*4.1.7*).

4.8 CYTOCHROME P450 DRUG METABOLISM

There are currently at least 58 known P450 enzymes, with numerous isoforms described, regulated by at least 684 genes. The main recognised P450s are 1A1, 1A2, 2A6, 2B6, 2C8, 2C9, 2C18, 2C19, 2D6, 2E1, 3A3, 3A4, 3A5, 3A6, 3A7, 3A43, 21A2. All have up to 70 variations each. These tables may be of use in determining actual or potential interactions. There are many discrepancies in the published literature and these tables may inadvertently perpetuate some inaccuracies or incomplete knowledge. The author would be happy to receive any advice on this.

Some points about P450/CYP interactions:

1. Most have ultrarapid (UM), extensive (EM), intermediate (IM) and poor (PM) metaboliser variations.
2. Some drugs are metabolised by several enzymes, so if one enzyme is inhibited, another may compensate.
3. A drug may inhibit or induce one enzyme, but be metabolised by another.
4. Onset and offset of inhibition is dependent on the half-life and time to steady state of the inhibitory drug (may be 24 hours to several months) and the drug to be metabolised, but onset is frequently rapid.
5. Onset and offset of induction may take days or several weeks to become apparent, dependent on the inducing drugs half-life, enzyme turnover, age (induction reduces with age) and concurrent liver disease (reduced induction ability).
6. Other enzyme systems are also important. The **UGT** (uridine diphosphate glucuronosyltransferase) enzymes are induced by phenytoin, valproate, phenobarbital and carbamazepine, and lamotrigine is a weak UGT inducer. The **FMO** (Flavin Monoxygenase) system is also important. Humans have FMO1, FMO3, FM04 and FM05 enzymes in the liver, intestine and kidney. Imipramine, chlorpromazine and orphenadrine are known to be metabolised by this enzyme system.

The general rules for avoiding metabolic interactions are:

1. Avoid reported and predictable interactions.
2. With potential interactions, use reduced doses where possible (start low, go slow).
3. Measure plasma levels of drugs with narrow therapeutic indices.

CYP1A2

Substrates (drugs metabolised by this enzyme) *

Agomelatine (90%)
Amiodarone
Anagrelide
Asenapine
Bortezomib
Caffeine
Carbamazepine (minor)
Chlordiazepoxide
Ciprofloxacin
Clarithromycin
Clopidogrel (minor)
Clozapine (most)
Dacarbazine
Dextropropoxyphene
Diazepam
Duloxetine
Erlotinib (minor)
Erythromycin
Escitalopram
Estradiol
Flecainide
Flutamine
Fluvoxamine (partly)
Haloperidol (partly)
Lefunomide
Lidocaine
Melatonin (partly)
Methadone (minor)
Mexiletine (minor)
Mirtazapine (partly)
Naproxen
Norfloxacin
Olanzapine (partly)
Omeprazole
Ondansetron
Oxfloxacin
Palonosetron (minor)
Paracetamol
Perphenazine
Pimozide (possibly)
Promazine
Propafenone
Propranolol
Ramelteon (95% first-pass effect)
Rasagiline (major)
Retinols
Ritonavir
Rofecoxib
Ropinirole
Sibutramine (partly)
Tacrine
Tamoxifen
Theophylline
Tizanidine (main)
Tricyclics (tertiary, e.g. amitriptyline, clomipramine, desipramine, trimipramine imipramine)
Verapamil
Warfarin-R (major)
Zotepine
Ziprasidone (minor)

Significant enzyme inducers (decrease levels of substrates) *

Cabbage
Caffeine (weak, animal studies)
Carbamazepine?
Charcoal-broiled food
Modafinil (small and dose-dependent)
Omeprazole
Phenobarbital (weak)
Phenytoin (weak)
Rifampicin
Ritonavir
Tipranavir (potent)
Tobacco smoke (polycyclic aromatic hydrocarbons are potent inducers of 1A2)

Significant enzyme inhibitors (increase levels of substrates)

Celery
Chlorpromazine
Cimetidine
Clarithromycin
Diet (low protein/ high carbohydrates)
Disulfiram (strong)
Erythromycin
Fluoroquinolones, e.g. ciprofloxacin and norfloxacin (strong)
Fluvoxamine (potent — other SSRIs only very weak inhibitors)
Grapefruit juice
Griseofulvin?
Isoniazid
Ketoconazole
Mirtazapine (very weak)
Moclobemide
Omeprazole
Parsley
Parsnip
Propafenone (major)
Quercetin (weak)
Sertraline (weak)
Ticlopidone

No effect

Anidulafungin
Asenapine
Bevacizumab
Benzodiazepines
Capecitibane
Cranberry juice
Duloxetine
Emtricitabine
Galantamine

No effect *continued*		
Isotretinoin	Nelarabine	Sunitinib
Lacosamide	Olanzapine	Telbivudine
Lanthanum	Palonosetron	Varenicline
Lenalidomide	Posaconazole	Venlafaxine
Levetiracetam	Pregabalin	Zoledronic acid
Lithium	Rasagiline	Zonisamide
Memantine	Rufinamide	Ziprasidone
Methylnaltrexone	Sitagliptin	
Mirtazapine	Sulpiride	

CYP1A2 *

1A2 accounts for about 13% of the total liver CYPs, and metabolises 20% of clinically used drugs (Wang and Zhou, *Curr Med Chem* 2009;**16**:4066–218), but may also bioactivate a number of biocarcinogens. Thus, 1A2 induction can increase carcinogenicity (Zhou *et al*, *Curr Drug Metab* 2009;**10**:713–29). Caffeine is the main substrate probe and fluvoxamine the inhibitor probe.

CYP2B6

Substrates (drugs metabolised by this enzyme)		
Alfentanil	Ifosfamide	Procarbazine
Bupropion	Ketamine	Promethazine
Carbamazepine	Lidocaine	Propofol (main)
Carteolol	S-methadone (major)	Rifampicin
Clopidogrel	R-methadone (minor)	Ropivacaine
Cyclophosphamide	Midazolam	Selegiline
Dexamethasone	Nevirapine	Sevoflurane
Diazepam	Nicotine	Tamoxifen
Ecstasy (MDMA)	Orphenadrine	Testosterone
Efavirenz	Pethidine	Thiotepa
Estrone	Phenobarbital	Valproic acid
Ethinylestradiol	Procainamide	

Significant enzyme inducers (decrease levels of substrates)		
Baicalin (significant)	Modafinil (minor and dose-dependent)	Rifampin
Efavirenz		

Significant enzyme inhibitors (increase levels of substrates)		
Clopidogrel (potent)	Ketoconazole	Thiotepa (potent),
Clotrimazole	Memantine	Ticopidine
Glabridin (a liquorice extract)	OCs (weak)	Tranylcypromine (modest)
HRT (potent)	Orphenadine	Zolpidem (very weak)
Itraconazole	Raloxifene	
	SSRIs (paroxetine, fluoxetine, fluvoxamine)	

No effect		
Anidulafungin	Bevacizumab	Isotretinoin
Benzodiazepines	Emtricitabine	Lacosamide

No effect *continued*		
Lamotrigine	Posaconazole	Telbivudine
Levetiracetam	Rasagiline	Venlafaxine
Lithium	Rufinamide	Zoledronic acid
Methylnaltrexone	Sertraline	Zonisamide
Nelarabine	Sulpiride	Ziprasidone
Palonosetron	Sunitinib	

CYP2B6 *

2B6 (general review by Zanger and Klein, *Front Genet* 2013:**5**;24; FFT) accounts for about 2–10% of the total hepatic CYP content and metabolises about 8% clinically used drugs. It is linked to 3A4 and UGT1A1. There are at least 28 known allelic variants, can be 20–250-fold interindividual variation in 2B6 expression and may be some ethnic variations as well (Mo *et al*, *Curr Drug Metab* 2009;**10**:730–53; Wang and Tompkins, *Curr Drug Metab* 2008;**9**:598–610; FFT). Probes for 2B6 include bupropion and thioTEPA (Turpeinen *et al*, *Drug Metab Dispos* 2004;**32**:626–31; FFT).

CYP2C9

Substrates (drugs metabolised by this enzyme) *		
Agomelatine (10%)	Fluoxetine	Phenytoin (major)
Alosetron	Flurbiprofen	Retinoids
Amiodarone	Fluvastatin	Rifampicin
Amitriptyline	Glipizide	Rosiglitazone
Arachidonic acid	Glyburide	Sibutramine (part)
Atorvastatin	Irbesartan	Sildenafil (partly)
Bortezomib	Losartan	Tolbutamide (8/9)
Bupropion (8/9)	Melatonin	Torasemide
Carbamazepine (minor)	Miconazole	Trimethoprim
Celecoxib	NSAIDs (e.g. diclofenac, naproxen, piroxicam, tenoxicam 8/9)	Valproate
Cimetidine		Valsartan
Etravirine		S-warfarin (major)
Fluconazole	Phenobarbital	

Significant enzyme inducers (decrease levels of substrates)		
Carbamazepine (weak)	Phenytoin (weak)	Tipranavir (minor)
Dexamethasone	Rifampicin	
Phenobarbital (weak)	St John's wort (weak?)	

Significant enzyme inhibitors (increase levels of substrates)		
Amiodarone	Fluvastatin	Paroxetine (weak)
Capecitibane	Fluvoxamine	Phenylbutazone
Cimetidine	Gingko biloba (weak)	Pomegranate juice (inhibits intestinal 2C9)
Cyclizine	Ginseng (weak)	
Disulfiram	Miconazole	Promethazine
Fluconazole	Modafinil	Sertraline (moderate)
Fluorouracil	Nilotinib (strong)	Suprofen
Fluoxetine	Omeprazole	Tamoxifen

Significant enzyme inhibitors (increase levels of substrates) *continued*

Tolcapone (minor)	Tranylcypromine (part)	Zafirlukast
Topiramate	Valproate	

No effect

Anidulafungin	Lenalidomide	Rufinamide
Aripiprazole	Lithium	Sitagliptin
Benzodiazepines	Memantine	Sulpiride
Bevacizumab	Methylnaltrexone	Sunitinib
Cranberry juice	Mirtazapine	Telbivudine
Emtricitabine	Nelarabine	Venlafaxine
Galantamine	Olanzapine	Varenicline
Isotretinoin	Palonosetron	Ziprasidone
Lacosamide	Posaconazole	Zoledronic acid
Lamotrigine	Pregabalin	Zonisamide
Lanthanum	Rasagiline	

CYP2C19 *

Substrates (drugs metabolised by this enzyme) *

Barbiturates	Flunitrazepam	Proguanil
Bortezomib	Fluoxetine	Promazine
Cannabis (minor)	Fluvoxamine	Propranolol (part)
Carisoprodol	Indometacin	Quazepam
Cimetidine	Lansoprazole	Rabeprazole
Citalopram (major 60%)	Melatonin (partly)	Ramelteon (minor)
Clobazam	Mephenytoin	Rifabutin
Clopidogrel (needs 2C19 to be metabolised from pro-drug)	Methadone	Rifampicin
Desmethylclobazam	Midazolam (minor)	Topiramate
Desvenlafaxine	Moclobemide (major)	Tranylcypromine
Diazepam (genotype important)	Nelfinavir	Tricyclics (3°, e.g. amitriptyline, clomipramine, doxepin, imipramine, trimipramine)
Etravirine	Omeprazole (major)	Venlafaxine
Etizolam	Perphenazine	R-warfarin (minor)
	Pethidine	
	Phenytoin (minor)	
	Piroxicam	

Significant enzyme inducers (decrease levels of substrates)

Carbamazepine (weak)	Ginkgo biloba (low dose, weak)	Rifampicin
Common sage (dose-dependent)	Phenobarbital (weak)	St John's wort (low dose)
		Valerian (weak)

Significant enzyme inhibitors (increase levels of substrates)

Cimetidine	Fluoxetine (moderate)	Isoniazid (potent)
Felbamate	Fluvoxamine	Ketoconazole
Fluconazole	Ginkgo biloba (higher dose, weak)	

Significant enzyme inhibitors (increase levels of substrates) *continued*		
Moclobemide	Paroxetine (weak)	Tipranavir (potent)
Modafinil	Phenytoin	Topiramate
Nilotinib (strong)	Sertraline (weak)	Tranylcypromine (weak)
Omeprazole	St John's wort (high dose)	Tricyclics (e.g. imipramine)
Oxcarbazepine	Ticlopidine	Valproate

No effect		
Anidulafungin	Levetiracetam	Rufinamide
Aripiprazole	Lithium	Sitagliptin
Benzodiazepines	Memantine	Sulpiride
Bevacizumab	Methylnaltrexone	Sunitinib
Cone flower	Mirtazapine	Telbivudine
Emtricitabine	Nelarabine	Varenicline
Horse chestnut	Olanzapine	Venlafaxine
Isotretinoin	Palonosetron	Ziprasidone
Lacosamide	Posaconazole	Zoledronic acid
Lanthanum	Pregabalin	Zonisamide
Lenalidomide	Rasagiline	

4

2C * is a sub-family, containing many closely related enzymes, e.g. 2C9, 2C10, 2C19, etc. About 20% Asians and 3–5% Caucasians are CYP2C19 poor metabolisers (PMs). Around 8% of the population are 2C19 PMs (Carlsson *et al*, *J Anal Toxicol* 2009;**33**:65–76; FFT). 2C9 accounts for around 20% total CYP in the liver, and metabolises about 15% of clinical drugs. It has at least 33 variants (Zhou *et al*, *Toxicology* 2010;**278**:165–88). Probes exist for 2C8 (substrate repaglinide, inhibitor gemfibrozil), 2C9 (substrate tolbutamide; no known inhibitor) and 2C19 (substrate omeprazole; inhibitor fluvoxamine).

CYP2D6

Substrates (drugs metabolised by this enzyme) *		
Amfetamines	Ciprofloxacin	Fluoxetine (partly)
Amprenavir	Citalopram (minor)	Fluvoxamine (partly)
Antiarrhythmics type 1c (encainide, flecainide, etc)	Clozapine (minor, unproven)	Gamma-hydroxybutyrate
	Codeine (to morphine)	Galantamine
Aripiprazole	Darifenacin (saturable)	Gefitinib
Asenapine (minor)	Debrisoquine	Haloperidol
Atomoxetine	Desvenlafaxine	Hydrocodone
Beta-blockers (especially lipophilic, metoprolol, nebivolol, propranolol, timolol)	Dexfenfluramine	Indoramin
	Dextromethorphan	Letrozole
	Diazepam	Loratadine
	Donepezil (partly)	Methadone (part)
Bortezomib	Duloxetine (partly)	Methamfetamine
Buprenorphine	Ecstasy	Mexiletine (main)
Carvedilol	Fenfluramine	Mianserin
Chloroquine	Fesoterodine (minor)	Mirtazapine (minor)
Chlorphenamine	Flecainide	Morphine derivatives
Cinnarizine	Fluphenazine	Imatinib (minor but can

Substrates (drugs metabolised by this enzyme) *continued* *

be major)
Nefazodone
Nicotine (partly)
Olanzapine (partly)
Ondansetron
Oxycodone (partly, to active oxymorphone)
Palonosetron (main)
Paroxetine
Phenothiazines (e.g. perphenazine, chlorpromazine, fluphenazine, thioridazine)
Propafenone
Quinidine
Risperidone (major)
Sertindole (partly)
Tamoxifen (pro-drug, metabolised to active drug)
Tolcapone (minor)
Tolterodine
Tramadol
Trazodone
Tricyclics — 2° and 3° tricyclics (e.g. nortriptyline, desipramine, doxepin, imipramine, amitriptyline, clomipramine, trimipramine)
Venlafaxine (major)
Vincristine
Vindesine
Vinorelbine
Zuclopenthixol

Significant enzyme inducers (decrease levels of substrates)

Carbamazepine (weak)
Ginseng (weak)
Phenobarbital (weak)
Phenytoin (weak)
Rifampicin (weak)
Ritonavir (weak)

Significant enzyme inhibitors (increase levels of substrates) *

Amiodarone
Asenapine (weak)
Buprenorphine (very weak)
Bupropion
Celecoxib
Chloroquine
Chlorphenamine
Chlorpromazine
Cimetidine
Citalopram (very weak/nil)
Clomipramine (moderate)
Cocaine
Cyclizine
Dextromethorphan
Dextropropoxyphene
Diltiazem (weak)
Diphenhydramine
Duloxetine
Escitalopram (weak)
Fenfluramine?
Flecainide
Fluoxetine (strong)
Fluphenazine
Fluvoxamine (very weak)
Haloperidol (dose-dependent)
Indinavir
Levomepromazine
Melperone
Methadone (moderate)
Metoclopramide
Metoprolol
Methylnaltrexone (weak)
Mexiletine
Mirtazapine (very weak/nil)
Moclobemide
Modafinil (small and dose-dependent)
Nicardipine
Nilotinib (strong)
Norfluoxetine (strong)
Oxycodone
Paroxetine (strong, dose-related)
Perphenazine
Pindolol
Primaquine
Promethazine
Propafenone
Propanolol
Quinidine
Quinine
Quetiapine
Ritonavir
Sertraline (weak, dose-related, moderate at 150mg/d)
Terbinafine (potent)
Thioridazine
Timolol
Tipranavir (potent)
Tricyclics (all, strong)
Yohimbine

No effect

Anidulafungin
Aripiprazole
Benzodiazepines
Bevacizumab
Emtricitabine
Galantamine
Isotretinoin
Lacosamide
Lamotrigine
Lanthanum
Lenalidomide
Levetiracetam
Memantine
Mirtazapine
Olanzapine
Palonosetron
Posaconazole
Pregabalin
Rasagiline
Rufinamide
Sitagliptin

No effect *continued*

Sulpiride	Varenicline	Zoledronic acid
Sunitinib	Venlafaxine (very weak, nil)	Zonisamide
Telbivudine	Ziprasidone	

CYP2D6 *

2D6 accounts for only about 2–4% of total liver CYPs but metabolises about 25% of current drugs (Zhou, *Clin Pharmacokinet* 2009;**48**:689–723). Metabolism occurs both in the liver and in the brain. An individual's CYP2D6 status (Zhou, *Clin Pharmacokinet* 2009;**48**:761–804) can be determined by giving the probes debrisoquine or dextromethorphan and measuring the ratios of drug and metabolite. Paroxetine is an inhibitor probe. Around 5–8% Caucasians, 8.5% African-Americans and 2–10% Asians are slow metabolisers. Up to 29% North Africans and Middle East people (de Leon *et al*, *Psychosomatics* 2006;**47**:75–85) are ultra-rapid metabolisers (three or more 2D6 alleles). All CYP2D6 inhibition is probably concentration-dependent and so inclusion in this list only predicts that an interaction could occur, not that it will.

CYP3A3/4

4

Substrates (drugs metabolised by this enzyme) *

Alfentanil	Chloramphenicol	Efavirez
Alitretinoin	Chloroquine	Exemestane
Alosetron	Ciclosporin	Ergotamine
Amiodarone (major)	Cimetidine	Erlotinib (major)
Amprenavir	Ciprofloxacin	Estradiol and estrogens
Androgens	Cisapride (restricted in UK)	Ethosuximide
Antihistamines, e.g. astemizole	Citalopram (minor, 30%)	Ethinylestradiol
Aripiprazole	Clindamycin	Etoposide
Asenapine (minor)	Clopidogrel	Etravirine
Benzodiazepines (e.g. alprazolam, clonazepam, clobazam, diazepam, flunitrazepam, midazolam, temazepam and triazolam, but not lorazepam)	Clotrimazole	Everolimus
	Clozapine (partly)	Fentanyl
	Cocaine (10%)	Fesoterodine (main)
	Codeine	Fexofenadine
	Colchicine	Fluconazole
	Cortisol	Fluoxetine
Bortezomib	Cyclophosphamide	Flutamine
Bromocriptine	Dapsone	Fluvoxamine
Budesonide	Darifenacin	Fosaprepitant
Buprenorphine	Dasatinib	Galantamine
Buspirone	Dexamethasone	Gefitinib
Busulfan	Dextromethorphan	Glibenclamide
Calcium-channel blockers (e.g. amlodipine, diltiazem, felodipine, isradipine, nicardipine, nifedipine, verapamil)	Digoxin	Glyburide?
	Disopyramide	Granisetron
	Docetaxol	Guanfacine
	Donepezil (part)	Haloperidol
	Doxorubicin	Ifosfamide
Cannabinoids (main)	Doxycycline	Imatinib (major)
Carbamazepine	Dutasteride	Indinavir

Substrates (drugs metabolised by this enzyme) *continued* *		
Irinotecan	Perphenazine	Steroids (e.g. dexamethasone)
Isoniazid	Pethidine	St John's wort
Isotretinoin	Phencyclidine	Sunitinib
Itraconazole	Phenobarbital	Tacrolimus
Ivabradine	Phenytoin	Tamoxifen
Ivermectin	Pimozide (mostly)	Temsirolimus
Ketamine	Prednisone	Testosterone
Ketoconazole	Progesterone	Theophylline
Lapatinib	Proguanil	Thiotepa
Levonorgestrel	Propafenone	Tiagabine
Lidocaine	Promazine	Tipranavir
Lisuride	Protein-pump inhibitors (lansoprazole [weak], omeprazole, rabeprazole)	Tolcapone (minor)
Lopinavir	Quetiapine (mostly)	Tolterodine
Loratadine	Quinidine	Tolvaptan
Losartan	Quinine	Topiramate (possibly)
Macrolides (e.g. erythromycin, clarithromycin)	Ramelteon (minor)	Toremifene
Maravoric	Reboxetine	Trabectedin
Meloxicam	Rifampicin	Tricyclics — tertiary (e.g. imipramine, amitriptyline, clomipramine)
Methadone (main)	Rimonabant	Valproate
Methylprednisolone	Risperidone (partly)	Vardenafil
Mianserin	Ritonavir	Venlafaxine
Mibefradil	Saquinavir	Vinblastine
Miconazole	Sertindole (partly)	Vincristine
Mifepristone	Sertraline	Vinorelbine (major)
Mirtazapine (partly)	Sibutramine (main)	R-warfarin (minor)
Modafinil	Sildenafil (partly)	Zaleplon (secondary route)
Nefazodone	Sirolimus	Ziprasidone (most)
Nelfinavir	Sitagliptin (limited except in renal failure)	Zolpidem (mainly)
Nilotinib	Sodium fusidate	Zonisamide (part)
Ondansetron	Sorafenib	Zopiclone (mostly)
Orphenadrine	Statins (e.g. atorvastatin, cerivastatin, lovastatin, pravastin, simvastatin)	Zotepine
Oxycodone (inactivation)		Zuclopenthixol
Paclitaxel		
Paracetamol		
Paricalcitol (?)		

Significant enzyme inducers (decrease levels of substrates)		
Armodafinil (weak)	Flucloxacillin	Prednisone
Barbiturates (all)	Modafinil (small and dose-dependent)	Primidone
Carbamazepine (induces 3A4 about 46% more than oxcarbazepine)	Nevirapine (?)	Rifampicin (rapid)
Cortisol	Omeprazole	Rufinamide (moderate effect)
Dexamethasone	Oxcarbazepine	St John's wort (moderate)
Efavirez	Phenobarbital	Topiramate (dose-dependent, especially at high doses)
Ethosuximide	Phenytoin	Troglitazone
	Pioglitazone	

Significant enzyme inhibitors (increase levels of substrates)		
Acetazolamide	Ginkgo biloba	Orange juice (weak)
Amiodarone	Grapefruit juice (weak)	Oxycodone
Atazaivir (moderate)	Imatinib	Paroxetine (weak)
Brivanib	Indinavir (moderate)	Pomegranate juice (inhibits intestinal 3A4)
Buprenorphine (weak/ moderate)	Isoniazid (potent)	Posaconazole (potent)
Cannabinoids	Itraconazole (strong)	Quinine
Cimetidine (moderate)	Ivabradine (very weak)	Ritonavir (moderate)
Citalopram (weak)	Ketoconazole (strong)	Saquinavir
Clotrimazole	Lopinavir	Sertraline (minor)
Danazol	Macrolides (some, e.g. clarithromycin, erythromycin [strong])	Statins (atorvastatin, fluvastatin)
Dextropropoxyphene	Methadone (weak?)	Stiripentol (variable)
Diltiazem (weaker)	Metronidazole	Terbinafine
Echinacea purpurea (weak)	Miconazole (strong)	Trazodone
Erlotinib	Mifepristone	Tricyclics (moderate)
Fluconazole (strong)	Nefazodone (strong)	Troleandomycin (strong)
Fluoxetine (weak)	Nelfinavir	Venlafaxine (very weak)
Fluvoxamine (moderate)	Nilotinib (moderate)	Verapamil (weak)
Fosaprepitant (minor)	Norfluoxetine (moderate)	Zafirlukast
Gestodene		

No effect		
Aliskiren	Ivabradine	Posaconazole
Anidulafungin	Lamotrigine	Pregabalin
Aripiprazole	Lanthanum	Rasagiline
Asenapine	Lenalidomide	Sitagliptin
Benzodiazepines	Levetiracetam	Sunitinib
Bevacizumab	Lithium	Telbivudine
Capecitibane	Memantine	Tofacitinib
Cranberry juice	Methylnaltrexone	Varenicline
Duloxetine	Mirtazapine	Zoledronic acid
Emtricitabine	Nelarabine	Zonisamide
Galantamine	Olanzapine	Ziprasidone
Honey	Palonosetron	
Isotretinoin	Pioglitazone	

CYP3A3/4 * (very similar structures, and are often grouped together). CYP3A4 is an important P450 enzyme, metabolising at least 50% of all marketed medications (Zhou, *Curr Drug Metab* 2008;**9**:310–22), and may account for up to 50–60% of the total liver P450. There is little generic polymorphism so little inter-individual variation exits. CYP3A4 occurs in the liver, gut, and possibly the brain. Ultra-rapid metabolisers have not yet been identified. Midazolam oral is a reliable substrate probe, although simvastatin, lovastatin and buspirone are alternatives (s = 113, Ohno *et al*, *Clin Pharmacokinet* 2007;**46**:681–96). Ketoconazole is the main inhibitor probe.

4

5 DRUG-INDUCED PSYCHIATRIC DISORDERS

Contents

5.1	Anxiety, agitation and nervousness	437
5.2	Aggression	440
5.3	Behavioural changes	440
5.4	Delirium and confusion	441
5.5	Depression	446
5.6	Hallucinations	452
5.7	Mania, hypomania or euphoria	456
5.8	Movement disorders	462
5.8.1	Pseudoparkinsonism	462
5.8.2	Akathisia	464
5.8.3	Dystonias	466
5.8.4	Dyskinesias	469
5.8.5	Other movement disorders	471
5.8.5.1	*Catatonia*	*471*
5.8.5.2	*Cataplexy*	*472*
5.8.5.3	*Choreas*	*472*
5.8.5.4	*Rabbit syndrome*	*473*
5.8.5.5	*Tics*	*474*
5.9.	Neuroleptic malignant syndrome	475
5.10	Obsessive-compulsive symptoms	477
5.11	Panic attacks	478
5.12	Paranoid or schizoprenic-like psychoses	480
5.13	Serotonin syndrome	490
5.14	Sleep problems	493
5.14.1	Sleep disturbances	493
5.14.2	Vivid dreams and nightmares	495
5.15	Suicidal ideation	496

The drugs listed in each section have been reported to cause those symptoms in some context (e.g. standard dose, high dose, prolonged courses, etc). The main references next to the drug should be consulted to ascertain the circumstances of reports. The references are offered without qualification and no indication of frequency or status of reports can be given, as this information is not really available, except where a side-effect is well recognised, e.g. BNF listed. For completeness, some drugs not available in every country are also listed.

The BNF side-effect categories generally mean:

- Very common = more than one in 10 people get this side-effect
- Common = one in 10 to one in 100 (1–10%)
- Uncommon or less common = one in 100 to one in 1,000 (0.1–1%)
- Rare = one in 1,000 to one in 10,000 (0.01–0.1%)
- Very rare = less than one in 10,000 (≤0.01%).

Each side-effect may be dose-related (the higher the dose, the more likely you are to get it, especially a higher starting dose) and may abate with time.

Sub-divisions are based on the BNF chapters: (although drugs may appear in several sections)

- CNS: sleep disorders and anxiety (BDZs, hypnotics, modafinil, sodium oxybate/GHB)
- CNS: antipsychotics (including lithium)
- CNS: antidepressants (including bupropion)
- CNS: analgesics
- CNS: anticonvulsants
- CNS: movement disorders (piracetam, neuroprotection, dystonias, Parkinson's)
- CNS: others
- Gastrointestinal drugs
- Cardiovascular drugs
- Respiratory drugs
- Anti-infection drugs
- Endocrine system drugs
- Malignancy and immunosuppressant drugs
- Musculoskeletal and analgesics
- Others

5.1 ANXIETY, AGITATION AND NERVOUSNESS

• CNS — sleep disorders and anxiety

Benzodiazepine withdrawal (n=43, d/b, p/c, 7/52, abrupt is much worse than gradual discontinuation, e.g. *Am J Psychiatry* 1984;**141**:848–52)

Buspirone (n=3, *J Clin Psychiatry* 1988;**49**:165–6)

Clomethiazole

Modafinil (BNF, common, n=2, *J Clin Psychopharmacol* 2005;**25**:628–9)

Sodium oxybate (BNF common; including GHB intoxication; n=66 with toxicity, 60% incidence, *Am J Emerg Med* 2005;**23**:316–20)

Temazepam

Zopiclone (n=1, *Ir Med J* 2007;**100**:511; n=1, *Prog Neurol Psychiatry* 2009;**13**:20–4)

• CNS — antipsychotics

Aripiprazole initiation (n=2, *J Clin Psychiatry* 2004;**65**:132–3; n=3, *Pharmacotherapy* 2007; **27**:1339–42)

~ high-dose (n=1, *J Neuropsychiatry Clin Neurosci* 2007;**19**:481–2)

~ after clozapine discontinuation (n=1, *J Clin Psychiatry* 2009;**70**:141–3)

Olanzapine (*Can J Psychiatry* 1998;**43**:1054)

Quetiapine (n=1, as adjunct, *Psychiatry Res* 2014;**216**:286–7)

Risperidone (e.g. n=1, *Psychiatry Clin Neurosci* 1999;**53**:682)

Zotepine (common)

• CNS — antidepressants *

Early worsening of anxiety and agitation with antidepressants is well-known, but very poorly researched (7% incidence, 10 x risk if first-degree relatives had a mood disorder; n=301, *Neuropsychiatr Dis Treat* 2014;**10**:2115–21; FFT).

Bupropion (incidence 9.7%; BNF, common)

Mianserin, abrupt discontinuation (n=1, *Jpn J Psychiatry Neurol* 1989;**43**:155–9)

Moclobemide (incidence 5–10%, *J Neural Transm Suppl* 1989;**28**:77–89)

Reboxetine (BNF, rare)

SSRIs (BNF, common)

→ citalopram

→ fluoxetine (incidence 9%? e.g. *J Clin Psychiatry* 1985;**46**(3 Pt 2):32–7)

→ paroxetine (incidence 11%? *Acta Psychiatr Scand Suppl* 1989;**350**:117–23)

→ paroxetine discontinuation (rebound anxiety, review, *Can J Clin Pharmacol* 2006;**13**:69–74; FFT)

→ SSRI discontinuation (BNF)

Tricyclics (e.g. amitriptyline, lofepramine at <2%, review in *Drugs* 1989;**37**:123–40)

• CNS — analgesics *

Buprenorphine (BNF, common)

Fentanyl (BNF, common)

Frovatriptan (BNF, less common)

Hydromorphone IV (n=1, *Ann Pharmacother* 2013;**47**:e34)

Morphine

Nefopam

Oxycodone (BNF, common)

Pentazocine (e.g. *Br Med J* 1974;**2**:224; FFT)

Pizotifen (BNF, rare)

Sumatriptan (in people with panic disorder, n=15, RCT, d/b, p/c, *Eur Neuropsychopharmacol* 2005;**15**:279–82)

• CNS — anticonvulsants

Carbamazepine (*J Am Acad Child Adolesc Psychiatry* 1988;**27**:500–3)

Clonazepam

Ethosuximide

Gabapentin (BNF, common)

Gabapentin discontinuation (e.g. n=1, *Am J Health Syst Pharm* 2010;**67**:910–2)

Lamotrigine

Levetiracetam (BNF, common)

Phenobarbital and other barbiturates

Rufinamide (BNF, common; 1–10% incidence, SmPC)

Topiramate (BNF, common)

Valproate (n=1, *J Neuropsychiatry Clin Neurosci* 2001;**13**:528–30)

Vigabatrin

Zonisamide (SmPC)

• CNS — movement disorders

Amantadine

Anticholinergics (BNF, common)

Baclofen (used in Parkinson's Disease, SmPC change 2009)

Botulinum toxin A injection (BNF, less common; e.g. *South Med J* 1999;**92**:738)

Bromocriptine

Levodopa (BNF, common)

Piracetam (BNF, uncommon)

Rotigotine (BNF, less common)

- **CNS — others** *

Alcohol (review, n=285, *Aggress Behav* 2007;**33**:327–38)
Anticholinesterases (n=4, *J Neuropsychiatry Clin Neurosci* 1992;**4**:189–94), e.g:
→ donepezil (n=1, *Int J Geriatr Psychiatry* 2003;**18**:657–8)
galantamine (n=1, *Consult Pharm* 2013;**28**:243–6)
→ rivastigmine (incidence <5%, inc transdermal patches; SmPC, common)
Aprepitant (BNF, less common)
Atomoxetine (BNF, common)
Caffeine (n=22 children, d/b, p/c, c/o, *J Am Acad Child Adolesc Psychiatry* 1994;**33**:407–15)
Cannabis (n=79, no association, *Psychiatry Res* 2003;**118**:1–8)
Dexamfetamine
Flumazenil (BNF, common)
Gamma-Hydroxybutyrate (GHB) — see sodium oxybate
Ginseng (reported, inc. abuse, see *Arch Gen Psychiatry* 1998;**55**:1033–44)
Granisetron (unconfirmed, e.g. *Eur J Cancer* 1990;**26**[Supp 1]:S19–23)
Heroin withdrawal (*Int J Addict* 1992;**27**:25–35)
LSD (n=16, responds to clonazepam, *Int Clin Psychopharmacol* 2003;**18**:101–5)
Memantine (5.6% incidence, n=196, *J Neuropsychiatry Clin Neurosci* 2015;**27**:e10–3)
Memantine abrupt discontinuation (n=2, *Geriatr Gerontol Int* 2009;**9**:203–5)
Methamphetamine (3% in people with psychosis, n=121, *Addict Health* 2015;**7**:37–46; FFT)
Metoclopramide (n=1, *Psychiatry Clin Neurosci* 2007;**61**:193–5)
Naltrexone (BNF, common)
Nicotine discontinuation (n=40, *Am J Psychiatry* 2011;**168**:395–9)
Orlistat (BNF, common)
Palonosetron (BNF, less common)
Rimonabant (BNF, common; see SmPC and *Lancet* 2007;**370**:1671–2)
Sibutramine (BNF, common)
Varenicline (lower risk, s=39, n=10761, RCTs, *BMJ* 2015;**350**:h1109; FFT; links with agitation but not substantiated, s=15, n=4,443, *Cochrane Database Syst Rev* 2012;**12**:CD006103)

- **Gastrointestinal drugs** *

Bismuth intoxication (*Postgrad Med J* 1988;**64**:308–10; FFT)
H2 blockers (BNF, rare) e.g:
→ cimetidine (*Adv Psychiatric Treat* 2005;**11**:68)
→ famotidine (mentioned in *Digestion* 1985;**32** [Suppl 1]:24–31)
Misoprostol
Omeprazole
Rabeprazole (n=1, *Ann Pharmacother* 2007;**41**:1315–7)

- **Cardiovascular drugs** *

Adrenaline/epinephrine (BNF, common)
Atenolol discontinuation (n=1, *Am J Psychiatry* 1994;**151**:1840)
Cilostazol (BNF, less common)
Doxazosin (incidence 2.4%)
Epoprostenol (BNF, common)
Fondaparinux sodium (BNF, rare)
Hydralazine (BNF, rare)
Methoxamine
Methyldopa (rare)
Metoprolol low-dose (n=1, *Gen Hosp Psychiatry* 2010;**32**:646.e5–7)
Moexipril (BNF, common)
Nicardipine (rare)
Nifedipine (*An Med Interna* 1992;**9**:362)
Ramipril (BNF, less common)
Sodium nitroprusside (BNF, common)
Streptokinase (see *Drugs* 1973;**5**:357–45)
Telmisartan (BNF, less common)

- **Respiratory drugs** *

Aminophylline
Cyproheptadine OD (n=57, *Clin Toxicol (Phila)* 2011;**49**:681–3)
Dextromethorphan + hydrocodone + propoxyphene (n=1, *J Psychopharmacol* 2009;**23**:989–91)
Ephedrine (BNF, common)
Mizolastine (BNF, common)
Montelukast (SmPC, FDA warning 2009; review, *Pharmacology* 2014;**94**:60–70; FFT)
Phenylpropanolamine OD (*Lancet* 1979;**314**:1367–8)
Pseudoephedrine (n=1, *Eur J Clin Pharmacol* 1978;**14**:253–9)
Salbutamol
Theophylline (*Med Clin [Barc]* 1987;**88**:549–50)

- **Anti-infection drugs** *

Atazanavir (BNF, less common)
Azithromycin (BNF, rare; n = 1, *Pediatr Neurol* 2011;**44**:311–3)
Chloroquine (*Adv Psychiatr Treat* 2005;**11**:66)
Clarithromycin (BNF, very rare)
Co-trimoxazole (n = 1, *J Clin Psychopharmacol* 1991;**11**:144–5)
Daptomycin (BNF, less common)
Darunavir (BNF, common)
Efavirenz (BNF, common)
Enfuvirtide (BNF, common)
Ertapenem (BNF, rare)
Ganciclovir (BNF, common)
Isoniazid (*Lancet* 1989;**334**:735–6)
Levamisole (rare, *N Engl J Med* 1990;**322**:352–8; FFT)
Levofloxacin (n = 3, *J Neurosci Rural Pract* 2012;**3**:212–4; FFT)
Lopinavir + ritonavir (BNF, less common)
Mefloquine (BNF, less common; *Pharm J* 1989;**243**:561)
Penicillins (*Adv Psychiatr Treat* 2005;**11**:66)
Piperazine (see *Trans R Soc Trop Med Hyg* 1976;**70**:358)
Quinine (*Adv Psychiatr Treat* 2005;**11**:66)
Quinupristin + dalfopristin (BNF, less common)
Ribavirin (BNF, common)
Ritonavir (BNF, common)
Stavudine (BNF, less common)
Voriconazole (BNF, common)
Zidovudine (BNF, common)

- **Endocrine system drugs**

Corticosteroids (BNF, less common; incidence may be as high as 5–6% in adults, usually emerges within a few days or weeks, risk may be higher with higher doses, *MHRA Drug Safety Update* 2007;1–9)
  - → dexamethasone (overall risks include dose (but not time, duration or severity), female gender and PMH (but only a weak association, see *Arch Gen Psychiatry* 1981;**38**:471–7)
  - → methyltestosterone
  - → prednisone

Danazol (BNF, common)
Levothyroxine
Testosterone and esters (BNF, common)
Zoledronic acid (BNF, less common)

- **Malignancy and immunosuppressant drugs** *

Buserelin (BNF, less common)
Ciclosporin (*Adv Psychiatr Treat* 2005;**11**:68)
Clofarabine (BNF, common)
Glatiramer acetate (BNF, common)
Imatinib (BNF, less common)
Interferons, e.g.:
  - → interferon alfa (responds to BDZs, n = 2, *J Psychopharmacol* 2004;**18**:41–6)
  - → peginterferon alfa 2a + ribavirin (n = 176, incidence < 36%, *Aliment Pharmacol Ther* 2008;**27**:257–65; FFT)

Letrozole (BNF, less common)
Octreotide
Trastuzumab (BNF, less common)
Tretinoin (BNF, common)

- **Musculoskeletal and analgesics**

Abatacept (BNF, less common)
Baclofen (BNF, common)
Etoricoxib (BNF, less common)
Leflunomide (BNF, common)
Methocarbamol (BNF, less common)
NSAIDs, e.g.:
  - → ibuprofen (overdose, *Am J Emerg Med* 1998;**16**:549–50)
  - → indometacin (n = 1, *South Med J* 1983;**76**:679–80)
  - → mefenamic acid
  - → naproxen
  - → naproxen + chloroquine (*Ann Pharmacother* 1993;**27**:1058–9)

- **Others** *

Atropine eye drops (n = 1, *J Ped Ophthalmol Strabis* 1985;**22**:38–9)
Cyclopentolate eye drops (n = 1, *Nervenarzt* 2009;**80**:967–9)
Deferasirox (BNF, less common)
Flunisolide
Hormone treatments for prostate cancer (n = 526, *Int J Clin Oncol* 2014;**19**:523–30)
Isotretinoin (BNF, rare; n = 45 [c = 23], no association with anxiety, *J Dermatolog Treat* 2004;**15**:153–7)
Ketamine (BNF, common; n = 2, *J Psychopharmacol* 2013;**27**:651–4)
Lead (higher levels, n = 1,987, *Arch Gen Psychiatry* 2009;**66**:1313–9; FFT)
Lidocaine (n = 15, incidence 73%, *Am J Psychiatry* 1987;**144**:159–63)

5

Neostigmine (cases in *Dtsch Med Wochenschr* 1966;**91**:699)
Organic solvents (n=77, up to 36% can develop anxiety clusters, *Psychosom Med* 2000;**62**:746–50)
Phenylephrine (rare)
Pyridostigmine (rare)
Ropivacaine (BNF, less common; n=3 after nerve block, *Reg Anesth Pain Med* 1999;**24**:175–8)
Sevoflurane (n=169, common, reduced by clonidine, *Anesth Analg* 2005;**101**:1619–22)
Sildenafil (BNF common)
Tacrolimus (BNF, rare)
Vardenafil (BNF, rare)
Yohimbine (mentioned in *Arch Gen Psychiatry* 1998;**55**:1033–44)
Zafirlukast (FDA warning 2009)

5.2 AGGRESSION, INCLUDING HOSTILITY AND VIOLENCE

Review: Shaw and Fletcher, *Adv Drug React Toxicolog Rev* 2000;**19**:35–45.

- CNS *

Alcohol (review, n=285, *Aggress Behav* 2007;**33**:327–38)
Alcohol withdrawal
Amantadine (cases in *Br Med J* 1972;**3**:50; FFT)
Amfetamine withdrawal
Anticholinesterases (n=4, *J Neuropsychiatry Clin Neurosci* 1992;**4**:189–94), e.g.:
→donepezil (many e.g. n=1, *Int J Geriatr Psychiatry* 2003;**18**:657–8)
Atomoxetine (*Pediatrics* 2004;**114**:895–6)
Barbiturate withdrawal
Benzodiazepines (incidence <1%, *J Clin Psychiatry* 1988;**49**:184–8; during prolonged BDZ use: *Can J Psychiatry* 2000;**45**:89–90; aggressogenic effect from diazepam, n=60 male, *Addict Behav* 2002;**27**:167–77), e.g.:
→alprazolam (greater response to provocation, n=23, RCT, p/c, 8/52, *J Affect Disord* 1995;**35**:117–23)
Cannabis (review, *J Drug Edu* 2011;**41**:369–89)
Carbamazepine
Gabapentin (n=1, *J Neuropsychiatry Clin Neurosci* 2001;**13**:424; n=2, *Epilepsia* 1996;**37**:501–2)
Lamotrigine (survey, n=19, *Epilepsia* 1998;**39**:280–2; n=2, murderous impulses, *Gen Hosp Psychiatry* 2014;**36**:451.e1–2)
Levetiracetam (SmPC, n=163, associated with depression, *Epilepsy Behav* 2015;**45**:64–7; see also n=1, *Epilepsy Behav Case Rep* 2015;**4**:79–81; FFT)
Methamphetamine dependence (n=76, *Arch Gen Psychiatry* 2011;**68**:271–82; FFT)
Modafinil (n=2, *J Clin Psychopharmacol* 2005;**25**:628–9)
Naloxone IV (n=2, *Ann Pharmacother* 1992;**26**:196–8)
Nicotine withdrawal (n=40, *Am J Psychiatry* 2011;**168**:395–9)
Olanzapine (*Can J Psychiatry* 1998;**43**:1054)
Paroxetine withdrawal (*Lancet* 1995;**346**:57)
Tricyclics (rare)
Varenicline (no effect, s=39, n=10761, RCTs, *BMJ* 2015;**350**:h1109; FFT)
Venlafaxine (n=1, *J Am Acad Child Adolesc Psychiatry* 2003;**42**:383–4)

- Others

Anabolic steroids, e.g. oxandrolone
Anabolic steroid discontinuation
Cyproheptadine (n=1, *J Am Acad Child Adolesc Psychiatry* 1998;**37**:668–70)
Omeprazole
Sildenafil (review, n=274, *Ann Pharmacother* 2002;**36**:1129–34)
Steroids high dose (n=71 and review; *Psychol Addict Behav* 2014;**28**:1096–104; *Lancet* 1987;**2**:750–1)
Testosterone (highly variable, n=56 men, RCT, p/c, c/o, 3x6/52, *Arch Gen Psychiatry* 2000;**57**:133–40)

5.3 BEHAVIOURAL CHANGES

- CNS

Barbiturates
Benzodiazepines:
→clonazepam (*Dev Med Child Neurol* 1991;**33**:362–5)
Carbamazepine (*J Paediatrics* 1982;**101**:785–7)
Donepezil (e.g. n=7, *Am J Psychiatry* 1998;**155**:1632–3)
Levetiracetam (n=553, incidence 7%, *Neurology* 2003;**61**:1218–21)
Sodium oxybate (as gamma-hydroxybutyrate/GHB intoxication; n=66 with toxicity, 60% incidence, *Am J Emerg Med* 2005;**23**:316–20)

- Others

Anabolic steroids (n = 1, bizarre after brief exposure, *Am J Psychiatry* 1992;**149**:271–2)
Bismuth (n = 99, *Acta Neurol Belg* 1979;**79**:73)
Prazosin (n = 1, bizarre behaviour, *Am J Psychiatry* 2008;**165**:774–5)
Prednisone discontinuation (*JAMA* 1989;**261**:1731–2)
Theophylline (disputed — not in children, *JAMA* 1992;**267**:2621–4)

5.4 DELIRIUM (ACUTE ORGANIC PSYCHOSIS) AND CONFUSION

Drug-induced delirium is usually an acute reaction and always with fluctuating levels of awareness of self and environment. It is most frequent in frail or dementing elderly, drug abusers and with pre-existing organic brain disease, and is strongly associated with anticholinergic activity:

- highest risk drug groups are tricyclics, phenothiazines and anticholinergics
- medium risk drugs include benzodiazepines, sedatives, dopamine-activating drugs, anticonvulsants, histamine H2 receptor blockers, digoxin, beta-blockers and analgesics. Most of these do not have direct anticholinergic effects but *in vitro* have been shown to bind to muscarinic receptors.

Reviews: general (Hufschmidt *et al*, *Acta Neurol Scand* 2009;**120**:436–8; Meyer *et al*, *Ther Umsch* 2010;**67**:79–83), systematic review (s = 14, Clegg and Young, *Age Ageing* 2011;**40**:23–9; FFT), drugs with anticholinergic properties (Cancelli *et al*, *Neurol Sci* 2009;**30**:87–92).

- CNS — sleep disorders and anxiety *

Benzodiazepine withdrawal
Benzodiazepines — new users over 65 (mean 78 years) have more chance of dementia (OR = 1.62) (n = 1796, 15 years, *BMJ* 2012; **345**: e6231), but a causal relationship has not been established and this may just be BDZs being used to treat early symptoms (*BMJ* 2012;**345**:e7986; n = 112, increased risk of delirium but limited to continuous infusion only;*Intensive Care Med* 2015;**41**:2130–7):
  → alprazolam (n = 1, *Clin Neuropharmacol* 1998;**21**:201–3)
  → diazepam as pre-med (n = 1, *Indian J Ophthalmol* 1989;**37**:35–6; FFT)

Chloral and derivatives
Clomethiazole
Clomethiazole withdrawal
Sodium oxybate (SmPC; as gamma-hydroxy butyrate/GHB; n = 1, *Gen Hosp Psychiatry* 2000;**22**:213–5; and GHB withdrawal; n = 1, *Ned Tijdschr Geneeskd* 2010;**154**:A1086)
Zolpidem (many cases, e.g. n = 1, elderly, *Psychosomatics* 2004;**45**:88–9; n = 1, *Indian J Pharmacol* 2011;**43**:729–30; FFT)
Zopiclone discontinuation (n = 1, *Age Ageing* 2005;**34**:526–7; FFT)

- CNS — antipsychotics *

Aripiprazole high-dose (n = 1, *J Neuropsychiatry Clin Neurosci* 2007;**19**:481–2)
Butyrophenones
Clozapine (may occur in 10%, especially in older people also taking other anticholinergics; n = 139, *Pharmacopsychiatry* 2003;**36**:156–60)
Clozapine discontinuation (n = 3, *J Clin Psychiatry* 1997;**58**:252–5)
Lithium (many e.g. n = 1, *Psychiatr Prax* 2000;**27**:296–7; n = 1, *Practitioner* 2009;**253**:28–30; n = 1, at therapeutic levels, *Prog Neurol Psychiatry* 2014;**18**:10–12)
Lithium discontinuation (n = 1, complicated by mania, *Gen Hosp Psychiatry* 2010;**32**:102–4)
Lithium + tricyclic (n = 1, Hayward and Luft, *Ther Adv Psychopharmacol* 2012;**2**:157–8)
Olanzapine (e.g. n = 1, *Psychiatry Investig* 2010;**7**:153–4; FFT; n = 1 elderly male, *J Neuropsychiatry Clin Neurosci* 2011;**23**:E54–5)
Olanzapine + opioid (n = 2, *J Pain Symptom Manage* 2005;**29**:330–2)
Phenothiazines (esp. sedative ones)
Quetiapine + lithium (n = 1, *Clin Neuropharmacol* 2008;**31**:176–9)
Quetiapine overdose (n = 1, *Pediatr Emerg Care* 2010;**26**:754–6) and toxicity (n = 1, *Aust N Z J Psychiatry* 2009;**43**:781)
Quetiapine + valproate (n = 2, *Gen Hosp Psychiatry* 2010;**32**:e1–2)
Risperidone (n = 1, *Can J Psychiatry* 1998;**43**:194; n = 1, *J Child Adolesc Psychopharmacol* 2005;**15**:520–5)

- CNS — antidepressants *

Agomelatine (n = 2, *Ann Clin Psychiatry* 2013;**25**: 67–8)

5

Bupropion (cases, e.g. *J Clin Psychiatry* 1990;**51**:307–8; n=1, *Int J Clin Pharm* 2012;**34**:9–12)
Bupropion + fluoxetine (n=1, *J Clin Psychopharmacol* 2006;**26**:677–9)
Bupropion + risperidone (*J Clin Psychopharmacol* 2014;**34**:161–2)
Duloxetine (n=1, *Psychiatry Clin Neurosci* 2012;**66**:166)
MAOIs, e.g.:
→ phenelzine (*J Clin Psychiatry* 1987;**48**: 340–1)
→ tranylcypromine (*J Clin Psychopharmacol* 1997;**17**:430–2)
→ tranylcypromine abuse (*J Clin Psychopharmacol* 2000;**20**:270–1)
→ tranylcypromine discontinuation (n=1, *J Clin Psychopharmacol* 2013;**33**:574–6)
Mianserin (n=5, *Eur Neuropsychopharmacol* 1995;**5**:147–9; in dementia, *J Clin Psychopharmacol* 2010;**30**:467–8)
Mirtazapine (n=3, *Int Clin Psychopharmacol* 2000;**15**:239–43; n=1 due to hyponatraemia, *Indian J Pharmacol* 2014;**46**:448–9; FFT)
SSRIs — a review suggested only 5 clear cases worldwide over last 20 years (*Psychiatr Danub* 2014;**26**:277–80; FFT) including:
→ citalopram IV (n=1, *Pharmacopsychiatry* 2013;**46**:37–38; n=1, *BMJ Case Rep* 2013; **2013**:bcr2013010511)
→ fluoxetine (n=1, *Am J Psychiatry* 1995;**152**:295–6)
→ paroxetine (n=1, *Pharmacopsychiatry* 2007;**40**:199–200)
→ paroxetine discontinuation (n=1, *J Neuropsych Clin Neurosci* 2004;**16**:119–20)
→ paroxetine + benzatropine (n=1, *Am J Psychiatry* 1997;**154**:581–2)
→ sertraline (n=1, *J Clin Psychopharmacol* 2014;**34**:527–9)
Trazodone (n=3, *Int Clin Psychopharmacol* 1998;**13**:225–8)
Tricyclics (n=10, *J Clin Psychiatry* 1983;**44**:173–6), e.g.:
→ imipramine (n=1, *Am J Psychiatry* 1983;**140**:1517–8)
Tricyclic discontinuation (n=1, *Aust N Z J Psychiatry* 2010;**44**:863)
Venlafaxine (n=1, *Aust NZ J Psychiatry* 2011;**45**: 606; n=1, *Can J Psychiatry* 2003;**48**:129)

- **CNS — analgesics** *

Buprenorphine patch (n=1, elderly, *Psychogeriatrics* 2013;**13**:118–23)
Dextropropoxyphene discontinuation
Ergotamine + caffeine (n=1, *Pharmacotherapy* 2002;**22**:126–9)
Fentanyl (*Anesthesiology* 1995;**83**:869–71)
Methadone (during switch from fentanyl, *J Pain Symptom Manage* 2001;**21**:177–8)
Nalbuphine
Narcotics
Opioids (n=1, *J Pain Symptom Manage* 2004;**27**:268–73)
Opioid discontinuation (*J Neuropsychiatry Clin Neurosci* 2011;**23**:E37)
Papaveretum
Tramadol (n=11, *Curr Problems* 1995;**21**:2; n=1, *Pharmacopsychiatry* 2006;**39**:194–9)

- **CNS — anticonvulsants** *

Barbiturate withdrawal
Barbiturates (dose-related)
Benzodiazepines (common cause, see anxiolytics)
→ clonazepam (*Mil Med* 1997;**162**:iii)
→ midazolam (alone and with propofol, n=1, *Anesth Prog* 2006;**53**:95–7; FFT)
Carbamazepine (especially early in therapy; as part of SIADH, *Psychiatr Prax* 2001;**28**:48–9)
Ethosuximide (*Psychiatr Neurol Med Psychol [Leipz]* 1990;**42**:513–37)
Gabapentin abuse (n=1, *J Psychiatr Pract* 2009;**15**:314–9)
Gabapentin discontinuation (n=1, *Am J Health Syst Pharm* 2010;**67**:910–2; n=1, *Can J Neurol Sci* 2013;**40**:126–7)
Lacosamide (common, SmPC)
Levetiracetam (n=1, *Am J Geriatr Pharmacother* 2010;**8**:170–4; n=1, *Am J Ther* 2013;**21**: 225–8)
Phenytoin (dose-related)
Phenytoin + temozolomide (n=1, *Psychosomatics* 2007;**48**:359–60)
Pregabalin (SmPC; common, *Clin Neuropharmacol* 2009;**32**:236–7; n=1, *Isr Med Assoc J* 2009;**11**:699–700; FFT; n=1, *Gen Hosp Psychiatry* 2012;**34**:436.e1–2; n=1, *Arq Neuropsiquiatr* 2012;**70**:960–1)
Topiramate (e.g. reversible dementia, n=1, *Clin Neuropharmacol* 2008;**31**:62; n=1, *Gen Hosp Psychiatry* 2010;**32**:647)

Valproate (n=272, usually in first 2/52, can be serious, more common in elderly, *Pharmacopsychiatry* 2009;**42**:61–5; n=1, rapidly reversible, *J Am Geriatr Soc* 2010;**58**:799–801; n=1, *Seizure* 2011;**20**:509–11; FFT)
Valproic acid loading dose (n=1, *J Clin Psychiatry* 2005;**66**:801–2)
Valproate + lamotrigine (n=1, *Am J Psychiatry* 2004;**161**:1128–9)
Valproate + high dose zotepine (n=1, *Br J Clin Pharmacol* 2012;**73**:486–8; FFT)
Zonisamide (SmPC very common, *J Clin Psychopharmacol* 2004;**4**:110–1)

- CNS — movement disorders

Amantadine (n=1, *Am J Psychiatry* 1980;**137**:240–2)
Amantadine discontinuation (n=3, *Neurology* 1998;**50**:1456–8)
Anticholinergic drugs (e.g. n=278, *Arch Intern Med* 2001;**161**:1099–105)
Biperiden IM (*J Neuropsychiatry Clin Neurosci* 2010;**22**:E15)
Bromocriptine
Levodopa (*Lancet* 1973;**ii**:929–31)
Lisuride
Pergolide discontinuation (*Clin Neuropharmacology* 1988;**11**:545–8)
Ropinirole (common, SmPC)
Selegiline

- CNS — others *

Alcohol (n=8,028, review, *Br J Psychiatry* 2010;**197**:200–6; FFT)
Alcohol + disulfiram (n=1, *Ann Pharmacother* 2001;**35**:32–5)
Alcohol withdrawal (n=1, persistent after heavy use, *Am J Psychiatry* 1997;**154**:846–51)
Amfetamines
Anticholinesterases, e.g.:
  → donepezil (n=1, *J Clin Psychiatry* 2002;**63**:250–1; n=1, *Iran J Psychiatry* 2013;**8**:59–60)
  → rivastigmine (incidence <5%)
  → rivastigmine transdermal patches (SmPC, common)
Baclofen (used in Parkinson's Disease, SmPC)
'Bath salts' (synthetic cathinones, *J Clin Psychiatry* 2013;**74**:518; summary, *Gen Hosp Psychiatry* 2012;**34**:647–50)
Betahistine (n=1, *Ned Tijdschr Geneeskd* 2004;**148**:2338–41)
Biperiden (n=1, *J Child Adolesc Psychopharmacol* 2011;**21**:499–500)
Caffeine (n=1, overdose and physical stress, *Am J Psychiatry* 1978;**135**:855–6)
Cannabis (in cookies, n=1, *CNS Spectr* 2006;**11**:262)
Cocaine (e.g. n=333, *Am J Forensic Med Pathol* 1999;**20**:120–7; n=3 deaths, *Ned Tijdschr Geneeskd* 2009;**153**:1014–7)
Disulfiram (n=5, *Am J Psychiatry* 1974;**131**:1281–2; n=1, *Nihon Arukoru Yakubutsu Igakkai Zasshi* 2006;**41**:535–40)
Disulfiram + alcohol (n=1, *Ann Pharmacother* 2001;**35**:32–5)
Disulfiram + griseofulvin (n=1, *J Clin Psychopharmacol* 2015;**35**:477–8)
Disulfiram + tranylcypromine (n=1, *Am J Psychiatry* 1995;**152**:296)
Ergotamine-caffeine (n=1, *Pharmacother* 2002;**22**;126–9)
Gamma-butyrolactone (GBL) withdrawal (n=1, *Pharmacopsychiatry* 2009;**42**:202–3; n=1, *Eur Addict Res* 2011;**17**:169–71)
Hyoscine, transdermal (e.g. n=1, *Lakartidningen* 2011;**108**:1508)
MDMA/ecstasy (n=3, *J Psychoactive Drugs* 1999;**31**:167–70)
Memantine (n=1, *J Clin Psychopharmacol* 2015;**35**:736–8)
Metoclopramide (*J Clin Psychopharmacol* 1987;**7**:281–2; SmPC)
Nabilone
Naltrexone (*Presse Med* 1999;**28**:1361–2)
Nicotine (*J Pain Symptom Manage* 1998;**16**:76–7)
Nicotine withdrawal (e.g. n=5, *Neurology* 2001;**57**:551–3)
Psilocybin in wild mushrooms (n=1, *Lakartidningen* 1995;**92**:3779–80)
Solvent intoxication
Varenicline (NZ monitoring; impaired memory, *Eur J Clin Pharmacol* 2013;**69**:1195–6)
Varenicline discontinuation (n=1, *Am J Psychiatry* 2010;**167**:720–1)

- Gastrointestinal drugs *

Bismuth toxicity (n=1, *W V Med J* 2013;**109**: 32–4)
H2 receptor antagonists e.g.:

→cimetidine (e.g. *Ann Intern Med* 1991;**114**:1027–34)
→famotidine (n=1, after switch from cimetidine; *Ann Pharmacother* 2001;**35**:1045–8; n=6, *Psychosomatics* 1996;**37**:349–55)
→nizatidine (n=1, *J Clin Psychiatry* 1997;**58**:327)
→ranitidine (*Ann Intern Med* 1991;**114**:1027–34)
Loperamide (*J Pediatr* 1991;**118**:656–7)
Methixene
Misoprostol (n=1, *DICP* 1991;**25**:133–4)
Omeprazole (several e.g. n=1, *Am J Emerg Med* 2008;**26**:519)
Rabeprazole (n=1, *Ann Pharmacother* 2007;**41**:1315–7)
Sulfasalazine (*Adv Psychiatr Treat* 2005;**11**:68)

- **Cardiovascular drugs** *

Alpha-adrenoceptor blockers, e.g. doxazosin, prazosin (*Adv Psychiatr Treat* 2005;**11**:66)
Amiloride
Amiodarone (several, e.g. n=1, *Am J Geriatr Pharmacother* 2010;**8**:170–4; n=1, *Psychosomatics* 2013;**54**:294–6)
Beta-blockers (e.g. *Postgrad Med J* 1990;**66**:1050–2; FFT)
→atenolol (n=1, *BMJ* 1988;**297**:1048; FFT)
→metoprolol (n=24, *Cardiovasc Drugs Ther* 2002;**16**:161–5; n=1, *Ned Tijdschr Geneeskd* 2005;**149**:2183–6)
→propranolol (*Can J Psychiatry* 2004;**49**:645; n=3, *Gaoxiong Yi Xue Ke Xue Za Zhi* 1994;**10**:40–7)
Calcium-channel blockers e.g.:
→diltiazem + fentanyl (n=1, *Gen Hosp Psychiatry* 2010;**32**:648)
→verapamil (n=1, *Am J Psychiatry* 1987;**144**:248)
Clonidine (n=7, *Int J Cardiol* 2006;**113**:276–8)
Digitalis (n=1, *Clin Cardiol* 1995;**18**:351–2)
Digoxin (*Am Heart J* 1983;**106**:419–20; n=4, *J Clin Pharmacol* 1979;**19**:747–50)
Diuretics (via severe K + loss)
Flecainide toxicity (n=1, *Ann Pharmacother* 2009;**43**:1366–9)
Hydralazine
Lidocaine
Mexilitine
Nitrates (*Adv Psychiatr Treat* 2005;**11**:66)
Procainamide
Sodium nitroprusside (*Psychosomatics* 1995;**36**:83–5)
Spironolactone
Statins (MHRA warning, *Drug Safety Update* 2008;**1**:10; *Anesthesiology* 2010;**113**:500–1)
Sulphonamide diuretics (*Adv Psychiatr Treat* 2005;**11**:66)

- **Respiratory drugs**

Aminophylline
Antihistamines, sedating (*Adv Psychiatr Treat* 2005;**11**:68)
Cyproheptadine OD (n=57, *Clin Toxicol (Phila)* 2011;**49**:681–3)
Dextromethorphan (n=1, *Am J Geriatr Pharmacother* 2005;**3**:17–20)
Diphenhydramine (*Psychosomatics* 1994;**35**:399–402)
Diphenhydramine + linezolid (n=1, *Ann Pharmacother* 2004;**38**:62–5)
Diphenhydramine + nefopam discontinuation (n=1, *Prog Neuropsychopharmacol Biol Psychiatry* 2010;**30**:705–6)
Doxapram
Mentholatum (n=1, *Am J Psychiatry* 2000;**157**:483–4)
Phenylpropanolamine O/D (*Br Heart J* 1982;**47**:51–4; FFT)
Promethazine/cyproheptadine overdose (n=1, *Australas Psychiatry* 2007;**99**:242–4)

- **Anti-infection drugs** *

These may indirectly cause delirium if inducing diarrhoea and dehydration.
Aciclovir (e.g. n=1, *Nervenarzt* 1998;**69**:1015–8; n=1, *Clin Infect Dis* 1995;**21**:435–6)
Amphotericin B (liposomal, n=1, *Am J Trop Med Hyg* 2011;**84**:566–8; FFT)
Azithromycin (several e.g. n=1, *Med Clin (Barc)* 2006;**126**:439; n=2, *Surg Neurol* 2003;**59**:509–11)
Cefazolin (n=1, *Br Med J* 1989;**299**:393–4; FFT)
Cephalexin (n=1, *J Adolesc Health* 2006;**39**:782–3)
Chloramphenicol (*Clin Pharmacol Ther* 1970;**11**:194)
Chloroquine
Ciprofloxacin (e.g. n=1, *Age Ageing* 2010;**39**:762; FFT; n=1, *Ann Pharmacother* 1997;**31**:252)
Clarithromycin (n=1, *Eur Respir J* 2006;**28**:671–

2; FFT; *J Antimicrob Chemother* 2007;**59**:331; FFT; n = 1 and review, *J Clin Neurosci* 2011;**18**:313–8)
Co-trimoxazole (n = 1, *Hum Exp Toxicol* 2000;**19**:149–51)
Cycloserine
Ertapenem (n = 2, *Ann Pharmacother* 2011;**45**:e6)
Fluconazole (*Gen Hosp Psychiatry* 2003;**25**:297–8)
Foscarnet sodium (*Adv Psych Treat* 2005;**11**:66)
Gancyclovir (n=1, *N Engl J Med* 1990;**322**:933–4; FFT)
Gatifloxacin (*Psychosomatics* 2003;**44**:85–6; n = 1, *J Am Geriatr Soc* 2006;**54**:871)
Isoniazid (n=1, *Br Med J* 1969;**i**:461; FFT; n = 1, *J Neuropsychiatry Clin Neurosci* 2013;**25**: E68–9)
Itraconazole (*Psychosomatics* 2003;**44**:260–1)
Levofloxacin (e.g. n = 1, *Gen Hosp Psychiatry* 2008;**30**:381–3; n = 1, *Curr Drug Saf* 2013; **8**:199–200; n = 1, *Indian J Palliat Care* 2015;**21**:76–8; FFT)
Mefloquine (e.g. *Lancet* 1993;**341**:632)
Moxifloxacin (*Psychosomatics* 2011;**52**:472–4)
Ofloxacin (*J Clin Psychiatry* 1992;**53**:137–8)
Oseltamivir (n = 1, *Int J Geriatr Psychiatry* 2007;**22**:935–6; n = 1, *Ther Umsch* 2010;**67**:613–5)
Penicillin
Piperacillin + tazobactam (n = 1, *Nephrol Dial Transplant* 2004;**19**:1341; FFT)
Piperazine
Quinine (n = 1, *Eur J Emerg Med* 2003;**10**:353–6)
Rifampicin
Streptomycin
Sulphonamides
Tobramycin (*JAMA* 1982;**248**:1971–2)
Voriconazole (n = 1, *J Oncol Pharm Pract* 2015; **21**:409–15)

- **Endocrine system drugs** *

Clomifene (n = 1, *Psychosomatics* 2007;**48**:65–6)
Corticosteroids (n = 1, *Gen Hosp Psychiatry* 1996;**18**:196–202)
Hypoglycaemics (oral)
Levothyroxine (n = 1, *Sao Paulo Med J* 2009;**127**:317–8; FFT)
Methylprednisolone
Triamcinolone
Zolendrate (n = 1, *J Pharmacol Pharmacother* 2014;**5**:217–9; FFT)

- **Malignancy and immunosuppressant drugs**

Acytokine
Ciclosporin (*Adv Psychiatr Treat* 2005;**11**:68)
Glucocorticoids (five times more likely with glucocorticoids, especially in older men; n = 372,696, *Am J Psychiatry* 2012;**169**:491–7)
Interferon alfa (several, e.g. n = 1, *Am J Psychiatry* 2000;**157**:1705–7)
Interleukin–2 + interferon alfa (n = 1, *Anticancer Res* 2001;**21**:3699–700)
Nelarabine (common, SmPC)
Tamoxifen (n = 273, no adverse effect on cognition, *J Clin Oncol* 2009;**27**:5144–52; FFT)

- **Musculoskeletal and analgesics**

Baclofen
Baclofen discontinuation (n = 1, *Aust N Z J Psychiatry* 2011;**45**:86–7 n = 23, review, *Psychosomatics* 2005;**46**:503–7; n = 1, *Gen Hosp Psychiatry* 2011;**33**:84.e1–2)
Corticosteroids (incidence may be up to 5–6% in adults, usually emerges within a few days or weeks, and the risk may be dose-related, *MHRA Drug Safety Update* 2007;1–9)
COX–2 inhibitors:
→ celecoxib (*J Neuropsychiatry Clin Neurosci* 2001;**13**:305–6)
→ rofecoxib (*J Neuropsychiatry Clin Neurosci* 2001;**13**:305–6; *Psychosomatics* 2004;**45**:361–3)
Etodolac (SmPC)
Hydroxychloroquine
NSAIDs e.g.:
→ aspirin toxicity (n = 1, *Ther Drug Monit* 2010;**32**:700–3)
→ fenoprofen
→ ibuprofen (*Arthritis Rheum* 1982;**25**:1013)
→ indometacin, including OD (*Drugs* 1980;**19**:220–42)
→ ketoprofen (*J Clin Psychopharmacol* 1999;**19**:95–6)
→ naproxen (cases)
→ salicylates? (*Psychosomatics* 1987;**28**:344)
→ sulindac (*JAMA* 1980;**243**:1630)
→ tiaprofenic acid (n=1, *CMAJ* 1987;**137**:1022–3; FFT)

- **Others** *

Anesthetic agents (incidence 56%, *Br J Psychiatry* 2001;**178**:360–6; FFT)

5

Atropine and homatropine eye drops
Cyclobenzaprine (n = 1, *BMJ Case Rep* 2013; **2013**:2013008997)
Cyclopentolate eye drops (n = 1, *Nervenarzt* 2009;**80**:967–9)
Herbal medicines (*Psychiatr Serv* 1999;**50**:969–70)
Homatropine eye drops (n = 1, *Clin Neurol Neurosurg* 1987;**89**:53–4)
Imiquimod (n = 2, *JAMA Dermatol* 2013;**149**: 500–1)
Iodoform gauze (n = 1, *Lancet* 1997;**350**:1294)
Lidocaine (n = 1, *Am J Emerg Med* 2015;**33**:603.e1–2)
Mercury intoxication (n = 1, *Appl Neuropsychol* 2008;**15**:79–91)
Mouthwash containing alcohol (n = 1, *Mil Med* 2009;**174**:828–31)
Nitrous oxide abuse (n = 1, *Arch Neurol* 1983;**40**:446–7)
Propofol (n = 1, *Can J Anaesth* 1996;**43**:877; review of risk, *Med Hypotheses* 2013;**81**: 536–9)
Sevoflurane (*Anesth Analg* 1999;**88**:1308–10; *Minerva Anestesiol* 2002;**68**:402–5; FFT; n = 1, *Anesth Prog* 2013;**60**:67–71)
Strontium (*Prescrire Int* 2009;**18**:216)
Tacrolimus (*Adv Psychiatr Treat* 2005;**11**:68)
Tolterodine + anticholinesterases (*J Am Geriatr Soc* 2002;**50**:1165–6)
Typewriter correction fluid (n = 1, *Psycho-somatics* 1986;**27**;665–6)
Valerian root discontinuation (*JAMA* 1998;**280**:1566–7)

5.5 DEPRESSION (SEE ALSO SUICIDAL IDEATION)

Occurs mainly in patients with a history of depression (Patten and Barbui, *Psychother Psychosom* 2004;**73**:207–99).

Reviews: * drug-induced depression and suicidal behaviour (Thomas *et al*, *BMC Pharmacol Toxicol* 2014;**15**:54; French Database n=474 from n=114,692, *Therapie* 2015;**70**:425–32)

- CNS — sleep disorders and anxiety

Benzodiazepines (BNF, common, especially resistant depression):
→ alprazolam (n = 15, incidence 33% at 3–10 mg/d, *Am J Psychiatry* 1987;**144**:664–5; n = 2, *J Clin Psychiatry* 1993;**54**(Suppl):78–84)
→ clobazam (n = 1, *BMJ* 1983;**286**:1246–7; FFT)
→ clonazepam
→ clorazepate
→ lorazepam (n = 8, incidence 27%, *Am J Psychiatry* 1989;**146**:1230–1)
Benzodiazepine discontinuation (several, e.g. n = 3, *Can J Psychiatry* 1988;**33**:626–7; diazepam abuse discontinuation, n = 1, *DICP* 1989;**23**:989–90)
Buspirone (incidence 3%? *J Clin Psychiatry* 1982;**43**[12 part 2]:100–2)
Hypnotics (n = 7,853, increased incidence with hypnotic use, 2% vs 0.9%, *BMC Psychiatry* 2007;**7**:42; FFT)
Modafinil (BNF, common)
Modafinil + sodium oxybate (n = 1, *Sleep Med* 2010;**11**:500–1)
Sodium oxybate (BNF, less common, SmPC)
Zaleplon (BNF, less common)
Zopiclone (BNF, rare)

- CNS — antipsychotics *

Switching to depression is less likely with olanzapine, quetiapine and ziprasidone than haloperidol, aripiprazole or risperidone (s = 6, RCT, Goikolea *et al*, *J Affect Disord* 2013;**144**: 191–8).

Aripiprazole (BNF, less common)
Clozapine (n = 1, managed successfully by SSRIs, *Eur Neuropsychopharmacol* 1998;**8**:239–40)
Fluphenazine decanoate (n = 1, *BMJ* 1969;**3**:564–7; FFT)
Pimozide (n = 4, *J Clin Psychiatry* 1997;**58**:433–6)
Quetiapine (n = 1, *Clin Neuropharmacol* 2005;**28**:133–5)
Risperidone (BNF, common; n = 17, incidence 29%, *J Clin Psychiatry* 2002;**63**:1040–4)
Ziprasidone (n = 3, *Clin Neuropharmacol* 2007;**30**:357–61)
Zuclopenthixol

- CNS — antidepressants

Bupropion (BNF, less common; rare during smoking cessation, *J Clin Psychiatry* 1999;**60**:436–41)
Citalopram (n = 1, comorbid panic, *Psychiatria Danubina* 2012;**24**:94–6; FFT)
Duloxetine (induction of ultra-rapid cycling,

n = 1, *J Clin Psychopharmacol* 2007;**27**:115–6; n = 2, *Clin Pract Epidemol Ment Health* 2008;**4**:18)
Tricyclics e.g.
→ nortriptyline (n = 2, *BMJ* 1964;**2**:1593; FFT)

- CNS — analgesics

Codeine — long-term use (n = 339, community survey, *J Clin Psychopharmacol* 1999;**19**:373–6)
Eletriptan (BNF, less common)
Fentanyl (transdermal)
Frovatriptan (BNF, less common)
Pentazocine (n=197, *South Med J* 1975;**68**:808)
Sumatriptan (n = 1, *J Clin Psychopharmacol* 1995;**15**:81–2)
Tramadol (n = 1, *Am J Psychiatry* 1996;**153**:843–4)

- CNS — anticonvulsants *

Barbiturates (BNF, less common)
Carbamazepine (BNF, less common)
Ethosuximide (BNF, less common)
Felbamate (FDA warning 2008)
Gabapentin (BNF, uncommon; FDA warning 2008; review, *Int J Psychiatry Med* 2015;**49**:245–8)
Lacosamide (common, SmPC)
Lamotrigine (rare, e.g. n = 1, *J Clin Psychiatry* 2006;**67**:1159–60)
Levetiracetam (BNF, common e.g. n = 163, 7-fold increased risk, *Epilepsy Behav* 2015;**45**:64–7)
Oxcarbazepine (BNF, uncommon)
Phenobarbital (*Pediatrics* 1990;**85**:1086–91)
Phenytoin (n = 2, *Arch Phys Med Rehab* 1990;**71**:422–3; n = 1, *Harefuah* 1993;**124**:762–4)
Pregabalin (BNF, uncommon)
Primidone (n = 241, incidence 42%, *Epilepsy Behav* 2005;**6**:413–6)
Tiagabine (BNF, rare)
Topiramate (BNF, common; e.g. n = 70, risk factors, *Epilepsia* 2003;**44**:1573–7; n = 1, responded to mirtazapine, *Psychosomatics* 2013;**54**:503–4)
Vigabatrin (BNF, common; incidence < 10%, *Neurology* 1991;**41**:363–4; n = 10, *J Neurol Neurosurg Psychiatry* 1993;**56**:925–8; FFT)
Zonisamide (BNF, common; *J Clin Psychopharmacol* 2004;**24**:110–1; n = 23, 4% incidence, *Epilepsy Behav* 2013;**29**:281–4)

- CNS — movement disorders

Amantadine (*JAMA* 1972;**222**:792–5)
Anticholinergics, e.g.:
→ benzatropine (BNF, less common)
Botulinum toxin A (n = 1, *South Med J* 1999;**92**:738)
Levodopa (BNF, common)
Piracetam (BNF, less common)
Rasagiline (BNF, common)
Tetrabenazine (BNF, common)

- CNS — others *

Amfetamine discontinuation (*Br J Hosp Med* 1993;**49**:361–3)
Anticholinesterases, e.g.:
→ galantamine (BNF, common)
→ rivastigmine (BNF, less common)
Atomoxetine (BNF, common)
Caffeine discontinuation (review in *N Engl J Med* 1992;**327**:1160–1)
Caffeine – reduced risk with caffeine intake between 68mg/d and 509mg/d (s = 11, n = 368900, *Aust N Z J Psychiatry* 2015;in press) with a non-linear J-shaped relationship between coffee and depression, peak protection at 400ml/d (s = 12, n = 346,913, *Mol Nutr Food Res* 2016;**60**:223–34)
Dexamfetamine withdrawal (BNF, uncommon)
Disulfiram (BNF, rare; case in *Arch Neurol* 1976;**33**:141)
Ergotamine (BNF, very rare)
Flumazenil (incidence < 1%)
Heroin withdrawal (*Int J Addict* 1992;**27**:25–35)
LSD (n = 1, responded to reboxetine, *Isr J Psychiatry Relat Sci* 2002;**39**:100–3)
MDMA/Ecstasy — former chronic users report higher levels of depression than matched controls (n = 29, *J Psychopharmacol* 2001;**15**:181–6; review, *J Psychoactive Drugs* 2007;**39**:31–9; n = 402, suggestion it does not lead to long-term depression, *J Psychopharmacol* 2008;**22**:47–54)
Memantine (BNF, very rare)
Methamphetamine (48% in people with psychosis, n = 121, *Addict Health* 2015;**7**:37–46; FFT)
Methamphetamine withdrawal (n = 145, *Addiction* 2010;**105**:1809–18; FFT)
Methylphenidate (BNF, common)
Nabilone (BNF, less common)
Nalbuphine

Naltrexone (probably not a cause, n=80, *J Psychiatry Neurosci* 2006;**31**:38–45; FFT)
Nicotine dependence and withdrawal (incidence 4%, *Addict Behav* 2003;**28**:461–70)
Ondansetron (n=1, *Am J Psychiatry* 1995;**152**:1101; n=1, *S Afr Med J* 1997;**87**:1013–4)
Orlistat (n=1, *Can J Psychiatry* 2000;**45**:87)
Oxetorone (n=1, *Cephalalgia* 1996;**16**:560–1)
Pizotifen (BNF, rare)
Rimonabant (BNF, common; but n=10,011, *Drug Saf* 2011;**34**:501–9; showed no difference in incidence of depression before and after 6/12 of rimonabant, but there might be a higher incidence in people with no PMH of depression; n=1, *Indian J Psychiatry* 2014;**56**:205; FFT)
Sibutramine (BNF, common)
Smoking (roughly doubles risk of depression in women; n=971, *Br J Psychiatry* 2008;**193**:322–6; FFT)
Smoking cessation, especially if previous MDD (n=304, *Am J Psychiatry* 2000;**157**:368–74; n=100 with history of MDD, *Lancet* 2001;**357**:1929–32; prospective cohort study; *BMJ* 2013;**347**:f5704)
Varenicline (no effect, s=39, n=10761, RCTs, *BMJ* 2015;**350**:h1109; FFT)

- **Gastrointestinal drugs**

Diphenoxylate
H2-blockers: (BNF, rare), e.g.:
→ cimetidine (several cases, e.g. n=2, *Can J Psychiatry* 1981;**26**:260–1)
→ famotidine (rare reports)
→ ranitidine (several e.g. n=3, *Aust NZ J Psychiatry* 1991;**25**:415–8)
Metoclopramide (BNF, less common; e.g. n=1, *Psychopharmacol Bull* 2002;**36**:82–93)
Proton pump inhibitors (BNF, rare), e.g.:
→ omeprazole (unproven reports)
Sulfasalazine (BNF, less common)

- **Cardiovascular drugs** *

Greater adherence to antihypertensives is associated with depression and anxiety in men but not women (n=926, two years, *J Am Geriatrics Society* 2012;**60**:2297–2301);
ACE inhibitors, e.g.:
→ enalapril (BNF, less common; n=1, *South Med J* 1989;**82**:402–3)
→ imidapril (BNF, less common)
→ lisinopril (rare)
→ quinapril (BNF, less common; n=1, *Am J Psychiatry* 1999;**156**:1114–5)
→ ramipril (BNF, less common)
Alpha-blockers (BNF, common; but a case–control study concluded no association, *Pharmacoepidemiol Drug Saf* 2002;**11**:55–61)
Amiodarone (n=1, *Br J Psychiatry* 1999;**174**:366–7)
Beta-blockers (n=381, concludes no increase in depression in first year, *J Am Coll Cardiol* 2006;**48**:2209–14; FFT) and a prospective study (n=5,104, Luijendijk *et al*, *J Clin Psychopharmacol* 2011;**31**:45–50) in elderly people, showed:
→ Beta-blockers in general were not associated with depression
→ Propranolol and other highly lipid soluble beta-blockers were associated with depressive symptoms in the first three months but not depression as such
→ Non-selective beta-blockers were not associated at all with depressive symptoms e.g.:
- acebutol (mentioned in *Am J Med* 1987;**83**:223–6)
- atenolol (*J Hum Hypertens* 1987;**1**:87–93; n=1, *Actas Esp Psiquiatr* 2006;**34**:352–4)
- celiprolol (BNF, less common)
- metoprolol (incidence 5%? review in *Drugs* 1977;**14**:321–48; n=1, *Gen Hosp Psychiatry* 2010;**32**:646.e5–7)
- nadolol (no difference cf. placebo, d/b, p/c, *J Neuropsychiatry* 1992;**4**:187–9)
- nebivolol (BNF, less common)
- propranolol (n=1, resolved with switch to atenolol, *Am J Psychiatry* 1982;**139**:1187–8)
- sotalol (*Ann Pharmacother* 2004;**38**:1321–2)
- timolol

Calcium-channel blockers, e.g.:
→ diltiazem (BNF, less common; *BMJ* 1989;**299**:796; FFT)
→ felodipine (*Br Heart J* 1987;**58**:122–8; FFT)
→ isradipine (BNF, rare)
→ nicardipine (BNF, uncommon; several cases e.g. n=2, *J Assoc Physicians India* 2002;**50**:1432–4)

→nifedipine (n = 1, *Br J Psychiatry* 1991;**159**:447–8; n = 1, *Br J Psychiatry* 1990;**156**;889–91)
Clonidine (BNF, common; 1% incidence, case study in *Postgrad Med J* 1993;**69**:327–8; FFT; when used for ADHD; *J Clin Psychopharmacol* 2008;**28**:725–6)
Cyclopenthiazide (BNF, rare)
Digoxin (BNF, less common)
Digoxin intoxication (*Psychosomatics* 2001;**42**:369–70)
Doxazosin (BNF, common)
Flecainide (BNF, rare)
Furosemide (BNF, caution in depression)
Hydralazine
Indoramin (BNF, less common)
Losartan (*Ugeskr Laeger* 1997;**159**:2106–8)
Methyldopa (BNF, common; review in *Am J Psychiatry* 1983;**140**:534–8)
Moxonidine (BNF)
Prazosin (BNF, uncommon)
Procainamide (BNF, common)
Statins and cholesterol (BNF, less common); Cholesterol levels seem to have a U-shaped curve effect and statins may reduce the incidence of depression (s = 7, n = 9187, *J Affect Disord* 2014;**160**:62–7):
In men: highest depression scores occur with low LDL-C (OR = 5) and high LDL-C (OR = 2.3) cf medium LDL-C (OR = 1)
In women: highest depression scores occur with low LDL-C (OR = 3) and high LDL-C (OR = 1.2) cf medium LDL-C (OR = 1) (n = 8,390, Tedders *et al*, *J Affect Disord* 2011;**135**:115–21). See also suicidal ideation *C5.15*
Review: * You *et al*, *Expert Opin Pharmacother* 2013;**14**:1467–76
Streptokinase (cases mentioned in *Drugs* 1973;**5**:357–445)
Telmisartan (BNF, rare)
Valsartan/hydrochlorothiazide overdose (n = 1, *Dtsch Med Wochenschr* 2003;**128**;2534–6)
Verapamil (*Can J Psychiatry* 1993;**38**:299–300)

- **Respiratory drugs** *

Alimemazine
Antihistamines (BNF, rare)
Astemizole (debatable, *Drugs* 1984;**28**:38–61)
Cinnarizine (*Br Med J* 1988;**297**:722; n = 1, *Rev Neurol* 1999;**28**:876–8)
Doxapram (BNF, C/I in depression)
Ephedrine (as part of a psychosis, *Br Med J* 1968;**2**:60; FFT)
Hydroxyzine (some reports)
Montelukast (BNF, rare; review, *Pharmacology* 2014;**94**:60–70; FFT)
Phenylpropanolamine (n = 1, persistent, *Am J Psychiatry* 1990;**147**:367–8; n = 1, *Mil Med* 1986;**151**:387–8)
Pulmicort Turbohaler (n = 1, *Lakartidningen* 1996;**93**:2083)
Theophylline (n = 2, *Br Med J* 1980;**281**:1322)
Zafirlukast (FDA warning 2009)

- **Anti-infection drugs** *

Amprenavir (BNF, less common)
Atazanavir (BNF, less common)
Cefradine (n = 1, *Med J Aus* 1973;**2**:742–3)
Chloramphenicol (BNF, less common)
Chloroquine (*Adv Psychiatr Treat* 2005;**11**:66)
Clofazimine (*Adv Psychiatr Treat* 2005;**11**:66)
Clotrimazole, oral (review in *Drugs* 1975;**9**:424)
Co-trimoxazole (BNF, very rare but severe cases, e.g. *DICP* 1988;**22**:267)
Cycloserine (BNF, less common)
Dapsone (n = 1, *Br Med J* 1989;**298**:1524; FFT)
Efavirenz (BNF, common; n = 355, same risk as placebo, *Clin Infect Dis* 2006;**42**:1790–9; FFT)
Ertapenem (BNF, rare)
Ethionamide (*Adv Psychiatr Treat* 2005;**11**:66)
Ganciclovir (BNF, common)
Griseofulvin (as part of psychosis, n = 1, *JAMA* 1974;**229**:1420)
Interferon alfa-2a (concurrent escitalopram for 12/52 does not seem to prevent any depression, n = 133, RCT, d/b, p/c, 12/52, *J Clin Psychiatry* 2011;**72**:522–8)
Levofloxacin (n = 1, *Conn Med* 2014;**78**:229–30)
Linezolid (BNF, common)
Lopinavir + ritonavir (BNF, less common)
Mefloquine (BNF, less common; e.g. n = 1, *J Clin Psychopharmacol* 2005;**25**:399–400; n = 1, *Encephale* 2011;**37**:393–6)
Metronidazole (n = 1, *Am J Psychiatry* 1977;**134**:329–30)
Oseltamivir (n = 1, *Psychiatry Investig* 2010;**7**:302–4; FFT)
Peginterferon alfa + ribavirin (n = 162, moderate to severe depression seems to be common, especially with higher doses of ribavirin; *J Clin Psychiatry* 2005;**66**:41–8; FFT)

5

Piperazine (cases, e.g. *J Indian Med Assoc* 1976;**66**:33)
Posaconazole (BNF, rare)
Primaquine (n=1, *Ann Intern Med* 1980;**92**:435)
Quinolones (BNF, less common)
→ ciprofloxacin (very rare)
Ribavirin (BNF, less common)
Stavudine (BNF, less common)
Sulphonamides
Trimethoprim (*Adv Psychiatr Treat* 2005;**11**:66)
Voriconazole (BNF, common)
Zidovudine (BNF, uncommon)

- **Endocrine system drugs** *

Buserelin (BNF, uncommon)
Cabergoline (BNF, less common)
Choriogonadotropin alfa (BNF, less common)
Clomifene (BNF, common)
Corticosteroids (BNF, rare but incidence may be as high as 5–6% in adults, usually emerges within a few days or weeks and the risk may be higher with higher doses, MHRA *Drug Safety Update* 2007;1–9; high dose in MS; c=88, *J Affect Disord* 2015;**187**:142–6):
→ deflazacort (SmPC)
→ dexamethasone (up to 40% incidence, *Arch Gen Psychiatry* 1981;**38**:471–7)
→ methyltestosterone (rare)
→ prednisolone (n=1, *J Assoc Physicians India* 1973;**21**:909)
→ prednisone
Cyproterone acetate (BNF, C/I in depression)
Depo-Provera (unlikely to be cause, n=495, *Contraception* 1998;**57**:237–40)
Dianette (SmPC)
Diethylstilbestrol (*in utero* exposure in females, n=1,612, *Am J Epidemiol* 2010;**171**:876–82)
Dopamine agonist discontinuation (n=2, *Sleep Med* 2013;**14**:696)
Estrogens for HRT (BNF, less common)
Finasteride (review, *J Cosmet Dermatol* 2010;**9**:331–2; n=128, *BMC Clin Pharmacol* 2006;**7**:7; FFT; n=90, 75% developed depression vs 10% controls, *J Clin Psychiatry* 2012;**73**:1220–3)
Flunisolide (inhaled, incidence 1–3%)
Gestrinone (BNF, common)
Iodine long-term (BNF, common)
Mecasermin (rare, SmPC)
Medroxyprogesterone acetate (Depo-Provera®; three years, 12% increase cf non-users, n=457, *Contraception* 2000;**61**:385–90)
Norplant implant (unlikely to cause or exacerbate, n=910, *Contraception* 1998;**57**:241–5)
Oral contraceptives, combined (BNF, rare; and a huge study in women 25–34 (1994–2008) showed hormonal contraceptive users were less likely to have depression or report a past-year suicide attempt, a stable longitudinal association (n=6654, *Am J Epidemiol* 2013;**178**:1378–88)
Progestogens (BNF, caution in depression)
Progestogen-only oral contraceptives (BNF, common)
Teriparatide (BNF, common)
Testosterone and esters (BNF, common)
Testosterone abuse cessation (n=1, *Can J Psychiatry* 1994;**39**:317–8)
Tibolone (BNF, rare)

- **Malignancy and immunosuppressant drugs** *

Review: cytokine-induced (Schiepers *et al*, *Prog Neuropsychopharmacol Biol Psychiatry* 2005;**29**:201–17)
Bicalutamide (BNF, less common)
Bortezomib (BNF, common)
Ciclosporin (n=1, *Lijec Vjesn* 2007;**129**:74–6)
Cyproterone (BNF, caution in depression)
Dasatinib (BNF, common)
Erlotinib (BNF, less common)
Exemestane (BNF, common)
Glatiramer (BNF, less common)
Glucocorticoids (twice as likely, n=372,696, *Am J Psychiatry* 2012;**169**:491–7)
Gonadorelin agonist therapy for ovarian suppression (treated with sertraline, d/b, p/c, *Fertil Steril* 2000;**74**:984–6)
Gonadorelin analogues (BNF, rare)
Goserelin (n=1, *Psychosomatics* 2006;**47**:360–1)
Hormone treatments for prostate cancer (n=526, *Int J Clin Oncol* 2014;**19**:523–30)
Imatinib (BNF, less common)
Interferons (prevalence and management, n=185 and review, *Dig Liver Dis* 2005:**37**:102–7; *Prog Neuropsychopharmacol Biol Psychiatry* 2005;**29**:808–18; *ibid* 201–17; n=50, review in *Rev Assoc Med Bras* 2014;**60**:35–9; FFT), e.g.:
→ aldesleukin
→ interferon + ribavirin (*Psychosomatics* 2006;**47**:254–6)

→ interferon alfa (BNF, uncommon; less likely in people with 5-HTTLPR gene; n=86, often preceded by insomnia, *Psychiatry Res* 2010;**177**:240–5; FFT; n=1,015, 20/52, *Psychosomatics* 2010;**51**:137–48; FFT; n=17 and review, *Int J Neuropsychopharmacol* 2011;**14**:247–53; can be treated with SSRIs [e.g. paroxetine; *N Engl J Med* 2001;**344**:961–6; FFT; escitalopram; n=2, Kajitani and Kanba, *Psychosomatics* 2013;**54**:506–7; or sertraline; *Med J Aus* 2000;**173**:359–61], omega-3 fatty acids [n=162[c=162], RCT, d/b, p/c, 2/52, *Biol Psychiatry* 2014;**76**:559–66] or methylphenidate [n=1, *J Psychopharmacol* 2006;**20**:687–9]; review of mechanisms and management, *Br J Hosp Med (Lond)* 2007;**68**:307–10)

→ interferon beta (BNF, caution in depression)

→ peginterferon 2-alfa-2 (prolonged low-dose maintenance is not associated with an increase in depression; n=129, 3.5 years, *J Affect Disord* 2011;**129**:205–12; FFT; 11; n=74, 6/12; incidence 20% for MDD, peaks at 12/52, *Psychiatr Danub* 2011;**23**:370–7; FFT)

Letrozole (BNF, common; n=1, *Bipolar Disord* 2006;**8**:516–8)

Leuprolide/leuprorelin (n=1, *J Clin Psychiatry* 2003;**64**:341–3)

→ leuprolide acetate (BNF, common)

Mesna (BNF, common)

Mithramycin

Mycophenolate mofetil (n=1, *Pharmacotherapy* 2008;**28**:136–9)

Nilotinib (BNF, less common)

Nilutamide (n=1, *Therapie* 1997;**52**:79–81)

Octreotide (rare)

Sorafenib (BNF, common)

Tacrolimus (BNF, common)

Tamoxifen (two large studies show no increased risk [n=2,943, *Psychosomatics* 2007;**48**:205–10; n=11,064, *J Natl Cancer Inst* 2001;**93**:1615–23; FFT], n=1, prevented by venlafaxine, *Psychosomatics* 2009;**50**:162–5)

Toremifene (BNF, less common)

Trastuzumab (BNF, common)

Tretinoin (BNF, common)

Triamcinolone (incidence up to 8%)

• Musculoskeletal and analgesics *

Baclofen (BNF, less common; rare cases, e.g. psychotic, n=1, *J Clin Psychiatry* 1992;**53**:211–2)

Cytokine modulators:

→ abatacept (BNF, uncommon)

→ adalimumab (BNF, uncommon)

→ etanercept (BNF, uncommon)

→ infliximab (BNF, uncommon)

→ rituximab (BNF, uncommon)

Dantrolene (BNF, common)

Etodolac (SmPC, rare)

Nabilone

NSAIDs (BNF, uncommon; poorer outcomes [n=1528, *Am J Psychiatry* 2012;**169**:1065–72] but not true with COX-2 or salicylates:

→ diflunisal (< 1% incidence)

→ flurbiprofen (> 1% incidence?)

→ ibuprofen (uncommon, *Arthritis Rheum* 1982;**25**:1013)

→ indometacin (BNF, rare; incidence 4%? *BMJ* 1972;**4**:398–400; FFT)

→ indometacin discontinuation (*Br J Rheumatol* 1992;**31**:211)

→ naproxen (rare)

→ sulindac

• Others *

Acetazolamide (BNF, common)

Acitretin (*J Drugs Dermatol* 2005;**4**:690–6)

Allopurinol

Anagrelide (BNF, less common)

Anesthetic agents (in elderly, n=140, *Br J Psychiatry* 2001;**178**:360–6; FFT)

Apraclonidine (BNF, common)

Betaine (BNF, less common)

Betaxolol eye drops (n=2, *Aust NZ J Psychiatry* 2001;**35**:569–71)

Brimonidine (BNF, common)

Brinzolamide (BNF, common)

Carbaryl (psychotic, n=1, *Am J Psychiatry* 1995;**152**:646–7)

Dorzolamide eye-drops (*Can J Ophthalmol* 1999;**34**:93–4)

Herbicides (but not insecticides or fungicides; n=567 farmers, *J Epidemiol* 2013;**178**:1051–8)

Lead (higher levels, n=1,987, *Arch Gen Psychiatry* 2009;**66**:1313–9; FFT)

Manganese (n=1, *Psychosomatics* 2011;**52**:74–7)

Mercaptamine (BNF, common)

Mothballs — see paradichlorobenzene
Nitrous oxide (possible risk factor, *J Clin Psychopharmacol* 2007;**27**:238–9)
Organophosphate pesticides (related to cumulative lifetime exposure, n=29,074, *J Occup Environ Med* 2006;**48**:1005–13; FFT)
Paradichlorobenzene (n=1, *Gen Hosp Psychiatry* 2010;**32**:341)
Pegaptanib (BNF, less common)
Retinoids e.g.:
- → etretinate (*Br Med J* 1989;**298**:964; FFT)
- → Isotretinoin (BNF, rare; be an incidence of 1–11%, *Semin Cutan Med Surg* 2007;**26**:210–20; and a statistically significant association, n=30,496, *J Clin Psychiatry* 2008;**69**:526–32; although it may abate over 6/12, n=100, *Psychol Rep* 2006;**99**:897–906; n=10, incidence up to 90% in bipolar patients, *J Affect Disord* 2010;**122**:306–8; has actually shown improvement in BDI-II scores, n=100, open, *Int J Dermatol* 2013;**52**:163–8)

Sodium phenylbutyrate (BNF, less common)
Tacrolimus (*Adv Psychiatric Treat* 2005;**11**:68)
Timolol eye drops (5–6 times more likely than placebo, n=312, *Ophthalmologica* 2011;**226**:157–60)
Vitamin A intoxication (*Psychosomatics* 1992;**33**:117–8)
Vitamin D (low levels have been associated with depression in generally healthy community-dwelling middle-aged and in older males there was an inverse relationship between serum 25-hydroxyvitamin D (25(OH) D) levels and depression, independent of lifestyle and other health factors; n=3,369, *J Psychopharmacol* 2011;**25**:1320–8)
Xylometazoline (n=1, child, *JAMA* 1970;**211**:123–4)

5.6 HALLUCINATIONS (INCLUDING VISUAL DISTURBANCES, SEE ALSO PSYCHOSIS)

Where known, the type of hallucination is mentioned.

• CNS — sleep disorders and anxiety *

Benzodiazepines (n=1, musical, *Can J Psychiatry* 1991;**36**:609–11), e.g.:
- → lorazepam overdose (n=65, *Ann Pediatr (Paris)* 1984;**31**:286–9)
- → midazolam IV (n=1, *DICP* 1989;**23**:671–2)
- → temazepam (n=1, visual, *J Am Geriatr Soc* 2006;**54**:1627–8)
- → triazolam (n=1 in dental surgery, *Anesth Prog* 2005;**52**:17–20; FFT)

Benzodiazepine discontinuation (n=1, visual, *Psychiatr Prax* 1997;**24**:309–10)
Modafinil (n=1, *J Clin Psychopharmacol* 2009;**29**:408 visual, n=1, *J Clin Psychopharmacol* 2010;**30**:347–50)
Ramelteon (n=1, *Asian J Psychiatr* 2015;**18**:111–2)
Sodium oxybate (SmPC)
Zaleplon (BNF, uncommon; n=1, dose-related, *Clin Toxicol (Phila)* 2008;**46**:344–5)
Zolpidem (n=5, *J Toxicol Clin Toxicol* 1998;**36**:195–203; distorted perception, n=1, *Ann Pharmacother* 2003;**37**:683–6; n=1, *Indian J Psychol Med* 2013;**35**:212–3)
Zolpidem overdose (n=1, command, *J Clin Psychiatry* 2010;**71**:92–3)
Zolpidem + fluvoxamine (n=1, *Int Psychogeriatr* 2006;**18**:749–51)
Zopiclone (BNF, rare; *Pharm J* 1990;**245**:210)

• CNS — antipsychotics *

Lithium (n=1, visual and auditory, *Nervenartz* 1993;**64**:747–9)
Olanzapine (BNF, common; n=1, hypno-pompic hallucinations, *Can J Psychiatry* 2004;**49**:496–7; adjunct, auditory, n=1, *BMJ Case Rep* 2014;**2014**:bcr2014205805)

• CNS — antidepressants *

Review: factors associated with visual hallucinations with antidepressants (*Hum Psychopharmacol* 2004;**19**:577–84).
Bupropion (BNF, very rare; tactile, n=2, *J Clin Psychiatry* 2006;**67**:1820–1; n=1, *J Neuropsychiatry Clin Neurosci* 2011;**23**:E53; n=1, *J Clin Psychopharmacol* 2013;**33**:717–9)
Bupropion + clozapine (n=1, *J Clin Psychopharmacol* 2015;**35**:97–9)
Bupropion + valproate (n=1, visual and auditory, *Can J Psychiatry* 2000;**45**:198–9)
Duloxetine (BNF, v rare; n=1, dose-dependent, *Clin Neuropharmacol* 2013;**36**:175–6)
MAOIs, e.g.:
- → phenelzine (BNF, rare; n=1, *Am J Psychiatry* 1994;**151**:450)
- → tranylcypromine (n=1, *Psychiatr Prax* 1993;**20**:116)

Mirtazapine (n = 3, *Int Psychogeriatr* 2010;**22**:837–9)
Moclobemide (pseudohallucinations, n = 1, *Pharmacopsychiatry* 2005;**38**:179–81)
Reboxetine (BNF, very rare)
SSRIs (BNF, uncommon), e.g.:
- →citalopram (e.g. n = 1, complex visual, *Prog Neuropsychopharmacol Biol Psychiatry* 2009;**33**:575–6; n = 1, *Aust N Z J Psychiatry* 2012;**46**:178; n = 1, *J Clin Psychopharmacol* 2013;**33**:583–4)
- →escitalopram (n = 1, *J Neuropsychiatry Clin Neurosci* 2012;**24**:E19)
- →fluoxetine (n = 1, *Am J Psychiatry* 1993;**150**:1750)
- →fluoxetine + dextromethorphan (n = 1, *Am J Psychiatry* 1992;**149**:1406)
- →fluoxetine + methylphenidate (n = 1, tactile, *J Child Adolesc Psychopharmacol* 2014;**24**:360–1)
- →fluoxetine + zolpidem (n = 1, *J Forensic Sci* 2004;**49**:392–3)
- →paroxetine (n = 1, *Psychiatry Clin Neurosci* 2010;**64**:666–7)
- →paroxetine, excessive use/OD (n = 1, *Psychiatry Clin Neurosci* 2003;**57**:548–9)
- →paroxetine discontinuation (n = 2, *Psychiatry Clin Neurosci* 2011;**65**:384–5)
- →paroxetine + zolpidem (n = 1, *Prim Care Companion CNS Disord* 2012;**14**: 12i01361; FFT)
- →sertraline (n = 1, *J Clin Psychiatry* 2004;**65**:446–7)

Trazodone (n = 1, *BMJ Case Rep* 2014;**2014**: bcr2014203865)
Tricyclics (musical, *Biol Psychiatry* 1996;**40**:309–10), e.g.:
- →amitriptyline low dose (visual, *J Clin Psychopharmacol* 1988;**8**:75–6)
- →clomipramine (n = 1, visual, *Acta Psychiatr Scand* 1999;**99**:388–90; n = 1, musical, *Br J Psychiatry* 1991;**159**:888–9)
- →doxepin (n = 1, visual, *Aust NZ J Psychiatry* 1982;**16**:295–6)
- →imipramine

Venlafaxine (BNF, uncommon, n = 1, *J Clin Psychiatry* 2009;**70**:601–3)

• CNS — analgesics

Buprenorphine (rare, incidence < 1%, *Br Med J (Clin Res Ed)* 1988;**296**:214; FFT)
Buprenorphine-epidural (n = 5, *BMJ* 1989;**298**:928–9; FFT)
Methadone (*J Am Acad Child Adolesc Psychiatry* 1999;**38**:355–6)
Morphine (n = 1, resolved when switched to oxycodone, *Cases J* 2009;**23**:9391; FFT)
Morphine SR + methadone (*Lancet* 1987;**2**:392)
Nefopam (BNF, uncommon; *Curr Probl* 1989;**1**:89)
Oxycodone (n = 1, musical, *Am J Geriatr Psychiatry* 2003;**11**:470)
Oxycodone + sertraline (n = 1, *J Clin Pharmacol* 2001;**41**:224–7)
Pentazocine
Tramadol (n = 1, visual and auditory, *Ann Med Interna* 2003;**20**:493; n = 1, visual, *Acta Clin Belg* 1996;**51**:184–6)
Tramadol + clarithromycin (n = 1, visual-auditory, *Neuropsychopharmacol Hung* 2010;**12**:309–12; FFT)

• CNS — anticonvulsants *

Carbamazepine hypersensitivity (n = 1, *Pharmacopsychiatry* 2006;**39**:192–3)
Gabapentin (BNF, rare; n = 1, parasitosis, *South Med J* 2010;**103**:711–2)
Lacosamide (n = 1, *J Neuropsychiatry Clin Neurosci* 2014;**26**:E8–9)
Lamotrigine (BNF, common; n = 1, *Am J Psychiatry* 2006;**163**:749–50; n = 1, *J Clin Psychiatry* 2014;**75**:e1330)
Levetiracetam (BNF, uncommon, n = 1, *Case Rep Med* 2012;**2012**:706243; FFT)
Midazolam (BNF, common; n = 1, visual, *DICP* 1989;**23**:671–2; oral n = 1, visual, *Rev Esp Anestesiol Reanim* 1995;**42**:76–7)
Phenobarbital (BNF, common)
Phenytoin (n = 1, *Eur J Paediatr Neurol* 2010;**14**:460–3)
Pregabalin (BNF, uncommon; n = 1, *Arq Neuropsiquiatr* 2012;**70**:960–1)
Primidone (n = 241, incidence 43%; *Epilepsy Behav* 2005;**6**:413–6)
Sodium valproate (BNF, rare)
Topiramate (n = 1, auditory, *J Clin Psychiatry* 2001;**62**:653; *Epileptic Disord* 2008;**10**:240; n = 1, *Gen Hosp Psychiatry* 2013;**35**:213.e1–3)
Valproate discontinuation (n = 2, *Pediatrics* 2012;**130**:236–8; FFT)
Vigabatrin (BNF, visual disturbance common)

Zonisamide (BNF, very rare; e.g. n = 3, *Pharmacotherapy* 2003;**23**:93–6)

- **CNS — movement disorders** *

Amantadine (BNF, common; e.g. n = 1, musical in PD, *Mov Disord* 2010;**25**:1505–6)
Amantadine overdose (n = 1, *Pediatr Emerg Care* 1991;**7**:89–92)
Anticholinergics, e.g.:
→ trihexyphenidyl (n = 1, tactile, *Rinsho Shinkeigaku* 2005;**45**:125–7; abuse, *Med Clin (Barc)* 1991;**97**:239)
COMT inhibitors:
→ entacapone (BNF, common)
→ tolcapone (BNF, common)
Dopamine agonists:
→ apomorphine (BNF, common)
→ bromocriptine (BNF, common; incidence < 1%, *Ann Int Med* 1984;**101**:149)
→ pergolide (BNF, common; in up to 13%, e.g. *Neurology* 1982;**32**:1181–4)
→ pergolide discontinuation (*Clin Neuropharmacology* 1988;**11**:545–8)
→ pramipexole (BNF, common; musical, n = 1, *Medicine (Baltimore)* 2014;**93**:e251; FFT)
→ ropinirole (BNF, common; n = 1, transient, *Prog Neuropharmacol Biol Psychiatry* 2008;**32**:1087–8)
→ rotigotine (BNF, common)
Levodopa (BNF, common; incidence < 26% in elderly, e.g. *Postgrad Med J* 1989;**65**:358–61; FFT)
Levodopa-carbidopa + paroxetine (n = 1, *Ned Tijdschr Geneeskd* 2002;**146**:1056–7)
MAO-B inhibitors:
→ rasagiline (BNF, common)
→ selegiline (BNF, common; esp. combined with levodopa and/or dopamine agonists, n = 94, *Parkinsonism Relat Disord* 2004;**10**:235–42)
Riluzole + memantine/bupropion (n = 1, *J Clin Psychopharmacol* 2006;**26**:218–20)

- **CNS — others**

Alcohol
Amfetamines (*Biol Psychiatry* 1980;**15**:749–57)
Anticholinesterases, e.g.:
→ donepezil (BNF, common; n = 1, hypnopompic, *J Psychopharmacol* 2000;**14**:303–4)
→ galantamine (BNF, rare)
→ rivastigmine (BNF, very rare)
Atomoxetine (MHRA warning 2009)
Ginseng (n = 1, *Acta Psychiatr Scand* 2002;**105**:76–8)
Guanfacine (n = 1, *J Am Acad Child Adolesc Psychiatry* 2003;**42**:1387)
Hyoscine patch (n = 1, *Lakartidningen* 1995;**92**:638)
Khat (n = 3, hypnagogic, *Acta Psychiatr Scand* 1988;**78**:458–61; n = 4, *Br J Hosp Med* 1995;**54**:322–6)
LSD (e.g. persistent n = 1, *Neurocase* 2010;**16**:106–18)
Meclizine + metaxalone (n = 1, *Ann Pharmacother* 2004;**38**:1968–9)
Memantine (BNF, uncommon; n = 3, *J Neurol Neurosurg Psychiatry* 2007;**78**:546; FFT exacerbation; n = 3, *Neurology* 2005;**65**:481–2)
Methylphenidate (*Neurology* 2004;**63**:753–4 US FDA warning in children; low-dose n = 1, *J Child Neurol* 2009;**24**:1005–7; visual, n = 1, *An Pediatr [Barc]* 2010;**72**:229–30; FFT; n = 1, *Neuropediatrics* 2011;**42**:30–1)
Methylphenidate + fluoxetine (n = 1, *J Clin Psychopharmacol* 2008:**28**:723–5)
Metoclopramide OD (SmPC)
Nabilone (BNF, uncommon)
Naltrexone (BNF, very rare)
Prolintane + diphenhydramine (n = 1, visual, *Pharmacopsychiatry* 2002;**35**:24–5)
Varenicline (SmPC; n = 1, *J Med Case Reports* 2009;**3**:7560; FFT)
Varenicline discontinuation (n = 1, *Am J Psychiatry* 2009;**166**:619–20)

- **Gastrointestinal drugs** *

Bismuth toxicity (n = 1, *Actas Luso Esp Neurol Psiquiatr Cienc Afines* 1984;**12**:427–33; n = 1, *W V Med J* 2013;**109**:32–4)
H2-antagonists (BNF, rare):
→ cimetidine (several, e.g. *Arch Intern Med* 1983;**98**:677)
→ famotidine (n = 1, *Pharmacotherapy* 1998;**18**:404–7)
→ ranitidine (n = 1, *Eur J Clin Pharmacol* 1985;**29**:375–6)
Proton-pump inhibitors (omeprazole, lansoprazole etc; BNF, very rare)
Sulfasalazine (BNF, uncommon)

- **Cardiovascular drugs**

ACE inhibitors (*Postgrad Med J* 1993;**69**:240; FFT), e.g.:
- → quinapril (*N Z Med J* 1999;**112**:83)

Beta-blockers, e.g.:
- → metoprolol (e.g. visual, *Psychosomatics* 2006;**47**:537–8; n=3, *J Med Case Rep* 2012;**6**:65; FFT)
- → pindolol (n=1, visual, *Harefuah* 1983;**104**:226–7)
- → propranolol (n=1, musical, *J Nerv Ment Dis* 1998;**186**:192–4; n=1, *Intensive Care Med* 1999;**25**:336–7)
- → timolol (*JAMA* 1980;**244**:768–9)

Calcium-channel blockers, e.g.:
- → diltiazem (n=1, *Psychiatr Prax* 1998;**25**: 91–2)

Clonidine (n=3, *Ann Intern Med* 1980;**93**:456–7; n=1, *Clin Ter* 2000;**151**:45–7)
Clopidogrel (BNF, very rare)
Digoxin (e.g. *Arch Neurol* 1983;**40**:386)
Disopyramide
Flecainide (BNF, rare; n=1, visual, *Postgrad Med J* 1986;**62**:61–2; FFT)
Isosorbide dinitrate (n=1, visual, *Psychosomatics* 1987;**28**:555–6)
Pentoxifylline (musical, *Neurology* 1993;**43**: 1621–2)
Prazosin (auditory, *J Clin Psychopharmacol* 1988;**8**:228)
Procainamide
Streptokinase (*Drugs* 1973;**5**:357–445)

- **Respiratory drugs** *

Cyproheptadine OD (n=57, *Clin Toxicol (Phila)* 2011;**49**:681–3)
Decongestants (containing pseudoephedrine and triprolidine; n=4, *Br Med J (Clin Res Ed)* 1984;**288**:1688; FFT; n=3, *Br Med J (Clin Res Ed)* 1984;**288**:1369; FFT)
Desloratidine (BNF, very rare)
Dextromethorphan (n=1, *Psychosomatics* 1996;**37**:71–4)
Doxapram (BNF, common post-op)
Montelukast (BNF, very rare; FDA warning 2009; review, *Pharmacology* 2014;**94**:60–70; FFT)
Phenylpropanolamine (*JAMA* 1981;**245**:601–2)
Promethazine (*Acta Paediatrica Scand* 1989;**78**:131–2)
Pseudoephedrine (BNF, rare, see decongestants)
Salbutamol (nebulised) (*Br Med J (Clin Res Ed)* 1986;**292**:1430; FFT; n=1, probably due to fluorocarbon propellant, *Pediatr Emerg Care* 1994;**10**:87–8)
Zafirlukast (FDA warning 2009)

- **Anti-infection drugs** *

Aciclovir (BNF, very rare)
Amoxicillin (e.g. n=1, *Br J Clin Pract* 1996;**50**:279)
Cefalosporins and other beta-lactams:
- → cefaclor (BNF, rare)
- → ertapenem (BNF, very rare)

Chloroquine (*Adv Psychiatr Treat* 2005;**11**:66)
Ciclosporin (visual, *Neurology* 1991;**41**:1156 *Transplantation* 1987;**43**:768–9)
Clarithromycin (n=1, *Farm Hosp* 2007;**31**:321–3; FFT; n=1, visual, *Int J Clin Pharmacol Ther* 2002;**40**:20–2; n=1, visual, *Am J Kidney Dis* 1996;**27**:143–6)
Co-trimoxazole (trimethoprim-sulfamethoxazole) BNF, rare (n=1, *Gen Hosp Psychiatry* 2014;**36**:7–6)
Efavirenz (significantly reduced with stepped dose increase, n=114, RCT, d/b, *Ann Intern Med* 2009;**151**:149–56)
Erythromycin + nitrazepam/triazolam (n=1, *Psychiatry Clin Neurosci* 1996;**50**:337–9)
Famciclovir (BNF, very rare)
Flucytosine (BNF, common)
Gatifloxacin (n=1, *Psychosomatics* 2006;**47**:360)
Gentamicin (*JAMA* 1977;**238**:53–4)
Isoniazid (n=1, *Presse Med* 2006;**35**:425–6; *Psychosomatics* 1993;**34**:537–9)
Maraviroc (uncommon, SmPC)
Mefloquine (BNF, uncommon; n=1, psychotic, *Psychiatr Prax* 1999;**26**:252–4)
Moxifloxacin (*Psychosomatics* 2011;**52**:472–4)
Osteltamivir (SmPC, <1% incidence)
Ofloxacin (n=1, *Indian J Pharmacol* 2013;**45**: 189–90)
Quinolones (BNF, uncommon; review, esp in elderly, *Prescrire Int* 2008;**17**:20), e.g.:
- → ciprofloxacin (e.g. n=1, visual, *Arch Soc Esp Oftalmol* 2007;**82**:299–301; FFT)
- → levofloxacin (n=2, visual, *Nihon Ronen Igakkai Zasshi* 1999;**36**:213–7; FFT)
- → nalidixic acid (*Nouv Presse Med* 1980;**9**:455)
- → norfloxacin (n=1, *J Assoc Physicians India* 1996;**44**:504)

Voriconazole (BNF, common; n=1, *Rev Clin*

5

Esp 2005;**205**:632–3; n = 1, musical, *Infection* 2004;**32**:293–5; n = 12, *Clin Infect Dis* 2008;**47**:e7–10; FFT)

- **Endocrine system drugs**

Alendronic acid (n = 1, auditory and visual, *Pharmacotherapy* 2004;**24**:799–802)
Cabergoline (BNF, common)
Corticosteroids (incidence may be as high as 5–6% in adults, usually emerges within a few days or weeks, risk may be higher with higher doses, *MHRA Drug Safety Update* 2007;1–9)
Disodium pamidronate (BNF, rare, *Ann Rheum Dis* 1992;**51**:927–8; FFT)
Estrogen (n = 1, visual, *Am J Ophthalmol* 2000;**129**:407)
Methylprednisolone IA (n = 1, *J Am Med Dir Assoc* 2011;**12**:609–10)

- **Malignancy and immunosuppressant drugs**

Bevacizumab (n = 1, visual, *Am J Ophthamol* 2007;**143**:169–70)
Chlorambucil (n = 1, *Ir Med J* 1984;**77**:288–9)
Hydroxycarbamide
Ifosfamide (n = 6, visual, *Cancer* 1994;**73**:1509–14; n = 5, *Drugs Aging* 2007;**24**:967–73)
Interferon alfa + ribavirin (n = 1, *Psychosomatics* 2010;**51**:1–7)
Vincristine (n = 2, visual, *Clin Lab Haematol* 1994;**16**:355–7)

- **Musculoskeletal and analgesics**

Baclofen (BNF, common; used in Parkinson's Disease, SmPC)
COX-2 inhibitors:
→celecoxib (auditory n = 1, *Am J Psychiatry* 2000;**157**:1022–3)
→etoricoxib (BNF, very rare)
Hydrochloroquine (n = 1, *Ann Dermatol Venereol* 2004;**131**:471–3)
NSAIDs, e.g.:
→fenbufen (*Br Med J (Clin Res Ed)* 1985;**290**:822; FFT)
→flurbiprofen (BNF, uncommon)
→indometacin (rare, e.g. n = 1, visual, *Int Clin Psychopharmacol* 1986;**1**:263–6; n = 32, *Can J Anaesth* 2003;**50**:586–8)
→piroxicam (visual, *Presse Med* 1995;**24**:504)
→salicylates
→sulindac (auditory and visual, *Psychosomatics* 1990;**31**:461–2)
Tizanidine (BNF, common)

- **Others** *

Anagrelide (n = 1, visual, *Eur J Haematol* 2004;**73**:223–4)
Atropine toxicity (n = 1, visual, *Can J Neurol Sci* 1991;**18**:18–27)
Benzydamine (as in Difflam, n = 78, 50% incidence, *Rev Bras Psiquiatr* 2009;**31**:208–12; FFT)
Erythropoietin (e.g. visual, *Psychosomatics* 1998;**39**:83–5; n = 5, *N Engl J Med* 1991;**325**:285; FFT)
Herbal products (overview for emergency departments, *J Emerg Nurs* 2010;**36**:594–6)
Isoflurane discontinuation (n = 1, *Acta Paediatr* 1993;**82**:885–6)
Ketamine (BNF, very common; n = 3, *Psychopathology* 2015;**48**:376–85)
Mercaptamine (BNF, rare)
Nitrous oxide (*J Am Dent Assoc* 1980;**101**: 595–7)
Phenylephrine nasal drops (*JAMA* 1982;**247**:1859–60)
Propofol (n = 1, *Acta Anaesthesiol Scand* 1998:**42**:739–41; n = 1, erotic, *Rev Esp Anestesiol Reanim* 2000;**47**:90–2)
Ranibizumab (n = 1, *Eye (Lond)* 2011;**25**:1374–5; FFT)
Radiographic contrast media (n = 2, review, *Br J Clin Pharmacol* 1999;**47**:226–7)
Strontium (*Prescrire Int* 2009;**18**:216)
Tolterodine (n = 1, *BJU Int* 1999;**84**:1109)

5.7 MANIA, HYPOMANIA OR EUPHORIA

- **CNS — sleep disorders and anxiety**

Benzodiazepines:
→alprazolam (*J Clin Psychiatry* 1987;**48**: 117–8)
→clorazepate (n = 5, *Ann Med Psychol [Paris]* 1987;**145**:855–60)
→midazolam (euphoria possible)
Benzodiazepine discontinuation (n = 1, abrupt, *Acta Psychiatr Scand* 1989;**79**:406–7)
→lorazepam discontinuation (n = 2, *J Affect Disord* 1989;**17**:93–5)
Buspirone (n = 1, *Br J Psychiatry* 1991;**158**: 136–7)

Modafinil (n=1, *Am J Psychiatry* 2005;**162**:813–4; n=1, *J Clin Psychiatry* 2006;**67**:1817; see also n=137, *Psychopharmacol Bull* 2008;**41**:37–47)
Zolpidem (n=1, *Psychosomatics* 2011;**52**:493–4)

- CNS — antipsychotics *

Reviews: mania has been reported to be induced by olanzapine, risperidone, quetiapine and ziprasidone, but only very rarely with clozapine or FGAs, including amisulpride (Rachid *et al, J Clin Psychiatry* 2004;**11**:1537–45 review of SGA cases, n=53, Benyamina and Samalin, *Int J Psychiatry Clin Pract* 2012;**16**:2–7)
Amisulpride (n=1, *Prog Neuropsychopharmacol Biol Psychiatry* 2009;**33**:1572–3; n=1, *Indian J Pharmacol* 2010;**42**:112–3; FFT; n=1, *Am J Health Syst Pharm* 2014;**71**:2038–41)
Aripiprazole (e.g. n=4, *Pharmacopsychiatry* 2011;**44**:78–81; n=1, first episode at 55 years, *Psychiatry (Edgmont)* 2010;**7**:37–9; FFT)
Lithium + imipramine (n=1, *Br J Psychiatry* 1988;**153**:828–30)
Lithium toxicity (n=3, *Drug Intell Clin Pharm* 1987;**21**:979–81)
Lithium discontinuation (n=1, complicated by delirium, *Gen Hosp Psychiatry* 2010;**32**:102–4)
Olanzapine (review, concludes half of reports are poorly documented but, in the others, mood-elevating effects were prominent, n=26, *J Clin Psychiatry* 2000;**61**:649–55. Lilly post-hoc analysis of two RCTs failed to show any evidence of olanzapine-induced mania; n=254, Baker *J Affect Disord* 2003;**73**:147–53)
Olanzapine/fluoxetine combination (no greater risk than olanzapine or placebo over 8/52, n=833, *J Clin Psychiatry* 2005;**66**:611–6)
Quetiapine (many, e.g. n=1, *Can J Psychiatry* 2003;**48**:349–50; n=1, *Rev Bras Psiquitr* 2009:**31**:286–7; FFT)
Paliperidone (n=1, *J Clin Psychopharmacol* 2010;**30**:202–4; n=1, *Prog Neuropsychopharmacol Biol Psychiatry* 2010;**34**:1351–2; n=1, oral to LAI, *Case Rep Psychiatry* 2015;**2015**:528370; FFT)
Risperidone (review concludes that half of the reports are poorly documented but, in the others, mood-elevating effects were prominent, n=26, *J Clin Psychiatry* 2000;**61**:649–55; n=2, *J Pharmacol Pharmacother* 2014;**5**:258–60; FFT)
Risperidone discontinuation (n=1, *J Clin Psychiatry* 1998;**59**:620–1)
Risperidone to paliperidone switch (n=1, *J Neuropsychiatry Clin Neurosci* 2011;**23**:E29)
Ziprasidone (n=14 worldwide, reviewed in *Clin Neuropharmacol* 2005;**28**:83–6; n=1, *CNS Spectr* 2007;**12**:578–9; n=1, *J Clin Psychopharmacol* 2008;**28**:711–3)
Ziprasidone + SSRI (n=1, *J Clin Psychiatry* 2003;**64**:1393–4)

- CNS — antidepressants

Probable antidepressant-induced mania is known (especially in bipolar III), as also is the spontaneous swing from depression to hypomania in bipolars. Depressed bipolar II patients may be less vulnerable than in bipolar I to switch to mania/hypomania when treated with an antidepressant and an adjunctive mood stabiliser (n=184, 10/52, Altshuler *et al, Am J Psychiatry* 2006;**163**:313–5). Risk factors include:

- → increased number of antidepressant trials
- → history of substance misuse (n=98, *J Clin Psychiatry* 2006;**67**:1341–5)
- → in bipolar depression, during acute and maintenance treatment. Venlafaxine appears worst, sertraline medium and bupropion lowest risk (n=159, RCT, 10/52, *Am J Psychiatry* 2006;**163**:232–9)
- → higher doses — SSRI-induced hypomania may be dose-related (n=2, *Acta Psychiatr Scand* 2001;**104**:236–9)

Switching can be reduced by using adjunctive lithium (n=44, review by Henry *et al, J Clin Psychiatry* 2001;**62**:249–55).
Reviews: extensive (meta-analysis, s=73, n=114,521, Iondo *et al, Acta Psychiatr Scand* 2010;**121**:404–14; FFT), general (Chen *et al, Curr Psychiatry Rep* 2010;**12**:512–21), antidepressant discontinuation (n=24, Narayan and Haddad, *J Psychopharmacol* 2011;**25**:306–13; Saatcioglu *et al, J Affect Disord* 2011;**134**:85–90).

Bupropion (rare, e.g. n=1, within a week, *Bipolar Disord* 2001;**3**:159–60; n=1, *Aust N Z J Psychiatry* 2008;**42**:746)
Bupropion discontinuation (n=1, *J Clin Psychiatry* 2004;**65**:277)
Desvenlafaxine (n=1, not bipolar, *J Psychiatr Pract* 2010;**16**:58–62)

5

Duloxetine (rare in unipolar depression; *J Affect Disord* 2005;**87**:115–9; n=1, *J Psychopharmacol* 2009;**23**:592–6)
Flupentixol (n=6, *Eur Psychiatry* 2002;**17**:349–52)
MAOIs, e.g.:
→ isocarboxazid (n=3, *J Clin Psychiatry* 1986;**47**:40–1)
→ isocarboxazid discontinuation (n=2, *J Clin Psychopharmacol* 1985;**5**:340–2)
→ phenelzine (e.g. *Biol Psychiatry* 1985;**20**:1009–14)
→ phenelzine discontinuation (n=1, see *J Psychopharmacol* 2011;**25**:306–13)
Mianserin
Mirtazapine (n=1, *Pharmacopsychiatry* 2010;**43**:37–8; n=1 after switch from fluoxetine, *J Psychopharmacol* 2009;**23**:220–2; n=1, *Aust NZ J Psychiatry* 2011;**45**:901)
Mirtazapine discontinuation (n=1, *Br J Psychiatry* 1999;**175**:390; see also *J Psychopharmacol* 2011;**25**:306–13)
Mirtazapine + fluoxetine (n=1, *Depress Anxiety* 2002;**15**:46–7)
Mirtazapine + sertraline (n=1, *J Clin Psychiatry* 1998;**59**:320)
Reboxetine (n=3, *J Clin Psychiatry* 2001;**62**:655–6)
SSRIs, e.g.:
→ citalopram (n=1, *Gen Hosp Psychiatry* 2007;**29**:374–6; n=1, *Psychosomatics* 2008;**49**:362–3)
→ citalopram + sibutramine (n=1, *J Clin Psychiatry* 2002;**63**:165)
→ escitalopram (n=1, *Eur Psychiatry* 2004;**19**:455–6; n=2, *Psychopharmacol Bull* 2009;**42**:89–91)
→ fluoxetine (e.g. n=3, *J Child Adolesc Psychopharmacol* 1998;**8**:73–80; n=1, *J Neuropsychiatry Clin Neurosci* 2011;**23**:E23–4)
→ fluvoxamine (n=1, *World J Biol Psychiatry* 2001;**2**:201–4; n=1, *J Psychiatry Neurosci* 2003;**28**:134–5; FFT)
→ fluvoxamine discontinuation (n=1, see *J Psychopharmacol* 2011;**25**:306–13)
→ paroxetine (n=1, psychotic mania, *Am J Psychiatry* 1995;**152**:1399–400; n=79, incidence 8.9%; *Hum Psychopharmacol* 2003;**18**:565–8)
→ paroxetine + methylphenidate (n=1, *Prog Neuropsychopharmacol Biol Psychiatry* 2010;**34**:719–20)
→ paroxetine discontinuation (n=3, see *J Psychopharmacol* 2011;**25**:306–13)
→ sertraline (n=1, *Acta Psychiatr Scand* 2003;**108**:70–4)
→ sertraline discontinuation (*Can J Psychiatry* 2002;**47**:584–5)
→ sertraline + TMS (n=1, *J Neuropsychiatry Clin Neurosci* 2011;**23**:E4–5)
St John's wort (n=12, review in *Int J Clin Pharmacol Ther* 2004;**42**:473–80)
Trazodone (several e.g. n=3, *Br J Psychiatry* 1991;**158**:275–8)
Tricyclics, e.g.:
→ amitriptyline (e.g. *Neurology* 1989;**39**:305)
→ amitriptyline discontinuation (n=1, *J Clin Psychiatry* 1980;**41**:33–4)
→ clomipramine (n=25, RCT, incidence 24%, *Arch Gen Psychiatry* 1979;**36**:560–5 inc. abuse; n=3, *Addiction* 2007;**102**:1166–7)
→ desipramine discontinuation (n=2, see *J Psychopharmacol* 2011;**25**:306–13)
→ dosulepin abuse (n=3, *Addiction* 2007;**102**:1166–7)
→ imipramine (n=25, RCT, incidence 4%, *Arch Gen Psychiatry* 1979;**36**:560–5)
→ imipramine discontinuation (n=1, *Am J Psychiatry* 1986;**143**:260)
→ nortriptyline discontinuation (n=1, see *J Psychopharmacol* 2011;**25**:306–13)
→ protriptyline discontinuation (n=1, see *J Psychopharmacol* 2011;**25**:306–13)
Venlafaxine (n=1, *Can J Psychiatry* 2004;**49**:496; n=1, *Can J Psychiatry* 2004;**49**:786–7)
Venlafaxine discontinuation (n=1, *Int J Neuropsychopharmacol* 2003;**6**:89–90; n=1, *Ann Pharmacother* 2007;**41**:359–60)
Venlafaxine + lithium + valproate (n=1, *Therapie* 2006;**61**:531–3)
Venlafaxine + TMS (n=1, *J Neuropsychiatry Clin Neurosci* 2010;**22**:E18–9)

• CNS — analgesics

Buprenorphine (incidence up to 1%, *Br J Clin Pract* 1980;**34**:144–6; n=1, *Aust N Z J Psychiatry* 2004;**38**:560–1)
Codeine + paracetamol (n=1, *Aust N Z J Psychiatry* 1998;**32**:586–8)
Frovatriptan (n=1, *J Neuropsychiatry Clin Neurosci* 2005;**17**:430–1)

Nefopam IM (euphoria, *Br J Anaesth* 1979;**51**:961–5)
Opioid discontinuation (n=9, *J Opioid Manag* 2012;**8**:67–72)
Pentazocine (*South Med J* 1975;**68**:808–11)
Tramadol (n=1, *Am J Psychiatry* 1997;**154**:1624)

- CNS — anticonvulsants *

Carbamazepine (*J Clin Psychiatry* 1984;**45**:272–4; n=1, *J Clin Psychiatry* 2015;**76**:e117–8)
Carbamazepine discontinuation (n=1, *Br J Psychiatry* 1995;**167**:698)
Clonazepam (*DICP* 1991;**25**:938–9)
Ethosuximide (n=1, *Epilepsy Behav* 2011;**21**:483–5)
Gabapentin (e.g. n=1, *Br J Psychiatry* 1995;**166**:679–80; n=1, *Br J Psychiatry* 1999;**175**:291)
Lamotrigine (n=1 as augmentation of duloxetine in unipolar depression, *Prim Care Companion CNS Disord* 2011;**13**:PCC.10l01064; FFT; n=2, *Prim Care Companion CNS Disord* 2011;**13**:PCC.10l01034; FFT; n=3, *Am J Psychiatry* 2006;**163**:159–60; n=1, *Aust N Z J Psychiatry* 2006;**40**:718; no increase in switch to mania in bipolar I, n=1,258, 6/12, open, p/c, *J Clin Psychiatry* 2009;**70**:1273–80)
Phenobarbital (*Pediatrics* 1984;**74**:1133)
Pregabalin (SmPC)
Topiramate (n=1, *J Neurol Neurosurg Psychiatry* 2002;**73**:208–9; FFT; *J Clin Psychopharmacol* 2005;**25**:196–7)
Vigabatrin (n=1, *Lancet* 1994;**343**:606–7)
Zonisamide (*J Clin Psychopharmacol* 2004;**24**:110–1; n=1, *J Clin Psychopharmacol* 2006;**26**:439–40)

- CNS — movement disorders

Amantadine (n=1, *J Clin Psychiatry* 1989;**50**:143–4; n=3, manic switch, *Rev Bras Psiquiatr* 2010;**32**:467–9; FFT)
Bromocriptine (n=600, incidence 1.3%, *Br Med J [Clin Res Med]* 1984;**289**:1101–3; FFT; postpartum mania, n=1, *J Gynecol Obstet Biol Reprod* [Paris] 2006;**35**:79–81; FFT)
Levodopa (e.g. *N Engl J Med* 1971;**285**:1326–7)
Levodopa + carbidopa (*J Clin Psychopharmacol* 1985;**5**:338–9)
Pramipexole (n=1, *Am J Psychiatry* 2007;**164**:351)
Procyclidine abuse (e.g. n=1 and review, *Br J Psychiatry* 1982;**141**:81–4)

- CNS — others *

Amfetamine discontinuation (*J Clin Psychiatry* 1980;**41**:33–4)
Anticholinesterases (n=2, relapses, *J Clin Psychopharmacol* 2011;**31**:254–6)
- donepezil (n=1, *Int Psychogeriatr* 2011;**23**:503–4)
- rivastigmine (n=1, *Int Psychogeriatr* 2012;**24**:1697–9)

Atomoxetine (MHRA warning 2009; n=1, *J Clin Psychopharmacol* 2004;**24**:567–8; n=1, *Pediatrics* 2004;**114**:895–6)
Bromide (n=1, *Am J Psychiatry* 1976;**133**:228–9)
Caffeine (*Gen Hosp Psychiatry* 2003;**25**:138–9; excess; n=1, *Am J Addict* 2015;**24**:289–91)
Cannabis (n=4,815, dose–related increased risk, *J Affect Disord* 2006;**95**:103–10; regular use increases illness severity, n=3,459, *J Nerv Ment Dis* 2009;**197**:35–40; n=1 and review, *Tijdschr Psychiatr* 2009;**51**:859–63; FFT)
Cannabis, synthetic (n=1, *Case Rep Psychiatry* 2015;**2015**:310930; FFT)
Cyclizine
Dexamfetamine (n=1 and review, *Am J Psychiatry* 1976;**133**:1177–80)
Disulfiram (*J Am Acad Child Adolesc Psychiatry* 1988;**27**:500–3; high dose; n=1, *J Clin Psychopharmacol* 2007;**27**:224–5)
Donepezil (n=2, undeclared use, *J Clin Psychopharmacol* 2014;**34**:753–5)
Fenfluramine (e.g. *Am J Psychiatry* 1997;**154**:711)
Ginseng (n=1, *Acta Psychiatr Scand* 2002;**105**:76–8)
Hydroxytryptophan via Internet + phenelzine (n=1, *de novo*, *Gen Hosp Psychiatry* 2012;**34**:102.e13–4; FFT)
LSD (n=1, *Am J Psychiatry* 1981;**138**:1508–9)
Marijuana (n=1, *Gen Hosp Psychiatry* 2011;**33**:640.e3–4)
Methamphetamine (16% in people with psychosis, n=121, *Addict Health* 2015;**7**:37–46; FFT)
Methylphenidate (e.g. n=137, *Psychopharmacol Bull* 2008;**41**:37–47; n=1, *Indian J Pharmacol* 2011;**43**:80–1; FFT)
Nicotine discontinuation (n=1, *Am J Psychiatry* 1992;**149**:708; n=1, *Am J Psychiatry* 1990;**147**:1254–5)

5

Sibutramine (in OTC diet aid, n = 1, *Turk Psikiyatri Derg* 2010;**21**:335–7; FFT; n = 1, *BMC Psychiatry* 2012;**12**:43; FFT)
Sibutramine + citalopram (n = 1, *J Clin Psychiatry* 2002;**63**:165)
Varenicline (n = 1, bipolar patient, *Clin Neuropharmacol* 2009;**32**:117–8; n = 1, first-episode, *Int J Geriatr Psychiatry* 2011;**26**:658–9; review of varenicline inducing manic relapse in bipolar; Knibbs and Tsoi, *Hosp Gen Psychiatry* 2011;**33**:641; n = 2, *Tijdschr Psychiatr* 2015;**57**:835–8; FFT)

- **Gastrointestinal drugs**

H2 blockers, e.g.:
→cimetidine (n = 2, *J Clin Psychiatry* 1983;**44**:267–8)
→famotidine (n = 1, *Pharmacopsychiatry* 2002;**35**:152–4)
→ranitidine IV (case in *South Med J* 1987; **80**:1467)
→ranitidine oral (n = 1, after 2/7, *Am J Psychiatry* 1988;**145**:271)
Metoclopramide (n = 1, *J Clin Psychiatry* 1984;**45**:180–1)

- **Cardiovascular drugs**

ACE inhibitors e.g.:
→captopril (several, e.g. n = 1, *Am J Psychiatry* 1993;**150**: 1429–30)
→lisinopril (n = 1, *Psychosomatics* 1995;**36**:508–9)
Beta-blockers, e.g.:
→propranolol (*South Med J* 1984;**77**:1603)
→propranolol discontinuation (n = 1, *Am J Psychiatry* 1986;**143**:1633)
Calcium-channel blockers, e.g.:
→diltiazem (n = 1, *Clin Cardiol* 1986;**9**:39)
Clonidine (n = 1, *Am J Psychiatry* 1982;**139**:1083)
Clonidine discontinuation (*J Clin Psychopharmacol* 1981;**1**:93–5; n = 1, *Am J Psychiatry* 1984;**141**:153)
Digoxin (*Med J Rec* 1929;**130**:381–2)
Hydralazine
Isosorbides (*Adv Psych Treat* 2005;**11**:66)
Methyldopa discontinuation (n = 1, *Am J Psychiatry* 1989;**146**:1075–6)
Omega-3 fatty acids (n = 1, *Arch Gen Psychiatry* 2000;**57**:715–6)
Procainamide (n = 1, *Am J Psychiatry* 1988;**145**:129–30)

- **Respiratory drugs**

Alimemazine (rare cases)
Aminophylline
Beclomethasone aerosol (n = 1, in stable bipolar person, *Am J Psychiatry* 1989;**146**:1076–7; n = 1, *Prim Care Companion CNS Disorders* 2011;**13**:10l01069; FFT)
Beclomethasone nasal spray (n = 1, *Br J Psychiatry* 1989;**155**:871–2)
Cyproheptadine (rare, e.g. *Am J Psychiatry* 1980;**137**:378–9)
Dextromethorphan (*Psychosomatics* 1996;**37**:71–4; *Psychosomatics* 1996;**37**; 571–3)
Dextromethorphan abuse (cases in *Br Med J (Clin Med Res)* 1986;**293**:597; FFT; *BMJ* 1993;**306**:896; FFT)
Ephedrine (*J Clin Psychopharmacol* 1983;**3**:97–100 and in a herbal diet supplement, n = 1, *Am J Psychiatry* 1995;**152**:647)
Phenylephrine (*Am J Psychiatry* 1981;**138**:837–8)
Phenylpropanolamine (n = 3, *Am J Psychiatry* 1981;**138**:392)
Pseudoephedrine (several e.g. n = 1, *Tijdschr Psychiatr* 2007;**49**:125–9; FFT; n = 1, *N Z Med J* 2002;**115**:86)
Salbutamol oral (n = 1, *Encelphale* 1981;**7**:45–9)

- **Anti-infection drugs** *

Generally low risk, most commonly with (in decreasing order) clarithromycin, ciprofloxacin, ofloxacin, then co-trimoxazole, metronidazole and erythromycin. It can be enduring in a very few people.
Review: n = 103, Abouesh *et al*, *J Clin Psychopharmacol* 2002;**22**:71–81.
Chloroquine (several e.g. n = 6, *Int J Psychiatry Med* 1993;**23**:349–56)
Ciprofloxacin (*Psychosomatics* 2007;**48**:363)
Clarithromycin (n = 1, *Acta Psychiatr Scand* 2010;**122**:267–8; n = 1, *Int J Neuropsychopharmacol* 2004;**7**:99–100; n = 1, *Acta Med Port* 2011;**24**:827–32; FFT; n = 1, *J Clin Psychopharmacol* 2014;**34**:416–7)
Dapsone (n = 1, *BMJ* 1989;**298**:1524; FFT)
Efavirenz overdose (n = 1, *Clin Infect Dis* 2001;**33**:270–1; FFT)
Ethambutol (n = 1, *Med J Aust* 1996;**164**:445–6)
Interferon alfa (*Aust N Z J Psychiatry* 2011;**45**:1004)
Isoniazid (n = 5, *Br Med J* 1957;**2**:743–6; FFT)

Isoniazid (isonicotinic acid hydrazine) + pyridoxine (*Can J Psychiatry* 1988;**33**:675–6)
Ketoconazole (*Adv Psychiatr Treat* 2005;**11**:66)
Mefloquine (e.g. n=2, *Encephale* 2011;**37**:393–6; n=1, child, *J Child Neurol* 2009;**24**:1008–9; n=1, *J Clin Psychopharmacol* 2010;**30**:339–41)
Mepacrine (*Mayo Clin Proc* 1989;**64**:129–30)
Oseltamivir (n=1, *Am J Psychiatry* 2010;**167**:350)
Quinacrine (n=1, *Mayo Clin Proc* 1989;**64**:129–30; n=1, *BMJ Case Rep* 2012;**2012**:bcr0220125842; FFT)
Tetracyclines (*Adv Psychiatr Treat* 2005;**11**:66)
Valaciclovir (n=1, *Psychosomatics* 2009;**50**:293–6)
Zidovudine (*JAMA* 1988;**259**:3406–7; n=2, *Med J Aust* 1989;**150**:339–41)

- **Endocrine system drugs** *

Review: steroid-induced mania (risk factors; *Can J Clin Pharmacol* 2001;**8**:109–12).
Androgens (*J Clin Psychiatry* 1985;**46**:354–5)
Clomifene (n=1, *Psychosomatics* 2007;**48**:65–6)
Corticosteroids (incidence may be as high as 5–6% in adults, usually emerges within a few days or weeks, risk may be greater at higher doses, *MHRA Drug Safety Update* 2007;1–9; high dose in MS; c=88, *J Affect Disord* 2015;**187**:142–6; may respond to quetiapine, *Can J Psychiatry* 2005;**50**:77–8):
→ cortisone (*Psychosomat Med* 1953;**15**:589–613)
→ deflazacort (SmPC)
→ dexamethasone (incidence up to 31%, *Arch Gen Psychiatry* 1981;**38**:471–7; n=1, *Psychopharmacol Bull* 2010;**43**:82–5)
→ hydrocortisone (e.g. n=1, *Postgrad Med J* 1992;**68**:41–3; FFT)
→ prednisolone + clarithromycin (n=1, *Can J Psychiatry* 1997;**42**:778)
→ prednisone (*J Affect Disord* 1983;**5**:319–32)
→ prednisone + bromocriptine (n=1, *Gen Hosp Psychiatry* 1991;**13**:345–6)
→ triamcinolone (rare cases)
Dehydroepiandrosterone DHEA (e.g. n=1, *Encephale* 2002;**28**:563–6; n=1, *Ann Pharmacother* 2000;**34**:1419–22)
Glucocorticoids (four times more likely than people not taking glucocorticoids, especially in younger people; n=372,696, *Am J Psychiatry* 2012;**169**:491–7)
HRT (n=1, *Am J Geriatr Psychiatry* 1997;**5**:179–81)
Leuprolide (n=1, *J Clin Psychiatry* 2010;**71**:1696–8)
Leuprolide acetate depot (n=1, relapse, *CNS Spectr* 2010;**15**:603–6)
Levothyroxine (n=1, *J Am Acad Child Adolesc Psychiatry* 2005;**44**:211)
Quinagolide (n=1, *Gen Hosp Psychiatry* 2007;**29**:464)
Testosterone patches (n=1, *Am J Psychiatry* 1999;**156**:969)
Triiodothyronine (*J Clin Psychiatry* 1986;**47**:521–2)

- **Malignancy and immunosuppressant drugs**

Anastrozole (n=1, *Bipolar Disord* 2006;**8**:516–8)
Ciclosporin (*Biol Psychiatry* 1984;**19**:1161–2)
Interferons (*J Postgrad Med* 2007;**53**:150; FFT; *Can J Psychiatry* 2004;**49**:867–8), e.g.:
→ interferon alfa (n=93, incidence 16%, *J Clin Psychiatry* 2005;**66**:1050–7; n=1, *Ir J Med Sci* 2007;**176**:137–9)
→ interferon alfa discontinuation (n=44, incidence 5%, *Arch Gen Psychiatry* 1998;**55**:88–9; n=1, *Psychiatry Clin Neurosci* 2002;**56**:647–8)
→ interferon alfa-2b (n=1, *J Postgrad Med* 2006;**52**:207–9; FFT; n=1, *Afr J Psychiatry (Johannesbg)* 2009;**12**:227–8; FFT)
→ peginterferon + ribavirin (n=1, *Am J Psychiatry* 2004;**161**:429–35)
Letrozole (n=1, *Bipolar Disord* 2006;**8**:516–8)
Procarbazine (*Br Med J (Clin Res Ed)* 1982;**284**:82–3; FFT)
Triptorelin (n=1, *Br J Psychiatry* 1999:**175**;290–1)

- **Musculoskeletal and analgesics** *

Baclofen (including high-dose, e.g. n=1, *J Clin Psychopharmacol* 1992;**12**:215–7; n=116, *Alcohol Alcohol* 2015;**50**:551–7)
Baclofen discontinuation (n=1, *Am J Psychiatry* 1980;**137**:1466–7)
Indometacin (*J Clin Psychopharmacol* 1987;**7**:203–4)
Infliximab (n=1, *Psychiatry Clin Neurosci* 2010;**64**:442–3)

- **Others** *

Aspartame high–dose (n = 1, *Psychosomatics* 1986;**27**:218–20)
Ayahuasca (n = 1, *Int J Bipolar DIsord* 2015;**3**:4; FFT)
Calcium IV (n=1, *J Nerv Ment Dis* 1980;**168**:562–3)
Decongestants
Energy drink containing caffeine, taurine and inositol (*Can J Psychiatry* 2001;**46**:454–5)
Herbal remedies (n = 1, *Am J Psychiatry* 1998;**155**:1627)
Horny Goat weed (n = 1, *Psychosomatics* 2004;**45**:536–7)
Inositol (n = 3, *Am J Psychiatry* 1996;**153**:839)
Ketamine (n=1, *Biol Psychiatry* 2011;**70**:e13–4)
Ma–hung (a herb in weight–loss supplements n = 1, *Pharmacotherapy* 2003;**23**:380–3)
Metrizamide (*N C Med J* 1984;**45**:759)
Nitrous oxide (n = 1, relapse, *Aust N Z J Psychiatry* 2011;**45**:1002)
Sildenafil (relapse, n = 1, *Int J Neuro-psychopharmacol* 2004;**7**:525)
Yohimbine (n = 3, *Am J Psychiatry* 1984;**141**:1267–8)

5.8 MOVEMENT DISORDERS, EXTRA-PYRAMIDAL DISORDERS

Four distinct types of drug-induced extra-pyramidal or movement disorders are known, especially with antipsychotics, i.e. dystonias, akathisias, pseudoparkinsonism and dyskinesias. All can occur acutely or be delayed (tardive). Acute reactions are usually at the start of treatment or after a dose increase and are usually reversible. The tardive forms are not invariably reversible on discontinuation or dose reduction and can be aggravated by anticholinergics.

Reviews: causes (Thanvi and Treadwell, *Postgrad Med J* 2009;**85**:322–6; Susatia and Fernandez, *Curr Treat Options Neurol* 2009;**11**:162–9).

5.8.1 PSEUDOPARKINSONISM

Pseudoparkinsonism is characterised by akinesia, tremor and rigidity, and generally occurs within a month of the start of treatment.

Reviews: postural induced-tremor in psychiatry (Arbaizar *et al*, *Psychiatry Clin Neurosci* 2008;**62**:638–45), extensive (Mena and de Yébenes, *Expert Opin Drug Saf* 2006;**5**:759–71), in the elderly (Esper and Factor, *Mov Disord* 2008;**23**:401–4).

- **CNS — antipsychotics**

Review: meta-analysis of SGA head-to-head studies (s = 54, Rummel-Kluge *et al*, *Schizophr Bull* 2012;**38**:167–77; FFT).

Aripiprazole (many cases, e.g. n = 2, *J Med Case Reports* 2009;**3**:6448; FFT; n = 1, *Tijdschr Psychiatr* 2011;**53**:299–303; FFT)
Aripiprazole + SSRIs (*Rev Med Chil* 2011;**139**:1517–8; FFT)
Chlorpromazine (n = 1, *Psychiatr Pol* 2007;**41**:495–501)
Clozapine (n = 1, *Ann Pharmacother* 2000;**34**:615–8)
Lithium:
- → short-term (*J Neurol Sci* 2000;**176**:78–9)
- → long-term (several, e.g. n = 2, *Tijdschr Psychiatr* 2009;**51**:123–7; FFT)
- → toxicity (n = 1, *Acta Neurol Taiwan* 2007;**16**;231–3; FFT)

Olanzapine overdose (n = 1, *Am J Psychiatry* 1998;**155**:1630–1)
Olanzapine after smoking cessation (n = 1, *Am J Health Syst Pharm* 2011;**68**:399–401)
Risperidone (may be plasma level/CYP2D6 phenotype dependent, n = 50, *Eur J Pharm Sci* 2010;**41**:289–98)
Ziprasidone (low incidence, e.g. n = 210, *Am J Psychiatry* 2003;**160**:741–8)

- **CNS — antidepressants** *

Review: n = 89, of which 66% were for duloxetine; *Ann Clin Psychiatry* 2010;**22**:148–56.

Bupropion (*J Clin Psychopharmacol* 2009;**29**:616–8; *Mov Disord* 2007;**22**:1830–1; n = 1, *Consult Pharm* 2011;**26**:665–71)
Duloxetine (see review above)
MAOIs
SSRIs (annual incidence may be around 0.1–0.2%; *Ann Pharmacother* 1998;**32**:692–8):
- → citalopram (n = 1, *Clin Neuropharmacol* 2011;**34**:92–3)
- → fluoxetine (n = 21, *Parkinsonism Relat Disord* 2002;**8**:325–7; mean latency for tremor 54 days, was mild and remitted in 50% over a mean of 35 days after discontinuation; n = 1, *Ann Gen Psychiatry* 2010;**9**:5; FFT)

→ fluoxetine discontinuation (n = 1, *Am J Psychiatry* 1991;**148**:1263)
→ paroxetine (cases reported in *Current Problems* 1993;**19**:1)
→ sertraline (n = 1, *Am J Psychiatry* 1994;**151**:288)
→ sertraline + oxycodone (n = 1, *J Clin Pharmacol* 2001;**41**:224–7)

Trazodone (e.g. n = 1, *Nephron* 2002;**90**:222–3; n = 1, *BMJ Case Rep* 2015;**2015**:bcr2015210726)
Tricyclics

- **CNS — analgesics**

Nabilone
Pethidine and other opioids

- **CNS — anticonvulsants**

Carbamazepine (incidence of tremor may be 22%, *N Engl J Med* 1992;**327**:765–71; FFT)
Carbamazepine + lithium (n = 1, *Clin Neuropharmacol* 2010;**33**:102–3)
Lacosamide (common, SmPC)
Lamotrigine (n = 1, *Mov Disord* 2006;**21**:2269–70)
Levetiracetam (n = 1, *Clin Neuropharmacol* 2005;**28**:188–90; n = 1, *Clin Neuropharmacol* 2006;**29**:303–4)
Oxcarbazepine (n = 1, *Parkinsonism Relat Disord* 2009;**15**:787–8)
Phenytoin (n = 1, *Singapore Med J* 2006;**47**:981–3; FFT)
Pregabalin (n = 1, *Clin Neuropharmacol* 2009;**32**:353–4)
Rufinamide (incidence 1–10%, SmPC)
Topiramate + fluvoxamine (n = 1, *Clin Neuropharmacol* 2008;**31**:366–7)
Valproate (incidence 5–10%, especially if taken for > 3 years, *Mov Disord* 2007;**22**:130–3; mechanism unclear as it is usually unresponsive to levodopa; n = 13 in elderly, *Am J Geriatr Pharmacother* 2011;**9**:405–12; n = 5, fully reversible on discontinuation, *Epilepsia* 2006;**47**:2183–5)
Zonisamide (SmPC)

- **CNS — movement disorders**

Bromocriptine
Levodopa
Tetrabenazine

- **CNS — others** *

Anticholinesterases:
→ donepezil (n = 1, *Ann Pharmacother* 1998;**32**:610–1)
→ rivastigmine

Atomoxetine + venlafaxine (n = 1, *Clin Toxicol [Phila]* 2007;**45**:182–5)
Cocaine abuse (*Arch Internal Med* 1997;**157**:241; as a risk factor, review, n = 106, *Psychopharmacol Bull* 2008;**41**:5–10)
Cyclizine
Dexamfetamine
Methamphetamine + haloperidol decanoate (n = 1, *Int J Psychiatry Med* 2015;**50**:405–11)
Metoclopramide (n = 1, *J Perianesth Nurs* 2008;**23**:292–9)
Ondansetron (n = 1, *Ann Pharmacother* 1994;**28**:280; n = 1, *Ann Pharmacother* 1996;**30**:196)
Varenicline (n = 1, *J Clin Psychopharmacol* 2015;**35**:355–7)

- **Gastrointestinal drugs**

Cimetidine (n = 1, possible, *Postgrad Med J* 1982;**58**:527–8; FFT)
Domperidone (rare, case in *Helv Paediatr Acta* 1984;**39**:285–8)
Metoclopramide (incidence 2–30%)
Prochlorperazine (common, e.g. *Lancet* 1984;**2**:1082–3)

- **Cardiovascular drugs**

Review: calcium-channel blockers as a cause of EPS (Simon *et al*, *Mov Disord* 2010;**25**:1818–22; FFT).

Amiodarone (n=1, *Ann Neurol* 1989;**25**:630–2)
Amlodipine (n = 1, *Mov Disord* 2002;**17**:833–5)
Diazoxide (n = 6, *Br Med J* 1973;**3**:474–5, FFT)
Diltiazem (*Am J Med* 1989;**87**:95–6; review, *Pharm J* 2012;**289**:209)
Flunarizine (n=26, *Arq Neuropsiquiatr* 2004;**62**:784–8; FFT)
Methyldopa (n=2, *Can Med Assoc J* 1966;**95**:928–9; FFT)
Metirosine
Mexilitine
Nifedipine (n=1, *Br Med J* 1978;**1**:1619; FFT)
Tocainide
Trimetazidine (8% incidence, n = 258, *Therapie* 2005;**60**:419–22; n = 21, *Fundam Clin Pharmacol* 2012;**26**:198–203)

5

- **Respiratory drugs**

Antihistamines:

→ brompheniramine (*N Engl J Med* 1975;**293**:486–7)

→ cinnarizine (n=26, *Arq Neuropsiquiatr* 2004;**62**:784–8; n=1, *Rev Neurol* 1999;**28**:876–8)

→ diphenhydramine (*N Engl J Med* 1977;**296**:111)

Montelukast (FDA warning 2009)
Orciprenaline
Promethazine (*Clin Pharm* 1984;**3**:83–5)
Salbutamol
Terbutaline
Zafirlukast (FDA warning 2009)

- **Anti-infection drugs**

Aciclovir
Cephaloridine
Chloroquine
Itraconazole (incidence 2%, n=216, 20/12, *J Neurol Neurosurg Psychiatry* 2010;**81**:327–9)

- **Endocrine system drugs**

Mecasermin (rare, SmPC)
Medroxyprogesterone
Prednisolone (increases incidence with antipsychotics, review in *JAMA* 1973;**224**:889–91)

- **Malignancy and immunosuppressant drugs**

Ciclosporin (n=1, *Transplant Proc* 2008;**40**:2823–4; 13% point prevalence, n=60, *Arq Neuropsiquiatr* 2005;**63**:592–6; FFT)
Interferons

→ peginterferon IFN-a 2a (n=1, *Arq Neuro Psiquiatr* 2009;**67**:715–6; FFT)

Nelarabine (very common, SmPC)
Octreotide high-dose (n=1, *Neurology* 2008;**70**:2345–6)

- **Musculoskeletal and analgesics**

Etodolac (SmPC)
Fenoprofen
Flurbiprofen (n=1, *BMJ* 1990;**300**:540–1; FFT)
Ibuprofen (n=1, *Postgrad Med J* 1987;**63**:593; FFT)
Indometacin
Mefenamic acid (n=1, *J R Soc Med* 1983;**76**:435)
Sulindac (n=1, *Ann Neurol* 1985;**17**:104–5)

- **Others** *

Distigmine bromide (n=1, *Rinsho Shinkeigaku* 2005;**45**:600–2)
Ethylene glycol + methanol (n=2, *Clin Pharmacol Ther* 2007;**81**:114–21)
Manganese intoxication (review, *Int J Environ Res Public Health* 2015;**12**:7519–40; FFT)
Organophosphates (chlorpyrifos overdose; n=1, *Clin Toxicol (Phila)* 2005;**43**:877–9; incl. pesticides; n=781, some association between PD and professional pesticide exposure, *Ann Neurol* 2009;**66**:494–504)

5.8.2 AKATHISIA

Akathisia is characterised by motor restlessness, with an inability to stay still. Onset is around 6–60 days and has been implicated with all antipsychotics, but especially with higher potency. **Reviews:** general (Kumar and Sachdev, *Curr Opin Psychiatry* 2009;**22**:293–99; Poyurovsky, *Br J Psychiatry* 2010; **196**:89–91).

- **CNS — sleep disorders and anxiety**

Alprazolam
Buspirone (several e.g. n=1, *J Clin Psychopharmacol* 1988;**8**:296–7)
Lorazepam (n=1, *Oncology* 1990;**47**:415–7)
Melatonin discontinuation (*Mov Disord* 1999;**14**:381–2)

- **CNS — antipsychotics** *

Review: akathisia has been observed with all antipsychotics, but is more common in bipolar than schizophrenia (s=77, Kane *et al*, *J Clin Psychiatry* 2009;**70**:627–43).

Amisulpride (10% incidence of acute akathisia, 21% incidence of delayed onset akathisia (n=56, *Indian J Pharmacol* 2011;**43**:460–2)
Aripiprazole (occurs early, is mild-to-moderate severity, leads to few discontinuations and does not compromise efficacy; e.g. n=4,967, *J Psychopharmacol* 2010;**24** 1019–29; n=1, *J Clin Pharmacol* 2012;**52**:1448–9)
Clozapine (incidence 6% claimed: *Psychopharmacology (Berl)* 1995;**118**:52–6; acute nocturnal, n=1, *J Clin Psychopharmacol* 2007;**27**:205; n=1 and review, *Indian J Pharmacol* 2015;**47**:234–5; FFT)
Haloperidol (review in *Psychopharmacol Bull* 1985;**21**:69–72)

Lithium (n = 1, *J Neurol Sci* 2000;**176**:78–9)
Olanzapine (incidence 6%; n = 1, switching from branded to generic, *J Clin Psychiatry* 2012;**73**:497)
Prochlorperazine (n = 140, incidence 44% with IV, *Ann Emerg Med* 1999;**34**:469–75)
Promazine
Quetiapine (e.g. n = 1, *Indian J Pharmacol* 2010;**42**:416–7; FFT; n = 1, *J Neuropsychiatry Clin Neurosci* 2012;**24**:E46–7)
Risperidone (SmPC)
Risperidone discontinuation (n = 1, *Am J Psychiatry* 1997;**154**:437–8; n = 2, *Actas Esp Psiquiatr* 2002;**30**:195–7)
Risperidone + levomepromazine (n = 1, *Eur Psychiatry* 2002;**17**:294–5)
Sulpiride (n = 1, *Clin Neuropharmacol* 1994;**17**:481–3)
Ziprasidone dose reduction (n = 5, *Am J Psychiatry* 2006;**163**:546)
Zuclopenthixol (*Pharmatherapeutica* 1989;**5**:380–6)

- CNS — antidepressants *

Agomelatine + duloxetine (n = 1, *Pharmacopsychiatry* 2012;**45**:162–3)
Mianserin (n = 1, *J Clin Psychopharmacol* 2010;**30**:338–9)
Mirtazapine (*Med J Aust* 2002;**176**:242; n = 1, *J Clin Psychopharmacol* 2008;**28**:467; after 20 years, n = 1, *Clin Neuropharmacol* 2010;**33**:50–1)
SSRIs (review by Koliscak and Makela, *J Am Pharm Assoc (2003)* 2009;**49**:e28–36):
→citalopram (n = 1, *J Clin Psychiatry* 1988;**49**[Suppl]:18–22; n = 1, *PM R* 2010;**2**:973–5)
→fluoxetine (e.g. *J Clin Psychiatry* 1991;**52**:491–3; n = 1, dose dependent, *J Psychopharmacol* 2003;**17**:451–2)
→paroxetine (n = 3, *Compr Psychiatry* 1996;**37**:122–4; *Can J Psychiatry* 2000;**45**:398)
→sertraline (n = 1, *Am J Psychiatry* 1993;**150**:986–7; mistaken for panic attack, n = 1, *Psychiatr Serv* 2002;**53**:1477–8)
Tricyclics e.g.:
→imipramine (n = 5, *J Clin Psychopharmacol* 1987;**7**:254–7)
→nortriptyline (*Am Fam Physician* 1993;**48**:1024–6)
→tricyclics and conjugated estrogens (n = 3, *Am J Psychiatry* 1984;**141**:696–7)
Venlafaxine (n = 1, *Indian J Pharmacol* 2014;**46**:660–1; FFT)
Venlafaxine discontinuation (n = 1, *Am Fam Physician* 1997;**56**:455–62)
Venlafaxine + methimazole (n = 1, *Gen Hosp Psychiatry* 2009;**31**:388–90)

- CNS — analgesics

Sumatriptan (n = 1, *J Neurol* 1997;**244**:131–2)

- CNS — anticonvulsants

Carbamazepine (n = 1, *Am J Psychiatry* 1986;**143**:1190–1; *N Z Med J* 1992;**105**:182)
Ethosuximide (n = 1, *Am J Dis Child* 1978;**132**:527–8)
Gabapentin discontinuation (n = 1, *Ann Pharmacother* 2011;**45**:e31)

- CNS — movement disorders

Levodopa (review in *Neurology* 1990;**40**:340–5)

- CNS — others

Alcohol (as trigger factor, *JAMA* 1976;**236**:2422–3)
Antiemetics, e.g. metoclopramide oral (e.g. n = 1, *Pharm World Sci* 2010;**32**:704–6; FFT), metoclopramide IV (n = 1, *Singapore Med J* 2011;**52**:e12–4; FFT) and prochlorperazine (many cases, e.g. n = 3, *Gan To Kagaku Ryoho* 2006;**33**:267–9; n = 56, *Acad Emerg Med* 2007;**14**:799–809)
Cocaine (recent use is a risk factor for antipsychotic-induced, n = 106, *Psychopharmacol Bull* 2008;**41**:5–10)
Methysergide (n = 1, *Clin Neuropharmacol* 1988;**11**:87–9)
Ondansetron (n = 1, *Cancer* 1992;**69**:1275)

- Cardiovascular drugs

Atenolol (n = 1, *J Clin Psychopharmacol* 1986;**6**:390)
Diltiazem (n = 1, *Ann Intern Med* 1983;**99**: 794–5)
Flunarizine (n = 1, *Rev Clin Esp* 1991;**188**: 384)
Midodrine + promethazine (n = 1, *JAMA* 2006;**295**:2000–1)
Trimetazidine (n = 1, *Therapie* 2005;**60**:603–5)

5

- **Respiratory drugs**

Alimemazine
Cinnarizine (n=1, *Rev Neurol* 1999;**28**:876–8)
Promethazine + midodrine (n=1, *JAMA* 2006;**295**:2000–1)

- **Malignancy and immunosuppressant drugs**

Interferon alfa (*Gen Hosp Psychiatry* 1999;**21**:134–5)

- **Others** *

Azithromycin (n=1, *Ann Pharmacother* 2015;**49**:609)

5.8.3 DYSTONIAS

Dystonias includes oculogyric crisis (OGC), trismus and torticollis. They may occur within 72 hours of start of therapy and occur more frequently with high-potency antipsychotics.
Review: general (van Harten *et al*, *BMJ* 1999;**319**:623–6; FFT).

- **CNS — sleep disorders and anxiety** *

Benzodiazepines, e.g.:
→ bromazepam (n=1, *Biomed Pharmacother* 1992;**46**:375–6)
→ diazepam (n=2, *J Emerg Med* 1988;**6**:491–3)
→ midazolam (*BMJ* 1990;**300**:614; FFT; n=1, *J Anaesthesiol Clin Pharmacol* 2012;**28**:368–70; FFT)
Buspirone (n=1, *Neurology* 1990;**40**:1904; discussion in *Neurology* 1991;**41**:1850)
Zolpidem discontinuation (n=1, *Parkinsonism Relat Disord* 2015;**21**:661–2)

- **CNS — antipsychotics** *

Review: n=43, Raja and Azzoni, *Int J Neuropsychopharmacol* 2001;**4**:393–7.

Amisulpride (e.g. n=1, *Prog Neuropsychopharmacol Biol Psychiatry* 2010;**34**:412–3; low dose n=1, *J Clin Psychopharmacol* 2008;**28**:573–4)
Aripiprazole (many cases, e.g. n=1, *J Clin Psychiatry* 2010;**71**:652–3; n=1, after single dose, *Am J Addict* 2007;**16**:244; n=1, *J Clin Pharmacol* 2012;**52**:1448–9; monotherapy, n=1, *J Clin Psychopharmacol* 2012;**32**:297–8)
Clozapine (rare, n=1, *Am J Psychiatry* 1995;**152**:647–8; OGC, n=3, *Clin Drug Investig* 2007;**27**:861–4)
Clozapine discontinuation, abrupt (n=4, *J Clin Psychiatry* 1998;**59**:472–7; OCG, n=1, *Aust N Z J Psychiatry* 2016;**50**:183–4)
Flupentixol decanoate (n=1, *Br Med J (Clin Res Ed)* 1981;**282**:1756; FFT)
Fluspirilene (n=1, *Nervenarzt* 1994;**65**:647)
Haloperidol (n=62, incidence 37%, in first episode, *Am J Psychiatry* 1994;**151**:1819–21; *Rev Esp Anetesiol Reanim* 2004;**51**:229–31)
Lithium (n=1, *Neurol India* 2002;**50**:473–5; FFT)
Loxapine
Olanzapine (e.g. n=1, *Am J Psychiatry* 1999;**156**:1662; tardive n=1, *Neurol Sci* 2001;**22**:331–2; n=1, *J Clin Psychopharmacol* 2006;**26**:431; *J Clin Psychiatry* 1998;**59**:384)
Olanzapine overdose (n=1, *J Emerg Med* 2006;**30**:311–7)
Paliperidone (dystonic dysphagia, n=1, *J Neuropsychiatry Clin Neurosci* 2010;**22**:451)
Paliperidone OD (n=1, *Psychosomatics* 2011;**52**:291–4)
Pimozide (low-dose n=1, *J Am Acad Child Adolesc Psychiatry* 1993;**32**:640–2; n=1, delayed by 12 hours in child, *J Toxicol Clin Toxicol* 2004;**42**:977–81)
Prochlorperazine
Quetiapine (several, e.g. n=1, *Aust N Z J Psychiatry* 2006;**40**:607–8; n=1, *J Am Geriatr Soc* 2009;**57**:918–9)
Risperidone (e.g. may be plasma level/CYP2D6 phenotype dependent, n=50, *Eur J Pharm Sci* 2010;**41**:289–98; persistent, n=1, *Psychiatr Danub* 2008;**20**:329–31)
Sulpiride (n=1, *Clin Neuropharmacol* 1991;**14**:463–4)
Ziprasidone (several, e.g. at 240 mg/d, n=1, *Prog Neuropsychopharmacol Biol Psychiatry* 2007;**31**:546–7; n=2, *J Clin Psychiatry* 2006;**67**:326–7)
Zuclopenthixol (study in *Acta Psychiatr Scand* 1991;**84**:14–21)
Zuclopenthixol acetate + fluoxetine (laryngeal, n=1, *Australas Psychiatry* 2010;**18**:174–6)

- **CNS — antidepressants** *

Amoxapine (n=1, *Indian J Psychiatry* 2009;**51**:327; FFT)
Bupropion (BNF, rare; cases e.g. n=1, *Ann Pharmacother* 2002;**36**:251–4; *J Clin*

Psychopharmacol 2009;**29**:616–8)
Bupropion abrupt discontinuation (n = 1, *Prog Neuropsychopharmacol Biol Psychiatry* 2007;**31**:766–8)
Duloxetine (n = 1, *Gen Hosp Psychiatry* 2010;**32**:646)
MAOIs, e.g.:
→ phenelzine (n = 1, *J Clin Psychopharmacol* 1990;**10**:144–5)
→ tranylcypromine (n = 1, *J Clin Psychopharmacol* 1989;**9**:229–30)
Mirtazapine (n = 1, *J Clin Psychiatry* 2002;**63**: 452–3; n = 1, *Tijdschr Psychiatr* 2006:**48**: 153–7; FFT)
SSRIs, e.g.:
→ citalopram (n = 9, *Global J Health Sci* 2014;**6**:295–9; FFT)
→ escitalopram (*Clin Neuropharmacol* 2007;**30**:124–6; n = 1, *Int Arch Allergy Immunol* 2006;**140**:27–9; n = 1, cervical, *Psychosomatics* 2015;**56**:572–5)
→ fluoxetine (e.g. n = 1, *Rev Neurol* 2004;**38**:99; FFT; n = 1, persistent, *Intern Med J* 2008;**38**:672–4)
→ fluvoxamine (*J Clin Psychopharmacol* 1993;**13**:220–1)
→ paroxetine (cases reviewed in *Curr Prob Pharmacovigilance* 1993;**19**:1; n = 1, *J Psychopharmacol* 2002;**16**:395–7)
→ paroxetine discontinuation (n = 1, *Rev Neurol* 2008;**46**:253–4; FFT)
→ sertraline (n = 1, *J Clin Psychopharmacol* 1999;**19**:98–100; mistaken for a panic attack, n = 1, *Psychiatr Serv* 2002;**53**: 1477–8)
Tricyclics, e.g.:
→ amitriptyline (*J Neurol Neurosurg Psychiatry* 1992;**55**:414; FFT)
→ amitriptyline (n = 1, *Am J Psychiatry* 1988;**145**:649)
→ clomipramine discontinuation (*Aust N Z J Psychiatry* 2001;**35**:696)
→ doxepin (n = 1, *Am J Psychiatry* 1988;**145**:649)
Venlafaxine (n = 1, *Mov Disord* 2010;**25**: 506–7)

• CNS — analgesics
Ergotamine (n=1, *Mov Disord* 1991;**6**:263–4; *Mov Disord* 1992;**7**:188–9)
Opioid withdrawal (n = 1, *Prog Neuropsychopharmacol Biol Psychiatry* 2011;**35**:640)
Sumatriptan (BNF, very rare; e.g. n = 1, *Ann Pharmacother* 1994;**28**:1199; n = 1, *Cephalagia* 1998;**18**:360–1)

• CNS — anticonvulsants
Carbamazepine (several, e.g. n = 1, *Gen Hosp Psychiatry* 2002;**24**:114–5; n = 1, OGC, *J Neurosurg* 2008;**109**:944–5)
Gabapentin (n = 1, *Ann Pharmacother* 2005;**39**:380–2; n = 1, possible case, *Br J Anaesth* 2007;**99**:218–20; FFT)
Midazolam (n = 1, *BMJ* 1990;**300**:614; FFT)
Phenobarbital (n = 1, *Clin Pediatr [Phila]* 1992;**31**:252)
Phenytoin (n = 1, *Dev Med Child Neurol* 1984;**26**:677–8)
Tiagabine (n = 3, *Epilepsia* 2001;**42**:944–6)

• CNS — movement disorders *
Benzatropine (n = 1, child, *Ann Emerg Med* 1986;**15**:594–6)
Bromocriptine (n = 5, *Neurology* 1993;**43**: 2319–22)
Entacapone (BNF, common)
Levodopa (BNF, common e.g. n = 1, *Parkinsonism Relat Disord* 2015;**21**:808)
Rotigotine (BNF, less common)
Tetrabenazine (n = 4, *Ann Neurol* 1985;**17**:200–2)
Tolcapone (BNF, common)
Trihexyphenidyl discontinuation (n = 1, *Mov Disord* 1989;**4**:349–53)

• CNS — others *
Amfetamine (risk factor with aripiprazole, *Prog Neuropsychopharmacol* 2008;**32**:1756–7)
Amfetamine + haloperidol (n = 2, *Br J Psychiatry* 1994;**165**:276)
Betahistine (n = 1, *Neurologia* 2000;**15**:417; n = 1, oromandibular dystonia after long-term use, *J Clin Neurosci* 2010;**17**:1330–1)
Cloperastine (a cough suppressant, *Dev Med Child Neurol* 2012;**54**:287)
Cocaine (including crack) in its own right or as a risk factor with dopamine-blocking drugs (n = 2, *Am J Emerg Med* 1997;**15**:513–5; n = 1, *South Med J* 1997;**90**:1050–2; n = 29 over two years, *J Clin Psychiatry* 1998;**59**:128–30)
Cocaine withdrawal (n=1, *Neurology*

1989;**39**:996–7; *Neurology* 1990;**40**:863–4)
Cyclizine (e.g. n=1, *Anaesthesia* 2004;**59**:413–4; n=1, *Anaesthesia* 2003;**58**:257–60)
Disulfiram overdose (n=1, *Mov Disord* 1991;**6**:166–70)
Domperidone (n=2, *Mov Disord* 1991;**6**:79–81)
Donepezil (n=1, cervical, *Rinsho Shinkeigaku* 2010;**50**:147–50)
MDMA/ecstasy (*Mov Disord* 2004;**19**:1386–7; n=1, *Mov Disord* 1995;**10**:353)
Methamphetamine (n=1, *Psychiatry Clin Neurosci* 2007;**61**:691–4)
Methylphenidate (n=1, *J Child Neurol* 1994;**9**:45–6)
Metoclopramide (BNF, less common; n=2, *Tidsskr Nor Laegeforen* 2001;**121**:2162–3; incidence 3%, see *N Engl J Med* 1983;**309**:433–4; cases in, e.g. *Ann Intern Med* 1989;**149**:2486–92)
Ondansetron (n=1, *Ann Pharmacother* 2011;**45**:e7; n=1, *J Clin Anesth* 2015;**27**:423–5; OCG, n=1, *Eur J Anaesthesiol* 2014;**31**:712–3)
Phencyclidine (OCG, n=1, *Case Rep Emerg Med* 2015;**2015**:506301; FFT)
Prochlorperazine (e.g. controlled by hyoscine patch n=1, *J Emerg Med* 2006;**30**:299–302; n=1, *Ir J Med Sci* 2007;**176**:53–4)
Rivastigmine (n=1, *Am J Health Syst Pharm* 2007;**64**:2468–70)

- Gastrointestinal drugs

Cimetidine (e.g. n=1, *J Emerg Med* 2001;**21**:27–9)
Ranitidine (e.g. n=1, *J La State Med Soc* 1997;**149**:36–8; n=1, *Am J Emerg* 1999;**17**:258–60)

- Cardiovascular drugs

Flecainide (n=1, *Mov Disord* 1992;**7**:62–3)
Midodrine + perphenazine (n=1, *J Neurol* 2008;**255**:767–8)
Midodrine + risperidone (n=1, *J Neuropsychiatry Clin Neurosci* 2000;**12**:285–6)
Nifedipine (*Ann Intern Med* 1986;**104**:125)
Propranolol (n=1, *Arch Neurol* 2000;**57**:570–1)
Verapamil (n=1, *J Clin Pharmacy Ther* 1998;**23**:79–80)

- Respiratory drugs

Alimemazine
Cetirizine (n=1, *Neurology* 2006;**66**:143–4; n=1, *Pediatr Emerg Care* 2008;**24**:627–8)
Cinnarizine (n=101, *Mov Disord* 1989;**4**:139–46)
Dextromethorphan (n=1, *J Toxicol Clin Toxicol* 1996;**34**:351–2)
Diphenhydramine:
→ oral (e.g. *Ann Intern Med* 1989;**111**:92–3; n=1, *Pharmacotherapy* 1994;**14**:492–6)
→ IV (*Ann Intern Med* 1989;**111**:92–3)
Flunarizine (n=101, *Mov Disord* 1989;**4**:139–46)
Phenylpropanolamine (*Clin Pediatr (Phila)* 1997;**36**:57–8)
Promethazine (n=1, *Clin Pharm* 1984;**3**:83–5; n=1, *Pediatr Emerg Care* 1987;**3**:91–2)

- Anti-infection drugs

Chloroquine + metronidazole (n=1, *Drug Intell Clin Pharm* 1988;**22**:308–10)
Erythromycin (n=1, *Am J Emerg Med* 1992;**10**:616)
Foscarnet (n=1, *Am J Ther* 2008;**15**:184–6)
Gemifloxacin (n=1, *Indian J Med Sci* 2009;**63**:557–60; FFT)
Lamivudine (n=2, *Clin Neuropharmacol* 2005;**28**:193–4)
Quinine (*An Med Interna* 2003;**20**:650–1)
Spiramycin (n=1, *Can J Psychiatry* 1997;**42**:665–6)

- Malignancy and immunosuppressant drugs

Capecitabine (n=1, *Acta Oncol* 2008;**47**:1161–5)
Etoposide (n=1, *Drug Intell Clin Pharm* 1988;**22**:41–2)
Peginterferon alfa (*Mov Disord* 2007;**22**:747–8)

- Musculoskeletal and analgesics

Azapropazone (n=1, *J Neurol Neurosurg Psychiatry* 1988;**51**:731–2; FFT)
Indometacin (rare reports)
Penicillamine (review, *Arch Neurol* 1987;**44**:490–3)

- Others

Acetazolamide (n=1, *Eur J Neurol* 2000;**7**:237–40)
Alfentanil (n=1, *Anesth Analg* 1991;**72**:557–8)
Contrast Media (n=1, *J Emerg Med* 2001;**21**:415–7)
Copper (n=1, *Lancet* 1990;**335**:410)

Cyanide (n = 1, *J Neurol Neurosurg Psychiatry* 1992;**55**:198–9; FFT)

Insecticides (cholinesterase inhibitors, n = 1, *Drug Intell Clin Pharm* 1988;**22**:311–2)

Ketamine abuse (n=1, *Ann Emerg Med* 1982;**11**:673–5)

Permethrin (n = 1, *Pharmacotherapy* 2005;**25**:448–50)

Propofol (BNF, very rare; n = 45, *Anesth Analg* 2002;**94**:1237–40; n = 1, *Paediatr Anaesth* 2005;**15**:597–601; *Parkinsonism Relat Disord* 2012;**18**:115–6)

Propofol + fentanyl (n = 1, *Br J Anaesth* 2000;**84**:828–9)

Sevoflurane (*Anaesthesiology* 1999;**90**:1215–6)

5.8.4 DYSKINESIAS

If (tardive) dyskinesia (TD) is of late onset, it can be a potentially irreversible movement disorder with a possible relationship to drug, dose and duration (see 6.7).

Review: non-therapeutic risk factors (s=8, Tenback *et al*, *Mov Disord* 2009;**24**:2309–15).

- CNS — sleep disorders and anxiety

Buspirone (n = 1, *J Clin Psychopharmacol* 1988; **8**:296–7; n = 1, *J Clin Psychiatry* 1988;**49**:322–3; n = 2, *Mov Disord* 1993;**8**:331–4)

Midazolam (*Palliat Med* 2000;**14**:435–6)

- CNS — antipsychotics *

A longitudinal study showed that FGAs and SGAs give a broadly similar incidence of tardive dyskinesia (n=352, four years, Woods *et al*, *J Clin Psychiatry* 2010;**71**:463–74; FFT), and that despite the rise in the use of SGAs, the incidence of TD has not dropped as much as would have been expected (Tarsy *et al*, *Handb Clin Neurol* 2011;**100**:601–16).

Amisulpride (e.g. n = 1, *Prog Neuropsychopharmacol Biol Psychiatry* 2010;**34**:728–9; n = 1, *J Neuropsychiatry Clin Neurosci* 2009;**21**: 104–5)

Aripiprazole (n = 1, after 18/12 for refractory depression, *CNS Spect* 2006;**11**:435–9; n = 2, *Prog Neuropsychopharmacol Biol Psychiatry* 2009;**33**:743–4; n = 8, usually irreversible on discontinuation, *Mov Disord* 2011;**26**:147–52; n = 1, *Curr Drug Saf* 2015;in press)

Aripiprazole + tamoxifen (n = 1, *Am J Psychiatry* 2007;**164**:1436–7)

Clozapine (e.g. very low incidence, n = 101, *World J Biol Psychiatry* 2009;**10**:919–24; n = 3, *Eur Psychiatry* 2003;**18**:260–1; n = 1, after 10 years, *Am J Psychiatry* 2003;**160**:588)

Clozapine, abrupt discontinuation (n=4, *J Clin Psychiatry* 1998;**59**:472–7)

Flupentixol decanoate (*Psychopharmacology [Berl]* 1983;**81**:359–62)

Haloperidol (many cases)

Lithium (n = 130, incidence 9%, *J Clin Psychiatry* 1996;**57**:22–8; n = 1, *J Neurol Sci* 2000;**176**:78–9)

Lithium + carbamazepine (n = 1, *J Clin Psychopharmacol* 1994;**14**:146–7)

Lithium + neuroleptics (n = 1, persistent, *Pharmacopsychiatry* 1998;**31**:201–4)

Loxapine

Olanzapine (e.g. n = 1, *J Clin Psychiatry* 1999;**60**:870; *J Neuropsychiatry Clin Neurosci* 2006;**18**:132; n = 1, *Psychiatry Clin Neurosci* 2003;**57**;605–6)

Paliperidone ER (n = 1, *Gen Hosp Psychiatry* 2011;**34**:578.e5–6)

Paliperidone palmitate (n = 1, *Gen Hosp Psychiatry* 2013;**35**:213.e5–7)

Pimozide (incidence 35% reported, probably rarer)

Quetiapine (several e.g. n = 1, oropharyngeal and facial dyskinesia, *J Clin Psychopharmacol* 2008;**28**:705–6; n = 1, *World J Biol Psychiatry* 2009;**10**:54–7; n = 1, low-dose, *Mov Disorder* 2011;**26**:2297–8)

Risperidone (many cases, e.g. n = 1, *Ann Pharmacother* 2000;**34**:1487–8; although a lower incidence has been reported in the elderly with low-dose, n = 330, RCT, open, 12/52, *Am J Psychiatry* 2000;**157**:1150–5)

Risperidone/citalopram abrupt discontinuation (n = 1, *Ann Pharmacother* 2000;**34**:269)

Sulpiride (*Clin Neuropharmacol* 1990;**13**:248–52)

Ziprasidone (e.g. n = 1, *Natl Med J India* 2007;**20**: 271–2; n = 1, *Am J Psychiatry* 2004;**161**:175–6; *Can J Psychiatry* 2005;**50**:567–8)

- CNS — antidepressants

Bupropion (n=1, *J Clin Psychiatry* 1997;**58**:218)

Duloxetine (n = 1, *Pharmacopsychiatry* 2006; **39**:237–8; n = 1, *Gen Hosp Psychiatry*

5

2010;**32**:646; n=1, *J Clin Psychopharmacol* 2012;**32**:723–4)
Mirtazapine (n=1, *Mov Disord* 2005;**20**:771; n=1, *Neurol India* 2010;**58**:672–3; FFT)
SSRIs:
→ citalopram (n=1, *J Clin Psychiatry* 2007;**68**:803; n=1, *PM R* 2010;**2**:973–5)
→ escitalopram + itopride (n=1, *Prog Neuropsychopharmacol Biol Psychiatry* 2009;**33**:380–1)
→ fluoxetine (e.g. n=5,555, incidence 0.2%, *Am J Psychiatry* 1991;**148**:1403; n=3, *Psychiatr Serv* 1996;**47**:991–3)
→ fluoxetine + low dose haloperidol (n=1, *Am J Psychiatry* 1991;**148**:683)
→ fluvoxamine (n=1, *J Clin Psychopharmacol* 1993;**13**:365–6)
→ paroxetine (*J Clin Psychopharmacol* 1996;**16**:258–9)
→ paroxetine + sumatriptan (n=1, persistent, *Biol Psychiatry* 1997;**42**:144–6)
→ sertraline (n=1, *J Clin Psychopharmacol* 1997;**17**:138–9)
Tricyclics, e.g.:
→ clomipramine (n=9, *Am J Psychiatry* 1993;**150**:165–6)
→ doxepin (n=50, 10% incidence in study in *J Clin Psychopharmacol* 1987;**7**:243–6)
Venlafaxine

• CNS — analgesics
Fentanyl (*Mov Disorder* 1995;**10**:679–80)

• CNS — anticonvulsants
Review: Zaatreh, *Expert Opin Drug Saf* 2003;**2**:385–93.
Carbamazepine (n=2, *Cleve Clin J Med* 1990;**57**:367–72)
Gabapentin (n=1, *J Clin Psychopharmacol* 2001;**21**:623–4; n=1, *Mov Disorder* 2007;**22**:288–9)
Lamotrigine (n=1, *Eur J Neurol* 2010;**17**:e37)
Lamotrigine overdose (n=1, *J Child Neurol* 2008;**23**:243)
Midazolam (*Palliat Med* 2000;**14**:435–6)
Oxcarbazepine (n=1, *J Pediatr Neurosci* 2010;**5**:85–6; FFT)
Phenytoin (n=1, *Arq Neuropsiquiatr* 1999;**57**:356–60; *Indian Pediatr* 1998;**35**:274–6; n=1, *Neurologia* 2013;**28**:193–4; FFT)

• CNS – movement disorders
Apomorphine abuse (n=1, *Mov Disord* 2005;**20**:105–8)
Benzatropine (n=10, 14/52, study showed worsening TD; *Neuropsychobiology* 1980;**6**:109–20)
Bromocriptine (n=1, low-dose, *Acta Med Port* 1992;**5**:347; FFT)
Levodopa (common)
Trihexyphenidyl (n=1, *Mov Disord* 1993;**8**:512–4)

• CNS — others *
Atomoxetine (n=2, with other drugs, *Clin Toxicol [Phila]* 2007;**45**:182–5)
Cannabis (n=51, *Schizophr Res* 1993;**11**:3–8)
Cocaine (recent use is a risk factor for antipsychotic-induced, n=106, *Psychopharmacol Bull* 2008;**41**:5–10; n=1, *Neurology* 2001;**56**:964–5)
Domperidone (n=1, *Ann Pharmacother* 2011;**45**:e51)
Donepezil (*Ann Pharmacother* 2000;**34**:1347)
Diphenhydramine (n=1, *Can J Psychiatry* 1985;**30**:370–1)
Methylphenidate (n=1, *Prim Care Companion J Clin Psychiatry* 2002;**4**:158–9; FFT; n=1, seven-year-old boy, *Pediatr Neurol* 2007;**37**:287–8; n=1, short-lived in six-year-old boy, *J Child Adolesc Psychopharmacol* 2007;**17**:378–81)
Metoclopramide (BNF, FDA warning, directly related to total dose taken; <1% incidence, review, *Aliment Pharmacol Ther* 2010;**31**:11–9; n=1 after 2/7, *Int J Clin Pharm* 2012;**34**:822–4)
Norpseudoephedrine (n=2, *J Neurol* 1994;**241**:167–9)
Prochlorperazine long-term (n=1, *South Med J* 1996;**89**:989–91)
Varenicline discontinuation (n=2, *Open Neurol J* 2015;**9**:7–8; FFT)

• Gastrointestinal drugs
Tiemonium (n=1, *Fundam Clin Pharmacol* 2007;**21**:657–8)

• Respiratory drugs
Aminophylline (*Pediatr Neurol* 1992;**8**:157)

• Anti-infection drugs
Ciprofloxacin (n=1, *Hosp Med* 2000;**61**:142–3;

n = 1, *J Neurol* 1996;**243**:616–7)
Ofloxacin (n = 1, *Mov Disord* 2004;**19**:731–2)

- Musculoskeletal and analgesics

Baclofen (n = 1, *Arch Phys Med Rehabil* 1993;**74**:766–7)

- Others

Phenylalanine (exacerbates TD, n = 18, d/b, p/c, *Neuropsychopharmacology* 1997;**16**:136–46; FFT)
Propofol (*Anesth Analg* 1996;**83**:420–2)
Sildenafil (n = 1, with Parkinson's Disease, *Int J Clin Pharmacol Ther* 2010;**48**:76–8)

5.8.5 OTHER MOVEMENT DISORDERS

5.8.5.1 CATATONIA

Reviews: general (Duggal and Singh, *Drugs Today [Barc]* 2005;**41**:599–607), in young people (Cohen *et al*, *J Am Acad Child Adolesc Psychiatry* 1999;**38**:1040–6), antipsychotics (n = 127, Lee, *J Clin Psychopharmacol* 2010;**30**:3–10).

- CNS — general *

Alcohol withdrawal (n = 1, *Med Sci Monit* 2009;**15**:CS129–31; n = 1, *Psychopathology* 2011;**44**:136)
Amfetamine (pseudocatatonia, *Postgrad Med* 1977;**61**:275–7)
Aripiprazole (possible case, *J Clin Psychopharmacol* 2009;**29**:503–4)
Benzodiazepine withdrawal (n = 5, *J Clin Psychopharmacol* 1996;**16**:315–9; *Pharmacopsychiatry* 2001;**34**:41–2):
→ alprazolam (n = 1, *J Clin Psychopharmacol* 2015;**35**:735–6)
→ clonazepam (n = 1, *Psychosomatics* 2009;**50**:289–92)
→ lorazepam (n = 1, *Ann Clin Psychiatry* 2012;**24**:170–1)
→ temazepam (n = 1, *Aust N Z J Psychiatry* 2011;**45**:1006–7)
Bupropion (n = 1, *J Clin Psychiatry* 1992;**53**:210)
Cannabis withdrawal (n = 1, *Subst Abus* 2015; in press)
Clozapine (*Can J Psychiatry* 2001;**46**:458)
Clozapine discontinuation (e.g. abrupt, n = 1, *Psychosomatics* 2010;**51**:355; n = 1, *Aust N Z J Psychiatry* 2011;**45**:499; *Aust N Z J Psychiatry* 2009;**43**:283–4; n = 1, *Afr J Psychiatry [Johannesbg]* 2010;**13**:402–4; FFT)
Clozapine + lorazepam discontinuation (n = 1, *Aust N Z J Psychiatry* 2012;**46**:795–6)
Cocaine (n = 1, *Am J Psychiatry* 1998;**155**:1629)
Disulfiram (e.g. n = 1, dose dependent, *J Clin Pharmacol* 2011;**51**:285–6)
Donepezil (n = 1, *No To Shinkei* 2004;**56**:881–4)
Fluphenazine (n = 1, *Br J Psychiatry* 1973;**122**:240–1)
Gabapentin (n = 1, *Am J Ger Pharmacother* 2009;**7**:220–4)
Haloperidol IV (n = 2, *J Pharm Pract* 2012;**25**:250–4)
Hydroxyzine (n = 1, *No To Shinkei* 2005;**57**:45–9)
Levetiracetam (n = 1, *Epilepsy Behav* 2006;**8**:303–7)
Lithium (n = 1, *J Clin Psychopharmacol* 2007;**27**:410–2)
Loxapine (n = 1, *J Clin Psychiatry* 1983;**44**:310–2)
LSD (n = 1, *Aust N Z J Psychiatry* 1995;**29**:324–7)
MDMA/ecstasy (several e.g. n = 1, *J Am Acad Child Adolesc Psychiatry* 2002;**41**:892)
Methadone overdose (delayed, n = 1, *Neurotoxicology* 2010;**31**:762–4; n = 1, *Prim Care Companion J Clin Psychiatry* 2009;**11**:275–6; FFT)
Morphine epidural (n = 1, *Lancet* 1980;**2**:984; n = 1, *Acta Anaesthesiol Scand* 1981;**25**:445–6)
Paliperidone (n = 1, *West J Emerg Med* 2010;**11**:186–8; FFT)
Paliperidone palmitate (n = 1, *J Clin Psychopharmacol* 2012;**32**:284–5)
Phenelzine + haloperidol (n = 1, *Can J Psychiatry* 1988;**33**:633–4
Pipotiazine (n = 1, *Br J Psychiatry* 1988;**152**:865–6)
Prochlorperazine (n = 1, *Postgrad Med* 1976;**60**:171–3)
Risperidone (n = 1, *Acta Psychiatr Scand* 1999;**99**:223–6)
Tramadol + pethidine (n = 1, *J Formos Med Assoc* 2007;**106**:323–6)
Valproate + risperidone (n = 1, *Neuropsychiatry Neuropsychol Behav Neurol* 1998;**11**:157–63)
Zolpidem (n = 1, *Psychosomatics* 2011;**52**:475–7)
Zotepine (n = 1, *Pharmacotherapy* 2005;**25**:1156–9)

- Others *

Allopurinol (n = 1, *BMJ* 1991;**302**:970)
ART (zidovudine/abacavir/efavirenz; n = 1, *J Pediatr Neurosci* 2014;**9**:293–5; FFT)
Azithromycin (n = 1, *J Clin Psychiatry* 2006;**67**:492–3)
Baclofen (*J Clin Psychopharmacol* 1986;**6**:387–8; n=37, *Clin Neuropharmacol* 1992;**15**:56–62)
Cefoxitin (n = 1, *Psychosomatics* 2011;**52**:379–83)
Ciprofloxacin (n = 1, *Psychosomatics* 2011;**52**: 379–83; *J Clin Psychiatry* 1993;**54**:115–6)
Cycloserine
Dexamethasone (n = 1, *Afr J Psychiatry (Johannesbg)* 2011;**14**:316–8; FFT)
Efavirenz (*AIDS* 2002;**16**:1841–2)
Lead intoxication (n = 1, *Cases J* 2009;**2**:8722; FFT)
Manganese (n = 1, *Psychosomatics* 2011;**52**:74–7)
Omeprazole + disulfiram (n = 1, *CMAJ* 1990;**143**:1207–8)
Oral contraceptive (n = 1, *Mov Disord* 2009;**24**:2166–7)
Paracetamol overdose (n = 1, *Prim Care Companion J Clin Psychiatry* 2010;**12**:PCC.09100790)
Phenylpropanolamine overdose (n = 1, *J Clin Psychiatry* 1985;**46**:288–9)
Piperazine (mentioned in *Trans Roy Soc Trop Med Hyg* 1976;**70**:358)
Prednisone (n = 1, *J Geriatr Psychiatry Neurol* 1989;**2**:41–4)
Sibutramine (n = 1, *J Psychosom Res* 2008;**64**:107–9)
Steroids (n = 1, *Br J Psychiatry* 1991;**158**:125–7)

5.8.5.2 CATAPLEXY

Cataplexy is a rare transient sudden loss of muscle tone, often triggered by emotions.

Clomipramine discontinuation (n = 3, *Neurologia* 2002;**17**:113–6)
Clozapine (e.g. *J Neuropsychiatry Clin Neurosci* 2007;**19**:87–8)
Fluoxetine discontinuation (n = 1, *Neurology* 2005;**65**:967–8)
Prazosin (n = 1, *Sleep* 1989;**12**:254–6)
Venlafaxine discontinuation (n = 2, *J Sleep Res* 2005;**14**:207–8; FFT)

5.8.5.3 CHOREAS

- CNS — antipsychotics

Chlorpromazine (n = 1, *Postgrad Med J* 1970;**540**:633–4)
Haloperidol (many cases)
Lithium toxicity (e.g. n = 1, *Eur J Neurol* 2003;**10**:743–4; n = 1, *Seishin Shinkeigaku Zasshi* 2003;**105**:1206–12)
Quetiapine discontinuation (n = 1, *Rev Neurol* 2004;**38**;1094; FFT)
Sulpiride (n = 1, *J Psychopharmacol* 1993;**7**:290–2; n = 6, *Clin Neuropharmacol* 1990;**13**:248–52)

- CNS — antidepressants

Fluoxetine (n = 1, *J Clin Psychiatry* 1999;**60**:868–9; n = 1, *Neurology* 1996;**46**;853)
Mianserin (n = 1, *Br J Psychiatry* 1989;**154**:113–4)
Paroxetine (n = 1, after a single dose, *Br J Psychiatry* 1997;**170**:193–4)
Trazodone low dose (n = 1, *Eur Neurol* 2006;**55**: 101–2)

- CNS — anticonvulsants

Review: choreas and anticonvulsants; Zaatreh *et al*, *Seizure* 2001;**10**:596–9; FFT).
Carbamazepine (*J Neurol Neurosurg Psychiatry* 1982;**45**:560; FFT; overdose; n = 4, *Neurology* 1988;**38**;755–9)
Gabapentin (e.g. n = 1, *Clin Rheumatol* 2008;**27**:389–90; *Neurology* 1996;**46**:851–2)
Lamotrigine (n = 1, *J Child Neurol* 2003;**18**:479–80; *J Child Neurol* 2006;**21**:357–8)
Lamotrigine overdose (n = 1, *J Child Neurol* 2008;**23**:243)
Lamotrigine + phenytoin (n = 3, *Seizure* 2001;**10**:596–9; FFT)
Phenytoin (e.g. n = 3, *Neuropediatrics* 2001;**32**: 231–5; *Postgrad Med J* 1990;**66**:1089; FFT)
Valproate (n = 1, *Pediatr Neurol* 2006;**35**:356–8; n = 3, *Arch Neurol* 1994;**51**:702–4; n = 1, *Seizure* 2002;**11**:205–6; n = 1, *Acta Neurol Belg* 2011;**111**:220–1)

- CNS — movement disorders

Anticholinergics (n = 1, *Med J Aust* 1979;**1**:465):
→ trihexyphenidyl (n = 1, *Nippon Ronen Igakkai Zasshi* 1992;**29**:686–9; FFT)
Levodopa (BNF)

- CNS — others *

Amfetamines (review, *Emerg Med Australas* 2005;**17**:277–80; n = 1, *Mov Disord* 2004;**19**;840–2)

Cocaine (cases in *Am J Emerg Med* 1991;**9**:618–20; including crack; *Med Clin [Barc]* 2006;**126**:555; n=9, *Biol Psychiatry* 1999;**45**:1630–5)
Donepezil (n=1, *Ann Pharmacother* 2000;**34**:1347; *J Neurol* 2007;**254**:1752–3)
Methadone (e.g. n=1, *J Pain Symptom Manage* 2003;**26**:688–91; n=1, *Clin J Pain* 2001;**17**:375–7)
Methamphetamine (*Ann Intern Med* 1994;**121**:986)
Methylphenidate (e.g. n=1, *J Neuropsychiatry Clin Neurosci* 2010;**22**:352)
Modafinil + tranylcypromine (n=1, *Am J Psychiatry* 2007;**164**:684)
Rivastigmine dose increase (n=1, *Medicine (Baltimore)* 2015;**94**:e1364; FFT)

- Gastrointestinal drugs

H2-blockers, e.g.:
→ cimetidine (n=1, *Ann Intern Med* 1982;**96**:126)
→ ranitidine (n=1, *Lancet* 1988;**2**:158)
Metoclopramide (n=1, *Am J Ther* 2006;**13**:543–4; *South Med J* 1986;**79**:1465)
Sulfasalazine (n=1, *Br Med J* 1991;**302**:1025; FFT)

- Anti-infection drugs

Azithromycin (n=1, *Pediatr Neurol* 2011;**44**:311–3)
Ciprofloxacin? (*Mov Disord* 2005;**20**:513–4)
Trimethoprim + sulfamethoxazole (n=1, *Paediatr Infect Dis J* 2005;**24**:934–5)
Valacyclovir + famciclovir (n=1, *South Med J* 2001;**94**:655)

- Others

Baclofen (n=1, *Mov Disord* 2010;**25**:959–60; *Ann Neurol* 1990;**28**:839)
Ciclosporin (n=1, *Ann Neurol* 1993;**33**:108–9)
Cyclizine (n=1, *J Neurol Sci* 1977;**31**:237–44)
Cyproheptadine (n=1, *Mov Disord* 1989;**4**:81–4)
Dienoestrol/dienestrol
Digoxin toxicity (n=1, *J Neurol Neurosurg Psychiatry* 1984;**47**:419; FFT; n=1, *Mov Disord* 1999;**14**:877–9)
Diphenhydramine (n=2, *Chudoku Kenkyu* 2007;**20**:125–9)
Estrogens:
→ conjugated (n=1, *BMJ* 1991;**302**:762; FFT)
→ topical vaginal cream (n=1, *Mov Disord* 1991;**6**:355–7)
Interferons:
→ interferon alfa (*Neurology* 2002;**58**:328–30; n=1, *Nippon Naika Gakkai Zasshi* 1997;**86**:1036–8)
Levofloxacin (n=1, *Nippon Ronen Igakkai Zasshi* 1999;**36**:213–7; FFT)
Luteinizing hormone–releasing hormone analog (n=1, *J Neurol* 2008;**255**:1264–5)
Oral contraceptives (BNF, rare; n=1, *J Neurol Neurosurg Psychiatry* 2004;**75**:327–8; n=2, *Rev Med Chil* 1999;**127**:468–71)
Oxymetholone (n=1, *Br Med J (Clin Res Ed)* 1981;**283**:349–50; FFT)
Propofol (n=1, *Anesth Analg* 1996;**82**:670)
Sildenafil (n=1, with Parkinson's Disease, *Int J Clin Pharmacol Ther* 2010;**48**:76–8)
Trimetazidine (*Rev Med Intern* 2008;**29**:512–5)

5.8.5.4 *RABBIT SYNDROME*

Rabbit syndrome is a distinct neuroleptic-induced EPSE, with fine, rapid, rhythmic movements of the mouth.

- CNS — antipsychotics

Reviews: Schwartz and Hocherman, *CNS Drugs* 2004;**18**:213–20; *Clin Pract Epidemiol Ment Health* 2007;**3**:6; FFT.
Amisulpride (n=1, *J Neuropsychiatry Clin Neurosci* 2010;**22**:352)
Aripiprazole (n=1, *J Psychopharmacol* 2010;**24**:429–31; n=1, *Schizophr Res* 2008;**103**:341–2; n=1, *Aust N Z J Psychiatry* 2004;**38**:561)
Chlorpromazine (n=2, *Clin Pract Epidemiol Ment Health* 2007;**3**:6; FFT)
Clozapine (n=1, *J Clin Psychiatry* 2003;**64**:219)
Fluphenazine (n=3; *Clin Pract Epidemiol Ment Health* 2007;**3**:6; FFT)
Haloperidol (n=1, *Indian J Psychiatry* 2001;**43**:279–80; FFT; n=12, *Clin Pract Epidemiol Ment Health* 2007;**3**:6; FFT)
Methotrimeprazine (n=1, *Clin Pract Epidemiol Ment Health* 2007;**3**:6; FFT)
Olanzapine (n=1, *Br J Psychiatry* 2000;**176**:193; FFT; *South Med J* 2008;**101**:1069–70; n=1, *Psychiatr Prax* 2005;**32**:202–4; n=1, *Clin Pract Epidemiol Ment Health* 2007;**3**:6; FFT)
Paliperidone (n=1, *J Clin Psychopharmacol* 2011;**31**:379–80)
Paliperidone discontinuation (n=1, *J Clin*

5

Psychopharmacol 2012;**32**:720–1)
Perphenazine (n = 1, *Clin Pract Epidemiol Ment Health* 2007;**3**:6; FFT)
Quetiapine (n = 1, *Prog Neuropsychopharmacol Biol Psychiatry* 2008;**32**:2002–3)
Risperidone (n = 8, *Clin Pract Epidemiol Ment Health* 2007;**3**:6; FFT; n = 1, *Pharmacotherapy* 2002;**22**:513–5; n = 1, *Eur Neuropsychopharmacol* 1999;**9**:137–9)
Risperidone discontinuation (n = 1, *Eur Neuropsychopharmacol* 2001;**11**:323–4)
Risperidone + lithium (n = 1, *Can J Psychiatry* 2005;**50**:369)
Sulpiride (n = 1, *Rinsho Shinkeigaku* 1982;**22**: 557–62)
Sulpiride (n = 4, *Clin Pract Epidemiol Ment Health* 2007;**3**:6; FFT)
Thioridazine (n = 3, *Clin Pract Epidemiol Ment Health* 2007;**3**:6; FFT)
Trifluoperazine (n = 3, *Clin Pract Epidemiol Ment Health* 2007;**3**:6; FFT)
Zuclopenthixol (n = 1, *Clin Pract Epidemiol Ment Health* 2007;**3**:6; FFT)
Zuclopenthixol decanoate (n = 1, *Br J Psychiatry* 2000;**176**:193; FFT)

- CNS — others

Citalopram (n = 1, *Clin Neuropharmacol* 2005;**28**:289–91)
Imipramine (n = 1, *J Psychiatry Neurosci* 1991; **16**.227–9, FFT)
Methylphenidate (n = 1, *Ann Pharmacother* 2006;**40**:2076)
Paroxetine + perphenazine + amitriptyline (n = 1, *Clin Neuropharmacol* 2004:**27**:299–300)

- Others

Phenol (n = 1, *J Toxicol Clin Toxicol* 1999;**37**: 509–11)

5.8.5.5 TICS (including exacerbation of Tourette's syndrome)

- CNS — general *

Amisulpride (n = 1, *Clin Neuropharmacol* 2006;**29**:163–4)
Aripiprazole + pimozide (n = 1, *J Clin Psychopharmacol* 2015;**35**:350–1)
Atomoxetine (many, e.g. n = 1, *CNS Spectr* 2008;**13**:301–3; n = 2, *Int J Psychiatry Med* 2007;**37**:415–24)
Atomoxetine + venlafaxine (n = 1, *Clin Toxicol [Phila]* 2007;**45**:182–5)
Bupropion (n = 1, *Clin Neuropharmacol* 2014;**37**:192–3)
Caffeine (n = 2, *Pediatrics* 1998;**101**:E4)
Carbamazepine (e.g. n = 1, *Epileptic Disord* 2000; **2**:39–40; n = 3, *Epilepsia* 1993;**34**:965–8)
Clozapine (e.g. n = 1, *Aust N Z J Psychiatry* 2005;**39**:202; n = 1, exacerbation, *Aust N Z J Psychiatry* 2008;**42**:1068–70)
Cocaine (several e.g. *N Engl J Med* 1986;**315**:398; n = 1, *Am J Psychiatry* 1996;**153**:965)
Escitalopram (n = 1, *Int Clin Psychopharmacol* 2005;**20**:177–8)
Fluoxetine (e.g. n = 1, Tourette's, *Am J Psychiatry* 1994;**151**:946–7; n = 1, child, *Turk Psikiyatri Derg* 2011;**22**:61–2)
Haloperidol (n = 2, tics, *Am J Psychiatry* 1986;**143**:1176–7)
Lamotrigine (several e.g. n = 5, *Epilepsia* 2000;**41**:862–7; n = 1, vocal and motor tics, *Am J Psychiatry* 2006;**163**:159; n = 1, *Curr Drug Saf* 2015; in press)
Quetiapine (n = 1, *J Clin Psychiatry* 2002;**63**:1184–5)
Risperidone discontinuation (n = 1, *J Am Acad Child Adolesc Psychiatry* 1997;**36**:162–3)
Sertraline (e.g. n = 1, *Int Clin Psychopharmacol* 2005;**20**:177–8; n = 1, *Pharmacopsychiatry* 2007,**40**.289–90)
Stimulants (frequent cause, especially in children treated for ADHD, incidence may be about 8% with methylphenidate, 6% with dexamfetamine; n = 555, chart review, Varley *et al, Compr Psychiatry* 2001;**42**:228–33):
→amfetamines (e.g. n = 1, *Mov Disord* 2004;**19**:840–2)
→methylphenidate
Sulpiride (review of n = 17, *Seishin Shinkeigaku Zasshi* 2006;**108**:459–65)
Tramadol abuse (n = 1, *J Clin Psychopharmacol* 2010;**30**:647–8)
Ziprasidone (n = 1, vocal, *J Clin Psychopharmacol* 2009;**29**:611–2)

- Others

Anabolic steroids (e.g. methandrostenolone, testosterone; *N Engl J Med* 1990;**322**:1674)
Clonidine (e.g. n = 1, *J Child Neurol* 2001;**16**: 380–1)

Human growth hormone (n = 1, *Eur Neurol* 2007;**57**:116–7)
Mercury poisoning (n = 1, *Arch Dis Child* 2000;**83**:174–5; FFT)
Ofloxacin (n = 1, *Ann Pharmacother* 1996;**30**:138–41)
Sibutramine (BNF, may exacerbate)
Prednisolone (n = 2, *Nervenarzt* 1998;**69**: 1111–4)

5.9 NEUROLEPTIC MALIGNANT SYNDROME

NMS is mostly related to the use of therapeutic or high doses of neuroleptics, particularly phenothiazines and higher potency drugs. It frequently occurs within 4–11 days of initiation, or alteration of dosages of neuroleptic therapy. See *6.8*.
Reviews: comparison of FGAs and SGAs causing NMS (Trollor *et al, Br J Psychiatry* 2012;**201**:52–6; FFT; Moscovich *et al, Arq Neuropsiquiatr* 2011;**69**; 751–5; FFT; over 11 years, Nielsen *et al, Can J Psychiatry* 2012;**57**:512–8).

- CNS — antipsychotics (including combinations with antipsychotics) *

Be aware that NMS with SGAs might actually be serotonin toxicity via 5HT1A partial agonism (Odagaki, *Curr Drug Saf* 2009;**4**:84–93).

Amisulpride (n = 1, *Clin Neuropharmacol* 2007;**30**:245–6; n = 1, *J Neuropsychiatry Clin Neurosci* 2007;**19**:488–9; n = 1, *Chang Gung Med J* 2011;**34**:536–40; FFT)
Amisulpride + oxcarbazepine (n = 1, *Gen Hosp Psychiatry* 2008;**30**:482–4)
Amisulpride discontinuation (n = 1, Ball *et al, Med Sci Law* 2009;**49**:298–300)
Aripiprazole (e.g. n = 1 without fever, *J Okla State Med Assoc* 2006;**99**:435–8; low dose, *J Psychiatr Pract* 2007;**13**:117–9; n = 1, *Mov Disord* 2010;**25**:2475–6; n = 1 in clozapine-intolerant patient, *Am J Health Syst Pharm* 2010;**67**:1254–9)
Aripiprazole + clozapine (n = 1, *Prog Neuropsychopharmacol Biol Psychiatry* 2010;**34**:427–8)
Aripiprazole + fluoxetine (n = 1, possible, *Am J Psychiatry* 2005;**162**:397–8)
Aripiprazole + lithium (n = 1, *J Clin Psychopharmacol* 2006;**26**:434–6)
Asenapine (n = 1, *Prim Care Companion J Clin Psychiatry* 2010;**12**:10l00966; FFT; n = 1, *J Neuropsychiatry Clin Neurosci* 2014;**26**:E36)
Bromperidol + donepezil (n = 1, *Nippon Ronen Igakkai Zasshi* 2001;**38**:822–4; FFT)
Chlorpromazine (e.g. n = 2, *Biol Psychiatry* 1983;**18**:1441–6; n = 1, *Trop Doct* 1992;**22**:92–3)
Clozapine (rare, but cases exist, e.g. long-term after 30 years uneventful treatment; n = 1, *Anasthesiol Intensivmed Notfallmed Schmerzther* 2006;**41**:125–7; after 10 years, n = 1, *Crit Care Resusc* 2007;**9**:338–40; n = 1, *J Child Adolesc Psychopharmacol* 2012:**22**:322–4)
Clozapine + aripiprazole (n = 2, *Int J Psychiatry Med* 2015;**49**:35–43)
Clozapine + paroxetine (n = 1, *Aging Clin Exp Res* 2006;**18**:266–70)
Clozapine + risperidone (n = 1, *Prog Neuropsychopharmacol Biol Psychiatry* 2002;**26**:407–9)
Clozapine + venlafaxine (n = 1, *Can J Psychiatry* 2004;**49**:497–8)
Flupentixol (SmPC, n = 1, possible case, *Br J Psychiatry* 1988;**152**:558–9)
Fluphenazine (reviewed in *Compr Psychiatry* 1985;**26**:63–70)
Fluphenazine decanoate (n = 1, *Ann Pharmacother* 2005;**39**:1131–5)
Haloperidol (many cases, e.g. in pregnancy, n = 1, *Obstet Gynecol* 2001;**98**:906–8; following clozapine discontinuation, n = 1, *Aust N Z J Psychiatry* 2005;**39**:947–8)
Haloperidol decanoate (n = 1, prolonged, *Acta Med Port* 2010;**23**:1155–9; FFT)
Haloperidol + lithium (n = 1, *Shanghai Arch Psychiatry* 2014;**26**:368–70; FFT)
Haloperidol + olanzapine (n = 1, *Am J Psychiatry* 2001;**158**:650–1)
Levomepromazine discontinuation (n = 1, *J Neuropsychiatry Clin Neurosci* 2010;**22**:E16)
Lithium (possible cases in *J Clin Psychopharmacol* 1987;**7**:339–41)
Lithium + amitriptyline (n = 1, *J Psychiatry Neurosci* 1995;**20**:305–6; FFT)
Lithium + risperidone (possible case in *Am J Psychiatry* 1995;**152**:1096)
Lithium + ziprasidone (n = 1, *Ann Pharmacother* 2006;**40**:139–42)
Loxapine (n = 1, *Br J Psychiatry* 1991;**159**:572–3)
Olanzapine (many e.g. atypical syndrome,

5

n = 1, *Pharmacotherapy* 2002;**22**:641–4; n = 1, with severe hypernatraemia, *Hum Psychopharmacol* 2001;**16**:279–81; n = 1, atypical with normal CK, *Acta Psychiatr Scand* 2005;**112**:238–40; n = 1, after one missed dose due to lung surgery, *Int J Clin Exp Med* 2015;**8**:11639–41; FFT; n = 1, stable, long-term, *Brain Inj* 2015;**29**:658–60)

Olanzapine + chlorpromazine overdose (n = 1, *J Med Toxicol* 2009;**5**:27–31; FFT)

Olanzapine + donepezil (n = 1, *Nat Clin Pract Neurol* 2008;**4**:170–4)

Olanzapine + fluphenazine (n = 1, *J Clin Psychopharmacol* 2003;**23**:672–4)

Olanzapine + levomepromazine (n = 1, *Acta Psychiatr Scand* 2000;**102**:231–3)

Olanzapine + lithium (n = 1, *Pharmacotherapy* 2003;**23**:255–9)

Olanzapine + paroxetine (n = 1, *J Clin Psychopharmacol* 2003;**23**:671–2)

Olanzapine + rivastigmine (n = 1, *Pharmacotherapy* 2008;**28**:403–5)

Paliperidone (many, e.g. n = 1, *J Clin Psychopharmacol* 2010;**30**:89–91; atypical, n = 1, *Prog Neuropsychopharmacol Biol Psychiatry* 2011;**35**:650–1; n = 1, *J Neuropsychiatry Clin Neurosci* 2011;**23**:E14–5)

Penfluridol + sulpiride (n = 1, *Acta Psychiatr Scand* 1987;**75**:335–6)

Perphenazine (e.g. n = 1, *Otolaryngol Head Neck Surg* 1992;**106**:206–8)

Promazine

Quetiapine (atypical n = 1, *J Clin Psychopharmacol* 2009;**29**:497–9; n = 1 after no dose changes and review of n = 13, *Ann Pharmacother* 2009;**43**:785–91; n = 1, in XYY syndrome, *Am J Health Syst Pharm* 2010;**67**:459–61; n = 1, fatal, *Am J Ther* 2015; in press)

Quetiapine + clarithromycin (n = 1, *Clin Neuropharmacol* 2015;**38**:36–7)

Quetiapine + fluvoxamine (n = 1, *Am J Psychiatry* 2005;**162**:812)

Risperidone (many cases, e.g. n = 1, *J Child Adolesc Psychopharmacol* 2005;**15**:844–5; n = 1, *J Natl Med Assoc* 2009;**101**:273–5; n = 1, misdiagnosed as status epilepticus, *Pediatr Rep* 2011;**3**:e19; FFT)

Risperidone + haloperidol (during switch, n = 1, *Ann Pharmacother* 2001;**35**:698–701)

Risperidone + lamotrigine (n = 1, *J Neuropsychiatry Clin Neurosci* 2012;**24**:E38–9)

Risperidone + lithium (*J Clin Psychopharmacol* 2003;**23**:315–7; n = 1, *J Clin Psychiatry* 2004;**65**:724)

Risperidone to paliperidone switch (n = 1, *J Neuropsychiatry Clin Neurosci* 2011;**23**:E16–7)

Risperidone + ritonavir/indinavir (n = 1, *Psychosomatics* 2000;**41**:453–4)

Trifluoperazine + venlafaxine (n = 1, *Lancet* 2000;**355**:289–90)

Ziprasidone (*J Clin Psychopharmacol* 2002;**22**:624–6; n = 1, adolescent, *Clin Ther* 2004;**26**:1105–8; n = 1, on second day, *World J Biol Psychiatry* 2007;**8**:42–4)

Zotepine + valproate + benzodiazepine (n = 2, *Psychiatr Clin Neurosci* 2003;**57**:369–71)

Zuclopenthixol (n = 1, *Br J Psychiatry* 1989;**154**:562–3)

- **CNS — antidepressants**

Amoxapine + lithium (n = 1, *Ann Clin Psychiatry* 2000;**12**:107–9)

SSRIs:

→ citalopram overdose (n = 1, *Can J Psychiatry* 2000;**45**:941–2)

→ fluoxetine monotherapy (n = 1, *Biol Psychiatry* 1990;**28**:518–21)

→ paroxetine monotherapy (n = 1, *Rinsho Shinkeigaku* 2006;**46**:575–8; n = 1, *Seishin Shinkeigaku Zasshi* 2004;**106**:723–6)

→ paroxetine + promethazine (n = 1, *Nervenartz* 1997;**68**:664–6)

→ paroxetine + alprazolam (n = 1, Naranjo = 6, *Prog Neuropsychopharmacol Biol Psychiatry* 2006;**30**:1176–8)

→ sertraline discontinuation (n = 1, *J Clin Psychopharmacol* 2009;**29**:300–1)

Tricyclics:

→ clomipramine (n = 1, *BMJ* 2004;**329**:1333–5; FFT)

→ desipramine (n = 1, *Neurology* 1990;**40**:1797–8)

→ imipramine discontinuation (n = 1, *J Clin Psychopharmacol* 1987;**7**:53–4)

→ nortriptyline (n = 1, *Am J Emerg Med* 1999;**17**:736–7)

→ trimipramine (n = 1, *J Clin Psychiatry* 1989;**50**:144–5)

Venlafaxine (n = 1, *J Formos Med Assoc* 2006;**105**:90–3; n = 1, *Lancet* 2000;**355**:2164–5)

- CNS — anticonvulsants

Carbamazepine (may also complicate symptoms, n= 1, *Br J Psychiatry* 1994;**164**:269–70; n= 1, *South Med J* 1991;**84**:1378–80)
Carbamazepine discontinuation (n= 1, *Am J Psychiatry* 1990;**147**:1687)
Phenytoin toxicity (n=1, *S Afr Med J* 1988;**73**:620–1)
Tiapride (n= 1, *Clin Neuropharmacol* 1996;**19**: 539–40; n= 1, *Rev Rhum Ed Fr* 1994;**61**:362)
Zonisamide + carbamazepine (n= 1, *Epilepsia* 2007;**48**:1999–2001)

- CNS — movement disorders

Amantadine (SmPC)
Amantadine discontinuation (e.g. n= 1, *Am J Psychiatry* 1994;**151**:451–2; n= 1, *Eur J Pediatr* 2001;**160**:401)
Anticholinergic discontinuation (n= 1, *Int Clin Psychopharmacol* 1996;**11**:207–9; n= 1, abrupt, *Asian J Psychiatr* 2014;**12**:158–9)
Bromocriptine to pergolide (rapid switch, n= 1, *Parkinsonism Relat Disord* 2002;**9**:115–6)
Fava bean abrupt discontinuation (n= 1, *Mov Disord* 2005;**20**:630–1; NB Fava beans contain appreciable amounts of levodopa)
Levodopa (n= 1, *Intern Med* 1992;**31**:1298–302; FFT)
Levodopa discontinuation (several e.g. n= 1, *Med J Aust* 1991;**155**:53–4; n= 1, *J Clin Anesth* 1995;**7**:652–6)
Levodopa/bromocriptine discontinuation (n= 1, *Singapore Med J* 2001;**42**:85–8)
Tetrabenazine long-term (n= 1, *Mov Disord* 1997;**12**:246–8; *Mov Disord* 1996;**11**:95)
Tolcapone discontinuation (n= 1, *Am J Med* 2000;**108**:517–8)

- CNS — others *

Anticholinesterases, e.g.:
- → donepezil (n= 1, *Int J Neuropsychopharmacol* 2004;**7**:101–3)
- → donepezil + maprotiline (n= 1, *Neurology* 2003;**60**:1050–1)

Cocaine (e.g. n= 1, *Tijdschr Psychiatr* 2006;**48**;399–404; FFT)
Cocaine + amfetamine overdose (fatal, n= 1, *Med Clin (Barc)* 1996;**106**:717–8)
Domperidone (n= 1, *Dig Dis Sci* 1992;**37**:946–8)
Hyoscine + antipsychotic (n= 1, *Psychiatr Danub* 2011;**23**[Suppl 1]:S43–5)
LSD (n= 1, fatal, *J Neurol Neurosurg Psychiatry* 1991;**54**:741–3; FFT)
LSD + alcohol (n= 1, *Br J Addict* 1990;**85**: 150–1)
Methylphenidate (n= 1, *Pediatr Neurol* 1998;**19**:299–301; n= 1, *Prim Care Companion J Clin Psychiatry* 2006;**8**:47; FFT)
Metoclopramide (e.g. *Ann Pharmacother* 1999;**33**:644–5; n= 1, *J Burn Care Res* 2006;**27**:237–41; n =1, child, *Turk J Pediatr* 2014;**56**:535–7; FFT)
Metoclopramide discontinuation (n= 1, *Aust N Z J Med* 1995;**25**:261)
Prochlorperazine (n= 1, *J Emerg Med* 1996;**14**:727–9; n= 1, *Ann Pharmacother* 2011;**45**:e61)

- Others

Alimemazine (n= 1, *Eur J Pediatr* 2002;**161**: 259–61)
Baclofen abrupt discontinuation (n= 1, *J Psychopharmacol* 2001;**15**:61–3; n= 1, *Med Clin (Barc)* 2006;**127**:79)
Diphenhydramine (n= 1, *Vet Hum Toxicol* 1988;**30**:58–9)
Diphenhydramine + diprophyllin overdose (n= 1, *J Neurol Sci* 1999;**162**:108–9)
Iron (low levels? *Lancet* 1987;**i**:1234–6)
Oral contraceptives (n= 1, *DICP* 1989;**23**:811 0)
Organophosphate poisoning (n= 1, *Can J Anesth* 1995;**42**:1027–30)
Promethazine (n= 1, *Aust N Z J Psychiatry* 2005;**39**:113–4)
Promethazine + lorazepam (n= 1, *Aust N Z J Psychiatry* 2001;**35**:250–1)
Rifampicin + chlorpromazine (n= 1, *J Korean Med Sci* 2008;**23**:734–6; FFT)
Simvastatin (complicated case, n= 1, *Clin Neuropharmacol* 2009;**32**:348–9)
Water, compulsive drinking (*Med J Aust* 1989;**150**:457–8)

5.10 OBSESSIVE-COMPULSIVE SYMPTOMS

- CNS — sleep disorders and anxiety

Benzodiazepine discontinuation (n= 1, *Br J Psychiatry* 1987;**150**:272; n= 1, *J Nerv Ment Dis* 1988;**176**:688–91)
Modafinil (n=2, exacerbation of symptoms, *Prim Care Companion J Clin Psychiatry* 2008;**10**:164–5; FFT)

5

- CNS — antipsychotics *

Antipsychotic-associated OCB or OCD may be related to antiserotonergic effects with e.g. clozapine and olanzapine (n=70, Schirmbeck et al, *Psychol Med* 2011;**41**:2361–73).

Reviews: antipsychotics (esp. clozapine and olanzapine, n=100, *Psychol Med* 2011;**41**:2361–73; review *Prog Neuropsychopharmacol Biol Psychiatry* 2012;**39**:75–9), FGA-induced OCD (*Prog Neuropsychopharmacol Biol Psychiatry* 2003: **27**;333–46). There is a 3% incidence with clozapine, olanzapine and risperidone in Asians (Mahendran et al, *J Clin Psychiatry* 2007;**68**:542–5).

Clozapine (e.g. n=40, 20% incidence, *Compr Psychiatry* 2009;**50**:437–42; n=59 on clozapine, 24% had OCD; *J Psychopharmacol* 2009;**23**:6–13; although clozapine might be of some use for OCD symptoms in people with schizophrenia; n=15, *Pharmacopsychiatry* 2004:**37**:52–6; n=7, *Clin Neuropharmacol* 2009;**32**:227–9)

Haloperidol (10% incidence, n=20, *Compr Psychiatry* 2009;**50**:437–42; n=1, *BMJ Case Rep* 2012;**2012**:bcr1120115161; FFT)

Olanzapine (e.g. severity associated with duration of treatment: n=113, *J Clin Psychiatry* 2002;**63**:104–7; review, n=9, *Int J Neuropsychopharmacol* 2004;**7**:375–7)

Paliperidone (n=1, *J Neuropsychiatry Clin Neurosci* 2011;**23**:E46)

Paliperidone LAI (n=1, *Ann Clin Psychiatry* 2014;**26**:301–2)

Quetiapine (a few cases e.g. n=1, *Aust N Z J Psychiatry* 2009;**43**:1185; n=5, *J Clin Psychopharmacol* 2006;**26**:396–400)

Risperidone (e.g. dose dependent case, *Aust N Z J Psychiatry* 1998;**32**:299–301; n=2, children, *J Child Adolesc Psychopharmacol* 2003;**13**[Suppl 1]:S89–92)

- CNS — antidepressants

Fluoxetine (n=3, *Am J Psychiatry* 1991;**148**:1262–3)

- CNS — analgesics

Codeine abuse (n=2, *Acta Psychiatr Scand* 1989;**79**:619–20)

- CNS — anticonvulsants

Gabapentin discontinuation (n=1, *J Clin Psychiatry* 1998;**59**:131)

Topiramate (n=1, *Psychiatry Clin Neurosci* 2006;**60**:394)

- CNS — others

Methamfetamine (*J Clin Psychiatry* 1999;**60**:337–8)

Methylphenidate (several e.g. n=1, *Can J Psychiatry* 2001;**46**:89; n=1, *CNS Spectr* 2003;**8**:612–3)

- Anti-infection drugs

Isoniazid (n=1, *J Clin Psychiatry* 1990;**51**:387)

- Endocrine system drugs

Corticosteroids (may respond to fluvoxamine, *Clin Neuropharmacol* 2009;**32**:176–7):

→cortisone (n=1, *Pharmacopsychiatry* 2002;**35**:72–4)

- Malignancy and immunosuppressant drugs

Interferons (*Gen Hosp Psychiatry* 2006;**28**:357–8)

Interferon alfa (n=1, *Pharmacopsychiatry* 2012;**45**:28–30)

- Others

Isotretinoin (n=1 after seven years, *Neuropsychiatr Dis Treat* 2010;**6**:719–22; FFT)

5.11 PANIC ATTACKS

- CNS — sleep disorders and anxiety

Benzodiazepines:

→alprazolam (n=1, *J Am Board Fam Pract* 2002;**15**:69–72; FFT)

→clobazam discontinuation (n=2, *BMJ* 1981;**282**:1931–2; FFT)

→diazepam discontinuation after long-term abuse (n=1, *DICP* 1989;**23**:989–90)

Buspirone (case + correspondence in *Lancet* 1989;**2**:46–7)

- CNS — antipsychotics

Review: long-term use of antipsychotics (n=45, incidence 20%, *Psychiatry Clin Neurosci* 1999;**53**:91–4).

Clozapine (n=1, *Am J Psychiatry* 2000;**157**:2056)

Olanzapine (e.g. hyperventilation, n=1, *J Psychiatry Neurosci* 2002;**27**:360–3; FFT)

Risperidone (in people with post-LSD visual disorder, n=3, *J Clin Psychopharmacol* 1996;**16**:238–41)

- **CNS — antidepressants**

Amitriptyline abrupt discontinuation (n=1, *Am J Psychiatry* 1981;**138**:117–8)
Duloxetine (n=1, *Psychiatr Danub* 2011;**23**:114–6; FFT)
Mianserin discontinuation (n=1, *Jpn J Psychiatry Neurol* 1989;**43**:115–9)
Mirtazapine discontinuation (*Can J Psychiatry* 2000;**45**:570–1)
SSRIs:
- → citalopram (n=1, *South Med J* 2002:**95**;1088–9)
- → fluoxetine (unless initial doses kept very low, e.g. n=1, *J Neuropsychiatry Clin Neurosci* 1989;**1**:219–20)
- → fluoxetine + bupropion (*J Clin Psychiatry* 1996;**57**:177–8)
- → sertraline (e.g. n=1, *Bol Asoc Med P R* 2009;**101**:59–60)

Trazodone

- **CNS — analgesics**

Opiate blockade (*J Clin Psychopharmacol* 1987;**7**:361–2;)
Sumatriptan (incidence 7.2%, although it can be confused for side-effects such as chest pain and palpitations, n=125, *Am J Psychiatry* 1996;**153**:1505; single dose n=15, RCT, d/b, p/c, *Eur Neuropsychopharmacol* 2005;**15**:279–82)

- **CNS — anticonvulsants**

Pregabalin (BNF, less common)
Topiramate (n=1, *J Clin Psychopharmacol* 2001;**21**:461–2; n=1, *J Clin Psychiatry* 2006;**67**:326–7; *Pharmacopsychiatry* 2008;**41**:79)

- **CNS — movement disorders** *

Amantadine (n=1, *J Clin Psychiatry* 1996;**57**:374)
Levodopa (n=31, *Acta Neurol Scand* 1993;**87**:14–8)
Pramipexole (*Eur J Neurol* 2007;**14**:e1; n=1, *J Neuropsychiatry Clin Neurosci* 2011;**23**:E21)
Selegiline (n=1, *Psychosomatics* 2015;**56**:583–7)

- **CNS — others** *

Amfetamines (e.g. n=1, *J Clin Psychopharmacol* 1998;**18**:95–6; methamphetamine n=1, *J Anxiety Disord* 1997;**11**:113–6)
Caffeine (s=8, RCT, d/b, *Expert Rev Neurother* 2011;**11**:1185–95)
Caffeine hyperreactivity (e.g. n=98, RCT, d/b, 1/52, *Psychiatry Res* 2009;**169**:149–53)
Cannabis (n=1, *Acta Psychiatr Scand* 1998;**98**:254–5; *J Am Acad Child Adolesc Psychiatry* 2000;**39**:1467)
Cocaine (e.g. reviews: *Am J Drug Alcohol Abuse* 1992;**18**:57–62; *Biol Psychiatry* 1996;**40**:938–40; *J Addict Dis* 1992;**11**:47–58)
Fenfluramine (n=1, *Braz J Med Biol Res* 1997;**30**:887–90)
MDMA/Ecstasy (n=3, *Biol Psychiatry* 1992;**32**:91–5)
Metoclopramide (n=1, *Psychopharmacol Bull* 2002;**36**:82–93)
Naltrexone (n=1, *Am J Psychiatry* 1998;**155**:447)
Phenylethylamine (n=1, *Psychosomatics* 2015;**56**:583–7)
Sibutramine (n=1, *Am J Psychiatry* 2002;**159**:1793–4; n=1, *Riv Psichiatr* 2009;**44**:64–7)
Smoking cessation (n=2, *J Clin Psychiatry* 2002;**63**:594–5)
Sumatriptan (n=125, incidence 7%, *Am J Psychiatry* 1996;**153**:1505)
Varenicline (BNF, less common)

- **Gastrointestinal drugs**

Pentagastrin (laboratory probe, n=14, incidence 86% in people with OCD, p/c, *Psychopharmacology [Berl]* 1996;**126**:339–44; n=25, RCT, p/c, d/b, c/o, *Psychoneuroendocrinology* 2002;**27**:417–29)

- **Cardiovascular drugs**

Carvedilol (n=1, *Ann Pharmacother* 2002;**36**:1736–40)
Isoproterenol (n=131, incidence 66%, p/c, d/b, *Biol Psychiatry* 1988;**24**:891–902)
Pentoxifylline (n=1, *Am J Psychiatry* 1994;**151**:290)

- **Respiratory drugs**

Doxapram (*Biol Psychiatry* 1993;**33**:295–7; n=10, s/b, *Psychiatry Res* 2005;**133**:253–61)
Epinephrine/adrenaline (n=25, incidence 67%, d/b, p/c, *J Affect Disord* 1996;**39**:133–40;

5

n=50, incidence 68%, RCT, d/b, *Biol Psychiatry* 1998;**44**:1017–26)
Salbutamol (n=1, *Eur Neuropsychopharmacol* 1997;**7**:241–2)
Theophylline (n=1, *An Med Interna* 1990;**7**:53; n=1, *Rev Clin Esp* 1988;**183**:280)

- **Anti-infection drugs**

Cefuroxime (n=1, *Prog Neuropsychopharmacol Biol Psychiatry* 2012;**36**:211)
Chloroquine + mefloquine
Co-trimoxazole (n=1, *J Clin Psychopharmacol* 1991;**11**:144–5)
Mefloquine (BNF, less common; incidence 0.3%, n=35,370, *Drug Saf* 2004;**27**:203–13)
Metronidazole (*South Med J* 1985;**78**:627)
Rifampicin (n=1, *Pharmacotherapy* 2005;**25**:435–7)

- **Endocrine system drugs**

Dexamethasone (e.g. *J Adolesc Health* 1994;**15**:345–7; n=1, *J Psychiatry Neurosci* 1997;**22**:346–7; FFT)
Estrogen (n=1, *Am J Psychiatry* 1994;**151**:1246; *Psychosomatics* 1988;**29**:433–5)
Glucocorticoids (oral courses, n=372,696, *Am J Psychiatry* 2012;**169**:491–7)
Levonorgestrel implant (n=2, *J Clin Psychiatry* 1994;**55**:478–80)
Oral contraceptive, combined (n=2, *J Clin Psychiatry* 1992;**53**:163–5; n=1, *Acta Obstet Gynecol Scand* 1992;**71**:78–80)
Prednisone (n=1, single dose, *Ann Pharmacother* 2011;**45**:1456–7)
TRH (n=99, *Depress Anxiety* 2003;**17**:78–87)

- **Malignancy and immunosuppressant drugs**

Interferons (n=1, *Gen Hosp Psychiatry* 2005;**27**:329–37)

- **Musculoskeletal and analgesics**

Infliximab (n=1, *Dig Dis Sci* 2006;**51**:1056)
Oxaprozin (n=1, *Am J Psychiatry* 1995;**152**:149)

- **Others**

Aspartame (n=1, unproven, high dose, *Lancet* 1986;**2**:631)
Carbon dioxide (mentioned in *Am J Psychiatry* 1994;**151**:292–3)
Flumazenil (n=36, incidence 9%, d/b, *J Psychopharmacol* 1998;**12**:146–50; n=1, given as part of ECT, *J ECT* 2009;**25**:145)
Isotretinoin (n=1, *Rev Med Chil* 2006;**134**:1565–7; FFT)
Lactate oral (e.g. in calcium lactate tablets, n=1, *Ann Pharmacother* 1995;**29**:539–40)
Lead (higher levels, n=1,987, *Arch Gen Psychiatry* 2009;**66**:1313–9; FFT)
Organic solvents (n=3, *Am J Psychiatry* 1987;**144**:1056–8)
Oxymetazoline discontinuation (n=1, *J Clin Psychiatry* 1987;**48**:293)
Phenylephrine (n=1, *Br J Psychiatry* 1980;**136**:297–9)
Procaine (in Penicillin G, n=3, *Am J Psychiatry* 1988;**145**:1317)
Sodium lactate (study in *Arch Gen Psychiatry* 1989;**46**:135–40)
Tyramine (*J S C Med Assoc* 2002;**98**:187–92)
Yohimbine (see *Arch Gen Psychiatry* 1998;**55**:1033–44; n=16, p/c, *Psychiatry Res* 1993;**48**:119–33)

5.12 PARANOID OR SCHIZOPHRENIC-LIKE PSYCHOSES (SEE ALSO HALLUCINATIONS 5.6)

This is characterised by paranoid delusions and hallucinations in a person with little clouding of consciousness. The literature on drug-induced psychosis is extensive but mainly case reports and short uncontrolled studies. A classification has been proposed.

- **Intoxication mimicking functional:** (e.g. drug-induced), e.g. stimulants and cannabis. Persists until the drug has cleared.
- **Psychoactive drugs altering the clinical presentation of a pre-existing psychosis:** e.g. cannabis/amfetamines, creating a more aggressive and disturbed person.
- **Chronic hallucinations induced by substance abuse:** insight usually present, no clouding of consciousness, and continue despite long-term abstinence, e.g. alcoholic hallucinosis, LSD or cannabis flashbacks.
- **Drug-induced relapse of functional psychosis:** e.g. schizophrenia.
- **Withdrawal states:** e.g. delirium tremens, benzodiazepine or barbiturate withdrawal.
- **Others:** acute intoxication/confusion with clouding of consciousness, post-intoxication depression, e.g. post-amfetamine crash, panic/anxiety attacks from hallucinogens, e.g. LSD.

- **True drug-induced psychosis:** any psychotic symptoms that occur with drug intoxication and then persist after elimination of the causing drug, e.g. one to two drug-free weeks.

Review: substance-induced psychosis (Mathias *et al*, *J Clin Psychiatry* 2008;**69**:358–67).

- **CNS — hallucinogens (major cause)** *

Cannabis — see box, *p. 482*
Cannabis, edible (*Am J Psychiatry* 2015;**172**: 911–2)
LSD (n=81, *Arch Gen Psychiatry* 1983;**40**:877–83)
Khat chewing (n=4, *Br J Hosp Med* 1995;**54**:322–6)
MDE/Eve (n=1, *Arch Gen Psychiatry* 1993;**50**:75)
MDMA/Ecstasy (e.g. n=1, *Br J Psychiatry* 1991;**159**:713–5; n=2, *J Psychopharmacol* 2003;**17**:342–5)
Petrol (n=2, *Am J Psychiatry* 1964;**120**:757–61)
Psilocybin (magic mushrooms) (*Neuroreport* 1998;**9**:3897–902)

- **CNS — stimulants (major cause)** *

Reviews: systematic (s=54, Curran *et al*, *Br J Psychiatry* 2004;**185**:196–204; FFT), illicit substances (Fiorentini *et al*, *Curr Drug Abuse Rev* 2011;**4**:228–40).

Adderall® (n=1, *J Am Board Fam Pract* 2002;**15**:498–500; FFT)
Amfetamines (e.g. *Gen Hosp Psychiatry* 1996;**18**:117–20; treatment for this, review *Cochrane Database Syst Rev* 2009;**1**:CD003026l; n=28; after six years 25% had schizophrenia and 25% had died, *Am J Addict* 2015;**24**:586–9)
Cocaine (n=50, incidence 68%, *Am J Psychiatry*, 1991;**148**:495–8; review, *J Dual Diagn* 2014;**10**:98–105)
Diethylpropion (e.g. n=1, *Int Clin Psychopharmacol* 1993;**8**:67–70)
Ephedrine (review in *Prim Care Companion J Clin Psychiatry* 2004;**6**:136–7; FFT)
Methamfetamine (n=42,412, 10 years, Callaghan *et al*, *Am J Psychiatry* 2012;**169**:389–96; n=21, 6/12 follow-up, *Zhonghua Yi Xue Za Zhi [Taipei]* 2001;**64**:388–94; incidence 13%, n=309, *Addiction* 2006;**101**:1473–8; n=39, *Psychiatry Res* 2008;**157**:273–7; review, *CNS Drugs* 2014;**28**:1115–26)
Methylphenidate (BNF, v rare; n=3 in adults, *Clin Neuropharmacol* 2010;**33**:204–6)
Methylphenidate + cocaine (n=1, *Gen Hosp Psychiatry* 2013;**35**:451.e7–9)
Phencyclidine (n=10, *South Med J* 1988;**81**: 565–7)
Phentermine (n=1, *Zhonghua Yi Xue Za Zhi [Taipei]* 1998;**61**:44–7)
Phenylephrine (e.g. *JAMA* 1982;**247**:1859–60)
Phenylpropanolamine (e.g. n=1, *Am J Psychiatry* 2000;**157**:1021–2)
Pseudoephedrine (many cases, e.g. *South Med J* 1990;**83**:64–5)
Solvents (e.g. review, *Nihon Arukoru Yakubutsu Igakkai Zasshi* 2005;**40**:471–84)

- **CNS — sleep disorders and anxiety**

Benzodiazepines (see also anticonvulsants):
→ alprazolam
→ lorazepam (e.g. *Br J Psychiatry* 1986;**148**:344; preoperative oral, n=1, *Anaesthesia* 2003;**58**:1036)
→ lormetazepam (n=1, *Pharmacopsychiatry* 1993;**26**:102–3)
→ midazolam (possible case in *DICP* 1989;**23**:671–2)
→ nitrazepam (BNF, C/I in psychosis)
→ nitrazepam normal-dose discontinuation (n=2, *J UOEH* 1988;**10**:337–40)
→ triazolam (e.g. *Pharmacopsychiatry* 1989;**22**:115–9)
→ triazolam discontinuation (n=1, *J Clin Psychiatry* 1987;**48**:168–9)
Benzodiazepine discontinuation (*Psychosomatics* 1997;**38**:160–1)
Buspirone (e.g. *J Psychopharmacol* 1993;**7**:295–300; n=1, *Psychosomatics* 1992;**33**:332–5)
Melatonin (n=1, *Ann Pharmacother* 1997;**31**:1408)
Modafinil (may exacerbate: e.g. n=1, *Am J Psychiatry* 2005;**162**:1983; n=1, *Intern Med J* 2008;**38**:677–8)
Sodium oxybate (BNF, less common, SmPC; n=1, *J Clin Sleep Med* 2011;**7**:665–6; FFT; n=4, *Front Neurol* 2014;**5**:136; FFT;
Sodium oxybate discontinuation (as gamma-hydroxybutyrate/GHB: n=8, *Ann Emerg Med* 2001;**37**:147–53; n=1, *Epilepsy Behav* 2011;**21**:203–5)
Zolpidem (e.g. n=2, *Ann Clin Psychiatry* 1996;**8**:89–91; n=1, *J Am Geriatr Soc* 1997;**45**:533–4)

The case for cannabis causing psychosis and/or schizophrenia *

- Earlier cannabis use is associated with a greater risk of developing psychosis (n=3,801, *Arch Gen Psychiatry* 2010;**67**:440–7; n=116, *Eur Psychiatry* 2009;**24**:282–6) and bringing onset forward by about a year (n=167, Power *et al*, *Aust N Z J Psychiatry* 2013;47:51–8; n=68, Dragt *et al*, *Can J Psychiatry* 2010;**55**:165–71) in high-risk individuals.
- People in the prodromal phase and at ultra-high risk for psychosis seem more vulnerable to the negative effects of cannabis (n=121, *Aust NZ J Psychiatry* 2009;**43**:1155–62).
- Regular use may increase illness severity (n=229, 10 years, Foti *et al*, *Am J Psychiatry* 2010;**167**:987–93; FFT; n=3,459, *J Nerv Ment Dis* 2009;**197**:35–40).
- Cannabis may reduce brain volume over five years (n=82, *Am J Psychiatry* 2008;**165**;490–6).
- The risk appears to be higher with skunk, if used for over five years (n=280[c=174], Di Forti *et al*, *Br J Psychiatry* 2009;**195**:488–91; FFT) and for over 10 years (Foti *et al*, *Am J Psychiatry* 2010;**167**:987–93; FFT).
- In someone with schizophrenia, stopping cannabis can lead to a clear improvement (n=92, González-Pinto *et al*, *Schizophr Bull* 2011;**37**:631–9; FFT).

The case against cannabis causing psychosis and/or schizophrenia *

- Cannabis use has risen steadily since the mid-1990s, but there is no evidence of an increasing incidence of schizophrenia or psychosis (n=600,000 a year, 2.3% UK population aged 16–44, Frisher et al, *Schizophr Res* 2009;**113**:123–8).
- Although cannabis could hasten the onset (n=116, Sugranyes *et al*, *Eur Psychiatry* 2009;**24**:282–6; n=766, De Hert *et al*, *Schizophr Res* 2011;**126**:270–6), many studies show no effect and one shows the opposite (s=11, van der Meer *et al*, *Curr Pharm Des* 2012;**18**:5036–44).
- Cannabis is neither a sufficient nor necessary cause for psychosis (Arseneault *et al*, *Br J Psychiatry* 2004;**184**:110–7; FFT; systematic review, s=35, *Lancet* 2007;**370**:319–28).
- The endocannabinoid system is a target for treatment of schizophrenia (e.g. review, Saito *et al*, *Neurobiol Dis* 2013;**53**:10–7; FFT; Zuardi *et al*, *Curr Pharm Des* 2012;**18**:5131–40).

Conclusion *

- There is a significant interindividual sensitivity (n=190, Goldberger *et al*, *Int J Neuropsychopharmacol* 2010;**13**:1145–54), especially if having the COMT Val(158)Met polymorphism (n=157, Estrada *et al*, *Acta Psychiatr Scand* 2011;**123**:485–92), or at ultra high risk (n=284, *Psychol Med* 2009;**39**:951–6; n=121, *Aust NZ J Psychiatry* 2010;**44**:230–6).
- Cannabis use may bring forward the onset of psychosis in vulnerable individuals (Casadio *et al*, *Neurosci Biobehav Rev* 2011;**35**:1779–87), reversibly impairs cognition (n=47, Rabin *et al*, *Psychiatry Res* 2013;**206**:158–65) and continued use makes the psychosis more difficult to treat (n=99, Leeson *et al*, *Schizophr Bull* 2012;**38**:873–80; FFT).
- Cannabis is a risk factor for the development or relapse of schizophrenia, but the effect is modest compared to other factors (n=124, two years, Faber *et al*, *J Clin Psychiatry* 2012;**73**: 632–8) and you would have to stop up to 5000 people smoking cannabis to prevent one case of schizophrenia (Hickman *et al*, *Addiction* 2009;**104**:1856–61).
- Use early in adolescence should be discouraged (n=245, *Acta Psychiatr Scand* 2012;**125**:45–53) and avoided if it makes psychotic symptoms worse. If antipsychotic compliance is good and positive symptoms unchanged on consumption, occasional modest use may carry a relatively lower risk. Absence of cannabis use is a protective factor for prevention of relapse (n=1,646, 6/12, San *et al*, *Int J Psychiatry Clin Pract* 2013;**17**:2–9).

Reviews: * meta-analysis (s=35, Koskinen *et al*, *Schizophr Bull* 2010;**36**:1115–30; FFT; Bugra *et al*, *Fortschr Neurol Psychiatr* 2012;**80**:635–43).

Zolpidem abuse (n = 1,500mg, *Addict Health* 2014;**6**:159–62; FFT)
Zolpidem discontinuation (n = 2, *Ugeskr Laeger* 1993;**155**:2711–3)
Zopiclone (some cases reported)

- **CNS — antipsychotics**

Antipsychotic discontinuation (rebound psychosis as opposed to relapse; n = 1, *Can J Psychiatry* 1989;**34**:227–9; in Tourette's; *Biol Psychiatry* 1993;**34**:341–2)
Aripiprazole (n = 1, *J Clin Psychiatry* 2005;**66**:1339; n = 4, *Int Clin Psychopharmacol* 2004;**19**:45–8)
Aripiprazole + clozapine (n = 1, *Prog Neuropsychopharmacol Biol Psychiatry* 2011;**35**:291–2)
Aripiprazole + haloperidol (n = 1, exacerbation, *Int J Psychiatry Clin Pract* 2012;**16**:153–6)
Aripiprazole + risperidone (as adjunct to risperidone, n = 1, *J Clin Psychiatry* 2007;**68**:1445–6)
Chlorpromazine (n = 1, *Can Med Assoc J* 1970:**102**:642; FFT; n = 1, *Brain Inj* 1993;**7**:77–83)
Clozapine discontinuation (e.g. rebound psychosis, study in *Psychopharmacol Bull* 1988;**24**:260–3; n = 3, *J Clin Psychiatry* 1997;**58**:252–5)
Clozapine + lorazepam discontinuation (n = 1, *Aust N Z J Psychiatry* 2012;**46**:795–6)
Haloperidol (n = 1, *Drug Intell Clin Pharm* 1981;**15**:209–13)
Olanzapine (psychotic mania, n = 1, *Eur Psychiatry* 1999;**14**:410–1)
Risperidone (n = 1, *J Child Adolesc Psychopharmacol* 2005;**15**:520–5)
Ziprasidone abrupt discontinuation (n = 1, *Eur Child Adolesc Psychiatry* 2012;**21**:165–8)

- **CNS — antidepressants**

Bupropion (a literature review notes many cases but data is incomplete and often contradictory; s = 23, *Gen Hosp Psychiatry* 2011;**33**:612–7; e.g. n = 1, *Prim Care Companion J Clin Psychiatry* 2010;**12**:09100943; FFT; n = 1, *Indian J Psychiatry* 2009;**51**:53–4; FFT; n = 2, *Pharm World Sci* 2009;**31**:238–40)
Mirtazapine (BNF, may aggravate psychosis; caused by dissociated sleep-wakefulness, n = 1, *Pharmacotherapy* 2010;**30**:145–50)
Phenelzine (BNF, rare; e.g. n = 1, *Br J Psychiatry* 1991;**159**:716–7)
SSRIs, e.g.:
→fluoxetine (e.g. n = 1, *J Am Acad Child Adolesc Psychiatry* 2007;**46**:944–5)
→fluvoxamine (e.g. n = 1, *Can J Psychiatry* 2000;**45**:762; n = 1, *Hum Psychopharmacol* 2003;**18**:477–8)
→paroxetine (case of psychotic mania, *Am J Psychiatry* 1995;**152**:1399–440)
→sertraline (n = 4, *Ann Clin Psychiatry* 1997;**9**:15–7)
→sertraline + TMS (n = 1, *J Neuropsychiatry Clin Neurosci* 2011;**23**:E4–5)
St John's wort (n = 1, *Hum Psychopharmacol* 2004;**19**:275–6; review, n = 17, possible association, *Int J Clin Pharmacol Ther* 2004;**42**:473–80)
Trazodone (n = 1, *J Neuropsychiatry Clin Neurosci* 2005;**17**:253–4)
Tricyclics (BNF, review concludes may exacerbate any psychosis is temporary and rare, s = 20, n = 177, *J Affect Disord* 2008;**106**:279–84)
Venlafaxine (n = 1, also occurred on rechallenge, *Indian J Psychiatry* 2009;**51**:308–9; FFT)
Venlafaxine + propafenone (n=1, *Int J Psychiatr Med* 2001;**31**:427–32)

- **CNS — analgesics** *

Buprenorphine (BNF, less common)
Buprenorphine discontinuation (n = 1, *Am J Psychiatry* 2008;**165**:400–1; n = 1, *J Clin Psychiatry* 2012;**73**:e756)
Butorphanol (*J Neuropsychiatry Clin Neurosci* 1998;**10**:236–7)
Codeine OD (n = 1, *Neurobehavioral Toxicol Teratol* 1985;**7**:193–4)
Diamorphine (BNF, caution in psychosis)
Dipipanone (BNF, uncommon)
Fentanyl (BNF, v rare)
Methadone withdrawal (e.g. n = 2, *J Clin Psychiatry* 1995;**56**:73–6)
Morphine intrathecal (*Anesth Analg* 1993;**77**:1298–9)
Naltrexone (after heroin detox, n = 1, *Am J Addict* 2005;**14**:486–7)
Oxycodone (BNF, caution in psychosis)
Paracetamol overdose (*Gen Hosp Psychiatry* 1997;**19**:149–50)

5

Pentazocine (esp. hallucinations, e.g. *Br Med J* 1974;**2**:224–5; FFT)
Ziconotide (n = 1, *Gen Hosp Psychiatry* 2015;**37**:e11–2)

• CNS — anticonvulsants *

Psychosis induced by anticonvulsants may be the result of 'forced normalisation'. Risk factors include temporal lobe epilepsy (TLE), treatment resistance, past history of psychosis or affective disorder, and becoming suddenly seizure-free (best to do this gradually). Drug regimens should be changed gradually and compliance should be maintained to prevent epileptic psychoses (n = 44, Matsuura, *J Neurol Neurosurg Psychiatry* 1999;**67**:231–3; FFT).

Barbiturates
Carbamazepine (BNF, rare)
Carbamazepine toxicity (*Lancet* 1989;**i**:167)
Carbamazepine discontinuation (n = 1, *Br J Clin Pract* 1996;**50**:350–1)
Clonazepam (n = 1, *J Nerv Ment Dis* 1982;**170**:117–9)
Clonazepam discontinuation (*J Clin Psychopharmacol* 1986;**6**:193)
Ethosuximide (BNF, rare)
Gabapentin (review, *Int J Psychiatry Med* 2015;**49**:245–8)
Lacosamide (n = 1, *Clin Neuropharmacol* 2015;**38**:198–200)
Lamotrigine (*Epilepsy Behav* 2007;**11**:476; n = 4, incidence 0.2%, *Epilepsy Behav* 2007;**11**: 133–9)
Levetiracetam (BNF, less common; cases within n = 517, *Neurology* 2003;**61**:704–6; n = 1, *Indian J Pharmacol* 2014;**46**:560–1; FFT; n = 1, enduring, *Actas Esp Psiquiatr* 2012;**40**:49; FFT; n = 1, *J Neuropsychiatry Clin Neurosci* 2011;**23**:E19–20)
Oxcarbazepine (n = 1, *Epilepsy Behav* 2008;**12**:492–3)
Phenytoin toxicity (e.g. n = 1 for trigeminal neuralgia, *Epilepsy Behav* 2003;**4**:771–2; *Clin Pediatr [Phila]* 1993;**32**:107–10)
Pregabalin (n = 1, *Seizure* 2006;**15**:208–10; FFT)
Tiagabine (BNF, rare; RCT shows no significant risk; n = 554, *Epilepsia* 2002;**43**:394–8; n = 1, *Neuropsychiatr* 2007;**21**:59–61; 1.5% incidence, esp. with previous episodes, n = 596, *Epilepsy Behav* 2003;**4**:548–52)
Topiramate (1.5% incidence, esp. with previous episodes, n = 596, *Epilepsy Behav* 2003;**4**:548–52; n = 1, migraine prophylaxis, *Am J Health Syst Pharm* 2010;**67**:1178–80; n = 2, *Clin Neuropharmacol* 2006;**29**:168–9)
Valproate (rare cases)
Vigabatrin (BNF, less common; e.g. n = 1, *Acta Med Port* 2000;**13**:111–4; FFT; review, *Acta Neurol Scand* 1996;**93**:1–8)
Vigabatrin discontinuation (*Med J Aust* 1992;**156**:291; letter in *Lancet* 1990;**335**:1279)
Zonisamide (BNF, less common; n = 74, incidence 13–18%, *Seizure* 2000;**9**:65–70; FFT; n = 1, *Am J Psychiatry* 2007;**164**:682; n = 1, *Am J Ther* 2014; **21**:e15–6; n = 1, *Am J Ther* 2014;**21**:e88–9)

• CNS — movement disorders *

The incidence with Parkinsonian treatments may be as high as 20–30% (see *C1*).

Amantadine (n = 2, exacerbation of schizophrenia, *Am J Psychiatry* 1986;**143**:1170–1; overdose, n = 1, *Ann Emerg Med* 1990;**19**:668–70)
Anticholinergics (in people with Alzheimer's, n = 230, *Clin Pharmacol Ther* 2008;**84**:63–8):
→ biperidin (*Med Clin (Barc)* 1992;**99**:79)
→ trihexyphenidyl
Dopamine agonists:
→ bromocriptine (BNF, rare; cases inc. *An Med Interna* 2003;**20**:50–1; low-dose n = 1, *Acta Obstet Gynecol Scand* 1991;**70**:375–6; n = 2, *Harefuah* 1990;**118**:203–4)
→ bromocriptine + pseudoephedrine (n = 1, *J Fam Pract* 1997;**45**:164–6)
→ cabergoline (BNF, caution in psychosis; n = 2, exacerbation of schizophrenia when used as adjunct, *Gen Hosp Psychiatry* 2008;**30**:378–80)
→ pergolide (BNF, caution in psychosis; esp. hallucinations, incidence ≤13%, e.g. *Neurology* 1982;**32**:1181–4)
→ pramipexole (BNF, *Psychiatry Clin Neurosci* 2008;**62**:245; n = 1, *Turk Psikiyatri Derg* 2014;**25**:212–4; FFT)
→ ropinirole (BNF, less common; n = 95, 14% incidence, *Ann Pharmacother* 2009;**43**:1426–32)
→ rotigotine (BNF, less common)

Levodopa (esp. hallucinations, n=214, *Med Clin (Barc)* 1999;**112**:245–50)
Lisuride (a few cases, e.g. *Lancet* 1986;**2**:349)
Selegiline (a few cases, e.g. *Neurology* 1981;**31**:19–23)

- **CNS — others (see also stimulants)** *

Alcohol (n=8,028, review, *Br J Psychiatry* 2010;**197**:200–6; FFT)
Alcohol, caffeine + 'vigueur fit' (n=1, *Med Sci Law* 2001;**41**:331–6)
Atomoxetine (n=1, transient, *J Child Adolesc Psychopharmacol* 2009;**19**:319–20)
Caffeine (n=1, *CNS Spectr* 2009;**14**:127–9; n=1, *Aust NZ J Psychiatry* 2011;**45**:179–80)
Cannabis (see box, p. 482)
Cocaine (reviews of risk factors, *Eur Psychiatry* 2013;**28**:141–6; e.g. low BMI, n=69, *Isr J Psychiatry Relat Sci* 2005;**42**:45–50; FFT; review, *Rev Med Leige* 2010;**65**:623–7)
Cocaine + OTC cold cure (*J Clin Psychiatry* 1989;**50**:147)
Dexamfetamine (BNF, less common; *Pediatrics* 2004;**113**:1466)
Dexfenfluramine (*Am J Psychiatry* 1997;**154**:1624–5)
Diethylpropion (n=1, *Int Clin Psychopharmacol* 1993;**8**:67–70; n=5, *Clin Neuropharmacol* 1988;**11**:183–8)
Disulfiram (BNF, rare; C/I in psychosis; e.g. n=1, *Ned Tijdschr Geneeskd* 2002;**146**:965):
→ low-dose (n=1, *Prog Neuropsychopharmacol Biol Psychiatry* 2008;**32**:311–2)
→ high-dose (n=1, *J Clin Psychopharmacol* 2007;**27**:224–5)
Disulfiram + methylphenidate (n=1, dose-dependent, *Subst Abus* 2012;**33**:186–8)
Domperidone discontinuation (n=1, *Ann Pharmacother* 2011;**45**:e51)
Donepezil (n=1, delusional parasitosis, *J Clin Psychopharmacol* 2011;**31**:781–2)
Ephedra alkaloids (in 'vigueur fit' tablets; n=1, *Med Sci Law* 2001;**41**:331–6; n=7, *South Med J* 2003;**96**:718–20)
Guanfacine (n=1, *Hosp Pharm* 2015;**50**:564–8)
Hyoscine (n=4 plus review, *Fortschr Neurol Psychiatr* 1998;**66**:289–95)
Hyoscine transdermal patches (e.g. Transderm®, *Neurology* 2000;**54**:1877)
Khat (n=1, *Tijdschr Psychiatr* 2007;**49**:763–7; FFT; review of association in Somalia, n=4,854, *BMC Med* 2005;**3**:5; FFT; n=1, *Ethiop Med J* 1997;**35**:137–9)
Khat + mushrooms (n=4, *World J Biol Psychiatry* 2004;**5**:167–8)
MDMA/ecstasy (n=1, *Lijec Vjesn* 2000;**122**:27–30; n=1, persistent after single dose, *Psychosomatics* 2001;**42**:525–7; n=1, very persistent, *Psychol Rep* 2004;**95**:192–6; n=32, *Eur Addict Res* 2002;**8**:133–40)
Memantine (BNF, less common; n=1, in bipolar, *J Clin Psychiatry* 2010;**71**:957; n=1, *J Clin Psychiatry* 2005;**66**:658–9; n=3, *Neurology* 2005;**65**:481–2)
Mephedrone (n=1, *Psychiatr Pol* 2011;**45**:431–7)
Methysergide (n=1, *Neuropsychobiology* 1989;**22**:125–7)
Metoclopramide (n=2, *Ann Pharmacother* 2002;**36**:1387–90)
Nabilone (BNF, common)
Naltrexone (after heroin detox, n=1, *Am J Addict* 2005;**14**:486–7)
Nandrolone (n=1, *Psychiatr Prax* 2003;**30**[Suppl 2]:S73–4)
Nicotine, abrupt withdrawal (n=1, *Am J Psychiatry* 1994;**151**:452)
Phentermine (n=1, *Aust N Z J Psychiatry* 2011;**45**:684–5)
Sibutramine (e.g. n=1, *Prog Neuropsychopharmacol Biol Psychiatry* 2010;**34**:1359–60; in OTC diet aid n=1, *Turk Psikiyatri Derg* 2010;**21**:335–7; FFT; n=1, *J Psychosom Res* 2008;**64**:107–9; n=16, *Clin Toxicol (Phila)* 2010;**48**:832–8)
Varenicline (no evidence for causal association between varenicline and criminal offending, suicidal behaviour, road accidents, traffic offences or psychosis in Sweden, n=69,757, *BMJ* 2015;**350**:h2388; FFT; review: *J Clin Psychiatry* 2012;**73**:1039–47; review of use in psychosis concludes it can be effective but must be used with careful monitoring; *J Addict Res Ther* 2011;**S4**:3045; FFT).
Varenicline discontinuation (n=1, *Am J Psychiatry* 2010;**167**:720–1)

- **Gastrointestinal drugs**

Antidiarrheals (OTC) (n=1, *Br J Psychiatry* 1990;**157**:758–9)
Bismuth toxicity (*Am Fam Physician* 1988;**38**:244–6)

5

Cimetidine (*Indian Pediatr* 1989;**26**:1061–2; n=1, *Am J Psychiatry* 1980;**137**:1112–3)
Dicycloverine

- **Cardiovascular drugs** *

ACE inhibitors, e.g.:
→ lisinopril (*Psychiatr Prax* 1998;**25**:204)
Beta-blockers (see under depression for differentials), e.g.:
→ atenolol (rare, n=1, *Am J Psychiatry* 1983;**140**:1382)
→ metoprolol (n=1, *Gen Hosp Psychiatry* 2013;**35**:102.e1–2; may be familial, n=3, *Gen Hosp Psychiatry* 2015;**37**:620.e5–6)
→ propranolol (well known, e.g. n=1, *Am J Emerg Med* 1995;**13**:536–7)
→ propranolol discontinuation (*Biol Psychiatry* 1989;**25**:351–4)
Calcium-channel blockers, e.g.:
→ diltiazem (n=1, *Arch Intern Med* 1991;**151**:373–4; *J R Soc Med* 1988;**81**:296–7; FFT)
→ enalapril (n=1, *DICP* 1991;**25**:558–9)
→ nifedipine (e.g. *Am J Med* 1987;**83**:389; n=1, *Am J Med* 1986;**81**:705–6)
→ quinapril (n=1, *J Am Geriatr Soc* 2000;**48**:1533)
Clonidine (n=1, *Prog Neuropsychopharmacol* 1980;**4**:211–3)
Clonidine discontinuation (n=3, *Am J Psychiatry* 1982;**139**:110–2)
Digoxin toxicity (BNF, v rare; *J Nerv Mental Dis* 1978;**166**:817–9; *Lijec Vjesn* 1991;**113**:417–9)
Disopyramide (BNF, very rare; e.g. *Lancet* 1978;**1**:858–9)
Dopamine infusion (*Biol Psychiatry* 1992;**31**:1225–7)
Doxazosin (n=1, *BMJ* 1997;**314**:1869)
Hydralazine (n=1, *J Am Med Assoc* 1953;**152**:1329–31)
Lidocaine IV (n=6, *Ann Intern Med* 1982;**97**:149–50)
Losartan (*Cardiology* 1996;**87**:569–70)
Methyldopa (BNF, mild psychosis is common)
Mexilitine (n=1, *Am Heart J* 1984;**107**:1091–8; n=1, *Int J Gen Med* 2011;**4**:765–6; FFT)
Nitrates, e.g. isosorbides
Pentoxifylline (*J Assoc Physicians India* 1992;**40**:479)
Procainamide (BNF, uncommon; *Crit Care Nurse* 1993;**13**:70–2)
Quinidine (n=1, *Med J Aust* 1990;**153**:47–9)
Simvastatin (n=3, *Ned Tijdschr Geneeskd* 1993;**137**:1312–5)
Tocainide (n=2, *Br Med J (Clin Med Res)* 1984;**288**:606–7)

- **Respiratory drugs**

Betamethasone (n=1, *No To Shinkei* 1992;**44**:913–6)
Chlorphenamine OD (n=1, *Med J Aust* 1973;**1**:382–6)
Coricidin cold medicine (*Ann Pharmacother* 2005;**39**:1577–8)
Cyproheptadine (*Indian J Pediatr* 1989;**56**:521–3; n=1, *Pediatr Emerg Care* 1986;**2**:183–5)
Dextromethorphan (review, *Addict Biol* 2005;**10**:325–7; n=1, *CJEM* 2011;**13**:53–6; FFT)
Dextromethorphan + hydrocodone + propoxyphene (n=1, *J Psychopharmacol* 2009;**23**:989–91)
Diphenhydramine (e.g. *Am J Emerg Med* 1997;**15**:548–9; n=2, *Chudoku Kenkyu* 2007;**20**:125–9)
Diphenhydramine overdose (n=1, *Dtsch Med Wochenschr* 1988;**113**;180–3)
Ephedrine (n=1, *Harefuah* 1994;**127**:166–8)
Phenylpropanolamine (e.g. with caffeine, *Biol Psychiatry* 1991;**30**:401–4; n=1, *Am J Psychiatry* 2000;**157**:1021–2)
Phenylpropanolamine + amantadine (n=1, *Gen Hosp Psychiatry* 1995;**17**:457–8)
Promethazine (n=1, *Psychosomatics* 2004;**45**:89–90)
Salbutamol (*Biol Psychiatry* 1989;**26**:631–3; as inhaler, n=1, *J Clin Psychopharmacol* 1995;**15**:446–7)
Theophylline (n=1, *J Clin Psychopharmacol* 1989;**9**:65–6)

- **Anti-infection drugs** *

Aciclovir (BNF, rare; *Adv Psych Treat* 2005;**11**:66)
Albendazole + ivermectin (n=1, *Gen Hosp Psychiatry* 2012;**34**:578.e9–578.e10)
Amoxicillin + clarithromycin (n=1, *Paediatr Anaesth* 2005;**15**:703–5)
Amoxicillin (co-amoxiclav; n=1, *Praxis (Bern 1994)* 2009;**98**:765–6)
Amoxicillin + clarithromycin + pantoprazole (n=1, *Neuropsychiatr* 2010;**24**:144–50)
Antifungals, e.g.:

→ griseofulvin
→ posaconazole (BNF, common)

Antimalarials, e.g.:
→ chloroquine (e.g. n = 1, *Am J Ther* 2007;**14**:406–7; n = 1, recurrent, *Indian J Med Sci* 1996;**50**:302–4; n = 1, *Presse Med* 2003;**32**:117)
→ lariam (severe is extremely low, e.g. one in 6000, *Pharm J* 1996;**256**:184)
→ mefloquine (BNF, less common; n = 179, more common in females and first-time users; *Eur J Clin Pharmacol* 2002;**58**:441–5; n = 1, after a single dose, responded to quetiapine, *Malar J* 2006;**5**:74; FFT)
→ quinine (*Br J Psychiatry* 1988;**153**:575–6)

Antiretrovirals, e.g.:
→ efavirenz (BNF, less common; e.g. n = 1, *Clin Infect Dis* 2007;**45**:e128–30; FFT; n = 1, *Clin Infect Dis* 2005;**40**:e22–3)

Antituberculous drugs (*Lancet* 1989;**2**:105):
→ cycloserine (BNF, common; e.g. n = 1, *Indian J Pharmacol* 2015;**47**:230–1; FFT; n = 1, *J Clin Diag Res* 2015;**9**:FD01–3; FFT)
→ ethambutol (n = 1, *Ann Thorac Med* 2008;**3**:149–51; FFT; toxicity n = 1, *Int J STD AIDS* 2007;**18**:287–8)
→ isoniazid (BNF, common; caution in psychosis; *Gen Hosp Psychiatry* 2007;**29**:85–6; n = 1, *Rev Pneumol Clin* 2011;**67**:118–20; n = 1, *Ann Thorac Med* 2008;**3**:149–51; FFT)
→ rifampicin (*Indian J Lepr* 1992;**64**:537–9)

Bleomycin/etoposide/cisplatin (n = 1, *BMJ Case Rep* 2015;**2015**:bcr2104208982)

Carbaryl (n = 1, *Am J Psychiatry* 1995;**152**:646–7)

Cephalosporins (*Aust N Z J Psychiatry* 2003;**37**:627–8), e.g.:
→ cefuroxime (*Lancet* 1984;**i**:965)
→ cephalexin (n = 1, *Med J Aust* 1973;**i**:497–8)

Colistin (BNF, rare)

Co-trimoxazole (several e.g. n = 1, *Pharmacopsychiatry* 2006;**39**:236–7; n = 4, *J Antimicrob Chemother* 2011;**66**:1117–9; FFT)

Dapsone (BNF, uncommon at low doses; e.g. n = 1, *J Trop Med Hyg* 1993;**96**:274–6; *Br Med J* 1989;**299**:324; FFT)

Ethionamide

Foscarnet (BNF, common)

Ganciclovir (BNF, less common; e.g. n = 1, *Pharmacother* 2000;**20**:479–83)

Gatifloxacin (n = 1, *Am J Geriatr Psychiatry* 2003;**11**:470–1; n = 1, *J Am Geriatr Soc* 2006;**54**:871; *Psychosomatics* 2007;**48**:87)

Ketoconazole (n = 1, idiosyncratic and v rare, *Am J Psychiatry* 1990;**147**:677)

Levamisole (*Ann Pharmacother* 1998;**32**:134–5)

Macrolides, e.g.:
→ clarithromycin (BNF, v rare; e.g. n = 1, *Med J Malaysia* 2006;**61**:263; FFT; n = 1, *Psychiatr Bull* 2004;**28**:98–9; n = 1, *J Nerv Ment Dis* 2015;**203**:149–51)
→ erythromycin (n = 2, *Arch Intern Med* 1986;**146**:897–9)
→ erythromycin + bromocriptine (n = 1, *Neurologia* 1997;**12**:429)
→ nalidixic acid (a few cases, e.g. CSM comment, *Br Med J* 1965;**2**:590)

Mefloquine (n = 1, child, *J Child Neurol* 2009;**24**:1008–9; n = 1, *Harefuah* 2010;**149**:583–4)

Mepacrine (BNF, rare, transient)

Methylenedioxypyrovalerone (n = 2, *Gen Hosp Psychiatry* 2011;**33**:640.e5–6)

Metronidazole (BNF, v rare; *J Fam Pract* 1988;**27**:323–5; n = 1, *Am J Psychiatry* 1997;**154**:1170–1)

Metronidazole + ofloxacin (*Br J Hosp Med (Lond)* 2009;**70**:236–7)

Nitrofurantoin (*Adv Psychiatr Treat* 2005;**11**:66)

Oseltamivir (no evidence for increased risk of neuropsychiatric ADRs in people aged 1–21; *Int J Adolesc Med Health* 2009;**21**:79–89)

Penicillin (several cases, e.g. *Br J Psychiatry* 1990;**156**:554–9)

Primaquine (n = 1, *Ann Intern Med* 1980;**92**:435)

Quinacrine (e.g. n = 1, *Hum Psychopharmacol* 2002;**17**:357–9)

Quinolones e.g.:
→ ciprofloxacin (many e.g. n = 1, *Eur Psychiatry* 2003;**18**:262–3; n = 1, *Psychosomatics* 2007;**48**:269)
→ levofloxacin (rare but can be serious, SmPC, n = 1, *Gen Hosp Psychiatry* 2008;**30**:381–3)
→ nalidixic acid (BNF, less common; injection n = 1, *J Forensic Sci* 1986;**31**:1145–9)
→ norfloxacin (*J Assoc Physicians India* 1994;**42**:844)
→ ofloxacin (*Psychiatr Prax* 1996;**23**:251; n = 2, *Int J STD AIDS* 2003;**14**:636–7)

5

→ pefloxacin (n = 1, *Prog Neuropsychopharmacol Biol Psychiatry* 1996;**20**:343–7)
Sulfadiazine (n = 2, *Clin Infect Dis* 1992;**15**:556–7)
Tobramycin (a few cases, e.g. *Pediatr Pulmonol* 1988;**4**:201–4)
Trimethoprim (*Adv Psychiatr Treat* 2005;**11**:66)
Triple therapy for H Pylori (n=1, *J Am Board Fam Pract* 2002;**15**:66–8: FFT; probably the clarithromycin, n = 1, *Case Rep Gastroenterol* 2012;**6**:381–6; FFT)
Valaciclovir (n = 1, *Psychosomatics* 2009;**50**:293–6)
Voriconazole (n = 1, *Indian J Pharmacol* 2015;**47**:332–3; FFT)

- **Endocrine system drugs** *

Review: brief psychosis with clomifene and related endocrine drugs (Seeman, *Gynecol Endocrinol* 2015;**31**;751–4).
Carbimazole (n = 1, *Br J Psychiatry* 1969;**115**:1181–3)
Clomifene (n = 1, *Hum Reprod* 1997;**12**:706–7; FFT; n = 2, *Am J Psychiatry* 1997;**154**:1169–70; see also review above)
Corticosteroid (oral courses can aggravate schizophrenia, incidence may be as high as 5–6% in adults, usually emerges within a few days or weeks, risk may be dose-related, *MHRA Drug Safety Update* 2007;1–9; review, *Gen Hosp Psychiatry* 2003;**25**:27–33):
→ corticosteroid discontinuation (*J Pain Symptom Manage* 2007;**34**:118–9)
→ deflazacort (aggravation of symptoms, SmPC)
→ dexamethasone (n = 1, *Afr J Psychiatry (Johannesbg)* 2011;**14**:316–8; FFT)
→ dexamethasone discontinuation (*Lijec Vjesn* 1988;**110**:94–6)
→ hydrocortisone IV 400mg/24hrs (n = 1, *Psychiatr Pol* 2015;**49**:673–81)
→ prednisolone + clarithromycin (n = 1, *Gen Hosp Psychiatry* 1998;**20**:325–6)
→ prednisone (usually > 40 mg/d, e.g. case and discussion in *Br J Psychiatry* 1993;**162**:549–51; low dose n = 1, *Endocr J* 2006;**53**:255–8; FFT)
→ triamcinolone (SmPC, dose-related; nasal spray, n = 1, *Prog Neurol Psychiatry* 2007;**11**:31–2)
Desmopressin (n = 1, *Lancet* 1981;**2**:808)
Estrogen discontinuation (review, n = 26, *J Acta Psychiatr Scand* 2001;**104**:323–31; n = 1, *Psychosomatics* 2012;**53**:285–8)
Iodine, radioactive (n = 1, *Am J Psychiatry* 2009;**166**:1067–8)
Insulin abuse (n=1, *Br Med J* 1971;**4**:792)
Methyltestosterone (*Lancet* 1987;**i**:863)
Oral contraceptive, combined (n = 1, *Gynecol Endocrinol* 2007;**23**:361–2)
Quinagolide (BNF, v rare)

- **Malignancy and immunosuppressant drugs**

Ciclosporin (*Psychosomatics* 1993;**34**:101–2; n = 1, *Lijec Vjesn* 2007;**129**:74–6)
5-fluorouracil (n = 1, *Clin Colorectal Cancer* 2009;**8**:166–8)
Glucocorticoids (review, *Psychosomatics* 2012;**53**:103–15)
Gonadorelin (*Br J Psychiatry* 1999;**175**:290–1)
Ifosfamide (BNF, common; e.g. n = 1, *Farm Hosp* 2006;**30**:315–6; n = 1, *Psychooncology* 2007;**16**:956–60)
Interferons e.g.:
→ interferon alfa (e.g. n = 1, psychotic depression, *J Psychopharmacol* 2005;**19**:102–5; n = 1, *Pharmacopsychiatry* 2007;**40**:146–8; n = 1, persistent, *J Clin Psychopharmacol* 2006;**26**:446–7)
→ interferon beta-1a (n = 1, *Psychiatry Clin Neurosci* 2012;**66**:462)
→ peginterferon alfa-2b + ribavirin (n = 1, *Int Clin Psychopharmacol* 2005;**20**:289–90; n = 1, *Braz J Infect Dis* 2006;**10**:406–7; FFT)
→ interferon alfa + ribavirin (n = 1, *Psychosomatics* 2009;**50**:538–421)
→ interferon beta-1b (n = 1, *Psychiatry Clin Neurosci* 2010;**64**:584–6)
Leuprolide s/c (n = 1, *J Clin Psychiatry* 2010;**71**:1696–8)
Leuprorelin acetate (n = 1, *Nervenarzt* 2007;**78**;694–5)
Paclitaxel infusion (n = 1, *Conn Med* 2011;**75**:465–6)
Sunitinib (n = 1, *Clin Genitourin Cancer* 2011;**9**:70–2)
Tacrolimus (BNF, rare; n = 1, *Int J Neuropsychopharmacol* 2006;**9**:493–4)

- **Musculoskeletal and analgesics**

Allopurinol (n = 1, causing relapse, *Schizophr Res* 2007;**93**:409)
Aspirin (*JAMA* 1965;**193**:555–8)
Baclofen (many, e.g. n = 1, *Ann Pharmacother*

2006;**40**:2071–3; intoxication, n = 18, *Przegl Lek* 2004;**61**:389–91)
Baclofen IT (n = 1, *Psychiatry Clin Neurosci* 2011;**65**:300–1)
Baclofen discontinuation (n = 1, *J Neuropsychiatry Clin Neurosci* 2009;**21**:476)
Carisoprodol discontinuation (n = 1, *Ann Clin Psychiatry* 2008;**20**:173–4)
Chloroquine (BNF, rare)
Hydroxychloroquine (BNF, rare)
Ibuprofen OTC (n = 1, *Prog Neurol Psychiatry* 2012;**16**:15–7)
Indometacin (rare, e.g. cases within n = 32, *Can J Anaesth* 2003;**50**:586–8; n = 1, *Postgrad Med J* 2000;**76**:736–7; FFT)
Indometacin + ciprofloxacin (n = 1, *Rev Clin Esp* 1992;**191**:401)
Sulindac (*JAMA* 1980;**243**:1420)

- **Others** *

Atropine (oral, IV, eye drops, e.g. *DICP* 1990;**24**:708–9; n = 4 plus review, *Fortschr Neurol Psychiatr* 1998;**66**:289–95)
'Bath salts' (synthetic cathinones, n = 18, 66% died, *Perspect Psychiatr Care* 2016;**52**:68–78)
Brimonidine eye drops (*Arch Ophthalmol* 2000;**118**:1132–3)
Butane (n = 1, *Psychiatry Clin Neurosci* 2001;**55**:163)
Colubrina — see Mabi bark tea
Cyanide (*Arch Environ Health* 1997;**52**:245–6)
Cyclobenzaprine (n = 1, *Can J Psychiatry* 2000;**45**:763–4)
Cyclopentolate eye drops (several e.g. n = 1, *J Cataract Refract Surg* 2003;**29**:1026–30)
Distigmine bromide (n = 1, *Eur Psychiatry* 2003;**18**:318–9)
Energy drinks (n = 1, *Am J Psychiatry* 2010;**167**:353)
Flumazenil (*Lancet* 1992;**339**:488–9)
Herbal preparations and supplements (n = 1, *Int J Psychiatry Med* 2007;**37**:279–82; n = 1, *S D Med* 2008;**61**:173–7)
Ibogaine (n = 1, *J Clin Psychopharmacol* 2011;**31**:659)
Inhalants (n = 40, responds to carbamazepine, *Psychiatr Serv* 1998;**49**:812–5)
Insect repellent (*Psychosomatics* 2001;**42**:78–80; n = 1, after 2/52 topical application of DEET, *Am J Psychiatry* 1987;**144**:1103–4)
Iohexol (n = 1, *Neuroradiology* 1994;**36**:141)
Isotretinoin (no evidence for causing psychosis or any other psychiatric disorder, n = 21,911, *Arch Dermatol* 2000;**136**:1231–6; n = 5, *Int Clin Psychopharmacol* 2005;**20**:39–41)
Ketamine (discussion, *Am J Psychiatry* 1997;**154**:805–11)
Ketorolac (BNF, less common)
Lactate oral (e.g. in calcium lactate tablets, case in *Ann Pharmacother* 1995;**29**:539–40)
Mabi bark tea (n = 1, *Br J Psychiatry* 1992;**161**:404–7; hotly disputed, *Br J Psychiatry* 1993;**162**:275)
Manganese (n = 1, *Psychosomatics* 2011;**52**:74–7; n = 1, *J Med Case Rep* 2011;**5**:146; FFT)
Methazolamide (n = 1, *Pharmacotherapy* 1997;**17**:387–9)
Metrizamide (n = 1, prolonged, *Psychosomatics* 1986;**27**:373–5)
Mouthwash containing alcohol (n = 1, *Mil Med* 2009;**174**:828–31)
Nitrous oxide abuse (n = 1, *J Med Toxicol* 2006;**2**:71–4; FFT; n = 1, *Can J Neurol Sci* 2015;**41**:672–4)
Nutmeg (n=1, *J R Soc Med* 1993;**86**:179–80; FFT; *Br J Psychiatry* 1993;**162**:131)
Organic solvents (n = 2, *Nihon Arukoru Yakubutsu Igakkai Zasshi* 2007;**42**:76–81)
Oxybutynin (n = 2, *Clin Drug Investig* 2006;**26**:603–6)
Oxymetazoline nasal spray (several e.g. n= 1, *CMAJ* 1994;**150**:375–6; FFT)
Peyote plant (n = 1, *J Clin Psychiatry* 2004;**65**:1433–4)
Phenylephrine (*JAMA* 1982;**247**:1859–60)
Pilocarpine (*Psychosomatics* 2005;**46**:88)
Procaine penicillin (n = 1, *Int J Dermatol* 1995;**34**:627–9)
Salvia divinorum (n = 1, *Am J Psychiatry* 2009;**166**:832)
Styrene exposure (n = 1, *J Clin Exp Neuropsychol* 1990;**12**:798–806)
Thallium poisoning (n = 1, *J Assoc Physicians India* 2006;**54**:53–5)
Timolol eye drops (n = 163 from National Registry, *J Clin Psychopharmacol* 1987;**7**:264–7)
Toluene (*Br J Psychiatry* 1991;**158**:578)
Trichloroethylene abuse (n = 1, *Arch Neurobiol [Madr]* 1989;**52**:198–202)
Yohimbine (unproven, see *Arch Gen Psychiatry* 1998;**55**:1033–44)

5

5.13 SEROTONIN SYNDROME (SS)

Serotonin syndrome (SS) is a predictable adverse consequence of excess serotonergic agonism. SS has been reported with a variety of medicines, usually in combination but can be monotherapy or in overdose. There has been an FDA alert on SS with SSRIs/SNRIs and triptans, but other data suggest SS is rare and the combination should not be prohibited (n=29, *MedGenMed* 2007;**9**:48; FFT). There were 7,349 reported cases of SS and 93 deaths in the USA in 2002 (Bush *et al, J Palliat Med* 2006;**9**:1257–9). Few SS reports have been fully documented or peer reviewed and so are not confirmed.

Reviews: prevention, recognition, management (Ables and Nagubilli, *Am Fam Physician* 2010;**81**:1139–42; FFT), misdiagnosis (n=7, Attar–Herzberg *et al, Isr Med Assoc J* 2009;**11**:367–70; FFT), SS vs NMS (Perry and Wilborn, *Ann Clin Psychiatry* 2012;**24**:155–62).

- Monotherapy *

Amantadine (n=1, *Am J Emerg Med* 2008;**26**:112.e5–6)

Bupropion OD (n=1, *J Med Toxicol* 2010;**6**:168–71; FFT)

Chlorphenamine? (comment, *Singapore Med J* 2006;**47**:1014)

Cyclobenzaprine (review; *Clin Pharmacol Ther* 2011;**90**:662–5; FFT)

Dexfenfluramine (n=1, *JAMA* 1996;**276**:1220–1)

Dextromethorphan (n=1, *Geriatr Gerentol Int* 2011;**11**:121–2)

Diphenhydramine OD (n=1, *Psychiatry Clin Neurosci* 2012;**66**:244–5)

Duloxetine (n=1, *Aust N Z J Psychiatry* 2009;**43**:581–2; n=1, *Clin Neuropharmacol* 2011;**34**:127–8)

Fentanyl (n=1, *Clin Neuropharmacol* 2015;**38**:206–8)

MDMA/ecstasy (review of risks; *Aust N Z J Psychiatry* 2007;**41**:649–55; *Pharmacol Biochem Behav* 2002;**71**:837–44)

MDPV (methylenedioxypyrovalerone, n=1, *Ann Emerg Med* 2012;**60**:100–2)

Methadone (n=1, *J Palliat Med* 2006;**9**:1257–9)

Methylene Blue (13 of 14 cases reported to 2011 met the criteria for SS; Gillman, *J Psychopharmacol* 2011;**25**:429–36; n=1, *J Oncol Pharm Pract* 2012;**18**:436–9)

Milnacipran (n=1, *Neurology* 2010;**74**:699–700; overdose, n=1, *J Med Toxicol* 2011;**7**:312–6; FFT)

Mirtazapine (n=1, *Rev Esp Anestesiol Reanim* 2009;**56**:515–6; n=1, *Clin Neuropharmacol* 2003;**26**:54–7)

Pethidine (n=1, *Br J Anaesth* 2009;**103**:369–70; FFT)

Phenelzine (n=1, *Case Rep Med* 2015; **2015**:931963; FFT)

Rasagiline (n=1, *Mov Disord* 2011;**26**:766–7)

Sibutramine (n=1, *Hum Exp Toxicol* 2012; **31**:414–7)

Sibutramine overdose (n=1, child, *Clin Toxicol [Phila]* 2009;**47**:598–601)

SSRIs, e.g.:

- →citalopram (n=1, *Kaohsiung J Med Sci* 2005;**21**:326–8; n=1, after a first-time low dose, *Neurotoxicology* 2007;**28**:1272–4; n=1, misdiagnosed as fibromyalgia, *Phys Ther* 2008;**88**:757–65; FFT)
- →escitalopram (n=1, restarted after five-day gap, *Neuropsychiatr Dis Treat* 2015;**11**:2505–7; FFT)
- →fluoxetine (several, e.g. n=1, *Psychopharmacol Bull* 2008;**41**:76–9; post-op in a secretive fluoxetine-user, n=1, *J Anaesthesiol Clin Pharmacol* 2011;**27**:233–5; FFT; n=1, breastfed neonate, *BMJ Case Rep* 2015;**2015**:bcr2015209418)
- →fluvoxamine (e.g. after single dose n=1, *Ann Emerg Med* 1999;**34**:806–7; mild syndrome may occur in 43% on fluvoxamine alone, n=37, *Int J Neurosci* 2001;**109**:165–72)
- →paroxetine (n=1, *Am J Ther* 2006;**13**:550–2; delayed effect, n=1, *Consult Pharm* 2009;**24**:64–8; OD n=1, fatal, *Psychosomatics* 2010;**51**:437–42)
- →sertraline (*J Clin Psychopharmacol* 2000;**20**:713–4; single 50mg dose in nine-year-old, *Clin Toxicol (Phila)* 2008;**46**:845–9; 25mg, n=1, *Seishin Shinkeigaku Zasshi* 2009;**111**:1041–6; overdose (n=1, *Arch Pediatr Adolesc Med* 1997;**151**:1064–7)

Suanzaorentang (*J Clin Psychopharmacol* 2008;**28**:113–4)

Tandospirone (n=1, *Rinsho Shinkeigaku* 2002;**42**:892–4)

Tramadol OD (n=1, *Pediatr Neurol* 2012;**46**:199)

Trazodone (*Int J Geriatr Psychiatry* 1997;**12**: 129–30)

Tricyclics e.g.:

- amitriptyline (n = 1, *Postgrad Med J* 2000;**76**:254–6; FFT)
- clomipramine (*J Clin Psychopharmacol* 1999;**19**:285–7; possible case after discontinuation of clozapine: n = 1, *Ann Pharmacother* 2001;**35**:180–2)
- dosulepin overdose (n = 1, *J Child Adolesc Psychopharmacol* 1998;**8**:201–4)

Venlafaxine (several e.g. n = 1, *Psychiatry Clin Neurosci* 2006;**60**:121–2; 37.5 mg/d, n = 1, *Ann Pharmacother* 2003;**37**:209–11)

Ziprasidone (n = 1, *Psychiatry Clin Neurosci* 2010;**64**:338–9)

- **Combinations, including SSRIs** *

A self-confessed expert in SS concludes that there is no evidence for serious SS with SSRIs and triptans, and that patients will be denied effective treatment if this combination is banned (Gillman, *Headache* 2010;**50**:264–72).

Amitriptyline + sertraline (*Ann Pharmacother* 1996;**30**: 1499–500)

Buspirone + citalopram (n = 1, *Int Clin Psychopharmacol* 1997;**12**:61–3)

Buspirone + fluoxetine (*Ann Pharmacother* 2000;**34**:871–4)

Buspirone + sertraline + loxapine (n = 1, *Therapie* 1999;**54**:269–71)

Bupropion + venlafaxine + sertraline (n = 1, *Clin Neuropharmacol* 2004;**27**:219–22)

Carbamazepine + fluoxetine (n = 1, *Lancet* 1993;**342**:442–3)

Clomipramine + sertraline (n = 1, *J Med Assoc Thai* 2005;**88**:993–6)

Cyclobenzaprine + escitalopram (n = 1, *Am J Emerg Med* 2008;**26**:1069)

Dextromethorphan + fluoxetine (n = 1, *Gen Hosp Psychiatry* 2006;**28**:78–80)

Dextromethorphan + SSRIs (supra-therapeutic dextromethorphan doses may be needed with an SSRI to create SS [n = 2, *Clin Toxicol (Phila)* 2008;**46**:771–3])

Dolasetron + sertraline (n = 1, *J Psychopharmacol* 2002;**16**:191)

Erythromycin + sertraline (n = 1, *Pharmacotherapy* 1999;**19**:894–6)

Fentanyl + SSRIs (n = 4538, symptom incidence 0.5%, full syndrome incidence 0.1%, *Pain Physician* 2015;**18**:E27–30)

Fluconazole + citalopram (n = 2, *Gen Hosp Psychiatry* 2008;**30**:372–7)

Hydromorphone + fluoxetine (n = 1, *Prescrire Int* 2004;**13**:57)

Indometacin + sertraline (n = 1, *J Clin Psychopharmacol* 2010;**30**:468–70)

Linezolid + citalopram (n = 1, *Ir J Med Sci* 2011;**180**:285–6; n = 1, *J Am Med Dir Assoc* 2004;**5**:111–3)

Linezolid + citalopram + mirtazapine (n = 1, *J Intensive Care Med* 2005;**20**:351–3)

Linezolid + citalopram + trazodone (n = 1, *Ann Pharmacother* 2005;**39**:956–61)

Linezolid + sertraline (n = 1, *Clin Infect Dis* 2002;**34**:1651–2; FFT; n = 1, *Pharmacotherapy* 2006;**26**:269–76)

Lithium + fluoxetine (n = 1, *Ugeskrift for Laeger* 1995;**157**:1204–5)

Lithium + paroxetine (n = 1, *Pharmacopsychiatry* 1997;**30**:106–7)

Metaxalone OD + escitalopram (n = 2, *Clin Toxicol [Phila]* 2015;**53**:185–7)

Methylene blue + citalopram (n = 1, *Med J Aust* 2008;**189**:534–5)

Methylene blue + paroxetine (n = 1, *Can J Anaesth* 2008;**55**:36–41)

Methylphenidate + paroxetine (n = 1, *Prog Neuropsychopharmacol Biol Psychiatry* 2010;**34**:719–20)

Methylphenidate + sertraline (n = 1, *Clin Neuropharmacol* 2015;**38**:65–6)

Metoclopramide + sertraline (n = 1, *Ann Pharmacother* 2002;**36**:67–71)

Miconazole + escitalopram (n = 1, *Int Psychogeriatr* 2012;**24**:845–7)

Mirtazapine + fluoxetine (*Int J Geriatr Psychiatry* 1998;**13**:495–6; n = 1, *Ann Pharmacother* 2001;**35**:1217–20)

Moclobemide + citalopram (*Med Clin [Barc]* 1999;**113**:677–8)

Moclobemide + citalopram overdose (many fatal e.g. n = 1, *Anaesthetist* 2006;**55**:1189–96; n = 1, *J Anal Toxicol* 2001;**25**:147–51; FFT)

Moclobemide + clomipramine + fluoxetine overdose (fatal case in *Anaesth Intensive Care* 1995;**23**:499–502)

Moclobemide + fluoxetine (e.g. *Pharmacopsychiatry* 1996;**29**:162; n = 1, *Can J Anaesth* 2000;**47**:246–50)

Moclobemide + fluoxetine overdose (n = 1,

5

Chang Gung Med 2011;**34**:644–9; FFT)
Moclobemide + paroxetine (n = 1, fatal, *J Anal Toxicol* 1997;**21**:518–20; FFT; *J Accid Emerg Med* 1999;**16**:293–5; FFT)
Moclobemide + paroxetine + selegiline (all low dose, n = 1, *J Chin Med Assoc* 2009;**72**:446–9)
Nefazodone + fluoxetine (n = 1, *J Clin Psychiatry* 2000;**61**:146)
Nefazodone + paroxetine (n = 1, *Ann Emerg Med* 1997;**29**:287–9)
OTC cold remedy + paroxetine (n=1, *Am J Emerg Med* 1994;**12**:642–4)
Oxcarbazepine + sertraline (n = 1, *Neurologist* 2012;**18**:204–5)
Oxycodone + citalopram (n = 1, *Case Rep Oncol Med* 2012;**2012**:261787; FFT)
Oxycodone + fluvoxamine (n = 1, *Ann Pharmacother* 2006;**40**:155–7)
Paroxetine + fluoxetine (n = 1, *Am Fam Physician* 1995;**52**:1475–82)
Pethidine + citalopram (n = 1, *Psychosomatics* 2007;**48**:361–3)
Pethidine + fluoxetine (n = 1, *Anesthesiology* 2003;**98**:1511–2)
Phenelzine + sertraline (n = 1, *Ann Pharmacother* 1994;**28**:732–5)
Quetiapine + citalopram (n = 1, *N Z Med J* 2006;**119**:2058)
Risperidone + paroxetine (*J Clin Psychopharmacol* 2000;**20**:103–5)
Risperidone + SSRI (n=2 [one fatal], *Ann Pharmacother* 2003;**37**:388–91)
Risperidone + trazodone + sertraline (n = 1, *CNS Spectr* 2007;**12**:596–8)
Selegiline + escitalopram (n = 1, *Indian J Pharmacol* 2010;**42**:418–9; FFT)
Sertraline + fluoxetine (n = 1, *Clin Pharmacol Ther* 1993;**1**:84–8)
St John's wort + citalopram (*Pharm J* 2007;**278**:487)
Tandospirone + fluvoxamine (n = 1, *Chudoku Kenkyu* 2011;**24**:305–10)
Tramadol + citalopram (n = 1, *Am J Psychiatry* 2004;**161**:1129; n = 1, *Am J Case Rep* 2014;**15**:562–4; FFT)
Tramadol + fluoxetine (n = 1, *J Royal Soc Med* 1999;**92**:474–5; FFT)
Tramadol + paroxetine (n = 1, *Int Clin Psychopharmacol* 1997;**12**:181–2)
Tramadol + sertraline (several e.g. n = 1, *Clin Neuropharmacol* 2004;**27**:150–1)
Tranylcypromine/trifluoperazine + fluoxetine (n = 1, *Anaesthesia* 1991;**46**:507–8)
Tranylcypromine + sertraline (n = 1, *Clin Pharm* 1993;**12**:222–5)
Tranylcypromine + tyramine + SSRI (n = 1, *Pharmacopsychiatry* 2010;**43**:284–5)
Trazodone + fluoxetine (*Biol Psychiatry* 1996;**39**:384–5)
Trazodone + paroxetine (*Psychosomatics* 1995;**36**:159–60)
Venlafaxine + fluoxetine (*Ann Pharmacother* 1998;**32**:432–6)

- **Combinations, including MAOIs/moclobemide (see also above) ***

Clomipramine + moclobemide (n = 1, *BMJ* 1993;**306**:248; FFT)
Clomipramine/moclobemide overdose (*Intensive Care Med* 1997;**23**:122–4; n=1, *J Toxicol Clin Toxicol* 1998;**36**:31–2)
Clomipramine + phenelzine (n = 1, *Clin Pharmacol Therap* 1993;**53**:84–8)
Cyclobenzaprine + phenelzine (n = 1, *Anesth Analg* 2006;**103**:1466–8)
Dextromethorphan + phenelzine (n = 1, *Clin Pharmacol Ther* 1993;**53**:84–8)
Modafinil + tranylcypromine (n = 1, *Am J Psychiatry* 2007;**164**:684)
Morphine + phenelzine (n = 1, *Pharmacotherapy* 2015;**35**:e102–5)
Quetiapine + phenelzine (n = 1, *CNS Spectr* 2007;**12**:596–8)
Pethidine + moclobemide (possible case, *Med J Aust* 1995;**162**:554)
Venlafaxine+ moclobemide overdose (n = 1, *Forensic Sci Int* 2009;**184**:16–20)
Venlafaxine + tranylcypromine (cases in *Vet Hum Toxicol* 1996;**38**:358–61; *Hum Exp Toxicol* 1997;**16**:14–7)

- **Other combinations (see also above) ***

Buprenorphine + naloxone (Suboxone® single dose, n = 1, *Am J Emerg Med* 2008;**26**:840)
Buspirone + linezolid (n = 1, *J Clin Pharm Ther* 2012;**37**:610–3)
Clomipramine + olanzapine (n = 1, *Minerva Anestesiol* 2008;**74**:41–5; FFT)
Dextromethorphan + chlorphenamine (n = 1, *Pediatr Emerg Care* 2007;**23**:829–31)
Duloxetine + cyclobenzaprine (n = 1, *Anesth Analg* 2006;**103**:1466–8)

Duloxetine + linezolid (n = 1, *J Clin Psychopharmacol* 2006;**26**:681–3)
Duloxetine + olanzapine, but only when olanzapine was discontinued (n = 1, *Pharmacopsychiatry* 2011;**44**:75–7)
ECT + bupropion/trazodone/quetiapine (n = 1, *Clin Neuropharmacol* 2015;**38**:112–3)
Fentanyl + 5HT3 antagonist (n = 1, *Psychosomatics* 2001;**42**:258–60)
Fentanyl + methadone (*Pharmacotherapy* 2015;**35**:112–7)
Fentanyl + trazodone/duloxetine (n = 1, *Case Rep Gastroenterol* 2015;**9**:132–6; FFT)
Fentanyl + ondansetron (n = 1, *J Clin Anesth* 2012;**24**:251–2)
Herbal detox cocktail (*Am J Emerg Med* 2004;**22**:625–6)
Lamotrigine + aripiprazole + cocaine (n = 1, *Case Rep Med* 2015;**2015**:769531; FFT)
Linezolid (shortly after stopping paroxetine, n = 1, *Clin Infect Dis* 2002;**34**:1651–2; FFT; review of cases, *Pharmacotherapy* 2006;**26**:1784–93)
Linezolid + pethidine (n = 1, *Clin Infect Dis* 2008;**46**:264–5; FFT; n = 1, *Farm Hosp* 2012;**36**:448–9)
Linezolid + tryptophan + metoclopramide (n = 1, *Med Intensiva* 2009;**33**:360–1; FFT)
MDPV (methylenedioxypyrovalerone, n = 1, *Ann Emerg Med* 2012;**60**:100–2)
Methylene blue (review, n = 25, *Psychosomatics* 2010;**51**:194–200)
Methylene blue + venlafaxine/trazodone (n = 1, *J Pharm Pract* 2015;**28**:207–11)
Metaxalone (n = 1, *Am J Emerg Med* 2015; in press)
Mirtazapine + tramadol + olanzapine (n = 1, *Am J Psychiatry* 2002;**159**:672–3)
Nortriptyline + selegiline (n = 1, *J Neurol* 2000;**247**:811)
St John's wort + buspirone (n = 1, *J Psychopharmacol* 2002;**16**:401)
Tramadol (review of SS; *Pain Physician* 2015;**18**:395–400; FFT)
Tramadol + venlafaxine + mirtazapine (n = 1, *Ann Pharmacother* 2004;**38**:411–3)
Tramadol abuse + sertraline/trazodone (n = 1, *Indian J Psychiatry* 2009;**51**:68; FFT)
Tramadol OD (n = 1, *Pediatr Neurol* 2011;**44**:72–4; n = 158, 5% incidence, *Clin Toxicol (Phila)* 2010;**48**:337–41)
Trazodone + amitriptyline (n = 1, *Int Clin Psychopharmacol* 1996;**11**:289–90)
Trazodone + nefazodone (n = 1, *Am J Psychiatry* 2000;**157**:1022)
Venlafaxine + amitriptyline (n = 1, *Postgrad Med J* 2000;**76**:254–6; FFT)
Venlafaxine + antiparkinsonian drugs (n = 1, *J Clin Psychopharmacol* 2010;**30**:620–2)
Venlafaxine + calcineurin inhibitors (e.g. tacrolimus, ciclosporin; n = 2, *Psychosomatics* 2011;**52**:286–90)
Venlafaxine + co-amoxiclav (n = 1, *J R Soc Med* 2003;**96**:233–4; FFT)
Venlafaxine + dexamfetamine (n = 1, *Med J Aust* 2002;**176**:240–1)
Venlafaxine + linezolid (n = 1, *J Antimicrob Chemother* 2004;**54**:289–90; FFT; n = 1, *Ann Pharmacother* 2005;**39**:956–61)
Venlafaxine + lithium + valproate (n = 1, *Therapie* 2006;**61**:531–3)
Venlafaxine + maprotiline + reboxetine (n = 1, *Eur Psychiatry* 2004;**19**:456–7)
Venlafaxine + methadone + ciprofloxacin (n = 1, *Psychosomatics* 2009;**50**:638–9)
Venlafaxine + metoclopramide (n = 1, *Ann Pharmacother* 2002;**36**:67–71)
Venlafaxine + mirtazapine (n = 1, *World J Biol Psychiatry* 2002;**3**:167; n = 1, well documented, *Int J Clin Pharm* 2012;**34**:686–8)
Venlafaxine + selegiline (n = 1, *J Clin Psychopharmacol* 1997;**17**:66–7)
Venlafaxine + sour date nut (n = 1, *Am J Psychiatry* 2004;**161**:1129–30)
Venlafaxine + St John's wort? (*Presse Med* 2000;**29**:1285–6)
Venlafaxine + trazodone (n = 1, *Am J Psychiatry* 2001;**158**:2088–9)

5.14 SLEEP PROBLEMS

5.14.1 SLEEP DISTURBANCES

Review: Foral *et al*, *Consult Pharm* 2011;**26**:414–25.

- CNS — sleep disorders and anxiety *

Lorazepam
Modafinil (SmPC)
Sodium oxybate (SmPC)
Zolpidem (hypnagogic, on temporary discontinuation, n = 1, *J Toxicol Clin Toxicol* 2003;**41**:869–72; sleep-walking, e.g. n = 1, *Indian J Psychol Med* 2015;**37**:105–6; FFT)

5

- **CNS — antipsychotics**

Chlorpromazine
Clozapine abrupt discontinuation (n = 1, *Eur Arch Psychiatry Clin Neurosci* 1996;**246**:79–82)
Olanzapine (somnambulism, n = 2, *Am J Psychiatry* 2001;**158**:1158)
Risperidone (sleep-related eating disorder, n = 1, *J Clin Psychiatry* 2004;**65**:273–4)
Sulpiride (SmPC, rare)

- **CNS — antidepressants**

Bupropion (incidence 11%)
Duloxetine (insomnia, BNF common)
MAOIs (hypersomnia, mainly with phenelzine tranylcypromine, *Am J Psychiatry* 1989;**146**:1078; n = 8, dose-related, *Am J Psychiatry* 1988;**145**:1552–6)
Mirtazapine (n = 1, *Br J Clin Pharmacol* 2009;**67**: 135–6; FFT)
SSRIs (all SSRIs can disrupt sleep architecture so are best taken in the morning, n = 14, RCT, *J Clin Psychiatry* 2001;**62**:642–52):
→fluoxetine
→paroxetine (somnambulism, n = 1, *J Clin Psychiatry* 2003;**64**:483)
Trazodone (suppresses REM, n = 8, *Psychopharmacology [Berl]* 1992;**107**:569–74)
Tricyclics

- **CNS — analgesics**

Nefopam (insomnia, SmPC less common)

- **CNS — anticonvulsants**

Lamotrigine (n = 109, incidence 6%, dose-related, *Epilepsia* 1999;**40**:322–5)
Levetiracetam (hypersomnia, n = 1, *Epilepsia* 2005;**46**:588–9)
Phenytoin (insomnia, SmPC)
Rufinamide (insomnia, incidence 1–10%, SmPC)

- **CNS — movement disorders**

Amantadine (4% incidence, *J Clin Psychiatry* 1981;**42**:344–5; *Rev Neurol* 1997;**25**:2062)
Biperiden discontinuation (n = 2, *Int Clin Psychopharmacol* 2000;**15**:357–9)
Bromocriptine
Pramipexole (n = 6, *Mov Disord* 2000;**15**:658–63; n = 40, 52% incidence of somnolence)
Ropinirole and/or pramipexole (n = 2, *Pharmacother* 2000;**20**:724–6)

- **CNS — others** *

Anticholinesterases:
→donepezil (n = 2, *J Am Geriatr Soc* 1998;**46**:119–20)
→rivastigmine (incidence < 5%)
Ginseng (common, *Drugs Exp Clin Res* 1996;**22**: 65–72)
Methylphenidate
Methysergide
Nicotine (n = 252, *J Clin Psychiatry* 2001;**62**:319–24)
Raltegravir (n = 2, *AIDS Patient Care STDS* 2009;**23**:689–90)
Sibutramine
Varenicline (n = 27 and review of WHO database, includes n = 17 abnormal dreams behaviour, *Sleep* 2015;**38**:833–7; FFT; slight increase in risk of insomnia, s = 39, n = 10761, RCTs, *BMJ* 2015;**350**:h1109; FFT)

- **Gastrointestinal drugs**

Bismuth toxicity (*Postgrad Med J* 1988;**64**: 308–10; FFT)
Propantheline
Ranitidine
Sulfasalazine

- **Cardiovascular drugs** *

Amiodarone (frequent, e.g. *Am J Cardiol* 1983;**52**:975–9)
Beta-blockers:
→atenolol (very common)
→carvedilol (n = 1, *Ann Pharmacother* 2002;**36**:1736–40)
→metoprolol low-dose (n = 1, *Gen Hosp Psychiatry* 2010;**32**:646.e5–7)
→propranolol (very common, *Adv Psychiatr Treat* 1999;**5**:30–8; sleep walking n = 1, *Can J Neurol Sci* 2014;**41**:787–8)
Calcium-channel blockers:
→diltiazem (see *Adv Psychiatr Treat* 1999;**5**:30–8)
→isradipine (up to 3%, *Am J Med* 1989;**86**[Suppl 4A]:98–102)
→nifedipine
Clonidine (for ADHD, *J Clin Psychopharmacol* 2008;**28**:725–6)
Digoxin
Statins (SmPCs), e.g.:
→lovastatin (*Lancet* 1994;**343**:973)

- **Respiratory drugs**

Aminophylline
Brompheniramine
Montelukast (FDA warning 2009)
Pseudoephedrine
Theophylline
Zafirlukast (FDA warning 2009)

- **Anti-infection drugs**

Cefalosporins
Chloroquine (*Presse Med* 1991;**20**:659)
Cinoxacin
Ciprofloxacin (n = 1, *Lancet* 1986;**1**:819–22)
Efavirenz (dose-related, *J Acquir Immune Defic Syndr* 2001;**28**:399–400)
Fleroxacin (n = 2, *Int Clin Psychopharmacol* 1994;**9**:295–6)
Ganciclovir
Griseofulvin
Interferon alfa (n = 86, insomnia often precedes depression, *Psychiatry Res* 2010;**177**:240–5; FFT)
Levofloxacin (n = 3, *J Neurosci Rural Pract* 2012;**3**:212–4; FFT)
Maraviroc (insomnia, common, SmPC)
Nitrofurantoin
Quinolones
Raltegravir (n = 1, severe insomnia, *AIDS* 2011;**25**:725–7)

- **Endocrine system drugs**

Clomifene
Corticosteroids (incidence may be as high as 5–6% in adults, usually emerges within a few days or weeks, risk may be higher with higher doses, *MHRA Drug Safety Update* 2007;1–9):
→ deflazacort (SmPC)
→ triamcinolone
Tolazamide

- **Malignancy and immunosuppressant drugs**

Review: chemotherapy and exacerbation of insomnia (Savard *et al*, *Cancer* 2015;**121**:1703–11).
Thalidomide cessation (n = 1, *Gastroenterology* 2001;**120**:1567–8)
Trabectedin (insomnia, common, SmPC)

- **Musculoskeletal and analgesics**

Diclofenac
Diflunisal
Etodolac (insomnia, SmPC)
Fenoprofen
Indometacin
Naproxen (*Eur J Rheumatol Inflamm* 1981;**4**:87–92)
Sulindac

- **Others**

Eculizumab (insomnia, uncommon, SmPC)
Mercury poisoning (n = 99, *Arq Neuropsiquiatr* 2000;**58**:32–8; FFT)
Sarin toxicity (n = 161, *Percept Mot Skills* 2005;**100**:1121–6)

5.14.2 VIVID DREAMS AND NIGHTMARES

A review noted that drugs affecting serotonin, noradrenaline and dopamine are clearly associated with reports of nightmares, and that immunological drugs and those affecting GABA, histamine and acetylcholine are also possible causative agents (Pagel and Helfter, *Hum Psychopharmacol* 2003;**18**:59–67).

Baclofen (SmPC, n = 10, RCT, d/b, p/c, c/o, *Eur Respir J* 1995;**8**:230–4; FFT)
Barbiturate withdrawal
Benzodiazepine withdrawal
Beta-blockers:
→ metoprolol low-dose (n = 1, *Gen Hosp Psychiatry* 2010;**32**:646.e5–7)
→ propranolol (*Adv Drug React Bull* 1983;**99**:364)
Ciprofloxacin (n = 1, *Indian J Psychiatry* 2008;**50**:305–6; FFT)
Clonidine (*Adv Drug React Bull* 1983;**99**:364)
Digoxin toxicity (*Ann Intern Med* 1980;**93**:639–40)
Famotidine (n = 1, *Pharmacother* 1998;**18**:404–7)
Galantamine (n = 1, nightmares, *J Am Geriatr Soc* 2009;**57**:565)
Indometacin (rare, n = 202, 2.5 years, incidence 0.5%, *Br Med J* 1965;**2**:1281–4)
Mirtazapine (SmPC at < 1 in 10,000; causing psychosis, n = 1, *Pharmacotherapy* 2010;**30**:145e–50e)
Nalbumetone (*Pharm J* 1990;**244**:764)
Nicotine patches (*Pharm J* 1992;**249**:384)
Opiate withdrawal
Paroxetine (n = 1, *Psychogeriatrics* 2012;**12**:54–7)

5

Pergolide (e.g. *Clin Neuropharmacol* 1986;**9**: 160–4)
Rivastigmine (REM sleep behaviour disorder, n = 1, *J Clin Sleep Med* 2010;**6**:192–5; FFT)
SSRI discontinuation (see *C2*)
Verapamil (*N Engl J Med* 1988;**318**:929–30)
Withdrawal from barbiturates, benzodiazepines, narcotics, etc

5.15 SUICIDAL IDEATION (SEE ALSO DEPRESSION)

Although suicidal ideation is not the same as actual suicide, more suicidal ideation is associated with more suicide attempts and completions (1,404,470 reports on 832 drugs, Robertson and Allison, *PLoS One* 2009;**4**:e7312). For example, up to 8.8% of 10–24-year-olds considered or attempted suicide in 2002, whereas the actual suicide rate was 0.0028% (Seemüller *et al*, *Acta Psychiatr Scand* 2009;**119**:166–7; reply by Castelpietra). **Review:** The European Psychiatric Association (EPA) guidance on suicide treatment and prevention (Wasserman *et al*, *Eur Psychiatry* 2012;**27**:129–41).

- **CNS — sleep disorders and anxiety**

Insomnia is an independent predictor of suicidal ideation in depression, so needs treating (n = 60, RCT, d/b, 9/52, *Sleep Med* 2010;**11**:822–7; FFT). Untreated anxiety disorders are also associated with increased suicide attempts, e.g. PTSD (AOR = 1.81) and panic (AOR = 1.3) increases the risk by 50%, and comorbid panic and personality disorder increase the risk to AOR = 5.76 (n = 34,653, Nepon *et al*, *Depress Anxiety* 2010;**27**:791–8; FFT).
Benzodiazepines (n = 1, *Br J Gen Pract* 2007;**57**:407–9; FFT):
→ alprazolam (caution in SmPC, n = 1, *Prim Care Companion J Clin Psychiatry* 2011;**12**:PCC.09l00865; FFT)
→ chlordiazepoxide (SmPC)
Modafinil (SmPC; BNF rare)
Sodium oxybate (SmPC; BNF less common; n = 1, *J Neuropsychiatry Clin Neurosci* 2010;**22**:352r)
Zaleplon (BNF caution)
Zolpidem (SmPC)

- **CNS — antipsychotics (including lithium)**

Antipsychotics can cause akathisia, with the associated risk of suicide (review, *Pharmacopsychiatry* 2012;**45**:292–6).
Aripiprazole (BNF very rare, SmPC states no increased risk of suicidality in bipolar disorder; n = 20,489, in schizophrenia, *Pharmacoepidemiol Drug Saf* 2010;**19**:1124–30; may actually be a reduced suicide rate as an adjunct in MDD, s = 2, n = 737, RCT, d/b, p/c, *J Clin Psychiatry* 2011;**72**:548–55; n = 1, *Am J Psychiatry* 2010;**167**:1535–6)
Asenapine (n = 2, *J Clin Psychopharmacol* 2011;**31**:534–5)
Clozapine (n = 1, dose-dependent, *Psychopharmacol Bull* 2011;**44**:65–9)
Flupentixol (SmPC; BNF)
Lithium (anti-suicide effect shown in numerous studies, see *Chapter 1* under Bipolar maintenance for the full review)
Ziprasidone (analysis of all valid trials shows only 52 events (1%), no completed suicides, and no difference to placebo, s = 22, n = 5,123, d/b, p/c, *J Clin Psychiatry* 2011;**72**:367–75; MS)

- **CNS — antidepressants**

Bupropion – no statistical difference cf. placebo (n = 15,473, *Prim Care Companion J Clin Psychiatry* 2010;**12**:09100894; FFT)
Duloxetine (SmPC; BNF rare; case series, *J Clin Psychopharmacol* 2008;**28**:101–2; n = 2, *Clin Pract Epidemiol Ment Health* 2008;**4**:18; FFT)
MAOIs:
→ isocarboxazid (SmPC; BNF in susceptible persons)
→ phenelzine (SmPC; BNF in susceptible persons)
Mirtazapine (SmPC; BNF rare; associated with statistically significantly lower suicide risk cf. placebo: s = 15, RCT, d/b, p/c, *World J Biol Psychiatry* 2010;**11**:36–44)
Moclobemide (SmPC)
SSRIs:
→ citalopram (SmPC, may be genetic link; incidence 8.6%, n = 1,447, *Arch Gen Psychiatry* 2007;**64**:689–97; n = 1,915, incidence 6%, 14/12, *Am J Psychiatry* 2007;**164**:1530–8)
→ escitalopram (SmPC; lower than with nortriptyline, n = 811, RCT, open, 12/52, *BMC Med* 2009;**7**:60; FFT; n = 1, but not

with five previous antidepressants; *Indian J Psychol Med* 2011;**33**:74–6; FFT)

→fluoxetine (SmPC; two analyses of FDA databases show no increase in the risk of treatment-emergent suicide with fluoxetine for MDD [s=18, n=3,751, *J Clin Psychopharmacol* 2007;**27**:682–6], or for non-MDD conditions [s=53, n=11,448, d/b, p/c, *Psychol Med* 2007;**37**:1585–93]. Reanalysis of all known relevant RCTs showed reduced suicidal thoughts and behaviour with fluoxetine or venlafaxine in adult and older people and no change in youths; [s=41, n=9,185, RCT, *Arch Gen Psychiatry* 2012;**69**:580–7; FFT]. Older data had suggested a possible problem [n=6, *Am J Psychiatry* 1990;**147**:1570–1])

→fluvoxamine

→paroxetine (SmPC, may be higher than reported, *BMC Psychiatry* 2006;**6**:55; FFT)

→paroxetine discontinuation (overall incidence of suicidal behaviour with paroxetine is the same as placebo but higher in adults <30 years old (s=57, n=14,911, p/c, *J Affect Disord* 2010;**120**:40–7; A meta-analysis of all known RCTs of treatment-emergent suicidality with paroxetine showed similar suicidality to placebo except in young adults, as with other antidepressants [s=61, n=14,911, *J Clin Psychiatry* 2011;**72**:1503–14; MS])

→sertraline (SmPC, but a meta-analysis showed that the 0.04% incidence of suicides with sertraline [n=4 from n=10,917] was similar to 0.03% with placebo [n=3 from n=9,006], s=126, n=19,923, d/b, p/c, *J Clin Psychiatry* 2009;**70**:674–83)

Reboxetine (SmPC; BNF rare)

Trazodone (SmPC)

Tricyclics:

→clomipramine (SmPC)

→lofepramine (SmPC)

→nortriptyline (SmPC)

→trimipramine (SmPC)

Tryptophan (SmPC; BNF)

Venlafaxine (SmPC; BNF very rare; has higher suicide rate than citalopram, fluoxetine and dosulepin, but there may be confounding factors, e.g. use in more severe MDD might explain this; n=219,088, *BMJ* 2007;**334**:242; FFT; reanalysis of all known relevant RCTs shows reduced suicidal thoughts and behaviour with fluoxetine or venlafaxine in adults and older people and with no change in youths, s=41, n=9,185, RCT, *Arch Gen Psychiatry* 2012;**69**:580–7; FFT)

• CNS — analgesics

Dihydrocodeine (SmPC)

Paracetamol

Tramadol (FDA warning 2010)

Ziconotide (SmPC, uncommon; IT, n=2, *Pain* 2011;**152**:235–7)

• CNS — anticonvulsants *

A meta-analysis claimed that an astonishing 32.5% of all deaths of people with epilepsy are from suicide and 13.5% of all registered suicides are committed by epileptics, so suicide in epilepsy appears to be disturbingly frequent (s=30, n=51,216, Pompili *et al*, *Epilepsy Behav* 2006;**9**:641–8). The BNF states that AEDs are associated with a small increase in risk of suicidal thoughts and behaviour, sometimes as soon as a week after starting, but there is no convincing evidence of a class effects (*Harv Rev Psychiatry* 2014;**22**:379–81) and the data is contradictory:

- Levetiracetam, tiagabine and topiramate use may lead to a 3-fold increase in suicidal behaviour, but not with older AEDs (n=9,415, *Neurology* 2010;**75**:335–40)
- Clonazepam, valproate, lamotrigine, phenobarbital seem to double the suicide risk, but only for a relatively short time after initiation (n=6,780, Olesen *et al*, *Pharmacoepidemiol Drug Saf* 2010;**19**:518–24)
- Compared to carbamazepine and topiramate, increased suicidal acts may occur with gabapentin (HR=1.42), lamotrigine (HR=1.84), oxcarbazepine (HR=2.07), tiagabine (HR=2.41) and possibly valproate (HR=1.65) (n=29,620, <180/7, *JAMA* 2010;**303**:1401–9), but:
  →there was no increase in suicide-related events in people with epilepsy or bipolar taking AEDs, but this *was* increased in people with depression taking AEDs and those taking AEDs but not having epilepsy, depression or bipolar (n=5,130,795,

5

Arana *et al, N Engl J Med* 2010;**363**:542–51; FFT), and AEDs do not cause suicidal ideation when psychiatric comorbidity and other factors are taken into account (n=131, *Seizure* 2011;**20**:280–4; FFT)

→ Consistent taking of AEDs is associated with a substantial reduction in risk of suicidal ideation (cf. lithium (n=16,645, *J Affect Disord* 2009;**117**:162–7)

→ The increase in suicidality with AEDs in epilepsy may be disease rather than AED-related (and may actually be protective in bipolars; n=47,918, *Arch Gen Psychiatry* 2009;**66**:1354–60; FFT).

CNS — antidepressants, including bupropion

The stats:

- **Depression is a risk factor for suicide:** Suicide practically does not occur without the presence of mental health problems, most commonly depression, then alcoholism.
- **Suicidal ideation is not necessarily the same as actual suicide or suicide attempt.**
- **The absolute risk of suicide during acute antidepressant treatment is about one in 3,000**, and serious suicide attempts is one in 1,000, with no evidence of a statistically significant increase in suicide or ideation in the first four weeks with newer antidepressants (n=65,103, Simon *et al, Am J Psychiatry* 2006;**163**:41–7).
- **Any suicidal ideation with antidepressants may have several causes:** e.g. increasing motivation, short-term akathisia and misdiagnosis of bipolar depression. Risk factors include drug abuse, severe MDD, melancholic features and younger age (n=1,090, Zisook *et al, J Affect Disord* 2009;**117**:63–73).
- **The risk with SSRIs is slightly increased in adolescents,** reduced in adults and much reduced in older adults (s=8, n>200,000, WHO systematic review, Barbui *et al, CMAJ* 2009;**180**:291–7; FFT; s=372, n=99,231, Stone *et al, BMJ* 2009;**339**:b2880; FFT):

Age	Suicidal behaviour	Suicidal ideation
<25	Increased (OR 2.3)	Increased (OR 1.6)
25–64	No significant change (OR 0.87)	Marginal reduced (OR 0.79)
>64	Decreased (OR 0.06)	Decreased (OR 0.37)

- **The risk in children and adolescents is in the first few weeks**: (meta-analysis, s=16, n=2,741, RCTs, Dubicka *et al, Br J Psychiatry* 2006;**189**:393–8; FFT), peaking at 3/52 and predicted by high baseline suicidal ideation, family conflict, and drug and alcohol use; the median time to non-suicidal event was 2/52, predicted by previous history of non-suicidal self-injury and venlafaxine (n=334, Brent *et al, Am J Psychiatry* 2009;**166**:418–26; FFT).
- **Antidepressants can cause akathisia** (see 5.8.2) and anxiety/jitteriness, but this is poorly defined and unproven (s=107, Sinclair *et al, Br J Psychiatry* 2009;**194**:483–90; FFT).

The case against antidepressants causing suicide:

- An analysis of all FDA trials for nine antidepressants was unable to find any link with increased suicide from any antidepressants compared to placebo (n=49,277; 77 suicides, Khan *et al, Am J Psychiatry* 2003;**160**:790–2).
- A meta-analysis of SSRIs showed no increased risk of suicide in adults (s=477, n=>40,000, RCTs, p/c, Gunnell *et al, Br Med J* 2005;**330**:385; FFT; see also n=146,095, Martinez *et al, Br Med J* 2005;**330**:389 FFT).
- Data from 29 European countries (1980–2009) shows an increased correlation between prescribing and suicide in all countries except Portugal (Gusmao *et al, PLoS One* 2013; **8**:e66455; FFT).

CNS — antidepressants, including bupropion (*continued*)

- In Denmark, the suicide rate (1995–1999) dropped, particularly in people treated with SSRIs or older antidepressants (n=438,625), compared to those not treated with antidepressants (n=1,199,057) (Søndergård *et al, Acta Psychiatr Scand* 2006;**114**:168–76).
- Improving diagnosis and treatment of MDD in Sweden (1995–2002) led to increased antidepressant use and decreased suicides (Henriksson and Isacsson, *Acta Psychiatr Scand* 2006;**114**:159–67).
- FDA and EMA warning (2003–6) led to a reduction in SSRI use in the under 19s in the Netherlands (22%) and USA (30%). This resulted in an increase in suicides in the Netherlands (49%, from 0.86 to 1.28 per 100,000 population) and USA (14%, from 2.83 to 3.23 per 100,000 population), an abrupt reversal of 20-year trends (Gibbons *et al, Am J Psychiatry* 2007;**164**:1356–63; see also n=943,313, Libby *et al, Arch Gen Psychiatry* 2009;**66**:633–9; disputed by Wheeler *et al, BMJ* 2008;**336**:542–5; FFT).
- For every extra DDD of antidepressant used per 1,000 population in Japan, the suicide rate reduced by 6% (Nakagawa *et al, J Clin Psychiatry* 2007;**68**:908–16; FFT).
- A Swedish study of suicides concluded the only explanation for the findings is that antidepressants reduce suicide (n=18,922 suicides, Isacsson *et al, Acta Psychiatr Scand* 2010;**122**:454–60).
- Of n=142,090 people in Germany prescribed antidepressants, there were only 33 (0.02%, 1 in 4,300) cases of suicide (14 probably antidepressant-related, 19 possibly) with 23 associated with akathisia (Stübner *et al, J Clin Psychiatry* 2010;**71**:1293–307).

Minimising the potential for antidepressants to cause suicidal ideation:

- **Be alert for bipolar depression presenting as unipolar depression, especially in the under-25s:** The increase in younger people may be because bipolar disorder is often (as yet) undiagnosed in younger people, and antidepressants without mood stabilisers may promote mixed states and hence suicidal ideation, although the actual antidepressant used seems to make no difference (n=20,906 on antidepressants, nine years, Schneeweiss *et al, Pediatrics* 2010;**125**:876–88; FFT), except venlafaxine (n=334, Brent *et al, Am J Psychiatry* 2009;**166**:418–26; FFT).
- **Avoid antidepressants toxic in overdose:** SSRIs and other newer agents have low toxicity in overdose but tricyclics and MAOIs can be toxic in overdose (seven years, Hawton *et al, Br J Psychiatry* 2010;**196**:354–8; FFT; n=287,543 adults on antidepressants, nine years, Schneeweiss *et al, Arch Gen Psychiatry* 2010;**67**:497–506; FFT).
- **Start antidepressants slowly,** especially in adolescents: there is a higher risk on initiation (OR=3.42) and dose titration (up OR=2.62; down OR=2.19) (n=52,261, Valuck *et al, J Clin Psychiatry* 2009;**70**:1069–77).
- **Take care early in treatment** and monitor for akathisia and agitation.
- **Avoid polypharmacy:** Three or more psychotropics from different classes may increase the risks (n=318, Fontanella *et al, Ann Pharmacother* 2009:**43**:1939–47).
- **Treat any insomnia:** see CNS — anxiolytics and hypnotics. SSRIs can disrupt sleep architecture so must be taken with breakfast.
- **Ensure antidepressants are not stopped prematurely or too abruptly:** Discontinuation (esp. within first 56 days) shows a slightly increased risk (OR=1.61) (n=52,261, Valuck *et al, J Clin Psychiatry* 2009;**70**:1069–77).
- **Not using antidepressants has its own risk:** People with MDD who have committed suicide have seldom been treated with antidepressants. If depression improves, suicidal ideation reduces (n=1,693, Olfson and Marcus, *J Clin Psychiatry* 2008;**69**:425–32).

5

Reviews: Mula *et al*, *Curr Neurol Neurosci Rep* 2010;**10**:327–32; n=163, *Epilepsy Behav* 2010;**19**;494–500.

Barbiturates (BNF uncommon)
Benzodiazepines, e.g.:
→ clobazam (SmPC, especially in elderly or children)
→ clonazepam, diazepam, flurazepam, loprazolam, lorazepam, midazolam, nitrazepam, temazepam (SmPC; BNF rare)
Carbamazepine (suicidality, FDA warning 2008)
Ethosuximide (SmPC)
Felbamate (suicidality, FDA warning 2008)
Gabapentin (BNF, uncommon; suicidality, FDA warning 2008; a pharmacoepidemiological study concluded that gabapentin reduced the risk of suicide attempts in people with psychiatric disorders [n=131,178, Gibbons *et al*, *Pharmacoepidemiol Drug Saf* 2010:**19**:1241–7; FFT], but another guarded appraisal came to the opposite conclusion [Ziemba *et al*, *Neurologist* 2010;**16**:325–8])
Lacosamide (SmPC)
Lamotrigine (suicidality, FDA warning 2008)
Levetiracetam (suicidality, FDA warning 2008; SmPC; BNF rare; n=1, *Epilepsy Behav Case Rep* 2015;**4**:79–81; FFT)
Oxcarbazepine (SmPC, FDA warning 2008)
Phenytoin (SmPC)
Pregabalin (FDA warning; SmPC addition; *Pharmacopsychiatry* 2011;**44**:119)
Rufinamide (as adjunct in bipolar, n=2, *Epilepsy Behav* 2011;**20**:386–9)
Tiagabine (suicidality, FDA warning 2008; SmPC)
Topiramate (SmPC; BNF less common, FDA warning 2008)
Valproate (SmPC addition, FDA warning 2008; but a large review showed no increased risk of suicide in a range of indications, s=13, n=1,327, p/c, *Ann Gen Psychiatry* 2011;**10**:1: FFT; the effect may vary according to indication, e.g. in bipolar, valproate may show similar suicidal ideation to lithium, and both are much less than with SGAs and than with no maintenance medication (n=1,306, Ahearn *et al*, *J Affect Disord* 2013;**145**:77–82; FFT)
Vigabatrin (BNF rare)
Zonisamide (SmPC; BNF less common, FDA warning 2008)
Zonisamide OD (n=1, *Epilepsy Behav* 2011;**21**:91–3)

- **CNS — movement disorders**

Levodopa (SmPC; BNF very rare)

- **CNS — others** *

Acamprosate (mentioned SmPC)
Alcohol (risk of suicide is primarily associated with the quantity of alcohol consumed per drinking day, but not with drinking frequency or overall alcohol consumption; n=47,654, *Soc Psychiatry Psychiatr Epidemiol* 2007;**42**:153–60)
Atomoxetine (SmPC; BNF less common, n=1, *J Paediatr Child Health* 2008;**44**:596–8)
Caffeine (in bipolars, high coffee consumption is significantly associated [OR 1.79] with suicidal acts; n=352, *Bipolar Disorder* 2009;**11**:494–503; from popular energy drink as consequence of sleep deprivation, n=1, *J Psychopharmacol* 2012;**26**:1502–10)
Cannabis (young users may possibly be more at risk, n=2,033, *Acta Psychiatr Scand* 2008;**118**:395–403; n=1, *Case Rep Med* 2009;**2009**:321456; FFT)
Disulfiram (SmPC)
Galantamine (SmPC, very rare)
Memantine (association, SmPC; BNF very rare)
Methylphenidate (SmPC; BNF less common; n=1, *Prim Care Companion CNS Disorder* 2015;**17**:17; FFT)
Naltrexone (BNF rare)
Nicotine dependence (n=34,653, OR 1.7, but drops to 0.15 on stopping, *Can J Psychiatry* 2011;**56**:161–70; high nicotine consumption is significantly associated [OR 2.42] with suicidal acts in bipolar people [n=352, *Bipolar Disorder* 2009;**11**:494–503] and in adolescent females [OR 4.7, n=508, *Compr Psychiatry* 2009;**50**:293–8])
Sibutramine (SmPC)
Varenicline (SmPC; BNF less common; large review concludes no effect, s=39, n=10761, RCTs, *BMJ* 2015;**350**:h1109; FFT; FDA review, *PLoS One* 2011;**6**:e27016; FFT; s=15, n=4443, *Cochrane Database Syst Rev* 2012;**4**:CD006103; no association, n=80,660, *BMJ* 2009;**339**:b3805; FFT; current depressive symptoms is highest predictor of suicidal ideation, n=72, 18/12,

retrospective, *Am J Addict* 2012;**21**:356–62)

- Cardiovascular drugs

ACE inhibitors (a review showed no additional risk of suicidal ideation with ACE inhibitors, n=58,529, *Br J Clin Pharmacol* 2001;**52**:313–8; FFT; n=743, *Eur J Clin Pharmacol* 2007;**63**:591–6)

Beta-blockers (a review showed medium and high lipid-soluble beta-blockers may be associated with an increased risk of suicide, n=58,529, *Br J Clin Pharmacol* 2001;**52**:313–8; FFT; but another study showed no increased risk; n=743, *Eur J Clin Pharmacol* 2007;**63**:591–6)

Calcium-channel blockers (reviews have shown no additional risk of suicidal ideation, n=58,529, *Br J Clin Pharmacol* 2001;**52**:313–8; FFT; n=743, *Eur J Clin Pharmacol* 2007;**63**:591–6; n=153,458, *BMJ* 2000;**320**:1251; FFT)

Omega-3 fatty acids (low plasma levels may be a risk factor for suicide or depression: *Am J Psychiatry* 2006;**163**:1100–2)

Statins — there is conflicting evidence as to whether low cholesterol is associated with an increased risk of suicidal ideation. Most data points out that the risk might actually be lower (n=2,813, *Arch Intern Med* 2003;**163**:1926–32; see also n=930, *J Clin Psychiatry* 2008;**69**:1920–7; high lipid levels are not linked to suicide risk in bipolar patients, n=220, *Prog Neuropsychopharmacol Biol Psychiatry* 2012;**37**:136–40), although some suggest the risk might be higher with low cholesterol (n=3,207, both genders, but no relationship with triglycerides so not due to malnutrition, *J Affect Disord* 2011;**133**:234–8). However, increased dietary intake may reduce impulsive and aggressive behaviours (*Pharmacopsychiatry* 2002;**35**:1–5) and there may be a high risk of violent suicide with high cholesterol (n=37,635, *Am J Psychiatry* 2000;**157**:648–50). Statins themselves have also been implicated (MHRA warning, *Drug Safety Update* 2008;**1**:10), e.g.:

→ atorvastatin (LDL cholesterol levels are not associated with increased suicide, n=10,001, *Am J Cardiol* 2007;**100**:747–52)

→ simvastatin (*Curr Problems* 1992;33: n=4, *Lancet* 1993;**341**:114)

- Respiratory drugs

Montelukast (FDA change 2009; SmPC, rare; BNF very rare; s=116, n=20,131 on montelukast, 17,633 controls, no completed suicides, only one suicidal ideation, and no evidence of a problem (*J Allergy Clin Immunol* 2009;**124**:691–6). A nested case control concluded no increased risk of suicidal ideation in people aged 5–24 with montelukast or zafirlukast (n=3,782, *J Allergy Clin Immunol* 2012;**130**:368–75)

Zafirlukast (see above)

- Anti-infection drugs

Antiretrovirals — multiple switching of agents is associated with higher distress and suicide than single or non-switchers in ART therapy (n=779, *Int J STD AIDS* 2007;**18**:700–4):

→ disoproxil (SmPC; BNF less common)

→ efavirenz (SmPC; BNF less common; not associated with increased suicide risk, n=355, 48/52, *Clin Infect Dis* 2006;**42**:1790–9; FFT)

→ emtricitabine (SmPC; BNF less common)

→ tenofovir (SmPC; BNF less common)

Ciprofloxacin (n=1, *Gen Hosp Psychiatry* 2011;**33**:82.e5–7)

Cycloserine (SmPC, psychosis with suicidal tendencies)

Fluoroquinolone (n=1, *Gen Hosp Psychiatry* 2010;**32**:108–10; n=1, *Psychosomatics* 2012;**53**:97–8)

Levofloxacin (SmPC, very rare)

Mefloquine (SmPC, rare; BNF rare; n=1, *Presse Med* 2006;**35**:789–92; n=1, successful, *Am J Forensic Med Pathol* 2010;**31**:378–81)

Ofloxacin (SmPC, very rare)

Ribavirin (SmPC; BNF oral, more common in children)

Ribavirin + interferon alfa-2a (n=1, *Indian J Pharmacol* 2011;**43**:210–1; FFT)

- Endocrine system drugs

Glucocorticoids (incidence 15.7 events per 100 person-years for all oral glucocorticoid courses cf. no glucocorticoid; sub-divided as 22.2 for first course, 14 for second courses, and 11.7 per 100 for third or fourth; more likely with higher doses and prior history, n=372,696, Fardet *et al*, *Am J Psychiatry* 2012;**169**:491–7)

Levothyroxine (n=1, *Sao Paulo Med J* 2009;**127**:317–8; FFT)

Systemic corticosteroids (SmPC; BNF especially high doses and during discontinuation):
- → beclomethasone (SmPC, BNF, as above)
- → cortisone (SmPC, BNF, as above)
- → deflazacort (SmPC, BNF, as above)
- → dexamethasone (SmPC, BNF, as above)
- → fludrocortisone (SmPC, BNF, as above)
- → hydrocortisone (SmPC, BNF, as above)
- → methylprednisolone (SmPC, BNF, as above)
- → prednisolone (SmPC, BNF, as above)
- → testosterone (an earlier study showed lack of clear association between high levels and suicide attempts, n=149, *Neuropsychobiology* 2011;**63**:125–30; FFT; but another suggests levels positively correlate with number of manic episodes and suicide attempts, n=67, *J Psychiatr Res* 2012;**46**:1267–71; FFT)
- → triamcinolone (SmPC, BNF as above)

• Malignancy and immunosuppressant drugs

Aldesleukin (suicide, n=1, *J Am Osteopath Assoc* 1993;**93**:799–800)

Interferons:
- → interferon alfa
- → interferon alfa + ribavirin (n=1, *Psychosomatics* 2009;**50**:538–42)
- → interferon beta-1a and 1b (n=11, *Clin Neuropharmacol* 2010;**33**:312–6)
- → interferon beta (n=11, *Clin Neuropharmacol* 2010;**33**:312–6)
- → peginterferon alfa (SmPC; BNF uncommon, contraindication for some in severe depression or suicidal ideation)

• Musculoskeletal and analgesics

Infliximab (n=1, *J Crohns Colitis* 2010;**4**:591–3)

• Others

Alitretinoin (SmPC, very rare)

Baclofen (SmPC)

Isotretinoin (SmPC; BNF rare; n=5,756, mean 15-year follow-up; 1.57 x increased risk for all attempts including repeat attempts, 1.36 x risk of first attempts occurring during treatment, and for 6/12 after treatment finishes (Sundström *et al*, *BMJ* 2010;**341**:c5812; FFT); prospective study showed that in fact depressive symptoms declined with isotretinoin and were not associated with treatment-emergent depression or suicidal ideation among young men, although idiosyncratic reactions could not be excluded (n=135 [c=126], 12/52, *J Eur Acad Dermatol Venereol* 2009;**23**:1294–7); retrospective chart review, no cases reported (n=1,743, *Australas J Dermatol* 2010;**51**:248–53); n=30,496, statistically significant association, (*J Clin Psychiatry* 2008;**69**:526–32); incidence 30% in bipolar patients (n=300, *J Affect Disord* 2010;**122**:306–8)

6 MANAGEMENT OF SIDE-EFFECTS

Contents

6.1 Anticholinergic and related side-effects 505
~ blurred vision 505
~ constipation 505
~ dry mouth 505
~ urinary retention 506
~ urinary hesitancy 506
~ urinary incontinence 506
6.2 Blood disorders 506
~ bleeding 506
~ blood dyscrasias; neutropenia, aganulocytosis 506
~ eosinophilia 507
6.3 Cardiac effects 507
~ hypertension 507
~ hypotension 507
~ myocarditis 508
~ postural hypotension 508
~ QTc prolongation 508
~ tachycardia 509
6.4 Central adverse effects 509
~ abnormal dreams 509
~ anorexia 509
~ ataxia 509
~ delirium 509
~ drowsiness 510
~ dysphoria 510
~ fatigue 510
· hypomania 511
~ insomnia 511
~ irritability, jitteriness or agitation 511
~ nausea 512
~ nocturnal enuresis 512
~ OCD 513
~ psychosis 513
~ sedation 513
~ seizures 513
6.5 Dermatological effects 514
~ acne 514
~ alopecia and hair loss 514
~ Darier's disease 515
~ exfoliative dermatitis 515
~ folliculitis 515
~ maculopapular eruption 515
~ photosensitivity 515
~ pigmentation 515
~ psoriasis 516
~ rash 516
~ seborrheic dermatitis 519
~ sweating 519
6.6 Endocrine effects 519
~ diabetes insipidus 519
~ diabetes mellitus 520
~ hepatotoxicity 520
~ hyperammonaemia 520
~ hypercalcaemia 521
~ hypercholesterolaemia 521
~ hyperglycaemia 521
~ hyperlipidaemia 521
~ hyperprolactinaemia 522
~ hyperthyroidism 524
~ hyponatraemia 524
~ hypothyroidism 525
~ polyuria and renal impairment 526
~ weight gain 526
6.7 Movement disorders 533
~ blepharospasm 533
~ bruxism 533
~ dysphagia 534
~ EPSE, akathisia 534
~ EPSE, dyskinesias 536
~ EPSE, Parkinsonism 538
~ EPSE, dystonia 539
~ laryngospasm 540
~ myoclonus 540
~ Pisa syndrome 541
~ restless legs 541
6.8 Neuroleptic malignant syndrome 542
~ neuroleptic rechallenge 542
6.9 Serotonin syndrome 544
~ Sternbach's diagnostic criteria 544
6.10 Sexual side-effects 544
~ libido 547
~ arousal 547

6

~ anorgasmia 548
~ ejaculation problems 550
~ priapism 551
6.11 Others, side-effects 551
~ gastric irritation or nausea 551
~ glaucoma 551
~ hypersalivation 551
~ incontinence 551
~ jaundice 552
~ mastalgia 552
~ megaloblastic anaemia 552
~ oedema 552
~ osteopenia 552
~ osteoporosis 552
~ pain at site of injection 552
~ raised LFTs 552
~ sialorrhoea 552
~ tremor 554
~ vomiting 554

All drugs have side-effects, which may range from being mild and transient to being intolerable or life-threatening. If switching from, or discontinuing, the causative agent is not clinically possible (e.g. patient preference, clinical response, risk of consequences of relapse), managing adverse effects may allow continued treatment, improved compliance and lead to better outcomes.

STANDARD STRATEGIES TO TRY FIRST INCLUDE:

- Drug — alter formulation (i.e. SR/MR, liquid, injection).
- Dose — adjust total daily dose (increasing rarely works, but a systematic and gradual decrease can be tried to determine the minimum effective dose).
- Dose — manipulate frequency and timings (e.g. split, or load to one particular time).
- Dose — consider drug holiday (e.g. omitting doses on particular days, although this is likely only to be helpful for some specific ADRs).
- Dose — consider slower dose escalation (including stopping and restarting more gently), particularly with buspirone, many tricyclics and SSRIs.
- Monitor plasma levels to optimise the dose if possible, e.g. tricyclic ADRs are clearly correlated with plasma levels.
- Switch to a drug from the same or a different chemical group.
- Discontinue completely.
- Discontinue any concurrent drugs that might be interacting.
- Wait for the side-effect to wear off, or at least to become more tolerable.
- Initiate adjunctive therapies (additional drugs, physical management strategies).

All of these routine strategies may be of some importance and relevance for each side-effect. This chapter comments on some of the above, along with additional strategies. Data in this area of therapy is notably sparse, and the author would be grateful for any additional ideas.

Disclaimers:

- Drug doses are quoted as total daily doses but many may benefit from divided doses.
- Drugs and strategies are not necessarily in any particular order within each section, and are in alphabetical order where possible.

6.1 Anticholinergic and related side-effects

Anticholinergic, blurred vision

Antidepressants	**Switch** to an antidepressant with less anticholinergic side-effects (see 2.1.2). Beware of glaucoma developing (see 3.5). **Bethanechol** 30–90 mg/d may be effective but is often poorly tolerated. **Pilocarpine** 1% drops QDS may restore pupilary responsiveness and has been used if desipramine-induced (Salah and Cameron, *Am J Psychiatry* 1996;**153**:579).

Anticholinergic, constipation

Antidepressants (usually tricyclics)

Ensure adequate fluid intake.

Bran or a bulking or lubricating laxative, e.g. lactulose or docusate may help.

Bethanechol 30–90 mg/d may be effective but often poorly tolerated.

Clozapine*

It is important to take this seriously as it may lead on to potentially fatal paralytic ileus (review, n = 102, Palmer *et al*, *J Clin Psychiatry* 2008;**69**:759–68) with or without previous abdominal symptoms.

Risk factors for clozapine-induced constipation:

- Recently starting clozapine
- High clozapine dose or plasma level
- Use of concomitant anticholinergics
- Intercurrent illness.

Additional actions:

- Regular physical monitoring, especially during higher risk times
- Appropriate and timely use of appropriate and gradually introduced non-stimulant laxatives e.g. lactulose or docusate
- Ensure adequate fluid intake
- Early referral before life-threatening pathological changes start
- Once resolved, preventative measures (high-fibre diet, adequate fluid intake, stool softeners and exercise) must be used to allow clozapine to continue safely (n = 1, Pelizza *et al*, *Acta Biomed* 2007;**78**:144–8).

Drug interventions:

Orlistat may help pain control as well as constipation, possibly in part by causing some diarrhoea (n = 54, RCT, p/c, 16/52, Chukhin *et al*, *Int Clin Psychopharmacol* 2013;**28**:67–70).

Pseudoephedrine up to 150 mg/d, 93% responded (n = 16, Hanes *et al*, *Innov Clin Neurosci* 2013;**10**:33–5).

Bethanecol (Poetter and Stewart, *J Clin Psychopharmacol* 2013;**33**:713–4).

***Lubiprostone** (a prostaglandin-derived bicyclic fatty acid; Wilson and Schey, *Ther Adv Chronic Dis* 2015;**6**:40–50) has been used (Meyer and Cummings, *Acta Psych Scand* 2014;**130**:71–2).

Anticholinergic, dry mouth (xerostomia)

General advice

- **Stimulate salivary flow** — sugarless gum and other confectionary (e.g. wine gums) stimulate salivary flow (avoid those with sugar as this can promote dental caries and weight gain).
- Artificial **saliva sprays** (most contain methylcellulose or glycerin).
- Ensure adequate **hydration**.
- **Distigmine** bromide, but this has its own notable adverse effects, e.g. digestive, urinary and dermatological (n = 25, open, Wolpert *et al*, *Fortschr Neurol Psychiatr Grenzgeb* 1980;**48**:224–33).
- **Pilocarpine** 10–30 mg/d, 2–3 times a day, may resolve the problem within a day, with no significant side-effects (overview, Masters, *Am J Psychiatry* 2005;**162**:1023).

SSRIs

Switching to fluvoxamine may be effective if paroxetine-induced (n = 1, Arima *et al*, *Ann Pharmacother* 2005;**39**:567–71).

6

	Stop any olanzapine, which may exacerbate the effect (n = 1, Hori *et al*, *Prog Neuropsychopharmacol Biol Psychiatry* 2006;**30**:758–60).
Tricyclics	**Coffee** — chewing 15 g cappuccino coffee for five minutes may help (n = 10, open, Chodorowski, *Przegl Lek* 2002;**59**:392–3). **Bethanechol** has been used at 5–10 mg at night, or up to 60 mg/d s/l to promote salivation (titrate dose slowly upwards, may be poorly tolerated). **Yohimbine** 4 mg/d may be effective for 3–4 hours (Bagheri *et al*, *Br J Clin Pharmacol* 1994;**37**:93–6; FFT).

Anticholinergic, urinary retention

SSRIs/tricyclics	Once physical causes have been excluded, the best option is probably to discontinue and/or switch. It can be a medical emergency and so must be taken seriously. **Mirtazapine** augmentation has reversed SSRI-induced retention (Lenze, *J Clin Psychopharmacol* 2012;**32**:434). **Bethanechol** 30–90 mg/d may be effective, albeit poorly tolerated (Hermesh *et al*, *Drug Intell Clin Pharm* 1987;**21**:877–9).
Antipsychotics*	**Switch to aripiprazole** 10 mg/d as an alternative (n = 1, Sahoo, *Isr J Psychiatry Relat Sci* 2007;**44**:74–5; FFT). **Paliperidone** has resolved amisulpride-induced retention (n = 1, Lai, *J Neuropsychiatry Clin Neurosci* 2012;**24**:E11–2).

Urinary hesitancy (see also anticholinergic effects)

Reboxetine	**Doxazosin** 1 mg/d (n = 1, Szabadi, *Br J Psychiatry* 1998;**173**:441–2). **Tamsulosin** 0.4 mg/d may be rapidly successful (within 20 minutes) and well tolerated (e.g. n = 8 males, Kasper and Wolf, *Eur Neuropsychopharmacol* 2002;**12**:119–22).

Urinary incontinence

Venlafaxine	**Sertraline**, switch to (n = 1, Polimeni *et al*, *Clin Neuropharmacol* 2005;**28**:247–8). **Duloxetine** might be an alternative if stress-related.

6.2 Blood disorders

Review: Haematological toxicity from psychotropics and how to treat it (Flanagan and Dunk, *Hum Psychopharmacol* 2008;**23**:27–41).

Bleeding

SSRIs	**Discontinuing**, or **switching** to a non-SSRI may be the best option. **Stop any NSAIDs** (including aspirin), prescribe a less gastrotoxic NSAID or co-prescribe gastroprotective drugs (Dalton *et al*, *CNS Drugs* 2006;**20**:143–51; Mort *et al*, *Pharmacotherapy* 2006;**26**:1307–13). **Vitamin C** 500 mg/d has been used (n = 1, Tielens, *Am J Psychiatry* 1997;**154**:883–4; Rasker, *Ned Tijdschr Genneesk* 1993;**137**:618).

Blood dyscrasias

Neutropenia, agranulocytosis

Clozapine*	**'Red result' — immediate cessation mandatory** Even a major **dose reduction** is unlikely to help in the short-term. **GCSF/filgrastim** may be effective (e.g. n=1, Gopalakrishnan *et al*, *J Postgrad Med* 2013;**59**:54–5; FFT; n=1, Munshi *et al*, *Neuropsychiatr Dis Treat* 2013;**9**:1267–71; FFT). GCSF can be used as a single rescue dose (n = 1), occasional (n = 1) or as long-term regular prophylaxis (n = 1) (Khan *et al*, *Ther Adv Psychopharmacol* 2013;**3**:266–71; n = 3, 11–48/12, Hagg *et al*, *Int Clin Psychopharmacol* 2003;**18**:173–4). Doses above 0.3 mg/wk may be more

successful, although any clozapine rechallenge still needs extreme care (n=5, Joffe *et al*, *Am J Psychiatry* 2009;**166**:236).

'Amber result' — advice on management

Exclude any interacting or contributing drugs, e.g. carbamazepine (Imbarlina *et al*, *Eur Psychiatry* 2004;**19**:506–9; see *Chapter 4.2.4* for list).

Take the blood sample in the afternoon: neutrophil levels have a diurnal variation and a transient and harmless morning pseudoneutropenia can occur, not requiring discontinuation (n=1, Esposito *et al*, *World J Biol Psychiatry* 2003;**4**:192–4).

Exercising before a sample can boost neutrophils, and **B12** and oral **folate** supplementation have also been used.

Lithium (e.g. n=1, Pinninti *et al*, *J Clin Psychopharmacol* 2010;**30**:219–21) has been used to prevent transition to 'red' by reversing a low wbc, e.g. during an 'amber' phase or raising baseline wbc where a low count exists, allowing clozapine to start. Lithium protects against neutropenia, but does not protect against progression to agranulocytosis (Paton and Esop, *Psychiatr Bull* 2005;**29**:186–8). Plasma levels of 0.4 mmol/l have been used.

After care and re-exposure:

After post-leucopenia or neutropenia clozapine rechallenge, 38% had a further dyscrasia and in most it was more severe, longer-lasting and occurred more quickly (peaking at 5.5 weeks), but 55% were rechallenged successfully and remained in treatment (n=53, Dunk *et al*, *Br J Psychiatry* 2006;**188**:255–63; FFT).

Reviews: rechallenge (Ghaznavi *et al*, *Am J Psychiatry* 2008;**165**:813–8), general (Herceg *et al*, *Psychiatr Danub* 2010;**22**:85–9; FFT).

Eosinophilia

Clozapine

The incidence with clozapine is 13%, and it nearly always resolves without intervention (n=160, Chatterton, *Aust N Z J Psychiatry* 1997;**31**:874–6). It is probably not a predictor of neutropenia (n=70, Ames *et al*, *J Clin Psychiatry* 1996;**57**:579–81), but monitor carefully anyway, especially in women (n=118, >3/52, Banov *et al*, *J Clin Psychiatry* 1993;**54**:466–9).

Switching to quetiapine can be a successful alternative (n=1, Zipris *et al*, *Isr J Psychiatry Relat Sci* 2007;**44**:54–6; FFT).

6.3 Cardiac effects

Hypertension

Antipsychotics

Beta-blockers and other standard strategies are often adequate, e.g. **propranolol** if aripiprazole-induced (n=1, Borras *et al*, *Am J Psychiatry* 2005;**162**:2392).

Clozapine

Hypertension is usually transient over the first month, so reduce the dose or the rate of upward titration.

Antihypertensives may be necessary if persistent or severe e.g. **pindolol** 5 mg BD has been used (e.g. n=82, review; Henderson *et al*, *J Clin Psychiatry* 2004;**65**:686–9).

MAOIs

For hypertensive crisis, refer to a specialist unit immediately for specialist care, e.g. using the British Hypertension Society guidelines for malignant hypertension (see also Elliot, *J Clin Hypertens [Greenwich]* 2004;**6**:587–92).

Hypotension (see also postural hypotension)

MAOIs

Hypotension occurs in about 10% of people on MAOIs (n=61, Remnick *et al*, *Prog Neuropsychopharmacol Biol Psychiatry* 1989;**13**:497–504) and usually needs specialist medical care.

Metoclopramide (Patterson, *J Clin Psychopharmacol* 1987;**7**:112–3).

Plasma expansion, e.g. salt tablets or fludrocortisone.

Myocarditis

Clozapine* — **Immediate stopping** is the only option. Myocarditis is most common (80%) in the first month (n=25, Hill and Harrison-Woolrych, *N Z Med J* 2008;**121**:68–75), but can occur at any time, e.g. even after six years of therapy (n=1, Tanner and Culling, *Postgrad Med J* 2003;**79**:412–3; FFT). There appear few obvious risk factors in fatal vs non-fatal clozapine-induced myocarditis, other than obesity (BMI > 30 kg/m2), CK > 1000 u/l (n=10 fatal cf n=666 non-fatal, Ronaldson *et al, Schizophr Res* 2011;**128**:161–5), which is doubled if used with valproate (n=401, Ronaldson *et al, Schizophr Res* 2012;**141**:173–8). The risk is reduced if clozapine is slowly dose titrated (26% increase for each additional 250mg administered in the first nine days).

Postural (orthostatic) hypotension (see also hypotension)

General strategies: (review by Freeman, *Semin Neurol* 2003;**23**:435–42)

- Self-care (e.g. if lying down, dangle legs for a minute before rising slowly and attempting to stand)
- Use of support stockings
- Slower dose titration
- Plasma volume expansion, e.g. increased fluid and sodium chloride intake
- **Desmopressin**, **indometacin** and **erythropoietin** can be used in extreme cases
- **Midodrine**, an alpha-adrenergic agonist, is licensed and available in some countries (review by McClellan *et al, Drugs Aging* 1998;**12**:76–86).

Additional strategies:

Tricyclics — **Fludrocortisone** has been used, but obviously has long-term side-effects (Chobanian *et al, N Engl J Med* 1979;**301**:68–73).

Yohimbine 12 mg/d (n=12, d/b, c/o, p/c, Lacomblez *et al, Clin Pharmacol Ther* 1989;**45**:241–51).

MAOIs — **Brewed coffee** (Pollack and Rosenbaum, *J Clin Psychiatry* 1987:**48**:3–8).

Fludrocortisone (Simonson, *Am J Psychiatry* 1964;**120**:1118–9).

Levothyroxine or liothyronine has been suggested (see review, Whybrow and Prange, *Arch Gen Psychiatry* 1981;**38**:106–13).

Methylphenidate 10–15 mg (case series, Feighner *et al, J Clin Psychiatry* 1985;**46**:206–9), but beware of ADRs.

Salt tablets 600–1800 mg BD (n=1, Munjack, *J Clin Psychiatry* 1984;**45**:89–90; mentioned in Pollack and Rosenbaum, *J Clin Psychiatry* 1987;**48**:3–8).

Review: general (Cockhill and Remick, *Can J Psychiatry* 1987;**32**:803–8).

Antipsychotics — The effect is probably alpha-adrenergic receptor related so slower dose titration and lower doses are logical. Tolerance usually develops.

Clozapine — **Bovril and moclobemide** have been used for severe clozapine-induced postural hypotension (n=1, Taylor *et al, Br J Psychiatry* 1995;**167**:409–10).

Fludrocortisone (n=1, Testani, *J Clin Psychiatry* 1994;**55**:497–8).

QTc prolongation

General strategies (see *Chapter 3.2* for risk factors and short review of management):

- **Switching** drugs is usually essential. If not possible, use the lowest doses in simple drug regimens. **Lurasidone** appears to have little or no effect on QTc (n=87, up to 555 mg/d, SmPC).
- Avoiding metabolic interactions minimises the impact.
- **Magnesium** ion (Mg^{++}) orally at a mean dose of magnesium oxide 15 mg/kg/d shortens QTc, and can be given long term with appropriate monitoring. Magnesium sulphate by IV injection has been recommended by the American Heart Association (n=24, Bachman, *J Clin Psychiatry* 2003;**64**:733–4).
- **Beta-blockers** are often ineffective (mentioned by Bachman, *J Clin Psychiatry* 2003;**64**:733–4).

Reviews: antipsychotics and QTc prolongation (Wenzel-Seifert *et al*, *Dtsch Arztebl Int* 2011;**108**:687–93), in the elderly (Vieweg *et al*, *Drugs Aging* 2009;**26**:997–1012).

Tachycardia

Antipsychotics	**Amisulpride** may be slightly safer than olanzapine for tachycardia (n=33, Wang *et al*, *Neuropsychobiology* 2008;**57**:200–5).
Clozapine*	Tachycardia is common (up to 67%) early in treatment, but usually resolves over 4–6 weeks (n=100, Marinkovic *et al*, *Prog Neuropsychopharmacol Biol Psychiatry* 1994;**18**;537–44). However, it may be the first, or only, presenting symptom of (often fatal) cardiomyopathy and so this must be fully excluded first. If tachycardia is persistent and/or associated with chest pain, this may also indicate myocarditis (review of n=26 where it was fatal in 46% of cases, Hagg *et al*, *J Clin Psychopharmacol* 2001;**21**:382–8). **Slower dose escalation** may help. **Manage nicotine and caffeine intake.** **Discontinuation** usually results in rapid resolution (e.g. n=1, Stampfer and Swanepoel, *Australas Psychiatry* 2005;**13**:80–2). **Beta-blockers** may help if the tachycardia is anticholinergic/noradrenergic-related, although the literature on this is minimal. Metoprolol is often used first-line as it has a short half-life, and can be converted to atenolol, which may be effective over five years with carvedilol and captopril (n=1, Rostagno *et al*, *Gen Hosp Psychiatry* 2008;**30**:280–3). * **Verapamil** has resolved clozapine-induced persistent sinus tachycardia (n=1, Das *et al*, *Psychosomatics* 2014;**55**:194–5).

6.4 Central adverse effects

Abnormal dreams and nightmares

Antidepressants	**Take in the morning,** especially if a serotonergic drug, as enhanced serotonin can disrupt sleep architecture **Discontinuing or switching** drugs may be the only option. **Switch** to e.g. bupropion if mirtazapine-induced dissociated sleep-wakefulness (n=1, Felthous *et al*, *Pharmacotherapy* 2010;**30**:145–50) **Discontinue any tramadol** (n=1, Devulder *et al*, *Acta Clin Belg* 1996;**51**:184–6) and possibly other similar drugs that may exacerbate the effect.

Anorexia

Valproate	Anorexia could be a sign of impending hepatic failure. Investigate immediately and discontinue if necessary.

Ataxia

Lithium	This is usually a sign of lithium toxicity and neurotoxicity, and requires immediate action, e.g. discontinuation or dose reduction. If acute, dialysis may be needed. Consider also the global clinical picture, as ataxia may occur with 'normal' therapeutic lithium plasma levels. **Discontinue** any exacerbating drugs, e.g. clozapine (Lee and Yang, *Zhonghua Yi Xue Za Zhi [Taipei]* 1999;**62**:184–7). **Buspirone** (high-dose) has been used for ataxia due to lithium toxicity (n=1, Megna and O'Dell, *Arch Phys Med Rehabil* 2001;**82**:1145–8).

Delirium

- Discontinue any causative agent (see 5.4).
- * There is very limited evidence for the use of antipsychotics to treat delirium (s=14, Seitz *et al*, *J Clin Psychiatry* 2007;**68**:11–21; n=90, Hale *et al*, *J Pharm Pract* 2015; [in press]).

Review: systematic review (Page *et al*, *Rev Bras Ter Intensiva* 2014;**26**:86–8; FFT).

Antidepressants	**Donepezil** may help if due to a tricyclic overdose (rapidly effective, n=1, Noyan *et al*, *Prog Neuropsychopharmacol Biol Psychiatry* 2003;**27**:885–7).
Antipsychotics	**Reduce** any concurrent anticholinergics. **Discontinue** if no clear indication. **Switch** to an antipsychotic with low anticholinergic effects (*Table 2.1.4*). **Quetiapine** has been used if risperidone-induced (n=1, Kato *et al*, *Psychosomatics* 2005;**46**:374–5) and **haloperidol** if clozapine-induced (Spisla and Bunter, *Psychiatr Prax* 1997;**24**:308). **Reduce dose**, e.g. clozapine-induced delirium appears to be dose-related (n=139, Centorrino *et al*, *Pharmacopsychiatry* 2003;**36**:156–60). **Propofol** has been used successfully for post-ictal delirium with clozapine-ECT therapy (n=1, Sienaert *et al*, *J ECT* 2004;**20**:254–7).

Drowsiness or sedation (see also fatigue)

Antipsychotics	**Wait**, as tolerance often partly develops. **Adjust dose**, e.g. use a lower dose, load the dose to night or early evening or spread out throughout the day. **Avoid any other concurrent CNS depressants.** **Methylphenidate** 20–40 mg/d has been used if clozapine-induced (with great care; Miller, *Am J Psychiatry* 1996;**153**:1231–2). **Modafinil** 200 mg/d has been used if sedation is caused by clozapine, risperidone or olanzapine, with no exacerbation of psychosis. A critical review concludes that the evidence is fairly poor but it may work in some (s=6, Saavedra-Velez *et al*, *J Clin Psychiatry* 2009;**70**:104–12).
Anticonvulsants	**Levetiracetam**-induced can be minimised by starting at a lower dose.
Topiramate	**Modafinil** (Berigan, *Prim Care Companion J Clin Psychiatry* 2002;**4**:249–50; FFT).
Valproate	**Investigate immediately** and discontinue if necessary. May be indicative of impending hepatic failure or encephalopathy. **Modafinil** (Berigan, *Can J Psychiatry* 2004;**49**:72–3).
Antidepressants*	*Sleepiness can be a residual or premorbid symptom of depression. *Any serotonin-enhancing antidepressant should be taken in the morning as night-time doses can disrupt sleep architecture. *Exercise can help sleep onset, waking and early morning wakening, but not hypersomnia (Rethorst *et al*, *Psychol Med* 2013;**43**:699–709).
SSRIs	**Modafinil,** used adjunctively to SSRIs at the start of treatment, may enhance the onset of action in people with MDD and fatigue (n=29, open, 6/52, Ninan *et al*, *J Clin Psychiatry* 2004;**65**:414–20, MS; n=16, open, 3/52, Schwartz *et al*, *J Clin Psychiatry* 2004;**65**:1223–7).
Mirtazapine	**Start at higher dose**: 30 mg/d may produce less drowsiness than 15 mg/d (mirtazapine is a highly potent H1 receptor blocker, and at 30 mg/d the noradrenergic enhancement may counteract some of the histamine blockade).
MAOIs	Triazolam (or presumably another short-acting hypnotic) can help sleep and reduced daytime somnolence caused by phenelzine (n=3, Gray, *Am J Psychiatry* 1989;**146**:1078).

Dysphoria

Antipsychotics	**Procyclidine** can help (n=51, King *et al*, *Br J Psychiatry* 1995;**167**:480–2). **Review:** Voruganti and Awad, *Can J Psychiatry* 2004;**49**:285–9.

Fatigue (see also drowsiness or sedation)

Antipsychotics	**Adjust dose** or spread the doses out throughout the day. **Modafinil** has limited efficacy, e.g. one study failed to show any differences vs. placebo on fatigue, attention, working memory and executive functioning

	(n=24[c=20], 8/52, d/b, p/c, Sevy *et al*, *J Clin Psychiatry* 2005;**66**:839–43), although it may be effective in some people (n=11, open, 4/52, Rosenthal and Bryant, *Clin Neuropharmacol* 2004;**27**:38–43).
Topiramate	**Modafinil** (Berigan, *Prim Care Companion J Clin Psychiatry* 2002;**4**:249–50; FFT).

Hypomania

Antidepressants	Any mania from antidepressants is restricted to people with bipolar disorder (previously diagnosed or not). It may be part of the natural course but **discontinuation** is the absolute priority, with acute management of mania. **Switch antidepressants if needed once resolved**; venlafaxine appears to have the highest risk of inducing mania, sertraline an intermediate risk and bupropion the lowest (n=159, RCT, 10/52, Leverich *et al*, *Am J Psychiatry* 2006;**163**:232–9). **Adjunctive mood stabilisers**, e.g. lithium, should be used.

Insomnia

Antidepressants (SSRIs, bupropion, venlafaxine)	**Standard hypnotic therapy** (time-limited) may be adequate, e.g. zolpidem 5–10mg/d if SSRI-induced (n=190, RCT, d/b, 5/52, Asnis *et al*, *J Clin Psychiatry* 1999;**60**:668–76). **Adjust time of doses**, e.g. the preferred morning doses, as all serotonergic antidepressants can disrupt sleep architecture. **Quetiapine** 50mg/d was effective for phenelzine-induced resistant insomnia (n=1, Sokolski and Brown, *Ann Pharmacother* 2006;**40**:567–70). **Trazodone** 50–75mg may be effective in people on MAOIs, SSRIs (n=12, d/b, p/c, c/o, 2x7/7, Kaynak *et al*, *Sleep Med* 2004;**5**:15–20), bupropion (67% improved, n=17, RCT, p/c, d/b, c/o, Nierenberg *et al*, *Am J Psychiatry* 1994;**151**:1069–72) and venlafaxine (especially in people with increased inner tension; n=50[c=42], open, 4/52, Bertschy *et al*, *Pharmacol Res* 2005;**51**:79–84).
MAOIs	**Adjust time of doses**, e.g. last dose of the day should be before 3.00 PM. **Switch** to isocarboxazid. **Hypnotics** may help sleep but have no effect on daytime somnolence (n=8, Teicher *et al*, *Am J Psychiatry* 1988;**145**:1552–6).
Aripiprazole	Add a hypnotic agent during the first days of treatment, administer in the morning or divide the dose of aripiprazole into two daily doses (AM and PM; Aitchison *et al*, *J Psychopharmacol* 2009;**23**:231–40).
Lamotrigine	Insomnia is probably dose-related so reduce the dose, switch (n=109, Sadler, *Epilepsia* 1999;**40**:322–5) or use hypnotics.
Methylphenidate*	**Mirtazapine** can be used (chart review, Adler *et al*, *Curr Psychiatry Rep* 2006;**8**:409–15). **Melatonin** add-on can partly improve sleep disturbance (n=60[c=50], RCT, d/b, p/c, 8/52, Mohammadi *et al*, *Iran J Psychiatry* 2012;**7**:87–92).
Beta-blockers	**Melatonin** can help as beta-blockers (except carvedilol) reduce the release of endogenous melatonin (n=15, RCT, d/b, p/c, c/o, Stoschitzky *et al*, *Eur J Clin Pharmacol* 1999;**55**:111–5), so oral melatonin may help correct this (Fares, *J Cardiovasc Dis Res* 2011;**2**:153–5; FFT).

Irritability, jitteriness or agitation *

SSRIs	**Slower dose titration** (or restarting more slowly) usually helps, especially if a first-degree relative has a mood disorder (n=3, Rietveld *et al*, *Gen Hosp Psychiatry* 2015;**37**:620.e5–6). **Valproate** has been used for fluoxetine-induced irritability in autism (Anagnostou *et al*, *J Clin Psychopharmacol* 2006;**26**:444–6).

Tricyclics	**Slower dose titration** (or restarting more slowly) usually helps. **Iron supplements** to resolve any contributing low serum iron (Yeragani *et al*, *Neuropsychobiology* 1992;**25**:8–10). **Perphenazine** has been used (n=2, Pohl *et al*, *J Clin Psychiatry* 1986;**47**:427).
Aripiprazole	Agitation is common when switching to aripiprazole and must be managed. **Benzodiazepines** (esp. lorazepam) can be used during the switch-over period, e.g. over 4/52 (Aitchison *et al*, *J Psychopharmacol* 2009;**23**:231–40). **Anticholinergic** drugs. **Antihistamines** (Aitchison *et al*, *J Psychopharmacol* 2009;**23**:231–40). **Valproic acid** or **gabapentin** as adjuncts. *__Chocolate__ — anecdotally taking aripiprazole with four or so squares of chocolate can reduce the adverse effects. **Review:** Cassano *et al*, *Clin Drug Invest* 2007;**27**:1–13.

Nausea

Antidepressants*	**Slower dose increases** help initially. See *Table 2.1.2* for comparative incidence of nausea. **Antiemetics** in the short term may be effective. **Slow-release** tablets/capsules (if available) reduce the peak plasma level effect, as would splitting doses throughout the day. **Gorei-san** (TJ-17), a Japanese herbal medicine may help if SSRI-induced (n=3, open, Yamada *et al*, *Psychiatr Clin Neurosci* 1999;**53**:681). **Mirtazapine** 15mg at night may be effective within four days (n=1, Caldis and Gair, *Can J Psychiatry* 2004;**49**:707) if the nausea is SSRI-induced (Pedersen and Klysner, *Int Clin Psychopharmacol* 1997;**12**:59–60). *__Olanzapine and milnacipran__ have been used for severe antidepressant-induced nausea (n=1, Yoshida *et al*, *Pharmacopsychiatry* 2007;**40**:84–5) e.g. from duloxetine .(n=268, open, 2/52, Zhong *et al*, *J Clin Psychopharmacol* 2014;**34**:495–4).
Antipsychotics	**Antiemetics**, e.g. ondansetron may be effective but **avoid** metoclopramide or prochlorperazine for the first 1–2 months, or if there is a history of EPSE. **Prochlorperazine** has been effective for quetiapine-withdrawal nausea, where ondansetron had failed (n=1, Kim and Staab, *Am J Psychiatry* 2005;**162**:1020), but see warning above.
Aripiprazole	Nausea is usually transient so administer aripiprazole with or after food, reduce the dose or add an antiemetic, e.g. domperidone (Aitchison *et al*, *J Psychopharmacol* 2009;**23**:231–40) if other measures fail (review, Cassano *et al*, *Clin Drug Invest* 2007;**27**:1–13).
Anticholinesterases*	**Galantamine** — **Switching** to the XL product has a disappointingly low impact on reducing nausea (n=965, RCT, d/b, p/c, 6/12, Dunbar *et al*, *Clin Ther* 2006;**28**:365–72, MS). Rivastigmine patches are an alternative. *__Domperidone__ 30mg has prevented GI disturbance from rivastigmine (n=30, open, 20/52, Kano *et al*, *Neuropsychiatr Dis Treat* 2013;**9**:1411–5; FFT)
Anticholinergics	Nausea appears more frequently with higher doses. **Patches** may be an option.
Atomoxetine*	Take after food (usually wears off with time, often within 1–8 weeks). Split dose into smaller amounts, e.g. 80mg once to 40mg twice a day. Eat with high protein or fatty food, e.g. toast with butter etc.

Nocturnal enuresis (see also urinary incontinence)

Antipsychotic-induced nocturnal enuresis is surprisingly common, e.g. clozapine (21%), olanzapine (10%), quetiapine (7%) and risperidone (6%) (n=497, Harrison-Woolrych *et al*, *Br J Psychiatry* 2011;**199**:140–4; FFT), and under-recognised (Barnes *et al*, *Br J Psychiatry* 2012;**200**:7–9; FFT).

Antipsychotics	**Imipramine** has been used for risperidone-induced enuresis (n = 1, Hergüner *et al, J Clin Psychopharmacol* 2011;**31**:782–3).
Clozapine	**Avoid or reduce fluids** at night or after 6.00 PM, have planned night awakenings, enuresis alarms, and full voiding before going to bed. **Adjust dose** and load towards morning if possible. **Desmopressin** can be used intranasally (10 mcg in each nostril) at bedtime (e.g. n = 1, Aronowitz *et al, Am J Psychiatry* 1995;**152**:472), although it risks hyponatraemia (n = 1, Sarma *et al, Aust N Z J Psychiatry* 2005;**39**:949). **Oxybutinin** (see Lurie and Hosmer, *J Clin Psychiatry* 1997;**58**:404). **Tolterodine** (there is one case where it did **not** work, whereas desmopressin did: n = 1, English *et al, Ann Pharmacother* 2001;**35**:867–9). **Trihexyphenidyl** 5 mg/d at bedtime (n = 2, Poyurovsky *et al, Int Clin Psychopharmacol* 1996;**11**:61–3). **Verapamil** 80 mg/d has been effective (n = 1, Poyurovsky *et al, Eur Psychiatry* 1995;**10**:413–5).
Methylphenidate	Nortriptyline has been used successfully (n = 43, RCT, d/b, p/c, 45/7, Ghanizadeh and Haghighat, *Pediatr Nephrol* 2012;**27**:2091–7).
Sertraline	**Switch** to fluoxetine (n = 1, Maalouf and Gilbert, *J Child Adolesc Psychopharmacol* 2010:**20**:161–2).

Obsessive-compulsive behaviour or symptoms

Antipsychotics*	**SSRIs** may be effective, e.g. **fluoxetine** if quetiapine-induced (n = 1, Ozer *et al, Prog Neuropsychopharmacol Biol Psychiatry* 2006;**30**:724–7). **Valproate** has been used as augmentation in clozapine-induced OCD (n = 1, Zink *et al, Pharmacopsychiatry* 2007;**40**:202–3). ***Aripiprazole** 10–30 mg/d adjunctively has been effective if clozapine-induced (n = 7, Englisch *et al, Clin Neuropharmacol* 2009;**32**:227–9; n = 4, Eryilmaz *et al, Ann Gen Psychiatry* 2013;**12**:40) and 5 mg/d for olanzapine-induced (n = 1, Schönfelder *et al, Clin Neuropharmacol* 2011;**34**:256–7). **Reduce dose** — **clozapine**-induced OCD symptoms may be related to high clozapine/norclozapine plasma levels, so try reducing the dose and/or measure plasma levels (n = 39, Lin *et al, Ther Drug Monit* 2006;**28**:303–7).
Benzodiazepines	Pregabalin has been successful if BDZ-induced (Oulis *et al, Prog Neuropsychopharmacol Biol Psychiatry* 2008;**32**:2000–1).

Psychosis

Methylphenidate	Monitor and use low-dose antipsychotics or switch to atomoxetine (n = 3, Kraemer *et al, Clin Neuropharmacol* 2010;**33**:204–6).

Sedation (see drowsiness)

Seizures

Clozapine*

The incidence of new-onset seizures with clozapine is about 5–6%. Risk factors include being male, aged 24–41, long duration of illness (> 10 years) and increasing plasma levels, e.g. 1–2% <300 mg/d, 3–4% 300–599 mg/d, 5% 600–900 mg/d (Iqbal *et al, J Pharm Technol* 2004;**20**:155–64; n = 222, Grover *et al, East Asian Arch Psychiatry* 2015;**25**:73–8; FT), so if seizures occur reduce the dose or rate of increase, or stop and restart. .

* Seizure-risk assessment:

- Has a gradual dose titration been used (including any re-titration)?
- Is person on any other seizure-threshold lowering drugs?
- Has person reported any drop attacks, myoclonic jerks or any similar events that may precede a GTC seizure?
- Are plasma levels above 1300 ng/ml?
- Does person have history of seizures (including febrile) or head injury?

6

- Is person on any drugs that might raise clozapine plasma levels, e.g. fluvoxamine, fluoxetine, high-dose sertraline, lamotrigine, erythromycin?
- Would a single seizure be potentially devastating (e.g. living alone, driver)?

If the answer to any of these is yes, or a seizure occurs, then:

- Reduce the dose so clozapine plasma levels fall below 1300 ng/ml.
- Carry out an EEG to test for ictal activity (n = 323, Centorrino *et al*, *Am J Psychiatry* 2002;**159**:109–15).
- Reduce/discontinue any seizure threshold-lowering or interacting drugs.
- Consider an add-on anticonvulsant, remembering that AEDs can be sedative, risks over-medicating if unnecessary and can risk agranulocytosis.

Valproate is standard management (e.g. n = 1, Foster and Olajide, *J Psychopharmacol* 2005;**19**:93–6), but the literature is remarkably sparse on this. It may be underused as only about 25% people on clozapine at risk of seizures receive prophylactic valproate (n = 81, Sparshatt *et al*, *Psychiatric Bull* 2008;**32**:262–5). **Other anticonvulsants** used include **gabapentin** (≤2100 mg/d, n = 1, Usiskin *et al*, *Am J Psychiatry* 2000;**157**:482–3), **lamotrigine** (n = 1, Muzyk *et al*, *J Psychiatr Pract* 2010;**16**:125–8) and **topiramate** (Navarro *et al*, *Am J Psychiatry* 2001;**158**:968–9).

Reviews: * management (Herceg *et al*, *Psychiatr Danub* 2010;**22**:85–9; FFT; Caetano, *Australas Psychiatry* 2014;**22**:78–82).

6.5 Dermatological effects

Lithium is a major cause of cutaneous reactions, often characterised by pathological findings of neutrophilic infiltration, which can cause or make it worse. The general advice with lithium is:

- Check for a personal or family history of skin diseases before prescribing; the incidence is also higher in males (n = 108, Chan *et al*, *J Affect Disord* 2000;**57**:107–13; review by Yeung and Chan, *Am J Clin Dermatol* 2004;**5**:3–8).
- For mild or moderate dermatoses — use specific or systemic therapy.
- For severe or persistent dermatoses — use specific or systemic therapy; try dose reduction or discontinuation or rechallenge at a lower dose.
- Exclude other factors, e.g. infections, other medication changes.
- Most reactions seem to be dose-related, usually not too serious and may resolve despite continuation. Dose reduction and discontinuation are obvious options.

Review: cutaneous reactions from lithium (Yeung and Chan, *Am J Clin Dermatol* 2004;**5**:3–8).

Acne

Lithium	**Systemic antibiotics** (avoid tetracycline because of an interaction; see Malt, *Br Med J* 1978;**2**:502; FFT). **Topical retinoids** (tretinoin; Remmer and Falk, *J Clin Psychiatry* 1986;**47**:48). **Reduce the dose or discontinue.** **Wait** (may spontaneously resolve even with continued treatment, n = 2, Kusumi, *Dis Nerv Sys* 1971;**32**:853–4).

Alopecia and hair loss

- Check trace minerals, as low plasma levels of copper and zinc may predispose to hair loss, so oral supplementation may be effective (Ftemi and Calabrese, *Ann Pharmacother* 1995;**29**:1302).
- Other standard management includes hair care techniques and minoxidil.

Review: hair loss in psychiatry (Mercke *et al*, *Ann Clin Psychiatry* 2000;**12**:35–42).

Carbamazepine	May occur in 6% and resolve after withdrawal, but can take several months.
Lithium	May occur in 12–19% people (Mercke *et al*, *Ann Clin Psychiatry* 2000;**12**:35–42), either *de novo* or exacerbation. It may occur in the first six months of treatment, and is more common in women.

	Alopecia may resolve with continued treatment (Ghadirian *et al*, *J Clin Psychiatry* 1986;**47**:212–3) or withdrawal (but might take several months). **Exclude hypothyroidism** as a causative factor (9%, Mortimer and Dawber, *Int J Dermatol* 1984;**23**:603–4) and other causes, e.g. stress, co-medication.
SSRIs	Occurs more in women and there may be an association with sertraline so switch if appropriate, e.g. to paroxetine or trazodone (may help if sertraline-induced; n = 1, Gautam, *Ann Pharmacother* 1999;**33**:631–7). **Review:** Hedenmalm *et al*, *Pharmacoepidemiol Drug Safety* 2006;**15**:719–25.
Venlafaxine	**Discontinue or switch**, and it may resolve within a month (Pitchot and Ansseau, *Am J Psychiatry* 2001;**158**:1159–60).
Valproate	The incidence is 5–6% (range 2.6–15%). It is usually transient and slight and may resolve without alteration of dose, although it may take 6/12 to regrow. * **Dose reduction** may help as alopecia is considered to be dose-dependent, e.g. 28% incidence at high dose, 5% at low dose (Mercke *et al*, *Ann Clin Psychiatry* 2000;**12**:35–42) or even plasma-level related (n = 1, Ramakrishnappa and Belhekar, *Indian J Pharmacol* 2013;**45**:187–8). **Check copper and zinc**, as low levels may predispose to hair loss (Ftemi and Calabrese, *Ann Pharmacother* 1995;**29**:1302; Tasaki *et al*, *J Dermatol* 1993;**20**:21–4).

Darier's disease

Lithium	Topical retinoids.

Exfoliative dermatitis

Lithium	**Discontinue** — although rare (e.g. Sarantidis and Waters, *Br J Psychiatry* 1983;**143**:42–50), it is serious and discontinuation is usually the only option.

Folliculitis

Lithium	**Observation** (as it is often transient, starting several months after starting lithium and resolving spontaneously), and keep lithium levels stable. **Topical antibiotics and corticosteroids.**

Maculopapular eruption

Lithium	Usually occurs within three weeks of starting treatment. **Topical corticosteroids.** **Oral antihistamines.** **Reduce dose or discontinue** (can recur on rechallenge).

Photosensitivity

Antipsychotics	**Exclude other causes**, e.g. SLE and porphyria. **Avoid direct sunlight** or sun-lamps. **Use a high factor** sun-block cream. **Reduce doses** or **switch drugs** (there is no reliable comparative information but chlorpromazine is almost certainly the worst). **Reviews:** antipsychotics (Warnock and Morris, *Am J Clin Dermatol* 2002;**3**:629–36), antipsychotics, antidepressants and anxiolytics (Harth and Rapoport, *Drug Saf* 1996;**14**:252–9).
Phenytoin	**Discontinue**, as this can be the presenting symptom of serious reactions (review by Scheinfeld, *Expert Opin Drug Saf* 2004;**3**:655–65). If mild, can reintroduce cautiously but discontinue immediately if it recurs.

Pigmentation

Imipramine	Blue-grey pigmentation, often facial, is probably due to melanin deposits. **Laser** (Q-switched alexandrite and ruby) treatment may be effective, and is better with higher doses (n = 1, Atkin and Fitzpatrick, *J Am Acad Dermatol* 2000;**43**:77–80).

Switch to an SSRI (e.g. sertraline, n = 1, Metelitsa *et al*, *J Cutan Med Surg* 2005;**9**:341–5).

Chlorpromazine

Withdrawal — chlorpromazine-pigmentation is almost completely reversible on withdrawal, although lenticular pigmentation may persist, whereas corneal changes may resolve slowly over several years on discontinuation.
Switching drugs, e.g. to haloperidol (n = 4, Thompson *et al*, *Acta Psychiatr Scand* 1988;**78**:763–5), levomepromazine (n = 4), trifluoperazine (n = 1) or combinations (n = 5) (Bloom *et al*, *Acta Psychiatr Scand* 1993;**87**:223–4).

Psoriasis

Lithium

Lithium takes about a month to exacerbate psoriasis (review, Skoven and Thormann, *Arch Dermatol* 1979;**115**:1185–7), and up to 10 months to induce it *de novo*.
Conventional topical therapy (e.g. topical corticosteroids and calcipotriol).
Oral retinoids.
Reduce dose (as it is apparently dose-dependent) or discontinue (rarely necessary and takes many weeks to resolve on discontinuation).

Rash

Anticonvulsants (general)

Switch AED: Skin rash with one AED seems to increase the risk of rash with another, especially combinations involving carbamazepine or phenytoin. Specific cross-sensitivity rates may be useful for AED selection and counselling of patients (n = 1,875, Hirsch *et al*, *Neurology* 2008;**71**:1527–34).

Rash with first AED	Second AED	Chance of rash with second AED
Carbamazepine	Lamotrigine	20% (n=50)
Carbamazepine	Oxcarbazepine	33% (n=15)
Carbamazepine	Phenobarbital	26.7% (n=30)
Carbamazepine	Phenytoin	57.6% (n=59)
Lamotrigine	Carbamazepine	26.3% (n=38)
Lamotrigine	Oxcarbazepine	20% (n=15)
Lamotrigine	Phenytoin	38.9% (n=36)
Oxcarbazepine	Carbamazepine	71.4% (n=7)
Oxcarbazepine	Lamotrigine	37.5% (n=8)
Phenobarbital	Carbamazepine	66.7% (n=12)
Phenobarbital	Phenytoin	53.3% (n=15)
Phenytoin	Carbamazepine	42% (n=81)
Phenytoin	Lamotrigine	18.9% (n=74)
Phenytoin	Phenobarbital	19.5% (n=41)

Oral corticosteroids (n = 1, Verrotti *et al*, *Int J Immunopathol Pharmacol* 2000;13:49–53).
Antihistamines, topical corticosteroids and **H2-blockers** have been used.
Avoid paracetamol — adverse cutaneous reactions with carbamazepine and valproate (e.g. EM, SJS and TEN) can be enhanced by paracetamol (n=72, Gau *et al*, *J Clin Psychopharmacol* 2008;**28**:509–17).
Review: ACHSS (anticonvulsant hypersensitivity syndrome; n = 32, Newell *et al*, *Pediatr Dermatol* 2009;**26**:536–46).

Carbamazepine

Occurs in about 10–13% of people. There may be a genetic susceptibility (Hung *et al*, *Pharmacogenet Genomics* 2006;**16**:297–306), e.g. in Chinese (n=24, Miller, *Epilepsy Curr* 2008;**8**:120–1; FFT).
If treating the rash rather than discontinuing, full laboratory test monitoring (including LFTs, FBC, U&E) must be carried out frequently to

exclude agranulocytosis, aplastic anaemia (n=10, Cates and Powers, *Ann Pharmacother* 1998;**32**:884–7) or internal organ involvement, which may occur in rare cases and is potentially fatal.

Slow increments (syrup 0.1 mg/d, doubling on alternate days over 4/52) have been successful in preventing recurrence of rash (n=1, Boyle and Lawlor, *Am J Psychiatry* 1996;**153**:1234).

Oral corticosteroids, e.g. prednisone (n=20, only four had to discontinue carbamazepine, Murphy *et al, Neurology* 1991;**41**:144–5).

Topicals corticosteroids — for CBZ-induced Lichen Plantus oxcarbazepine can be used instead, with topical steroids (n=1, Hajnsek *et al, Epilepsy Behav* 2012;**24**:269–71).

Lamotrigine*

Take very seriously: Although relatively rare, rash may be the first sign of a potentially fatal Stevens-Johnson syndrome (n=1175, RCT, Ketter *et al, J Clin Psychiatry* 2006;**67**:400–6) or toxic epidermal necrolysis (review by Antai-Otong, *Perspect Psychiatr Care* 2005;**41**:193–6).

Prevention:

Risk factors: It is more common in females (relative risk of 1.8; Wong *et al, Ann Pharmacother* 1999;**33**:1037–42), people with a previous anticonvulsant rash and in the under 13s (n=988, Hirsch *et al, Epilepsia* 2006;**47**:318–22).

Slow dose titration — the risk of rash is almost abolished by following the recommended titration schedule (n=254, Huang *et al, Kaohsiung J Med Sci* 2002;**18**:66–72), especially the initial dose (n=1,955, Calabrese *et al, J Clin Psychiatry* 2002;**63**:1012–9). The starting dose in adults should be 25 mg/d for two weeks, 50 mg/d for two weeks, then increasing every 1–2 weeks, halved if added to valproate (where rash is also more likely to occur) or if allergic to trimethoprim, and doubled if combined with concurrent enzyme-inducing drugs, e.g. phenytoin, carbamazepine, etc.

* **Vitamin B complex** must be stopped as it may exacerbate TEN (n=1, Fegade *et al, J Clin Diagn Res* 2012;**6**:1571–3).

Preventative dermatological advice should be given, e.g. avoid other new medicines, foods, cosmetics, deodorants, detergents and fabric softeners, and avoid sunburn or exposure to poison ivy/oak (n=100, Ketter *et al, J Clin Psychiatry* 2005;**66**:642–5).

Valproate adjunctively is currently not contraindicated but lamotrigine must be added to valproate only if started at very low initial doses (n=108, Faught *et al, Epilepsia* 1999;**40**:1135–40), as the risk is 3–4 times more common with the combination (n=103, Li *et al, Arq Neuropsiquiatr* 1996;**54**:47–9).

Management:

Corticosteroids for mild non-progressive types.

IV immunoglobulins (n=1, Schwartz *et al, Arch Dermatol* 2008;**144**:724–6) e.g. IgG IV for lamotrigine hypersensitivity (n=1, Comfere *et al, J Am Acad Dermatol* 2012;**66**:249–50) and **corticosteroids** are essential in specialist care settings for more severe reactions.

Switching may be the best option in epilepsy (long-term follow-up, n=2, Feliciani *et al, Int J Immunopathol Pharmacol* 2003;**16**:89–93).

Aftercare:

Very careful rechallenge may be possible in some (88% successful rechallenge, n=44, Lorberg *et al, Int J Neuropsychopharmacol* 2009;**12**:257–65) but with a much slower dose escalation. Leave a gap of 1–2 months, restart at 0.1 mg/d (n=7, Besag *et al, Seizure* 2000;**9**:282–6; FFT), then

2.5–5 mg/d for 2/52, increasing by 5 mg/d every 2/52 to 25 mg/d, then as per SmPC (n = 52, P-Codrea Tigaran *et al*, *Acta Neurol Scand* 2005;**111**:191–4).

Phenytoin Rash can be the presenting symptom of serious reactions (review by Scheinfeld, *Expert Opin Drug Saf* 2004;**3**:655–65).
If mild, can re-introduce cautiously but discontinue immediately if it recurs.

Antipsychotics **Clozapine** — slow introduction, starting at 0.0125 mg/d doubled over four days, reaching 250 mg/d after 105 days has been successful (n = 1, Raju, Southern *et al*, *Progress Neurol Psychiatry* 2010;**14**:30–1).

Antidepressants **Fluoxetine** — care is needed, as rash can develop into the more serious Stevens-Johnson syndrome or toxic epidermal necrolysis (Lyell syndrome).
Switching may not be effective as there can be cross-reactivity with other SSRIs (e.g. n = 1, Sannicandro *et al*, *Pharmacotherapy* 2002;**22**:516–8; paroxetine and sertraline n = 1, Warnock and Azadian, *Ann Pharmacother* 2002;**36**:631–3).
Avoid chocolate, which might be a precipitant (n = 1, Cederberg *et al*, *BMC Psychiatry* 2004;**4**:36;FFT), although this could be a tough call for many.
Antihistamines and topical steroids are widely mentioned as effective where the rash is mild and self-limiting, e.g. fluoxetine and paroxetine rash has responded to oral diphenhydramine and a topical hydrocortisone cream (n = 1, Sannicandro *et al*, *Pharmacotherapy* 2002;**22**:516–8).

Rivastigmine patches Rash and itchiness with rivastigmine patches is a well recognised ADR and is common with all transdermal preps. The two mechanisms are allergic dermatitis (tends to spread out from the patch) and irritant dermatitis (just the patch area itself). A review showed 27% had adverse skin reactions, leading to discontinuation in 19%. Perspiration due to high temperature and low humidity in the first month of treatment can lead to poorer tolerance and rash, so try to manage this as far as possible (Segers *et al*, *J Clin Psychopharmacol* 2012;**32**:412–5). Management includes:
Varying the site — the best areas compared to the back are the upper arm and chest, with the lower back better than the upper back. Do not apply to excessively hairy, broken, burned, cut or irritated skin; move the patch application site daily and do not use the exact same site for at least 14 days.
Skin care: If cleaning the skin before patch application, gently wash with water and dab dry with a cloth or towel.

- Avoid shaving, vigorous rubbing or use of alcohol-based cleansers or gels on the area, as they may damage the integrity of the stratum corneum, the thin outer layer of skin.
- Remove the patch carefully to avoid surface damage to frail skin.
- Gently clean the skin and apply moisturisers after every patch removal to reduce irritation and promote healthy skin.
- Any irritant dermatitis (localised to the patch) should be left to resolve spontaneously, usually occurring in a few days without any intervention.

Treat any allergic dermatitis (hypersensitivity to patch adhesive or rivastigmine, presenting as localised redness that can spread beyond the edge of the patch) or leave to resolve spontaneously, usually within two weeks once the patch is removed. However, once allergic, people will continue to experience skin reactions with subsequent use.

- **Use moisturising creams** and lotions for skin irritation (dryness, scaling, fissures or cracks).
- **Antihistamines and calamine lotion** can help itchiness but have no effect on irritant or allergic dermatitis.

- **Potent topical corticosteroids** may help severe allergic dermatitis, with referral to a dermatologist and discontinuation considered.

Review: general (Greenspoon *et al*, *CNS Drugs* 2011;**25**:575–83).

Seborrheic dermatitis

Lithium — Ketoconazole shampoo.
Topical or systemic antifungal agents.

Sweating

Antidepressants — **Discontinuation** or **dose-reduction** usually improves this rapidly.

Adjunctive therapies

- **Aripiprazole** 10–20mg/d has been used for SSRI/duloxetine-induced sweating in women (Lu *et al*, *J Clin Psychopharmacol* 2008;**28**:710–1).
- ***Anticholinergics** e.g. benzatropine 0.5mg PRN for venlafaxine-induced (n=1, Kolli and Ramaswamy, *Innov Clin Neurosci* 2013;**10**:10–1).
- **Beta-blockers** (propranolol, atenolol, labetalol) should be excluded as they probably make sweating worse (n=1, Butt, *J Clin Psychiatry* 1989;**50**:146–7).
- **Benzatropine** 0.5–1 mg/d if venlafaxine-induced (Pierre and Guze, *J Clin Psychopharmacol* 2000;**20**:269).
- **Clonidine** 0.2mg/d may help dramatically within 24 hours, (n=1, Feder, *J Clin Psychiatry* 1995;**56**:35; n=1, Mago and Monti, *J Clin Psychiatry* 2007;**68**:639–40), although stopping it sometimes helps (Leeman, *J Clin Psychiatry* 1990;**51**:258–9).
- **Cyproheptadine** 4mg either BD or at night (n=5, open, Ashton and Weinstein, *Am J Psychiatry* 2002;**159**:874–5).
- **Mirtazapine** has been successful for 'hot flushes' in women (n=22 [c=16], Perez *et al*, *J Support Oncol* 2004;**2**:50–6), although sedation was a tolerance problem (n=27 [c=20]), open, 12/52, Biglia *et al*, *Breast J* 2007;**13**:490–5). It may be dose-dependent, perhaps via 5HT2/3 antagonism and influence on regulation of body temperature and diaphoresis (n=1, Buecking *et al*, *Eur J Clin Pharmacol* 2005;**61**:543–4).
- **Oxybutinin** 5–15mg (n=2, Grootens, *Am J Psychiatry* 2011;**168**:330–1).
- **Terazosin** 2mg/d (e.g. very effective if venlafaxine or sertraline-induced, n=1, Mago and Monti, *J Clin Psychiatry* 2007;**68**:639–40).

Review: Marcy and Britton, *Ann Pharmacother* 2005;**39**:748–52.

6.6 Endocrine effects

Metabolic syndrome is a term used to describe a series of endocrine disturbances such as weight gain, hypertriglyceridemia and increased insulin, glucose, and low-density lipoprotein cholesterol levels. These are associated with antipsychotic use and raise the risk of diabetes and cardiac problems.

Reviews: Hert *et al*, *World Psychiatry* 2009;**8**:15–22; FFT; Meyer and Stahl, *Acta Psychiatr Scand* 2009;**119**:4–14.

Diabetes:

Diabetes insipidus

Diabetes insipidus (not related to diabetes mellitus) is caused by poor kidney function or inadequate antidiuretic hormone production. It is becoming more common anyway, and often undiagnosed. Screening before prescribing psychotropics helps exclude pre-existing diabetes, for which any medication would obviously get the blame.

- Discontinuing or replacing the causative drug is the obvious first strategy if possible, plus standard management, e.g. thiazides and/or amiloride or sometimes NSAIDs (e.g. indometacin).

6

Diabetes mellitus

Type 1: Person is unable to produce any insulin (previously known as insulin-dependent diabetes).

Type 2: Person is unable to produce enough insulin, or insulin fails to work (insulin resistance):
- May be caused by decreased insulin sensitivity and weight gain
- Monitor carefully if there is a family history or risk factors exist.

General management includes:
- Lifestyle adjustment and related changes, e.g. weight, smoking, exercise and diet.
- Sleep loss or deprivation increases the risk of diabetes and weight gain and is a novel independent risk factor, through altered leptin and ghrelin signals, decreased glucose tolerance and insulin sensitivity (n=12, RCT, 2x2/7, c/o, Spiegel *et al*, *Ann Intern Med* 2004;**141**:846–50), especially if associated with activation of the stress system which leads to consumption of comfort food (n=21, Pejovic *et al*, *J Sleep Res* 2010;**19**:552–8; FFT).
- Oral hypoglycaemics, e.g. metformin (increases utilisation, but not production, of insulin; n=40, RCT, d/b, 14/52, Baptista *et al*, *Can J Psychiatry* 2006;**51**:192–6) or insulin can be considered.

Clozapine

Discontinue (although it may not always resolve, n=2, Tovey *et al*, *J Psychopharmacol* 2005;**19**:207–10).

Orlistat has been used (Pavlovic, *Eur Psychiatry* 2005;**20**:520).

Review: Henderson, *CNS Drugs* 2002;**16**:77–89.

Olanzapine

Discontinue (although it may not always resolve, see Koller and Doraiswamy, *Pharmacotherapy* 2002;**22**:841–52).

Reduced dosage may help (n=237, Koller and Doraiswamy, *Pharmacotherapy* 2002;**22**:841–52) as the effect seems to be dose-related (n=49,946, Ulcickas Yood *et al*, *BMC Psychiatry* 2011;**11**:197; FFT).

Switch to an alternative antipsychotic, e.g. quetiapine (n=6 and review, Ashim *et al*, *J Psychopharmacol* 2004;**18**:128–32), risperidone (n=1, Wu *et al*, *Psychiatry Clin Neurosci* 2006;**60**:115–6), aripiprazole (De Hert *et al*, *Diabetes Care* 2006;**29**:2329–30), or ziprasidone (n=84, Montes *et al*, *Prog Neuropsychopharmacol Biol Psychiatry* 2007;**31**:383–8).

Rosiglitazone 4–8mg/d improved glycaemic control in olanzapine metabolic disturbance but not HbA1c or lipids (n=30, RCT, d/b, p/c, 12/52, Baptista *et al*, *Pharmacopsychiatry* 2009;**42**:14–9), and 4mg/d non-significantly improved glucose utilisation and insulin sensitivity, and reduced LDL in clozapine metabolic disturbance (n=18, RCT, d/b, p/c. 8/52, Henderson *et al*, *Acta Psychiatr Scand* 2009;**119**:457–65; FFT).

Risperidone

Telmisartan has been used successfully as an adjunct (n=1, Yamaguchi and Tsutsumi, *Intern Med* 2010;**49**:919–23; FFT).

Hepatotoxicity

Valproate

Early discontinuation and supportive therapy is usually vital (Konig *et al*, *Epilepsia* 1999;**40**:1036–40), although **dose reduction** may be possible if monitored with extreme care (n=1, Lackmann, *Pharmacology* 2004;**70**:57–8).

L-carnitine can help, especially if given IV and within the first five days (e.g. n=92, Bohan *et al*, *Neurology* 2001;**56**:1405–9). It can also be used prophylactically (review by Leheureux *et al*, *Crit Care* 2005;**9**:431–40; FFT).

Garlic organosulfur and **ginkgo biloba** use has been postulated (Sabayan *et al*, *Med Hypotheses* 2007;**68**:512–4).

Hyperammonaemia

Valproate *

Discontinue, as it can lead to coma and is usually rapidly reversible (e.g. n=2, Carlson *et al*, *J Am Acad Child Adolesc Psychiatry* 2007;**46**:356–61).

Dose reduction, as it may be plasma level related (n=2, Wadzinski *et al*, *J Am Board Fam Med* 2007;**20**:499–502; FFT), e.g. above 20mg/kg/d (n=2,724, Yamamoto *et al*, *Epilepsy Res* 2012;**101**:202–9). Alternatively stop and add

lactulose (n=1) or IV normal saline (n=1) (Shan *et al, J Psychopharmacol* 2010;**24**:943–5).
Stop other drugs that may exacerbate, e.g. concomitant phenytoin (11x more likely), phenobarbital (4.3x), carbamazepine (2.8x) and topiramate (2.8x) (n=2,724, Yamamoto *et al, Epilepsy Res* 2012;**101**:202–9), or pivmecillinam (n=1, Lokrantz *et al, Acta Neurol Scand* 2004;**109**:297–301).
* **Carglumic acid** (orphan drug in Europe for hyperammonaemia) has been used successfully (e.g. n=1, Fernández Polomer *et al, An Pediatr [Barc]* 2014;**81**:251–5; n=2, Kasapkara *et al, J Pediatr Neurosci* 2013;**8**:250–2).
* **L-carnitine** can correct valproate-induced carnitine depletion (which results in high ammonia plasma levels; Vázquez *et al, Biomed Res Int* 2014;**2014**:217269) and is well tolerated (e.g. n=1, Martín-Del Rincón *et al, Med Intensiva* 2014;**38**:124–5; review by Mock and Schwetschenau, *Am J Health Syst Pharm* 2012;**69**:35–9).
Peritoneal dialysis (n=1, Kumar *et al, Indian J Crit Care Med* 2014;**18**:461–3).
Review: Vivekanandan and Nayak, *Ann Indian Acad Neurol* 2010;**13**:145–7.

Hypercalcemia (hyperparathyroidism)

Lithium

Although relatively rare, hypercalcemia/hyperparathyroidism is a recognised ADR (reviews, Broome and Solorzano, *Endocr Pract* 2011;**17**Suppl 1:31–5; Saunders *et al, World J Surg* 2009;**33**:2314–23).
Surgery (bilateral or unilateral parathyroidectomy) may only be effective in <50% of people (n=71, 6/12, Järhult *et al, Br J Surg* 2010;**97**:1680–5).
Calcimimetic therapy (a potential alternative to parathyroidectomy).

Hypercholesterolaemia

Antipsychotics

Standard treatments for reducing cholesterol, e.g. statins (n=28, Ojala *et al, J Psychopharmacol* 2008;**22**:33–8).
Switching drugs, e.g. ziprasidone (n=84, Montes *et al, Prog Neuropsychopharmacol Biol Psychiatry* 2007;**31**:383–8), aripiprazole or lurasidone for people on olanzapine, quetiapine or risperidone, may improve weight and non-HDL cholesterol but there may be a higher rate of discontinuation than in people staying on the first drug (n=215, RCT, Stroup *et al, Am J Psychiatry* 2011;**168**:947–56; FFT), but not for lurasidone.
Discontinue any beta-blockers, as these may enhance clozapine's effect on cholesterol (n=50, Batmiller *et al, Schizophr Res* 2003;**59**:49–57).

Hyperglycaemia

Clozapine

Standard hypoglycaemic therapies
Orlistat has been used (Pavlovic, *Eur Psychiatry* 2005;**20**:520).
Amisulpride has a lower hyperglycaemic effect compared to clozapine (n=22, 12–16/52, Rettenbacher *et al, J Psychopharmacol* 2007;**21**:400–4), although unlikely to be therapeutically equivalent.
Review: Ramaswamy *et al, Ann Clin Psychiatry* 2006;**18**:183–94.

Hyperlipidaemia

Antipsychotics

Hyperlipidaemia has been reported with all antipsychotics (decreasing incidence from clozapine, olanzapine, risperidone, quetiapine, ziprasidone to first generation) except aripiprazole and lurasidone.
Manage risk factors, such as weight gain, dietary changes and glucose intolerance (Koro and Meyer, *Essent Psychopharmacol* 2005;**6**:148–57).
Discontinue any beta-blockers which may enhance the effects on lipids (n=50, Batmiller *et al, Schizophr Res* 2003;**59**:49–57).
Lipid-lowering therapy, e.g. rosuvastatin (n=100, 3/12, De Hert *et al, J Clin Psychiatry* 2006;**67**:1889–96).

Switch drugs:

- **Amisulpride, lurasidone** or **ziprasidone** (Rettenbacher *et al, Int Clin Psychopharmacol* 2006;**21**:369–72) and **risperidone** (n=15, Su *et al, Psychopharmacology* [Berl] 2005;**183**:383–6) may be alternatives if olanzapine or clozapine-induced.
- **Aripiprazole** has resolved clozapine (n=1, Ball *et al, Ann Pharmacother* 2005;**39**:1570–2) and olanzapine-induced hyperlipidaemia (s=3, n=546, RCT, Newcomer *et al, Schizophr Res* 2008;**106**:300–7; FFT) and may be the best option (n=13,133 vs 17,240, Olfson *et al, Am J Psychiatry* 2006;**163**:1821–5; mean –6.2mg/dL in triglycerides, n=84, Montes *et al, Prog Neuropsychopharmacol Biol Psychiatry* 2007;**31**:383–8), but not all improve and the switch has a significant risk of worsening symptoms (n=52, 52/52, Chen *et al, J Psychopharmacol* 2012;**26**:1201–10).
- **Fluvoxamine** 50mg/d has been used for clozapine-induced hyperlipidaemia, partly by altering the clozapine:norclozapine ratio and possibly by facilitating a reduced clozapine dose via CYP1A2 inhibition (n=68, RCT, 12/52, Lu *et al, J Clin Psychiatry* 2004;**65**:766–71).

Hyperprolactinaemia *

Hyperprolactinaemia is more common in bipolar disorder and schizophrenia (Bushe and Shaw, *J Psychopharmacol* 2007;**21**:768–73), higher dose and female gender (n=268, Suzuki *et al, Schizophr Res* 2013;**145**:116–9) and is linked to longer-term clinical sequelae, such as osteoporosis, hip fractures and possibly breast cancer.

Reviews: * general (Peuskens *et al, CNS Drugs* 2014;**28**:421–53; FFT; Besnard *et al, Encephale* 2014;**40**:86–94), drug causes (review, Torre and Falorni, *Ther Clin Risk Manag* 2007;**3**:929–51; FFT).

Antidepressants

Switching seems the safest option.

In decreasing order, fluvoxamine (ROR=4.5), citalopram (ROR=3.9), fluoxetine (ROR=3.6) and paroxetine (ROR=3.1) were most likely to cause hyperprolactinaemia, whereas duloxetine, milnacipran and sertraline are not associated with an increased risk (n=187 from 11,863, Trenque *et al, Drug Saf* 2011;**34**:1161–6).

Antipsychotics *

Reducing the dose of the causative agent may help.

Check the clinical relevance or importance (remembering the potential long-term effects of raised prolactin), especially if it is resulting in amenorrhoea in women or testosterone deficiency in men.

Test for a lesion by stopping the drug temporarily (or switching to a prolactin-sparing antipsychotic) to see if prolactin returns to normal, and/or by performing a CT scan (Molitch, *Mayo Clin Proc* 2005;**80**:1050–7).

HRT/combined oral contraceptive in women and **exogenous testosterone** in men (see Molitch, *Mayo Clin Proc* 2005;**80**:1050–7) may help, and avoid the need to switch drugs (Miller, *CNS Spectr* 2004;**9**[8 Suppl 7]:28–32).

Smoking — this is not a suggestion to take up smoking, but in people stabilised on risperidone, prolactin was higher in females than males, but smoking led to a lower prolactin in females but no difference in males (n=154, >4/52, Ohta *et al, Prog Neuropsychopharmacol Biol Psychiatry* 2011;**35**:573–6), a robust association (n=228, Mackin *et al, J Psychopharmacol* 2011;**25**:698–703).

Switch drugs:

Switching to a prolactin-sparing antipsychotic (*Table 2.1.4*) is first-line strategy. In children and adolescents quetiapine, lurasidone and clozapine are best and amisulpride and risperidone worst, but there is insufficient data on the others (s=29, Roke *et al, J Child Adolesc Psychopharmacol* 2009:**19**:403–14).

- * **Aripiprazole** may be an alternative as it can reduce prolactin in its own right, albeit not always successful. Augmenting with aripiprazole or switching to aripiprazole significantly has reduced prolactin levels within a week, maintained for eight weeks (n=269, 8/52, Byerly *et al*, *Schizophr Res* 2009;**107**:218–22; n=555, RCT, open, 26/52, Hanssens *et al*, *BMC Psychiatry* 2008;**8**:95; FFT). 60% may get subnormal prolactin levels with aripiprazole cf 8% with placebo so beware of this during monotherapy (Safer *et al*, *J Child Adolesc Psychopharmacol* 2013;**23**:282–9; FFT).
- * **Lurasidone** has almost no effect on prolactin levels (n=609, RCT, d/b, 12/12, Citrome *et al*, *Int Clin Psychopharmacol* 2012;**27**:165–76).
- **Olanzapine** has been used if risperidone-induced (n=17, c/o, Lin *et al*, *J Clin Psychiatry* 2006;**67**:1470–1).
- **Quetiapine** has a low incidence of hyperprolactinaemia (20%; n=70, Stevens *et al*, *J Child Adolesc Psychopharmacol* 2005;**15**:893–900) and switching to quetiapine from FGAs may be successful in about 65% of cases (n=69, Nakajima *et al*, *Pharmacopsychiatry* 2005;**38**:17–9).
- * **Risperidone** — switching people from oral to RLAI may reduce prolactin levels, possibly by reducing surges in 9-OH-risperidone levels (35% reduction, n=25, open, 12/52, Bai *et al*, *J Clin Psychopharmacol* 2007;**27**:306–8). **Paliperidone** and **risperidone** cause the same amount of prolactin elevation (n=76, 6/7, RCT, d/b, Berwaerts *et al*, *J Psychopharmacol* 2010;**24**:1011–8), although switching to paliperidone LAI can significantly decrease serum prolactin with a four-fold reduction in sexual dysfunction (n=11, 3/12, Montalvo *et al*, *Int Clin Psychopharmacol* 2013;**28**:46–9).

Adjunctive therapies: *

- * **Aripiprazole** augmentation may be useful (see also above). The optimum dose appears to be 5 mg/d, as this produces the optimum effect with least dose-related side-effects (s=5, n=639, RCT, p/c, Li *et al*, *PLoS One* 2013;**8**:e70179):
  - ~ **Benzamides**: only 10% had normalised prolactin with aripiprazole augmentation (n=10, 8/52, open, Chen *et al*, *Prog Neuropsychopharmacol Biol Psychiatry* 2010;**34**:1495–9).
  - ~ **Haloperidol:** aripiprazole 15–30 mg/d can reduce prolactin levels, with 88% normal after 8/52 (cf. 4% with placebo) and reversal of symptoms in most (n=56, p/c, 8/52, Shim *et al*, *Am J Psychiatry* 2007;**164**:1404–10), albeit with some risk of exacerbation of hallucinations (n=7, Lee *et al*, *Prog Neuropsychopharmacol Biol Psychiatry* 2006;**30**:714–7).
  - ~ **Olanzapine:** aripiprazole 15 mg has produced complete resolution (n=1, Aggarwal *et al*, *Indian J Pharmacol* 2010;**42**:58–9; FFT).
  - ~ **Paliperidone** - aripiprazole 5mg/d reversed the effect within 4/52 (e.g. n=1, Basterreche *et al*, *Actas Esp Psiquiatr* 2012;**40**:290–2).
  - ~ * **Risperidone:** aripiprazole 5–20 mg/d normalised prolactin in 93% (n=15, 8/52, open, Chen *et al*, *Prog Neuropsychopharmacol Biol Psychiatry* 2010;**34**:1495–9) in 4–6 weeks (n=113[c=107], RCT, open, 8/52, Zhao *et al*, *PLoS One* 2015;**10**:e0139717; FFT). 5 mg/d (range 3–6 mg/d) seems an effective dose as an adjunct to RLAI (n=13, open, 3/12, Trives *et al*, *J Clin Psychopharmacol* 2013;**33**:538–41; n=16, Yasui-Furukori *et al*, *J Clin Psychopharmacol* 2010;**30**:596–9).

Dopamine agonists should generally be avoided as they may precipitate psychosis, but with careful monitoring and dose adjustment may be successful in selected cases where other strategies have failed (review; Colao *et al*, *Nat Clin Pract Endocrinol Metab* 2006;**2**:200–10). There may be significant differences in tolerability of dopamine agonists and a systematic review and meta-analysis suggested **carbergoline** as preferable to bromocriptine (s=4, Dos Santos Nunes *et al*, *Pituitary* 2011;**14**:259–65).

- **Amantadine** has been successful in 90% people (n=10, open, 7/52, Correa *et al*, *J Clin Psychopharmacol* 1987;**7**:91–5).
- **Bromocriptine** 2.5–10mg/d reduces prolactin over four weeks then plateaus, with no relapses (n=60 [c=48], RCT, s/b, p/c, 8/52, Lee *et al*, *Psychiatry Clin Neurosci* 2010;**64**:19–27).
- * **Cabergoline** is longer-acting, better tolerated and may be superior to bromocriptine in efficacy. Cabergoline 0.125–0.25mg/d has been used if risperidone-induced (statistically significant reduction in 58%, with no adverse affects nor deterioration in psychosis; n=19, 8/52, Cavallaro *et al*, *J Clin Psychiatry* 2004;**65**:187–90). Use a carefully chosen lower dose as the standard starting dose of 0.5mg/d or higher might cause psychosis (n=2, Chang *et al*, *Gen Hosp Psychiatry* 2008;**30**:378–80).
- **Pergolide** – mentioned in some reviews (see below).
- **Peony-glycyrrhiza decoction** (PGD, a herbal medicine) 45g/d was as effective as bromocriptine 5mg/d for risperidone-induced hyperprolactinaemia in women with schizophrenia, and also improved symptoms of raised prolactin (n=20, RCT, c/o, 3x4/52, Yuan *et al*, *J Clin Psychopharmacol* 2008;**28**:264–70).

Reviews: management (Madhusoodanan *et al*, *Hum Psychopharmacol* 2010;**25**:281–97), general (Verhelst and Abs, *Treat Endocrin* 2003;**2**:23–32).

Hyperthyroidism

Lithium

Lithium can raise TSH levels, which has been linked strongly with an increased risk of depression, so monitor regularly and manage (s=2, n=32, RCT, d/b, p/c, 18/12, Frye *et al*, *Acta Psychiatr Scand* 2009;**120**:10–3), e.g. with **carbimazole** (n=9 and review, Barclay *et al*, *Clin Endocrinol* [Oxf] 1994;**40**:759–64).

Radioactive iodine (n=3, Dwarakanathan, *Endocr Pract* 1998;**4**:201–3).

Hypocalcaemia (see hyperparathyroidism)

Hyponatraemia*

Risk factors for hyponatraemia include older age, female gender, low body weight, concurrent drugs (e.g. diuretics, NSAIDs, carbamazepine, cancer chemotherapy), reduced renal function, smoking, comorbidity (e.g. hypothyroidism, diabetes, COPD), previous hyponatraemia, bleeding, urinary loss, CHF, cirrhosis, SIADH, psychosis, and hotter weather (review by Jacob and Spinler, *Ann Pharmacother* 2006;**40**:1618–22), so monitor serum sodium over the high risk period of the first 14 days in higher risk patients. Rapid correction is extremely hazardous.

- If withdrawing a causative drug, sodium usually returns to normal within two weeks (e.g. with bupropion, n=1, Kate *et al*, *Gen Hosp Psychiatry* 2013;**35**:681.e11–2).
- Rechallenge may be possible without recurrence (review, Kirby and Ames, *Int J Geriatr Psychiatry* 2001;**16**:484–93). If necessary, restart at low dose, increase slowly and monitor carefully.
- If sodium is >125mmol/l, monitor daily until above 135mmol/L. If <125mmol/L, refer for urgent specialist medical care.
- Loop diuretics have been used (Jacob and Spinler, *Ann Pharmacother* 2006;**40**:1618–22).
- Restrict fluid intake (to around 800ml/d).

Review: Management (Munger, *Am J Health Syst Pharm* 2007;**64**:253–65).

Antidepressants *

May be due to inappropriate antidiuretic hormone secretion (SIADH).
Use a lower risk antidepressant. According to CSM data the risks are as follows (although there is doubtless under-reporting for all drugs):

- Highest risk (> 1% incidence): (es)citalopram, fluoxetine, sertraline.
- Medium risk (0.5–1% incidence): amitriptyline, clomipramine, dosulepin, doxepin, imipramine, lofepramine, moclobemide, paroxetine, venlafaxine.
- Lowest risk (< 0.5% incidence): mirtazapine and agomelatine (see below), reboxetine, nortriptyline, trazodone, phenelzine, tranylcypromine.

Mirtazapine appears to have the lowest risk based on current evidence and case reports (isolated cases; n = 2, Cheah *et al*, *Am J Geriatr Pharmacother* 2008;**6**:91–5).
Agomelatine has no case reports.
Bupropion 150 mg/d has been a successful alternative if sertraline-induced (n = 1, Cerimele and Robinson, *Prim Care Companion CNS Disorders* 2011;**13**:PCC.11l01175; FFT).
Tolvaptan (a vasopressin-2-receptor antagonist) has rapidly resolved venlafaxine-induced hyponatraemia non-responsive to discontinuation or fluid restriction (n = 1, Meyer *et al*, *Dtsch Med Wochenschr* 2012;**137**:1096–9), but cannot be recommended yet.
Water restriction and/or careful use of demeclocycline can be considered if hyponatraemia is recurrent although **demeclocycline** use is controversial and some texts recommend avoiding it with antidepressants.
Review: Cawley, *Ann Pharmacother* 2007;**41**:840–50.

Antipsychotics

This can be caused by water intoxication, SIADH or severe hyperlipidaemia and/or hyperglycaemia.
If caused by water intoxication (serum and urine osmolality both low):

- **Fluid restriction** (refer to acute medical care if sodium is < 125 mmol/L).
- **Switch drugs**, e.g. clozapine (may reverse hyponatraemia/hypoosmolemia; n = 8, 18–24/52, open, Canuso and Goldman, *J Neuropsychiatry Clin Neurosci* 1999;**11**:86–90), olanzapine, risperidone or quetiapine.
- There is no evidence yet that reducing doses is effective.

If caused by SIADH (high urine but low serum osmolality):

- **Fluid restriction** (refer to acute care if sodium < 125 mmol/L).
- **Switch** antipsychotic as soon as possible. A low incidence has been reported with aripiprazole (Bachu *et al*, *Am J Ther* 2006;**13**:370–2).
- **Demeclocycline** probably directly blocks the renal tubular effect of antidiuretic hormones (usual dose range is 0.9–1.2 g daily, reduced to 600–900 mg/d for maintenance, see standard texts).
- **Discontinue any concurrent desmopressin** (n = 1, Sarma *et al*, *Aust N Z J Psychiatry* 2005;**39**:949).
- **Lithium** has been used (mentioned in Madhusoodanan *et al*, *Adverse Drug React Toxicol Rev* 2002;**21**:17–29).

Hypothyroidism

Lithium

Lithium inhibits thyroid release but compensatory mechanisms operate in most people. It is more common in people with circulating thyroid antibodies (n = 150, Bocchetta *et al*, *J Endocrinol Invest* 2007;**30**:363–6). Refer to an endocrinologist if TSH levels are repeatedly abnormal.
Lithium withdrawal tends to resolve euthyroid or hypothyroid goitres.
Supplementary levothyroxine/liothyronine therapy is indicated for overt hypothyroidism, but use for subclinical hypothyroidism is controversial.
Manage weight, especially during the first year, as this is highly predictive

of hypothyroidism (Henry, *J Psychiatry Neurosci* 2002;**27**;104–7; FFT).
Reviews: general (Fagiolini *et al*, *Epidemiol Psichiatr Soc* 2006;**15**:123–7), mechanisms (Bocchetta and Loviselli, *Clin Pract Epidemol Ment Health* 2006;**12**:23; FFT).

Polyuria and renal impairment (often a symptom of diabetes insipidus)

Lithium* Renal impairment may be due to lithium's effect on vasopressin at a hypothalamic level, a decrease in GFR, or the aging process as there are no properly documented cases of lithium alone causing renal damage if maintained within normal plasma limits. Closer monitoring in recent decades may have reduced the incidence (Aiff *et al*, *J Psychopharmacol* 2014;**28**:151–4), although perhaps not completely (n=630, Aiff *et al*, *J Psychopharmacol* 2015;**25**:608–14). The main strategies are:

- **Reduce dose** to the lowest possible, making it **once daily** (if not already).
- * **Ensure plasma levels are robustly kept below 0.8 mmol/L** (n=699, 10 years, Kirkham *et al*, *BMJ Open* 2014;**4**:e006020; FFT) by monitoring every 3/12 and ignoring NICE's Bipolar Guidelines (2014) utterly inexplicable six-monthly monitoring recommendation change.
- **Switch** to an alternative drug if possible (e.g. valproate has been used; n=7, Stoll *et al*, *J Clin Psychiatry* 1996;**57**:356–9).
- **Discontinue** any other drugs that might be contributing.
- **Stop any serotonergic antidepressants** that may enhance polyuria (n=75, Movig *et al*, *Br J Psychiatry* 2003;**182**:319–23; FFT).
- **Diuretics** such as amiloride have been used (n=1, Finch *et al*, *Pharmacotherapy* 2003;**23**:546–50), but great care is needed with interactions, see *Chapter 4.4* (mentioned in van Gerven and Boer, *Ned Tijdschr Geneeskd* 2006;**150**:1705–9).
- **NSAIDs** such as ketoprofen 100mg IV have been used in acute lithium toxicity presenting as severe nephrogenic diabetes mellitus (n=1, Tran-Van *et al*, *Presse Med* 2005;**34**:1137–40), as has indometacin 150mg (rapidly effective, within 36 hours; e.g. n=1, Lam and Kjellstrand, *Ren Fail* 1997;**19**:183–8), probably by blocking lithium's prostaglandin-inducing activity. Adequate hydration is essential.
- **Refer** to renal specialists for advice (although they are likely to recommend discontinuation).

Review: systematic review and meta-analysis (s=385, McKnight *et al*, *Lancet* 2012;**379**:721–8).

Weight gain *

Numerous mechanisms for drug-induced weight gain have been proposed, including:

- Sedation — leading to decreased activity.
- Thirst — anticholinergic dry mouth may lead to an increased intake of fluids and calories.
- Reduced metabolism — fat and carbohydrate oxidation.
- Increased appetite, e.g. via blockade of receptors such as 5HT2A, 5HT2C (n=30, RCT, d/b, Kluge *et al*, *J Clin Psychopharmacol* 2007;**27**:662–6), H1 or H2, perhaps D2, and polypeptides such as CCK.
- Increased leptin (which controls food intake) levels are consistently associated with increases in BMI (s=28, Potvin *et al*, *Can J Psychiatry* 2015;**60**[3 Suppl 2]:S26–34;FFT).
- Other polypeptides may also be implicated, e.g. reductin and cytokines, neuropeptide Y, tumour necrosis factor alpha (TNF-alpha), NPY and AMPK pathways (Lian *et al*, *Psychoneuroendocrinology* 2014;**48**:77–86) and ghrelin (n=112, Esen-Danaci *et al*, *Prog Neuropsychopharmacol Biol Psychiatry* 2008;**32**:1434–8).
- Induction of abdominal fat deposition, combined with a dysfunction of the normal leptin control of weight (n=46, 10/52, Zhang *et al*, *Br J Psychiatry* 2004;**184**:58–62; FFT).
- Fluid retention — via peripheral oedema, a minor effect.

- Endocrine effects — increased prolactin levels (which may promote adiposity and variation in cortisol or altered insulin secretion).
- Poor sleep or sleep deprivation leads to increased hunger and opportunities to eat plus increased fatigue and altered thermoregulation (reducing energy need), leading to obesity. More than seven hours sleep per day has the lowest and less than 5.5 hours sleep per day has the highest prevalence of adiposity. Evening watching of back-lit screens (TV, PCs etc) may inhibit the release of melatonin, which does not trigger the normal sleep-wake cycle (unless wearing yellow or orange glasses).

Reviews: overview (s=248, Gentile, *Obes Rev* 2009;**10**:527–42), therapeutic options (Cordes *et al, Fortschr Neurol Psychiatr* 2008;**76**:703–14), in bipolar (Torrent *et al, Acta Psychiatr Scand* 2008;**118**:4–18), in younger people (Maayan and Correll, *J Child Adolesc Psychopharmacol* 2011;**21**:517–35).

Antidepressants * — Weight changes in depression can be part of the presenting symptoms, although weight gain with antidepressants may be the reversal of a pre-treatment weight loss in some (heavier people are more likely to gain weight if they become depressed).

* **Switching** is an option. A meta-analysis and review concludes that tricyclics (due to carbohydrate craving; Paykel, *Br J Psychiatry* 1973;**123**:501–7; and a decreased metabolic rate; Fernstein *et al, Biol Psychiatry* 1985;**20**:688–92), mirtazapine and paroxetine are associated with the greatest weight gain, fluoxetine and bupropion with some weight loss and the others seem weight neutral, with any weight gain more evident over long-term (Blumenthal *et al, JAMA Psychiatry* 2014;**71**:889–96). There is no effect on weight from **vortioxetine** (SmPC).

SSRIs — There is a tendency for weight loss over the first six weeks (increased metabolic rate, suppressed appetite, and increased basal body temperature; n=20, RCT, p/c, Bross and Hoffer, *Am J Clin Nutrition* 1995;**61**:1020–5; FFT), gradually regained over six months. Many may then gain weight over the longer term.

Topiramate up to 250 mg/d has produced a mean 4 kg loss of weight (n=15, open, 10/52, Van Ameringen *et al, J Clin Psychiatry* 2002;**63**:981–4).

Bupropion has been used for SSRI-induced weight gain (see review by Demyttenaere and Jaspers, *J Psychopharmacol* 2008;**22**:792–804).

Review: review and meta-analysis (s=116, Serretti and Mandelli, *J Clin Psychiatry* 2010;**71**:1259–72).

Mirtazapine — Weight gain is difficult to manage and so switching may be the only option. **Starting at 30 mg/d** may reduce weight gain (manufacturer's global data). **Ranitidine** at night is probably of no use.

Antipsychotics * — **Education:** WWW (warn, weigh, watch):

Warn: Counsel people with a higher risk of weight gain (see risk factors below) because, let's face it, no one wants to look like Miss Piggy.

* **Weigh:** Take a baseline weight, warn of the unpredictable nature of the weight gain, that the effect plateaus after several months, and the need to optimise calorie intake, e.g. weight gain with olanzapine is greatest in the first two months, slows in months 2–4, but still continues over six months (s=86, n=12,425, Millen *et al, J Psychopharmacol* 2011;**25**:639–47) or longer (n=170, Pérez-Iglesias *et al, Int J Neuropsychopharmacol* 2014;**17**:41–51) and increases visceral fat (Salviato Balbão *et al, Ther Adv Psychopharmacol* 2014;**4**:30–6).

Watch: As most weight is gained in the first few months, ensure dietetic advice is sought early on as it is easier to prevent weight gain than lose it once it has happened. Moderate physical exercise may be helpful. Intake of high calorie fluids should be avoided. Weight management includes all variations on 'eat less, move more', but should also include 'sleep better'.

Manage more carefully where risk factors exist:

- Higher parental BMI.
- Pre-morbid BMI (higher predicts 12.5% of gain with olanzapine), e.g. being underweight or normal weight predicts weight gain, but being overweight predicts weight loss, and is not dose-related (n=374, RCT, 1 year, Xiang *et al*, *Pharmacopsychiatry* 2011;**44**:135–41).
- Age (negative correlation, more common in younger, gain is reduced by 0.6 kg for every extra 10 years of age).
- Other risk factors include being female, lower baseline body weight (Musil *et al*, *Expert Opin Drug Saf* 2015;**14**:73–96), prone to overeating under stress, narcissistic personality traits, family or personal history of obesity, schizophrenia spectrum disorder and a greater than 6.5 kg difference between adult maximum and minimum weights (e.g. n=65, Gebhardt *et al*, *J Psychiatr Res* 2009;**43**:620–6).
- High cumulative olanzapine dose (n=118; 12/52, Smith *et al*, *Int Clin Psychopharmacol* 2008;**23**:130–7; n=164, <24/52, Ujike *et al*, *J Clin Psychiatry* 2008;**69**:1416–22).

Cochrane concludes that modest weight loss can be achieved with some drug and non-drug therapies, but the data is limited by small samples, duration and intervention variety (s=23, Faulkner *et al*, *Cochrane Database Syst Rev* 2007:**1**:CD005148; FFT).

Behavioural interventions:

Dietary interventions and nutritional education may be effective, e.g:

- Regular dietician appointments and self-directed dieting (n=35 [c=29], 15/12, Kalarchian *et al*, *J Clin Psychiatry* 2005;**66**:1058–63).
- Individual nutritional education for the 3–6/12 after starting olanzapine may be successful, although studies are small and excluded obese people (e.g. Evans *et al*, *Aust N Z J Psychiatry* 2005;**39**:479–86).
- Weight management programmes and groups may be effective (e.g. n=48 [c=36], RCT, 12/52, Kwon *et al*, *J Clin Psychiatry* 2006;**67**:547–53; n=93, 1yr, Pendlebury *et al*, *Acta Psychiatr Scand* 2007;**115**:286–94).
- * **Exercise** may help. Light jogging for 30 minutes three times a week plus reducing food intake by 500 kcal/d leads to 2 kg less gained with olanzapine (n=28, RCT, 8/52, Milano *et al*, *Adv Ther* 2007;**24**:123–34). The STRIDE weight loss programme and Lifestyle Interventions may help (Green *et al*, *Am J Psychiatry* 2015;**172**;71–81).

Medication interventions: *

Reduce the dose. There is evidence that weight gain with clozapine and olanzapine is related to **plasma** levels, but reducing the dose may reduce plasma levels. However, there is insufficient evidence on other second generation antipsychotics (Simon *et al*, *J Clin Psychiatry* 2009;**70**:1041–50).

Slower introduction has been postulated to lead to a lower final weight gain.

Switching drugs: (see *Table 6.6.1* for the relative risks; review s=4, n=636, Mukundan *et al*, *Cochrane Database Syst Rev* 2010;**12**:CD006629).

- **Aripiprazole** (see also adjunctive) — a meta-analysis in schizophrenia showed a mean 2.55 (+1.5) kg weight loss when switching to aripiprazole from other antipsychotics (s=9, n=784, Barak and Aizenberg, *J Obes* 2011;**2011**:898013; FFT). Another systematic review concluded aripiprazole had less impact on weight and dyslipidemia and diabetes than other SGAs (s=22, Citrome *et al, Curr Med Res Opin* 2014;**30**:1629–41), albeit with higher drop-outs.

- **Asenapine** only causes a mean weight gain of less than 1 kg over a year (Potkin, *J Clin Psychiatry* 2011;**72**[suppl 1]:14–18).
- * **Lurasidone** has a very low potential for weight gain (over 12/12, s=6, c=593, Meyer *et al, Int Clin Psychopharmacol* 2015;**30**:342–50; s=63, n=24083, RCT, d/b, De Hert *et al, CNS Drugs* 2012;**26**:733–59), with weight loss as likely as weight gain and weight gained with other antipsychotics being lost on switching.

Adjunctive therapies:

Might outperform placebo (in order; s=32, n=1482, p/c, Maayan *et al, Neuropsychopharmacology* 2010;**35**:1520–30; FFT):

- * **Metformin** only increases the utilisation of insulin not the production, so it can be safe in the long-term but is not without the risk of, e.g. lactic acidosis. If used at the start of treatment it significantly reduces weight gain and waist circumference (s=6, n=336, RCT, p/c, Ehret *et al, J Clin Psychiatry* 2010;**71**:1286–92). In people stable on clozapine, adjunctive metformin 500–1000mg/d can lead to a mean weight loss of 1.87kg (n=61 [c=56], RCT, d/b, p/c, 14/52, Carrizo *et al, Schizophr Res* 2009;**113**:19–26) and improved BMI, weight, fasting blood sugar and HDL levels with no effect on BPRS or other metabolic measures (n=37, RCT, d/b, p/c, 20/52, Hebrani *et al, J Res Med Sci* 2015;**20**:364–71; FFT). In EIS/first episode psychosis in women, metformin reversed the weight gain from antipsychotics (n=84 [c=76], RCT, d/b, p/c, 6/12, Wu *et al, Am J Psychiatry* 2012;**169**:813–21). A meta-analysis suggested metformin may produce a short-term weight loss with olanzapine-induced weight gain (s=4, n=104, RCT, p/c, 12/52, Praharaj *et al, Br J Clin Pharmacol* 2011;**71**:377–82; FFT). Metformin is modestly effective at reducing weight in overweight people with chronic schizophrenia (n=148[c=116], RCT, d/b, p/c, 16/52, Jarskog *et al, Am J Psychiatry* 2013;**170**:1032–40).
- **Sibutramine** 15mg/d significantly reduced olanzapine-induced weight gain (8lb vs 2lb), but increased bp and disturbed sleep (n=37, RCT, d/b, p/c, 12/52, Henderson *et al, Am J Psychiatry* 2005;**162**:954–62). Addition of sibutramine (10–20mg/d) to metformin (850–1700mg/d) was no more effective than metformin alone for reducing olanzapine-induced weight gain (n=28, d/b, p/c, 12/52, Baptista *et al, Psychiatry Res* 2008;**159**:250–3). It is contraindicated in 'psychiatric illness' so care is needed. However, it was ineffective for clozapine-induced weight gain (n=21, RCT, d/b, p/c, 12/52, Henderson *et al, Acta Psychiatr Scand* 2007;**115**:101–5).
- * **Topiramate** may be effective. A meta-analysis concluded that adjunctive topiramate can prevent or reduce the weight gain from antipsychotics (s=8, n=336, RCTs, Mahmood *et al, J Clin Psychopharmacol* 2013;**33**:90–4). The most effective dose may be 100–200mg/d (n=66, RCT, d/b, p/c, 12/52, Ko *et al, Clin Neuropharmacol* 2005;**28**:169–75).
- **Modafinil** 200mg/d has reduced the weight gained with olanzapine by 50% (n=50 [c=40], RCT, d/b, p/c, 3/52, Roerig *et al, Biol Psychiatry* 2009;**65**:607–13), but a pilot study failed to show any evidence that modafinil would routinely counteract clozapine-induced weight gain and metabolic effects (n=35, RCT, d/b, p/c, 8/52, Henderson *et al, Schizophr Res* 2011;**130**:53–6).

- * **Melatonin** as an adjunctively to olanzapine resulted in less weight gain, and lower increase in waist circumference and triglyceride levels cf placebo (n=48[c=36], RCT, d/b, p/c, 8/52, Modabbernia *et al, J Psychiatr Res* 2014;**53**:133–40), especially in bipolar disorder (n=44, RCT, d/b, p/c, 8/52, Romo-Nava *et al, Bipolar Disord* 2014;**16**:410–21).
- * **Naltrexone** significantly reduced the increase in weight gain when started with olanzapine (n=30, RCT, d/b, p/c, 12/52, Taveira *et al, J Psychopharmacol* 2014;**28**:395–400) and 25 mg/d induced significant weight loss in overweight women with schizophrenia/schizoaffective disorder (n=24, RCT, p/c, 8/52, Tek *et al, J Clin Psychopharmacol* 2014;**34**:608–12; FFT).
- * **Reboxetine** started with olanzapine may help (n=26[c=20], RCT, p/c, d/b, 6/52, Poyurovsky *et al, Am J Psychiatry* 2003;**160**:297–302) and may be enhanced if used with betahistine 48 mg/d (n=43[c=32], RCT, d/b, p/c, 6/52, Poyurovsky *et al, Psychopharmacology [Berl]* 2013;**226**:615–22).
- **Ziprasidone** can reduce the weight gain from olanzapine and other antipsychotics (e.g. n=25[c=18], open, 12/52, Wang *et al, J Psychiatr Res* 2011;**45**:1128–32), but not without the cost of cognitive impairment as an ADR (n=42, RCT, p/c, 16/52, McElroy *et al, J Clin Psychopharmacol* 2012;**32**:165–72).

***Newer options and case reports:* ***

- **Acetazolamide** has been used as an alternative to topiramate (n=1, Schneiderhan and Marvin, *Am J Ther* 2007;**14**:581–4).
- * **Alpha-lipoic acid** (ALA) is a potent antioxidant and was effective in reducing weight (-2.2 kg) especially in people taking strongly antihistaminic antipsychotics (n=10, open, 10/52, Ratliff *et al, Clin Schizophr Relat Psychoses* 2015;**8**:196–200).

Table 6.6.1: Relative weight gain with antipsychotics

Drug	Long-term change †	Range (95% CI)	Change at 10/52 ‡
Perphenazine	5.8	0.4–11.1	–
Clozapine	5.7	4.3–7	4 (2.7–5.3)
Chlorpromazine	4.2	2.9–5.4	2.1 (0.9–3.4)
Olanzapine	4.2	3.7–4.6	3.5 (3.3–3.7)
Quetiapine	2.5	<1.5–3.5	(0?)
Risperidone	1.7	1.4–2	2 (1.6–2.4)
Fluphenazine	1.1	0.1–2.2	0.4 (-0.7–1.5)
Non-drug controls	0.8	0.1–1.6	1.3 (0.8–1.8)
Polypharmacy	0.5	0.2–0.7	1.2 (0.4–2.1)
Haloperidol	0.5	0.2–0.8	0.5 (0.1–1)
Ziprasidone	0.3	-0.3–0.8	0 (-0.5–0.6)
Trifluoperazine	0.3	-0.9–1.5	–
Placebo	-1	-1.8–0.1	0.4 (-1.3–1.5)

(Allison *et al, Am J Psychiatry* 1999;**156**:1686–96; n=427; Brecher *et al, In J Psychiatr Clin Pract* 2000;**4**:287–91)

† longer-term weight change in kg (random effects mode)

‡ weight change at 10 weeks (fixed effects mode)

Please bear in mind that this is aggregated data, so is subject to error; weight was often measured at a different time and there may be a dose-relationship and a huge inter-individual variation.

- **Amantadine** 100–300mg/d may be well tolerated and attenuate the weight gain from olanzapine (n=125, RCT, d/b, p/c, 16/52, Deberdt *et al*, *Eur Neuropsychopharmacol* 2005;**15**:13–21), but not in all studies (n=25, Bahk *et al*, *Psychiatr Clin Neurosci* 2004;**58**:163–7).
- **Aripiprazole** 15mg/d (see also switching) significantly reduced the gain in weight and BMI from olanzapine (n=15, d/b, p/c, c/o, 10/52, Henderson *et al*, *J Clin Psychopharmacol* 2009;**29**:165–9; FFT) and clozapine (mean -2.5kg vs -0.4kg; n=207, RCT, d/b, p/c, 16/52, Fleischhacker *et al*, *Int J Neuropsychopharmacol* 2010;**13**:1115–25).
- **Bofu-tsusho-san** (an Oriental herbal medicine) can attenuate weight gain from olanzapine (Yamamoto and Inada, *Psychiatry Clin Neurosci* 2008;**62**:747).
- **Bupropion** 150–300mg/d as an adjunct to olanzapine produces modest weight loss (n=8 [c=7], open, 24/52, Gadde *et al*, *J Clin Psychopharmacol* 2006;**6**:409–13; review by Gadde and Xiong, *Expert Rev Neurother* 2007;**7**:17–24).
- * **Dehydroepiandrosterone** (DHEA) as adjunct in olanzapine-induced weight gain stabilised BMI, waist circumference and fasting glycaemia values (n=55[c=45], RCT, d/b, p/c, 12/52, Holka-Pokorska *et al*, *Psychiatr Pol* 2015;**49**:363–76;FFT).
- **Memantine** augmentation had a significant effect on clozapine-induced weight gain (n=1, Scharfer *et al*, *Pharmacopsychiatry* 2007;**40**:149–51).
- **Mifepristone** 600mg/d can attenuate weight gain from olanzapine (n=57, RCT, d/b, 2/52, Gross *et al*, *Adv Ther* 2009;**26**:659–69).
- **Switching to orodispersible olanzapine** — two RCTs have failed to show any loss of weight with orodispersible compared to plain tablets (e.g. n=23, RCT, open, Bobo *et al*, *Ann Clin Psychiatry* 2011;**23**:193–201), but there are case reports (e.g. especially in males and Americans, n=149, 16/52, Karagianis *et al*, *Int J Clin Pract* 2010;**64**:1520–9).
- * **Zonisamide** when started with a SGA resulted in a net weight loss (-1.9kg) cf placebo (+2.2kg) and was well tolerated (n=41, RCT, d/b, p/c, 10/52, Ghanizadeh *et al*, *Schizophr Res* 2013;**147**:110–5).

Not significantly superior to placebo:*

- **Appetite suppressants** may exacerbate psychosis or fail to work.
- **Atomoxetine** is ineffective if olanzapine or clozapine-induced (n=37 [c=26], RCT, p/c, d/b, 24/52, Ball *et al*, *Clin Schizophr Relat Psychoses* 2011;**5**:17–25).
- **Fluoxetine** is ineffective if olanzapine-induced (e.g. n=31, RCT, d/b, Bustillo *et al*, *Neuropsychopharm* 2003;**28**:527–9; FFT).
- * **H2-antagonists** such as **famotidine** (n=14, d/b, p/c, 6/52, Poyurovsky *et al*, *Eur Neuropsychopharmacol* 2004;**14**:332–6) and **nizatidine** are ineffective for olanzapine-induced weight gain (n=175, d/b, p/c, 16/52, Cavazzoni *et al*, *Eur Neuropsychopharmacol* 2003;**13**:81–5), but may have some effect in a few (n=59, RCT, d/b, 8/52, Atamaca *et al*, *Hum Psychopharmacol* 2003;**18**:457–61). **Ranitidine** may stop the weight gain with quetiapine (n=47, RCT, Atmaca *et al*, *Hum Psychopharmacol* 2004;**19**:37–40) or olanzapine (n=52, RCT, p/c, 16/52, Ranjbar *et al*, *Biomed Res Int* 2013;**2013**:639391).
- **Orlistat** has a modest effect that may only be seen in men (n=71 [c=63], RCT, d/b, p/c, 16/52, Joffe *et al*, *J Clin Psychiatry* 2008;**69**:706–11).

6

- **Phenylpropanolamine** is ineffective if clozapine-induced (n=16, RCT, d/b, 12/52, Borovicka *et al*, *J Clin Psychiatry* 2002;**63**:345–8).
- **Quetiapine** has been used as an alternative of adjunct to clozapine (review by Werneke *et al*, *Int Clin Psychopharmacol* 2002;**17**:145–60) but in olanzapine-induced weight gain, switching to quetiapine led to increased relapses and no significant weight improvements (n=133, 13/52, Deberdt *et al*, *Ther Clin Risk Manag* 2008;**4**:713–20; FFT).

Reviews: * general (s=21, n=3391, RCT, d/b, p/c, Parsons *et al*, *Schizophr Res* 2009;**110**:103–10), interventions to reduce weight in obese people with schizophrenia (Hjorth *et al*, *Acta Psychiatr Scand* 2014;**130**:279–89).

Lithium *

Weight gain is a very common reason for non-compliance with lithium (RR=1.89; s=385, McKnight *et al*, *Lancet* 2012;**379**:721–8). It occurs predominantly during the first two years of treatment, more often in people already overweight and in women than men.

Manage increased thirst, which is common, and may correlate with weight gain through increased intake of high-calorie drinks.

Thyroid status should be assessed as a possible contributory cause.

Counselling, e.g. use of plain/low-calorie beverages, along with normal sodium intake, dietary advice and monitoring, particularly during the first year, may be adequate.

Lamotrigine may be an alternative as it is associated with weight loss, there being no significant differences in non-obese people (n=554, s=2, d/b, p/c, 12/12, Bowden *et al*, *Am J Psychiatry* 2006;**163**:1199–201).

Topiramate added to lithium or valproate in bipolar I mania or mixed episodes may significantly reduce weight (n=287, RCT, d/b, p/c, 12/52, Chengappa *et al*, *J Clin Psychiatry* 2006;**67**:1698–1706; MS).

Methylphenidate *

Melatonin as an adjunct can improve increases in height and weight, probably by modifying circadian cycles, increasing sleep and allowing more growth hormone to be released (n=50, RCT, d/b, p/c, 8/52, Mostafavi *et al*, *Iran J Psychiatry* 2012;**7**:114–9).

Anticonvulsants

There is less likelihood of gaining weight with AEDs if physical activity is included as well as dieting (n=66, <8/12, Gaspari and Guerreiro, *Arq Neuropsiquiatr* 2010;**68**:277–81; FFT).

Gabapentin should be avoided as weight gain can be a significant ADR (n=44, 12/12, DeToledo *et al*, *Ther Drug Monit* 1997;**19**:394–6).

Levetiracetam at normal doses is usually weight neutral (s=4, n=970, RCT, p/c, Gidal *et al*, *Epilepsy Res* 2003;**56**:121–6).

Topiramate can produce weight loss (n=76, open, Ghaemi *et al*, *Ann Clin Psychiatry* 2001;**13**:185–9) and has even been abused to try to promote weight loss (n=1, Colom *et al*, *J Clin Psychiatry* 2001;**62**:475–6). The effect appears dose-related, with average amounts lost ranging from 1.1 kg/1.5% (up to 200mg/d) to 5.9kg/7% (800mg/d or above). The effect peaks at 12–15 months, is greater in people with higher starting weights, and is at least partially reversible.

Carbamazepine

Weight gain may be due to increased appetite.

It is reversed by discontinuation but not by dieting (n=4, Lampl *et al*, *Clin Neuropharmacol* 1991;**14**:251–5).

Pregabalin

Early management is important as 82% stay within 7% of their starting weight over one year, whereas 15% gain >7% weight but only in months 3–12, and 3% gain >7% weight in first 2/12, and continue gaining (s=41, n=3,187, 1 year, Cabrera *et al*, *Curr Med Res Opin* 2012;**28**:1027–37).

Valproate * — Weight gain with valproate (especially abdominal adiposity during maintenance therapy; n = 19 twins, Petty *et al*, *Epilepsia* 2014;**55**:1551–7) may be more common in people with normal or below normal weight before starting (n = 70, Corman *et al*, *Can J Neurol Sci* 1997;**24**:240–4) and so warning people in advance may be advantageous (review of mechanisms, Verrotti *et al*, *Obes Rev* 2011;**12**:32–43).
Get a new set of genes (n = 5 twin pairs, Klein *et al*, *Obes Res* 2005;**13**:1330–4). OK, it's not realistic, but may help to explain to some people that weight gain with valproate isn't all their 'fault'.

6.7 Movement disorders

Blepharospasm (see also tardive dystonia)

Blepharospasm is a sustained, forced, involuntary closing of the eyelids, often a presenting symptom of tardive dystonia.

Antipsychotics — **Switching** antipsychotics is usually the main effective strategy, e.g. to **clozapine**, (n = 4, Levin and Reddy, *J Clin Psychiatry* 2000;**61**:140–3) or **quetiapine** (n = 1, Reeves and Liberto, *Mov Disord* 2003;**18**:1072–3).
ECT has been used (n = 1, Sienaert and Peuskens, *J ECT* 2005;**21**:132–4).

Bruxism (teeth grinding)

Bruxism is defined as grinding, clenching and forceful teeth or jaw movements, usually during sleep. Almost everyone bruxes, but bruxism is where it is severe enough to cause damage or distress.

Review: * general (Reddy *et al*, *J Int Oral Health* 2014;**6**:105–9).

Antidepressants — **Dose reduction** usually leads to resolution (n = 4, Ellison and Stanziani, *J Clin Psychiatry* 1993;**54**:432–4) but this can take several months (n = 1, Alonso-Navarro *et al*, *Clin Neuropharmacol* 2009;**32**:111–2).
* **Switching antidepressants** — paroxetine, venlafaxine and duloxetine may be the most likely to cause bruxism (n = 807, open, Uca *et al*, *Clin Neuropharmacol* 2015;**38**:227–30)
Buspirone has been used if bruxism is induced by venlafaxine (40mg/d, significantly effective over 4/52: Pavlovic, *Int J Neuropsychopharmacol* 2004;**7**:523–4; n = 1, Kuloglu *et al*, *J Psychopharmacol* 2010;**24**:627–8), duloxetine (n = 1, Alhayrak and Ekinci, *Clin Neuropharmacol* 2011;**34**:137–8) or SSRIs e.g. fluoxetine (n = 1, Sabuncuoglu *et al*, *Spec Care Dentist* 2009;**29**:215–7) or paroxetine (n = 1, Milanlioglu, *Clinics (Sao Paulo)* 2012;**67**:191–2; FFT).
* **Gabapentin** has been used if venlafaxine-induced (e.g. n = 1, Soyata and Oflaz, *J Clin Psychopharmacol* 2015;**35**:481–3).
* **Aripiprazole** low-dose can help if SSRI-induced (Oulis *et al*, *J Neuropsychiatry Clin Neurosci* 2012;**24**:E39).
ECT, if fluvoxamine-induced (n = 1, Miyaoka *et al*, *J ECT* 2003;**19**:170–2).
* **Trazodone** has helped nocturnal bruxism caused by escitalopram (n = 1, Grinshpoon *et al*, *J Clin Psychopharmacol* 2014;**34**:662).

Antipsychotics — **Dose reduction** usually leads to resolution.
Switch to low-dose clozapine (n = 1, 16/52, Mendhekar and Andrade, *J Neuropsychiatry Clin Neurosci* 2009;**21**:105–6).
Lamotrigine has been successful (n = 1, McMeekin, *J S C Med Assoc* 2007;**103**:69–73).
Propranolol (case where concurrent akathisia also improved; n = 2, Amir *et al*, *Clin Neuropharmacol* 1997;**20**:86–9).

Atomoxetine * — **Buspirone** 5mg (n = 1, Yüce *et al*, *J Child Adolesc Psychopharmacol* 2013:**23**:634–5; FFT).

6

Dysphagia

Difficulty in swallowing or painful swallowing has been reported with many antipsychotics.

Review: * dysphagia in mental health (Aldridge and Taylor, *Dysphagia* 2012;**27**:124–37).

Antipsychotics

Discontinuation is usually rapidly successful (e.g. n = 1, Stewart, *Dysphagia* 2003;**18**:274–5).

Benzodiazepines (clonazepam) or oral **anticholinergics** may be effective in life-threatening dysphagia (trihexyphenidyl, n = 2, Hayashi *et al*, *Clin Neuropharmacol* 1997;**20**:77–81; benzatropine, n = 1, Nair *et al*, *Gen Hosp Psychiatry* 2001;**23**:231–2), although if used regularly, anticholinergics may be a causative or exacerbating factor.

EPSE, akathisia

Neuroleptic-induced akathisia (NIA) is a subjective unpleasant feeling of inner restlessness and the urge to move, with rocking while standing or sitting, lifting feet as if marching on the spot, and crossing and uncrossing legs while sitting. NIA has been associated with suicidal behaviour (s = 83, Hansen, *Hum Psychopharmacol* 2001;**16**:495–505) and subjective cognitive dysfunction and so needs managing. It is probably an imbalance of cortical and nigrostriatal dopaminergic innervation and has been reported with drugs other than antipsychotics.

Reviews: use of serotonin-based drugs (Poyurovsky and Weizman, *Br J Psychiatry* 2001;**179**:4–8; FFT; including an algorithm).

Antidepressants

Dose reduction, as it is dose-related at least for fluoxetine (n = 1, Hansen, *J Psychopharmacol* 2003;**17**:451–2).

Switch antidepressants, e.g. **paroxetine** for fluoxetine-induced (n = 1, Bauer *et al*, *J Clin Psychiatry* 1996;**57**:593–4).

Propranolol has also been used if fluoxetine-induced (Fleischhacker, *Biol Psychiatry* 1991;**30**:531–2).

Review: SSRI-induced akathisia (Koliscak and Makela, *J Am Pharm Assoc* 2009;**49**:28–36).

Antipsychotics

Reducing the dose or switching antipsychotics can be an effective strategy (prospective naturalistic trial, n = 3,861, 6/12, Schuster *et al*, *J Clin Psychopharmacol* 2012;**32**:672–7), e.g. switch to risperidone or quetiapine if olanzapine-induced (n = 1, Peritogiannis and Tsouli, *J Psychopharmacol* 2010;**24**:1121–5).

For **aripiprazole**, reduce dose, use benzodiazepines as 'glue', adrenoceptor antagonists (propranolol), gabapentin, pregabalin, mirtazapine or anticholinergic agents (review, Cassano *et al*, *Clin Drug Invest* 2007;**27**:1–13; Aitchison *et al*, *J Psychopharmacol* 2009;**23**:231–4). Anecdotally taking aripiprazole with about four squares of chocolate can reduce akathisia.

Adjunctive therapies:

The following drugs may be useful in the short or long-term if the dose or antipsychotic cannot be changed:

- **Anticholinergics** may have some efficacy (e.g. biperiden IV, n = 23, open, Hirose and Ashby, *Int J Psychiatry Med* 2000;**30**:185–94) but Cochrane concludes that there is no reliable evidence to support or refute their use for acute NIA (s = 0, n = 0, RCT. Rathbone *et al*, *Cochrane Database Syst Rev* 2006;**4**:CD003727).
- **Benzodiazepines**, e.g. clonazepam 0.5–3 mg/d have been used with 81% improved in two days (n = 21, open, Horiguchi *et al*, *Acta Psychiatr Scand* 1989;**80**:106–7). Diazepam 10–17 mg IV (at 5 mg/30 seconds) has also provided rapid relief of acute NIA (n = 18, open, Hirose and Ashby, *J Clin Psychiatry* 2002;**63**:524–7).
- **Beta-blockers** have been used, but Cochrane concludes there is

insufficient data to show an effect on NIA (s=3, n=51, Lima *et al*, *Cochrane Database Syst Rev* 2004;**4**:CD001946). Lipophilic beta-blockers, e.g. **metoprolol** (RCT, Adler *et al*, *Biol Psychiatry* 1990;**27**:673–5; n=1, Kurzthaler *et al*, *Am J Psychiatry* 1997;**154**:1316) and **propranolol** 30–80 mg/d can be effective but may take up to three months to act in chronic cases (d/b, p/c, Kramer *et al*, *Biol Psychiatry* 1988;**24**:823–7). Nadolol, sotalol and atenolol are probably ineffective.

- **Cyproheptadine** 16 mg/d may be effective, supported by a robust trial (n=30, RCT, d/b, 7/7, Fischel *et al*, *J Clin Psychopharmacol* 2001;**21**:612–5).
- **Diphenhydramine** IV may rapidly (over 30 minutes) reduce the symptoms of acute NIA from IV prochlorperazine (n=87, open, Vinson, *J Emerg Med* 2004;**26**:265–70).
- **Gabapentin**, where a dose-related effect has been reported (n=1, Pfeffer *et al*, *Int Clin Psychopharmacol* 2005;**20**:179–81).
- **Mianserin** 5 mg/d may produce a significant improvement in NIA and dysphoria (n=15, RCT, 5/7, Poyurovsky *et al*, *Br J Psychiatry* 1999;**174**:238–42; n=1, Stryjer *et al*, *Eur Psychiatry* 2004;**19**:237–8).
- * **Mirtazapine** — a systematic review and meta-analysis concludes 25% show a partial response and 20% show complete remission with mirtazapine (s=2, n=86, RCT, d/b, p/c, Praharaj *et al*, *Ther Adv Psychopharmacol* 2015;**5**:307–13; FFT).
- **Ropinirole** 18 mg/d has helped aripiprazole-induced tardive NIA (n=1, Hettema and Ross, *J Clin Psychiatry* 2007;**68**:1814–5).
- **Thiamine** (vitamin B1) high-dose (1.2 g/d) may be useful for acute NIA (n=20, RCT, p/c, d/b, 5/7, Lerner *et al*, *J Clin Psychiatry* 2004;**65**:1550–4).
- **Trazodone** 100 mg/d showed definite and statistically significant activity against NIA, probably by 5HT2A postsynaptic receptor antagonism, in a small but perfectly-formed study (n=13, RCT, d/b, p/c, c/o, 6/7, Stryjer *et al*, *Clin Neuropharmacol* 2010;**33**:219–22).
- **Zolmitriptan** (a selective 5HT1D agonist) 7.5 mg/d has produced a significant and rapid improvement in resistant NIA (n=8, open, 3/7, Gross-Isseroff *et al*, *Int Clin Psychopharmacol* 2005;**20**:23–5).

Less useful:

Other drugs tried, usually without success, include:

- **Amantadine** (n=4, Zubenko *et al*, *J Clin Psychopharmacol* 1984;**4**:218–20).
- **Apomorphine** low dose may reduce objective (movement) effects but not subjective distress (Karstaedt and Pincus, *Neurology* 1993;**43**:611–3).
- **Buspirone** has only a minor effect, with only 20% showing any benefit (n=10, Poyurovsky and Weizman, *Int Clin Psychopharmacol* 1997;**12**:263–8).
- **Fluvoxamine** for aripiprazole-induced (n=2, Furuse and Hashimoto, *Ann Gen Psychiatry* 2010;**9**:11; FFT).
- * **Gabapentin** 1200 mg/d has helped for olanzapine or quetiapine-induced (n=1, Jumar *et al*, *Asian J Psychiatr* 2014;**9**:89–90; n=2, Sullivan and Wilbur, *Ther Adv Psychopharmacol* 2014;**4**:100–2).
- **Granisetron** is ineffective (n=10, 4/7, Poyurovsky and Weizman, *Int Clin Psychopharmacol* 1999;**14**:357–60).
- **Iron supplements** — although there is no relationship between plasma iron and chronic akathisia (Barnes *et al*, *Br J Psychiatry* 1992;**161**:791–6), IV iron has been used successfully in iron-deficient akathisia (n=1, Cotter and O'Keeffe, *J Neurol Neurosurg Psychiatry* 2007;**78**:548; FFT).
- **Lorazepam** (Yassa and Grouix, *J Clin Psychopharmacol* 1989;**9**:70–1).

- **Moclobemide** (n=1, Ebert and Demling, *Pharmacopsychiatry* 1991;**24**:229–31).
- * **Pregabalin** for aripiprazole-induced tardive akathisia (n=1, De Berardis *et al*, *J Neuropsychiatry Clin Neurosci* 2013;**25**:E9–10).

EPSE, dyskinesia (acute or tardive)

Tardive dyskinesia (TD) is an involuntary hyperkinesia, which increases with anxiety, goes away during sleep and in some cases may be irreversible. Symptoms include choreas, tics, dystonias and orolingual dyskinesias, but not tremor. It is generally seen as repetitive, involuntary and purposeless movements of, e.g. the tongue, neck and jaw. It may be a late symptom of schizophrenia and antipsychotics might in fact just bring such symptoms forward (rather than cause them), e.g. brain structures are similar (n=93, McCreadie *et al*, *Arch Gen Psychiatry* 2002;**59**:332–6) and TD fluctuates with time (n=37, McCreadie *et al*, *Br J Psychiatry* 2002;**181**:135–7; FFT).

Risk factors include the length of exposure to antipsychotics in the elderly, alcohol consumption, older age, being male, previous head injury, organic brain disease, structural brain damage, any earlier EPSE, being left-handed, being diabetic, concurrent affective or negative symptoms and having a parent with schizophrenia who themselves has or had a dyskinesia.

Reviews: * general (Aia *et al*, *Curr Treat Options Neurol* 2011;**13**:231–41; Correll and Schenk, *Curr Opin Psychiatry* 2008;**21**:151–6), in children (Correll and Kane, *J Child Adolesc Psychopharmacol* 2007;**17**:647–56), 'miscellaneous' treatments (s=7, Soares-Weiser and Joy, *Cochrane Database Syst Rev* 2003;**2**:CD000208).

Antidepressants

Mirtazapine has been used for bupropion-induced TD (n=1, Kohen and Sarcevic, *Movement Disord* 2006;**21**:584–5).

* **Fluvoxamine** for duloxetine-induced TD (n=1, Albayrak and Ekinci, *J Clin Psychopharmacol* 2012;**32**:723–4).

Antipsychotics

Withdrawal or **dose reduction** are the usual strategies, although the risk of relapse may be high.

'Drug holidays' seem detrimental, and a lot less fun than they sound.

Transient dose increases may help occasionally, but only in the short-term.

Withdraw or reduce any anticholinergic drugs if possible, as these can provoke or exacerbate TD, although are not a risk factor as such (Soares and McGrath, *Cochrane Database Syst Rev* 2000;**2**:CD000204).

Switching antipsychotics:

Switching to a SGA is usually considered the main strategy, e.g. switching to risperidone or olanzapine can be equally effective (n=60, RCT, s/b, 24/52, Chan *et al*, *J Clin Psychiatry* 2010;**71**:1226–33) assuming it is drug-related.

- **Aripiprazole** may be effective if induced by quetiapine (n=1, Rizos *et al*, *World J Biol Psychiatry* 2009;**10**:54–7), risperidone (Caykoylu *et al*, *Prog Neuropsychopharmacol Biol Psychiatry* 2009;**33**:571–2) or haloperidol (n=3, Osorio *et al*, *Neurotox Res* 2010;**17**:432–4).
- * **Clozapine** may improve TD, especially with dystonic features, over the short-term (n=7, open, Bassitt *et al*, *Eur Arch Psychiatr Clin Neurosci* 1998;**248**:209–11) and longer term (n=7, open, five years, Louza and Bassitt, *J Clin Psychopharmacol* 2005;**25**:180–2), although in a Chinese in-patient cohort the incidence of TD was actually higher with clozapine (49%, n=341) than FGAs (39%, n=243, n=584, Ye *et al*, *Int Clin Psychopharmacol* 2014;**29**:318–21).
- **Olanzapine** may markedly reduce pre-existing symptoms of TD (e.g. n=2, Agarwal and Kumar, *J Clin Psychiatry* 2001;**62**:298–9).
- **Quetiapine** — a switch study showed it maintained antipsychotic efficacy but reduced TD compared to haloperidol (n=45, RCT, 12/12, s/b, Emsley *et al*, *J Clin Psychiatry* 2004;**65**:696–701) and aripiprazole

(n=1, Ono *et al*, *J Clin Pharm Ther* 2012;**37**:370–2). Adjunctive quetiapine has been used for risperidone (n=1, Nelson *et al*, *Clin Neuropharmacol* 2003;**26**:297–8) and olanzapine-induced TD (n=1, Peritogiannis and Tsouli, *J Psychopharmacol* 2010;**24**:1121–5).

- **Risperidone** — the response may occur in a few weeks and then be maintained (n=40, 48/52, Bai *et al*, *Int Clin Psychopharmacol* 2005;**20**:79–85; n=49, RCT, d/b, p/c, 16/52, Bai *et al*, *J Clin Psychiatry* 2003;**64**:1342–8; MS). Paliperidone has helped aripiprazole-induced dyskinesia (n=1, Lai, *J Neuropsychiatry Clin Neurosci* 2011;**23**:E18).

Adjunctive therapies:

Adjunctive therapies are usually considered to be of low efficacy, although tetrabenazine is licensed:

- ***Tetrabenazine** is licensed in the UK, starting at 12.5 mg/d and titrated to 25–75 mg/d (maximum 200 mg/d). In refractory TD, tetrabenazine (mean 58 mg/d) has significantly improved AIMS scores (n=20, 20/52, Ondo *et al*, *Am J Psychiatry* 1999;**156**:1279–81). It may have long-term efficacy (n=448, mean 2.3 years, Kenney *et al*, *Mov Disord* 2007;**22**:193–7; review by Fasano and Bentivoglio, *Expert Opin Pharmacother* 2010;**10**:2883–96). However, a review concluded that the evidence for tetrabenazine is thin and it can only be recommended as a final option (Leung and Breden, *Ann Pharmacother* 2011;**45**:525–31). One report used tetrabenazine (mean 142 mg/d), clonazepam (mean 4.3 mg/d) and clozapine (mean 125 mg/d) in combination, where all patients were symptom-free after 4/52 and thereafter (n=6, four years, Kimiagar *et al*, *J Neurol* 2012;**259**:660–4).
  Review: * Chen *et al*, *Clin Ther* 2012;**34**:1487–504.
- **Amantadine** was superior to placebo in one study (d/b, c/o, p/c, 18/52, Angus *et al*, *J Clin Psychopharmacol* 1997;**17**:88–91).
- **Anticholinesterases** e.g. **donepezil** 5–10 mg/d (n=10, open, 8/52, Caroff *et al*, *J Clin Psychiatry* 2001;**62**:772–5) and **galantamine** 8–24 mg/d adjunctively have reduced AIMS-rated scores slightly, with a statistically significant deterioration on discontinuation (n=35, RCT, d/b, p/c, c/o, 2 x 12/52, Caroff *et al*, *J Clin Psychiatry* 2007;**68**:410–5).
- **Buspirone** at up to 180 mg/d may be useful (n=8, open, 12/52, Moss *et al*, *J Clin Psychopharmacol* 1993;**13**:204–9).
- **Gabapentin** has improved long-term TD, with an average improvement of 47.5% (n=25, open, 12/12, Hardoy *et al*, *J Affect Disord* 2003;**75**:125–30).
- **Ginkgo biloba** significantly reduced AIMS scores cf placebo, with no effect on PANSS scores in a Chinese cohort (n=157 [c=152], RCT, d/b, p/c, 12/52, Zhang *et al*, *J Clin Psychiatry* 2011;**72**:615–21).
- **Levetiracetam** (500–3000 mg/d) was well tolerated and significantly reduced AIMS scores (43% vs 19%) compared to placebo (n=50, RCT, d/b, p/c, 12/52, Woods *et al*, *J Clin Psychiatry* 2008;**69**:546–54; n=1, Chen and Liu, *J Clin Psychopharmacol* 2010;**30**:205–7).
- **Melatonin** 10 mg/d has been shown to decrease AIMS scores in TD (n=22, d/b, p/c, c/o, 6/52, Shamir *et al*, *Arch Gen Psychiatry* 2001;**58**:1049–52).
- **Naltrexone** plus clonazepam have reduced TD scores (n=23, RCT, d/b, p/c, Wonodi *et al*, *J Clin Psychopharmacol* 2004;**24**:441–5).
- **Ondansetron** (a 5HT3 antagonist) 12 mg/d has been used successfully (n=12, open, 12/52, Sirota *et al*, *Am J Psychiatry* 2000;**157**:287–9, although this could have been an interaction).

6

- **Piracetam** (mean 4800 mg/d) may be effective (n=40, RCT, d/b, p/c, c/o, 2×4/52, Libov *et al*, *J Clin Psychiatry* 2007;**68**:1031–7).
- **Sodium oxybate** resolved olanzapine-induced TD, with a 2/52 latency of onset (n=1, Berner, *J Clin Psychiatry* 2008;**69**:862).
- **Thiamine** was effective in one small but careful study (n=15, RCT, d/b, p/c, 4/52, Lerner *et al*, *Am J Psychiatry* 2001;**158**:1511–4).
- * **Vitamin B6 (pyridoxine)** may reduce the severity of severe TD but the evidence is considered weak, small and inadequate (s=3, n=80, RCT, p/c, Adelufosi *et al*, *Cochrane Database Syst Rev* 2015;**4**:CD010501).
- **Yi-gan san**, a Japanese herbal medicine, may help (n=22, open, 12/52, Miyaoka *et al*, *Prog Neuropsychopharmacol Biol Psychiatry* 2008;**32**:761–4).
- **Zonisamide** may be safe and effective for TD (n=11 [c=11], open, 4/52, Iwata *et al*, *J Neurol Sci* 2012;**315**:137–40).
- **Zopiclone** has been used (n=1, Sugawara *et al*, *Prog Neuropsychopharmacol Biol Psychiatry* 2009;**33**:727–8).

Less useful:

Many adjunctive therapies have been tried, but few have any real use. The following are not in the useful group:

- **Baclofen**, see GABA agonists.
- **Benzodiazepines** have been used but Cochrane concludes that they have no proven advantage over placebo (s=3, n=56, Bhoopathi and Soares-Weiser, *Cochrane Database Syst Rev* 2006;**3**:CD000205).
- **Calcium-channel blockers** are not supported by any robust studies (s=0, n=0, Essali *et al*, *Cochrane Database Syst Rev* 2011;**1**:CD000206).
- **Cholinergic drugs** (e.g. choline, lecithin) are probably ineffective (see systematic review; s=11, n=261, RCTs, Tammenmaa *et al*, *Prog Neuropsychopharmacol Biol Psychiatry* 2004;**28**:1099–107).
- **Citalopram** was ineffective in one study (n=13, Korsgaard *et al*, *Clin Neuropharmacol* 1986;**9**:52–7).
- **GABA agonists/enhancers (e.g. baclofen, progabide and valproate)**. Cochrane concludes the evidence is inconclusive and unconvincing (s=8, n=547, Soares *et al*, *Cochrane Database Syst Rev* 2011;**4**:CD000203).
- **Insulin** (low-dose) has been suggested to be as superior to placebo (see Soares-Weiser and Joy, *Cochrane Database Syst Rev* 2003;**2**:CD000208).
- **Lithium** has no consistent positive effect (e.g. Yassa *et al*, *Can J Psychiatry* 1984;**29**:36–7) and may even be detrimental.
- **Valproate**, see GABA agonists.
- **Vitamin E** may protect against deterioration but does not improve symptoms once established (s=11, n=427, Soares-Weisler *et al*, *Cochrane Database Syst Rev* 2011;**2**:CD000209).

EPSE, Parkinsonism

Pseudoparkinsonism or Parkinsonian side-effects include akinesia, rigidity, bradykinesia and coarse tremor at rest. They can occur with many drugs but particularly antipsychotics (see *Chapter 5.8.1*).

Antidepressants, (especially tricyclics)	**Switch drugs** (e.g. to reboxetine if paroxetine-induced; n=1, Kuloglu *et al*, *J Psychopharmacol* 2010;**24**:623–4), or treat as per antipsychotics. **Benzodiazepines**, e.g. diazepam (mentioned in Pollack and Rosenbaum, *J Clin Psychiatry* 1987;**48**:3–8). **Propranolol** 40–120 mg/d has been used (mentioned in Pollack and Rosenbaum, *J Clin Psychiatry* 1987;**48**:3–8).
Antipsychotics	**Dose reduction** of any antipsychotic. **Switching to another antipsychotic** with lower EPS.

Anticholinergics (antimuscarinics) are first-line treatments. They include **benzatropine** (also has antihistaminic properties and a long half-life of up to 24 hours), **orphenadrine** (which is probably more toxic: Slørdal and Gjerden, *Br J Psychiatry* 1999;**174**:275–6), **procyclidine** (with a disputed abuse potential) and **trihexyphenidyl** (benzhexol; with a reported abuse and dependence potential; Frauger *et al*, *Therapie* 2003;**58**:541–7). They may improve survival (n=88, 10-year prospective study, Waddington *et al*, *Br J Psychiatry* 1998;**173**:325–9) and compliance, and may actually only be detrimental to positive symptoms during acute phases (when excess dopaminergic activity is thought to occur) but not during stable phases (Tandon and Dequardo, *Am J Psychiatry* 1995;**152**:814–5). Anticholinergics may adversely affect memory, exacerbate TD, and abrupt withdrawal can produce rebound EPS and cholinergic rebound. They are best prescribed only for overt symptoms and discontinued gradually after three months, reinstated only if symptoms reappear. However, if they aid long-term compliance, it may be a benefit that outweighs the risks.

Adjunctive therapies:

- **Diphenhydramine** 25–300mg (oral or parenteral) may be effective within minutes. Maintenance with 25–50mg TDS has been used (n=5, RCT, Granana *et al*, *Medicina [B Aires]* 1999;**59**:38–42).
- **Donepezil** may have some use in treating EPSE in the elderly (n=7, open, Bergman *et al*, *J Clin Psychiatry* 2005;**66**:107–10).
- **Estrogen** at high plasma levels has been reported to reduce hyperkinetic symptoms of EPSE in women with psychosis (n=25, RCT, Thompson *et al*, *Acta Psychiatr Scand* 2000;**101**:130–4).
- **Iron supplementation** may help EPSE if it is associated with iron-deficient anaemia (n=1, Yoshida *et al*, *Nihon Shinkei Seishin Yakurigaku Zasshi* 2004;**24**:29–31).
- **Kava special extract** WS1490 has been claimed to be effective (n=42, open, Boerner and Klement, *Wien Med Wochenschr* 2004;**154**:508–10).
- **Zolpidem** 5mg QDS has been used for persistent and refractory EPSE (n=1, Farver and Khan, *Ann Pharmacother* 2001;**35**:435–7).

Less useful:

Some drugs that have been tried but failed include:

- **Amantadine** is not recommended for EPSE but may be effective (d/b, c/o, Silver *et al*, *J Clin Psychiatry* 1995:**56**;167–70; review by Mamo *et al*, *Drug Saf* 1999;**20**:269–75).
- **Mianserin** is ineffective (Korsgaard and Friis, *Psychopharmacol [Berl]* 1986;**88**:109–11).

6

EPSE, dystonia (including oculogyric crisis)

Dystonia is a syndrome of sustained or slow involuntary muscular contractions, resulting in twisting of the neck, limbs, trunk or face. Acute dystonia from antipsychotics is more likely to occur in younger and more severely ill people, especially if antipsychotic-naïve. It can present as an oculogyric crisis (review by Abe, *World J Biol Psychiatry* 2006;**7**:70–4).

Review: general (Balash and Giladi, *Eur J Neurol* 2004;**11**:361–70).

Antidepressants

Switching drugs is the main strategy.

* **Aripiprazole low-dose** (e.g. 1.5mg/d) has been used for orofacial and buccal dystonias from SSRIs (Oulis *et al*, *Psychiatry Clin Neurosci* 2012;**66**:462–3), and amitriptyline 10mg/day and trazodone 25mg/day (n=1, Huh and Lee, *Psychiatr Danub* 2015;**27**:195–7; FFT).

Epinephrine/adrenaline 0.3mg s/c has been used for escitalopram-induced

oculogyric dystonia (n = 1, Patel and Simon, *Int Arch Allergy Immunol* 2006;**140**:27–9).
Mianserin has been used at low dose for fluoxetine-induced dystonia (Poyurovsky et al, *Mov Disord* 1997;**12**:1102–5).

Antipsychotics

Acute dystonia:

- **Anticholinergics** are usually effective for acute dystonias (e.g. laryngeal dystonia: Christodoulou and Kalaitzi, *J Psychopharmacol* 2005;**19**:307–11) and **procyclidine** is the standard UK treatment.
- **Diphenhydramine** (oral or parenteral) has rapidly reversed dystonic reactions, e.g. oculogyric crisis (Leigh et al, *Ann Neurol* 1987;**22**:13–7).

Tardive dystonia:

Switching antipsychotic is the first choice strategy:

- **Aripiprazole** 3 mg/d has abolished sulpiride-induced tardive oromandibular dystonia (n = 1, Imai and Ikawa, *Intern Med* 2011;**50**:635–7; FFT).
- **Clozapine** may improve severe and persistent dystonias (e.g. Sieche and Giedke, *J Clin Psychiatry* 2000;**61**:949).
- **Olanzapine** may have some role (n = 4, s/b, Lucetti et al, *Clin Neuropharmacol* 2002;**25**:71–4).
- **Quetiapine** has been used if induced by risperidone, olanzapine (n = 2, Gourzis et al, *Clin Neuropharmacol* 2005;**28**: 195–6), aripiprazole (n = 1, Ono et al, *J Clin Pharm Ther* 2012;**37**:370–2) or amisulpride (n = 1, Fountoulakis et al, *Schizophr Res* 2006;**88**:232–4).

Others:

In resistant cases, other strategies may be worth trying:

- **Benzodiazepines** — a multiple drug-resistant disabling dystonia responded partly to clozapine and virtually completely when clonazepam was added (n = 1, Shapleske et al, *Br J Psychiatry* 1996;**168**:516–8).
- **Botulinum toxin** may possibly relieve the pain and symptoms of dystonia (n = 34, open, Tarsy et al, *Clin Neuropharmacol* 1997;**20**:90–3).
- **Levodopa** combined with an anticholinergic has been used (n = 1, Looper and Chouinard, *Can J Psychiatry* 1998;**43**:646–7).
- **Levetiracetam** has helped generalised dystonia (n = 1, 20/52, Sullivan et al, *Parkinsonism Relat Disord* 2005;**11**:469–71).
- * **Tetrabenazine** has been used for olanzapine-induced tardive dystonia (n = 1, Rauchverger et al, *J Neuropsychiatry Clin Neurosci* 2007;**19**:484–5; review by Chen et al, *Clin Ther* 2012;**34**:1487–504).

Less useful:

- **Anticholinergics** are less effective in tardive dystonia (e.g. n = 32, Wojcik et al, *Am J Psychiatry* 1991;**148**:1055–9).
- **Carbamazepine** is ineffective (Perényi and Sztaniszláv, *Psychopharmacol Bull* 1985;**21**;345–6).

Other drugs tried include baclofen and bromocriptine.

Benzodiazepines

Diazepam has been rapidly effective if midazolam-induced (n = 1, Komur et al, *J Anaesthesiol Clin Pharmacol* 2012;**28**:368–70; FFT).

Laryngospasm (see also dystonia)

Benzodiazepines

Flumazenil may be effective in 25 minutes if midazolam-induced (n = 1, Davis et al, *Ann Emerg Med* 1998;**32**:263–5).

Myoclonus

Myoclonus presents as shock-like, involuntary movements. It can also be caused by CNS infections, systemic metabolic disorders or neurodegenerative disorders. General management includes:

- **Exclude serotonin syndrome and akathisia**, as myoclonus can be a symptom of these.

- **Discontinuation, switching** or **dose reduction** usually resolves myoclonus.
- **Discontinue any other causative drugs**, e.g. levodopa, tricyclics, lamotrigine (n = 1, Rosenhagen *et al, J Clin Psychopharmacol* 2006;**26**:346–7) and bismuth salts (including OTC products).

Reviews: * Mills and Mari, *Curr Neurol Neurosci Rep* 2015;**15**:512; Caviness, *Neurotherapeutics* 2014;**11**: 188–200; FFT.

Other strategies:

Antidepressants	**Valproate** has been used if sertraline-induced (n = 1, Ghaziuddin *et al, J Child Adolesc Psychopharmacol* 2001;**11**:199–202).
Antipsychotics	**Carbamazepine** has been used if clozapine-induced, but beware of the potential interaction (n=5, Bak *et al, J Clin Psychiatry* 1995;**56**:418–22).
	Haloperidol may be an alternative if olanzapine-induced (n = 1, Camacho *et al, Clin Neuropharmacol* 2005;**28**:145–7).
	Valproate has been used if clozapine-induced (n = 1, Meltzer and Ranjan, *Am J Psychiatry* 1994;**151**:1246–7).

Pisa syndrome (antipsychotic-induced pleurothonus)

Persistent dystonia of the trunk is a rare ADR from long-term antipsychotics.

Antipsychotics	**Switching** to olanzapine has worked if risperidone-induced (n = 1, Nishimura *et al, J Neuropsychiatry Clin Neurosci* 2007;**19**:202–3).
	Switching to clozapine has worked over six weeks if olanzapine-induced (n = 1, Arora *et al, Ann Pharmacother* 2006;**40**:2273–5).
	Anticholinergics may help (n = 1, Bhattacharya *et al, Mov Disord* 2000;**15**:1285–7; Suzuki *et al, J Clin Psychopharmacol* 1999;**19**:277–80).
Galantamine	**Memantine** has been used as an alternative (Chen *et al, Int J Geriatr Psychiatry* 2008;**23**:660–1).

Restless legs (may also be akathisia)

Standard treatments include correcting any low ferritin with iron, plus gabapentin or clonidine.

Antidepressants	Although there are anecdotal reports, there is no clear association with restless legs (n=200, Brown *et al, Sleep Med* 2005;**6**:443–50).
	Exclude other drugs as a cause, e.g. D2 receptor antagonists (e.g. domperidone, n = 1, Chang *et al, Prog Neuropsychopharmacol Biol Psychiatry* 2006;**30**:316–8), tramadol and dopamine-blockers, plus possibly antihistamines and non-opioid analgesics (n = 14, Kim *et al, Hum Psychopharmacol* 2008;**23**:615–20).
	Re-exposure may be possible without recurrence with **mirtazapine** (n = 1, Pae *et al, Psychiatry Clin Neurosci* 2004;**58**:669–70).
	Bupropion 150 mg/d does not appear to exacerbate RLS and is a suitable alternative (n=60, RCT, d/b, p/c, 6/52, Bayard *et al, J Am Board Fam Med* 2011;**24**:422–8; FFT), but it is unclear if it a primary treatment as such.
	* **Pramipexole** has been used for mirtazapine-induced restless legs (n = 1, Makiguchi *et al, J Neuropsychiatry Clin Neurosci* 2015;**27**:e76)
Antipsychotics	* **Switching** — olanzapine-induced restless legs may resolve on stopping or dose reduction (n = 11, Zhao *et al, J Clin Neurosci* 2014;**21**:1622–5), or if switched to risperidone, quetiapine or **aripiprazole** (n=3, Aggarwal *et al, Curr Drug Saf* 2010;**5**:129–31) if clozapine-induced (n = 1, Raveendranathan *et al, J Neuropsychiatry Clin Neurosci* 2013;**25**:E62–3).
	Benzodiazepines, e.g. clonazepam have been used (n = 1, Horiguchi *et al, Int Clin Psychopharmacol* 1999;**14**:33–6; (n = 11, Zhao *et al, J Clin Neurosci* 2014;**21**:1622–5).
	* **Pramipexole** for clozapine-induced (n = 1, John *et al, J Clin Psychopharmacol* 2014;**34**:764–6).
	Ropinirole has been used if caused by olanzapine (n=5, Kang *et al, J*

	Psychopharmacol 2009;**23**:597–601; n = 11, Zhao *et al*, *J Clin Neurosci* 2014;**21**:1622–5) or quetiapine (n = 2, Urbano and Ware, *J Clin Psychopharmacol* 2008;**28**:704–5).
Carbamazepine	**Vitamin D** deficiency can be a cause (n = 1, Prakash *et al*, *Gen Hosp Psychiatry* 2010;**32**:228).

Tremor (see EPSE, Parkinsonism and under 'others')

6.8 Neuroleptic malignant syndrome (NMS)

NMS is a rare and potentially fatal idiosyncratic dose-independent ADR resulting in a sudden loss in control of body temperature. The main symptoms are hyperthermia or fever and severe muscle rigidity, with two or more of: diaphoresis, dysphagia, tremor, incontinence, altered consciousness, tachycardia, altered blood pressure, leucocytosis and raised CPK concentration. Body temperature rises rapidly and it can be fatal in 1–3 days, although death rates have reduced due to increased awareness, early intervention, and the use of newer antipsychotics. It is probably caused by a sudden over-blockade of dopaminergic function, disrupting the thermoregulatory centre.

Risk factors include:

- **History** (previous NMS, known cerebral compromise, previous ECT).
- **Mental state** (agitation, overactive, in need of restraint or seclusion, catatonia, affective disorders [Berardi *et al*, *Hum Psychopharmacol* 2002;**17**:99–102] or mental retardation).
- * **Physical state** (dehydration, postpartum, Parkinson's disease, young and male, low serum iron [Patil *et al*, *Int J Appl Basic Med Res* 2014;**4**:117–8; FFT], high serum creatinine phosphokinase [n = 32, Hermesh *et al*, *J Clin Psychopharmacol* 2002;**22**:252–6]).
- **Drugs** (see *Chapter 5.9*, e.g. high potency antipsychotics, IM therapy, high doses over short periods, abrupt or recent changes, rapid neuroleptisation, and concurrent carbamazepine).
- **Genetic** vulnerability (n = 2 siblings, Ziegenbein *et al*, *Ann Pharmacother* 2006;**40**:574–5).
- **Catatonia**, also a prodromal state (n = 17, White and Robins, *CNS Spectr* 2000;**5**:58–65).

Neuroleptic rechallenge:

Rechallenge may show a high rate of recurrence, although most people may be able to tolerate antipsychotics again if monitored carefully and a two-week recovery period is allowed (n = 15, Rosebush *et al*, *J Clin Psychiatry* 1989;**50**:295–8). Rechallenge with clozapine has been successful (Weller and Kornhuber, *Br J Psychiatry* 1992;**161**:855–6). Depots are contraindicated.

Reviews: risk factors (Gupta *et al*, *Int J Psychiatry* 2003;**45**:30–5; FFT; n = 15, controls n = 45, Viejo *et al*, *Acta Psychiatr Scand* 2003;**107**:45–9), general (Strawn *et al*, *Am J Psychiatry* 2007;**164**:870–6).

Antipsychotics

Immediate management is essential.

Withdraw any antipsychotics, lithium or antidepressants.

Correct any dehydration and hyperpyrexia, e.g. using ice packs, re-hydration, and sedation with benzodiazepines if necessary.

Measure WCC, U&E, LFT and CPK to assess diagnosis, cause and response.

Manage acute symptoms, initially using a first-line agent below:

First line strategies:

- **Dantrolene** IV (a skeletal muscle relaxant used for malignant hyperthermia) is usually the treatment of choice. It reduces the duration and mortality of NMS (n = 9, Nisijima and Ishiguro, *Biol Psychiatry* 1993;**33**:45–8) and reduces body temperature in 2–24 hours.
- * **Bromocriptine** 7.5–60 mg/d reduces the duration and mortality of NMS (Sakkas *et al*, *Psychopharmacol Bull* 1991;**27**:381–4), e.g. for

aripiprazole/imipramine-induced NMS (n = 1, Lopez *et al*, *Med Clin (Barc)* 2013;**141**:273–4).

- **Amantadine** 100 mg BD may be the third-line choice (mentioned by Waldorf, *AANA J* 2003;**71**:389–94).

Other strategies:

- **Anaesthetics** have been used for emergency treatment (n = 1, Parke and Wheatley, *Anesthesia* 1992;**47**:908–9).
- **Complete anticoagulation** has been used as adjunctive therapy to reduce death as a result of pulmonary embolism (van Harten and van Agtmael, *Am J Psychiatry* 1995;**152**:1103).
- **Apomorphine** s/c can improve NMS significantly (n = 1, Lattanzi *et al*, *Am J Psychiatry* 2006;**163**:1450–1).
- * **Benzodiazepines** (e.g. high-dose lorazepam and diazepam; n = 1, Tsai and Huang, *Chang Gung Med J* 2010;**33**:576–80; FFT; n = 1, Kishimoto *et al*, *J Anesth* 2013;**27**:768–70) can be used if dantrolene and bromocriptine have failed. Predominantly catatonic symptoms may rapidly respond to diazepam, including via continuous IV administration (Miyaoka *et al*, *Am J Psychiatry* 1997;**153**:882), although its longer half-life may complicate recovery (Velamoor, *Br J Psychiatry* 1992;**160**:135–6).
- **ECT** has been used for low-dose quetiapine-induced NMS (e.g. n = 1, Patel *et al*, *J Assoc Physicians India* 2008;**56**:49–50).
- **Levodopa IV plus bromocriptine** may be an effective alternative to dantrolene (Nisijima *et al*, *Biol Psychiatry* 1997;**41**:913–4), as may carbidopa/levodopa (Shoop and Cernek, *Ann Pharmacother* 1997;**31**:119).
- * **Methylprednisolone** pulse therapy has been used in Parkinson's (n = 40, d/b, p/c, Sato *et al*, *J Neurol Neurosurg Psychiatry* 2003;**74**:574–6; FFT; Clarke, *J Neurol Neurosurg Psychiatry* 2004;**75**:510–1; FFT).
- **Nifedipine** 25 mg s/l has been used (Talley and Taylor, *Psychosomatics* 1994;**35**:168–70).

Post-NMS care:

1. Review NMS symptoms to confirm diagnosis.
2. Review psychiatric diagnosis and the need for further antipsychotics.
3. Consider alternative management strategies.
4. Leave as long a gap as possible before restarting antipsychotics (e.g. 14 days), considering also the risks of untreated psychosis.
5. Choose an antipsychotic from a different group to the causative agent, particularly any previously used without problem. Start low and go slow. Contraindicate depots.
6. Alternate day CPK monitoring.
7. Perform daily temperature, pulse and muscle tone measures, weekly wbcs and ensure adequate hydration and nutrition.
8. Obtain an informal or formal second opinion, as informed consent for re-exposure may not be possible. Inform family and carers of the decisions and risks (and document this).
9. Educate patients, carers and care team of the symptoms of early NMS and of the appropriate action to take, i.e. seek urgent medical advice.

Reviews: general (Ambulkar *et al*, *J Anaesthesiol Clin Pharmacol* 2012;**28**:517–9; FFT; Ananth *et al*, *J Clin Psychiatry* 2004;**65**:464–70).

6

6.9 Serotonin syndrome

This potentially fatal syndrome is attributed to a toxic hyperserotonergic state from hyper-stimulation of the brain stem and spinal cord 5HT1A and 5HT2 receptors. Onset is usually within a few hours of drug or dose changes and usually resolves in about 24 hours.

Sternbach's diagnostic criteria

1. At least three of the following: mental state changes (e.g. confusion), agitation/restlessness, sweating, diarrhoea, fever, hyperreflexia, tachycardia, myoclonus, lack of co-ordination, shivering, and tremor. Other symptoms can include nausea, vomiting, tachycardia, myoclonus, hypertension, convulsions and multiple organ failure.
2. Other causes ruled out, e.g. infection, metabolic disturbances, substance abuse or withdrawal.
3. No concurrent antipsychotic dose changes.

The Hunter Serotonin Toxicity Criteria (Dunkley *et al*, *QJM* 2003;**96**:635–42; FFT) may be more specific and is an alternative to Sternbach's criteria.

Reviews: general (Isbister *et al*, *Med J Aust* 2007;**187**:361–5; Boyer and Shannon, *N Engl J Med* 2005;**352**:1112–20; Gillman, *Biol Psychiatry* 2006;**59**:1046–51).

All drugs

Discontinue all serotonergic drugs (see *Chapter 5.13*), including over-the-counter sympathomimetics (usually adequate management in mild cases).

Symptomatic support, e.g. cooling blankets and fans.

Benzodiazepines, e.g. lorazepam (1–2 mg by slow IV injection every 30 minutes until excessive sedation occurs) may be superior to clonazepam, which has a lower affinity for peripheral benzodiazepine receptors (e.g. Nierenberg and Semprebon, *Clin Pharmacol Ther* 1993;**53**:84–8).

Cyproheptadine (a non-specific 5HT blocker) at 4–8 mg orally (but perhaps as high as 10–20 mg), repeated every 2–4 hours up to 0.5 mg kg/d maximum (beware of urinary retention) has been claimed to be the best antiserotonergic drug strategy, with case reports of rapid success (n = 3, McDaniel, *Ann Pharmacother* 2001;**35**:870–3; Baigel, *Eur J Anaesthiol* 2003;**20**:586–8; n = 2, Levin *et al*, *Gen Hosp Psychiatry* 2008;**30**:372–7).

Lipids (20% lipid emulsion IV bolus) have been used for venlafaxine, lamotrigine and diazepam OD (n=1, *Minerva Anestesiol* 2011;**77**:93–5; FFT).

Mirtazapine blocks 5HT2 and 5HT3 receptors and may reduce serotonergic toxicity (Hoes, *Pharmacopsychiatry* 1996;**29**:81).

Nitroglycerin (2 mg/kg/min) has been rapidly successful in severe SS (e.g. n = 1, Brown and Skop, *Ann Pharmacother* 1996;**30**:191; n = 1, Brown, *Am J Emerg Med* 2004;**22**:510).

Propranolol (1–3 mg every five minutes, up to 0.1 mg/kg) may be useful, as it blocks 5HT1A and 5HT2 receptors (Guze and Baxter, *J Clin Psychopharmacol* 1986;**6** 119–20).

6.10 Sexual side-effects

General

The main stages of sexual activity that can be affected by mental health problems and by psychotropics are libido, arousal/lubrication, erectile issues and orgasmic disorders. Many published studies do not differentiate between these stages and refer to generic 'sexual dysfunction'. This section includes general advice and then stage-specific strategies to improve sexual problems.

Review: female sexual dysfunction (Clayton, *J Clin Psychiatry* 2006;**67**:991–2), general (Lombardi *et al*, *BJU Int* 2015;**115** Suppl 6:47–56).

General sexual dysfunction

Anticonvulsants

Switching drugs:

- **Lamotrigine** improves sexual function, testosterone levels and gonadal efficiency (cf. to carbamazepine and phenytoin; n=85, Herzog *et al*, *Neurology* 2005;**65**:1016–20), including when starting on lamotrigine as a first anticonvulsant (n=79) and when switching (n=62) to it (n=141, open, 8/12, Gil-Nagel *et al*, *Seizure* 2006;**15**:142–9; FFT).
- **Levetiracetam** has no apparent adverse sexual or endocrine effects in men or women (n=136, p/c, Svalheim *et al*, *Epilepsy Behav* 2009;**16**:281–7).
- **Oxcarbazepine** — in 228 males with epilepsy and pre-existing sexual dysfunction, 79% improved when switched to oxcarbazepine with the effect more marked if they had previously been on an enzyme-inducing AED (n=673, 12/52, Luef *et al*, *Acta Neurol Scand* 2009;**119**:94–9).
- * **Carbamazepine** should be avoided as, compared to controls, men are 17x more likely to have ED, lower sperm motility and poor sperm morphology/quality (93% vs 35%) with reduced sexual activity and reproductive chances (n=118, Reis *et al*, *J Sex Med* 2013;**10**:493–9), partly by reducing testosterone and androgen levels (n=160, RCT, d/b, 12/12, Lossius *et al*, *Epilepsia* 2007;**48**:1875–82).

Adjunctive therapies:

* **Exogenous testosterone** (review, s=41, RCTs, Corona *et al*, *J Sex Med* 2014;**11**:1577–92) and **aromatase inhibitors** (to reduce testosterone's metabolism) have been tried for male sexual dysfunction.

Antidepressants

Untreated depression has a greater impact on global sexual functioning than antidepressants (e.g. n=70, RCT, d/b, 8/52, Lanza di Scalea *et al*, *J Clin Psychiatry* 2009;**70**:423–8; with duloxetine, n=288, d/b, p/c, 52/52, Montejo *et al*, *J Sex Med* 2011;**8**:773–82), so treating depression improves sexual satisfaction more than antidepressants unimprove it (n=2280, Ishak *et al*, *J Clin Psychiatry* 2013;**74**:256–61).

Testosterone gel can significantly improve sexual function in men with low or low-normal testosterone levels, with an almost zero placebo response (n=63, RCT, d/b, p/c, 6/52, Amiaz *et al*, *J Sex Marital Ther* 2011;**37**:243–54).

* **General interventions** include behavioural strategies, psychotherapy, delaying drug intake until after sexual activity, reduction in dosage, omitting doses, adjuncts and switching. Sexual side-effects from SSRIs rarely seem to abate with time (n=119, Landén *et al*, *J Clin Psychiatry* 2005;**66**:100–6).

Switching drugs:

Switching antidepressants is often the main strategy. The adverse sexual effects in decreasing order is sertraline, venlafaxine, citalopram, paroxetine, fluoxetine, imipramine, phenelzine, duloxetine, escitalopram, and fluvoxamine, with no difference from placebo with agomelatine, vortioxetine (5–15mg/d), bupropion, moclobemide and mirtazapine (meta-analysis by Serretti and Chiesa, *J Clin Psychopharmacol* 2009;**29**:259–66).

- **Agomelatine** has minimal effect compared to placebo (n=25, 12/52, Sapatti, *J Sex Marital Ther* 2012;**38**:190–7; n=193, Montejo *et al*, *Hum Psychopharmacol* 2011;**26**:537–42), paroxetine (n=92 males, RCT, p/c, d/b, 8/52, Montejo *et al*, *J Psychopharmacol* 2010;**24**:111–20) and venlafaxine (n=276, d/b, 12/52, Kennedy *et al*, *J Clin Psychopharmacol* 2008;**28**:329–33).
- * **Bupropion** has statistically less sexual dysfunction than other antidepressants on a range of scales (meta-analysis and systematic review, s=63, n>26000, Reichenpfader *et al*, *Drug Saf* 2014;**37**:19–31).
- **Mirtazapine** has lower sexual ADRs than other antidepressants, apart

6

from the potentially counter-productive sedation (e.g. n=78, open, 6/12, Saiz-Ruiz *et al*, *Hum Psychopharmacol* 2005;**20**:435–40).

- **Moclobemide** may have low sexual ADRs (n=5, open, Ramasubbu, *J Psychiatry Neurosci* 1999;**24**:45–50; FFT).
- **Reboxetine** lacks serotonin-related sexual ADRs (e.g. n=357, RCT, d/b, 24/52, Langworth *et al*, *J Clin Psychopharmacol* 2006;**26**:121–7).
- * **Trazodone** has less adverse effects than fluoxetine and sertraline (n=195, RCT, s/b, 14/52, Khazaie *et al*, *Gen Hosp Psychiatry* 2015;**37**:40–5).
- * **Vortioxetine** has less sexual ADRs than escitalopram, citalopram, paroxetine and sertraline (n=447, RCT, 8/52, Jacobsen *et al*, *J Sex Med* 2015;**12**:2036–48) and no effect cf. placebo except at 20mg/d (SmPC).

Adjunctive therapies:

- **Aripiprazole** as an adjunct may improve sexual functioning especially libido and satisfaction, which is independent of improvement in depression (s=3, n=1,092, RCT, d/b, p/c, Fava *et al*, *Prim Care Companion CNS Disorders* 2011;**13**:PCC.10m00994).
- **Ephedrine** 50mg was shown to be effective for SSRI-induced sexual dysfunction but, then again, so was placebo (n=19 women, RCT, p/c, c/o, 8/52, Meston, *J Sex Marital Ther* 2004;**30**:57–68).
- **Ginkgo biloba** has produced some spectacular individual responses but nothing statistically significant different (n=24[c=11], RCT, t/b, p/c, 12/52, Wheatley, *Hum Psychopharmacol* 2004;**19**:545–8).
- **Pregabalin** has reversed citalopram-induced sexual dysfunction (n=2, Oulis *et al*, *J Clin Psychopharmacol* 2008;**28**:362–3).
- * **Quetiapine** — a bit of a long shot but an analysis of depression studies showed quetiapine XR 50–300mg/d had placebo-level sexual ADRs (s=6, RCT, p/c, 6-10/52, Clayton *et al*, *CNS Spectr* 2014;**19**:182–96).
- **Ropinirole** up to 2–4mg/d was effective in 54% (n=13[3F, 10M], open, 4/52, Worthington *et al*, *Int Clin Psychopharmacol* 2002;**17**:307–10).
- **Sildenafil** 50–100mg may help all domains of sexual function in women (n=49, RCT, d/b, p/c, 8/52, Nurnberg *et al*, *JAMA* 2008;**300**:395–404).
- **Trazodone**, a 5HT2A antagonist, may help as an adjunct in SSRI-induced sexual dysfunction in all four domains (n=20[c=15], Stryjer *et al*, *Clin Neuropharmacol* 2009;**32**:82–4).

No efficacy:

- * **Escitalopram** has been claimed to have less sexual ADRs but an extensive review concludes that it is probably among the worst (s=63, n>26000, Reichenpfader *et al*, *Drug Saf* 2014;**37**:19–31).
- **Granisetron** does not help (n=12, RCT, d/b, p/c, 14/7, Jespersen *et al*, *Int Clin Psychopharmacol* 2004;**19**:161–4).
- **Methylphenidate** is ineffective but at least it did not exacerbate the problem (Pae *et al*, *Clin Neuropharmacol* 2009;**32**:85–8).

Reviews: * antidepressant-induced sexual dysfunction (Taylor *et al*, *Cochrane Database Syst Rev* 2013;**5**:CD003382; Keks *et al*, *Australas Psychiatry* 2014;**22**:525–8; Clayton *et al*, *Expert Opin Drug Saf* 2014;**13**:1361–74).

Antipsychotics

Sexual dysfunction occurs at higher rates in schizophrenia (86–96%) than in the general population (n=179, MacDonald *et al*, *Br J Psychiatry* 2003;**182**:50–6; FFT), and is higher with antipsychotics, especially in men (n=243, Montejo *et al*, *J Sex Med* 2010;**7**:3404–13), but with only 37% spontaneously reporting it. Hyperprolactinaemia appears to be the predominant cause (n=101, Smith *et al*, *Br J Psychiatry* 2002;**181**:49–55;

FFT), but is not necessarily the only cause as, in first episodes, sexual dysfunction may occur despite normal prolactin levels (n = 74, open, van Bruggen *et al*, *Psychoneuroendocrinology* 2009;**34**:989–95).

General principles:

Normalise prolactin, e.g. by switching to a prolactin-sparing antipsychotic, e.g. lurasidone, quetiapine, ziprasidone and aripiprazole have a lower incidence of sexual dysfunction (incidence 16–27%) than olanzapine, risperidone, haloperidol and clozapine (40–60%) (Serretti and Chiesa, *Int Clin Psychopharmacol* 2011;**26**:130–40). **Cabergoline** can also improve overall sexual function without adversely affecting symptoms (n = 80, 6/12, Kalkavoura *et al*, *Exp Clin Psychopharmacol* 2013;**21**:332–41). **Aripiprazole** 3–6 mg/d has helped either as an alternative (45%) or adjunct (55%) to another antipsychotic, with prolactin reducing significantly, improvement in libido, and reduced erectile, ejaculation and menstrual dysfunction, established from 12/52 and maintained for 6/12 (n = 27 [c = 22], 26/52, open, Mir *et al*, *J Psychopharmacol* 2008;**22**:244–53; see also n = 555, RCT, open, 26/52, Hanssens *et al*, *BMC Psychiatry* 2008;**8**:95; FFT).

Reviews: * in women (Smith, *J Clin Psychopharmacol* 2003;**23**[3 Suppl 1]:S27–32), general (Park *et al*, *World J Men's Health* 2012;**30**:153–9).

Lithium * — **Poor compliance** is a risk factor for sexual dysfunction in people taking lithium (mean 10 years, dose 800mg/d; n = 100, Grover *et al*, *J Clin Psychopharmacol* 2014;**34**:475–82).

Opiates * — **Buprenorphine** (13% incidence) causes less sexual dysfunction than methadone (52% incidence) in males in a meta-analysis suggesting switching to buprenorphine should difficulties occur (s = 16, n = 1570, Yee *et al*, *J Sex Med* 2014;**11**:22–32). The main risk factors are age, hormone levels, treatment duration, methadone dose, medical status, co-morbid psychiatric illness and other SMS (s = 16, n = 2619, Yee *et al*, *Int J Impot Res* 2014;**26**:161–6).

1. Libido (see also general advice section)

Libido and desire is controlled by the mesolimbic dopamine reward pathway and facilitated by noradrenaline and serotonin. Testosterone is essential for male and estrogen and progesterone for female sexual behaviour. It is unclear to what extent psychotropics effect libido specifically.

Antidepressants — **Switch drugs** to, e.g. **agomelatine, moclobemide** (n = 5, open, Ramasubbu, *J Psychiatr Neurosci* 1999;**24**:45–50), **bupropion, vortioxetine** or **mirtazapine.**

Antipsychotics — **Raised prolactin** may be a significant factor, so check and, if raised, see the hyperprolactinaemia section for options (review, Zeitlin and Rajfer, *Rev Urol* 2000;**2**:39–42; FFT).

2. Arousal (lubrication and erection) — see also general advice section

Arousal mechanisms involve acetylcholine (erection/lubrication), adrenergic fibres (detumescence), cAMP (smooth muscle relaxation), dopamine (stimulates arousal especially in females), and nitric oxide (activates the production of cGMP).

Antidepressants — **Switching drugs** is the main strategy, e.g. to:

- **Agomelatine** (no reported problems; see general advice).
- **Bupropion** (n = 18 ethnic minority women, open, 10/52, Dobkin *et al*, *J Clin Psychopharmacol* 2006;**26**:21–6).
- **Moclobemide** (n = 5, open, Ramasubbu, *J Psychiatr Neurosci* 1999;**24**:45–50).
- **Mirtazapine** (no reported problems unless sedation is significant).
- ***Vortioxetine** up to 15 mg/d (SmPC).

6

Adjunctive therapies:
- **Bupropion** is effective in women, but the overall evidence is limited (s=23, n=1886, RCT, Taylor *et al, Cochrane Database Syst Rev* 2013;**5**:CD003382).
- * **PDE-5 inhibitors**, e.g. sildenafil. Cochrane concludes that sildenafil and tadalafil are effective for antidepressant-induced ED but that overall the evidence is limited (s=23, n=1886, RCT, Taylor *et al, Cochrane Database Syst Rev* 2013;**5**:CD003382).
- * **Saffron** 30 mg/d can help SSRI-induced impaired arousal (n=38[c=34], RCT, d/b, p/c, 4/52, Kashani *et al, Hum Psychopharmacol* 2013;**28**:54–60).
- **Yohimbine** given 1–2 hours pre-intercourse has been shown to improve ED (review by Labbate *et al, J Clin Psychiatry* 2003;**64**[Suppl 10]:11–9; n=140, Pushkar' Dlu *et al, Urologiia* 2002;**6**:34–7).

Antipsychotics

Switching drugs is the main strategy, e.g. to:
- **Olanzapine**, if haloperidol-induced (n=570, Bitter *et al, Int Clin Psychopharmacol* 2005;**20**:19–21; part of the SOHO study).
- **Quetiapine** may improve erectile function and lubrication compared to other antipsychotics (n=86, 6/12, open, Montejo-Gonzalez *et al, J Clin Psychopharmacol* 2005;**25**:533–8).
- * **Aripiprazole** and **lurasidone** have nothing specific reported.

Adjunctive therapies:
- **Amantadine** 100 mg/d has helped (n=6, open, 6/52, Valevski *et al, Clin Neuropharmacol* 1998;**21**:355–7).
- * **PDE-5 inhibitors**, e.g. sildenafil can be effective for ED induced by olanzapine (n=10, 4/52, Atmaca *et al, Int J Impot Res* 2002;**14**:547–9; FFT) or risperidone (n=32[c=31], RCT, d/b, p/c, c/o, Gopalakrishnan *et al, Am J Psychiatry* 2006;**163**:494–9). Cochrane concludes that sildenafil may be useful but the data is very limited (Berner *et al, Cochrane Database Syst Rev* 2012;**11**:CD003546). Vardenafil 10 mg is also well tolerated and effective (n=25[c=21], open, 12/52, Mitsonis *et al, J Clin Psychiatry* 2008;**69**:206–12).

Carbamazepine

Switching to oxcarbazepine (n=4, Sachdeo and Sathyan, *Curr Med Res Opin* 2005;**21**:1065–8).

Pregabalin*

Switching to levetiracetam or lacosamide (n=3, Calabrò *et al, Epileptic Disord* 2013;**15**:358–61; FFT).

Buprenorphine*

Wait, as users show improvement over three months (n=111 males, RCT, d/b, p/c, 3/12, Cioe *et al, J Subst Abuse Treat* 2013;**45**:451–6).

3. Anorgasmia (see also general advice section)

Noradrenaline exerts an excitatory or facilitatory action on orgasm. Serotonin 5HT2A receptor agonism is inhibitory on orgasm.

Antidepressants

Anorgasmia is a common phenomenon and while a minor effect can be advantageous in some men (by delaying ejaculation), it is almost invariably considered disadvantageous in women.

Main strategies:

Dose adjustment:
- Reduce dose (there may be some relationship to dose or plasma levels)
- Use a single daily dose, e.g. a dose taken at night will give trough levels the next evening, useful if that is when sexual activity occurs
- Partial drug holiday i.e. missing specific doses (although, as David Baldwin once said, you'd need a sabbatical for fluoxetine, due to its long half-life).

Wait for spontaneous resolution (occurs in less than a third).

Withdraw drug as anorgasmia is rapidly reversible on drug withdrawal.

Switching drugs:

Switching drugs is an option but is obviously a major problem if the person has responded to the causative agent:

- **Agomelatine** (no reported problems; see general advice).
- **Bupropion** (with a low serotonergic effect) may be successful if the anorgasmia is SSRI-induced (s=2, n=830, RCT, d/b, p/c, 8/52, Clayton *et al, J Clin Psychiatry* 2006;**67**:736–46).
- **Duloxetine** may have a lower anorgasmic effect (s=4, n=1,466, RCT, d/b, p/c, Delgado *et al, J Clin Psychiatry* 2005;**66**:686–92), but is still serotonergic.
- **Mirtazapine** has placebo-level effects because although it increases serotonin, it blocks serotonin's anorgasmic effect on 5HT2A receptors.
- **Trazodone** 50–200mg/d may help men with psychogenic ED, if they can stay awake long enough (s=6, n=396 men, RCTs, >1/52, Fink *et al, BJU Int* 2003;**92**:441–6).
- **Venlafaxine** 75mg/d may have no effect on premature ejaculation (n=31, p/c, s/b, c/o, Kilic *et al, Int J Androl* 2005;**28**:47–52).
- ***Vortioxetine** up to 15mg/d (SmPC).

Adjunctive therapies:

Many adjunctive therapies have been tried and may work for some individuals. They are presented in alphabetical order as there is no robust way of assessing their relative efficacies:

- **Bupropion** was effective in 46% of women and 75% of men, in an open study (n=24, 7/52, Gitlin *et al, J Sex Marital Ther* 2002;**28**:131–8), but an RCT failed to show any effect (n=30, RCT, p/c, Masand *et al, Am J Psychiatry* 2001;**158**:805–7).
- **Buspirone** 20–60mg/d has improved anorgasmia in 58% people cf. 30% on placebo if SSRI-induced (n=117, p/c, >4/52, Landen *et al, J Clin Psychopharmacol* 1999;**19**:268–71).
- **Cyproheptadine** 2–4mg 30–60 minutes before sex (provided you can then stay awake) may help SSRI-induced anorgasmia, although relapse of depression has been reported (see 4.3.2.2). 4mg (but not 2mg) the day before has been used (being referred to by the male patient as 'the catapult pills' Lauerma, *Acta Psychiatr Scand* 1996;**93**:69–70).
- **Dronabinol**, a synthetic cannabinol, one hour pre-sex has increased libido, arousal, lubrication, orgasm and overall quality, but warn people wandering around with a grin on their face in case they get tested for illicit drug use (n=1, Salerian, *J Clin Psychiatry* 2004;**665**:1146–7).
- * **Loratadine** 10–15mg/d has rapidly reversed SSRI-induced anorgasmia in men and women (n=10, case series, Brubaker, *J Clin Psychiatry* 2002;**63**:534; n=9, 2/52, Aukst-Margetic and Margetic, *Prog Neuropsychopharmacol Biol Psychiatry* 2005;**29**:754–6).
- **Methylphenidate** (Roeloffs *et al, J Clin Psychiatry* 1996;**57**:548) and **dexamfetamine** (15–20mg/d) have been used successfully for SSRI-induced anorgasmia (n=5, Bartlik, *J Sex Marital Ther* 1995;**21**:264–71).
- **Mirtazapine** may help in premenopausal females (n=148, RCT, p/c, 6/52, Michelson *et al, J Psychiatr Res* 2002;**36**:147–52). Stimulation of the 5HT2A receptor via SSRIs inhibits orgasm, but mirtazapine blocks 5HT2A receptors, reversing the anorgasmic effect. This may happen at relatively low doses, e.g. 7.5–15mg/d.

6

- **PDE-5 inhibitors,** e.g. **sildenafil** 50–100mg, taken 30–60 minutes pre-sex, may help SSRI-induced anorgasmia in men (n=90, RCT, p/c, 6/52, Nurnberg *et al*, *JAMA* 2003;**289**:56–64) and in women (n=98 [c=89], RCT, d/b, p/c, 8/52, Nurnberg *et al*, *JAMA* 2008;**300**:395–404), but high doses 50–200mg/d may be needed (n=21, open, Seidman *et al*, *J Clin Psychiatry* 2003;**64**:721–5).

Less useful:

- **Amantadine** 200–300mg/d is generally ineffective (n=57, RCT, p/c, 8/52, Michelson *et al*, *Am J Psychiatry* 2000;**157**:239–43), but there are cases of successful use (n=596, Keller Ashton *et al*, *J Sex Marital Ther* 1997;**23**:165–75).
- **Ginkgo biloba** has failed to show any significant effect (n=37, RCT, p/c, 2/12, Kang *et al*, *Hum Psychopharmacol* 2002;**17**:279–84).
- * **Granisetron** (5HT3 antagonist) has been used for SSRI-induced anorgasmia but was ineffective in two studies (n=20, p/c, c/o, Nelson *et al*, *J Clin Psychiatry* 2001;**62**:469–73; n=12 [c=11], RCT, d/b, p/c, Jespersen *et al*, *Int Clin Psychopharmacol* 2004;**19**:161–4).
- **Mianserin** 7.5–15mg/d may be successful in 65% within 1–2 weeks (n=17, open, 3/12, Dolberg *et al*, *Psychopharmacol* [Berl] 2002;**161**:404–7), although the only RCT showed no significant difference in women (n=75, RCT, d/b, p/c, 4/52, Michelson *et al*, *J Psychiatr Res* 2002;**36**:147–52).
- **Yohimbine** 5.4–10.8mg has been used if SSRI-induced, although it was no better than placebo in the main RCT (n=148, RCT, p/c, 6/52, Michelson *et al*, *J Psychiatr Res* 2002;**36**:147–52) and it can cause insomnia, so rolling over and going to sleep afterwards may be trickier.

Antipsychotics

Switching drugs:

- **Aripiprazole** (nothing relevant published).
- **Quetiapine** has a lower incidence of problems than risperidone and fluphenazine (n=27, RCT, d/b, Kelly and Conley, *Psychoneuroendocrinology* 2006;**31**:340–6).
- * **Lurasidone** seems to have a low incidence of problems.

Opiates

Methadone produces a dose-dependent anorgasmia (n=92, Brown *et al*, *J Addict Disord* 2005;**24**:91–106), so reduce the dose (Chekuri *et al*, *Addict Behav* 2012;**37**:124–6) or switch to **buprenorphine,** which causes less suppression of plasma testosterone (n=105, Bliesener *et al*, *J Clin Endocrinol Metab* 2005;**90**:203–6).

Anticonvulsants

Reduce the dose or discontinue as it may be dose-related for topiramate (n=7, Sun *et al*, *Headache* 2006;**46**:1450–3) and oxcarbazepine (e.g. n=1, Calabrò *et al*, *Epilepsy Behav* 2010;**17**:287–8; n=1, Boora *et al*, *Prim Care Companion J Clin Psychiatry* 2009;**11**:173–4; FFT).

4. Ejaculation problems (see also general advice section)

All drugs

Discontinue or reduce the dose, e.g. retrograde ejaculation from risperidone 8mg/d promptly responds to dose reduction (n=1, Loh *et al*, *Int Clin Psychopharmacol* 2004;**19**:111–2). Discontinuation generally works for clozapine (n=3, Talmon *et al*, *Harefuah* 1994;**126**:509–10).

Tamsulosin may help (n=405, Goktas *et al*, *J Urol* 2006;**175**:650–2).

Reboxetine

Switching drugs, e.g. inappropriate ejaculation with reboxetine resolved when switched to sertraline (n=1, Sivrioglu *et al*, *Prog Neuropsychopharmacol Biol Psychiatry* 2007;**31**:548–50).

Tamsulosin has helped painful ejaculation (n=2, Demyttenaere and Huygens, *Eur Neuropsychopharmacol* 2002;**12**:337–41).

5. Priapism

Early treatment (within 4–6 hours, before local hypoxemia) reduces morbidity and the need for invasive procedures, and may prevent or minimise long-term complications e.g. impotence.

- Immediate short-term treatment includes conservative measures, e.g. pain control, vigorous hydration, and cold compress before urology consultation.
- Active treatments include cavernosal penile aspiration, irrigation, instillation of vasoactive agents, intracavernosal phenylephrine and, if necessary, shunting procedures.

Terbutaline orally may be effective for about 40% (cf. 15% with placebo) (n=68, RCT, p/c, Priyadarshi, *Int J Impot Res* 2004;**16**:424–6).
Switching if antipsychotic related, switch to one with a lower propensity to cause priapism (highest with chlorpromazine, and risperidone; see review by Compton and Miller, *J Clin Psychiatry* 2001;**62**:362–6).
* **Goserelin** 3.5 mg every 4/52 has been used for clozapine-induced recurrent priapism (Kashyap *et al*, *Ther Adv Psychopharmacol* 2013;**3**:298–300).

Reviews: general (Wang *et al*, *Int Clin Psychopharmacol* 2006;**21**:245–8), antipsychotics (Sood *et al*, *Int Clin Psychopharmacol* 2008;**23**:9–17).

6.11 Others, side-effects

Gastric irritation (see also nausea)

Valproate	**Take with or after food.** **Slow-release or enteric-coated tablets** may help. **Avoid fizzy drinks** with the liquid or soluble tablets.

Glaucoma (see also glaucoma section in *Chapter 3*)

Topiramate	**Discontinuation** usually quickly leads to reversal. **Laser surgery** or peripheral iridectomy may be longer-term options (n=83, Fraunfelder *et al*, *Ophthalmology* 2004;**111**:109–11). **Methylprednisolone** and **mannitol** may be rapidly effective if acute (n=1, Rhee *et al*, *Am J Ophthalmol* 2006;**141**:1133–4).

Hypersalivation (see also sialorrhoea)

Lithium	**Propantheline** may give some symptomatic relief (n=1, Donaldson, *Am J Psychiatry* 1982;**139**:1350–1). * **Dose reduction** may be effective as it may be dose-related (Rampes and Bhandari, *J Psychopharmacol* 1994;**8**:261).

Incontinence (see also nocturnal enuresis)

Clozapine	**Wait** as nearly all cases, usually resolves spontaneously within 3/12 (n=16, Warner *et al*, *Int Clin Psychopharmacol* 1994;**9**:207–9). It may be due to alpha-adrenergic antagonism with an incidence of up to 44% (persistent in 25%) (n=61, >3/12, Lin *et al*, *Acta Psychiatr Scand* 1999;**100**:158–61). **Reducing fluid intake** during the evening may help. **Alpha-adrenergic agonists; ephedrine** 150mg at night maintained over 12/12 (n=57, Fuller *et al*, *J Clin Psychiatry* 1996;**57**:514–8). **Aripiprazole** 10–15 mg/d as an adjunct may be useful (n=2, Lee and Kim, *J Korean Med Sci* 2010;**25**:333–5; FFT). **DDAVP® (Ferring)/Desmopressin** intranasally has been used symptomatically (n=1, English *et al*, *Ann Pharmacother* 2001;**35**:867–9). **Oxybutinin** has been used (Lurie and Hosmer, *J Clin Psychiatry* 1997;**58**:404). **Tolterodine** has been used, albeit unsuccessfully (n=1, English *et al*, *Ann Pharmacother* 2001;**35**:867–9). * **Pseudoephedrine** 30 mg QDS has helped (n=1, Hanes *et al*, *Innov Clin Neurosci* 2013;**10**:33–5).

Jaundice (see also hepatotoxicity)

Valproate	Could be a sign of impending hepatic failure. Investigate immediately and discontinue if confirmed.

Mastalgia (see also hyperprolactinaemia)

Venlafaxine	**Check prolactin** and take appropriate action. **Bromocriptine** 5 mg/d has been used with no recurrence on discontinuation (n = 1, Bhatia *et al*, *J Clin Psychopharmacol* 2000;**20**:590–1).

Megaloblastic anaemia

Anticonvulsants	**Folic acid** may be used if caused by, e.g. phenytoin or phenobarbital.

Oedema

Antidepressants	**Vitamin B6** (pyridoxine) has been used if isocarboxazid or mirtazapine-induced (Larsen *et al*, *Acta Psychiatr Scand* 2011;**124**:76–7) **Reduction in dose or discontinuation** may be rapidly successful (n = 10, Barrnett *et al*, *J Clin Psychopharmacol* 1985;**5**:161–4).
Lithium	**Reduce the dose**, as this common effect may be dose-related. **Diuretics** may be useful but see *Chapter 4.4* for interactions.
Valproate	**Discontinuation** — oedema can occur after long-term treatment (but can be after short-term use), can fluctuate and rapidly improve if valproate is stopped (n = 2, Lin *et al*, *Int J Neuropsychopharmacol* 2009;**12**:991–3).

Osteopenia (see also osteoporosis and hyperprolactinaemia)

Antipsychotics	**Correct** any raised prolactin. **Standard therapies**, e.g. alendronic acid 5 mg/d has improved spine and hip T-scores by 7% and 9% respectively over a year (n = 1, Howes and Smith, *Am J Psychiatry* 2004;**161**:756). **Switching to clozapine** — women on clozapine have better bone density than women taking prolactin-raising antipsychotics (Lin *et al*, *Int J Neuropsychopharmacol* 2012;**15**:897–906).

Osteoporosis (see also osteopenia)

General	**Beer drinking** — quantitative bone ultrasound values for women (pre-, peri- and post-menopausal) are greater in beer drinkers (in moderation of course), compared to non-beer or non-wine drinkers, possibly due to the phytoestrogen content (n = 1,697, Pedrera-Zamorano *et al*, *Nutrition* 2009;**25**:1057–63). So, a double benefit then.

Pain at site of injection

Depots/LAIs	**Warm baths** and regular exercise can help. **Change site** or systematically alternate injection sides. **Check injection technique**, as Z-tracking technique may not always be meticulously followed (Bélanger-Annable, *Canadian Nurse* 1985;**81**:41–3). **Switch** to a depot/LAI with a different needle size, bore, length or frequency.

Raised LFTs

Valproate	**Wait**, as raised LFTs are usually transient, so monitor LFTs (including prothrombin time) until they return to normal. **Discontinue** if the prothrombin time is abnormally prolonged. **Salicylates** (inc. OTC) may exacerbate so these should be discontinued.

Sialorrhoea (hypersalivation)

Clozapine	Hypersalivation with clozapine may be an inhibition of the swallowing reflex (rather than excess saliva production; n = 17, Rabinowitz *et al*, *Biol Psychiatry* 1996;**40**:1132–4), or due to clozapine's pharmacology, e.g. M4 activation or alpha-2 blockade, so hypersalivation may be an inaccurate term for this side-effect, albeit descriptive. **Reviews:** Cochrane concludes there is insufficient evidence for any treat-

ment (s = 15, Syed *et al, Cochrane Database Syst Rev* 2008;**3**:CD005579; FFT), as does Bird (s = 13 + n = 13, Bird *et al, Ann Pharmacother* 2011;**45**:667–75).

More useful:

Physical strategies:

- **Propping pillows** up at night helps a little in some people.
- **Absorbent pillows.**
- **Reduce caffeine intake** (n = 1, Odom-White and de Leon, *J Clin Psychiatry* 1996;**57**:175–6).

Adjunctive therapies:

Adjunctive therapies are usually the only realistic option.

- ***Atropine 1% eye drops**, one drop given sub-lingually (Mustafa *et al, Aft J Psychiatry (Johannesbrg)* 2013;**16**:242) at bedtime may be rapidly effective (n = 3, Antonello and Tessier, *J Psychiatry Neurosci* 1999;**24**:250; FFT; Comley *et al, Aust N Z J Psychiatry* 2000;**34**:1033–4).
- **Glycopyrrolate** (glycopyrronium) was superior to biperiden and placebo, and had minimal effect on cognitive function, unlike biperiden (RCT, d/b, c/o, 3×4/52, Liang *et al, Schizophr Res* 2010:**119**:138–44).
- **Hyoscine** hydrobromide 300 mcg up to TDS. Hyoscine is erratically absorbed and so tablets should be **sucked and swallowed** to optimise efficacy.
- **Moclobemide** 150–300 mg/d showed a beneficial effect in 66% patients (n = 53, 6/52, c/o, Kreinin *et al, World J Biol Psychiatry* 2011;**12**:620–6).
- **Pirenzepine** (M1/M4 blocker) 25–100 mg/d is frequently used (e.g. n = 29, Schneider *et al, Pharmacopsychiatry* 2004;**37**:43–5).
- **Quetiapine** may allow a reduced clozapine dosage.
- **Sulpiride** (150–300 mg/d) may have some efficacy (n = 18, open, 3/52, Kreinin *et al, Isr J Psych Relat Sci* 2005;**42**:61–3; FFT), as may **amisulpride** 150mg/d (a 'strong ameliorating effect'; n = 20, RCT, d/b, p/c, c/o, Kreinin *et al, Int Clin Psychopharmacol* 2006;**21**:99–103; n = 53, 6/52, c/o, Kreinin *et al, World J Biol Psychiatry* 2011;**12**:620–6).

Less useful:

- **Anticholinergics** or antimuscarinics are generally ineffective (s = 0, n = 0, RCT, Essali *et al, Cochrane Database Syst Rev* 2013;**12**:CD009546), although there are a few cases of success with **trihexyphenidyl** (n = 14, open, Spivak *et al, Int Clin Psychopharmacol* 1997;**12**:213–5; n = 1, Aggarwal *et al, Indian J Med Sci* 2009;**63**:470–1; FFT; n = 1, Praharaj *et al, Psychopharmacol Bull* 2010;**43**:73–5). **Biperiden** was just superior to placebo but significantly reduced MMSE scores (RCT, d/b, c/o, 3×4/52, Liang *et al, Schizophr Res* 2010:**119**:138–44). **Scopolamine** patches have been used (Gaftanyuk and Trestman, *Psychiatr Serv* 2004;**55**:318).
- **Botulinum toxin** (injected into the parotid gland) has been successful (n = 9, p/c, 16/52, Steinlechner *et al, Psychopharmacology [Berl]* 2010;**207**:593–7), although the evidence was weak (s = 6, Lim *et al, Clin Otolaryngology* 2006;**31**:267–72).
- **Bupropion** has helped (n = 1, Stern *et al, Prog Neuropsychopharmacol Biol Psychiatry* 2009;**33**:1578–80).
- **Chewing gum** has been used to stimulate salivation and swallowing.
- **Clonidine** 50–100 mcg/d increases adrenergic tone and reduces hypersalivation (n = 12, open, 4/52, Parharaj *et al, J Psychopharmacol* 2005;**19**:426–8), although it might exacerbate depression and psychosis. Clonidine patches (0.1 mg/week) have been used.

- * **Diphenhydramine** has worked if induced by risperidone (n = 1, Usta *et al, J Child Adolesc Psychopharmacol* 2012:**22**:254–5) or aripiprazole (n = 1, Kılınç *et al, J Child Adolesc Psychopharmacol* 2015; in press)
- **Guanfacine** has been used (Webber *et al, J Clin Psychopharmacol* 2004;**24**:675–6) and is clonidine-like.
- **Ipratropium** (s/l or intranasal) has limited efficacy (e.g. Freudenreich *et al, J Clin Psychopharmacol* 2004;**24**:98–100). The only RCT showed no sublingual efficacy compared to placebo (n=20, RCT, d/b, p/c, 6/52, Sockalingam *et al, J Clin Psychiatry* 2009;**70**:1114–9).
- **Lofexidine** 0.2 mg BD has been used as an alpha-2 agonist in the short-term (testing the theory that hypersalivation is due to clozapine's alpha-2 antagonism; n = 1, 1/12, Corrigan *et al, Br J Psychiatry* 1995;**167**:412; rebuttal by Szabadi, *Br J Psychiatry* 1996;**169**:380–1).
- **Oxybutinin** IR 5 mg/d resolved clozapine-induced sialorrhoea, with the suggestion that ER would be less effective (n = 1, Leung *et al, Ann Pharmacother* 2011;**45**:e45).
- **Propantheline** 7.5 mg/d has been used.
- **Septoplasty** was dramatically successful in one patient with a deviated septum causing him to breathe through his mouth (n = 1, Conry *et al, Am J Psychiatry* 1996;**153**:444).
- **Tricyclics** (e.g. amitriptyline; n = 1, Praharaj and Arora, *Br J Clin Pharmacol* 2006;**63**:128–9; FFT) can be useful, mainly for their anticholinergic effect.

Reviews: general (Praharaj *et al, Psychopharmacol [Berl]* 2006;**185**:265–73; Freudenreich, *Drugs Today* [Barc] 2005;**41**:411–8).

Tremor (see also EPSE, Parkinsonism)

Lithium

* **Dose reduction** is appropriate since tremor is dose or plasma level related and classed as a postural tremor (s=64, Baek *et al, Acta Psychiatr Scand* 2014;**129**:17–23).

Beta-blockers are standard therapy, e.g. **propranolol** 30–40 mg/d (n=5, Lapierre, *Can Med Assoc J* 1976;**114**:619–20; FFT), **metoprolol** (comparison with propranolol, Zubenko *et al, Psychiatry Res* 1984;**11**:163–4), **atenolol** and **nadolol** (for a hepatically-compromised patient; n = 1, Dave and Langbart, *Ann Clin Psychiatry* 1994;**6**:51–2).

Pregabalin (n = 1, Marks *et al, Int J Neuropsychopharmacol* 2008;**11**:879–81).

Vitamin B6 (pyridoxine) 900–1200 mg/d was completely effective in 80% people (open, n=5, Miodownik *et al, Int J Psychiatr Med* 2002;**32**:103–8).

Linoleic acid is ineffective (Schou, *Prostaglandins Med* 1980;**5**:343–4; Anton, *Prostaglandins Med* 1980;**5**:321–2).

Review: * general (s=64, Baek *et al, Acta Psychiatr Scand* 2014;**129**:17–23).

Vomiting (see also nausea)

Valproate

This could signal impending hepatic failure so investigate immediately and discontinue if necessary.

7 PSYCHOTROPIC DRUGS

This section details currently and formerly available psychotropic drugs in the UK. The dates are rarely definitive. A drug may be licensed but not launched, it may be different in different countries, may be launched but not promoted, different salts or presentations may exist; medicines may be discontinued but not withdrawn, or there may be much stock left so continues to be used. Patents may exist for the drug, manufacturing process, different salts, presentation/formulation appearance, packaging or license. Patent extension or protection may be gained and subject to appeal. The author would be grateful to hear of any clarifications and/or corrections.

NAME (UK GENERIC, TRADE AND OTHERS)	UK LAUNCH	UK PATENT EXPIRY	UK STATUS	COMMENTS
Acamprosate (Campral EC®)	1996	Expired 2002	Available	
Acetazolamide (Diamox®)	1953	Expired	Available	
Agomelatine (Valdoxan®)	2009	Expired February 2016	Available	
Alprazolam (Xanax®)	1983	Expired 1990	Available	Black list in UK
Amisulpride (Solian®)	1997	Expired 2001	Available	
Amitriptyline (Tryptizol®, Lentizol®)	1961 SR caps 1971	Expired	Available	SR caps discontinued 2000
Amobarbital (amylobarbital, amylobarbitone, Amytal®)	c1923	Expired	Tablets discontinued 2006 Injection 2000	Low use
Amoxapine (Asendis®)	1989	Expired	Discontinued 2006	Low use
Asenapine (Saphris®, Sycrest®)	2012	Expires February 2020	Available	Available USA 2009
Aripiprazole (Abilify®)	2004 IM inj 2008 LAI 2014	Expired April 2015	Available	
Atomoxetine (Strattera®)	2004 Adult license 2013	Expires 2019	Available	
Beclamide (Nydrane®)	c1956	Expired	Discontinued 1987	Low use
Benperidol (Anquil®)	1973	Expired	Available	
Benzatropine, benztropine (Cogentin®)	1950s	Expired	Discontinued 2008	Injection available only, as UK import
Benzoctamine (Tacitin®)	1971	Expired	Discontinued 1983	Low use

7

NAME	UK LAUNCH	UK PATENT EXPIRY	UK STATUS	COMMENTS
Biperiden (Akineton®)	c1957	Expired	Discontinued 2003	Low use
Bromazepam (Centrax®)	1984	Expired	Discontinued 2002	Low use
Buprenorphine (Subutex®, Suboxone®, Temgesic®)	1980 (USA 2003) 1999 for SM	Expired 2006	Available	Suboxone 2007 (with naloxone)
Bupropion (Zyban®, Welbutrin®)	2000 (US 1985 for depression)	Expired 2009	Available	
Buspirone (Buspar®)	1987	Expired 2000	Available	
Butobarbitone (Sonergan®)	1931	Expired	Discontinued 2012	Low use
Butriptyline (Evadyne®)	1975	Expired	Discontinued 1993	Low use
Carbamazepine (Tegretol®, Carbatrol®)	1962 (1965 for epilepsy), SR tabs 1989 Rectal 1994	Expired	Available	
Chloral hydrate (Noctec®)	1870s	Expired	Available	First made 1832, first medical use 1869. Noctec capsules discontinued 1996
Chlordiazepoxide (Librium®)	1960	Expired	Available	Injection discontinued 1988
Chlormethiazole, clomethiazole (Heminevrin®)	First used 1938 First used for DTs in 1959 Syrup 1972	Expired	Available	Infusion discontinued 2000 Syrup discon-tinued 2009
Chlormezanone (Trancopal®)	c1961	Expired	Withdrawn 1996 worldwide	Toxic epidermal necrolysis
Chlorpromazine (Largactil®, Thorazine®)	1954	Expired	Available	
Chlorprothixene (Taractan®)	1959	Expired	Discontinued 1987	Low use
Citalopram (Cipramil®, Celexa®)	1995 Drops 2000	Expired 2002	Available	
Citrated calcium carbimide (Abstem®)	1977	Expired	Discontinued 1984	Low use

NAME	UK LAUNCH	UK PATENT EXPIRY	UK STATUS	COMMENTS
Clobazam (Frisium®)	1979	Expired 1997	Available	
Clomipramine (Anafranil®)	1970	Expired	Available	Injection discontinued 2002, syrup 2001
Clonazepam (Rivotril®)	1974	Expired c1995	Available	
Clorazepate Dipotassium (Tranxene®)	1973	Expired c1988	Discontinued 2005	Low use
Clozapine (Clozaril®, Zaponex®, Denzapine®, Leponex®, Clopine®, Klozapol®, Faxaclo®)	1990	Expired	Available	
Cyclobarbitone (Rapidal®, Phanodorm®)	c1920s	Expired	Discontinued 1988	Lack of use and toxicity
Deprol® (meprobamate and benactyzine)	1965	Expired	Discontinued 1970s	Low use
Desipramine (Pertofran®)	1963	Expired c1988	Discontinued 1997	Low use/toxicity
Dexamfetamine (dexamphetamine, dextroamphetamine) (Dexadrine®)	1937	Expired	Available	First made 1887. Marketed 1932 for nasal congestion, as stimulant 1935 and Dexadrine® launched 1937
Diazepam (Valium®)	1963	Expired	Available	
Dibenzepine (Noveril®)	1970	Expired	Discontinued 1981	Low use
Dichloralphena-zone (Welldorm®)	1940s?	Expired	Discontinued 1992 (converted to chloral betaine)	Production problems
Disulfiram (Antabuse®)	1949 (1951 in USA)	Expired	Available	First synthesised 1881
Donepezil (Aricept®)	1997	Expired 2012	Available	
Dosulepin, dothiepin (Prothiaden®)	1969	Expired	Available	
Doxepin (Sinequan®, Adapin®)	1969	Expired	Available	
Droperidol (Droleptan®)	c1980	Expired	Available	IV for nausea
Duloxetine (Cymbalta®, Yentrene®)	2004 for stress incontinence 2005 for depression	Expired 2014	Available	
Escitalopram (Cipralex®, Lexapro®)	2002	Expired 2014	Available	

7

NAME	UK LAUNCH	UK PATENT EXPIRY	UK STATUS	COMMENTS
Eslicarbazepine (Zebinix®)	2009	Expires 2021	Available	
Ethosuximide (Zarontin®, Emeside®)	1982ish	Expired	Available	
Ethotoin (Peganone®)	1957	Expired	Discontinued 1985	Low use
Fencamfamin (Reactivan®)	c1965	Expired	Withdrawn 1986	Abuse and dependency
Fenfluramine (Ponderax®)	1968	Expired	Withdrawn 1997	Toxicity (deaths) and abuse
Flumazenil (Anexate®)	1988	Expired 2002	Available	
Flunitrazepam (Rohypnol®)	1982	Expired	Withdrawn 1986	Abuse
Fluoxetine (Prozac®)	1989 Liquid 1992 Dispersible 2014	Expired 2000	Available	
Flupentixol (Fluanxol®, Depixol®)	1965	Expired	Available	
Flupentixol decanoate (Depixol®)	1972 Low vol 1992	Expired	Available	
Fluphenazine decanoate (Modecate®)	1968	Expired	Available	
Fluphenazine enanthate (Moditen®)	1966	Expired	Discontinued 1991	Low use
Fluphenazine HCl (Moditen®)	c1967	Expired	Discontinued 2008	Low use
Flurazepam (Dalmane®)	1973	Expired	Available	
Fluspirilene (Redeptin®)	1975	Expired	Discontinued 1995	Low use, import in UK
Fluvoxamine (Faverin®, Luvox®)	1987	Expired 1996	Available	
Fosphenytoin (Pro-Epanutin®)	1998	Expired US 2007	Available	
Gabapentin (Neurontin®)	1993	Expired 2000	Available	
Galantamine (Reminyl®, Nivalin®, Razadyne®)	2000 Syrup 2003 XL 2004	Expired 2012	Available	
Glutethimide (Doriden®)	1954	Expired	Discontinued 1983	Low use
Guanfacine (Intuniv®)	2016	TBC	Available	
Haloperidol (Haldol®, Serenace®)	1959	Expired	Available	

NAME	UK LAUNCH	UK PATENT EXPIRY	UK STATUS	COMMENTS
Haloperidol decanoate (Haldol Decanoate®)	1982	Expired 2000	Available	
Heptabarbitone (Medomin®)	c1950s	Expired	Discontinued 1985	Low use
Hexobarbital (Citopan®)	c1940	Expired	Discontinued 1960s	Low use
Hydergine® (codergocrine)	c1975	Expired	Discontinued 2005	Low use
Hydroxyzine (Atarax®, Vistaril®)	c1958	Expired	Available	
Imipramine (Tofranil®)	1959	Expired	Available	
Iprindole (Prondol®)	c1972	Expired	Discontinued 1995	Low use
Iproniazid (Marsilid®)	1958	Expired	Discontinued 1987	Low use
Isocarboxazid (Marplan®)	1959–60	Expired	Available	
Ketazolam (Anxon®)	1980	Expired	Discontinued 1990	Low use
Lacosamide (Vimpat®)	2008	2023	Available	
Lamotrigine (Lamictal®)	1991 Dispersible tablets 1994	Expired 2005	Available	
Levetiracetam (Keppra®)	2000 Syrup 2005	Expired 2010	Available	
Levomepromazine/ methotrimeprazine (Nozinan®)	c1950s	Expired	Available	
Limbitrol® (amitriptyline and chlordiazepoxide)	c1966	Expired	Discontinued 1994	Low use
Lisdexamfetamine *	2013	Expires 2023	Available	
Lithium carbonate (Camcolit®, Priadel®, Liskonum®, Phasal®)	c1955 (mania license 1970) Priadel 1968 Liskonum 1980	Expired	Available	
Lithium citrate tablets (Litarex®)	1982	Expired	Discontinued 2001	Low use
Lofepramine (Gamanil®)	1983	Expired	Available	
Lofexidine (Britlofex®)	1992	Expired 2003	Available	
Loprazolam (Dormonoct®)	1983	Expired 1995	Available	
Lorazepam (Ativan®, Temesta®)	1971	Expired 1982	Available	

NAME	UK LAUNCH	UK PATENT EXPIRY	UK STATUS	COMMENTS
Lormetazepam (Noctamid®)	1980	Expired	Available	
Loxapine (Loxapac®)	1989 (oral)	Expired 1996	Oral discontinued 2003	Low use
Lurasidone (Latuda®) *	2014	Expires c2026	Available	
Maprotiline (Ludiomil®)	1975	Expired c1989	Discontinued UK 2005	Low use Available in NZ
Mazindol (Teronac®)	1960s (1973 USA)	Expired	Discontinued 1992	Low use
Meclofenoxate (Lucidril®)	1966	Expired	Discontinued 1982	Low use
Medazepam (Nobrium®)	1968	Expired	Discontinued 1994	Lack of use after black-listing
Memantine (Ebixa®, Axura®)	2002	Expired 2014	Available	
Meprobamate (Equanil®)	1955	Expired	Discontinued 2002	Low use
Methadone (Physeptone®, Methadose®)	c1947 (as analgesic)	Expired	Available	First synthesised 1937
Methixene (Tremonil®)	1970s	Expired	Discontinued 1994	Low use
Methohexitone (Brietal®)	c1957	Expired	Discontinued 1999	Low use
Methoin (Mesontoin®)	1940s	Expired	Discontinued 1981	Low use
Methylphenidate (Ritalin®, Concerta®, Medikinet®, Equasym®, Xenidate®, Matoride®, Daytrana®)	1954 (for fatigue and depression) Equasym 2000 Concerta 2002 Medikinet 2007 Matoride 2014 Xenidate 2014	Expired	Available	First synthesised 1944, off market in mid-1980s, reintroduced 1995
Methylphenobarbitone (Prominal®)	1935	Expired	Discontinued 2001	Low use
Methyprylon(e) (Noludar®)	c1958	Expired	Discontinued 1989	Adverse effects and low use
Mianserin (Norval®, Bolvidon®)	1976	Expired	Available	
Midazolam (Hypnovel®)	1982	Expired 1995	Available	
Mirtazapine (Zispin®, Remeron®, Avanza®)	1997	Expired 2005	Available	
Moclobemide (Manerix®, Aurorix®)	1993	Expired 2002	Available	
Modafinil (Provigil®, Modavigil®)	1998	Expired 2003	Available	
Motipress® (fluphenazine 1.5mg and nortriptyline 30mg)	1976	Expired	Discontinued 2003	Low use

NAME	UK LAUNCH	UK PATENT EXPIRY	UK STATUS	COMMENTS
Motival® (fluphenazine 0.5mg and nortriptyline 10mg)	1973	Expired	Discontinued 2006	Low use
Nalmefene (Selincro®) *	2013	TBC	Available	
Naltrexone (Nalorex®, Opizone®, Adepend®, Revia®)	1988, alcohol license 2012	Expired 2007	Available	
Nefazodone (Dutonin®)	1995	Expired 2007	Withdrawn 2002	Hepatic ADRs
Nialamide (Niamid®)	1950s	Expired	Discontinued 1970s	Low use
Nitrazepam (Mogadon®, Remnos®, Somnite®)	1965	Expired	Available	
Nomifensine (Merital®)	1977	Expired	Withdrawn worldwide 1986	Haemolytic anaemia
Nortriptyline (Allegron®, Aventyl®, Pamelor®)	1963	Expired c1988	Available	
Olanzapine (Zyprexa®, Zalasta®, Zolafren®)	1996 Velotabs 2001 IM injection 2005 Depot 2010	Expired 2011	Available	
Olanzapine pamoate/ embonate (Zypadhera®)	2010	TBC	Available	
Opipramol (Insidon®)	1970s	Expired	Discontinued 1981	Available in Germany
Orphenadrine (Disipal®, Norflex®, Biorphen®)	c1951	Expired	Available	Injection discontinued 1990
Oxazepam (Serenid®)	c1965	Expired c1987	Available	
Oxcarbazepine (Trileptal®)	2000	Expired 2000	Available	
Oxprenolol (Trasicor®)	c1968 1983 for anxiety	Expired	Available	
Oxypertine (Integrin®)	c1950s	Expired	Discontinued 2002	Low use
Paliperidone (Invega®)	2007	Expired 2014	Available	
Paliperidone palmitate (Xeplion®, Invega Sustenna®)	2011	Expires 2018	Available	
Paraldehyde	First used as AED in 1882	Expired	Discontinued UK 2009	Available as special only in UK
Paramethadione (Paradione®)	1970s?	Expired	Discontinued UK 1984	Low use

7

NAME	UK LAUNCH	UK PATENT EXPIRY	UK STATUS	COMMENTS
Paroxetine (Seroxat®, Aropax®, Paxil®)	1991 (liquid 1997)	Expired 2006	Available	
Parstelin® (tranylcypromine 10mg, trifluoperazine 1mg)	<1964	Expired	Discontinued 1999	Low use
Pemoline (Volital®, Kethamed®, Ronyl®)	1975 in USA	Expired	Withdrawn 1997	Withdrawn worldwide 2005 due to hepatotoxicity
Pentobarbital (Nembutal®)	c1919	Expired	Discontinued 1986	Low use
Pericyazine (Neulactil®)	1966	Expired	Available	
Perphenazine (Fentazin®, Triafon®)	1957	Expired 1987	Available	Injection discontinued 1990
Phenelzine (Nardil®)	1959–60	Expired	Available	
Phenobarbitone sodium (Gardenal®)	1912	Expired	Available	
Phenytoin (Epanutin®, Dilantin®)	1938	Expired	Available	
Pimozide (Orap®)	1971	Expired	Available	
Pipothiazine palmitate (Piportil®)	1983	Expired	Discontinued worldwide 2015	Low use and production issues
Piracetam (Nootropil®)	1992	Expired	Available	
Pramindole	1968	Expired	Discontinued 1981	Low use
Prazepam (Centrax®)	1982	Expired c1988 in US	Discontinued 1988	Lack of use after black-listing
Pregabalin (Lyrica®)	2004 (epilepsy) 2007 (GAD)	Expired 2014 for epilepsy and GAD, 2018 for neuropathic pain	Available	
Primidone (Mysoline®)	1952	Expired	Available	Suspension discontinued 2000
Prochlorperazine (Stemetil®, Buccastem®)	1950s	Expired	Available	
Procyclidine (Kemadrin®)	1951 UK	Expired	Available	
Promazine (Sparine®)	1955	Expired	Available	
Promethazine (Phenergan®)	c1951 (USA)	Expired	Available	OTC in UK from 1985

NAME	UK LAUNCH	UK PATENT EXPIRY	UK STATUS	COMMENTS
Propranolol (Inderal®)	1965 Anxiety 1973	Expired	Available	
Protriptyline (Concordin®)	1967	Expired	Discontinued 2000	Low use
Quetiapine (Seroquel®)	1997, Bipolar 2009 XL 2009 Bipolar depression 2010	Expired 2012	Available	
Reboxetine (Edronax®)	1997	Expired 2004	Available	
Remoxipride (Roxiam®)	1990	Expired	Suspended 1993, withdrawn 1994	Aplastic anaemia
Risperidone (Risperdal®, Ridal®, Sizodon®)	1993 Quicklets 2003 Consta 2002	Expired 2007 Consta expired 2014	Available	
Rivastigmine (Exelon®)	Oral 1998, Liquid 2001 Patches 2007	Expired 2012	Available	
Secobarbital (Seconal sodium)	1934	Expired	Discontinued 2009	Was quinalbarbitone
Sertindole (Serdolect®, Serlect®)	1996	Expired 2011	Discontinued UK 2010, Australia 2014	Voluntarily withdrawn 1998, reintroduced 2003 as named-patient only.
Sertraline (Lustral®, Zoloft®)	1991	Expired 2005	Available	
Sodium oxybate (Xyrem®)	2006	Expires 2019 (USA)	Available	
Sodium valproate (Epilim®, Episenta®, Depakene®)	1977 1988 injection 1994 Chrono	Expired	Available	
Sulpiride (Dolmatil®, Sulpitil®, Dogmatil®, Modal®)	1983	Expired	Available	
Sulthiame (Ospolot®)	c1965	Expired	Discontinued 1986	Low use
Tacrine (Cognex®)	Licensed 1997 in UK	Expired	Never marketed in UK	
Temazepam (Normison®, Euhypnos®, Restoril®)	1969	Expired	Available	

NAME	UK LAUNCH	UK PATENT EXPIRY	UK STATUS	COMMENTS
Tetrabenazine (Nitoman®, Xenazine®)	1950s	Expired	Available	
Thiopropazate (Dartalan®)	c1950s	Expired	Discontinued 1984	Low use
Thioproperazine (Majeptil®)	1950s	Expired	Discontinued 1981	Low use
Thioridazine (Melleril®, Mellaril®, Thoril®)	1958	Expired	Voluntarily withdrawn 2005 (liquids 2004)	Restricted due to QTc prolongation
Thiothixene (Navane®)	1967	Expired	Discontinued c1980	Low use
Tiagabine (Gabitril®)	1998	Expired 2011	Available	
Topiramate (Topamax®)	1995	Expired 2009	Available	
Tranylcypromine (Parnate®)	1959–60	Expired	Available	
Trazodone (Molipaxin®, Desyrel®, Trittico®)	1980 SR tabs 1992	Expired	Available	
Triazolam (Halcion®)	1978	Expired	UK license revoked 1993	Adverse effects. Available NZ/Australia
Triclofos sodium	1962	Expired	Discontinued 2010	Lack of availability of ingredient
Trifluoperazine (Stelazine, Eskazine®)	1958 Spansules 1967	Expired	Available	Injection discontinued 1995
Trifluperidol (Triperidol®)	1967	Expired	Discontinued 1981 Reintroduced c1986 Discontinued 1995	Low use
Trihexyphenidyl, benzhexol (Artane®)	c1955	Expired	Available	
Trimipramine (Surmontil®)	1966	Expired c1988	Available	
Triptafen® preps perphenazine/amitriptyline	1970s	Expired	Still available	
Troxidone (Triodone®)	1960s	Expired	Withdrawn 1985	Toxicity (especially teratogenicity) and low use
Tryptophan (Optimax®, Pacitron®)	Licensed for depression Optimax® 1971 Pacitron® 1976	Expired	Discontinued 2015	Discontinued 1990 due to Eosinophilia-myalgia syndrome. Relaunched 1994

Name	UK launch	UK patent expiry	UK status	Comments
Tybamate (Solacen®)	1966	Expired	Discontinued 1970s	Low use
Valproate semisodium (Depakote®)	2000	Expired 2008	Available	
Valproic acid (Convulex®)	1993	Expired	Available	
Venlafaxine (Efexor®, Effexor®, Foraven®, Polirid®)	1995	Expired 2008 XL expiry 2012	Available	
Vigabatrin (Sabril®)	1989	Expired 2001	Available but restricted	
Viloxazine (Vivalan®)	1974	Expired	Discontinued 2000	Low use and toxicity
Vortioxetine (Brintellix®, Trintellix®)	2015	N/K	Available	NICE TA367
Zaleplon (Sonata®)	2000	Expired 2011	Available	
Zimelidine (Zelmid®)	1982	Expired	Withdrawn 1983	Guillaine-Barré syndrome
Ziprasidone (Zeldox®, Geodon®)	Licensed but never launched	N/K	Never launched in UK	SPC restrictions made non-viable
Zolpidem (Stilnoct®, Ambien®)	1994	Expired 2002	Available	
Zonisamide (Zonegran®)	2005	Expired 2008	Available	
Zopiclone (Zimovane, Imovane®)	1999	Expired 1993	Available	
Zotepine (Zoleptil, Nipolept®)	1998	Expired	Discontinued December 2010	Japan since 1982
Zuclopenthixol acetate (Clopixol Acuphase®)	1990	Expired	Available	Clopenthixol until 1985
Zuclopenthixol decanoate (Clopixol®)	1978	Expired	Available	Clopenthixol until 1985
Zuclopenthixol oral (Clopixol®, Cisordinol®)	1982	Expired 1994	Available	Clopenthixol until 1985

NEW DRUGS OR PRODUCTS EXPECTED

Name, trade name and manufacturer	Details
Aripiprazole LAI *	Alkermes have an aripiprazole lauroxil one or two monthly injection formulation of aripiprazole in development.
Armodafinil (Nuvigil®, Waklert®, Cephalon) *	Armodafinil is the r-enantiomer of modafinil, presumably with similar effects but a longer half-life (12–15 hours). Approved USA 2007. Adjunctive efficacy in bipolar depression has been shown (n=433, d/b, p/c, RCT, 8/52, Calabrese *et al*, *J Clin Psychiatry* 2014;**75**:1054–61).

7

Name, trade name and manufacturer	Details
Asenapine (Sycrest) *	A daily transdermal patch is in Phase III trials (Shreya *et al*, *J Liposome Res* 2015; [in press]).
Bitopertin (Roche) *	Development discontinued for negative symptoms of schizophrenia. Still being investigated for OCD, currently in Phase II.
Blonanserin (Lonasen®, Dainippon) *	Blonanserin is a D2 and 5HT2A antagonist antipsychotic, compared successfully to haloperidol (s=4, Kishi *et al*, *J Psychiatr Res* 2013;**47**:149-54). Launched 2010 in Japan and Korea.
Brexpiprazole (Otsuka/ Lundbeck) *	A D2, D3 and 5-HT1A partial agonist developed from aripiprazole and being investigated for schizophrenia (d/b, p/c, 6/52, RCT, Correll, *Am J Psychiatry* 2015;**172**:870–80), depression and ADHD. USA have accepted an application for schizophrenia and as an adjunct for depression.
Brivaracetam (Rikelta®, UCB) *	In phase III for partial-onset and myoclonic seizures. It is an analogue of levetiracetam. FDA and EMA have granted orphan drug status for myoclonus. Submitted for approval as an adjunct in USA in 2015.
Buprenorphine implants (Probuphine®, Titan) *	Buprenorphine s/c solid rod implant for opioid dependence. US study showing a possible relapse prevention effect (n=163 [c=88], RCT, d/b, p/c, 24/52, Ling *et al*, *JAMA* 2010;**304**:1576–83) was insufficient for FDA approval. Further studies underway 2015.
Cariprazine (Vraylar®, Forest and Gedeon Richter) *	Potent D2/D3 partial agonist, with low potency for other receptors. Six RCTs show efficacy. FDA approved and launched in September 2015 for schizophrenia and mania.
Desvenlafaxine (Pristiqs®, Pfizer) *	Metabolite of venlafaxine, for depression, anxiety and non-hormonal vasomotor symptoms associated with menopause. Launched USA in 2008 and Spain in 2012. See *Chapter 1* (depression, unlicensed).
Edivoxetine (Lilly) *	Development for depression discontinued 2014.
Gantenerumab (Roche) *	Human antibody for prodromal AD, dose-dependent reduction in cerebral beta-amyloid peptide burden in AD. The SCarlet RoAD trial failed to show efficacy (December 2014).
Iloperidone (Zomaril®, Fanapt®, Novartis/Vanda)	Antipsychotic approved in USA for schizophrenia. UK application withdrawn 2013 after a negative opinion from EMA due to modest acute efficacy, lack of data on long-term efficacy and QTc prolongation concerns.
Leuco-thiomethoninium *	In phase III for Alzheimer's Disease (2017 or later). It is a Tau protein aggregation inhibitor (first-in-class).
Leuprolide acetate or leuprorelin (Lupron®, Eligard®, Pfizer) *	Licensed for prostate cancer, in phase III for Alzheimer's disease (2015), where memory loss was reported to be stabilised for a year, although ADRs are a problem.
Levomilnacipran (Fetzima®) *	SNRI enantiomer of milnacipran. Approved in USA 2013. Also being investigated for Alzheimer's Disease.
Loxapine nasal spray (Adasuve) *	See APE in *chapter 1*. Possible UK launch 2016–7 if a company takes it on.
Methylphenidate transdermal (Daytrana®) *	Daytrana® is a daily patch with a nine-hour duration (n=282, RCT, d/b, p/c, 7/52, Findling *et al*, *J Clin Psychiatry* 2008;**69**:149–59). Licensed in USA but yet to be launched in UK or Europe.

Name, trade name and manufacturer	Details
Mifepristone *	Development for psychotic depression discontinued.
Naltrexone depot (Vivitrol®, Alkermes) *	Naltrexone extended-release depot suspension, licensed in USA in 2011 as long-term relapse prevention in alcohol and opioid dependence (n=306, RCT, d/b, p/c, 6/12, Krupitsky *et al*, *Arch Gen Psychiatry* 2012;**69**:973–81; FFT). UK license stalled.
Nicergoline (Sermion®, Farmitalia) *	Ergot derivative in phase III studies for Alzheimer's disease, and may help protect cells against beta-amyloid toxicity. Available in over 50 countries for some years.
Nilvadipine (Archer) *	This calcium-channel blocker is in phase III trials for mild-to-moderate AD (NILVAD trial, plus n=86, open, 6/52, Kennelly *et al*, *Int J Ger Psychiatry* 2011;**26**:1038–45).
Paliperidone palmitate (Janssen) *	An FDA application was made for a three-monthly (quarterly) injection in November 2014 (n=305, d/b, p/c, RCT, Berwaerts *et al*, *JAMA Psychiatry* 2015;**72**:830–9).
Pitolisant (Wakix®, Bioproject)*	Pitolisant (also called tiprolisant) was approved by the EMA in November 2015 for narcolepsy, with or without cataplexy. It is an H3 inverse agonist/antagonist that increases histamine release, enhancing wakefulness and alertness (e.g. n=78, Leu-Semenescu *et al*, *Sleep Med* 2014;**15**:681–7).
Ramelteon (Rozerem®, Takeda) *	An MT1, MT2 and MT3 receptor agonist for insomnia, with no abuse potential in previous sedative abusers, even at massive doses (s=13, n=5812, Kuriyama *et al*, *Sleep Med* 2014;**15**:385–92). It is available in USA, but the European license application has been withdrawn.
Selegiline Transdermal System (Emsam®, BMS) *	Selegiline Transdermal System (6–12mg/24 hours) is licensed in USA for depression (NNT for response=11, Remission=9; s=2, Citrome *et al*, *J Affect Disord* 2013;**151**:409–17). Available on named patient basis in UK.
Solanezumab (Lilly) *	Solanezumab is a beta-amyloid monoclonal antibody, with disease modifying potential. It failed two phase 3 trials (EXPEDITION1 and EXPEDITION2) but showed 34% less decline in memory over 18/12 cf placebo. Due 2018 at earliest if EXPEDITION3 is positive.
Suvorexant (Belsomra®, Merck) *	Suvorexant is a novel orexin OX1 and OX2 receptor antagonist for insomnia (n=522+259[c=322+162], RCT, d/b, p/c, 12/12, Michelson *et al*, *Lancet Neurology* 2014;**13**:461–71). It was approved by the FDA in August 2014, and launched in USA in February 2015. Review by Owen, *Drugs of Today* 2016;**52**:29–40
Tasimelteon (Hetlioz®, Vanda) *	Melatonin agonist acting on M1 and M2 receptors. Licensed by EMA in April 2015 for the treatment of non-24-hour sleep-wake disorder in totally blind adults (s=2, n=450, RCT, d/b, p/c, Rajaratnam *et al*, *Lancet* 2009;**373**:482–91). Phase III trials starting for MDD.
Vilazodone (Viibryd®) *	Vilazodone is similar to trazodone (SSRI and 5HT1A partial agonist), although it is unclear if it has any advantages over other antidepressants (s=24, n=2898, Laughren *et al*, *J Clin Psychiatry* 2011;**72**:1166–73). Launched in USA 2011.
Zicronapine (Lundbeck) *	D1, D2 and 5HT2A antagonist underwent phase III trials in USA for schizophrenia but development seems to have been discontinued (2016).

7

INDEX

All the main psychotropic drugs are indexed according to their BNF or other main indications in *Chapter 1*, but obviously may appear elsewhere. In order to keep the index down to a manageable size, you are then referred to the index listing for that drugs chemical or therapeutic group. Individual drugs should be looked up under their drug group.

Acamprosate
for alcohol dependence 10
interactions 406
perinatal use 281, 312
use in cardiac disease 240, 250
use in diabetes 251, 255
use in epilepsy 256, 259
use in glaucoma 260, 262
use in hepatic impairment 263, 267
use in Parkinson's disease 276, 279
use in renal impairment 316, 321
use in sleep apnea 325
Acute psychiatric emergency 2
Aggression
drug-induced 440
treatment of 7
Agitation
drug-induced 437
Agomelatine
for depression 91–92
pharmacokinetic and receptor effects 198
switching 228, 231, 235
perinatal use 280, 296
use in cardiac disease 240, 241
use in diabetes 251, 254
use in epilepsy 256, 258
use in glaucoma 260, 261
use in hepatic impairment 263, 265
use in old age 268, 272
use in Parkinson's disease 276, 277
use in renal impairment 316, 318
use in sleep apnea 322, 323
Agoraphobia
treatment of 9
Akathisia
drug-induced 464
management of 534
Alcohol dependence 10
Alcohol interactions 420
Alcohol withdrawal syndrome 17
Alprazolam
for anxiety 22
see also benzodiazepines
Alzheimer's disease
treatment of 67
Amisulpride
for psychosis 145
see also antipsychotics
Amitriptyline
for depression 91
see also tricyclics
Anorexia nervosa
treatment of 114
Anorgasmia
drug effects 548
Anticholinergics
for extra-pyramidal side-effects 534
interactions 406
switching 216
perinatal use 281, 312
use in cardiac disease 240, 249
use in diabetes 251, 255
use in epilepsy 256, 259
use in glaucoma 260, 262
use in hepatic impairment 263, 267
use in Parkinson's disease 276, 279
use in renal impairment 316, 321
use in sleep apnea 322, 325
Anticholinesterases
for Alzheimer's disease 67
interactions 407
perinatal use 281
use in cardiac disease 240, 249
use in diabetes 251, 255
use in epilepsy 256, 259
use in Parkinson's disease 276, 278
use in renal impairment 316, 321
use in sleep apnea 322, 325
Anticonvulsants
interactions 395
sexual side-effects 544–545
perinatal use 281, 307–310
use in cardiac disease 240, 248
use in diabetes 251, 254
use in glaucoma 262
use in hepatic impairment 263, 266
use in old age 268, 275
use in Parkinson's disease 276, 278
use in renal impairment 316, 320–321
use in sleep apnea 322, 324
weight changes 532
Antidepressants
for agoraphobia 9–10
for anxiety disorder 21
for benzodiazepine dependence and

withdrawal 40
for bulimia 116
for depression 85
for OCD 126–131
for panic 132–135
for PTSD 136
for social phobia 182
interactions 348–381
pharmacokinetics 197–198
relative side-effects 195–196
sexual side-effects 545
switching or stopping 228
perinatal use 280, 289–299
use in bariatric surgery 238
use in cardiac disease 240, 245–247
use in diabetes 251, 253
use in epilepsy 256, 257–258
use in glaucoma 260, 261
use in hepatic impairment 263, 265
use in old age 268, 271–273
use in Parkinson's disease 276, 277
use in renal impairment 316, 318
use in sleep apnea 322, 323
weight changes with 527

Antihistamines
for insomnia 121

Antimuscarinics
see anticholinergics

Antipsychotics
for acute psychiatric emergencies 3
for anxiety 24
for mania 48
for Tourette's syndrome 185
for psychosis 142
equivalent doses 213
injections, depot 156–159
injections, depot kinetics 156
interactions 335–348
relative receptor blockades 201
relative side-effects 199
sexual side-effects 546
switching or discontinuing 205
perinatal use 280, 284–289
use in bariatric surgery 238
use in cardiac disease 240, 245
use in diabetes 251, 252
use in epilepsy 256, 257
use in glaucoma 260, 261
use in hepatic impairment 263, 264
use in old age 268, 269
use in Parkinson's disease 276, 277
use in renal impairment 316, 317
use in sleep apnea 322, 323
weight changes with 527–528

Anxiety
drug-induced 437
treatment of 21

Anxiolytics
for anxiety 21
interactions 327
relative side-effects 203
perinatal use 280, 303–307
use in bariatric surgery 239
use in cardiac disease 240, 248
use in diabetes 251, 254
use in epilepsy 256, 259
use in hepatic impairment 263, 266
use in old age 268, 274
use in Parkinson's disease 276, 277
use in renal impairment 316, 320
use in sleep apnea 322, 324

Aripiprazole
for acute psychiatric emergency 3
for bipolar disorder 43
for mania 48
for psychosis 145–146
for psychosis (LAI) 152
interactions 338
see also antipsychotics
perinatal use 280, 285
use in bariatric surgery 238
use in cardiac disease 240, 242
use in diabetes 251, 252
use in epilepsy 256, 257
use in glaucoma 260
use in hepatic impairment 263, 264
use in old age 268, 270
use in Parkinson's disease 276
use in renal impairment 316, 317
use in sleep apnea 322, 323

Asenapine
for mania 49
for psychosis 163
interactions 339
relative side-effects 200
switching or discontinuing 210
perinatal use 281, 299
use in cardiac disease 240, 247
use in diabetes 251, 254
use in epilepsy 256, 258
use in glaucoma 260, 262
use in hepatic impairment 263, 266
use in old age 268, 273
use in Parkinson's disease 276, 277
use in renal impairment 316, 319
use in sleep apnea 322, 324

Atomoxetine
for ADHD 27
interactions 408
perinatal use 281, 310
use in bariatric surgery 239
use in cardiac disease 240, 248
use in diabetes 251, 255
use in epilepsy 256, 259
use in glaucoma 260, 262
use in hepatic impairment 263, 267
use in old age 269, 275
use in renal impairment 316, 321
use in sleep apnea 322, 324

Attention deficit disorder 26

Autism
see autistic spectrum disorder

Autistic spectrum disorder
treatment of 36
Barbiturates
for insomnia 121
interactions 397
perinatal use 281, 308
use in cardiac disease 240
use in diabetes 251, 254
use in hepatic impairment 263, 266
use in old age 268
use in Parkinson's disease 276, 278
use in renal impairment 316
Bariatric surgery
drug use in 238
Behavioural toxicity
drug-induced 440
Benperidol
for psychosis 144
for sexual deviancy 180
see also antipsychotics
Benzodiazepine dependence 40
Benzodiazepine withdrawal 40
Benzodiazepines
dependence 40
for acute psychiatric emergency 2
for agoraphobia 10
for aggression 8
for alcohol dependence 15
for alcohol withdrawal 17
for anxiety 22
for insomnia 120
for panic disorder 133
equivalent doses 216
interactions 327
relative side-effects 203
switching/equivalent doses 226
perinatal use 280, 303–304
use in cardiac disease 240, 248
use in diabetes 251, 254
use in epilepsy 256, 259
use in hepatic impairment 263, 266
use in old age 268, 274
use in Parkinson's disease 276, 278
use in renal impairment 316, 320
use in sleep apnea 324
withdrawal 40
Benzhexol
see trihexyphenidyl
Benzatropine
for extra-pyramidal side-effects 534
see also anticholinergics
Beta-blockers
for anxiety 22
perinatal use 280, 305
use in cardiac disease 248
use in epilepsy 259
use in Parkinson's disease 278
Binge-eating disorder
treatment of 117
Bipolar mood disorder
bipolar depression, treatment of 42
prophylaxis, treatment of 42
rapid-cycling, treatment of 59
Body dysmorphic disorder
treatment of 131
Borderline personality disorder 61
Bromazepam
see also benzodiazepines
Bulimia nervosa
treatment of 115
Buprenorphine
interactions 409
perinatal use 281, 312
use in cardiac disease 240, 250
use in diabetes 251, 255
use in epilepsy 256, 259
use in hepatic impairment 263, 267
use in old age 275
use in Parkinson's disease 276, 279
use in sleep apnea 322, 325
Bupropion
interactions 410
perinatal use 280, 296
use in cardiac disease 240, 246
use in diabetes 251, 254
use in epilepsy 256, 258
use in glaucoma 260, 261
use in hepatic impairment 263, 265
use in Parkinson's disease 276, 277
use in renal impairment 316, 318
use in sleep apnea 322, 323
Buspirone
for anxiety 22
interactions 330
see also anxiolytics
Caffeinism 187
Cannabis
interactions 423
Carbamazepine
dermatological side-effects 514
for aggression 8
for alcohol dependence 14
for alcohol withdrawal 19
for bipolar disorder 43
for mania 49
for rapid-cycling 60
interactions 381
sexual side-effects 548
perinatal use 281, 299
use in cardiac disease 240, 247
use in diabetes 251, 254
use in epilepsy 256, 259
use in glaucoma 260, 262
use in hepatic impairment 263, 266
use in old age 268, 273
use in Parkinson's disease 276, 277
use in renal impairment 316, 319
use in sleep apnea 324
weight changes with 532
see also anticonvulsants
Cardiovascular disease
drugs in 240
Catatonia
drug-induced 471

treatment of 64
Chloral hydrate
for insomnia 121
interactions 331
see also hypnotics
Chlordiazepoxide
for anxiety 22
see also benzodiazepines
Chlormethiazole
see clomethiazole
Chlorpromazine
for acute psychiatric emergency 3
for psychosis 143
see also antipsychotics
Choreas
drug-induced 472
Citalopram
for agoraphobia 9–10
for depression 88
for panic disorder 133
interactions 352
see also SSRIs
Clobazam
for anxiety 22
see also benzodiazepines
Clomethiazole
for alcohol withdrawal 18
for insomnia 121
interactions 412
perinatal use 281, 306
relative side-effects 194
use in cardiac disease 240, 248
use in diabetes 251, 255
use in epilepsy 256, 259
use in glaucoma 260, 262
use in hepatic impairment 263, 266
use in old age 268, 274
use in Parkinson's disease 276, 278
use in renal impairment 316, 320
use in sleep apnea 324
see also anticonvulsants
Clomipramine
for depression 91
for OCD 126–127
for panic disorder 134, 135
see also tricyclics
Clonazepam
for panic disorder 133
see also benzodiazepines
Clorazepate
see benzodiazepines
Clozapine
for schizophrenia 146–150
for psychosis in Parkinson's disease 176, 177
interactions 339
use in bariatric surgery 238
use in ECT 190–191
see also antipsychotics
Cocaine
interactions 423–424
Confusion
drug-induced 441
Cyproterone
for sexual deviancy 180
Cytochrome P450 enzymes 426
CYP1A2 427
CYP2B6 428
CYP2C9 429
CYP2C19 430
CYP2D6 431
CYP3A4 433
Delirium
drug-induced 441
Dementia
treatment of 66
Depression
bipolar, treatment of 54
drug-induced 446
in Parkinson's disease 110
postpartum, treatment of 107
unipolar, treatment of 85
Depot injections
see antipsychotics
Dexamfetamine
for ADHD 28
for narcolepsy 124
see also stimulants
Diabetes
drugs in 251
Diazepam
for acute psychiatric emergency 5
for anxiety 22
for benzodiazepine withdrawal 40
see also benzodiazepines
Disulfiram
for alcohol dependence 11–13
interactions 412
perinatal use 281, 312
use in cardiac disease 240, 250
use in diabetes 251, 255
use in epilepsy 256, 259
use in glaucoma 260, 262
use in hepatic impairment 263, 267
use in Parkinson's disease 276, 279
use in renal impairment 316, 321
use in sleep apnea 325
Dose equivalents 213
Donepezil
for Alzheimer's disease 67
interactions 407
see also anticholinesterases
Dosulepin
for depression 91
see also tricyclics
Dothiepin
see dosulepin
Doxepin
for depression 91
see also tricyclics
Drug-induced disorders 436
Drug interactions
acamprosate 406
agomelatine 364
alcohol 420
anticholinesterases 407
anticholinergics 406
anticonvulsants 395
antidepressants 348
antipsychotics 335
anxiolytics 327
aripiprazole 338
atomoxetine 408
benzodiazepines 327
buprenorphine 409
bupropion 410
buspirone 330
cannabis 423

carbamazepine 381
chloral hydrate 331
citalopram 352
clomethiazole 412
clozapine 339
cocaine 423
disulfiram 412
donepezil 407
escitalopram 352
fluoxetine 354
fluvoxamine 357
gabapentin 395
galantamine 406
guanfacine 413
hypnotics 327
lamotrigine 387
levetiracetam 396
lisdexamfetamine 413
lithium 389
lurasidone 342
MAOIs 376
melatonin 332
memantine 413
methadone 414
methylphenidate 417
mianserin 366
mirtazapine 366
moclobemide 368
modafinil 417
nalmefene 418
olanzapine 343
oxcarbazepine 396
paroxetine 360
phenobarbital 397
phenytoin 400
pregabalin 332
primidone 397
quetiapine 345
reboxetine 369
risperidone 346
rivastigmine 408
sertraline 362
smoking 424
SSRIs 352
St John's wort 373
topiramate 405
trazodone 370
tricyclics 348
valproate 393
venlafaxine 371
vortioxetine 373
zaleplon 333
ziprasidone 348
zolpidem 333
zopiclone 334

Duloxetine
in anxiety 23
in depression 92
drug interactions 365
see also antidepressants

Dystonia
drug-induced 466
management of 539

Eating disorders 114

ECT 189

Epilepsy
drug use in 256

Escitalopram
for agoraphobia 10
for anxiety 23
for depression 89
for OCD 127
for panic disorder 133
for social anxiety 182
interactions 352
see also SSRIs

Equivalent doses 194–203

Ethosuximide
see anticonvulsants

Extra-pyramidal side-effects
drug-induced 462
management of 533

Flunitrazepam
for insomnia 120
see also benzodiazepines

Fluoxetine
for bulimia 116
for depression 89
for OCD 127
interactions 354
see also SSRIs

Flupentixol
for depression 92
for psychosis 145
see also antipsychotics

Flupentixol decanoate
for psychosis 153, 156
see also antipsychotics

Fluphenazine decanoate
for psychosis 153, 156
see also antipsychotics

Flurazepam
for insomnia 120
see also benzodiazepines

Fluspirilene
for psychosis 153
see also antipsychotics

Fluvoxamine
for depression 89
for OCD 127
interactions 357
see also SSRIs

Gabapentin
interactions 395
see also anticonvulsants

Galantamine
for Alzheimer's disease 67
interactions 408
see also anticholinesterases

Glaucoma
drug use in 260

Guanfacine
for ADHD 28, 34
for autistic spectrum disorders 39
for psychosis 173
for PTSD 140
interactions 413
perinatal use 281, 311
use in cardiac disease 240, 249
use in diabetes 251, 255
use in epilepsy 256, 259
use in glaucoma 260, 262
use in hepatic impairment 263, 267
use in old age 269, 275
use in renal impairment 316, 321
use in sleep apnea 324

Hallucinations
drug-induced 452

Haloperidol
for acute psychiatric emergency 4
for psychosis 144
for Tourette's syndrome 184
see also antipsychotics

Haloperidol decanoate
for psychosis 153, 157
see also antipsychotics

Hepatic impairment
drugs in 363

Hydroxyzine
for anxiety 23
see also anxiolytics
Hyperactivity
see attention deficit disorder
Hypomania
see mania
Hypnotics
for insomnia 119
interactions 327
relative side-effects 194
perinatal use 280, 303–307
use in bariatric surgery 239
use in cardiac disease 240, 248
use in diabetes 251, 254
use in epilepsy 256, 259
use in hepatic impairment 263, 266
use in old age 268, 274
use in Parkinson's disease 276, 277
use in renal impairment 316, 320
use in sleep apnea 322, 324
Imipramine
for depression 91
for panic disorder 134
see also tricyclics
Insomnia
drug-induced 493
treatment of 119
Interactions
see drug interactions 326
Isocarboxazid
for depression 94
see also MAOIs
Lamotrigine
for bipolar depression 43
for depression 101
dermatological side-effects 517
interactions 387
see also anticonvulsants
Levetiracetam
interactions 396
see also anticonvulsants
Levomepromazine
for psychosis 144
see also antipsychotics
Libido
drug effects on 547
Lisdexamfetamine
for ADHD 28
for binge-eating disorder 118
see also stimulants
Lithium
dermatological side-effects 516
for aggression 7
for bipolar disorder 43
for depression 95
for mania 49
for rapid-cycling 60
interactions 389
perinatal use 281, 301
use in bariatric surgery 239
use in cardiac disease 240, 247
use in diabetes 251, 254
use in ECT 191
use in epilepsy 256, 259
use in glaucoma 260, 262
use in hepatic impairment 263, 266
use in old age 268, 273
use in Parkinson's disease 276, 277
use in renal impairment 316, 319
use in sleep apnea 322, 324
weight changes with 532
Liver impairment
drugs in 316
Lofepramine
for depression 91
see also tricyclics
Long-acting injections
equivalent doses 215
for psychosis 151–160
frequency changes and missed doses 217–225
pharmacokinetics 199–202
switching 205–216
Loprazolam
for insomnia 120
see also benzodiazepines
Lorazepam
for acute psychiatric emergency 5
for anxiety 22
see also benzodiazepines
Lormetazepam
for insomnia 120
see also benzodiazepines
L-tryptophan
see tryptophan
Loxapine
for acute psychiatric emergency 3
Lurasidone
for bipolar depression 57
for psychosis 147
interactions 342
see also antipsychotics
Mania
drug-induced 456
treatment of 48
Manic-depression
see bipolar mood disorder
MAOIs
for depression 94
interactions — drugs 376
interactions — food 379–380
patient information 377
switching 232
perinatal use 280, 299
use in cardiac disease 240, 241
use in diabetes 251, 254
use in ECT 191
use in epilepsy 256, 258
use in glaucoma 260, 262
use in hepatic impairment 263, 266
use in old age 268, 273
use in Parkinson's disease 276, 277
use in renal impairment 316, 319
use in sleep apnea 324
Melatonin
for insomnia 121
interactions 332
see also hypnotics
Memantine
for Alzheimer's disease 68
for BPSD 72
interactions 413
perinatal use 281, 311

use in cardiac disease 240, 249
use in diabetes 251, 255
use in epilepsy 256, 259
use in glaucoma 260, 262
use in hepatic impairment 263, 267
use in Parkinson's disease 276, 279
use in renal impairment 316, 321
use in sleep apnea 322, 325

Methadone
interactions 414
perinatal use 281, 312, 313
use in bariatric surgery 239
use in cardiac disease 240, 250
use in diabetes 251, 255
use in epilepsy 256, 259
use in glaucoma 260, 262
use in hepatic impairment 263, 267
use in Parkinson's disease 276, 279
use in pregnancy 291
use in sleep apnea 322

Methotrimeprazine
see levomepromazine

Methylphenidate
for ADHD 30
interactions 417

Mianserin
for depression 92
interactions 366
see also antidepressants

Midazolam
see benzodiazepines

Mirtazapine
for anxiety 25
for depression 92
for insomnia 122
for panic disorder 134
interactions 366
pharmacokinetics 198
sexual side-effects 545
switching to and from 231, 233
perinatal use 280, 297
use in bariatric surgery 238
use in cardiac disease 240, 247
use in diabetes 251, 254
use in ECT 190
use in epilepsy 256, 258
use in glaucoma 260, 262
use in hepatic impairment 263, 265
use in old age 268, 272
use in Parkinson's disease 276, 277
use in renal impairment 316, 318
use in sleep apnea 322, 323
see also antidepressants

Moclobemide
for depression 93
interactions 368
pharmacokinetics 198
see also antidepressants

Modafinil
for narcolepsy 125
interactions 417
perinatal use 281, 315
use in cardiac disease 240, 250
use in diabetes 251, 255
use in epilepsy 256, 259
use in hepatic impairment 263, 267
use in Parkinson's disease 276, 279
use in renal impairment 316, 321
use in sleep apnea 325

Movement disorders
drug-induced 462
management of 533

Nalmefene
for alcohol dependence 12
interactions 418
perinatal use 281, 312
use in cardiac disease 240, 250
use in diabetes 251, 255
use in epilepsy 256, 259
use in glaucoma 260, 262
use in hepatic impairment 263, 267
use in Parkinson's disease 276, 279
use in renal impairment 316, 321
use in sleep apnea 322, 325

Naltrexone
for alcohol dependence 12
for self-injurious behaviour 180–181
interactions 419
perinatal use 281, 312
use in cardiac disease 240, 250
use in diabetes 251, 255
use in epilepsy 256, 259
use in glaucoma 260, 262
use in hepatic impairment 263, 267
use in Parkinson's disease 276, 279
use in renal impairment 316, 321

Narcolepsy
treatment of 124

Nervousness
drug-induced 437

Neuroleptic malignant syndrome
drug-induced 475
management of 542

Neuroleptics
see antipsychotics

Nightmares
drug-induced 495

Nitrazepam
for insomnia 120
see also benzodiazepines

Nortriptyline
for depression 91
see also tricyclics

Obsessive-compulsive disorder
drug-induced 477
treatment of 126

Olanzapine
for acute psychiatric emergency 4
for bipolar 56
for mania 49
for psychosis and schizophrenia 150
interactions 343

see also antipsychotics
Olanzapine pamoate
for schizophrenia 153, 157
see also olanzapine
Old age
drug use in 268
Orphenadrine
for extra-pyramidal side-effects 539
see also anticholinergics
Oxazepam
for anxiety 22
see also benzodiazepines
Oxcarbazepine
interactions 396
see also anticonvulsants
Oxprenolol
see beta-blockers
P450 enzymes
see Cytochrome P450
Panic disorder
drug-induced 478
treatment of 132
Paliperidone
for schizophrenia 150
see also antipsychotics
Paliperidone palmitate
for schizophrenia 154
see also antipsychotics
Parkinson's disease
depression in, treatment 110
drug use in 276
Parkinsonian side-effects
drug-induced 462
management of 538
Paroxetine
for agoraphobia 10
for anxiety 23
for depression 89
for OCD 127
for panic disorder 133
for PTSD 136
for social anxiety 182
interactions 360
see also SSRIs
Pericyazine
for psychosis 144
see also antipsychotics
Perinatal period
drug use in 280
Perphenazine
for psychosis 144
see also antipsychotics
Phenelzine
for depression 94
see also MAOIs
Phenobarbital
interactions 397
see also barbiturates
Phenobarbitone
see phenobarbital
Phenytoin
interactions 400
see also anticonvulsants
Pimozide
for psychosis 145
see also antipsychotics
Pirenzepine
for EPSE 553
interactions 419
Postpartum depression
treatment of 107
Post-traumatic stress disorder
treatment of 135
Potassium clorazepate
see benzodiazepines
Pregabalin
for anxiety 23
for benzodiazepine dependence 41
interactions 332
see also anticonvulsants
Priapism 551
Primidone
interactions 397
see also barbiturates
Prochlorperazine
for psychosis 144
see also antipsychotics
Procyclidine
for extra-pyramidal side-effects 539, 540
see also anticholinergics
Promazine
for psychosis 144
see also antipsychotics
Promethazine
for acute psychiatric emergencies 6
Propranolol
for anxiety 22
see also beta-blockers
Psychosis
drug-induced 480
treatment of 143
Quetiapine
for acute psychiatric emergency 4
for bipolar disorder 45
for bipolar depression 54
for psychosis 150
for unipolar depression 98
interactions 345
see also antipsychotics
Rabbit syndrome
drug-induced 473
Rapid-cycling bipolar disorder 59
Rapid tranquillisation 1
Reboxetine
for depression 93
interactions 369
see also antidepressants
Renal disease
drug use in 316
Risperidone
for autistic spectrum disorder 36
for bipolar disorder 46
for BPSD 72
for mania 50
for psychosis 151
interactions 346
see also antipsychotics
Rivastigmine
for Alzheimer's disease 67
for dementia in Parkinson's disease 79
interactions 408
see also anticholinesterases
Schizophrenia
drug-induced 480
treatment of 140
Seasonal affective disorder
treatment of 178
Selegiline
for depression 93
Self-injurious behaviour
treatment of 179
Serotonin syndrome
drug-induced 490

management of 544
Sertraline
for depression 89
for OCD 127
for PTSD 136
interactions 362
see also SSRIs
Sexual deviancy disorders
treatment of 180
Sexual side-effects 544
Sleep apnea
drug use in 322
Sleep disorders
drug-induced 493
treatment of 124
Smoking
interactions 424
Social anxiety (phobia)
treatment of 181
Sodium oxybate
for narcolepsy 125
interactions 419
perinatal use 281, 315
use in cardiac disease 240, 250
use in diabetes 251, 255
use in epilepsy 256, 259
use in hepatic impairment 263, 267
use in old age 275
use in Parkinson's disease 276, 279
use in renal impairment 316, 321
use in sleep apnea 325
Sodium valproate see valproate
Somnolence
drug-induced 493
SSRIs
for agoraphobia 9
for anxiety 21
for bulimia 116
for depression 88–91
for OCD 126–129
for panic disorder 133–135
for PTSD 136–138
for social phobia 182
interactions 352
relative side-effects 195
sexual side-effects 545
switching or stopping 228–230
perinatal use 280, 318
use in bariatric surgery 238
use in cardiac disease 240, 245
use in diabetes 251, 253
use in ECT 192
use in epilepsy 256, 258
use in glaucoma 260, 261
use in hepatic impairment 263, 265
use in old age 268, 271
use in Parkinson's disease 276, 277
use in renal impairment 316, 318
use in sleep apnea 323
weight changes with 527
Stimulants
for ADHD 27, 33
perinatal use 281, 310
use in cardiac disease 249, 250
use in diabetes 251, 255
use in epilepsy 256, 258, 259
use in glaucoma 260, 262
use in hepatic impairment 263, 267
use in old age 269, 275
use in Parkinson's disease 276, 278
use in renal impairment 316, 321
use in sleep apnea 322, 324
Sulpiride
for psychosis 145
see also antipsychotics
Suicidal ideation 496
Switching psychotropics
ADHD treatments 226
anticholinergics 216
anticholinesterases 226
antidepressants 228–236
antipsychotics 205–216
benzodiazepines 216
narcotics, etc 216
opiates 216
Tardive dyskinesia
drug-induced 469
management of 536
Tardive dystonia
drug-induced 466
management of 539
Temazepam
for insomnia 120
see also benzodiazepines
Tetrabenazine
for dystonias 540
for psychosis 166
Tics
drug-induced 474
management of 536
Topiramate
interactions 405
see also anticonvulsants
Tourette's syndrome
drug-induced 474
treatment of 184
Tranylcypromine
for depression 95
see also MAOIs
Trazodone
for depression 93, 112
for insomnia 124
interactions 370
sexual side-effects 546, 549
switching or discontinuing 230
see also antidepressants
use in ECT 192
Trichotillomania
treatment of 186
Tricyclic antidepressants
for depression 91
for OCD 129, 131
for panic disorder 134
interactions 348
pharmacokinetics 197
perinatal use 280, 295
relative side-effects 195
use in bariatric surgery 239
use in cardiac disease 240, 246
use in diabetes 251, 253
use in ECT 192
use in epilepsy 256, 258
use in glaucoma 260, 261
use in hepatic impairment 263, 265
use in old age 268, 272

use in Parkinson's disease 276, 277
use in renal impairment 316, 318
use in sleep apnea 323
weight changes with 527
Trifluoperazine
for acute psychiatric emergency 5
for psychosis 144
see also antipsychotics
Trihexyphenidyl
for extra-pyramidal side-effects 539
see also anticholinergics
Trimipramine
for depression 91
see also tricyclics
Triptorelin pomoate
for sexual deviancy disorders 180
Tryptophan
for depression 95
see also antidepressants
Unipolar depression
treatment of 85
Valproate
for bipolar disorder 45
for mania 50
interactions 393
see also anticonvulsants
Valproic acid
see valproate
Valproate semisodium
see valproate
Venlafaxine
for anxiety 24
for depression 93
interactions 371
pharmacokinetics 198
relative side-effects 203
sexual side-effects 545, 549
switching or discontinuing 234
see also antidepressants
Vitamins
for alcohol withdrawal 18
Vortioxetine
for anxiety 25
for depression 94
interactions 373
pharmacokinetics 198
perinatal use 280, 296–297
relative side-effects 196
switching or discontinuing 233, 236
use in cardiac disease 240, 247
use in diabetes 251, 254
use in ECT 192
use in epilepsy 256, 258
use in glaucoma 260, 262
use in hepatic impairment 263, 265
use in old age 268, 272
use in Parkinson's disease 276, 277
use in renal impairment 316, 318
weight changes with 527
Zaleplon
for insomnia 120
interactions 333
see also hypnotics
Ziprasidone
for psychosis 151
interactions 348
see also antipsychotics
Zolpidem
for insomnia 120
interactions 333
see also hypnotics
Zopiclone
for insomnia 121
interactions 334
use in ECT 192
see also hypnotics
Zuclopenthixol
for psychosis 145
see also antipsychotics
Zuclopenthixol acetate
for acute psychiatric emergency 5
for psychosis 159
see also antipsychotics
Zuclopenthixol decanoate
for psychosis 160
see also antipsychotics

Abbreviations

FOR DETAILS OF STUDIES:

* = new or updated entry
n = number of patients
RCT = randomised controlled trial
d/b = double-blind
c/o = cross-over
o/p = out-patient
s/b = single blind (trial)
p/c = placebo-controlled
MS = manufacturer's study
S = number of studies

OTHER ABBREVIATIONS:

AAPCD = American Academy of Pediatrics Committee on Drugs
ABC-C = aberrant behaviour checklist — community
ACh = acetylcholine
ACEI = ACE inhibitors
Ad = adult
AD = Alzheimer's disease
ADHD = attention deficit hyperactivity disorder
ADD = attention deficit disorder
ADL = activities of daily living
ADME = absorption, distribution, metabolism and excretion
ADR = adverse drug reaction
AED = anti-epileptic drug
AFP = alpha-fetoprotein
AIMS = abnormal involuntary movement scale
ALDH = hepatic aldehyde-NAD reductase
AN = anorexia nervosa
APE = acute psychiatric emergency
APA = American Psychiatric Association
ASD = autistic spectrum disorders
AWS = alcohol withdrawal syndrome
BAP = British Association for Psychopharmacology
BD = twice a day
BDD = body dysmorphic disorder
BDI = Beck Depression Inventory
BDZ = benzodiazepine(s)
BEN = benign ethnic neutropenia
BMA = British Medical Association
BMI = body mass index
BN = bulimia nervosa
BNF = British National Formulary
BPD = borderline psychiatric disorder
BPRS = Brief Psychiatric Rating Scale
BPSD/BPSSD = behavioural and psychological (signs and) symptoms of dementia
bp = blood pressure
BP = British Pharmacopoeia
CA = care above
CBT = cognitive behavioural therapy
CBZ = carbamazepine
CBZ-E = carbamazepine-epoxide
CCK = cholecystokinin
CGI = clinical global impression
ChEIs = cholinesterase inhibitors
CHD = coronary heart disease
CNS = central nervous system
CPK = creatinine phosphokinase
CSE = convulsive status epilepticus
CSM = Committee on the Safety of Medicines
CVAE = cerebrovascular adverse events
D1 = dopamine-1 (receptor)
D2 = dopamine-2 (receptor)
DA = dopamine
DDD = defined daily dose
DHA = docosahexaenoic acid
DHEA = Dehydro-epiandrosterone
DLB = lewy body dementia
DSM-IV = Diagnostic Statistical Manual IV
DT = delirium tremens
DUP = duration of untreated psychosis
e/c = enteric-coated
ECG = electrocardiogram
ECT = electroconvulsive therapy
ED = erectile dysfunction
EDNOS = eating disorders not otherwise specified
EBMH = Evidence-Based Mental Health (Journal)
EEG = electro-encephalogram
EPA = eicosapentaenoic acid
E-EPA = ethyl-eicosapentaenoic acid
EPO = evening primrose oil
EPSE = extra-pyramidal side-effects
ERT = estrogen replacement therapy
FBC = full blood count
FDA = Federal Drug Agency
GABA = gamma-aminobutyric acid
GAD = generalised anxiety disorder
GB = Ginkgo biloba
G-CSF = granulocyte colony stimulating factor
GFR = glomerular filtration rate
GHB = gamma-hydroxybutyrate
GTC = generalised tonic-clonic (seizure)
HAL-PRO = haloperidol + promethazine

5-HT = 5-hydroxytryptamine
HF = heart failure
IED = intermittent explosive disorder
IV = intravenous
IM = intramuscular
INR = international normalised ratio
IPT = interpersonal therapy
ISE = ion-selective electrode
ITT = intention to treat
L/A = long-acting
LAI = long-acting injection
LD = low dose
LDX = lisdexamfetamine
LFT = liver function tests
LSD = lysergic acid diethylamide
LTG = lamotrigine
MAOI = mono-amine oxidase inhibitor
MCM = major congenital malformations
MDD = major depressive disorder
MHRA = Medicines and Healthcare products Regulatory Agency (was CSM/MCA)
MI = manufacturers' information
MMSE = mini-mental state examination
MS = mood stabiliser
NA = noradrenaline
NARI = Noradrenaline reuptake inhibitor
NCSE = non-convulsive status epilepticus
NE = norepinephrine
NICE = National Institute for Health and Clinical Excellence
N/K = not known
NMDA = N-methyl-D-aspartate receptor
NMS = neuroleptic malignant syndrome
NPI = Neuropsychiatric Inventory
NNH = numbers needed to harm
NNT = numbers needed to treat
NPSA = National Patient Safety Agency
NSAIDs = non-steroidal anti-inflammatory drugs
OCD = obsessive-compulsive disorder
O/C = oral contraceptive
OD = overdose
OFC = olanzapine-fluoxetine combination
OR = odds ratio
OTC = over-the-counter (medicine)
O3FA = omega-3 fatty acids
PD = Parkinson's disease and personality disorders
PKC = protein kinase C
PMH = previous medical history
PMS = pre-menstrual syndrome
PP = paliperidone palmitate
PPD = postpartum depression
PPD = psychosis in Parkinson's disease
PPHN = persistent pulmonary hypertension in the newborn
PT = prothrombin time
PTs = psychological therapies
PTSD = post-traumatic stress disorder
PUFA = polyunsaturated fatty acid
QoLS = Quality of Life Scale
QTc = corrected QT interval
REM = rapid eye movement
RIMA = reversible inhibitor of monoamine-A
RPS = Royal Pharmaceutical Society
RR = relative risk
RT = rapid tranquillisation
SA = short-acting
SAD = seasonal affective disorder
SAM = S-adenosyl-L-methionine
s/c = subcutaneous
SDS = Severity of Dependence scale
SF = sugar-free
SFQ = sexual functioning questionnaire
SIB = self-injurious behaviour
SIDS = sudden infant death syndrome
SJW = St John's wort
SmPC = summary of product characteristics
SSRI = serotonin-selective reuptake inhibitor
STEP-BD = systematic treatment enhancement program for bipolar disorder
SUD = substance use disorders
t½= half life
TCA = tricyclic antidepressant
TD = tardive dyskinesia
TDM = therapeutic drug monitoring
TEAEs = treatment emergent adverse events
THC = tetrahydrocannabinol
TIA = transient ischaemic attack
TRD = treatment-resistant depression
TRS = treatment-resistant schizophrenia
U&E = urea and electrolytes
UPDRS = unified Parkinson's disease rating scale
USP = United States Pharmacopoeia
VaD = vascular dementia
WE = Wernicke's encephalopathy
YMRS = Young Mania Rating scale